Praise for

The Treatment of Modern Western Medical Diseases with Chinese Medicine

This book represents another major step in the development of a more comprehensive view of East Asian medicine. The authors help students and practitioners begin to think their way around frequently seen clinical scenarios that are not covered in other English language sources.

—**Greg Bantick**, B.Ac., MTOM,
Senior Lecturer, Pacific College of Oriental Medicine

These two unanimously recognized and appreciated specialists in their field have managed to combine the nosology of modern Western medicine with the subtle, multidimensional modes of thousands-year-old traditional Chinese medicine. This powerful textbook is a rich, invaluable, and totally accessible source of diagnostic and therapeutic teachings, even for experts of Chinese medicine.

—**Patrick Basmadjian**, M.D. & acupuncturist (Belgium)

Written by two of the West's most prolific teachers, writers, researchers, *and* clinicians of Chinese medicine and written specifically for Western practitioners of Chinese medicine, this book is the first comprehensive clinical resource of its kind. Its detailed Chinese medical discussions of more than 60 diseases, including concise Chinese medical disease mechanisms and detailed medicinal in acupuncture treatment protocols, as well as an Introduction that will improve every practitioner's clinical skills in treating the complicated Western diseases we see in real-life practice are sure to make this superb work the most valuable textbook and clinical manual on the shelves of every Western practitioner of Chinese medicine.

—**Simon Becker**, Dipl. Ac. & C.H.,
Author of *A Handbook of Chinese Hematology*

This book skillfully combines a clear and complete approach to each disease by both Western and Chinese medicine. Physiopathology, clinical aspects, and therapeutics are described thoroughly and precisely in both systems. It is a bridge that will enable MD's to understand the Chinese medical point of view and Chinese medical practitioners to gain clear access to the Western medical approach. A brilliant synthesis!

—**Florence Bouvelot-Brézillon**, M.D. & acupuncturist (France)

It must be said with great verve: There is no other book like this one in the cross-cultural bibliography of East-West healing. It is destined to quench the yearning of many seasoned practitioners that uncomfortably straddle both healing realms. It is like finally having a bilingual encyclopedic clinical dictionary that adroitly renders obeisance to both languages. Bravo!!

—**Robert J. Casanas**, M.A., M.D.,
Board-certified Internist, Assistant Clinical Professor, School of Medicine, University of California

This excellent text provides a sophisticated response to one of the more pressing concerns facing practitioners of Traditional Chinese Medicine today: how to integrate contemporary clinical experience with ancient therapeutic wisdom. The authors systematically analyze a comprehensive range of modern diseases and syndromes from both a Western and Chinese medical perspective using intelligent and well-researched interpretations of etiology, pathophysiology, and diagnosis, including classical and contemporary reference materials. The result is a serious clinical manual of internal medicine which focuses on modern, recalcitrant disease and the relevance of Traditional Chinese Medicine in both understanding and treating it. This is a text that any practitioner, faced with their more challenging cases, from chronic fatigue syndrome to irritable bowel syndrome to multiple sclerosis, will be excited about. It will enhance not only their therapeutic endeavors, but also their ability to integrate Western and Eastern interpretations of disease. As such, any committed practitioner of TCM will want it in their library immediately.

—**Nigel Dawes**, M.A., L.Ac.,
Dean, Graduate School of Oriental Medicine
New York College of Wholistic Medicine, New York, USA

The Treatment of Modern Western Medical Diseases with Chinese Medicine represents a major contribution to the professional literature of TCM. Bob Flaws and Philippe Sionneau have crafted a brilliant text based on scholarly review of the contemporary medical literature and their own clinical insights and wisdom. This volume provides a wealth of clinically relevant information which will be of immediate use to both students and professional practitioners of TCM. This text is destined to become a standard reference in the practice of TCM in the West.

—**Steve Erickson**, Dipl. Ac. & C.H.,
Assistant Professor, Northwestern Health Sciences University

While this may not be the first book to describe the Chinese pattern discrimination and treatment of modern Western diseases, this one is the most helpful in that it addresses the complexity of the mixed patterns we tend to see in our patients with ever increasing frequency these days. Rather than simple patterns with one root cause, we tend to see even the most apparently simple conditions complicated by layers of chronic illness which must be considered and appropriately dealt with in order for full and lasting function and balance to be restored. . . All in all, this is a very practical text.

—**Gary Klepper**, D.C., Certified Chiropractic Acupuncturist

Every book published by Blue Poppy Press is exceptional in its material, and now *The Treatment of Modern Western Medical Diseases with Chinese Medicine* joins its predecessors as one of the most knowledgeable and informative resources for medical practitioners. It is refreshing to have both the Chinese and Western medical approaches to disease readily available under one cover and to have the current medical literature from both ends of the spectrum at one's fingertips. Thank you again, Blue Poppy Press, for your innovative, thorough, and unparalleled approach.

—**Lynn Kuchinski**, M.I.M., L.Ac., Dipl. Ac. & C.H.,
Author of *Controlling Diabetes Naturally with Chinese Medicine*

In order for Chinese medicine, and in particular, Traditional Chinese Medicine (TCM), to become more integrated into medical practice in the West, there is a need to bridge the many conceptual and practical differences between Western medicine and Chinese medicine. In his latest work, *The Treatment of Modern Western Medical Diseases with Chinese Medicine*, Bob Flaws, along with Philippe Sionneau, have produced a text that is, I believe, a major step in the integration of these two medicines. Written in a clear style and very well organized and produced, this book will provide practitioners with much valuable information both for understanding these two medicines as well as for using Chinese medicine in caring for Western patients who have Western medical diagnoses. Western medical practitioners with an interest in professional level Chinese medicine will find a great abundance of information to further their understanding. Practitioners of Chinese medicine in Western countries have within this text a multitude of invaluable clinical insights and, perhaps more importantly, an excellent source for an overall approach to utilizing Chinese medicine/TCM in approaching patients who have been diagnosed and treated with Western medicine. As a Western-trained physician practicing Chinese medicine, I applaud the publication of this text and heartily recommend it to any practitioner desiring a more harmonious fusion of Chinese and Western medical practice.

—**Charles May**, M.D., DOM
Acupuncture and Chinese Herbology Diplomate, American Boards of Family Practice & Emergency Medicine, former instructor and board member, American Academy of Medical Acupuncture

This volume will serve not only as a valuable reference for all experienced practitioners but, more importantly, its detailed analytical approach will serve to teach and inspire less accomplished practitioners to begin to manage complex Western diseases.

—**John Pan**, M.D., Clinical Professor & Director,
Center for Integrative Medicine, George Washington University Medical Center

Hyperthyroidism, essential hypertension, and fibromyalgia are Western medical terms, while qi goiter, wasting thirst, and seasonal epidemics are traditional Chinese medical terms, and all have their own reality. This work represents a magnificent bridge between these different medicines which is solidly constructed on clear, precise, profound, and impeccable exposition of these different terms. This is an indispensable book for all those who hope to encounter harmony on the path of medicine.

—**José A. Roquet**, M.D.,
President of the Scientific Association of Medical Acupuncturists of Barcelona (Spain)

The Treatment of Modern Western Medical Diseases with Chinese Medicine

The Treatment of Modern Western Medical Diseases with Chinese Medicine

A Textbook & Clinical Manual

By

Bob Flaws & Philippe Sionneau

Published by:
BLUE POPPY PRESS
A Division of Blue Poppy Enterprises, Inc.
5441 Western Ave., Suite 2
Boulder, CO 80301
www.bluepoppy.com

First Edition, September 2001

ISBN 1-891845-20-9

Page design: Eric J. Brearton
Cover design: Frank Crawford

COMP Designation: Original work

10 9 8 7 6 5 4 3 2 1

Printed at Bang Printing, Brainerd, Minnesota

Library of Congress Cataloging-in-Publication Data

Flaws, Bob, 1946-
The treatment of modern Western diseases with Chinese medicine: a textbook & clinical manual: including indications for referral to Western medical services / by Bob Flaws & Philippe Sionneau.
p. ; cm.
Includes bibliographal references and index.
ISBN 1-891845-20-9
1. Medicine, Chinese. I. Sionneau, Philippe. II. Title.
[DNLM: 1. Medicine, Chinese Traditional. WB 50.1 F591t 2001]
R601. .F583 2001
610'.951–dc21

2001035418

PREFACE

WHAT THIS BOOK IS

This book is a textbook and clinical manual on the treatment of modern Western medical diseases with Chinese medicine. By modern Western medical diseases, we mean the disease categories of modern Western medicine excluding gynecology and pediatrics. By Chinese medicine, we mean standard contemporary professional Chinese medicine as taught at the two dozen or so provincial Chinese medical colleges in the People's Republic of China. The two main therapeutic modalities used in the practice of this style of Chinese medicine are acupuncture-moxibustion and the internal administration of multi-ingredient Chinese medicinal formulas, and treatment plans for each disease discussed herein are given for each of these two main modalities.

Since the middle of the 20th century at least, Chinese doctors in China have been working out the most commonly seen Chinese medical patterns of modern Western diseases. This book follows in that tradition. We have taken this approach because this book is meant primarily for use by Western practitioners, and Western medicine's diagnostic nosology is the dominant one in this milieu. Most Western patients come to Western practitioners of acupuncture and Chinese medicine with a pre-established Western medical diagnosis. This is what they are seeking treatment for and this is what they feel most comfortable talking about. It is the *lingua franca* of the Western health care marketplace. It is our experience that, rightly or wrongly, even most Western Chinese medical practitioners themselves mainly think in terms of Western disease diagnoses. Thus the need for textbooks such as this.

HOW THIS BOOK WAS CREATED

In creating this book, we based its materials on two main sources: 1) the contemporary Chinese language Chinese medical literature and 2) our own clinical experience as Western practitioners treating Western patients. As far as we know, this is the first time that the treatment based on pattern discrimination of some of these diseases, such as fibromyalgia syndrome, interstitial cystitis, celiac disease, and Lyme disease, has been discussed in the Chinese medical literature. Under each disease, we have included short introductory sections on its Western medical etiology, pathophysiology, diagnosis, and treatment. However, these short sections are in no way meant to replace more complete Western medical discussions of these conditions. We are also not suggesting that Western Chinese medical practitioners can or should make such Western medical disease diagnoses, nor that every practitioner can or should treat every case of every disease presented herein. Some of the conditions contained in this book or some of the stages of some of these diseases go beyond the clinical skills of most Western Chinese medical practitioners. Therefore, readers are warned to be circumspect about what they choose to treat, neither exceeding their legal scope of practice or the bounds of good judgement.

In general, Bob Flaws is responsible for most of the Introduction as well as the Western medical introductions to each disease, their Chinese medical disease categorization, and their Chinese medical disease causes and mechanisms. Signs and symptoms for each pattern under each disease and their treatment principles were a joint effort by Bob Flaws and Philippe Sionneau. In most cases, Bob Flaws is responsible for the guiding formula under each pattern, Philippe Sionneau is responsible for the formula's analysis, and both Bob and Philippe worked together on the additions and subtractions. Philippe Sionneau is responsible for the majority of the acupuncture protocols presented in this book, including the basic formulas, formula analyses, and additions and subtractions. The concluding Remarks section to each disease was likewise a joint effort on the part of Flaws and Sionneau.

How this book is arranged

The diseases in this book are arranged in alphabetical order for ease of use by busy clinicians. However, a second Table of Contents is provided arranging these same diseases under the main subspecialties of internal medicine, such as cardiovascular disorders, gastrointestinal disorders, respiratory disorders, neurological disorders, musculoskeletal disorders, etc. A bibliography of Chinese, English, and French language sources is given at the back as well as both a general and a separate formula index.

How the diseases included were chosen

As the title of this book makes clear, all the diseases in it are modern Western medical diagnoses. In chosing what to include and what not to include, we constantly found ourselves juggling what is commonly seen by Western practitioners of Chinese medicine, what there is information on in the Chinese language Chinese medical literature, and what already exists in the English language Chinese medical literature. Some of the diseases in this book are not so commonly seen in the West, such as idiopathic thrombocytopenic purpura and aplastic anemia, not to mention Behçet's syndrome. However, these diseases are routinely included in Chinese language texts of this type. Although Western practitioners may not need daily access to the information on these diseases, when they do, this information will be available to them. In addition, they also give evidence of how Chinese medical practitioners think about and treat such Western medical diseases. Therefore, they serve as a model of a methodology as well as a clinical repertoire. If one understands how the Chinese medical materials under these diseases was arrived at, then one should also be able to do the same thing when faced with a Western medical disease not currently included in this or other books on Chinese medicine.

As the reader will see, some Western medical diseases which are very common in the everyday clinical practice are not included in this book. Mostly this is because good information on their Chinese medical treatment already exists in other English language sources and there were size constraints on how big a single volume such as this can be. For instance, constipation is dealt with exhaustively in Philippe Sionneau's *The Treatment of Disease in TCM*, impotence is dealt with in Anna Lin's *A Handbook of TCM Urology & Male Sexual Dysfunction*, colic, otitis media, and strep throat are dealt with in Bob Flaws's *A Handbook of TCM Pediatrics*, depression and anxiety are dealt with in Bob Flaws and James Lake's *Chinese Medical Psychiatry*, and psoriasis and eczema are dealt with in Liang Jian-hui's *A Handbook of TCM Dermatology*, all available from Blue Poppy Press.

Terminological standards

As with other Blue Poppy Press books, the Chinese-English translational terminology for all Chinese medical technical terms used in this book is based on the work of Nigel Wiseman as it has appeared in *Glossary of Chinese Medical Terms and Acupuncture Points* (1990), *English-Chinese Chinese-English Dictionary of Chinese Medicine* (1995), and, more recently, Wiseman and Feng Ye's *A Practical Dictionary of Chinese Medicine* (1998). Readers wanting a definition of any of the Chinese medical technical terms used in this book should refer to the last title listed above. We believe it is the single best Chinese medical dictionary existing in English at the present time. Departures from Wiseman *et al.*'s suggested terminological standards are footnoted with explanations. Chinese medicinals are identified first by pharmcological Latin followed by the Pinyin romanization of their Chinese names in parentheses. However, after identifying a medicinal within a particular section in this dual manner, only Pinyin is used when the same medicinal is discussed in subsequent paragraphs. Similarly, Chinese medicinal formulas are also identified dually throughout this text. We first give their Chinese name in Pinyin romanization followed by our own translation of that Chinese name in parentheses. In terms of acupuncture points, these are identified first by their Chinese name rendered in Pinyin followed by a channel-numeric notation. These notations are based on the World Health Organization's suggested acupoint nomenclature system. However, as in other Blue Poppy Press books, we have chosen to abbreviate the channel names thus: Lu = lungs, LI = large intestine, St = stomach, Sp = spleen, Ht = heart, SI = small intestine, Bl = bladder, Ki = kidneys, Per = pericardium, TB = triple burner, GB = gallbladder, Liv = liver, GV = governing vessel, and CV = conception vessel.

What this book is meant to do & where it fits in the Chinese medical literature

As a textbook and clinical manual, this book is an example of a particular genre within the Chinese medical literature. In this genre, diseases are broken down into a number of discrete patterns and then treatment protocols are given for each pattern. While such a simplistic approach is not reflective of real-life clinical practice, it is a necessary step in one's Chinese medical education. Textbooks such as this are meant as the first step in a process leading to a more mature and complete understanding of clinical reality. They are not meant as stand-alone bibles, and no such book can fulfill all a clinician's needs. After familiarizing oneself with the information in a book such as this, the Chinese medical student or practitioner is expected to go on to read various case histories, research reports, and medical essays exemplifying and elucidating how this material is actually used. More importantly, one's clinical mentors are meant to demonstrate and embody the real-life use of this information.

However, by and large, Western practitioners do not have access to this supplementary literature, nor do most of us have on-going mentoring relationships with "old Chinese doctors" with 20-50 years clinical experience. Therefore, this book is arranged somewhat differently from most Chinese language examples of this genre. It is divided into two parts. The first part is a general introduction to the theories and principles that we believe are most important in treating the types of complex diseases contained in this book. Most Western patients with chronic diseases do not present a single, neatly circumscribed pattern. Instead, they typically present anywhere from a minimum of three simultaneous patterns to 10 or more. While textbooks such as this must present the discrete patterns under each disease, these patterns do not appear in such a stark and simple manner. Rather they combine in complicated multipattern presentations. This is why the kinds of diseases described in this book are often referred to as "knotty," meaning that they are complicated knots of several disease mechanisms bound together. When it comes to the Chinese medical treatment of such knotty, multipattern conditions, there are certain Chinese medical theories and principles which can help one understand and untie such complicated webs. These include Liu Wan-su's theory of similar transformation, Li Dong-yuan's theory of yin fire, and Zhu Dan-xi's theory of the six depressions. Thus, unlike most such treatment manuals, the first part of this book is devoted to an explanation of these extremely useful theories.

The second part of this book is the treatment formulary section. Like most textbooks of this genre, each disease or condition is divided into a number of patterns with treatment principles and protocols given for each pattern. This method of presentation is a convention meant to demonstrate the main disease mechanisms at work in each disease in as "high relief" as possible. However, the reader is advised to always keep in mind that this method of presentation is *only* a convention. Although we have tried to include as many complicated, multipart patterns under each condition as possible, the patterns that appear in Chinese medical textbooks such as this are only building blocks which must be combined and modified in order to more accurately match each individual patient. In Chinese medicine, patients are not squeezed into patterns to make them fit. Rather, patterns are modified around the patient to completely reflect each patient as they actually are in any given moment of time. In an attempt to underline this fact, the reader is reminded in the "Remarks" section at the end of each disease that the real situation is typically more complicated than any one pattern presented above.

Readers unfamiliar with the Chinese medical literature and the process of Chinese medical education may ask, "Why create such a textbook if it is not congruent with clinical reality?" The answer, or at least our answer, is that no words can completely encompass reality. As Lao Zi said, "The dao that can be spoken of is not the dao." However, one can hint at reality by approaching it from several directions until a fuller, more complete picture is at least intimated. Presenting simple patterns under each disease is a necessary first step in gaining clarity into the treatment of diseases by Chinese medical pattern discrimination even though it is not the definitive or last step. If one understands that textbooks such as these only provide a sort of bare-bones map or groundwork, then one can gratefully accept them for what they are worth as part of a multipart process of maturation.

OUTCOMES STUDIES & CASE HISTORIES

Stastical outcomes studies and representative case histories for most of the diseases covered in this text are available from Blue Poppy Press. Blue Poppy Press currently publishes over 275 Research Reports on almost as many Western diseases, with new Research Reports being added on a regular basis. Each Blue Poppy Research Report contains abstracts of one or more clinical audits or other outcomes studies published in Chinese medical journals in the last 10 years. Many of these reports also contain representative case histories as per Chinese medical convention. In addition, Blue Poppy Press publishes a quarterly on-line Chinese medical journal. Typically, abstracts of 8-12 Chinese outcomes studies are published in each issue of this on-line journal. Subscriptions to this journal are free, and the journal can be accessed at: www.bluepoppy.com.

We hope this book will be useful to many Western practitioners of Chinese medicine. The authors take full responsibility for any errors contained herein and ask our readers to send us their corrections, amendments, and advice. We would also like to thank Drs. John Pan and Robert J. Casanas and Chinese medical practitioners Greg Bantick and Simon Becker for their review of our working manuscript and their many pieces of valuable advice which were included in our finished product.

TABLE OF CONTENTS
(ALPHABETICAL)

TABLE OF CONTENTS
(BY MEDICAL SPECIALTIES)

Pulmonary Disorders

Ear, Nose & Throat Disorders

Ophthalmologic Disorders

Dental & Oral Disorders

Dermatologic Disorders

Hematologic Disorders

Immunologic & Allergic Disorders

Infectious Disorders

Neurologic Disorders

Cardiovascular Disorders

Genitourinary Disorders

INTRODUCTION

This book is a clinical manual on the treatment of modern Western diseases with traditional Chinese medicine. However, any clinician who thinks that one can practice Chinese medicine out of a book like this as easy as one copies recipes from a cookbook is mistaken. After practicing Chinese medicine, in Bob Flaws's case, for more than 20 years and having written, translated, and edited scores of similar clinical manuals in both English and French, we can tell you this is just not possible. At least it is not possible if your goal is to practice Chinese medicine skillfully at the professional level. Books such as this are meant to and can only act as starting places for thinking about and applying the Chinese medical methodology to one's patients' clinical dilemmas. Every patient is unique, and, therefore, in professional Chinese medicine, every patient is supposed to get their own individualized treatment plan. It is such individually tailored treatment plans which make Chinese medicine the safe, effective, and holistic medicine it is.

It is the prescriptive and problem-solving methodology of Chinese medicine which is its most valuable attribute. Professional Chinese medicine is a way of thinking, not a bag of clinical tricks from the mysterious East. Clinical manuals such as this suggest this or that formula or this or that group of acupuncture points for various patterns of various diseases. However, because of the constraints of language and the printed page, no author can give a categorically complete set of treatment protocols for every manifestation of every disease. Therefore, at some point, the reader must fall back on their own understanding of and proficiency in Chinese medicine's prescriptive methodology. Hence, unlike most other clinical manuals of Chinese medicine, we feel that it is important to take some time to clarify this methodology in order to help the reader understand what books such as this can and cannot do.

1. PREREQUISITES

First of all, before being able to use the information in this book, we must presuppose that our readers have successfully completed certain basic courses in their Chinese medical training. In terms of acupuncture, those prerequisite courses are shown in the table below. In terms of Chinese herbal medicine, the necessary preliminary courses are shown in the table on top of the next page.

In China today, entry-level students study either acupuncture or Chinese internal medicine. Each is its own five year, 4,000 hour, full-time course of study.[1] Chinese students do not attempt to master both these arts. While some of the course

BASIC PREREQUISITES FOR TREATING MODERN WESTERN DISEASES WITH ACUPUNCTURE

• Basic Chinese medical physiology	• Point theory
• Basic Chinese medical pathophysiology	• Combining points
• The four examinations	• Needle technique (including moxibustion, bleeding, cupping, etc.)
• Basic Chinese medical pattern discrimination	• The acupuncture treatment of two dozen or more traditional Chinese diseases
• Basic Chinese medical treatment principles	
• Channel & network vessel theory	

BASIC PREREQUISITES FOR TREATING MODERN WESTERN DISEASES WITH CHINESE MEDICINALS

- Basic Chinese medical physiology
- Basic Chinese medical pathophysiology
- The four examinations
- Basic Chinese medical pattern discrimination
- Basic Chinese medical treatment principles
- Materia medica (not less than 160 individual Chinese medicinals)
- Formulas & prescriptions (not less than 70 basic formulas)
- Processing Chinese medicinals
- Combining Chinese medicinals
- Modifying formulas with additions & subtractions
- The Chinese medicinal treatment of two dozen or more traditional Chinese diseases

work overlaps, each modality has its own huge body of information which must be memorized and mastered. This contemporary separation in the practice of these two modalities mirrors the situation in most Asian countries throughout the majority of historical periods.[2] In the West, most students try to learn both modalities in 3-4 years of often part-time training conducted at night and on weekends. Because most Western practitioners of Chinese medicine practice both modalities concurrently on the majority of their patients, we have given both Chinese medicinal and acupuncture protocols for each pattern of each disease discussed. However, to practice either modality competently requires a great deal of study and practice. Further, some diseases respond better to internal medicine than to acupuncture, while other diseases are adequately treated by acupuncture alone. When one is truly competent in either of these modalities, then one understands what one can and cannot treat efficiently and effectively. Those conditions which fall outside the scope of one's personally practiced modality should be referred to a specialist expert in the other modality.

If one has not completed the above elementary courses in Chinese medicine, then one cannot reasonably and responsibly use the material in this or similar Chinese medical clinical manuals. Chinese medicine is not safe and effective because its modalities are either Chinese or natural. Chinese medicine is safe and effective because of its prescriptive methodology, and one cannot apply this prescriptive methodology in a professionally standard, competent way until or unless one has mastered the foregoing course work.[3]

2. THE CHINESE MEDICAL PRESCRIPTIVE METHODOLOGY

Basically, the Chinese medical prescriptive methodology can be summed up in four Chinese words: *bian zheng lun zhi*. This means that, no matter what the patient's disease diagnosis, professionally administered Chinese medical treatment is primarily predicated on the patient's Chinese pattern discrimination. When Chinese doctors say that treatment should be based on the patient's personal pattern discrimination, they are implicitly juxtaposing this methodology with that of basing treatment primarily on the patient's disease diagnosis. In Chinese, this other methodology is called *bian bing lun zhi*. Basing treatment primarily on disease diagnosis is the prescriptive methodology of both modern Western medicine and most Chinese folk medicine. According to this latter methodology, patients with the same disease get the same treatment. However, in standard professionally practiced Chinese medicine, patients with the same disease do not always get the same treatment. Thus it is said:

> Different diseases, same treatment (*yi bing tong zhi*)
> Same disease, different treatment (*tong bing yi zhi*)

This means that two patients with different named disease diagnoses will receive different Chinese medical treatments *if their Chinese patterns are different*. In fact, not only will the treatment for one patient not help the other, it may, in fact, cause serious harm. Conversely, two patients with different disease diagnoses will receive the same treatment in Chinese medicine if their Chinese patterns are the same. For instance, one patient may be diagnosed as suffering from systemic lupus erythmatosus and another from Lyme disease. In Western medicine, these are two different disease diagnoses. One is an autoimmune disease and the other is an infectious disease. Nevertheless, if these two patients both exhibit the same Chinese patterns, their Chinese medical treatment will be essentially the same and possibly even identical.

THE RELATIONSHIP BETWEEN DISEASES & PATTERNS

Both diseases and patterns have their pathognomonic or defining signs and symptoms. However, the defining signs and symptoms of patterns are always more inclusive than the defining signs and symptoms of a disease. Said the other way round, the defining signs and symptoms of a disease are always only part of the signs and symptoms of the patient's pattern. The defining signs and symptoms of a patient's pattern are all those deviations in all bodily functions and appearances from the norms of Chinese medicine as gathered by the four examinations. Thus the relationship between diseases and patterns is that between figure and ground or tree and forest. The signs and symptoms defining a patient's disease are like a figure existing against the backdrop of its ground or like a tree or clump of trees standing in a forest.

Take for instance the Western disease diagnosis of migraine headache. For a patient's headache to be diagnosed as a migraine, it must last from 4-72 hours, be throbbing in nature, moderate to severe in intensity, unilateral in location, worse with exertion, and associated with nausea, vomiting, or sensitivity to light, sound, or smell.[4] These are the pathognomonic signs and symptoms of the disease category of migraine headache. If one does not have preponderance of these signs and symptoms, *ipso facto*, one does not have a migraine headache. However, migraineurs may be male or female, ectomorphic or endomorphic, old or young. They may have constipation or diarrhea. They may have large or small appetites. They may have dry mucus membranes or secrete excessive mucus and phlegm. They may be thirsty and crave chilled drinks, thirsty and like warm drinks, be thirsty and yet not desire to drink, or they may not be thirsty at all. In fact, they may be averse to drinking. If female, their migraines may come before, during, or after menstruation, and such women's menses may be either early, late, erratic, scanty, or profuse, bright red, pale red, or dark red. All these signs and symptoms are in addition to the defining signs and symptoms of migraine headache. These other signs and symptoms make up the totality of the patient's diseased condition. They are what individuate one migraineur from another, making each patient a unique clinical conundrum.

When treatment is focused primarily on the disease diagnosis, that treatment may or may not fit the totality of the patient's unique condition. If it does happen to fit, there will be healing without side effects. If not, either the patient will not get completely better or there may be unwanted side effects. Side effects are always due to a medicine's or treatment's not completely fitting the totality of a patient's condition, at least as defined by Chinese pattern discrimination. Within Chinese medicine, because the body is seen as a single, integrated, organic whole, eliminating one symptom while producing some other symptom is like robbing Peter to pay Paul. Except in very limited circumstances, such as Herxheimer reactions discussed below, this kind of shortsighted, myopic treatment is considered unacceptable to Chinese doctors. Symptoms, no matter how they are produced, are always a sign that something is out of balance in the bodymind, and the goal of professional Chinese medicine is to bring the entire organism back into a state of healthy, dynamic balance. Therefore, because it is pattern discrimination which allows us to see the larger picture or the whole person, it is treatment based on pattern discrimination which allows Chinese doctors to provide safe and effective treatment without side effects.

THE 10 TYPES OF PATTERN DISCRIMINATION

In contemporary standard professional Chinese medicine, 10 types of pattern discrimination are used in order to describe the totality of a patient's condition. These 10 are shown in the table below.

Each of these 10 systems of pattern discrimination is studied and learned as a self-contained system at Chinese medical schools. Those people who characterize modern Chinese practitioners as using only eight principle pattern discrimination simply do not know what they are talking about. No one of these 10 systems is pre-eminent or privileged above any other. The issue is using that system which best describes the patient's mixture of signs and symptoms.

In real-life clinical practice, these different systems are usually combined to achieve as comprehensive and accurate description of the patient's imbalance as possible. For instance, when

THE 10 TYPES OF CHINESE PATTERN DISCRIMINATION

1. Eight principles pattern discrimination
   (*ba gang bian zheng*)
2. Five phases pattern discrimination
   (*wu xing bian zheng*)
3. Qi & blood pattern discrimination
   (*qi xue bian zheng*)
4. Fluid & humor pattern discrimination
   (*jin ye bian zheng*)
5. Viscera & bowel pattern discrimination
   (*zang fu bian zheng*)
6. Channel & network vessel pattern discrimination
   (*jing luo bian zheng*)
7. Disease cause pattern discrimination
   (*bing yin bian zheng*)
8. Six divisions pattern discrimination
   (*liu fen bian zheng*)
9. Four divisions pattern discrimination
   (*si fen bian zheng*)
10. Three burners pattern discrimination
   (*san jiao bian zheng*)

one says that a patient's pattern was liver depression qi stagnation with transformative heat, one is using three different systems of pattern discrimination. By saying liver and not heart or stomach, one is using viscera and bowel pattern discrimination. Saying that there is transformative heat is a type of eight principles pattern discrimination since the discrimination of heat from cold is part of that system. In addition, liver depression is a species of repletion, and the discrimination of repletion from vacuity is another part of eight principles pattern discrimination. As another example, if one says that the patient's pattern is liver wood assailing and damaging the spleen, one has specifically used viscera bowel pattern discrimination and five phases pattern discrimination. One has also implied eight principles pattern discrimination, since liver assailing spleen means that, due to the liver being replete, the spleen has become vacuous.

Of these 10 systems, only the last three tend to be used as stand-alone systems, and even the last two are typically combined. System No. 8 refers to the six divisions of cold damage originated by Zhang Zhong-jing. Of these six divisions, only the *shao yang* division is still regularly used in Western clinical practice.[5] Systems No. 9 and 10 are both parts of Qing dynasty warm disease theory. The four divisions are the defensive, qi, constructive, and blood. These describe the common routes of transmission of externally contracted warm heat evils in the body. Three burner pattern discrimination offers yet further elaboration on the routes of transmission of such warm heat evils through the three burners.

THE THREE CONSTITUENTS OF A CHINESE MEDICAL PATTERN

Chinese medical patterns are made up of three groups or streams of information gathered by the four examinations. Those three groups of information are 1) general signs and symptoms, 2) tongue signs, and 3) pulse signs. First of all, *only* information gathered by the four examinations is germane with making a Chinese pattern discrimination. Although research is currently being conducted in the People's Republic of China trying to ascertain what Western medical laboratory tests reliably correspond to Chinese patterns[6], no such test is yet considered standard in professional Chinese medicine. Secondly, it is the coordination of signs and symptoms, tongue signs, and pulse signs which make up a Chinese medical pattern. No single sign or symptom equals a pattern. By its very nature, a pattern must be made up of more than a single element.[7] The meaning of any single sign or symptom only becomes apparent in the light of the other signs and symptoms with which it appears. If any element of these three groups of information is materially different, then one is dealing with a different pattern. If all three groups of information are the same, then the patterns are the same, and their different names are only that, different names for essentially the same diagnostic entity.

THE STEPS IN THE CHINESE MEDICAL PRESCRIPTIVE METHODOLOGY

Professional Chinese medicine is a rational medicine, and there is a definite step-by-step process taught at Chinese medical schools for arriving at correct treatment plans.[8] The table below outlines the steps in this logical process.

This step-by-step methodology is the standard of care in professionally practiced Chinese medicine in the People's Republic of China, and it is only by reliance on such a codified prescriptive methodology that one can have a national

THE STEPS IN THE CHINESE MEDICAL PRESCRIPTIVE METHODOLOGY

1. Gather information via the four examinations
2. Analyze that data according to Chinese medical theory
3. Determine the modern Western disease diagnosis (or write down such a pre-established diagnosis)
4. Determine the traditional Chinese medical disease diagnoses
5. Determine the Chinese pattern discrimination
6. State the treatment principles necessary to rebalance the imbalance implied in the name(s) of the patient's pattern(s)
7. Choose treatment methods logically derived from those treatment principles
8. Administer that treatment
9. Assess the outcome of that treatment
10. Reframe the patients' pattern discrimination based on that assessment
11. Reframe the treatment principles based on the new pattern discrimination
12. Modify the treatment plan to embody these new or revised treatment principles
13. Continue with steps 9-13 until the patient is cured or stabilized

or even international profession with confidence of referral, peer review, and third party payment. As Birch and Felt say, "Bluntly stated, if practitioners who are trained in the same system of practice cannot examine the same group of patients without statistically significant agreement on diagnosis and treatment, those diagnoses will not be considered valid."[9]

THE FOUR EXAMINATIONS

The four examinations are looking, listening-smelling, palpating, and questioning. Looking means to assess the spirit by looking at the clarity of the eyes, the affect, and the facial complexion. It also means to inspect the carriage and physical movement, the body type, the skin, and any physical lesions, sites of injury, or diseased body parts. Listening-smelling refers to listening to the breathing and any pathological respiratory sounds as well as to listening to the volume, tone, and timbre of the voice and the quality of coherence of the speech. Listening-smelling also refers to smelling any abnormal body or excretory odors, although, nowadays, such abnormalities in smell are mostly reported by the patient themself or their close family members. Palpating primarily means palpating the pulse at the radial arteries on each wrist. For a thorough exposition of Chinese pulse examination, the reader should see Bob Flaws's *The Secret of Chinese Pulse Diagnosis* also published by Blue Poppy Press. In addition, practitioners typically palpate any diseased area or body part to detect changes in temperature, tone, articulation, and anatomy.

Questioning means asking the patient about the cause, onset, duration, and symptoms of their disease as well as the result of any previous treatment for their current complaint. In addition, questioning includes asking the patient about all their bodily functions, such as appetite, diet, energy, memory, mood, excretion (*i.e.*, perspiration, defecation, and urination), and sleep. Women are further asked about their menstruation and any history of conception, gestation, and lactation. All patients are typically asked to furnish a basic medical history, including any medications they are currently taking. Nowadays in the West, some of this questioning is accomplished by the use of in-take questionnaires. An example of the one used by Bob Flaws, available in packets of 50 from Blue Poppy Press, is presented in Fig. 1, on the next two pages.

When questioning, it is extremely important to only add to one's Chinese medical analysis of the patient's case those answers that a traditional Chinese doctor might have elicited in the mid-19th century. In other words, one must mentally set aside information conveyed by the patient regarding Western medical tests. For instance, patients may tell their Chinese medical practitioner that they are anemic. By itself, this information is meaningless in terms of Chinese pattern discrimination. If the practitioner mistakenly hears the word anemia and immediately turns that into the Chinese pattern of blood vacuity, this is a mistake in Chinese medical methodology. While anemia may manifest as blood vacuity, it never manifests as only blood vacuity. In fact, its first clinical manifestation is typically fatigue, a qi vacuity symptom, not a blood vacuity symptom. Patients in the 21st century may tell their Chinese medical practitioners all sorts of Western medical information about their blood analyses, ovulation, or peristalsis, and their Chinese medical practitioner must be very careful to set this information in abeyance in terms of making their Chinese pattern discrimination. Only signs and symptoms gathered and knowable by the traditional four examinations may be used to establish a Chinese pattern.

In order to do Chinese medical pattern discrimination, one must unambiguously know the signs and symptoms which are considered the standard definitive ones for each of the major patterns of Chinese medicine. In addition, one should also understand the basic Chinese disease mechanisms responsible for the production of these signs and symptoms. By understanding these disease mechanisms, one can then understand other possible signs and symptoms which may also be produced by these same mechanisms.

In addition, it is very important that Western practitioners be sure to use the technically correct English language equivalents for signs and symptoms used to define the professionally standard patterns of Chinese medicine. Often this requires clarifying and reframing a patient's response to a Chinese medical query. For instance, the Chinese medical concepts of *xiong men*, chest oppression, and *mei he qi*, plum pit qi, are not common Western concepts. Therefore, Western patients never spontaneously use these terms. Thus, when a Western patient says that they are short of breath, the Chinese medical practitioner must be sure to clarify whether that means that they struggle for breath with short, rapid, shallow breaths after slight exertion (*qi duan*, shortness of breath) or they feel a sense of constriction and stuffiness in their chest which makes them want to take a deep breath from time to time (*xiong men*, chest oppression). Likewise, a patient who says they have postnasal drip must be further questioned to ascertain whether this means that they have a chronic sore throat (*yan tong*, throat pain) or plum pit qi *(mei he qi)* in terms of Chinese medical symptoms. In either of these two cases, lack of clarification and reframing of these linguistic equivalents would lead to quite different, possibly even diametrically opposed patterns and, therefore, erroneous treatments. For more information on the definitive signs and symptoms of the main patterns of Chinese medicine, readers are referred to Bob Flaws and Daniel Finney's *A Compendium of TCM Patterns & Treatments* (Blue Poppy Press).

New Patient Intake Form

Today's Date____/____/____

Name | SS# | Birthdate / /
Marital Status | Age
Address | ❑M ❑ F | Ht | Wt

City, State, Zip
Home Phone | Work Phone | Occupation
Emergency Contact Name & Phone
Referred by
Reason for visit today | Have you had acupuncture before? ❑ Yes ❑ No | Chinese herbal medicine? ❑ Yes ❑ No
How long have you had this condition?
Is it getting worse? Does it bother your: ❑ Sleep ❑ Work ❑ C (what?)
What seemed to be the initial cause?
What seems to make it better?
What seems to make it worse?
Are you under the care of a physician now? ❑ Ye ❑ ...or what?
Who is your physician? Phy...ian's Phone
Other concurrent therapies

Health Insurance Info:
Insurance Co. Name | Policy #
Address | Phone
City, State, Zip

Medicare Info:
Insurance Co. Name | Policy #
Address | Phone
City, State, Zip

Family Medical H...ory

❑ Allergies ❑ Arteriosclerosis ❑ Asthm... ❑ Cancer ❑ Diabetes ❑ Heart Disease ❑ High Blood Pressure ❑ Seizures ❑ Stroke

Your Past Medical Histor...

(Check any of the following conditions you currently ...e, or have had in the past. Please also check if you feel any of the following are a significant part of your medical history.)

❑ AIDs/HIV
❑ Alcoholism
❑ Allergies
❑ Appendicitis
❑ Arteriosclerosis
❑ Asthma
❑ Birth Trauma (your own birth)
❑ Cancer
❑ Chicken Pox
❑ Diab...
❑ Emphy...sema
❑ Epilepsy
❑ Goiter
❑ Gout
❑ Heart Disease
❑ Hepatitus
❑ Herpes
❑ High Blood Pressure
❑ Measles
❑ Multiple Sclerosis
❑ Mumps
❑ Pacemaker
❑ Pleurisy
❑ Pneumonia
❑ Polio
❑ Rheumatic Fever
❑ Scarlet Fever
❑ Seizures
❑ Stroke
❑ Surgery (list)
❑ Thyroid Disorders
❑ Major Trauma (Car, fall, etc--list)
❑ Tuberculosis
❑ Typhoid Fever
❑ Ulcers
❑ Venereal Disease
❑ Whooping Cough
❑ Other (Specify)

Your Diet

Appetite ❑ Low ❑ High | ❑ Coffee ❑ Soft Drinks | ❑ Artificial Sweetener | ❑ Sugar ❑ Salty Food | Thirst for water: # glasses per day:________

Average Daily Menu

Morning | Snack | Noon | Snack | Evening | Snack

Pharmaceuticals taken in last 2 months:
Vitamins/supplements taken in last 2 months:

FIGURE 1

Your Lifestyle

❑ Alcohol
❑ Tobacco
❑ Marijuana
❑ Drugs
❑ Stress
❑ Occupational Hazards

Regular Exercise
Type__________ Frequency__________
Type__________ Frequency__________

General Symptoms

❑ Poor appetite
❑ Heavy appetite
❑ Strongly like cold drinks
❑ Strongly like hot drinks
❑ Recent weight loss/gain
❑ Poor sleep
❑ Heavy sleep
❑ Dream-disturbed sleep
❑ Fatigue
❑ Lack of strength
❑ Bodily heaviness
❑ Cold hands or feet
❑ Poor circulation
❑ Shortness of breath
❑ Fever
❑ Chills
❑ Night sweats
❑ Sweat easily
❑ Muscle cramps
❑ Vertigo or dizziness
❑ Bleed or bruise easily
❑ Peculiar taste (describe)
____
____
____

Head, Eyes, Ears, Nose, Throat

❑ Glasses
❑ Eye strain
❑ Eye pain
❑ Red eyes
❑ Itchy eyes
❑ Spots in eyes
❑ Poor vision
❑ Blurred vision
❑ Night blindness
❑ Glaucoma
❑ Cataracts
❑ Teeth problems
❑ Grinding teeth
❑ TMJ
❑ Facial pain
❑ Gum problems
❑ Sores on lips or tongue
❑ Dry mouth
❑ Excessive saliva
❑ Sinus problems
❑ Excessive phlegm
Color of phlegm
____
❑ Recurrent sore throat
❑ Swollen glands
❑ Lumps in thro
❑ Enlarged th d
❑ Nose ble
❑ Ringi s
❑ Poor he
❑ Earaches
❑ Headaches
❑ Migraines
❑ Concussions
Other head or neck problems
____
____
____

Respiratory

❑ Difficulty breathing when lying down
❑ Shortness of breath
❑ Tight chest
❑ Asthma/wheezing
❑ Cough
Wet or Dry?__________
Thick or thin?__________
or of phlegm
____
❑ Coughing blood
❑ Pneumonia

Cardiovascular

❑ High blood pressure
❑ Blood clots
❑ Low blood pressure
❑ Fainting
❑ Chest pain
❑ Difficulty breathin
❑ Tachycar
❑ Heart palpitations
❑ Phlebitis
❑ Irregular heartbeat

Gastrointestinal

❑ Nausea
❑ Vomiting
❑ Acid regurgitation
❑ Gas
❑ Hiccup
❑ Bloating
❑ Bad breath
❑ Diarrhea
❑ Constipation
❑ Laxative use
❑ Black stools
❑ Bloody stools
❑ Mucous in stools
❑ Intestin mping
❑ Itchy anu
❑ Burning a
❑ Rectal pain
hoid
Bowel movements:
Frequency__________ Texture/form__________
Color__________ Odor__________

Musculoskeletal

❑ Neck/shoulder pain
❑ Muscle pain
❑ Upper back pai
❑ Low back pain
❑ Join n
ib pain
❑ Limited range of motion
❑ Limited use
Other (describe)
____

Skin and Hair

❑ Rashes
❑ Hives
❑ Ulcerations
❑ Eczema
Psori
❑ Dandruff
❑ Itching
❑ Hair loss
❑ Change in hair/skin texture
❑ Fungal infections
Other hair or skin problems
____
____

Neuropsychological

❑ Seizures
❑ Numbness
❑ Tics
❑ Poor me
❑ Depressio
❑ Anxiety
❑ Irritability
❑ Easily stressed
❑ Abuse survivor
❑ Considered/attempted suicide
❑ Seeing a therapist
Other (specify)
____
____

Genito-urinary

❑ Pain on urination
❑ Frequent urination
❑ Urgent urination
❑ Blood in urine
❑ Unable to hold urine
❑ Incomplete urination
❑ Venereal disease
❑ Bedwetting
❑ Wake to urinate
❑ Increased libido
❑ Decreased libido
❑ Kidney stone
❑ Impotence
❑ Premature ejaculation
❑ Nocturnal emission

Gynecology

❑ Age menses began
____
Length of cycle (day 1 to day 1)
____
❑ Duration of flow
____
❑ Irregular periods
❑ Painful periods
❑ PMS
❑ Vaginal discharge (color)__________
❑ Vaginal sores
❑ Vaginal odor
❑ Clots
❑ Breast lumps
Pregnancies__________
Live births__________
Premature births__________
Age at Menopause__________
Date of last PAP
____
Date last period began
____

Other

____
____
____
____

FIGURE 1 (CONTINUED)

TREATMENT PRINCIPLES

In Chinese medicine, it is said that the treatment principles are the bridge between the patient's pattern and their treatment. We cannot overemphasize the over-riding guiding importance of always stating, in writing on the patient's chart, the requisite treatment principles after arriving at the patient's pattern discrimination. First, these treatment principles should always be stated according to the terminological norms of standard professional Chinese medicine. In standard professional Chinese medicine, only certain principles are accepted as the logical remedies to certain patterns. For instance, for the pattern of spleen qi vacuity, we can say either fortify the spleen and supplement the qi, fortify the spleen and boost the qi, or supplement the spleen and boost the qi. We can even say to bank up earth. But to say warm the spleen and transform dampness is categorically wrong. The next table lists the most commonly seen patterns and the most common statement of their treatment principles as well as the corresponding chapters of materia medica and formulas and prescriptions books to these principles.

COMMON PATTERNS AND TREATMENT PRINCIPLES

Corresponding chapters of materia medica and formulas are noted in italic.

1. Liver depression qi stagnation

Course the liver & rectify the qi
Course the liver & resolve depression
Soothe the liver
Move the qi

Pick treatment from qi-rectifying chapter.

2. Spleen qi vacuity weakness

Fortify the spleen & boost the qi
Fortify the spleen & supplement the qi
Supplement the spleen & boost the qi
Bank earth

Pick treatment from qi-supplementing chapter.

3. Blood vacuity

Nourish the blood
Supplement the blood

Pick treatment from the blood-supplementing chapter.

4. Yin vacuity

Enrich yin
Nourish yin
Supplement yin
Supplement the kidneys & enrich yin
Engender fluids (for lung and/or stomach yin vacuity or intestinal dryness)

Pick treatment from yin-supplementing chapter.

5. Yang vacuity

Invigorate yang
Strengthen yang
Assist yang
Warm yang
Supplement yang
Supplement the kidneys & invigorate, strengthen, or assist yang

Pick treatment from yang-supplementing chapter.

6. Heat

Clear heat
Drain heat
Discharge heat
Out-thrust heat
Precipitate heat
Recede or abate heat

Pick treatment from heat-clearing chapter for clearing, discharging, draining, and abating heat. Pick treatment from exterior-resolving or qi-rectifying chapter for out-thrusting heat. Pick treatment from precipitating chapter for precipitating heat.

7. Dampness

Eliminate dampness
Dry dampness
Transform dampness
Disinhibit dampness
Percolate or seep dampness

Pick treatment from dampness-eliminating chapter.

8. Blood stasis

Quicken the blood & transform stasis
Quicken the blood & dispel stasis
Quicken the blood & free the flow of the network vesels
Break the blood (or stasis)

Pick treatment from blood-rectifying chapter.

9. Phlegm

Transform phlegm
Disperse phlegm
Scatter nodulation

Pick treatment from the phlegm-dispelling chapter.

10. Wind

External wind:

Dispel wind

Expel wind
Course wind
Scatter wind

Pick treatment from exterior-resolving or wind-dispelling chapter.

Internal wind:

Extinguish wind
Search or track down wind
Level the liver & extinguish wind

Pick treatment from the liver-leveling, wind-extinguishing chapter.

11. Food stagnation

Abduct stagnation
Disperse stagnation (or food)
Transform food
Abduct or disperse accumulation

Pick treatment from the dispersing, abducting, transforming accumulation chapter.

12. Liver-spleen disharmony (*i.e.*, liver depression-spleen vacuity)

Harmonize the liver & spleen
Course the liver & rectify the qi, fortify the spleen & boost the qi

Pick treatment from the harmonizing chapter.

13. Liver-kidney yin vacuity

Nourish the liver & enrich the kidneys
Nourish the liver & supplement the kidneys
Supplement the liver & kidneys, nourish the blood & enrich yin

Pick treatment from the yin-supplementing chapter.

14. Liver-kidney yang vacuity

Supplement the liver & kidneys, nourish the blood & warm or invigorate yang
Nourish the liver, supplement the kidneys and warm or invigorate yang

Pick treatment from the yang-supplementing chapter.

Secondly, always state the treatment principles in the same order as the listing of the patient's patterns. If one says, "liver depression qi stagnation with spleen vacuity and dampness," this implies that liver depression is primary, spleen vacuity is secondary, and dampness is third in importance. Therefore, the treatment principles should also be stated in the same order as the patient's pattern, thus reflecting the priorities in treatment. In our preceding example, this means that we should say, "Course the liver and rectify the qi, fortify the spleen and eliminate dampness," in this order. In standard professional Chinese medicine, any other order is considered categorically wrong. Having stated the treatment principles in this way, one immediately knows that the patient's treatment will be made up of three different groups of points or classes of medicinals. There will be points or medicinals to course the liver and rectify the qi, points or medicinals to fortify the spleen, and points or medicinals to eliminate dampness.

As long as one always states the requisite treatment principles for each pattern in the patient's case in the same order as their patterns, it does not matter how many patterns the patient is manifesting simultaneously. One simply chooses appropriate treatments for each of the stated principles, remembering to weight these treatments in the proportions implied by the order of these principles' statement. In terms of Chinese medicinals and formulas, most contemporary materia medicas and formulas and prescriptions books categorize medicinals and formulas using the same terminology as the main treatment principles. Therefore, there are qi-rectifying chapters, blood-supplementing chapters, exterior-resolving chapters, wind-extinguishing chapters, etc. Typically, one will find their guiding prescription in the chapter of their formulas and prescriptions book with the same title as the first treatment principle in their list. Then medicinals added for the sake of addressing complicating patterns are usually found in the chapters titled similarly to the succeeding treatment principles. Because of the overlapping use of the same terminology from treatment principles to materia medicas and formulas and prescriptions books, it is very important to use this terminology correctly. When one uses this terminology correctly, it makes it extremely easy to find guiding formulas and modifying medicinals.

In addition, when stating the treatment principles, one should include at least one principle for each of the patient's patterns as well as be careful not to add any principles not strictly derived from the statement of the patient's pattern. In this sense, the treatment principles are the practitioner's warrant. In law, a warrant allows someone to do something which is otherwise illegal. A warrant gives a person permission to do something. Likewise, our treatment principles allow us to administer certain treatments. Therefore, unless our patient's patterns include the pattern of kidney yang vacuity, we may not decide to supplement the kidneys and invigorate yang. Without the presence of that pattern, we cannot posit that principle, and without positing that principle, supplementation of the kidneys and invigoration of yang is unwarranted. Hence the statement of treatment principles act not only as a bridge or funnel to the treatment plan, it also acts as a check or balance against unwarranted and erroneous treatment.

When one moves from signs and symptoms → pattern discrimination → treatment principles → treatment plan, the logic and correctness of this progression can be checked at every stage. Do the signs and symptoms truly add up to the stated pattern? Are the treatment principles ones which are generally accepted as standard within the profession? Is each point of the treatment plan logically derived from one or more of the treatment principles? Because there are generally accepted standards of care within professionally practiced Chinese medicine (at least as practiced in the People's Republic of China), this step-by-step methodology allows for peer review.

When one follows this step-by-step process in a very careful, methodical way, one is funneled to the correct Chinese medical treatment plan *as long as one has mastered the prerequisite information to make this process work.* For example, if a patient's Chinese pattern discrimination is liver depression qi stagnation, then the treatment principles are to course the liver and rectify the qi. As soon as one has stated those principles, one knows that anything which courses the liver and rectifies the qi will be good for this patient. In terms of acupuncture points, one will generally (though not always) begin by choosing a point or points on the liver channel. Secondly, one will narrow their choice of points on that channel down to those which A) course the liver and rectify the qi (as opposed to clearing heat or supplementing yin), and B) are empirically known to treat the patient's major complaints which are the manifestation of liver depression qi stagnation. In terms of Chinese medicinals, as soon as one sees the words "course the liver and rectify the qi," one knows that, as long as that is the only pattern stated, one should find the guiding formula in the qi-rectifying chapter of their formulas and prescriptions book. If liver depression qi stagnation is the patient's only pattern, to look for a guiding formula in any other chapter is categorically incorrect. Then, within that chapter, one must find a formula which A) addresses liver depression and B) is empirically known to treat the patient's major complaints due to liver depression.

Because of the reliability of this step-by-step methodology, when Bob Flaws was studying Chinese herbal medicine at the Shanghai College of Chinese medicine, Prof. Chen Wei said, "In clinical practice, if the emphasis is on correct pattern discrimination and strict deduction of treatment principles, then the choice of formulas is easy and the therapeutic effect will be good."[10] This is Chinese medical methodology in a nutshell.

WHAT ABOUT THE WESTERN & CHINESE DISEASE DIAGNOSES?

Above, we said that steps number three and four in this step-by-step methodology are to first state the patient's Western medical disease diagnosis and then state their traditional Chinese disease diagnosis. If treatment is primarily predicated on the patient's pattern(s), what difference does it make whether we state these disease diagnoses or not? On the one hand, it does not make any difference. It is true, no matter what the disease diagnosis, the bottom line in standard professionally practiced Chinese medicine is that treatment is primarily based on the patient's pattern discrimination. On the other hand, both the Western and Chinese disease diagnoses do supply us with useful information.

First of all, each Western medical disease does have its own unique natural history. Chinese patterns are not very useful for prognosis or determining the severity of a condition. One person may manifest yin vacuity with vacuity heat and only have a little pale red, diffuse papular acne on their forehead plus a tendency to poor sleep and easy excitability, while another person with the same pattern may have severe Cushing's syndrome. Similarly, one person with liver depression qi stagnation may suffer from irritability and a tendency to hiccups, while another person may be diagnosed with breast cancer. It is the Western disease diagnosis which helps understand the severity of the patient's condition and alerts us to their probable course. Knowing that a person is suffering from hyperthyroidism, we can be on guard for thyroid storms. Knowing that one person has fibromyalgia and another has MS, tells us that one person's disease is not progressive and potentially life-threatening, while the other person's is.

Secondly, knowing a patient's Chinese disease diagnosis can help us determine what their patterns are. For over 2,000 years, Chinese doctors have been writing down which patterns are the main ones for each traditional Chinese disease. In Chinese internal medicine or *nei ke,* there is an open-ended, indefinite list of Chinese diseases. Because there is no single unifying principle grouping these together, as in gynecology or pediatrics, they are referred to as *za bing* or "miscellaneous diseases." Some of these "diseases" are common symptoms, such as headache, stomachache, low back pain, tinnitus, dizziness, cough, diarrhea, and bloody nose. Others are Chinese categories which have no exact equivalents in modern Western medicine. The Chinese disease of mounting includes hernias of various kinds but also covers other ingenuinal and genital region conditions which are not hernias *per se,* such as hydrocele, scrotal cysts, scrotal infections, testicular tumors, epididymitis, and orchitis. Wasting and thirsting covers diabetes mellitus, but it also covers the cachexia of AIDS and end-stage cancer. Strangury covers gonorrhea, cystitis, prostatitis, and even urinary tract stones. There are hundreds, if not thousands, of Chinese books, both premodern and contemporary, which discuss the commonly seen patterns and their treatments under each of these Chinese disease categories.

Therefore, if one comes across a modern Western disease which one has never seen before and knows nothing about, the first thing one should do is determine what are the main Chinese disease categories which correspond to the Western diseases main clinical manifestations.[11] For instance, two of the main clinical manifestations of Lyme disease, a disease not yet discussed in the Chinese language Chinese medical literature as far as we know, are joint pain and fatigue. Joint pain corresponds to the Chinese disease category of impediment, while fatigue is simply fatigue. Each of these is a traditional Chinese disease category in its own right about which there is voluminous Chinese literature. Therefore, every Chinese medical book and journal article dealing with a modern Western disease always begins by identifying the Chinese disease categories covering the same clinical manifestations.

Every entry level student of either acupuncture or Chinese internal medicine is supposed to have studied the disease causes, disease mechanisms, pattern discrimination, treatment principles, and treatments of 20 or more of these Chinese disease categories. This is basic, foundational material which all professional practitioners are supposed to have well memorized and at their fingertips. If one knows that the chronic symptoms of Lyme disease revolve mostly around impediment and fatigue and one knows how to pattern discriminate and treat impediment and fatigue, then, *voilá!*, one knows how to pattern discriminate and treat Lyme disease. This is why the reader will see that the first category of Chinese medical information after the Western medical description of each disease covered in this book is a statement of the Chinese diseases which correspond to that Western disease. For more information on these traditional Chinese diseases, the reader is recommended to Philippe Sionneau and Lü Gang's seven volume series, *The Treatment of Disease in TCM* also published by Blue Poppy Press. This is the largest and most complete collection of patterns and treatments of Chinese disease categories yet to appear in English.

Further, most Western diseases are covered by more than one Chinese disease. If one knows the patterns for each of the Chinese diseases manifesting in a given patient, this can help one determine the patient's most likely core patterns. For instance, let us say that a systemic lupus erythmatosus patient has joint or impediment pain and periodic eruptions of a red, macular rash which, as a disease entity, is called cinnabar toxins in Chinese medicine. The most common patterns describing the Chinese disease of impediment are:

A. Wind damp cold
B. Wind damp heat
C. Qi & blood vacuity not nourishing the sinews & vessels
D. Liver-kidney yin vacuity
E. Kidney yang vacuity
F. Blood stasis blocking the network vessels

The Chinese patterns covering cinnabar toxins are always some kind of evil heat which has entered the blood division. Although it is possible for a person to have two different disease mechanisms for two different but simultaneous Chinese diseases, this is not the most likely scenario, especially when both Chinese diseases are pathognomonic symptoms of a single Western disease. Since, according to Chinese medicine, the entire human bodymind is a single integrated whole, it makes more sense to suppose that there is a single disease mechanism at work causing both disease manifestations. Therefore, when one looks at the above list of patterns (and hence disease mechanisms) at work in the above conditions, only some kind of evil heat is common to both Chinese diseases. Therefore, we should immediately suspect that there is evil heat.

We can further complicate this scenario by saying that this patient also has occasional bouts of diarrhea. The main patterns associated with the Chinese disease of diarrhea are:

A. Wind cold
B. Cold & dampness
C. Damp heat (including summerheat)
D. Food stagnation
E. Spleen qi vacuity
F. Spleen vacuity with damp encumbrance
G. Spleen-kidney yang vacuity
H. Lingering heat evils damaging yin

Since heat toxins (*i.e.*, cinnabar toxins) may develop from damp heat and since damp heat may cause both diarrhea and impediment, it makes sense that the most likely pattern in this patient's case is damp heat. Armed with that supposition, we should then examine and question the patient to confirm or deny that hypothesis.

We refer to this method of determining the most likely hypothetical pattern from which to begin our pattern discrimination as "triangulation." In geometry and, therefore, surveying, triangulation means working from what you know in order to figure out what you do not know. When we attempt to discriminate any patient's pattern, we should have some basic hunches about the most likely patterns based on the patient's sex, age, body type, coloring, carriage, affect, and voice. Determining which patterns are common to all the patient's named Chinese disease categories should further refine the most likely list of suspects. Then questioning and examination merely confirm or deny those working hypotheses. On the next page, Fig. 2 shows this method of triangulation in visual form.

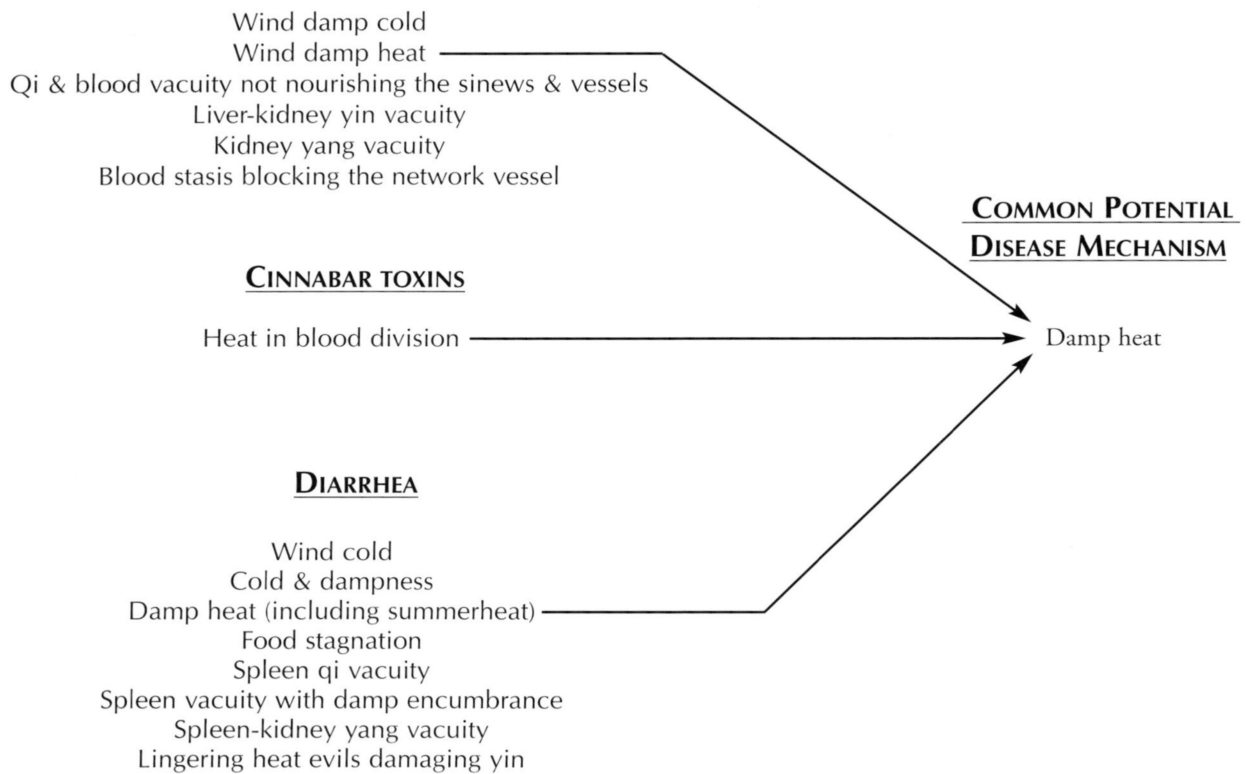

FIGURE 2

3. DIFFICULT TO TREAT, KNOTTY DISEASES

In modern Chinese medicine, the kinds of Western diseases discussed in this book are mostly referred to as "difficult to treat, knotty diseases." This means that they are chronic, complex conditions commonly developed over decades due to faulty diet, lifestyle, and mental-emotional habits compounded by constitution and aging.[12] According to Wan Wen-rong:

> So-called knotty, difficult diseases mean diseases which present-day practitioners in clinical practice feel thorny. The question revolves around knottiness [due to their complicated nature] in discriminating patterns and, [therefore,] difficulty in determining treatment.[13]

These conditions are mostly not self-limiting, and they rarely present as a single, discrete pattern. In fact, based on our clinical experience treating Western patients with these kinds of diseases, we would say that most patients will display not less than three, often five, and sometimes eight or more patterns concomitantly. This means that one cannot rely on the simple formulas for simple patterns which tend to be the norm in textbooks such as this. However, that does not mean that such multipattern presentations are insoluble. Complex combinations are made up of nothing but simple aggregates. In order to treat such complex presentations, all one ever has to do is tease apart the individual patterns, state the treatment principles for each pattern, and insure that the treatment plan (whether acupuncture or Chinese medicinal) addresses each of these stated principles.

Wan Wen-rong lists five keys for improving one's treatment of difficult, knotty diseases:

1. Strengthening one's proficient mastery of basic theory

To us, this means memorizing verbatim the key statements of fact in Chinese medicine and understanding what those facts mean. The more of these facts one has memorized and understands, the easier it is to think in and problem solve with Chinese medicine.

2. Being flexible in one's application [of that theory] in clinical practice

There is no unified ground theory of Chinese medicine. Chinese medicine has developed over not less than 2,500 years and a large land mass encompassing many different peoples. Each theory or statement of fact in Chinese medicine developed in a certain time and place due to particular factors. While many of these theories fit together to form a larger whole, not all do. In fact, certain theories are mutually contradictory. For instance, one theory states that the defensive qi issues from the lower burner, while another theory says it issues from the upper burner. Therefore, one must be flexible in the use of Chinese medical theories, using the appropriate theory in the appropriate situation and not allowing oneself to be abused by these theories as if they were anything other than tools. As every mechanic knows, it is important to use the right tool for the right situation, and, when not in use, no tool is inherently better than any other tool. Therefore, sometimes it is appropriate to use five phase theory, while, in other situations, it is more useful to use yin and yang, viscera and bowel, or qi and blood theory. Similarly, sometimes the six divisions or aspects of the *Shang Han Lun (Treatise on Damage [Due to] Cold)* describe a particular patient most precisely, while other times it is the four divisions of warm disease theory which most accurately organize a patient's presenting signs and symptoms.

3. Unceasingly exploring and refining pattern discrimination and treatment determination

This means incessantly refreshing one's memory of the pathognomonic signs and symptoms, tongue and pulse signs of all the major patterns. It also means understanding the disease mechanisms which produce each sign or symptom as well as the most important signs and symptoms which are dependable markers in real-life patients. For instance, while all Chinese textbooks list poor appetite as a symptom of spleen vacuity, when spleen vacuity is complicated by stomach heat, the appetite is either not poor or may actually be excessive. Further, one should pickle oneself in the treatment principles for the various patterns at the same time as continually searching for the most effective formulas and medicinals for the main patterns that modern Western patients present.

4. Looking for the essence of the pattern

In Chinese medicine, it is said, "[When] treating disease, first seek [its] root." In most Western patients with chronic diseases, the root is a liver-spleen disharmony which is then complicated by any number of other disease mechanisms. For instance, if damp heat is due to spleen vacuity engendering dampness and liver depression transforming heat, simply clearing heat and eliminating dampness will not achieve the desired results and may actually aggravate the situation.

5. Developing a high level of excellence in the prescription of Chinese medicinal formulas[14]

Developing a high degree of excellence in the prescription of Chinese medicinal formulas begins with thoroughly understanding the Chinese materia medica. The basic repertoire of 270-350 Chinese medicinals is the ABCs of this art. One cannot create words or sentences if one does not have a firm grasp of the alphabet. Likewise, one cannot create and modify formulas if one does not have a firm grasp of the natures, flavors, channel entries, functions, indications, combinations, dosages, and contraindications of the basic Chinese materia medica. Armed with such a basic understanding, one can then proceed to memorizing a core repertoire of 70-100 Chinese medicinal formulas, including each formula's ingredients, their standard dosages or proportions, their roles in the formula, the formula's functions and indications, its best known modifications, and its contraindications. This core repertoire of formulas provides the models upon which an infinite number of variations and new formulas can be created to meet the exigencies of each individual patient.

Unfortunately, there are simply no shortcuts to learning all the above information to the degree necessary to make it really work as a well-honed system. This is why great Chinese doctors are referred to as *lao yi sheng*, "old doctors." However, in terms of Wan's first key, there are some theories within Chinese medicine that are particularly helpful in explaining why certain patterns group together and how one pattern evolves into other patterns. If one understands these important theories, it is our experience both as teachers and clinicians that they can take years off one's process of maturation in Chinese medicine. As it so happens, a number of these theories stem from the Jin-Yuan dynasties and the four great masters of that time.

LIU WAN-SU'S THEORY OF SIMILAR TRANSFORMATION

Liu Wan-su, a.k.a. Liu He-jian, was, chronologically speaking, the first of the four great masters of medicine of the Jin-Yuan dynasties. Liu is remembered today as the founder of the School of Cold & Cool (Medicine). Liu Wan-su's theory of similar transformation says that the righteous or ruling qi of the living human organism is yang and, therefore, warm in nature. Hence, any guest qi, whether externally invading or internally engendered, will tend to transform into a warm evil over time no matter what its original nature. As an extension of this, the more habitually yang exuberant a person is, the more likely and the quicker this similar transformation will be. This theory helps explain why most pathologies tend to transform into heat patterns even if their original disease causes or manifestations were not hot in nature.

ZHU DAN-XI'S THEORY OF THE SIX DEPRESSIONS

Zhu Dan-xi, a.k.a. Zhu Zhen-heng, was, chronologically speaking, the last of the four great masters of the Jin-Yuan dynasties. Zhu is remembered today as the founder of the School of Enriching Yin. Zhu Dan-xi's six depressions are qi, blood, dampness, phlegm, food, and fire. Zhu's theory explains why, if one has any one of these six depressions, one will probably have more than one. In addition, his theory also uses Liu's theory of similar transformation to explain why five of these six depressions tend to transform into heat or become mixed with evil heat.[15]

To begin with, qi is responsible for moving and transforming blood, body fluids, and food. If, for any reason, the qi becomes depressed or stagnant, the blood will become static, fluids will stop and accumulate, and food will also become stagnant and accumulate. If damp evils linger and endure, they will tend to congeal into phlegm. Therefore, qi stagnation is often complicated by blood stasis, damp accumulation, phlegm obstruction, and/or food stagnation.

Vice versa, if, for any reason, blood, dampness, phlegm, or food depressions are engendered in the body, because these are yin evils consisting of physical substance, any of these may hinder and obstruct the free flow of qi. Therefore, even

Six Depressions		Modern Terminological Equivalents
Qi Depression	=	Qi Stagnation
Blood Depression	=	Blood Stasis
Damp Depression	=	Damp Accumulation
Phlegm Depression	=	Phlegm Obstruction
Food Depression	=	Food Stagnation
Fire Depression	=	Depressive Heat

FIGURE 3

THE FIVE DEPRESSIONS & FIRE

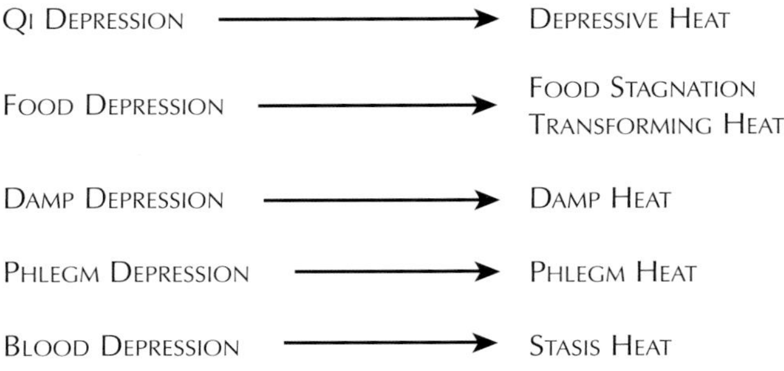

FIGURE 4

if qi stagnation has not caused the engenderment of any of these yin depressions, over time, these yin depressions will give rise to qi stagnation.

Further, because qi is yang in nature, qi stagnation tends to transform into depressive heat or fire. Because qi stagnation is commonly mixed with blood stasis, damp accumulation, phlegm obstruction, and food accumulation, these four yin depressions also commonly become mixed with evil heat. Hence, blood stasis commonly becomes stasis heat, damp accumulation becomes damp heat, phlegm obstruction becomes phlegm heat, and food stagnation becomes complicated or mixed with stomach and intestinal heat. Thus, in real-life clinical practice, when one has one of these six depressions, one typically has more than one.

LI DONG-YUAN'S YIN FIRE THEORY

Li Dong-yuan, a.k.a. Li Gao, was arguably the greatest of the four great masters of the Jin-Yuan dynasty, at least in terms of understanding how to treat the "difficult to treat, knotty diseases" most Western practitioners of acupuncture and Chinese medicine are called on to treat as our daily fare. In Chinese, there is a saying, "For external diseases, [Zhang] Zhong-jing; for internal diseases, [Li] Dong-yuan." Li is remembered today as the founder of the *Bu Tu Pai*, the School of Supplementing the Spleen and Stomach, and his greatest literary masterpiece is the *Pi Wei Lun (Treatise on the Spleen & Stomach)*, available in translation from Blue Poppy Press. However, if, judging from the title of Li's book, one thinks that it is about nausea, indigestion, diarrhea, and constipation, one will be greatly mistaken. If one knows the common clinical manifestations of modern Western diseases, one will immediately recognize that the clinical examples Li presents primarily correspond to allergies and autoimmune diseases.

Li's main theory is called the theory of yin fire. Like Liu Wan-su, Li thought that most diseases eventually display heat patterns. However, Li's vision of where this heat comes from and how it is engendered is somewhat different from Liu's. Although Li accepted Liu's theory of similar transformation, he felt that, at least in the case of chronic, enduring diseases, heat is typically mixed with vacuity and especially spleen vacuity. The term yin fire has several meanings in Li's work. First, yin fire develops from the lower burner, the yin part of the body. Secondly, yin fire is commonly associated with damp or yin evils. And third, this heat or fire is pathological and, therefore, also yin.[16] Yin fire is a pathological transformation, hyperactivity, and upward stirring of ministerial fire. According to Chinese medical theory, ministerial fire or lifegate fire is only healthy and beneficial when it remains calm or level in the lower burner, its lower source. The Chinese word *ping* (平) means both calm in an abstract

QI & 4 YIN DEPRESSIONS

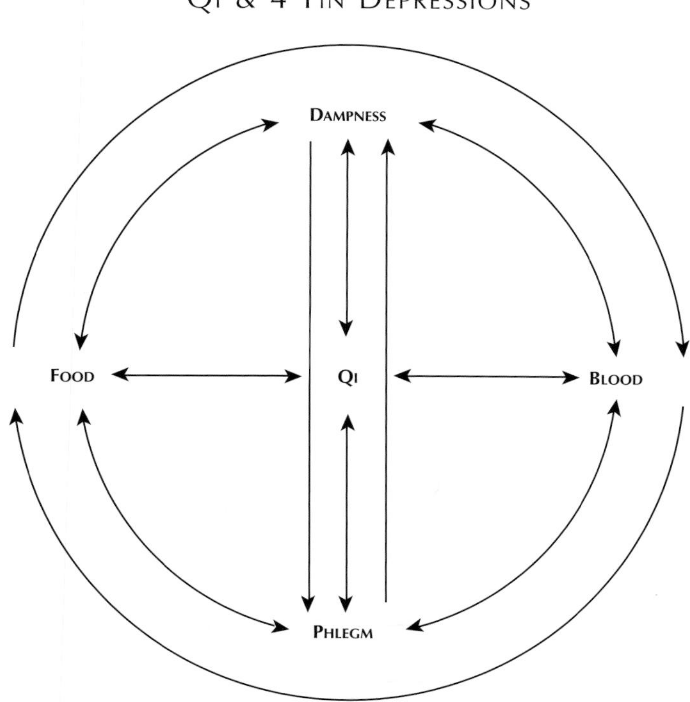

FIGURE 5

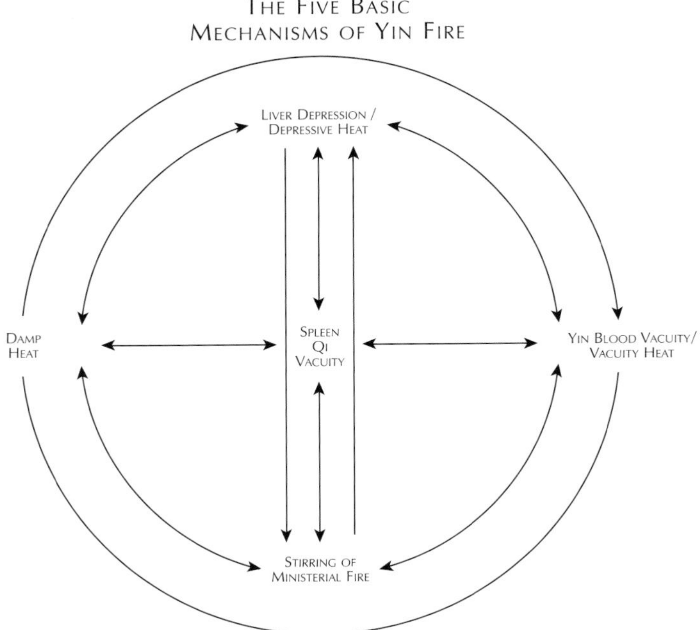

FIGURE 6

sense and level in a spatial sense. If ministerial fire stirs, A) it loses its calm and B) it counterflows upward. When ministerial fire counterflows upward, it damages the spleen or central qi. As Li says, "Ministerial fire and the source qi [here meaning the central or latter heaven source qi] are enemies; both cannot exist in the same place." If one reads Li's *Pi Wei Lun*, Li posits five basic disease mechanisms for the development of yin fire. These are:

1. Spleen qi vacuity
2. Damp heat
3. Liver depression/depressive heat
4. Yin & blood vacuity
5. Stirring of ministerial fire

Although we must explain these one after the other in a linear fashion, the reader should understand that these five disease mechanisms are all mutually interdependent. This means that *any one of these mechanisms can result in the creation of any of the others.* Because of this, real-life patients do not typically exhibit only one or another of these five, but rather three, four, or all five *at one time.* However, Li begins his explanation of yin fire with the spleen, and that is where we will also begin.

If, due to overthinking, anxiety and worry, under-exercise, overtaxation, faulty diet, or erroneous medical treatment, the spleen qi is damaged and becomes vacuous and weak, then the spleen will not be able to do its various duties and functions. One function of the spleen is to upbear clear yang. If clear yang is not upborne properly, it may fall downward to the lower burner. Because it cannot upbear and out-thrust, it becomes depressed. Because yang qi is warm in nature, this downwardly fallen central qi transforms into depressive heat which mutually engenders upward stirring of ministerial fire. Because heat is yang, it always travels upward, harassing and disturbing the viscera and bowels above it. Such evil heat can further damage the spleen qi and mutually engender depressive heat in the liver as well as damage and consume yin fluids in the stomach, lungs, heart, and eventually the kidneys. In addition, this upwardly counterflowing evil heat may also harass and disquiet the heart spirit.

A second function of the spleen is to move and transform body fluids. If the spleen qi becomes vacuous and weak and, thus, cannot move and transform water liquids, these may gather and accumulate and transform into dampness. This dampness may then hinder and obstruct the free flow of yang qi. Because yang qi is inherently warm, it too becomes stagnant and depressed. The yang qi backs up and transforms into depressive heat. If this depressive heat mutually binds with accumulated dampness, this will give rise to damp heat. Although this damp heat may be engendered in the middle burner, dampness, being turbid and heavy, typically seeps or percolates downward to the lower burner. However, because heat is yang, it tends to counterflow upward. If this heat mutually engenders stirring, hyperactivity, and upward counterflow of ministerial fire, it may damage yin fluids and the qi of the spleen, stomach, heart, and/or lungs. In addition, damp heat pouring downward damages the yin and/or yang of the liver and kidneys below.

A third function of the spleen is to engender and transform the blood. If the spleen becomes vacuous and weak, it may, therefore, fail to engender the blood. Blood and essence share a common source. Hence, blood vacuity may lead to yin vacuity. Yin is supposed to control yang. Therefore, if yin becomes vacuous and insufficient, it may fail to control yang which becomes exuberant and hyperactive. This may lead to upward counterflow of hyperactive ministerial fire and/or to the engenderment of internal heat. In addition, if blood fails to nourish the liver or yin fails to moisten the liver, the liver will not be able to perform its function of coursing and discharge. Hence the liver will become depressed and the qi will become stagnant. If qi depression transforms depressive heat, this heat may mutually engender stirring of ministerial fire.

On the other hand, if, due to unfilled desires or anger damaging the liver, the liver loses its command over coursing and discharge, the liver will become depressed and the qi become stagnant. Once again, because the qi is inherently yang and, therefore, warm, qi depression may transform into depressive heat and mutually engender stirring of ministerial fire. These heat evils will also counterflow upward to accumulate in and damage the spleen, stomach, heart, and/or lungs. Because liver depression is a repletion and replete liver wood may counterflow horizontally to assail the spleen, liver depression typically results in concomitant spleen qi vacuity. Over time, enduring depressive heat will also damage and consume yin fluids with consequent loss of balance between yin and yang. Further, since the qi moves and transforms water fluids in the body, qi stagnation may give rise to damp accumulation which may then transform into damp heat.

Damp heat may not only be engendered as a result of spleen vacuity and liver depression. It may also be directly caused by external invasion of damp heat evils or overeating hot, acrid, peppery, spicy foods, and thick-flavored, sweet, fried, fatty foods, or drinking alcohol. Since the spleen is averse to dampness, the dampness of damp heat damages the spleen, leading to spleen vacuity, while the heat of damp heat damages yin, blood, and fluids, leading to yin and blood vacuity. This is especially so since dampness is transformed out of righteous fluids which then become unavailable to the body to enrich and moisten. In addition, dampness, being a yin evil, hinders and obstructs the free flow of qi, thus inhibiting the qi mechanism and ultimately damaging the liver, leading to its depression. Therefore, damp heat may lead to or aggravate spleen vacuity, liver depression, or yin and blood vacuity.

Similarly, blood vacuity may be due directly to excessive blood loss, and yin vacuity may be due to excessive fluid loss or simply due to the consumption of yin due to aging. As it says in the *Nei Jing (Inner Classic)*, "At 40 years [of age], yin is half consumed." Since blood is primarily engendered and transformed by the spleen, blood vacuity may lead to damage and detriment of the spleen. As mentioned above, if blood and yin do not nourish and enrich the liver, the liver will not be able to do its duty of governing coursing and discharging. Hence the liver will become depressed and may transform heat. Thus it is easy to see that spleen qi vacuity, liver depression/depressive heat, and damp heat are all mutually engendering.

While spleen qi vacuity, liver depression/depressive heat, damp heat, and yin blood vacuity with vacuity heat may all lead to hyperactivity and frenetic stirring of ministerial fire, ministerial fire may also be stirred directly on its own. All physical, verbal, and mental-emotional activity are species of stirring. Chinese medicine's view of health and disease is based on the Confucian Doctrine of the Mean (*zhong yong*). That means that any matter or function in the body which is too much or too little is pathological. Although the ministerial fire, as the yang expression of the lifegate or stirring qi between the kidneys, must stir to fulfil its duty, hyperactive stirring of ministerial fire is pathological. Because the moving qi between the kidneys is the root of all the bodymind's stirring, any excessive stirring, be it mental-emotional, verbal, or physical may mutually engender stirring of ministerial fire. However, sex, most recreational drugs, and some over-the-counter and prescription drugs especially stir ministerial fire, easily leading to it becoming frenetically hyperactive and flaming upward.

Further, because ministerial or lifegate fire is the root of all yang qi in the body, it is connected to all other viscera and bowels and tissues in the body. If heat is engendered in any of these viscera and bowels or tissues, it may mutually inflame ministerial fire and all other viscera and bowels and tissues connected to ministerial fire. In particular, ministerial fire connects to the liver-gallbladder below and the heart-pericardium above. Therefore, flaring of ministerial fire can engender or exacerbate depressive liver heat or fire, and it can also cause harassment by heat evils of the heart spirit above. In particular, it was Zhu Dan-xi, in his *Ge Zhi Yu Lun (Extra Treatises Based on Investigation & Inquiry)*, who further elaborated the Chinese medical theory of excessive stirring and ministerial fire.

Since ministerial fire is rooted in the kidneys and the kidneys are the root of yin and yang of the entire body, stirring of ministerial fire may cause loss of balance of the yin and yang of the entire system. When ministerial fire stirs and counterflows upward, A) it leaves its lower source which becomes vacuous and cold, and B) it commonly results in evil heat above. Hence yin fire scenarios are often associated with hot above-cold below patterns.[17]

As the reader should by now understand, no matter how any one of the above five basic disease mechanisms of yin fire are engendered, once one of these disease mechanisms is put in process, it will tend to create one or more of the other four. In real-life patients with yin fire scenarios, one will virtually always have a liver-spleen disharmony with some form of evil heat leading to upward stirring of ministerial fire. Because all these five disease mechanisms are so closely inter-related, it is impossible to treat them separately. Even if one could get rid of a single mechanism (which one cannot in any case), the remaining disease mechanisms would quickly re-establish it. Therefore, one must address all the disease mechanisms that make up a yin fire scenario in a given patient all at one go. If one analyzes the majority of Li Dong-yuan's formulas, we can describe Li's treatment protocols as being made up of five principles:[18]

1. Fortify the spleen and boost the qi
2. Rectify the qi mechanism
3. Clear heat
4. Do anything else necessary based on the presence of concomitant patterns or branch symptoms
5. Prioritize among the preceding four principles.

According to Li Dong-yuan, a strong, healthy spleen can keep ministerial fire calm or level in its lower source, while a vacuous, weak spleen may allow ministerial or yin fire to counterflow upward. Because spleen vacuity plays a part in virtually all yin fire scenarios, one will always have to fortify or supplement the spleen and boost the qi. Because there will be some kind of inhibition to the qi mechanism, one will have to rectify the qi. Usually, this means coursing the liver and rectifying the qi, but it may also mean harmonizing the center or rectifying the qi of the stomach and intestines. Because there will be some kind of evil heat, one will have to clear that heat. Evil heat in the case of yin fire is mainly depressive heat, damp heat, or vacuity heat. However, it may also involve summerheat, heat toxins, and phlegm heat. Because of the inter-relationships between the qi and blood, qi and body fluids, blood and body fluids, qi and yang, blood and yin, and all the viscera and bowels, when there is three or more of the five basic mechanisms of yin fire, there will undoubtedly be other related disease mechanisms also at work. Because the qi moves the blood, if there is liver depression qi stagnation, over time, there is likely to be blood stasis. Because the blood and body fluids flow together, if there is damp accumulation or damp heat, there is also likely to be blood stasis. Because the defensive qi issues from the middle burner due to the upbearing function of the spleen, if there is spleen vacuity, there is likely to be a defensive qi insecurity with easy contraction of external evils. Whatever other disease mechanisms there are which are intimately related to yin fire, these must also all be treated at the same time.

However, by saying that the first principle of treating yin fire scenarios is to fortify the spleen and boost the qi does not mean that one should always begin with a qi-supplementing formula. In some cases, heat may be most prominent. In other cases, liver depression may be most prominent, and in yet other cases, phlegm may be most pronounced. Therefore, one should pick as their guiding formula whatever is appropriate based on the treatment principles of the first pattern stated in the list of requisite treatment principles. That may mean the guiding formula is a heat-clearing formula, a phlegm-transforming formula, a wind damp treating formula, or a yang-supplementing formula. However, if the case is a yin fire scenario, those formulas will have to be modified to include fortification of the spleen and supplementation of the qi, rectification, freeing the flow, or movement of the qi, and the clearing of some kind of heat somewhere in the body. As stated above, if one does not treat all the disease mechanisms associated with yin fire altogether in a single protocol, the disease mechanisms which are not addressed will quickly re-establish the one that was addressed.

The benefit of understanding Li Dong-yuan's yin fire theory is that it explains why the most commonly seen combined patterns do combine so readily with one another. If one knows that, in real-life clinical practice, if one has liver depression, they will have spleen vacuity and *vice versa*, then seeing signs and symptoms of the one, they can immediately check for the presence of a few key signs and symptoms of the other. If one knows there is spleen vacuity, then one should immediately check to see if there is either dampness or blood vacuity. If there is dampness, is there damp heat? If there is blood vacuity, there will probably be liver depression. If blood vacuity endures, it may evolve into yin vacuity, etc. In addition, Li's formulas serve as excellent models, if not guiding formulas, for the creation of Chinese medicinal formulas for such complicated scenarios. Readers interested in looking at a collection of Li's representative formulas can find such a collection at www.bluepoppy.com in the articles section under Blue Poppy Press at that Website.

A LARGER VISION OF LIFEGATE FIRE

In our experience, most Western practitioners of Chinese medicine equate the lifegate fire with kidney yang or kidney fire and leave it at that. We regard this as the little view of lifegate fire. Although lifegate fire is rooted in kidney yang, its ramifications affect the entire body. Lifegate or ministerial fire is the source of all yang qi in the human body, and all yang qi in the body connects with the lifegate fire. This means that the yang qi of the entire body is, in a sense, unitary. Various statements of fact in Chinese medicine emphasize the fundamental importance of the lifegate[19] in human physiology:

> The lifegate is the root of nature and destiny [or life], the sea of essence and blood, the source of engenderment and transformation, and the mother of the spleen and stomach.
>
> The lifegate is the root of the original qi. Without it, the yin qi of the five viscera is not able to enrich. Without it, the yang qi of the five viscera is not able to emit.
>
> The lifegate governs the 12 channels. If the kidneys are without it, there is no making strong and skill cannot exit. If the bladder is without it, the qi of the three burners cannot be transformed and the water passageways cannot move. If the spleen and stomach are without it, they are not able to rotten and ripen water and grains and the five flavors cannot exit. If the liver and gallbladder are without it, the general has no decisiveness and decision-making cannot exit. If the large and small intestines are without it, change and transformation do not move and the two excretions are blocked. If the heart is without it, the spirit brilliance is clouded and it is not able to react to the tens of thousands of affairs.
>
> The heart receives the lifegate and the spirit brilliance is primary. It is the first to respond to things. The liver receives the lifegate and engenders strategems and considerations. The gallbladder receives the lifegate and [there is] decision-making. The stomach receives the lifegate and is capable of reception and assimilation. The spleen receives the lifegate and is capable of movement and transformation. The lungs receive the lifegate and govern the regulation [of qi of the entire body]. The large intestine receives the lifegate and transforms and guides. The small intestine receives the lifegate and disseminates and transforms. The kidneys receive the lifegate and [there is] vigor. The triple burner receives the lifegate and establishes the sluiceways. The bladder attains the lifegate and receives and stores [the urine].

As these various sayings imply, it is the lifegate fire that warms and steams all the viscera and bowels, channels and network vessels, and tissues of the body, including the sinews and bones, muscles and flesh, skin and hair. Therefore, the lifegate is the root of all warm transformations in the body. However, certain viscera and bowels have a closer relationship to the lifegate than others. In particular, the influence and activities of the lifegate fire are most clearly seen in the workings of the heart-pericardium, liver-gallbladder, spleen-stomach, kidneys-bladder, and triple burner. When the lifegate fire promotes the yang function of these viscera and bowels in a normal, healthy way, it is also referred to as lesser fire. If this lesser fire becomes excessively effulgent and flames upward, it becomes vigorous fire, a species of evil qi.

In terms of the clinical implications of the above theory, since the yang qi of these viscera and bowels are all connected via the lifegate, flaming and hyperactivity of lifegate fire may cause flaming and hyperactivity of the yang qi of any of these viscera and bowels. *Vice versa*, flaming of heat or hyperactivity of yang in any of these viscera and bowels may lead to flaming and hyperactivity of the lifegate or ministerial fire. In Chinese medicine, this ability of heat or hyperactivity in one part of the body to cause flaming of heat or hyperactivity of yang in another part of the body is called "mutual engenderment," and the viscus with the closest (pathological) relationship to lifegate fire is the liver. The following two sayings underscore the especially close relationship between lifegate fire/ministerial fire and the liver (gallbladder): "[If] the five minds become excessively exhausted, ministerial fire may rise up internally within the liver and gallbladder," and, "Ascending and upbearing of the qi may join with liver-gallbladder ministerial fire." Thus this theory helps explain why liver depressive heat, fire, and ascendant hyperactivity of yang may cause heat and hyperactivity in the heart, stomach, and/or kidneys, while heat in the heart, stomach, and/or kidneys may cause or aggravate heat or hyperactivity in the liver.

QING DYNASTY GU WORM THEORY

Heiner Fruehauf, Dean of Chinese Medical Studies at the Northwest College of Naturopathy in Portland, OR, has recently published some interesting research on gu worm theory and therapy.[20] The concept of gu worms and gu poisoning is a very ancient one within Chinese medicine, stemming from shamanistic beginnings. However, over the centuries, this concept has evolved from a shamanistic one to a more mainstream Chinese medical one. In particular, this

CHARACTERISTICS OF *GU CHONG* OR GU WORM DISEASES

1. Gu toxins spread throughout the body like oil mixing with flour.
2. Gu worms cause polysystemic pathologies with multiple symptoms.
3. Gu evils primarily enter the body through food.
4. Gu evils severely harm the body's source qi (meaning the spleen or spleen *and* kidney qi).
5. *Chong* worms include intestinal parasites *and* invisible organisms which cause skin diseases.
6. *Candida albicans* is classified as a type of *chong* or worms in modern Chinese medicine.

COMMONLY USED ANTI-GU MEDICINALS ACCORDING TO MODERN STANDARD CATEGORIZATION

QI SUPPLEMENTS: Radix Astragali Membranacei (*Huang Qi*), Radix Glycyrrhizae (*Gan Cao*), Rhizoma Polygonati (*Huang Jing*), Radix Panacis Quinquefolii (*Xi Yang Shen*)

BLOOD SUPPLEMENTS: Radix Angelicae Sinensis (*Dang Gui*), Radix Albus Paeoniae Lactiflorae (*Bai Shao*), Radix Polygoni Multiflori (*He Shou Wu*)

HEAT-CLEARING MEDICINALS: Fructus Forsythiae Suspensae (*Lian Qiao*), Flos Lonicerae Japonicae (*Jin Yin Hua*), Flos Chrysanthemi Morifolii (*Ju Hua*), Radix Sophorae Flavescentis (*Ku Shen*), Herba Artemisiae Apiaceae (*Qing Hao*), uncooked Radix Rehmanniae (*Sheng Di*), Radix Scrophulariae Ningpoensis (*Xuan Shen*)

QI-RECTIFYING MEDICINALS: Radix Auklandiae Lappae (*Mu Xiang*), Pericarpium Citri Reticulatae (*Chen Pi*), Fructus Meliae Toosendan (*Chuan Lian Zi*)

BLOOD-QUICKENING MEDICINALS: Tuber Curcumae (*Yu Jin*), Squama Manitis Pentadactylis (*Chuan Shan Jia*), Radix Ligustici Wallichii (*Chuan Xiong*), Rhizoma Curcumae Zedoariae (*E Zhu*), Rhizoma Sparganii (*San Leng*), Herba Lycopi Lucidi (*Ze Lan*)

EXTERIOR-RESOLVING MEDICINALS: Herba Menthae Haplocalycis (*Bo He*), Folium Perillae Frutescentis (*Zi Su Ye*), Radix Angelicae Dahuricae (*Bai Zhi*), Radix Et Rhizoma Ligustici Chinensis (*Gao Ben*), Rhizoma Cimicifugae (*Sheng Ma*), Radix Bupleuri (*Chai Hu*)[23]

INTERIOR-WARMING MEDICINAL: Flos Caryophylli (*Ding Xiang*)

YIN-SUPPLEMENTING MEDICINALS: Radix Glehniae Littoralis (*Sha Shen*), Bulbus Lilii (*Bai He*)

YANG-SUPPLEMENTING MEDICINALS: Fructus Cnidii Monnieri (*She Chuang Zi*)[24]

DAMPNESS-ELIMINATING MEDICINALS: Sclerotium Poriae Cocos (*Fu Ling*)

WIND DAMPNESS TREATING MEDICINALS: Cortex Radicis Acanthopancis Gracistylis (*Wu Jia Pi*)

PHLEGM-TRANSFORMING, ORIFICE-OPENING MEDICINALS: Rhizoma Acori Graminei (*Shi Chang Pu*)

SECURING & ASTRINGING MEDICINALS: Fructus Terminaliae Chebulae (*He Zi*), Fructus Pruni Mume (*Wu Mei*)

BLEEDING STOPPING MEDICINALS: Flos Immaturus Sophorae Japonicae (*Huai Hua Mi*), Radix Pseudoginseng (*Tian San Qi*), Lignum Dalbergiae Odoriferae (*Jiang Xiang*)

WORM-DISPELLING MEDICINAL: Semen Arecae Catechu (*Bing Lang*)

---

concept seemingly became the central one of a whole school of Chinese medicine by the Qing dynasty. Within contemporary Chinese medicine, gu are a species of *chong* or worms. However, they are unlike the more pedestrian form of worms in Chinese medicine. Gu worms are, unlike roundworms, pinworms, and tapeworms, invisible and tend to cause multi-symptom, complex, chronic, and enduring diseases. Such gu worm diseases are hard to treat. They typically cause a simultaneous combination of chronic digestive complaints, musculoskeletal complaints, and psychiatric and/or neurological complaints, and are often associated with dermatological conditions. The table on page 19 shows some of the key characteristics of gu worm diseases.

According to Heiner Fruehauf, many patients with intestinal dysbiosis, polysystemic chronic candidiasis, and intestinal parasitosis should be diagnosed as suffering from gu worms, and it is our experience that many patients suffering from a number of the allergies and autoimmune diseases discussed in this book also suffer from polysystemic chronic candidiasis or intestinal dysbiosis at the least. Therefore, we believe that it is important to understand something about gu worm disease when discriminating such patients' patterns and erecting Chinese medical treatment plans.

According to gu worm theorists, formulas for the treatment of gu worm conditions should be made up of five groups of Chinese medicinals:

1. Toxin-scattering medicinals
2. Worm-killing medicinals
3. Spirit-quieting medicinals
4. Qi & blood supplementing medicinals
5. Qi & blood moving & quickening medicinals

Although these five categories of medicinals sound very similar to modern standard Chinese medicinal categories, they are not the same. Nevertheless, most of the medicinals in these five categories are commonly used Chinese medicinals in standard contemporary Chinese medicine. If one chooses medicinals from all five of these categories of anti-gu Chinese medicinals, one will typically wind up with what is also essentially a Li Dong-yuan yin fire protocol.

Beginning with Zhu Dan-xi[21] and continuing up to today, [22] the main disease mechanisms at work in gu worm diseases are a marked spleen qi vacuity with dampness and/or damp heat and liver depression qi stagnation. Therefore, the main disease mechanisms of gu worm disease are essentially the same as Li Dong-yuan's yin fire theory. However, as mentioned above, Qing dynasty gu worm school practitioners have identified certain Chinese medicinals that are especially effective for treating such conditions. The previous table shows the most commonly used anti-gu medicinals according to modern Chinese medicinal categorization.

Therefore, whenever treating complex chronic diseases associated with intestinal dysbiosis or polysystemic chronic candidiasis, we recommend choosing at least some of the medicinals in one's formula based on their specific anti-gu functions and abilities.

HERXHEIMER REACTIONS

Herxheimer reactions refer to die-off reactions when large yeast and fungi populations are suddenly killed off.[25] Many of the anti-gu medicinals described above are described by Western pharmacologists as having pronounced fungicidal ability. Therefore, it is not uncommon to provoke such die-off reactions when first administering a yin fire/anti-gu based formula to a patient with marked intestinal dysbiosis. In that case, there will be nausea and vomiting, headache, possible fever, possible body aches, and a general sense of malaise. These symptoms are caused by the toxicity of the breakdown products produced by the dying yeast and fungi and the body's attempt to purge these toxins by any means possible. Although such Herxheimer reactions can be intense, they are usually of short duration, typically lasting 6-12 hours and not more than a maximum of 36 hours. If one does provoke a Herxheimer reaction, see suggestions below for what to do.

1. Stay calm (both patient *and* practitioner)
2. Drink plenty of water
3. Soak in an Epsom salts bath
4. Purge the bowels using Magnesium citrate purchased from the local pharmacy or add Mirabilitum (*Mang Xiao*) and/or Radix Et Rhizoma Rhei (*Da Huang*) to the patient's formula
5. Keep taking the Chinese medicinals

Although one may think that a Herxheimer reaction is a sign that one has prescribed the wrong Chinese medicinal formula, in this particular case, that is not so. The formula is correct. It is just that the patient's yeast and fungi populations are very large. If one stops administering the Chinese medicinal formula for fear that it is an erroneous formula which is causing these unwanted side effects, then one will stop killing these yeast and fungi. Although all side effects are normally considered a sign of inaccurate, erroneous treatment in Chinese medicine, this is one instance where a "healing crisis" is truly warranted. One will know that these symptoms are a Herxheimer reaction due to the limited length of time they persist and by the fact that all the patient's signs and symptoms take a great leap forward in terms of improvement as these flu-like symptoms abate. If these reactions continue beyond 36 hours or are not followed by across-the-board improvement in the patient's condition, then these symptoms were not a Herxheimer reaction. The formula was indeed wrong, and it should be stopped while one re-evaluates the patient's pattern discrimination from top to bottom.

When treating either a yin fire or gu worm condition, it is imperative that the patient eat a yeast-free, hypoallergenic, clear bland diet. For more information on these aspects of Chinese dietary therapy, the reader should see Bob Flaws's *The Tao of Healthy Eating* (Blue Poppy Press). Trying to treat these kinds of conditions without proper dietary therapy is like bailing water from a sinking boat without plugging the leak. Such a clear bland diet should be adhered to strictly for the first 3-6 months at the very least and moderately strictly for a year to 18 months after that. Further, the patient should be advised that they should not completely revert to their previous diet or their condition will surely relapse. It is our experience that, in clinical practice, most relapses of chronic, remittent diseases are due to dietary indiscretions. For further information on yin fire and gu worms, please see Bob Flaws's freely downloadable articles at www.bluepoppy.com.

LIVER DEPRESSION

Because the primary immediate cause of liver depression is unfulfilled desires and everyone with a chronic disease has unfulfilled desires, we agree with the famous Chinese geriatric specialist Yan De-xin that, even if liver depression did not cause the disease, liver depression does complicate every chronic disease.[26] In addition, in Chinese gynecology there is the saying, "In adults, blame the liver." This is because all adults living in civilized societies must have unfulfilled desires. In fact, delayed gratification or non-gratification of desires is most peoples' definition of being an adult. Therefore, it is very important to understand all the causes of liver depression. Some of these have been touched on above. However, since this is such an important aspect of pattern discrimination in real-life patients, we believe it bears reiterating.

While unfulfilled desires are the primary immediate cause of liver depression, there are a number of indirect causes of liver depression. First of all, anger may damage the liver. If anger is unexpressed, that itself is a very powerful unfulfilled desire. However, if anger is expressed, that results in over-coursing and over-discharging. Since any activity which is extreme, being too much or too little, may damage its corresponding Chinese organ, the secondary result of this over-coursing is that the liver loses its normal control over-coursing and discharge. Hence the liver becomes depressed and the qi becomes stagnant.

DISEASE CAUSES & MECHANISMS RESULTING IN LIVER DEPRESSION

1. Unfulfilled desires
2. The sequelae of anger
3. Insufficient nourishment and emolliation by blood
4. Insufficient enrichment and moistening by yin
5. Insufficient warming and steaming by yang
6. Any of the four yin depressions
7. Anything which inhibits or damages the lungs' diffusion & downbearing
8. Any evil qi which hinders and obstructs the free flow of qi

If the liver does not receive sufficient blood, the liver will also not be able to maintain its proper control over coursing and discharge. This is based on the idea from the *Nei Jing (Inner Classic)* that, if the eyes obtain blood, the eyes can see; if the hands obtain blood, the hands can grasp; and if the feet obtain blood, the feet can step. Likewise, all tissues and organs in the body can only do their function if they receive sufficient blood to nourish them. This theory has large implications for women which we will discuss below under "Sex & Age."

Since "blood and essence share a common source," blood and yin are part and parcel of a single entity. Therefore, just as the liver cannot function if it does not receive nourishment by sufficient blood, it also cannot function if it does not receive adequate emolliation and moistening. Further, the function of the liver is also empowered, at least in part, by the warming and steaming of kidney yang/ministerial fire. Therefore, if kidney yang becomes vacuous and debilitated, this may also cause or aggravate liver depression qi stagnation.

The liver is only one of the two primary viscera which control the movement and free flow of the qi. The other viscus is the lungs. "The lungs control the qi of the entire body." This means that it is the lungs' downward depuration and diffusing that supply the pushing power for the movement of the qi. "The liver governs coursing and discharge." This means that the liver allows or permits the free and easy flow of qi. In order for the qi to flow freely, both viscera must work in a coordinated fashion. Therefore, anything which hinders or obstructs the lungs' downward depuration and diffusion may cause or aggravate liver depression qi stagnation. Lung failure to depurate and diffuse may be due to either vacuity or repletion. If the lung qi (derived primarily from the spleen's upbearing of clear yang) is vacuous and weak, it cannot do its function of depurating and diffusing. Likewise, if evil qi lodge in and obstruct the lungs' qi mechanism, the lungs will also fail to depurate and diffuse properly. Such evil qi can either be externally invading or internally engendered.

And finally, the presence of any evil qi and especially the other four yin or material depressions may also hinder and obstruct the free flow of qi. Because the qi cannot flow freely, the liver cannot do its duty of coursing and discharge. This means that, short-term, the presence of evil qi may aggravate any pre-existing liver depression qi stagnation, but, long-term, it also means that the continued, enduring presence of evil qi may actually cause liver depression qi stagnation in cases where it was not already present.

Hence, there are numerous causes for the engenderment and aggravation of liver depression qi stagnation. This is why this pattern rarely presents in its simple, discreet textbook form. It is also why this pattern complicates virtually all adult chronic diseases. In that case, either liver depression is the main pattern, and therefore, one should pick their guiding formula from the qi-rectifying chapter or category, or it is a

COMMONLY USED CHINESE MEDICINALS WHICH FREE THE FLOW OF THE NETWORK VESSELS

1. WORMS (MEANING ANNALIDS, INSECTS, ARACHNIDS, AMPHIBIANS & REPTILES)

Buthus Martensis (*Quan Xie*)
Scolopendra Subspinipes (*Wu Gong*)
Lumbricus (*Di Long*)
Euployphaga Seu Ophisthoplatia (*Di Bie Chong*)
Hirudo (*Shui Zhi*)
Bombyx Batryticatus (*Jiang Can*)
Periostracum Cicadae (*Chan Tui*)
Zaocys Dhumnades (*Wu Shao She*)
Squama Manitis Pentadactylis (*Chuan Shan Jia*)
Plastrum Testudinis (*Gui Ban*)
Carapax Amydae Sinensis (*Bie Jia*)

2. RESINS

Resina Olibani (*Ru Xiang*)
Resina Myrrhae (*Mo Yao*)
Sanguis Draconis (*Xue Jie*)
Succinum (*Hu Po*)

3. RETICULAR, NETWORK VESSEL SHAPED MEDICINALS

Fasciculus Vascularis Luffae Cylindricae (*Si Gua Luo*)
Fasciculus Vascularis Citri Reticulatae (*Ju Luo*)
Herba Asari Cum Radice (*Xi Xin*)

secondary pattern, and one will have to add acupuncture points or medicinals based on the principles of coursing the liver and rectifying the qi.

BLOOD STASIS

Just as Old Doctor Yan De-xin mentioned above believes that liver depression complicates all chronic diseases, Dr. Yan also believes that blood stasis complicates all geriatric disease[27], and a large proportion of the chronic diseases discussed in this book primarily affect older middle-aged and elderly patients. In part, Dr. Yan derives this idea from the Chinese statement of fact, "New diseases are in the channels; enduring diseases enter the network vessels." The traditional explanation of the second half of this axiom is that chronic, enduring diseases are typically complicated by blood stasis in the network vessels. Above, we have seen how liver depression qi stagnation is such a common, almost universal component to chronic disease. Therefore, it is no large leap to understand why blood stasis also complicates most chronic diseases. This is explained by the following Chinese medical syllogism: The qi moves the blood. If the qi moves, the blood moves. If the qi stops, the blood stops. In fact, blood stasis is such a fundamental part of the aging process that liver spots, a sign of blood stasis in the grandchild network vessels, are also called age spots.

As we have seen above, the qi moves the blood. Therefore, qi stagnation may lead to blood stasis. However, blood and body fluids also flow together. Therefore, either evil dampness or phlegm congelation may also result in blood stasis. Likewise, so may long-standing food stagnation. Of course, blood stasis may be caused by the severing of the channels and vessels by traumatic injury. It may also be the sequela of any pathological bleeding. Bleeding is, *ipso facto*, a sign of blood moving outside its channels and vessels, and the blood can only flow freely as long as it is canalized by these channels and vessels. Therefore, all enduring or repeated pathological bleeding results in blood stasis.

Other causes of blood stasis are scars which impede the free flow of qi, blood, and body fluids, qi vacuity which fails to move the blood, blood vacuity which fails to nourish the vessels, and any type of cold, either vacuity or repletion. According to Chinese medicine, cold's nature is constricting and contracting. Therefore, the blood can only flow as long as adequate yang qi warms and steams it. Further, there is a particular reflexive relationship between fresh or new blood and static blood which is also called dead blood. As we have seen above, blood vacuity may fail to nourish the vessels, thus resulting in blood stasis. However, it is also just as true that static blood impedes the engenderment and transformation of fresh or new blood. Hence, blood vacuity may lead to blood stasis and blood stasis may lead to blood vacuity. In actual fact, if either exist for any length of time, there must be both.

Because blood stasis complicates most chronic diseases, most if not all protocols for chronic diseases must be modified by the inclusion of one or more points or medicinals to quicken the blood and transform or dispel stasis even if the main pattern is not blood stasis. If the stasis has entered the network vessels, then medicinals which specifically free the flow of the network vessels must be used. These tend to come from three groups of Chinese medicinals shown in the previous table.

PHLEGM

Phlegm is likewise a complicating factor in many difficult, knotty diseases. Phlegm is nothing other than congealed fluids, and fluids are moved and transformed by the qi. Therefore, phlegm may be engendered by either qi vacuity or qi depression. Phlegm may also be congealed if there is cold constricting and congealing body fluids or heat brewing and stewing fluids and humors. Thus it is said:

> Phlegm is root in water and dampness.
> [If] these obtain qi and fire, this leads to
> binding making phlegm.

In addition, as we have seen above, because blood and fluids flow together, phlegm stagnation may lead to blood stasis, while blood stasis may lead to phlegm stagnation. Therefore, when it comes to the treatment of phlegm in difficult, knotty diseases, Zhu Liang-chun thought that, besides transforming phlegm:

> To treat phlegm, it is essential to treat the
> blood. Quickening the blood leads to the
> transformation of phlegm.[28]

This means that there are a number of disease mechanisms, any one of which may engender phlegm internally. Hence phlegm may be either the cause or result of other disease mechanisms in the body. Futher, phlegm is not always overt. One species of phlegm is called hidden or deep-lying phlegm. This refers to phlegm which is lodged in the body but which is not seen under normal circumstances. However, when the right combination of disease mechanisms concur, then phlegm becomes visible and overt. For instance, everyone with allergic rhinitis and asthma has deep-lying phlegm. During periods of remission, there may be few or no signs and symptoms of this phlegm. When external wind evils inhibit the lungs' diffusion and downbearing of fluids and the lung qi counterflows upward, this deep-lying phlegm is drafted upward with this counterflow and becomes manifest.

It is also important to remember that any palpable, round, rubbery nodulation is considered phlegm nodulation in Chinese medicine no matter what the make-up of this tissue is according to Western biology. Examples of such phlegm nodulation include lymphadenopathy, lipomas, fibrocystic lumps in the breast, thyroid enlargement and lumps, hepato- and/or splenomegaly, and even small, unattached calcifications many people develop along the edges of their bones, especially their tibia. Whenever one feels such a nodulation, one knows that phlegm is playing a part in that patient's overall pattern discrimination.

Because phlegm may mist or confound the orifices of the heart, thus blocking the spirit brilliance, many psychoemotional disorders are due to or complicated by phlegm. In fact, the more severe the psychiatric disturbance, the more likely phlegm is blocking the patient's clear orifices. When phlegm blocks the clear orifices of the heart, it mostly results in symptoms of withdrawal. However, because phlegm commonly combines with heat, if heat harasses the heart spirit, this may result in mania. As Wan Wen-rong states:

> If phlegm drool hinders and obstructs, the qi pathways will not be cleared and the mansion of the spirit brilliance will be misted and encumbered by phlegm. The upper [burner] will not be able to flow freely, the lower [burner] will not be able to spread, and this may lead to withdrawal, mania, and epilepsy. If this recurs and becomes insidious, the patient's withdrawal, mania, and epilepsy do not get less [but rather get more day by day].[29]

Ironically, the more phlegm becomes profuse, the more fluids and humors are consumed. This is because fluids and humors are bound up as phlegm dampness and are not available to the body to moisten and emolliate. Thus, it is not at all unusual to have conditions with profuse phlegm and dampness complicated by yin fluid dryness and insufficiency.

CONSTITUTION & DISEASE

In Chinese medicine, there are four basic body types or constitutions. These are *tai yang, shao yang, tai yin*, and *shao yin*. In Chinese, the term for constitution is *chang ti*, "habitual bodily." This means a body that is habitually a certain way. Such a habitual body type may be genetic or it may be due to diet, lifestyle, aging, or disease. In other words, it is not necessarily something we are born with and stays the same throughout our life. It may and usually does change over time and with aging. In terms of the causation of illness, different body types predispose one to different disease mechanisms and, therefore, different patterns of disease.

The tai yang is a yang exuberant body type. The person has a well-developed upper body and less well-developed lower body. They may be obese in the upper half of their body, but this obesity overlies a well-developed musculature. Tai yang persons typically have a red facial complexion due to yang exuberance, and they easily develop replete heat. Because this body type also tends to exhibit phlegm damp signs and symptoms, replete heat is often complicated by dampness and/or phlegm. In general, patients with this body type should eat less meaty, fried, fatty, oily foods, acrid, hot peppery foods, and not drink too much alcohol. More men tend to be habitually bodily tai yang than women, but women can also exhibit this body type.

THE FOUR YIN-YANG BODY TYPES

***TAI YANG*:** Large, beefy, red-faced, overdeveloped upper body, underdeveloped lower body

***SHAO YANG*:** Healthy mesomorphic, neither fat nor thin, normal muscular tone

***TAI YIN*:** Endomorphic, obese, pale-faced, lack of tone, overdeveloped lower body

***SHAO YIN*:** Ectomorphic, thin, nervous, restless

The shao yang body type is the body type of the healthy young adult of either sex. From a Western somatotyping point of view, this is the mesomorphic body type. The shao yang body type is an outward sign that yin and yang are in relative balance and the viscera and bowels are functioning relatively normally. Because shao yang body types tend not to be either greatly yin or greatly yang, depending on disease causes and mechanisms as well as their severity and duration, they can become either yin or yang vacuous or replete. However, because this is inherently a yang body type, most often these patients transform heat when ill.

The tai yin body type is endomorphic. The person is obese, often grossly so, and the tissue is flaccid and without tone. The facial complexion is typically pale, and the lower body is often more obese than the upper body. More women exhibit this body type than men, but either sex can manifest it. This body type is a result of insufficient yang qi to move and transform phlegm and dampness. In most cases, the spleen is vacuous and weak, and so there is also often qi and blood vacuity. This means that people with this body type often suffer from phlegm damp conditions and qi and blood vacuity conditions. Tai yin body types need more exercise, should not eat too much, should mostly eat, warm cooked foods, and should not eat chilled, uncooked foods. Because they easily engender phlegm, they also need to be careful about fluid-engendering foods.

The shao yin body type is ectomorphic. The person does not have enough muscle and flesh. Shao yin persons tend towards yin vacuity and, therefore, easily develop vacuity heat. In addition, these people often manifest liver depression qi stagnation due to the liver's not obtaining sufficient blood and yin to nourish and moisten it. Shao yin body types need to get adequate rest and to control their impulse to constantly stir. They also need to stay away from stimulating foods and drinks as well as acrid, hot, drying foods and flavors. Instead, they should take care to eat enough "bloody, meaty foods" so as to get enough *wei* to supplement their essence. People with serious cachectic disease, the anorectic, and many of the elderly develop this body type even though they were not born ectomorphic.

Just as in Sheldon somatotyping, no one is a pure type, similarly, the above four body types are only rough guidelines for disease tendencies. While most healthy young adults exhibit the shao yang body type, even within that type there may be mixtures. Therefore, one can talk about mixed shao yang-tai yang types, mixed shao yang-tai yin, and mixed shao yang-shao yin body types. Typically as we age, we move from a more shao yang type to more of one of these other three.

SEX & AGE

Sex and age both play major parts in the disease mechanisms of complex, chronic diseases and, therefore, typically must be factored into any pattern discrimination. It is said in Chinese medicine that men and women are essentially the same except that women have a uterus and thus they menstruate, gestate, and lactate. Further, ever since the Song dynasty, it has been said that, "[In] men the main [thing is] qi, [while in] women, the main [thing is] blood." Since menstruation, at least according to Chinese medicine, is a function primarily associated with blood, the fetus is nourished and constructed by the mother's blood, and breast milk is transformed out of the blood, blood is the central concept for understanding differences in disease mechanisms between men and women.

Because the spleen is the latter heaven root of engenderment and transformation of the qi and blood and because, A) women lose blood each month with menstruation, and B) huge amounts of blood are consumed by gestation, birthing, and lactation, women's spleens are more prone to overtaxation and, therefore, vacuity than men's. In particular, most Western women begin showing the clinical signs and symptoms of spleen vacuity at around 35 years of age, if not before. Because the spleen is the latter heaven root and the kidneys are the former heaven root, the spleen and kidneys share a close reciprocal relationship wherein they bolster and support each other. Thus, it is not hard to understand that spleen vacuity in the mid 30s may and usually does lead to kidney vacuity in the 40s. This can be a spleen qi-kidney yang vacuity, a spleen qi-liver-blood-kidney yin vacuity (a.k.a. a qi and yin vacuity), or a spleen qi-kidney yin and yang vacuity. Because menopause puts a stop to this monthly loss of blood, after menopause, assuming that the change of life has taken place completely, a woman's spleen and kidneys have the opportunity to recuperate. The above theories explain why women develop premenstrual and perimenopausal complaints and also why many chronic diseases either relapse or worsen each month during the premenstruum. Blood vacuity, spleen qi vacuity and, therefore, lung qi vacuity, and kidney yin and/or yang vacuity all cause or aggravate liver depression qi stagnation.

According to the *Nei Jing (Inner Classic)*, yin is half used up in both men and women by around 40 years of life. Since men are not as constitutionally predisposed to spleen vacuity as women, their spleen qi vacuity leading to kidney yang vacuity tends to happen a little later in life and is typically not attended by such overt and obvious symptoms as in women. Nevertheless, as we age, we all become qi and blood, yin and yang vacuous and insufficient. Since all four of these vacuities may cause or aggravate liver depression, this is why many older persons become depressed and irritable.

THE MOST COMMON SYMPTOMS OF THE MOST COMMON PATTERNS

As we have said, in complex, chronic diseases in Western patients, one should expect to see the signs and symptoms of not less than three and frequently as many as eight or more patterns simultaneously. When the disease mechanisms which produce individual patterns react with other disease mechanisms, they change the signs and symptoms of those patterns. Therefore, one will typically not see all of the textbook signs and symptoms of a pattern when that pattern is combined with another pattern. For instance, in real-life practice with Western patients, one rarely sees both a spleen and stomach vacuity weakness. More often, when the spleen becomes vacuous and damp, the stomach becomes hot and possibly either disharmonious or dry. Although torpid intake or lack of appetite is a textbook symptom of spleen vacuity, when spleen vacuity combines with stomach heat, either the appetite will be normal or may even be excessive. Therefore, one must know the key symptoms which you can always count on in Western patients to confirm the core set of patterns most patients manifest. These are shown on the next page.

The following patterns are the most commonly seen building blocks of complex patterns in chronic diseases. The signs and symptoms given under each pattern are, in our experience, the most reliable signs and symptoms in Western patients. In particular, the tongue and pulse are not good indicators of cold in the body. First of all, because of our

THE MAIN SIGNS & SYMPTOMS OF THE MOST COMMONLY SEEN PATTERNS

SPLEEN VACUITY

Fatigue which is often worse after large meals
A tendency to loose stools
Cold hands and nose
Orthostatic hypotension
A craving for sweets
A swollen tongue with teeth-marks on its edges

LIVER DEPRESSION

A bowstring pulse
Irritability
Emotional depression
PMS and/or dysmenorrhea in women
A dark-hued tongue

LIVER DEPRESSION-DEPRESSIVE HEAT

A bowstring, rapid pulse
A dark red tongue, red tongue edges, or inflated tongue edges
More marked irritability
A bitter taste in the mouth on arising in the morning

BLOOD VACUITY

Dry skin
Dry hair
Brittle nails
Night-blindness
A pale white or sallow yellow facial complexion
A pale tongue
A fine pulse

KIDNEY YIN VACUITY

Low back and knee soreness and weakness
Dizziness
Tinnitus
Matitudinal insomnia (*i.e.*, waking from sleep in the early morning)[30]
Night sweats
A red tongue or red tongue tip with scanty, dry, no, or peeled fur
A fine rapid, fine floating, or surging pulse

KIDNEY YANG VACUITY

Low back and knee soreness and weakness
Decreased sexual desire
Nocturia
Cold feet

STOMACH HEAT

A large appetite with rapid hungering
Red blemishes on the course of the *yang ming* on the face
Yellow tongue fur

STOMACH DRYNESS

Thirst
A dry mouth and throat with a desire to drink
Dry tongue fur

STOMACH & INTESTINAL DAMP HEAT

Diarrhea with dark or bright colored stools
Foul-smelling diarrhea
Burning around the anus with or after defecation
Slimy, yellow tongue fur, at least at the root

PHLEGM

Profuse phlegm from any body orifice
Plum pit qi
Phlegm nodulation
Obesity
Oily skin
Mental abstraction or depression
A fat, enlarged tongue with slimy or powdery fur
A slippery, bowstring or moderate (*i.e.*, slightly slow) pulse

FOOD STAGNATION

Bad breath
Slimy tongue fur
A slippery pulse
Possible reduced desire to eat and/or abdominal fullness

BLOOD STASIS

Severe, fixed, and/or lancinating pain
Pain which is worse at night
Visible venous thrombosis or varicosities, *e.g.*, cherry hemangiomas, spider nevi, varicose legs, etc.
Liver or age spots
A sooty facial complexion
A bowstring and/or choppy pulse

HEART-SPLEEN DUAL VACUITY

Fatigue
Heart palpitations
Insomnia
Poor memory
A pale, swollen tongue with teeth-marks on its edges
A moderate (*i.e.*, slightly slow) pulse between 50-60 bpm

GALLBLADDER-STOMACH DISHARMONY

Plum pit qi
Profuse phlegm
Waking in the middle of the night with nightmares and/or anxiety
Heart palpitations
A slippery, bowstring pulse

HEART-GALLBLADDER QI VACUITY

Same as above plus signs and symptoms of qi and/or blood vacuity, such as:

Lassitude of the spirit
Fatigue
Lack of strength
A fat, swollen tongue with teeth-marks on its edges
A fine, bowstring pulse

HEART FIRE

A red tongue tip with possible sores or sensitivity
Anxiety and restlessness
Insomnia
Heart palpitations
A rapid pulse

HEART FIRE SHIFTED TO THE SMALL INTESTINE AND BLADDER

The same symptoms as above plus:

Urinary frequency and urgency
Short, choppy urination
Burning, painful urination
Darker than normal urine

WIND COLD DAMP IMPEDIMENT

Sore, painful joints which are *not* red or hot
Worse pain on exposure to cold and dampness
Relief or lessening of pain on exposure to warmth

WIND DAMP HEAT IMPEDIMENT

Sore, painful, possibly swollen joints which are hot and may be red
Worse pain on exposure to heat or after eating hot, acrid, spicy, greasy, fried, fatty foods or drinking alcohol
Worse pain in hot, damp weather or environments
A slippery, rapid pulse

MALNOURISHMENT OF THE SINEW VESSELS

Worse pain after inactivity or on arising in the morning
Relief of pain after several minutes of movement and activity
Generalized qi and blood vacuity signs and symptoms

Western diet and lifestyle, replete cold is not so often seen in our patients. Secondly, most Western patients will have some evil heat somewhere in their body even if there is either replete or vacuity cold. In that case, because heat travels upward and the tongue and pulse at the radial artery are both in the upper burner, the tongue and pulse will tend to show the signs of this heat rather than the signs of cold.

In particular, when there is a dual kidney yin and yang vacuity, the tongue and pulse typically show the signs of the vacuity heat rather than the vacuity cold. In that case, one must rely on the four basic symptoms listed under kidney yang vacuity above. As long as the patient has three of these four and one of those three is decreased sexual desire, they do, in our opinion, manifest sufficient signs and symptoms to qualify for kidney yang vacuity. Since this diagnosis is likely in perimenopausal women, a woman's age may also be taken into account. In that case, kidney yang vacuity is always an evolution from spleen vacuity. Therefore, the actual pattern will be a spleen-kidney dual vacuity.

TONGUE CRACK PATTERNS INDICATING SPLEEN VACUITY

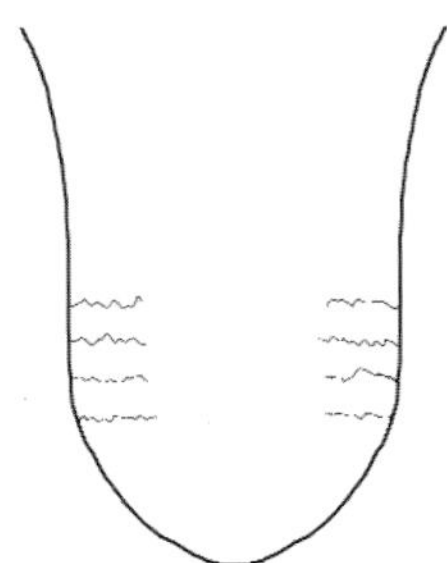

Transverse cracks on the sides

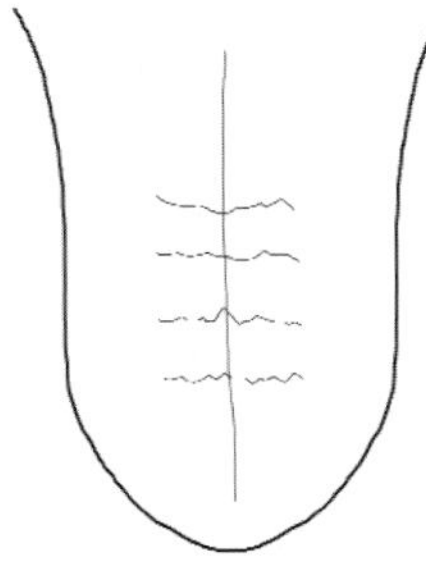

Vertical midline crack with transverse cracks

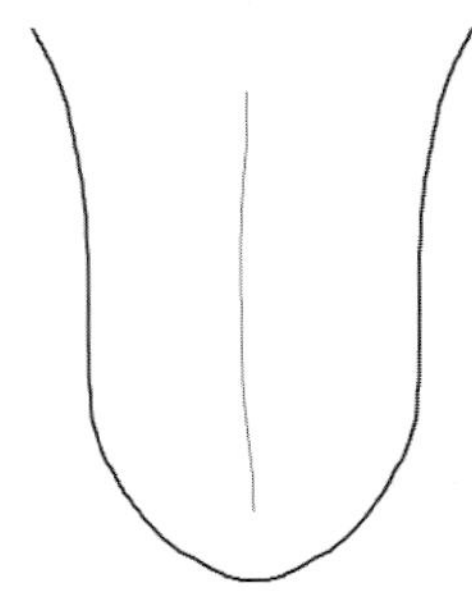

Vertical midline crack

FIGURE 7

One last piece of diagnostic information: Cracks on the tongue, whether large or small, are more often a sign of deep-seated, chronic spleen vacuity than yin vacuity. Such cracks should only be read as yin vacuity signs if there is a dry, red tongue with scanty fur and other clear-cut symptoms of yin vacuity. Figure 7 shows some common patterns of cracks on the surface of the tongue which indicate a long-standing, deep-seated spleen vacuity.

When treating difficult, knotty diseases, there are several Chinese medical statements of fact that should always be kept in mind. These statements all have to do with the most common complicating factors of other, often more obvious patterns. They are:

1. Enduring diseases are mostly [associated with] vacuity.
2. Enduring diseases are mostly [associated with] stasis.
3. Enduring diseases enter the network vessels.
4. Enduring [diseases] must reach the kidneys.

4. CASE HISTORIES EXEMPLIFYING TREATMENT BASED ON PATTERN DISCRIMINATION IN COMPLEX, MULTIPATTERN CASES

The following case histories and their analyses are based on actual cases treated by Bob Flaws. These are presented as examples of how the step-by-step methodology of professional Chinese medicine is used in real-life practice. While they do not show how the original pattern discrimination and, therefore, the treatment was modified during succeeding visits, they do show how to discriminate complicated combinations of patterns with a confusing welter of signs and symptoms and how to write complex Chinese medicinal prescriptions for these patterns.

CASE 1

The patient was a 39 year-old female who had had genital herpes since she was in her early 20s. These erupted as several, small slightly red papules which eventually ruptured and then transformed into wet ulcers. These arose on her perineum. They occurred before, during, or after her menstruation. They also occurred if she became fatigued. The lesions tended to linger but were not very painful. In addition, the patient had a diminished appetite, fatigue, lack of strength, lack of warmth in her four limbs, a tendency to loose stools, premenstrual breast distention, lower abdominal bloating, and irritability. Her tongue fur was thin and white, while the tongue substance was pale and swollen with teeth-marks on its edges. Her pulse was soggy in the right bar and fine and bowstring overall. It was neither fast nor slow.

PATTERN DISCRIMINATION: Spleen vacuity complicated by liver depression and damp heat in the lower burner

TREATMENT PRINCIPLES: Fortify the spleen and supplement the qi, course the liver and rectify the qi, clear heat and eliminate dampness

RX: *Dan Zhi Xiao Yao San Jia Wei* (Moutan & Gardenia Rambling Powder) with added flavors, *i.e.*, Rhizoma Smilacis Glabrae (*Tu Fu Ling*), Radix Sophorae Flavescentis (*Ku Shen*), Cortex Radicis Dictamni Dasycarpi (*Bai Xian Pi*)

ANALYSIS:

The patient was 39 years old. Therefore, her condition was probably a mixed repletion-vacuity one based simply on age alone. The spleen typically begins to become vacuous, if it is not already so, around 35 years of age, while the kidneys become vacuous in women sometime after that, based on the interdependence of the former and latter heaven roots. Thus, one should be looking for evidence of spleen and kidney vacuity. She had had genital herpes since her early 20s. This means that her condition was a recurrent, chronic one. That means that, although the branch manifestation may be a repletion, the root condition was probably a vacuity one. Small lesions suggest vacuity as opposed to repletion. *Slightly* red lesions also suggest not very strong heat. That they did rupture and then were wet indicates the presence of dampness.

So, up to this point, we know that the woman's condition probably involved a mixture of repletion and vacuity, that there was dampness and heat, but that the heat was not as important as the dampness. That the lesions occurred on the perineum is linked to dampness being a yin evil which is heavy and turbid and tends to sink downward. The fact that they might occur before, during, or after menstruation indicates that the condition was also not a simple repletion. Since women are relatively vacuous and empty after menstruation, repletions are not so common then.

As stated above, women in their late 30s typically suffer from some element of spleen vacuity. The spleen is the latter heaven root of qi and blood engenderment and transformation. It is the decline and vacuity of spleen qi and kidney yang cyclically each month which result in the onset of the menses. The menstrual blood flows out of the body due to the spleen not being able to restrain the blood nor the kidneys being able to seal and secure the lower yin. We also know that the spleen is the single most important viscera in the engenderment of dampness. The fact that these attacks also occurred when the patient was fatigued shows that they were due to vacuity. Fatigue is a main symptom of qi vacuity and the spleen is the main viscus involved in the engenderment and transformation of the qi. The facts that the lesions lingered and were not very painful also show that they were associated with vacuity. In repletion patterns, the disease course is usually short but dramatic. Since replete evils obstruct the qi and in repletion patterns there is a lot of qi and blood to obstruct, thus there is more pain. In this case, there was very little.

Next come the signs and symptoms that confirm that we are dealing with a spleen qi vacuity as the source of the dampness. Poor appetite, lack of or diminished, scanty appetite, fatigue, lack of strength, lack of warmth in the four limbs, and a tendency to loose stools, *when taken together as a pattern*, are the standard signs and symptoms of spleen qi vacuity. Thin, white tongue fur is considered normal in Chinese medicine. It shows there is no obvious repletion and little if any heat. If there is heat, it is not affecting the yang ming. The tongue substance being pale suggests blood vacuity. Immediately we should think that the spleen is the main viscus associated with the engenderment and transformation of blood. In that case, we should then immediately think that the spleen is responsible for engendering and transforming not only the blood but also the qi. The fact that the tongue was swollen with teeth-marks on its edges shows that the qi was vacuous and was not moving and transforming body fluids. Since the tongue was pale, pointing to the spleen, a swollen, indented tongue tells us that it was spleen qi vacuity which was not moving and transforming fluids which were then gathering and producing water dampness. This is further confirmed by the soggy pulse on the right bar. The soggy pulse is defined as a floating, fine, and forceless pulse. The right bar corresponds to the spleen and stomach. A soggy pulse in the right bar, therefore, indicates spleen qi vacuity with spilling over of water dampness. The fact that the pulse was fine overall also confirms that we are dealing primarily with a vacuity condition. Fine means finer than normal. The fine pulse means that there is not as much qi and blood flowing through the vessels as there should be. Based on all the other signs and symptoms, this points back again to spleen vacuity.

The bowstring pulse is an indication of liver depression qi stagnation. This is then confirmed by the premenstrual breast distention, lower abdominal bloating, and irritability. The fact that the pulse was neither fast nor slow shows that there was no heart or yang vacuity (a slow pulse) nor exuberant heat (a fast pulse).

Ergo, the case was one of spleen qi vacuity with liver depression and dampness and heat, with more dampness than heat. Hence the treatment principles in the case were to supplement the spleen and boost the qi, course the liver and rectify the qi, and clear heat and eliminate dampness with the emphasis on eliminating dampness. The formula, *Dan Zhi Xiao Yao San*, is based on the harmonizing formula, *Xiao Yao San* (Rambling Powder), which harmonizes the liver and spleen, supplements the spleen, and eliminates dampness. With the addition of *Dan Pi* and *Zhi Zi*, it clears heat and eliminates dampness at the same time as it resolves depression. To this base, *Tu Fu Ling*, *Bai Xian Pi*, and *Ku Shen* were added to clear heat and eliminate dampness more effectively, especially in the genital region.

CASE 2

The patient was a 35 year-old female with external vaginal itching and profuse vaginal discharge. The discharge was a creamy, opaque white. It did not have any particularly bad smell. This discharge was worse when the patient ate sugar or sweets. She was also fatigued, tended to have loose stools, and tended to have cold hands and feet. She frequently got dizzy when she stood up rapidly. She also often experienced white, clear to opaque nasal mucus after eating sweets or dairy. Her tongue was somewhat swollen with thin, white fur. Her right bar position was soft. Otherwise, her pulse tended to be fine and just a little bowstring. She did not have much PMS. She did tend to have two to three bowel movements per day which occurred after meals.

PATTERN DISCRIMINATION: Spleen vacuity leading to dampness pouring downward, possibly with a slight element of heat and only very, very minor qi stagnation

TREATMENT PRINCIPLES: Fortify the spleen and boost the qi, eliminate or transform dampness and stop vaginal discharge

RX: *Bu Zhong Yi Qi Tang Jia Wei* (Supplement the Center & Boost the Qi Decoction) with added flavors, *i.e.*, Rhizoma Dioscoreae Hypoglaucae (*Bi Xie*), Semen Coicis Lachryma-jobi (*Yi Yi Ren*), Rhizoma Acori Graminei (*Shi Chang Pu*), Fructus Tribuli Terrestris (*Bai Ji Li*)

ANALYSIS:

The patient was 35. "At 35 years, the yang ming declines in women and so they get wrinkles on their face." So says the *Nei Jing (Inner Classic)*, or at least something very close to that. The woman had external vaginal itching and profuse vaginal discharge. Excessively profuse vaginal discharge *always* involves dampness. The discharge was creamy and opaque white. White usually means that there is no heat. However, because it is somewhat thick and opaque, we cannot rule heat out altogether yet. It did not have any particularly bad smell. Offensive odor is mostly associated with heat. That this discharge was immediately worse if the woman ate sweets shows that it was associated with excessive dampness in turn associated with spleen vacuity. The sweet flavor inherently engenders fluids and enters the spleen channel. A little sweet supplements the spleen, but concentrated, excessive sweet damages the spleen causing vacuity detriment. She was also fatigued. This is *always* a symptom of qi vacuity. Her stools were loose and she tended to have cold hands and feet. Taken together, these are standard textbook symptoms adding up to spleen qi vacuity. She frequently got dizzy when she stood up too rapidly. This is spleen qi not upbearing the clear. Thus the brain loses its clarity and dizziness occurs. She also experienced white (no heat), clear (no heat) to opaque nasal phlegm after eating sweets or diary. Phlegm is nothing other than congealed dampness. This again leads back to dampness due to spleen vacuity. Her tongue was somewhat swollen with thin, white fur. Swollen equals gathered fluids due to spleen qi vacuity. Thin, white fur equals no particular heat or other repletions affecting the yang ming or upper burner, remembering that the tongue is in the upper part of the body and heat travels upward due to its inherently yang nature. Her right bar was soft. The soft pulse is another name for the soggy pulse. It means that the pulse is floating, fine, and forceless. The meaning is the same as in case number one. Her pulse was also a little fine and bowstring. Again the meaning is the same as in case one. That she *does not have much PMS* also confirms that liver depression qi stagnation is not an important part of this case, since one does not have PMS signs and symptoms without some element of liver depression. Two to three bowel movements per day are considered somewhat excessive by Chinese medical standards. When they occur after meals, this shows that the spleen qi is too vacuous and weak to separate the clear and turbid. Thus the clear and turbid get mixed up and descend.

Itching can be due to blood vacuity causing internal stirring of wind locally; it can be due to heat causing stirring of wind locally; and it can be due to blood stasis impeding the nourishment of the skin locally which then results in stirring of wind locally. One might make a case for a little heat based on the creamy, opaque vaginal discharge. The thicker and more opaque a discharge is, the more likely an element of heat is also involved. However, this would be the only sign of heat. Since it was so minimal, it probably does not need to be cleared. If one eliminates the dampness, then one eliminates the damp depression and probably automatically the local depressive heat. Given the other signs and symptoms of spleen vacuity and the fact that there were no other corroborating signs and symptoms of heat, this itching was more probably due to blood vacuity aggravated by local damp depression giving rise to stirring of wind in the skin.

Ergo, the pattern discrimination was spleen qi vacuity with dampness (and maybe a tiny bit of heat, but you need not to nor even should you say this). The treatment principles for this pattern are to supplement the spleen and boost the qi, transform dampness, stop vaginal discharge and stop itching. Since the woman had orthostatic hypotension due to spleen qi vacuity, one should pick *Bu Zhong Yi Qi Tang* as their guiding formula. *Bi Xie*, *Shi Chang Pu*, and *Yi Yi Ren* are all good choices for additions to transform dampness and stop excessive vaginal discharge. *Bai Ji Li* is the best choice for stopping itching associated with vacuity.

CASE 3

A 45 year old woman had fibrocystic breasts. She had had this condition for 20 years. However, it always got worse before each menstruation. She also had night sweats, cold feet, nocturia, occasional hot flashes, low back pain, and decreased libido. Her menses tended to come on day 24 or 25, down from 28-30 days when she was younger. There were nodular lumps in her breasts which were present throughout her cycle. However, these got larger and sore to pressure premenstrually. The patient was fatigued, had a tendency to loose stools, and bloated after eating a heavy meal. She also had postnasal drip or phlegm in the back of her throat which was clear to white when she was able to spit it out. Her tongue was light red with a redder tip and thin, white fur. Her pulse was bowstring and a little rapid overall. Her left cubit was fine and floating or soft. Her right cubit was deep, slipppery, and bowstring. Both inch positions were slippery, large, and floating.

PATTERN DISCRIMINATION: *Chong* and *ren* loss of harmony, *i.e.*, liver-kidney yin and yang vacuity, with liver depression, spleen vacuity, blood stasis, and phlegm nodulation

TREATMENT PRINCIPLES: Nourish the liver and supplement the kidneys, enrich yin and invigorate yang, course the liver and rectify the qi (or loosen the chest), fortify the spleen and supplement the qi, quicken the blood, soften the hard, and scatter nodulation

RX: *Er Xian Tang Jia Wei* (Two Immortals Decoction) with added flavors, *i.e.*, Radix Astragali Membranacei (*Huang Qi*), Radix Panacis Ginseng (*Ren Shen*), Sclerotium Poriae Cocos (*Fu Ling*), Rhizoma Pinelliae Ternatae (*Ban Xia*), Pericarpium Citri Reticulatae (*Chen Pi*), Bulbus Fritillariae Thunbergii (*Zhe Bei Mu*), Spica Prunellae Vulgaris (*Xia Ku Cao*), Radix Scrophulariae Ningpoensis (*Xuan Shen*), Concha Ostreae (*Mu Li*), Herba Sargassii (*Hai Zao*), Semen Citri Reticulatae (*Ju He*), Squama Manitis Pentadactylis (*Chuan Shan Jia*), Semen Vaccariae Segetalis (*Wang Bu Liu Xing*)

ANALYSIS:

A 45 year-old woman had fibrocystic breasts for 20 years. In Chinese medicine there is a saying that, "Breast disease in younger women or new breast diseases are due to the liver, while breast disease in older women or enduring breast diseases are due to the chong mai." Functionally, the chong mai is connected with the liver and kidneys. The breast condition got worse before each menstruation. Women this age commonly suffer from a spleen qi-kidney yang vacuity before their menses. They may also often suffer from liver blood-kidney yin vacuities premenstrually as they move towards the exhaustion of their *tian gui*. This patient had night sweats and hot flashes. This suggests yang counterflowing upward. Why was it counterflowing upward? It could be blood and/or yin vacuity; it could be due to damp heat; it could be due to liver depression transforming into depressive heat resulting in ascendant hyperactivity of liver yang. She had cold feet, decreased libido, and low back pain. This confirms kidney yang vacuity. Her menses were early. In women this age, we primarily look for spleen qi-kidney yang vacuity resulting in early menstruation, and we have confirmed an element of kidney yang vacuity. Nodular lumps throughout her cycle tell us there is phlegm nodulation. Phlegm nodulation does not come and go. These lumps got larger and sorer premenstrually. This shows that premenstrually there was depressed qi and possibly static blood. She often had a runny nose. This confirms the presence of phlegm. The fact that she had plum pit qi also confirms that she had both phlegm and liver depression. Her fatigue, bloating after heavy meals, and tendency to loose stools confirm spleen qi vacuity. Her tongue was light red. This means that any heat was a vacuity heat associated with some element of blood vacuity. The tip was red. This tells us that this heat was rising upward. The thin, white fur tells us there was no replete heat and that even the vacuity heat was not too severe in that it had not damaged fluids. Her pulse was bowstring. This confirms liver depression. It was slightly rapid. This confirms the presence of heat. Her left cubit was fine and floating or soft. This shows that yin was too vacuous to control yang which was counterflowing upward. Her right cubit was deep, slippery, and bowstring. The bowstring quality confirms that there was liver depression. The slippery quality in this case suggests stirring of ministerial fire. This means that yang had lost its root in its lower source. Actually in this case, the two cubits should be read together as a single pulse picture of stirring yang (right cubit) with vacuous yin (left cubit). Both inch positions are slippery, large, and floating. This equals the surging pulse. The slippery quality points to the phlegm and the heat. The floating and large images show upward and outward counterflow of yang. A floating and large pulse in the inch position is one of the characteristics of a yin fire scenario.

Ergo, the pattern was one of liver blood and kidney yin and yang vacuity with liver depression and phlegm nodulation. There were also signs and symptoms of spleen qi vacuity and blood stasis (soreness of the lumps with pressure premenstrually). Therefore, the treatment principles are to supplement the kidneys and invigorate yang, supplement the spleen and boost the qi, nourish the blood (or liver) and rectify the qi, quicken the blood, transform phlegm, and scatter nodulation. If one wanted to include leading yang back down to its lower source, coursing the liver, and/or softening the hard, that would also be OK but not absolutely necessary.

THE FIVE TYPES OF DISHARMONY

1. A constructive-defensive, *i.e.*, interior-exterior, disharmony
2. A liver-spleen disharmony
3. A liver-stomach disharmony
4. A spleen-stomach disharmony
5. A stomach-intestine disharmony

In terms of the formula, *Er Xian Tang* is the textbook guiding formula for chong and ren loss of harmony with a liver-kidney yin and yang vacuity. Therefore, it addressed the core pattern. *Huang Qi* and *Ren Shen* were added to supplement the spleen and boost the qi. *Ban Xia* and *Fu Ling* were added to fortify the spleen and transform phlegm. *Chen Pi* was added to rectify the qi, transform phlegm, and loosen the chest. *Xia Gu Cao* was added to clear the liver and scatter nodulation; *Zhe Bei Mu* transforms phlegm and scatters nodulation; *Xuan Shen* clears heat and scatters nodulation; and *Ju He* rectifies the qi and scatters nodulation. *Mu Li* subdues yang, constrains yin, and softens the hard. *Hai Zao* transforms phlegm and softens the hard. And *Chuan Shan Jia* and *Wang Bu Liu Xing* both quicken the blood and free the flow of the network vessels, free the flow of the breasts and dispel stasis.

5. THE IMPORTANCE OF HARMONIZING FORMULAS

Because most cases of difficult, knotty diseases revolve around a core disease mechanism of liver-spleen disharmony and tend to exhibit cold and heat, dampness and dryness, repletion and vacuity at the same time, the single most useful category of Chinese medicinal formulas for the treatment of these disorders is the harmonizing formulas. Harmonizing formulas harmonize any of five different pairs of disharmony. The table above shows these five different types of disharmony.

It is important not to think of harmonizing formulas as only harmonizing the constructive and defensive. In fact, harmonizing the constructive and defensive is the least often used of the harmonizing methods in the Western practice of Chinese medicine, and, even when harmonizing of the constructive and defensive is indicated, harmonizing one of the other four disharmonies is also usually indicated as well.

At least one harmonizing formula, *Xiao Chai Hu Tang* (Minor Bupleurum Decoction), has the potential for harmonizing all five of these disharmonies. This is why this is one of the most commonly prescribed formulas in all of Chinese medicine. It consists of: Radix Bupleuri (*Chai Hu*), Radix Panacis Ginseng (*Ren Shen*) or Radix Codonopsitis Pilosulae (*Dang Shen*), Radix Scutellariae Baicalensis (*Huang Qin*), Rhizoma Pinelliae Ternatae (*Ban Xia*), mix-fried Radix Glycyrrhizae (*Gan Cao*), Fructus Zizyphi Jujubae (*Da Zao*), and uncooked Rhizoma Zingiberis (*Sheng Jiang*). If one understands how to modify this formula in numerous different ways, it can be used to treat a large proportion of patients in real-life clinical practice. Some of the most famous independently named modifications of *Xiao Chai Hu Tang* include:

Chai Hu Gui Zhi Tang (Bupleurum & Cinnamon Decoction)
Chai Hu Wu Ling Tang (Bupleurum & Five [Ingredients] Poria Decoction)
Chai Hu Jia Long Gu Mu Li Tang (Bupleurum Plus Dragon Bone & Oyster Shell Decoction)
Chai Hu Jia Mang Xiao Tang (Bupleurum Plus Mirabilitum Decoction)
Chai Hu Si Wu Tang (Bupleurum Four Materials Decoction)
Chai Ping Tang (Bupleurum Calm [or Level the Stomach] Decoction)
Chai Hu Qing Zao Tang (Bupleurum Clear Dryness Decoction)
Chai Xian Tang (Bupleurum Bogged Down Decoction)
Chai Hu Gui Zhi Gan Jiang Tang (Bupleurum, Cinnamon & Dry Ginger Decoction)
Chai Shao Liu Jun Zi Tang (Bupleurum, Peony & Six Gentlemen Decoction)

Other famous harmonizing formulas include:

Xiao Yao San (Rambling Powder) and all its modifications
Dan Zhi Xiao Yao San (Moutan & Gardenia Rambling Powder)
Hei Xiao Yao San (Black Rambling Powder), etc.
Ban Xia Xie Xin Tang (Pinellia Drain the Heart Decoction) and all its modifications
Gan Cao Xie Xin Tang (Licorice Drain the Heart Decoction)
Sheng Jiang Xie Xin Tang (Uncooked Ginger Drain the Heart Decoction), etc.
Huang Lian Tang (Coptis Decoction)
Tong Xie Yao Fang (Painful Diarrhea Essential Formulas)

Xiao Yao San treats a liver-spleen disharmony with concomitant blood vacuity and some dampness. *Ban Xia Xie Xin Tang* treats a spleen-stomach and stomach and intestines disharmony. *Huang Lian Tang* also treats a spleen-stomach/stomach and intestines disharmony. *Tong Xie Yao Fang* treats a liver-spleen disharmony specifically resulting in abdominal cramping and diarrhea. All these formulas can be modified in many, many ways.

Although *Bu Zhong Yi Qi Tang* (Supplement the Center & Boost the Qi Decoction) is not categorized as a harmonizing formula, it can easily become one by raising the dosage of Radix Bupleuri (*Chai Hu*). In that case, it treats a liver-spleen disharmony in which spleen vacuity is more marked than liver depression. When *Bu Zhong Yi Qi Tang* is added into the list of potentially harmonizing formulas, it is our experience that this core group of formulas and their modifications can treat 7-8 out of 10 patients with chronic, complicated, difficult to treat disorders. For numerous modifications to the above formulas, please see Bob Flaws's *Seventy Essential Chinese Medicinal Formulas* (Blue Poppy Press, 2001).

6. Why decoctions are the standard of care in professional Chinese medicine

Here in the West, acupuncturists and practitioners of Chinese medicine are frequently care-givers of last resort. That means we get all the difficult to treat diseases which other health care providers have failed to treat successfully. Our patients typically only come to us after having seen one or more MDs, their DC, and often one or more other alternative health care practitioners, from *bona fide* NDs to the clerk at their local health food store. This means that our patients suffer from functional syndromes of unknown etiology, such as PMS, chronic fatigue syndrome, and fibromyalgia, allergies, autoimmune diseases, such as RA, MS, and SLE, and various malignancies. *In China, these kinds of conditions are never treated professionally, at least not in their active phase, by patent medicines.* They are always treated by polypharmacy, internally administered, water-based decoctions. We say this based on three sources of information: 1) our teachers' classroom lectures at the Shanghai and Hubei Colleges of Chinese Medicine, 2) our own observations at a number of Chinese hospitals and clinics in various parts of China, and 3) the modern published Chinese medical literature, both book and journal. What we were taught in school, what we saw in clinic, and what we have consistently read in the Chinese medical literature is that, in treating these kinds of "difficult to treat, knotty diseases," the professional standard of care in Chinese medicine in China is the prescription of relatively large, complex, and frequently modified bulk-dispensed decoctions.

The issue of modifiability

The issue of modifiability is an important one in professional Chinese medicine. In the Yuan dynasty, Zhu Dan-xi reported that, when he studied with Luo Tai-wu, "During a year and a half, there was not [one] set formula [prescribed]."[31] In our own times, Qin Bo-wei has said, "When I say to use *Liu Wei Di Huang Wan* (Six Flavors Rehmannia Pills), I don't mean for you to use the ingredients of *Liu Wei Di Huang Wan* but rather the *idea* of *Liu Wei Di Huang Wan.*"[32] Rarely in professional clinical practice in China is a standard formula prescribed in its standard form. Either medicinals are added to the standard ingredients (*jia wei*, added flavors) or some ingredients are added while others are subtracted (*jia jian*, additions and subtractions). It is the modification of standard formulas which allows professionally prescribed Chinese medicine to cure without side effects. Such modifications are made on the basis of the patient's individualized pattern discrimination plus their personal presenting signs and symptoms. Ingredients are typically added to prevent side effects and also to extend and strengthen a formula's clinical effects.

Most standard Chinese medicinal formulas are keyed to only one or two basic patterns. Because Western patients with chronic, difficult to treat diseases typically present with 5-8 patterns simultaneously, most standard Chinese formulas fall well short of comprehensively treating these kinds of patients. However, taking out unwanted medicinals is just as important as adding missing ingredients. Take *Liu Wei Di Huang Wan* for example. Three of these six ingredients are supplementing (cooked Radix Rehmanniae, *Shu Di,* Fructus Corni Officinalis, *Shan Zhu Yu*, and Radix Dioscoreae Oppositae (*Shan Yao*), while three are draining (Sclerotium Poriae Cocos, *Fu Ling*, Rhizoma Alismatis, *Ze Xie*, and Cortex Radicis Moutan, *Dan Pi*). The first two of the draining medicinals seep dampness, while the third clears heat and quickens the blood. If any three of these draining medicinals are not indicated, they must be removed. Because they are draining, they attack the righteous qi. In other words, if they are prescribed when they are unwanted, they can actually damage the patient and cause problems. Therefore, one simply cannot make up a shortfall in ingredients by piling one ready-made formula on top of another. If one does this, one is bound to be prescribing unwanted medicinals, and these eventually will take their toll.[33]

Because our Western patients present with such complex, multipattern diagnoses, simple, ready-made formulas rarely match them. In addition, these complex pattern discriminations are themselves not static. They tend to shift constantly. Unlike disease diagnoses, patients' patterns (or at least their relative proportions) tend to shift every week or so in relationship to the weather, phases of the moon, changes in season, fluctuations in diet, rest, activity, mood, and in reaction to medical treatment. This is why most patients in China check with their Chinese medical doctors once per week. Depending on the doctor's reassessment of their patient's pattern, the prescription will be modified further on an ongoing basis. Because treatment based on pattern discrimination is the very definition of high quality, professionally practiced Chinese medicine and patterns are so fluid and ever-changing, treatment must allow for easy modification. Ready-made medicines do not allow for this.

THE ISSUE OF PROCESSING

In Chinese, the processing of Chinese medicinals prior to decoction is called *pao zhi.* Within Chinese medicine, there are a number of different methods of this processing. Some of these methods are only for ease of storing or handling. Other methods are nothing more than cleaning, while yet other methods are, when all is said and done, not much more than cosmetic. However, many of these methods actually change the properties (*i.e.*, nature and/or flavor), functions, and indications of medicinals. According to Philippe Sionneau, one should not regard uncooked and honey mix-fried Radix Astragali Membranacei (*Huang Qi*) as the same medicinal any more than *Huang Qi* and Radix Angelicae Sinensis (*Dang Gui*) are the same medicinals. Once a medicinal has undergone processing, it becomes a different medicinal with different indications.

Although we have tried to keep the use of processed medicinals to a minimum in this text, processing does add a whole other level of sophistication and efficacy to the prescription of Chinese medicinals. Some ready-made medicines are made with properly processed medicinals, but others are not, and, when using a ready-made medicine, one cannot process a particular ingredient so that it can have an even stronger, more targeted effect with less potential side effects. The fact that one cannot further refine and tailor a prescription via processing is yet another drawback of ready-made medicines. For most common processing methods, all one needs is a wok, a hot plate, some water, and a handful of common household foodstuffs, such as salt, bran, rice, honey, vinegar, and alcohol. In addition, many Chinese medicinal suppliers, at least in the U.S., sell already processed versions of the most commonly processed Chinese medicinals. Therefore, it is not that difficult to use processed Chinese medicinals in most Western clinical practices. For more information on processing and the use of processed Chinese medicinals, readers should see Philippe Sionneau's *Pao Zhi: An Introduction to the Use of Processed Chinese Medicinals* also available from Blue Poppy Press.

THE ISSUE OF DOSE

When we said above that the kinds of difficult to treat, knotty conditions which are the stock in trade of Western practitioners commonly require "large" prescriptions, we meant two things. First, Chinese formulas for these kinds of conditions typically have more than 12 ingredients and often 15, 18, or even more than 20. If our average patient has 5-8 patterns simultaneously and most practitioners use at least two ingredients per disease mechanism, most Chinese medicinal formulas for these kinds of conditions will have at least a dozen ingredients. Formulas with lots of ingredients in them are called *da fang* in Chinese, "large prescriptions."

Secondly, although some of these ingredients may be dosed at the standard 9-10 grams per ingredient per day, many of them are dosed much higher than nine. For instance, it is not uncommon to see Radix Astragali Membranacei (*Huang Qi*) prescribed at anywhere from 18-60 grams *per day* in the contemporary Chinese literature. In other words, within a 15 ingredient formula, it is not uncommon to find a half dozen or more of these ingredients dosed at 15 grams or more. Even if the average dose of these ingredients is 10 grams, that means a total of somewhere between 150-180 grams per day. This is what the overwhelming majority of Chinese clinical audits published in the 30 or more Chinese medical journals suggest, and this is also my own (BF) experience of what reliably works in a cost effective manner here in the U.S. In our experience, many of the clinical failures of Western practitioners are due to using too small doses. We have many cases in our files where patients had been given the correct formula for their pattern by some previous practitioner, however, in the form of Chinese patent medicines, and the doses had simply been too low. When the doses were brought up to modern Chinese standards of care in the form of water-based, bulk-dispensed decoctions, their symptoms immediately improved.

This is not just our own experience. Recently another practitioner told Bob Flaws the following story. When this practitioner herself takes a particular ready-made formula as a 15:1 extract, it works fine. However, taking this formula as a 15:1 extract costs $50 per week (at least from her supplier). Therefore, on several occasions, she has tried to use the same formula as a less expensive 5:1 extract. At those times, the ingredients and their proportions have been the same. The only difference is the total daily dosage of medicinals. Whenever she has tried to use the less potent extract, her symptoms have come back. When she switches back to the more potent extract, her symptoms go away. As this story shows, the dosage of Chinese medicinals is extremely important in terms of getting the correct clinical outcome.

We cannot stress this fact too strongly. Students and practitioners in our classes both in the U.S. and Europe often ask us how to treat RA, SLE, MS, breast cancer, colon cancer, etc. with patent medicine. Where did we ever get the notion that these things could be treated by patent medicines? In Chinese, the word *wan* means pill. According to the Chinese medical definition, *wan* are made up of powdered Chinese medicinals (not extracts) held together by honey, water, or some other binder.[34] [35] The average stated dose of most Chinese ready-made pills is eight pills three times per day for a total of 24 pills. That equals four grams *per day*. Since they are 1:1 powders, that is all they are. Compare that to 150-180 grams of medicinals per day administered in decoction. Also consider that decocted medicinals are more efficiently absorbed than are swallowed powdered medicinals.

Pian in Chinese means tablets. *Pian* are made from powdered medicinal extracts. So are *chong ji*, soluble granules. Therefore, tablets and soluble granules tend to be more potent than pills. However, the overwhelming majority of desiccated, powdered extracts on the market today are only 3:1-5:1 extracts. That means a daily recommended dosage of three grams of extract still only equals nine to a maximum 15 grams of Chinese medicinals, and that is still only 1/10 of the average professionally prescribed daily dose for the kinds of diseases which are most Western practitioners' standard case load. If, on the other hand, one visits the dispensary at a typical Chinese hospital, one can easily tell the prescriptions for the patients with RA, SLE, MS, CFS, FMS, etc. They are all in the largest bags!

That being said, we are not necessarily advocating that every Western patient should be treated with the same daily standard doses of Chinese medicinals as in the People's Republic of China. In our experience, in many cases, a daily dose of 80-100g of a polypharmacy formula seems to work quite well. In addition, many Westerners simply cannot afford the full standard Chinese daily dose of Chinese medicinals. It is also true that the best grades (and, therefore, the most potent) Chinese medicinals are sold to the West for hard currency. Hence, while it is our experience that many Westerners are not receiving adequate doses of Chinese medicinals for quick and efficient healing, a lower dose may, for a number of reasons, be acceptable and even preferable in Western patients. Not the least of these reasons is that most Western patients seeking Chinese medical treatment are routinely treated by both Chinese medicinals and acupuncture, and such bimodal therapy is not the standard of care in the People's Republic of China. In raising this issue of dose, we are primarily asking our fellow practitioners to ask themselves what is the optimal daily dose of Chinese medicinals in each individual instance while keeping in mind the standards of care in the PRC.

THE ROLE OF READY-MADE PILLS IN PROFESSIONAL MEDICINE IN CHINA

When Bob Flaws studied *fang ji xue* (*i.e.*, formulas and prescriptions) at the Shanghai College of Chinese Medicine, Prof. Chen Wei gave a lecture on the clinical uses and indications of different forms of medicinal administration. In that lecture, Prof. Chen said:

> The merits of decoctions are that they are quickly absorbed, easy to modify and customize, and are the most practical form of administration for complicated cases. They are indicated for both chronic

> and acute diseases and are the most commonly used form of medicinal administration [read, the standard of care] in China.[36]

In contradistinction, Xu Ji-qun *et al.*, the authors of *Fang Ji Xue (A Study of Formulas & Prescriptions)*, the textbook for this course, have this to say about pills:

> Pills are slow to absorb. Therefore, their medicinal power is continuous and enduring. . . .They are appropriate for chronic [literally, slow] conditions and for vacuity weakness diseases.[37]

This means that, in the People's Republic of China, pills and decoctions each have their own particular indications and uses. They are not considered interchangeable. This is supported by the fact that the only times we have seen ready-made pills prescribed by professional practitioners of Chinese medicine in China was in order to "secure treatment efficacy" after treatment by decocted medicinals had achieved the therapeutic effect or when the practitioner wanted to increase the dosage of certain medicinals. In that case, pills were prescribed *along with* decocted medicinals as if the pills where themselves a single medicinal.[38] In other words, ready-made pills are primarily prescribed by professional practitioners for preventive as opposed to remedial treatment. For remedial treatment of active disease processes, individually prescribed, bulk-dispensed, water-based decoctions are the professional standard of care.

Further, ready-made pill medicines in China are available "over the counter" without a prescription. Laypeople in China often attempt to treat themselves with such OTC medications the same way laypeople do here in the West. When Bob Flaws was an intern in China, he often saw patients who began their case history saying that they had used this or that ready-made medicine and that it had not helped or had made them worse. So now they were there to get a proper professional prescription. Likewise, Philippe Sionneau has never seen professional practitioners of Chinese medicine prescribe ready-made pills for the remedial treatment of disease, even, as he says, for minor diseases. As Dr. Chen also said in her *fang ji xue* lectures, many people in China take supplementing ready-made pills. However, this is on their own initiative and does not constitute the professional practice of Chinese medicine. Rather, it is analogous to how Westerners take vitamin and mineral supplements.

Compliance vs. convenience

As every real-life clinician knows, when determining any course of therapy, one has to weigh the relative costs versus benefits (not just risks versus benefits). Ease of administration helps insure patient compliance, especially over a protracted course of treatment. However, when patients fail to see results, they do not stay with therapy no matter how easy it is. Many practitioners say that Western patients will not take decoctions. Although some Western patients will not, most will if: A) they are not given a choice in the matter and, B) the decoctions achieve better results than any other treatments they have tried. If practitioners tell patients they can either take easy pills or somewhat more difficult decoctions and voice this choice as if these two forms of administration were equal, then, of course, patients will chose the easier pills. However, it is my experience that, when patients are told how much more effective decoctions tend to be, most patients want to do what is going to work best.

In order to make this choice a realistic one for the patient, the practitioner also has to be willing and comfortable with taking decoctions. Placebo studies confirm that how a practitioner feels about a therapy influences how their patients also feel. Otherwise, double-blind studies would not be necessary. Practitioners who themselves do not like taking decoctions will have a hard time convincing their patients that they should take decoctions. However, when the practitioner themself takes decoctions when they are ill and also is firm in stating that 1) decoctions are the standard of care in professional Chinese medicine, 2) they are more effective than most pills and powders, and 3) they are no more difficult to make than cooking a pot of rice, then Western patients serious about their health *are willing* to drink bad-tasting Chinese medicinal decoctions.

Dr. Christopher, a famous American naturopath in the 1970s, said, "Good doctors require good patients." Paracelsus, several hundred years earlier, said, "The good doctor attracts patients who are ready to be cured." If a patient refuses to spend the time and energy on making and taking decoctions even though they are more potent and can be tailored to fit their case exactly, then that patient is not serious about their health and is probably not going to get a satisfactory outcome anyway. Patients who are unwilling to make and take decoctions are also not likely to make the substantial, long-term diet and lifestyle changes that are also necessary to get a good result.

Comparing apples to apples

While pills are still the most commonly used form of ready-made Chinese medicine, desiccated powdered extracts taken in the form of infused teas or swallowed capsules are also extremely popular. However, no matter what the form of the ready-made medicine, the single most important question to ask is, "What are the dosage equivalencies?" Most Chinese-made pills equal one gram of ground, powdered medicinals per gram of pills. Thus their equivalency ratio is 1:1. As we have seen above, that means their daily recommended dose is only a small fraction of the standard daily dose of typical decoctions. A 3:1 extract means that each gram of extract equals three grams of bulk-dispensed medicinals. A 5:1 extract means that each gram of extract equals five grams of bulk medicinals. As we have mentioned above, a few companies are beginning to introduce higher powered extracts, 8-15:1. However, at this time, there is a manufacturing limit as to the upper potencies of these extracts. In any case, when determining what dosage of any medicine to prescribe, be it pill, powder, or decoction, one *must* know what are the equivalencies to bulk-dispensed medicinals. If the standard daily dose of a decocted formula in China is 180 grams per day, then giving 3-5 grams per day of Chinese medicinals is nothing. Even the equivalent of 15-45 grams per day is still several times lower than the standard of care set in the People's Republic of China, and, in our experience, those standards are the ones we should be following if we want to get comparable results.

It is disingenuous to hold out to the public that we practice a 2,000 year old medicine and then not follow the professional standards of care that have evolved over that 2,000 years. When we say that Chinese medicine works because it has been proven to work over not less than 100 generations of literate, professional practitioners, then we the authors believe that we as a profession have an obligation to actually do what has been shown to work. If we choose to do something else, then we believe it is incumbent upon us to disclose to our patients that we are experimenting on them.

7. Some thoughts on the practice of acupuncture in the West

In China, acupuncture is mainly used for musculoskeletal diseases, such as impediment conditions, neurological conditions, such as post-stroke sequelae and neuritis, pain conditions, and traumatic injuries. Although, in theory, acupuncture can treat many more diseases than just musculoskeletal, neurologic, and pain disorders, the efficient scope of application of acupuncture is more narrow than that of Chinese medicinals. That is not to say that acupuncture and moxibustion are inferior to Chinese medicinals. What we mean here is that, in China, acupuncture has a different scope of application. Based on 2,000 plus years of Chinese clinical experience, only certain diseases are routinely referred to the acupuncture department. For treating a herniated disk or migraine headache, acupuncture works very well in a time and cost efficient manner, but, for infectious diseases or chronic, complicated metabolic or functional diseases such as diabetes mellitus, acupuncture is often not time and/or cost effective.

Based on the normative standards in the People's Republic of China and our own clinical experience in the West, we believe that acupuncture should only be used as an adjunctive treatment for the majority of the difficult to treat, knotty diseases discussed in this book. For such complex, enduring, multifaceted disorders as myasthenia gravis, hypo- and hyperglycemia, hyperlipoproteinuria, and chronic active hepatitis, internally administered Chinese medicinals are the standard of care. When even better than average Chinese acupuncturists are faced with these kinds of diseases, they rarely use only acupuncture. Mu La-mei, one of Philippe Sionneau's teachers, is considered as one of the best acupuncturists at the Hubei College of Chinese Medicine in Wuhan. Dr. Mu has more than 30 years of clinical experience. She has lots of patients and gets excellent clinical results. But she always prescribes not less than 200g of Chinese medicinals per day on top of acupuncture whenever the patient presents with a chronic, complicated metabolic or functional disease.

Secondly, there is the question of the effective spacing of acupuncture treatments. Here in the West, most acupuncturists perform one treatment per week regardless of the disease being treated as if their patient was coming for a weekly massage or psychoanalysis session. In China, even very experienced acupuncturists treat acute diseases, such as common cold, diarrhea, and traumatic injuries, 1-3 times per day for several days in a row. For enduring diseases, such as asthma, impediment conditions, and peptic ulcers, patients are routinely treated 2-3 times per week for at least several weeks. Thus, in China where the bulk of experience in the use of acupuncture is found, patients receive far more treatments spaced much more closely together than is the norm here in the West where many patients are even only treated 1-2 times per month.

There are no good comparative studies addressing this issue. Why do we, as Western practitioners, assume that a single acupuncture treatment per week is adequate? Certainly, there is little if any precedent for this practice in Asia. The authors of this text have heard again and again from Westerners who were treated for relatively long periods of time with acupuncture but only once a week or less and who did not get the result they were hoping for. Therefore, when Western practitioners choose to perform acupuncture on a particular patient, we advise that, first, they determine whether or not acupuncture is a or the preferred treatment modality in the case at hand and, secondly, that they schedule treatments close enough together so that the patient's time and money are truly well spent. Until or unless well-designed studies show that once weekly acupuncture is as effective as the more closely spaced acupuncture which is the norm in China, we believe Western patients would be best served by Western practitioners emulating the standards of care for acupuncture developed in the People's Republic of China, at least regarding the frequency of treatment. It is our experience that more closely spaced treatments are often more effective than routine once weekly treatments, at least during the active remedial phase of care.

Similarly, the duration of each acupuncture session also affects the outcome of treatment. According to Chinese acupuncture theory, how long the needles are left in place depends on whether the disease is manifesting a vacuous or replete pattern and whether it is an acute or chronic one. Based on a comparison of protocols reported on in recent Chinese medical journals, it is apparent that the more difficult a disease is to treat, the more painful it is, and/or the longer the disease has lasted, the longer should be the acupuncture session. For instance, for acute cholecystitis, acute nephrolithiasis, and acute gout, the standard 20 minute needle retention may be stretched to 90 minutes. When it comes to the duration of acupuncture treatments, one size, or rather length, does not fit all. It is the authors' experience that adjusting the length of needle retention for the specific condition being treated can make a big difference in the outcomes in some diseases.

CONCLUSION

As stated in the opening paragraph of this introduction, no single textbook or clinical manual can cover all the exigencies of clinical practice. The reader should keep in mind that patients with chronic, enduring diseases will have more than a single pattern. Therefore, other formulas may be more efficient in a given patient's case then the ones recommended in this book. As mentioned above, Qin Bo-wei, one of the architects of modern Chinese medicine said, "When I say to use *Liu Wei Di Huang Wan* (Six Flavors Rehmannia Pills), I don't mean for you to use the ingredients of *Liu Wei Di Huang Wan* but rather the *idea* of *Liu Wei Di Huang Wan.*" These formulas are not meant for rote application. They are only meant as examples. Likewise, the dosages for the ingredients in these formulas are only meant as starting places for thinking about dosages. Depending on a particular patient's combination of patterns and the severity of their various symptoms, one may come up with variations that look very different than the formulas in this book. Since every formula is meant to be written *ad hoc* in Chinese medicine, this is just the way it is. If one understands the method of formulating treatment plans based on patterns and treatment principles and one has a firm grasp of points and medicinals, this is not a difficult task. It is what makes professional Chinese medicine an art as well as a science.

ENDNOTES

[1] Li, Wei-dong, "A Brief Report on Traditional Chinese Medical Education in China," *AATOM Newsletter*, American Association for Teachers of Oriental Medicine, Austin, TX, Nov. 1998, p. 5

[2] Birch, Stephen J. & Felt, Robert L., *Understanding Acupuncture*, Churchill Livingstone, Edinburgh, 1999, p. 33

[3] By standard professional Chinese medicine, we mean that style of Chinese medicine taught as the core curriculum at the provincial schools of Chinese medicine in the People's Republic of China. Although these standards of care have been established over the last 40 years or more in a host of national symposia and conventions, this style of Chinese medicine has evolved over not less than a recorded 2,500 years.

[4] *The Merck Manual of Diagnosis & Therapy*, 17th edition, Mark H. Beers & Robert Berkow, ed., Merck Research Laboratories, Whitehouse Station, NJ, 1999, p. 1376

[5] In China, amongst general practitioners, the *tai yang* and *yang ming* divisions are also sometimes still used. It is also true that some Chinese doctors only use the six divisions methodology of the *Shang Han Lun (Treatise on Damage [Due to] Cold)* as well as the teachings of its companion, the *Jin Gui Yao Lue (Essentials of the Golden Cabinet).* Often these doctors are especially famous and respected.

[6] *E.g.*, the work of Xie Zhu-fan conducted at the Beijing College of Chinese Medicine described by Birch & Felt, *op. cit.*, p. 175

[7] *Webster's New World Dictionary of the American Language*, The World Publishing Co., Cleveland & NY, 1966, p. 1073, gives this meaning of the word pattern as a "grouping or distribution [of elements], as of a number of bullets fired at a mark, [or] a diagram showing such distribution."

[8] According to Philippe Sionneau, in China, doctors are legally required to give the name of the patient's disease according to Western medicine, the name of the Chinese disease, the pattern discrimination, the treatment principles, and the treatment plan.

[9] Birch & Felt, *op. cit.*, p. 175

[10] Chen Wei, based on Bob Flaws's lecture notes, "Formulas & Prescriptions," Shanghai College of Chinese Medicine, Shanghai, April, 1986

[11] In actuality, one must first determine if the disease in question is amenable to Chinese medical treatment and, if so, if the practitioner is personally qualified to treat that disease.

[12] The word "knotty" in this context means that there are a number of disease mechanisms bound together and, therefore, a number of simultaneously presenting patterns.

[13] Wan Wen-rong, "Zhu Liang-chun's Thoughts on the Treatment of Knotty, Difficult Diseases," *Zhong Yi Za Zhi (Journal of Chinese Medicine)*, #1, 2000, p. 14

[14] *Ibid.*, p. 14

[15] Depressive heat or fire is itself the sixth of Zhu's six depressions.

[16] In yin yang theory, disease evils are yin as compared to the righteous qi which is yang.

[17] In terms of diagnostic signs, yin fire is commonly indicated by a combination of spleen vacuity symptoms, liver depression symptoms, a fat tongue with teeth-marks on its edges, and a surging pulse. The surging pulse indicates heat counterflowing upward, however, due to vacuity below. In that case, the surging pulse is primarily or especially prominent in the inch position and is easily misread as a sign of repletion in neophytes.

[18] We are indebted to Charles (Chip) Chace for first identifying these five principles in this way.

[19] Strictly speaking, the lifegate and lifegate fire are two different things. The lifegate is the moving qi between the kidneys which encompasses both true yin and true yang. Lifegate fire is the ministerial fire or simply the true yang.

[20] Fruehauf, Heiner, "Driving Out Demons and Snakes: Gu Syndrome and a Forgotten Clinical Approach to Chronic Parasitism," *The Journal of Chinese Medicine*, UK, #57, 1998, p. 10-17

21 Zhu Dan-xi, *The Heart & Essence of Dan-xi's Methods of Treatment*, trans. by Yang Shou-zhong, Blue Poppy Press, Boulder, CO, 1993, p. 142

22 Wiseman, Nigel & Feng, Ye, *A Practical Dictionary of Chinese Medicine*, Paradigm Publications, Brookline, MA, 1998, p. 249

23 Although Bupleurum is categorized as an acrid, cool exterior-resolver, it is primarily used in modern Chinese medicine and in gu therapy as a qi-rectifier.

24 Although *She Chuang Zi* is categorized as a yang-supplementing medicinal, it is mostly used for damp heat itching and skin lesions, especially of the genitalia.

25 Jarisch-Herxheimer reactions were first identified in and are also seen in patients treated with antibiotics for syphilis.

26 Yan De-xin, *Aging & Blood Stasis*, trans. by Tang Guo-shun & Bob Flaws, Blue Poppy Press, Boulder, CO, 1995, p. 39-40, 46-47

27 *Ibid.*, p. 33-48

28 Zhu Liang-chun, quoted by Wan Wen-rong, *op. cit.*, p. 14

29 Wan Wen-rong, *op. cit.*, p. 14

30 If yin vacuity is severe or yin vacuity is combined with marked yang hyperactivity, there may also be onset insomnia. This means difficulty falling asleep initially.

31 Yang Shou-zhong, "Editor's Preface," *Extra Treatises Based on Investigation & Inquiry, A Translation of Zhu Dan-xi's Ge Zhi Yu Lun*, Blue Poppy Press, Boulder, CO, 1994, p. vi

32 Qin Bo-wei, *Qin Bo Wei Yi Wen Ji (A Collection of Qin Bo-wei's Writings)*, Hunan Science & Technology Press, Changsha, 1991, p. 34

33 While some Western practitioners believe that Chinese herbs are safe and free from side effects because they are "natural," this is just not the case. If something is strong enough to push the body into balance, it only stands to reason that same thing must be strong enough to push a person out of balance if they don't need it. Such naturally occurring substances as fresh water and salt can kill when taken to excess. Thus there is no such thing as a medical panacea, and those Western practitioners who say that Chinese medicinals are safe because they are natural are dangerously naïve.

34 Bensky, Dan & Barolet, Randall, *Chinese Herbal Medicine: Formulas & Strategies*, Eastland Press, Seattle, 1990, p. 19 and Chen Wei, lecture notes, "Formulas & Prescriptions," Shanghai College of Chinese Medicine, April, 1986. According to Prof. Chen, tablets are made from extracts, while pills are not.

35 According to Philippe Sionneau, the popular Lanzhou Brand of ready-made Chinese medicinal pills is made from a low potency extract combined with a large amount of inert binder.

36 Chen Wei, lecture notes, "Formulas & Prescriptions," Shanghai College of Chinese Medicine, April, 1986. However, this essentially same teaching also appears in Bensky & Barolet, *op. cit.*, p. 18.

37 Xu Ji-qun *et al.*, *Fang Ji Xue (A Study of Formulas & Prescriptions)*, Shanghai Science & Technology Press, Shanghai, 1986, p. 10

38 It is true that Chinese acupuncturists often recommend or prescribe Chinese ready-made medicines as adjunctive therapy to their acupuncture. However, when more than adjunctive treatment is required, Chinese acupuncturists typically refer patients to other Chinese doctors in the internal medicine department specifically qualified to write bulk-dispensed, individualized prescriptions.

1

Acne Vulgaris

Acne vulgaris or common acne (as opposed to acne rosacea) is a common inflammatory disease of the pilosebaceous glands characterized by comedones, papules, pustules, inflamed nodules, superficial pus-filled cysts, and, in extreme cases, canalizing and deep, inflammed, sometimes purulent sores. The pathophysiology of this condition is a complex interaction between hormones, keratinization, sebum, and bacteria. Acne usually begins at puberty when an increase in androgens causes an increase in the size and activity of pilosebaceous glands. Intrafollicular hyperkeratosis leads to blockage of the pilosebaceous follicles which then leads to the formation of comedones. These comedones are composed of sebum, keratin, and microorganisms, particularly *Propionibacterium acnes.* These microorganisms break down triglycerides in the sebum to free fatty acids which then irritate the follicular wall. Superficial acne refers to blackheads (*i.e.*, open comedones) and whiteheads (closed comedones), inflamed papules, pustules, and superficial cysts. Deep acne refers to the form characterized by deep, inflamed nodules and pus-filled cysts which often rupture and become abscesses. This is sometimes also referred to as cystic acne. While scarring is not common with superficial acne, it is common with deep acne.

Acne lesions mostly appear on the face, chest, and upper back where the sebaceous follicles are largest. Acne usually remits spontaneously. However, the time or age of remittance is unpredictable. Acne is somewhat more common in males than in females. However, in females the incidence and severity of acne is often tied to the menstrual cycle, with outbreaks occurring especially during the premenstruum. Acne may also improve or worsen in women during pregnancy. In general, acne is often worse in winter and better during the summer. This is probably due to the benefits of sunlight.

The Western medical diagnosis of acne is primarily dependent on visual examination of the characteristic lesions. Differential diagnosis includes acne rosacea and corticosteroid-induced acneiform lesions. The Western medical treatment of acne includes the topical application of clindamycin or erythromycin, azelaic acid cream, topical tretinoin, benzoyl peroxide, and various sulfur-resorcinol combinations. Recalcitrant cases or deep acne is treated by oral administration of broad-spectrum antibiotics. The most commonly prescribed of these is tetracycline. Unfortunately, because relapse ordinarily follows short-term treatment, therapy must contine for months to years. Side effects of such antibiotics include gastrointestinal problems, dizziness, and pigmentation of the skin and mucous membranes. Oral isotretinoin is used in those in whom antibiotics have proved unsuccessful or in patients with very severe deep acne. However, side effects occur in virtually 100% of patients treated with this approach and include dryness of the conjunctivae and mucosae of the genitalia, chapped lips, and musculoskeletal stiffness and/or low back pain.

Chinese disease categorization: The most common Chinese name for acne vulgaris is *fen ci*, white thorns. This describes the protruding shape of whiteheads. Acne is also called *fei feng fen ci*, lung wind white thorns, *jiu ci*, wine thorns, and *qing chun li*, green spring (*i.e.*, pubescent) granules. *Cuo chuang*, another common name for acne, means pimples.

Disease causes: Natural endowment repletion or insufficiency, stirring of ministerial fire due to maturation, the cyclic waxing and waning of yin and yang in women, faulty diet, and emotional stress and frustration

Disease mechanisms: This disease primarily involves heat and dampness. The red color of acne lesions indicates the existence of heat evils, while the white matter and pus inside the lesions indicate dampness and phlegm. More men experience acne than women because men tend to be constitutionally more yang exuberant. Acne tends to begin at puberty because of the stirring and hyperactivity of lifegate fire at that time. This upward flaming of ministerial or lifegate fire aggravates any tendency to heat in the lungs, stomach, and liver, the main organs involved in acne. The lungs govern the skin and are the florid canopy of the five viscera and six bowels. This means that any heat counterflowing upward will tend to gather and accumulate in the lungs. Thus the *Yi Zong Jin Jian (The Golden Mirror of Ancestral Medicine)* says, "This illness is produced by blood heat in the lung channel." The fact that this disease is ascribed primarily to the lungs, at least in terms of its proximate cause, is corroborated by the *Wai Ke Zheng Zong (Correct Ancestral [or Gathered] External Medicine)* which says, "Acne pertains to the lungs." The yang ming channels are the places on the face where acne lesions often tend to cluster, and it is liver depression giving rise to depressive heat which often tends to stir and inflame both the lifegate fire below and stomach heat above. Heat may stew the juices and congeal phlegm which is drafted upward with the counterflowing heat. A tendency to engender phlegm is all the more pronounced if there is liver depression, spleen vacuity, or overeating of fluid-engendering foods, such as oils and fats. When this lodges in the space between the skin and muscles in the upper body, it may give rise to phlegm nodulations. If heat is severe, it may also brew toxins which then putrefy the blood and fluids, engendering pus and welling abcesses. Either phlegm or toxins may inhibit the free flow of qi and blood in the affected area. In that case, enduring diease may also give rise to blood stasis. When acne is due to adolescent hyperactivity of lifegate fire, sex, drugs, and alcohol may all aggravate this stirring and hyperactivity. In women who experience premenstrual acne, this is usually due to aggravation of liver depression due to blood vacuity leading to transformation of depressive heat. Last but not least, it is also possible for a constitutional yin vacuity to fail to control hyperactive yang.

TREATMENT BASED ON PATTERN DISCRIMINATION:

1. LUNG CHANNEL WIND HEAT PATTERN

MAIN SYMPTOMS: The face tends to be red with red lesions which feel hot and may be painful and there may be pustules. The tongue is red with yellow fur, and the pulse is rapid and floating.

NOTE: The "wind" in the name of this pattern means that, traditionally, the cause of this condition was invisible. Other names for this pattern include lung-stomach depressive heat and lung channel blood heat. While essentially all patients with acne have lung heat, most have other disease mechanisms as well. Therefore, the pure form of this pattern is not commonly met.

TREATMENT PRINCIPLES: Diffuse the lungs, drain heat, and cool the blood

RX: *Pi Pa Qing Fei Yin* (Eriobotrya Clear the Lungs Drink)

INGREDIENTS: Folium Eriobotryae Japonicae (*Pi Pa Ye*), Cortex Radicis Mori Albi (*Sang Bai Pi*), and Cortex Phellodendri (*Huang Bai*), 9g each, and Rhizoma Coptidis Chinensis (*Huang Lian*), uncooked Radix Glycyrrhizae (*Gan Cao*), and Radix Panacis Ginseng (*Ren Shen*), 6g each

ANALYSIS OF FORMULA: Within this formula, *Pi Pa Ye* and *Sang Bai Pi* drain heat from the lungs. *Huang Bai* and *Huang Lian* drain fire from the heart, stomach, liver, and kidneys. They also clear and resolve heat toxins. Uncooked *Gan Cao* clears heat and resolves toxins at the same time as it harmonizes the rest of the ingredients in this formula. *Ren Shen* supplements the spleen and engenders fluids, thus protecting the spleen and stomach from the other harshly attacking medicinals.

ADDITIONS & SUBTRACTIONS: If heat is more pronounced, remove *Ren Shen* and add 30 grams of uncooked Gypsum Fibrosum (*Shi Gao*) and 15 grams each of Radix Lithospermi Seu Arnebiae (*Zi Cao*) and Flos Immaturus Sophorae Japonicae (*Huai Hua Mi*). If there is concomitant constipation, also add 3-15 grams of Radix Et Rhizoma Rhei (*Da Huang*). If there is marked blood stasis, remove *Ren Shen* and add 12 grams each of Spina Gleditschiae Chinensis (*Zao Jiao Ci*) and Semen Vaccariae Segetalis (*Wang Bu Liu Xing*), nine grams of Flos Carthami Tinctorii (*Hong Hua*), and 1.5-3 grams of Hirudo Seu Whitmania (*Shui Zhi*). If there is marked dampness and turbidity, remove *Ren Shen* and add 21 grams of Semen Coicis Lachryma-jobi (*Yi Yi Ren*) and nine grams each of Radix Sophorae Flavescentis (*Ku Shen*) and Rhizoma Smilacis Glabrae (*Tu Fu Ling*). If there is phlegm nodulation, remove *Ren Shen* and *Gan Cao* and add nine grams each of Rhizoma Sparganii (*San Leng*), Rhizoma Curcumae Zedoariae (*E Zhu*), Thallus Algae (*Kun Bu*), and Herba Sargassii (*Hai Zao*).

For marked heat entering the blood division or aspect, replace *Pi Pa Qing Fei Yin* with *Liang Xue Qing Fei Yin* (Cool the Blood & Clear the Lungs Drink): uncooked Radix Rehmanniae (*Sheng Di*) and Gypsum Fibrosum (*Shi Gao*), 30g each, Cortex Radicis Moutan (*Dan Pi*), Radix Rubrus Paeoniae Lactiflorae (*Chi Shao*), Radix Scutellariae Baicalensis (*Huang Qin*), Rhizoma Anemarrhenae Aspheloidis (*Zhi Mu*), Cortex Radicis Mori Albi (*Sang Bai Pi*), and Folium Eriobotryae Japonicae (*Pi Pa Ye*), 9g each, and uncooked Radix Glycyrrhizae (*Gan Cao*), 6g.

For lung heat with heat toxins and blood stasis, replace *Pi Pa Qing Fei Yin* with the following unnamed formula: uncooked Radix Rehmanniae (*Sheng Di*), 30-45g, Herba Violae Yedoensitis Cum Radice (*Zi Hua Di Ding*), 30g, uncooked Gypsum Fibrosum (*Shi Gao*), 15g, Folium Daqingye (*Da Qing Ye*), Cortex Radicis Mori Albi (*Sang Bai

Pi), and Flos Lonicerae Japonicae (*Jin Yin Hua*), 18g each, Folium Eriobotryae Japonicae (*Pi Pa Ye*), Radix Scutellariae Baicalensis (*Huang Qin*), Radix Rubrus Paeoniae Lactiflorae (*Chi Shao*), and Flos Carthami Tinctorii (*Hong Hua*), 15g each, and Radix Glycyrrhizae (*Gan Cao*), 9g.

ACUPUNCTURE & MOXIBUSTION: *Qu Chi* (LI 11), *Shen Zhu* (GV 12), *Fei Shu* (Bl 13)

ANALYSIS OF FORMULA: Needling and draining *Qu Chi* clears heat from the upper burner and clears heat from the blood division or aspect. Needling with draining technique *Shen Zhu* and *Fei Shu* followed by bleeding and cupping clears heat from the lungs.

ADDITIONS & SUBTRACTIONS: For more severe blood heat, add *Xue Hai* (Sp 10) and *He Gu* (LI 4). For concomitant blood stasis, add *Xue Hai* (Sp 10) and *San Yin Jiao* (Sp 6). For concomitant yin vacuity, add *San Yin Jiao* (Sp 6) and *Tai Xi* (Ki 3). For concomitant liver depression transforming heat, add *Xing Jian* (Liv 2) and *Yang Ling Quan* (GB 34). For concomitant phlegm dampness, add *Feng Long* (St 40) and *Shang Qiu* (Sp 5).

2. INTESTINE & STOMACH DAMP HEAT PATTERN

MAIN SYMPTOMS: Red lesions with nodular papules, especially located on the course of the yang ming, oily skin, strong appetite, easy hungering, bad breath, oral thirst with a desire for chilled drinks, dry, bound stools, short voidings of scanty, dark-colored urine, a red tongue with slimy, yellow fur, and a rapid, slippery pulse

NOTE: This pattern rarely presents in its pure form. Rather, it tends to complicate other patterns of acne. It is also called damp heat smoldering and binding pattern.

TREATMENT PRINCIPLES: Clear heat and eliminate dampness from the stomach and intestines

RX: *Dan Di Tang* (Salvia & Rehmannia Decoction)

INGREDIENTS: Radix Salviae Miltiorrhizae (*Dan Shen*), 30-60g, uncooked Radix Rehmanniae (*Sheng Di*), Radix Glycyrrhizae (*Gan Cao*), and Rhizoma Polygoni Cuspidati (*Hu Zhang*), 30g each, Radix Et Rhizoma Rhei (*Da Huang*), 3-15g

ANALYSIS OF FORMULA: *Dan Shen* quickens and cools the blood, as does *Sheng Di*. *Hu Zhang* clears heat and resolves toxins. It is especially useful for treating hot skin lesions. *Da Huang* precipitates the stools and discharges heat from the stomach and intestines. It also resolves toxins. In addition, a large dose of uncooked *Gan Cao* clears heat and resolves toxins.

ADDITIONS & SUBTRACTIONS: If there is damp heat, remove *Da Huang* and add 30 grams of Semen Coicis Lachyrma-jobi (*Yi Yi Ren*), 15 grams of Sclerotium Poriae Cocos (*Fu Ling*), and nine grams each of Herba Eupatorii Fortunei (*Pei Lan*) and Herba Agastachis Seu Pogostemi (*Huo Xiang*). If heat is severe, add nine grams each of Flos Immaturus Sophorae Japonicae (*Huai Hua Mi*) and Cortex Radicis Moutan (*Dan Pi*). If there are pus-filled lesions, add bitter, cold medicinals, such as 30 grams of Herba Houttuyniae Cordatae Cum Radice (*Yu Xing Cao*) and 15 grams each of Herba Taraxaci Mongolici Cum Radice (*Pu Gong Ying*) and Folium Daqingye (*Da Qing Ye*). If there are nodulations, add 12 grams each of Radix Angelicae Sinensis (*Dang Gui*), Concha Ostreae (*Mu Li*), Spina Gleditschiae Chinensis (*Zao Jiao Ci*), and Flos Chrysanthemi Indici (*Ye Ju Hua*). If there is blood stasis, add six grams each of Radix Ligustici Chinensis (*Gao Ben*), Radix Angelicae Dahuricae (*Bai Zhi*), and Radix Ledebouriellae Divaricatae (*Fang Feng*).

ACUPUNCTURE & MOXIBUSTION: *Qu Chi* (LI 11), *Ling Tai* (GV 10)

ANALYSIS OF FORMULA: Needling and draining *Qu Chi* clears heat from the upper burner and from the blood division. Needling with draining method *Ling Tai* followed by cupping and bleeding discharges heat from the stomach and intestines which is counterflowing upward to accumulate in the lungs.

ADDITIONS & SUBTRACTIONS: For more severe blood heat, add *Xue Hai* (Sp 10) and *He Gu* (LI 4). For concomitant blood stasis, add *Xue Hai* (Sp 10) and *San Yin Jiao* (Sp 6). For concomitant yin vacuity, add *San Yin Jiao* (Sp 6) and *Tai Xi* (Ki 3). For concomitant liver depression transforming heat, add *Xing Jian* (Liv 2) and *Yang Ling Quan* (GB 34). For concomitant phlegm dampness, add *Feng Long* (St 40) and *Shang Qiu* (Sp 5).

3. BLOOD STASIS PATTERN

MAIN SYMPTOMS: Purple scars, enduring, recalcitrant disease, a dark, purple tongue and/or static spots or macules, possible menstrual irregularities in women, clots in the menstruate, and a bowstring pulse

NOTE: This pattern mainly complicates other patterns of acne.

TREATMENT PRINCIPLES: Quicken the blood and dispel stasis

RX: *Tao Hong Si Wu Tang* (Persica & Carthamus Four Materials Decoction)

INGREDIENTS: Uncooked Radix Rehmanniae (*Sheng Di*), 12g, and Radix Rubrus Paeoniae Lactiflorae (*Chi Shao*), Radix Angelicae Sinensis (*Dang Gui*), Radix Ligustici

Wallichii (*Chuan Xiong*), Semen Pruni Persicae (*Tao Ren*), and Flos Carthami Tinctorii (*Hong Hua*), 9g each

ANALYSIS OF FORMULA: Within this formula, *Sheng Di, Tao Ren, Hong Hua,* and *Chi Shao* quicken the blood and dispel stasis. *Dang Gui* primarily nourishes the blood and secondarily quickens it, and *Chuan Xiong* moves the qi within the blood division or aspect.

ADDITIONS & SUBTRACTIONS: If there is concomitant blood vacuity, add 12 grams of cooked Radix Rehmanniae (*Shu Di*) and nine grams Radix Albus Paeoniae Lactiflorae (*Bai Shao*). If there is dual qi and blood vacuity, add 15 grams each of Radix Astragali Membranacei (*Huang Qi*) and Caulis Milletiae Seu Spatholobi (*Ji Xue Teng*). If there is concomitant liver depression and/or perimenstrual acne, add nine grams each of Radix Bupleuri (*Chai Hu*) and Rhizoma Cyperi Rotundi (*Xiang Fu*).

ACUPUNCTURE & MOXIBUSTION: *Ge Shu* (Bl 17)

ANALYSIS OF FORMULA: Needling with draining method *Ge Shu* followed by bleeding and cupping quickens the blood and dispels stasis as well as clears heat from the blood division.

ADDITIONS & SUBTRACTIONS: If blood stasis is severe, also drain *Xue Hai* (Sp 10). If there is concomitant phlegm, add *Feng Long* (St 40). If there is a yin blood vacuity, add *San Yin Jiao* (Sp 6) with even supplementing-even draining method.

4. HEAT TOXINS PATTERN

MAIN SYMPTOMS: Pustules on a erythmatous base, larger, more inflamed, angrier lesions, pussy abscesses, possible pain, lesions also on the chest and upper back, a red tongue with dry, yellow fur, and a bowstring, slippery, rapid pulse

NOTE: This pattern simply describes more exuberant heat. It can combine with any of the other patterns.

TREATMENT PRINCIPLES: Clear heat and resolve toxins

RX: *Wu Wei Xiao Du Yin Jia Wei* (Five Flavors Disperse Toxins Drink with Added Flavors)

INGREDIENTS: Herba Violae Yedoensitis (*Zi Hua Di Ding*), Flos Chrysanthemi Indici (*Ye Ju Hua*), Fructus Forsythiae Suspensae (*Lian Qiao*), uncooked Radix Rehmanniae (*Sheng Di*), and Radix Rubrus Paeoniae Lactiflorae (*Chi Shao*), 15g each, Radix Scutellariae Baicalensis (*Huang Qin*), Cortex Radicis Moutan (*Dan Pi*), Semen Citri Reticulatae (*Ju He*), Folium Eriobotryae Japonicae (*Pi Pa Ye*), and Radix Platycodi Grandiflori (*Jie Geng*), 9g each, and Radix Glycyrrhizae (*Gan Cao*), 6g

ANALYSIS OF FORMULA: *Zi Hua Di Ding, Ye Ju Hua,* and *Lian Qiao* all clear heat and resolve toxins. *Huang Qin* clears heat specifically from the lungs, stomach and intestines, and liver, all main organs in the site and engenderment of these heat evils. Likewise, *Pi Pa Ye* clears heat from the lungs and stomach. *Sheng Di, Chi Shao,* and *Dan Pi* all cool and quickens the blood. *Jie Geng* and *Ju He* transform phlegm and scatter nodulation. In additon, *Jie Geng* guides the other medicinals upward to the head and face region. *Gan Cao* clears heat and resolves toxins at the same time as it harmonizes all the other medicinals in this formula.

ADDITIONS & SUBTRACTIONS: If there is phlegm nodulation, add 12 grams each of Spica Prunellae Vulgaris (*Xia Gu Cao*), Bulbus Fritillariae Thunbergii (*Zhe Bei Mu*), and Radix Scrophulariae Ningpoensis (*Xuan Shen*). If there is liver depression and/or perimenstrual acne, add nine grams each of Radix Bupleuri (*Chai Hu*) and Rhizoma Cyperi Rotundi (*Xiang Fu*). If there is greasy, oily skin, add nine grams each of Semen Sinapis Albae (*Bai Jie Zi*) and Herba Artemisiae Capillaris (*Yin Chen Hao*).

ACUPUNCTURE & MOXIBUSTION: *Ge Shu* (Bl 17), *Xue Hai* (Sp 10), *Qu Chi* (LI 11), *He Gu* (LI 4)

ANALYSIS OF FORMULA: Draining *Ge Shu* and *Xue Hai* clears heat from the blood division as well as quickens the blood. Draining *Qu Chi* and *He Gu* strongly drains heat.

ADDITIONS & SUBTRACTIONS: If there is phlegm nodulation, add *Feng Long* (St 40).

5. SPLEEN VACUITY-PHLEGM DAMPNESS PATTERN

MAIN SYMPTOMS: Deep cystic nodules under the skin, oily skin, possible profuse phlegm, possible loose stools, a fat, enlarged tongue with slimy, white fur, and a slippery or moderate (*i.e.*, relaxed or slightly slow) pulse

NOTE: As with the above pattern, this pattern really only complicates other patterns. It often coexists with blood stasis based on the saying, "Phlegm stagnation leads to blood stasis; blood stasis leads to phlegm stagnation."

TREATMENT PRINCIPLES: Fortify the spleen and eliminate dampness, soften the hard, transform phlegm, and scatter nodulation

RX: *Si Jun Zi Tang* (Four Gentlemen Decoction) plus *Er Chen Tang* (Two Aged [Ingredients] Decoction)

INGREDIENTS: Processed Rhizoma Pinelliae Ternatae (*Ban Xia*) and Sclerotium Poriae Cocos (*Fu Ling*), 12 each, Radix Codonopsitis Pilosulae (*Dang Shen*) and Radix Atractylodis Macrocephalae (*Bai Zhu*), 9g each, mix-fried Radix

Glycyrrhizae (*Gan Cao*) and Pericarpium Citri Reticulatae (*Chen Pi*), 6g each, and uncooked Rhizoma Zingiberis (*Sheng Jiang*), 2 slices

ANALYSIS OF FORMULA: *Ban Xia*, *Chen Pi*, and *Sheng Jiang* transform phlegm and rectify the qi mechanism. *Dang Shen*, *Bai Zhu*, *Fu Ling*, and *Gan Cao* fortify the spleen and supplement the qi. *Bai Zhu* aromatically dries dampness, while *Fu Ling* blandly seeps dampness.

ADDITIONS & SUBTRACTIONS: If there are phlegm nodulations which are hard to disperse, add 12 grams each of Spica Prunellae Vulgaris (*Xia Gu Cao*) and Concha Ostreae (*Mu Li*) and nine grams of Bulbus Fritllariae Thunbergii (*Zhe Bei Mu*).

If there is spleen damp heat internally brewing without marked phlegm, replace *Si Jun Zi Tang* plus *Er Chen Tang* with the following unnamed formula: uncooked Semen Coicis Lachyram-jobi (*Yi Yi Ren*) and Cortex Radicis Dictamni Dasycarpi (*Bai Xian Pi*), 30g each, and Semen Dolichoris Lablab (*Bai Bian Dou*), Rhizoma Atractylodis Macrocephalae (*Bai Zhu*), Sclerotium Poriae Cocos (*Fu Ling*), Rhizoma Dioscoreae Oppositae (*Bie Xie*), Cortex Phellodendri (*Huang Bai*), Fructus Citri Aurantii (*Zhi Ke*), Semen Euryalis Ferocis (*Qian Shi*), Cortex Magnoliae Officinalis (*Hou Po*), Rhizoma Cyperi Rotundi (*Xiang Fu*), and Radix Sophorae Flavescentis (*Ku Shen*), 9g each.

If there is phlegm heat, replace *Si Jun Zi Tang* plus *Er Chen Tang* with *Liu Jun Zi Tang* (Six Gentlemen Decoction) plus *Xiao Xian Xiong Tang* (Minor Bogged Down Chest Decoction) with added flavors: processed Rhizoma Pinelliae Ternatae (*Ban Xia*) and Sclerotium Poriae Cocos (*Fu Ling*), 12 each, Semen Trichosanthis Kirlowii (*Gua Lou Ren*), 9-12g, Radix Codonopsitis Pilosulae (*Dang Shen*), Radix Atractylodis Macrocephalae (*Bai Zhu*), and Radix Scutellariae Baicalensis (*Huang Qin*), 9g each, mix-fried Radix Glycyrrhizae (*Gan Cao*) and Pericarpium Citri Reticulatae (*Chen Pi*), 6g each, and Rhizoma Coptidis Chinensis (*Huang Lian*), 3g.

If there is phlegm heat combined with blood stasis but no marked spleen vacuity, replace *Si Jun Zi Tang* plus *Er Chen Tang* with *Tao Hong Er Chen Tang Jia Wei* (Persica & Carthamus Two Aged [Ingredients] Decoction with Added Flavors): Pericarpium Citri Reticulatae (*Chen Pi*), Rhizoma Pinelliae Ternatae (*Ban Xia*), Sclerotium Poriae Cocos (*Fu Ling*), Rhizoma Cyperi Rotundi (*Xiang Fu*), Bulbus Fritillariae Thunbergii (*Zhe Bei Mu*), Semen Citri Reticulatae (*Ju He*), Spica Prunellae Vulgaris (*Xia Ku Cao*), Flos Carthami Tinctorii (*Hong Hua*), Radix Salviae Miltiorrhizae (*Dan Shen*), Radix Angelicae Sinensis (*Dang Gui*), Radix Scutellariae Baicalensis (*Huang Qin*), Fructus Forsythiae Suspensae (*Lian Qiao*), and Folium Eriobotryae Japonicae (*Pi Pa Ye*), 9g each, and Radix Glycyrrhizae (*Gan Cao*), 6g.

If there is phlegm heat with nodulations, blood stasis, and no marked spleen vacuity but the heat is even greater, replace *Si Jun Zi Tang* plus *Er Chen Tang* with *Nei Xiao Lou Li Wan Jia Jian* (Internally Dispersing Scrofula Pills with Additions & Subtractions): Herba Taraxaci Mongolici Cum Radice (*Pu Gong Ying*) and uncooked Gypsum Fibrosum (*Shi Gao*), 30g each, Spica Prunellae Vulgaris (*Xia Ku Cao*), Bulbus Fritillariae Thunbergii (*Zhe Bei Mu*), Flos Lonicerae Japonicae (*Jin Yin Hua*), Fructus Forsythiae Suspensae (*Lian Qiao*), Rhizoma Smilacis Glabrae (*Tu Fu Ling*), Radix Rubrus Paeoniae Lactiflorae (*Chi Shao*), Radix Salviae Miltiorrhizae (*Dan Shen*), Radix Sophorae Flavescentis (*Ku Shen*), 15g each, Herba Sargassii (*Hai Zao*) and Radix Angelicae Sinensis (*Dang Gui*), 9g each, stir-fried Squama Mantidis Pentadactylis (*Chuan Shan Jia*), 6g, and uncooked Radix Et Rhizoma Rhei (*Da Huang*), 3-6g.

ACUPUNCTURE & MOXIBUSTION: *Feng Long* (St 40), *Shang Qiu* (Sp 5)

ANALYSIS OF FORMULA: Draining *Feng Long* transforms phlegm. Draining *Shang Qiu* drains dampness. This combination is based on the saying that, "The spleen is the root of phlegm engenderment."

ADDITIONS & SUBTRACTIONS: If spleen vacuity is marked, add *Zu San Li* (St 36). To clear heat from the lungs, add *Qu Chi* (LI 11). If there is liver depression transforming heat, add *Xing Jian* (Liv 2). If heat exists in the stomach, add *Nei Ting* (St 44). If heat exists in the lungs, add *Fei Shu* (Bl 13). If heat is severe, add *He Gu* (LI 4). If there is concomitant blood stasis, add *Ge Shu* (Bl 17), *Xue Hai* (Sp 10), and/or *San Yin Jiao* (Sp 6). If there is yin vacuity, add *San Yin Jiao* (Sp 6) and *Tai Xi* (Ki 3).

6. YIN VACUITY-FIRE EFFULGENCE PATTERN

MAIN SYMPTOMS: Small, light red papules spread diffusely, often primarily over the forehead, a flushed red face, especially in the afternoon and early evening, dry skin, dry lips, a thin body, possible perimenstrual acne in females, a tendency to vexation and agitation, possible late menarche, scanty or delayed menstruation in females, a red tongue or red tongue tip with scanty fur, and a fine, bowstring, rapid pulse

TREATMENT PRINCIPLES: Supplement the kidneys and enrich yin, drain fire and cool the blood

RX: *Zhi Bai Di Huang Wan* (Anemarrhena & Phellodendron Rehmannia Pills)

INGREDIENTS: Uncooked Radix Rehmanniae (*Sheng Di*), 25g, Fructus Corni Officinalis (*Shan Zhu Yu*), Radix Dioscoreae Oppositae (*Shan Yao*), Rhizoma Anemarrhenae Aspheloidis (*Zhi Mu*), and Cortex Phellodendri (*Huang Bai*), 18g each, and Cortex Radicis Moutan (*Dan Pi*), Rhizoma Alismatis (*Ze Xie*), and Sclerotium Poriae Cocos (*Fu Ling*), 15g each

ANALYSIS OF FORMULA: Within this formula, *Zhi Mu* and *Huang Bai* primarily clear heat and drain fire. *Zhi Mu* also enriches yin, while *Huang Bai* also clears heat and eliminates dampness. *Sheng Di* and *Dan Pi* clear heat and cool the blood. *Sheng Di* also enriches yin, while *Dan Pi* also quickens the blood. *Shan Zhu Yu* and *Shan Yao* both supplement the kidney qi. *Fu Ling* and *Ze Xie* both seep dampness. Seeping dampness and disinhibiting urination lead ministerial fire back downwards to its lower source. The combination of *Shan Yao* and *Fu Ling* also supplements the spleen, and the spleen and kidneys are mutually engendering and supporting.

ADDITIONS & SUBTRACTIONS: For more marked yin vacuity, add 15 grams each of Fructus Ligustri Lucidi (*Nu Zhen Zi*) and Herba Ecliptae Prostratae (*Han Lian Cao*). For more marked blood heat, add 15 grams each of Radix Rubrus Paeoniae Lactiflorae (*Chi Shao*) and Radix Salviae Miltiorrhizae (*Dan Shen*). In case of insomnia, add 12 grams each of Caulis Polygoni Multiflori (*Ye Jiao Teng*) and Radix Polygalae Tenuifoliae (*Yuan Zhi*). For puss-filled lesions, add 15 grams each of Radix Ilicis Pubescentis (*Mao Dong Qing*), Spica Prunellae Vulgaris (*Xia Gu Cao*), and Herba Oldenlandiae Diffusae Cum Radice (*Bai Hua She She Cao*). For greasy, oily skin due to dampness, add 15 grams each of Herba Artemisiae Capillaris (*Yin Chen Hao*) and Radix Sophorae Flavescentis (*Ku Shen*). If there is intestinal fluid dryness with constipation, add 20 grams of Semen Cannabis Sativae (*Huo Ma Ren*) and 12 grams of Semen Pruni Persicae (*Tao Ren*). For concomitant blood stasis, add 9 grams each of Radix Rubiae Cordifoliae (*Qian Cao Gen*) and Flos Carthami Tinctorii (*Hong Hua*).

ACUPUNCTURE & MOXIBUSTION: *Ge Shu* (Bl 17), *Qu Chi* (Li 11), *San Yin Jiao* (Sp 6), *Tai Xi* (Ki 3)

ANALYSIS OF FORMULA: Draining *Ge Shu* and *Qu Chi* clear heat from the blood division. Supplementing *San Yin Jiao* and *Tai Xi* supplement the kidneys and enrich yin.

ADDITIONS & SUBTRACTIONS: If there are heart palpitations, add *Nei Guan* (Per 6) and *Jian Shi* (Per 5). If there is vexation and agitation, add *Shen Men* (Ht 7) and *Da Ling* (Per 7). If there is concomitant liver blood vacuity, add *Qu Quan* (Liv 8).

REMARKS

1. Like all dermatological diseases, the pattern discrimination of acne begins with and mainly rests on visual inspection of the lesions themselves. Red always indicates heat. The redder the red, the more heat. Thus bright or dark red indicates replete heat, while pale red tends to indicate vacuity heat. Purple indicates stasis. Hence, purplish red indicates stasis heat. Nodulations under the skin are a sign of phlegm nodulation. The white matter extruded from comedones is nothing other than phlegm, dampness, and turbidity. Actual pus indicates damp heat toxins. Oily, greasy skin also indicates dampness or damp heat. Large lesions suggest repletion, and multiple small, widely diffuse lesions suggest vacuity.

In addition, the location of the lesions is also important. Some of the most common areas for pimples are around the mouth, along the nasolabial sulcus, along the chin line, and in front of the ears and up into the lateral corners of the forehead. All of these locations describe the course of the hand and foot yang ming on the head and face. Therefore, pimples in these locations strongly suggest heat in the stomach (and possibly the intestines).

In most cases of acne, there are varying proportions of heat, dampness, and phlegm. The heat is mostly depressive heat which may or may not be associated with hyperactivity of ministerial fire. If fire is extreme, there may be heat toxins. If the disease is enduring, there may be blood stasis. By analyzing the exact physical descriptions and locations of acne, one should be able to determine the relative proportions of each of these disease mechanisms and, hence, craft an appropriate treatment.

2. While the above are the patterns most commonly discriminated in Chinese textbooks such as this, in real--life practice, most patients with acne have liver depression/depressive heat along with phlegm dampness. This then causes heat in the stomach (and intestines), phlegm nodulation, and/or blood stasis. When liver depression transforms heat, this heat may cause mutual engenderment of heat or hyperactive yang in the lungs, heart, or stomach. If this heat combines with pre-existing dampness, it may cause damp heat. If a replete liver counterflows horizontally onto spleen earth, there may be a liver-spleen disharmony. In women, such a liver-spleen disharmony is commonly complicated by blood vacuity.

In this case, *Xiao Chai Hu Tang* (Minor Bupleurum Decoction) often makes a good guiding formula: Radix Scutellariae Baicalensis (*Huang Qin*), 12g, Radix Bupleuri (*Chai Hu*), Radix Codonopsitis Pilosulae (*Dang Shen*),

Rhizoma Pinelliae Ternatae (*Ban Xia*), 9g each, mix-fried Radix Glycyrrhizae (*Gan Cao*), 3-6g, Fructus Zizyphi Jujubae (*Da Zao*), 2-3 pieces, and uncooked Rhizoma Zingiberis (*Sheng Jiang*), 2-3 slices. If there is more serious heat evils, add 3 grams of Rhizoma Coptidis Chinensis (*Huang Lian*). If there are heat toxins, add 12-15 grams each of Herba Taraxaci Mongolici Cum Radice (*Pu Gong Ying*), Flos Lonicerae Japonicae (*Jin Yin Hua*), Fructus Forsythiae Suspensae (*Lian Qiao*), Flos Chrysanthemi Indici (*Ye Ju Hua*), and/or Herba Violae Yedonensitis Cum Radice (*Zi Hua Di Ding*). If there is blood stasis and/or blood heat, add 9-12 grams each of Radix Rubrus Paeoniae Lactiflorae (*Chi Shao*), Cortex Radicis Moutan (*Dan Pi*), and/or uncooked Radix Rehmanniae (*Sheng Di*). If there is phlegm nodulation, add 15 grams each of Spica Prunelliae Vulgaris (*Xia Gu Cao*), Radix Scrophulariae Ningpoensis (*Xuan Shen*), and Bulbus Fritillariae Thunbergii (*Zhe Bei Mu*) and consider adding 9-12 grams each of Concha Ostreae (*Mu Li*) and/or Herba Sargassii (*Hai Zao*). If dampness is marked, add 9-12 grams of Sclerotium Poriae Cocos (*Fu Ling*) and 6-9 grams of Pericarpium Citri Reticulatae (*Chen Pi*). If there is simultaneous blood vacuity, add 12 grams of cooked Radix Rehmanniae (*Sheng Di*) and nine grams of Radix Albus Paeoniae Lactiflorae (*Bai Shao*). If enduring heat has damaged lung and stomach yin, add 12 grams of Tuber Ophiopogonis Japonici (*Mai Men Dong*) and possibly nine grams of Radix Trichosanthis Kirlowii (*Tian Men Dong*). If there is stomach and intestinal heat constipation, add 3-12 grams of Radix Et Rhizoma Rhei (*Da Huang*) and 3-6 grams of Mirabilitum (*Mang Xiao*). For hyperactivity of lifegate fire, combine with *Zhi Bai Di Huang Wan* (Anemarrhena & Phellodendron Rehmannia Pills).

Although some Chinese textbooks give a liver depression pattern of acne, we have chosen not to because, unless there is depressive heat, liver depression by itself does not cause acne. Therefore, we have chosen to discuss this pattern under the remarks section where we typically discuss real-life complicated patterns.

3. Because Radix Scutellariae Baicalensis (*Huang Qin*) clears heat from the lungs, liver-gallbladder, and stomach and intestines, it is a main medicinal in the treatment of many patterns of acne. It is generally considered a statement of fact that acne is due to heat accumulating in the lungs and entering the blood. This medicinal is especially good for depressive heat rooted in the liver but ramifying to the lungs and stomach, and this is the most commonly seen proximate disease mechanism of acne vulgaris. In our experience, *Huang Qin* has a low propensity for damaging the stomach. Therefore, it can typically be administered for relatively long periods of time.

4. Some Chinese authors also identify a chong and ren disharmony pattern of acne. This describes acne which is cyclically associated with the menstruation (or premenstruum). In that case, *Dan Zhi Xiao Yao San* (Moutan & Gardenia Rambling Powder) is frequently recommended as the guiding formula. This pattern is nothing other than a liver-spleen disharmony complicated by blood vacuity and depressive heat. For that, we prefer *Xiao Chai Hu Tang* (Minor Bupleurum Decoction) with Radix Angelicae Sinensis (*Dang Gui*) and Radix Albus Paeoniae Lactiflorae (*Bai Shao*) added over *Dan Zhi Xiao Yao San.* This is because Fructus Gardeniae Jasminoidis (*Zhi Zi*) is better for depressive heat entering the blood and causing bleeding as opposed to depressive heat accumulating in the lungs and entering the blood causing acne.

5. For cystic nodules and large, inflamed pustules, use fire needle technique locally. This consists of needling perpendiculary into the center of a cyst or pustule and then heating the shaft of the needle with an open flame. Continue until the center of the pustule or cyst around the shaft of the needle turns a yellow color. This technique does not typically cause a scar and, paradoxically, helps to avoid a scar if the cyst or pustule were left to ripen and rupture on its own.

6. Another acupuncture treatment for acne (regardless of pattern) is to use a three-edged needle to bleed a nonchannel point located five fen lateral and five fen inferior to the spinous process of the 7th cervical vertebra. This method clears heat from the lungs. Three to five treatments are usually sufficient.

7. Most of the topical Chinese remedies for acne are messy powders and washes. Since most patients with acne are adolescents, they are rarely willing to go to the fuss and mess of such traditional topical applications. Therefore, our advice is to use Western medical topical medicines combined with acupuncture and/or internally administered Chinese medicinals.

One can also use Aloe Vera gel applied topically to the face. In Chinese medicine, Herba Aloes (*Lu Hui*) is bitter, cold, and nontoxic. It enters the jue yin channel (when taken internally), and its functions are to kill worms and clear heat. Modern pharmacological research has shown that *Lu Hui* contains emodin glycosides which are anti-inflammatory, bacteriostatic, and bacteriocidal. Other research has shown that *Lu Hui* has an exceptionally powerful ability to permeate the skin, thus giving this medicinal the ability to reach deep layers of the skin. Since *Lu Hui* also contains saccharides, amino acids, vitamins, and trace minerals, not only does it kill bacteria and resolve toxins, it also helps in tissue regeneration.[1]

8. Chinese medicinals can be used to offset the side effects of internally administered broad-spectrum antibiotics, such as tetracycline. In that case, one simply does a pattern discrimination of the side effects and either adds medicinals to the patient's formula to address the drug-induced pattern or administers a Chinese medicinal formula based on the entirety of the patient's pattern(s), including the side effects.

9. Acne is one of the common signs of polycystic ovarian or Stein-Leventhal syndrome. In this case, there is usually liver depression with depressive heat in the lungs and stomach and phlegm dampness plus kidney yin, yang, or yin and yang vacuity not uncommonly complicated by blood stasis. In that case, one should determine the relative proportions of each of these, state their requisite treatment principles in their order of prominence, and then combine medicinals to address each treatment principle.

10. Some Chinese doctors believe that all adolescent acne is due to a loss of regulation between yin and yang. Thus ministerial fire becomes excessively effulgent and it is this which causes lung and stomach fire and heat to steam upward to the face. In this case, using *Zhi Bai Di Huang Wan* (Anemarrhena & Phellodendron Rehmannia Pills) as the main treatment is an example of "treating disease [by] seeking the root." When using this approach, either *Zhi Bai Di Huang Wan* becomes the main formula or these pills are given along with another formula in decoction designed to address the tips or branches.

11. While Western medicine largely denies diet as a main factor in the cause of acne, Chinese medicine definitely does consider faulty diet to be an important disease cause. Overeating fatty, greasy foods easily causes the internal engenderment of dampness and heat as does drinking alcohol. Acrid, hot, peppery foods may also aggravate internal heat. Pepperoni pizza is not a good food for most patients with acne from the Chinese medical point of view.

ENDNOTES

[1]Liu Ying, "Clinical Observations of the Treatment of Common Acne with Herba Aloes (*Lu Hui*)," *Si Chuan Zhong Yi (Sichuan Chinese Medicine)*, #12, p. 40

2

Allergic Rhinitis

Allergic rhinitis refers to a complex of symptoms characterized by seasonal or perennial sneezing, rhinorrhea, nasal congestion, itching, and often conjunctivitis and pharyngitis in response to airborne allergens. Seasonal allergic rhinitis, more often called hayfever, is divided into three types: 1) spring type, 2) summer type, and 3) fall type. In spring allergic rhinitis, the allergens are usually tree pollens. In summer allergic rhinitis, the allergens are usually grass pollens, and in fall allergic rhinitis, the allergens are usually weed pollens, of which the most common is ragweed. Allergic rhinitis may also occur in some patients without regard to season. This is referred to as perennial allergic rhinitis. The most common allergens in this type of rhinitis are fungus spores, dust containing insect feces and proteins, and animal dander.

The symptoms of allergic rhinitis include itching of the nose, roof of the mouth, pharynx, and eyes. This is accompanied by lacrimation, sneezing, and a clear, watery nasal discharge. In addition, there may be frontal headache, irritability, anorexia, depression, and insomnia. Coughing and asthmatic wheezing may develop if the condition is more severe. Its Western medical diagnosis is based on the clinical symptoms and history, allergen skin patch tests, and many eosinophils in the nasal secretions. Western treatment mainly relies on antihistamines and sympathomimetic type drugs, such as ephedrine and pseudoephedrine. However, both of these types of drugs have side effects which many people find unacceptable. Glucocorticoids and corticosteroids may be resorted to if antihistamines are inadequate. Desensitization treatment is possible if antihistamines are poorly tolerated or if steroids are necessary.

As many as one in 10 Americans are affected by hayfever or allergic rhinitis. Both males and females may suffer from allergic rhinitis. Children may grow out of allergic rhinitis after puberty. However, as the patient ages, this condition may recur. Most patients with allergic rhinitis have a history of being treated with repeated antibiotics as children as well as eating a diet high in sugars and sweets, dairy products, fruit juices, and yeasted grain products. Stress may also play a part in this condition. Allergic asthma and sinusitis are dealt with separately in their own chapters.

Chinese disease categorization: Allergic rhinitis is mainly categorized as *liu bi ti*, runny nose, *bi sai*, nasal congestion, and *pen ti* or *ti pen*, sneezing. Frontal headache is *tou tong*, headache, irritability is *yi nu*, easy anger, anorexia is *na dai*, torpid intake, or *na shao*, reduced (food) intake, depression is *yu zheng*, depressive condition, and insomnia is *shi mian*, loss or lack of sleep.

Disease causes: Former heaven natural endowment insufficiency, habitual bodily vacuity due to faulty diet, iatrogenesis, taxation fatigue, and internal damage by the seven affects, and external invasion of wind evils.

Disease mechanisms: Unseen airborne pathogens are categorized as external wind evils in Chinese medicine. Therefore, during the acute attack of allergic rhinitis, all patients are classified as displaying a wind cold exterior pattern. This accounts for the itching, nasal congestion, sneezing, and clear, watery nasal discharge. The lungs are the delicate viscus. This means that they are typically the first viscus affected by externally invading evils and especially those entering through the nose, the orifice of the lungs. These wind evils hinder and obstruct the lungs' diffusing and downbearing. If the lung qi does not downbear but rather stagnates and accumulates, it will eventually counterflow upward. This results in sneezing. Because the lungs are the upper source of water in the body, if the lungs fail to diffuse and downbear fluids, these may collect and accumulate, transforming into dampness and phlegm. When these spill over or are drafted upward by counterflowing lung qi, they result in nasal discharge and nasal congestion. Wind evils themselves cause the itching based on the Chinese medical saying, "No wind, no itching." Basically, all patients with allergic rhinitis are believed to have deep-lying or hidden phlegm in their lungs which only becomes apparent when lung function is damaged by the presence of some evil qi.

However, for these wind evils to invade, there must be an underlying defensive qi vacuity. In fact, the patient is being invaded by wind evils with which other, healthier people have no problem. The defensive qi issues from the middle burner. This means that all patients with allergic rhinitis have, *ipso facto*, a spleen qi vacuity. In addition, it is a spleen qi vacuity which causes deep-lying or hidden phlegm. As it is said, "The spleen is the root of phlegm engenderment; the lungs are (merely) the place where phlegm is stored." This spleen vacuity may be due to immaturity, aging, worry and anxiety, or taxation fatigue. However, in Western patients, its two main causes are faulty diet and iatrogenesis. Faulty diet means two things. First, it refers to improper feeding of infants, *i.e.*, feeding infants too many uncooked, chilled foods, too many, hard to digest foods which are high in *wei* or flavor, or simply over-feeding, even if this is breast milk as in "feeding on demand." Secondly, it means eating too many sugars and sweets, eating too many uncooked, chilled foods (including chilled drinks), and eating too many foods which strongly engender fluids, such as dairy products and fruits and fruit juices. Iatrogenesis refers to over or inappropriate use of antibiotics which are described in Chinese medicine as similar to bitter, cold medicinals which damage the spleen.

Because the latter heaven spleen qi and the former heaven kidney yang are mutually promoting and also because the lungs, spleen, and kidneys are the three viscera involved in fluid movement and transformation, many patients with allergic rhinitis also have a kidney yang vacuity. Kidney yang does not become exuberant until puberty. Therefore, many children with allergic rhinitis have a spleen-kidney dual vacuity. However, when we age, first the spleen becomes vacuous and weak and then spleen vacuity reaches the kidneys. Therefore, many older patients also have a spleen-kidney dual vacuity. If kidney yang is not sufficient, the spleen is not warmed and fluids are not transformed and steamed (*i.e.*, vaporized).

Because the lungs and liver share a close inter-relationship via the five phase control cycle and both viscera participate in promoting and controlling the flow of qi, lung-spleen qi vacuity often results in or aggravates liver depression qi stagnation. On the other hand, liver depression due to emotional upset and frustration may result in A) damage of the spleen with subsequent phlegm damp engenderment and non-engenderment of the defensive qi, and B) upwardly counterflowing qi which affects the diffusing and downbearing of the lungs.

If the qi flow becomes retarded and stagnant due to hindrance and obstruction by phlegm dampness and/or liver depression, over time this may result in blood stasis. Therefore, static blood may part in allergic rhinitis. In particular, if the orifice of the nose is congested and blocked for some time, stasis may enter the network vessels surrounding the nose. Stagnant qi may also transform into depressive heat. However, when this occurs, it is mostly diagnosed as either deep source nasal congestion, *i.e.*, sinusitis, or panting and wheezing, *i.e.*, asthma.

TREATMENT BASED ON PATTERN DISCRIMINATION:

1. WIND COLD INVADING THE LUNGS PATTERN

MAIN SYMPTOMS: Profuse, clear nasal discharge accompanied by nasal congestion, frequent sneezing, loss of smell, itchy eyes, nose, and throat, aversion to wind and cold, possible headache, possible cough, absence of sweating, a pale tongue with thin, white fur, and a floating, tight or bowstring pulse

NOTE: This pattern describes the acute attack of allergic rhinitis.

TREATMENT PRINCIPLES: Resolve the exterior with warm, acrid ingredients, course wind and scatter cold

RX: *Cang Er Zi San Jia Jian* (Xanthium Powder with Additions & Subtractions)

INGREDIENTS: Fructus Xanthii Sibirici (*Cang Er Zi*), Flos Magnoliae Liliflorae (*Xin Yi Hua*), Herba Agastachis Seu Pogostemi (*Huo Xiang*), and Radix Angelicae Dahuricae (*Bai Zhi*), 9g each, and Herba Asari Cum Radice (*Xi Xin*), 3g

NOTE: This formula is for symptomatic use only.

ANALYSIS OF FORMULA: *Cang Er Zi, Xin Yi Hua, Huo Xiang, Bai Zhi,* and *Xi Xin* all course wind and scatter cold as well as free the flow of the orifices of the nose. All these ingredients have a well-known action on the nose, especially for nasal discharge, nasal congestion, itchy nose, and loss of smell.

ADDITIONS & SUBTRACTIONS: For profuse clear, runny nose, add nine grams each of Fructus Terminaliae Chebulae (*He Zi*) and Fructus Schisandrae Chinensis (*Wu Wei Zi*). For sneezing, add nine grams each of Lumbricus (*Di Long*) and Periostracum Cicadae (*Chan Tui*). For itchy eyes, add nine grams each of Radix Ligustici Wallichii (*Chuan Xiong*) and Herba Seu Flos Schizonepetae Tenuifoliae (*Jing Jie*). For nasal congestion, add six grams of Rhizoma Acori Graminei (*Shi Chang Pu*) and nine grams of Ramulus Cinnamomi

Cassiae (*Gui Zhi*). If there is enduring nasal congestion with purple-blue nasal mucosa, add nine grams of Fructus Liquidambaris Taiwaniae (*Lu Lu Tong*) and 15 grams of Radix Ligustici Wallichii (*Chuan Xiong*). For marked wind cold symptoms, add nine grams each of Herba Ephedrae (*Ma Huang*) and Herba Schizonepetae Tenuifoliae (*Jing Jie*). For concomitant severe qi vacuity, add 15 grams of Radix Astragali Membranacei (*Huang Qi*) and nine grams of Rhizoma Atractylodis Macrocephalae (*Bai Zhu*).

Acupuncture & moxibustion: *Shang Xing* (GV 23), *Ying Xiang* (LI 20), *Feng Men* (Bl 12), *Lie Que* (Lu 7)

Analysis of formula: Draining *Shang Xing* and *Ying Xiang* diffuses and frees the flow of the nose. Moxibustion should be used on *Shang Xing*. Draining *Feng Men* and *Lie Que* courses wind, scatters cold, and resolves the exterior.

Additions & subtractions: For marked wind cold symptoms, add *He Gu* (LI 4) and, if necessary, *Feng Chi* (GB 20). One can also alternate *Shang Xing* with *Yin Tang* (M-HN-3).

2. Defensive qi vacuity-exterior insecurity & deep-lying phlegm dampness pattern

Main symptoms: Frequent and easy contraction of wind evils, a pale facial complexion, aversion to wind and cold, possible chilled extremities, fatigue, lack of strength, disinclination to speak and spontaneous perspiration if severe, a pale, fat tongue with possible teeth-marks on its edges and thin, possibly slimy, white fur, and a fine, soggy pulse

Note: Defensive qi vacuity may also be described as a spleen-lung qi vacuity pattern. This pattern describes the underlying root imbalance of this condition.

Treatment principles: Fortify the spleen and boost the qi, supplement the defensive and secure the exterior

Rx: *Bu Zhong Yi Qi Tang* (Supplement the Center & Boost the Qi Decoction), *Yu Ping Feng San* (Jade Wind-screen Powder) & *Er Chen Tang* (Two Aged [Ingredients] Decoction)

Ingredients: Radix Astragali Membranacei (*Huang Qi*), 15g, Rhizoma Atractylodis Macrocephalae (*Bai Zhu*), 12g, Radix Codonopsitis Pilosulae (*Dang Shen*), Radix Ledebouriellae Divaricatae (*Fang Feng*), Sclerotium Poriae Cocos (*Fu Ling*), Rhizoma Pinelliae Ternatae (*Ban Xia*), and Pericarpium Citri Reticulatae (*Chen Pi*), 9g each, Radix Angelicae Sinensis (*Dang Gui*) and mix-fried Radix Glycyrrhizae (*Gan Cao*), 6g each, Rhizoma Cimicifugae (*Sheng Ma*), 4.5g, Radix Bupleuri (*Chai Hu*), 3g, and uncooked Rhizoma Zingiberis (*Sheng Jiang*), 3 slices

Analysis of formula: *Huang Qi, Dang Shen, Bai Zhu, Fu Ling*, and mix-fried *Gan Cao* fortify the spleen and boost the qi, supplement the lungs and the defensive qi. In addition, *Huang Qi* and *Bai Zhu* secure the exterior to avoid further damage by evils. *Fang Feng* gently out-thrusts any lingering or retained evils in the exterior without damaging the righteous. *Ban Xia, Chen Pi, Fu Ling*, and mix-fried *Gan Cao* together compose *Er Chen Tang* (Two Aged [Ingredients] Decoction), the major formula in Chinese medicine for transforming phlegm dampness and treating stubborn phlegm or deep-lying, hidden phlegm. *Dang Gui* nourishes and quickens the blood. In this formula, it harmonizes the blood to promote the regulation of the qi. *Chai Hu* and *Sheng Ma* upbear the clear in order to more effectively supplement the spleen and lungs. *Chai Hu* also courses the liver and rectifies the qi. *Sheng Jiang* and mix-fried *Gan Cao* harmonize the center as well as the other medicinals in this formula.

Additions & subtractions: If there is concomitant kidney qi vacuity with enuresis in a child or enduring, clear, chilly, white vaginal discharge in a woman, add nine grams each of Fructus Alpiniae Oxyphyllae (*Yi Zhi Ren*), Radix Linderae Strychnifoliae (*Wu Yao*), and Radix Dioscoreae Oppositae (*Shan Yao*). If there is concomitant kidney yang or kidney yin and yang vacuity, combine with *Shen Qi Wan* (Kidney Qi Pills, a Chinese ready-made medicine). If there is a spleen qi-kidney yin vacuity, combine with *Liu Wei Di Huang Wan* (Six Flavors Rehmannia Pills) or *Zhi Bai Di Huang Wan* (Anemarrhena & Phellodendron Rehmannia Pills) if yin vacuity is complicated by effulgent fire. Both of these are also Chinese ready-made medicines. If liver depression qi stagnation is marked, increase the dose of *Chai Hu* to nine grams and add nine grams of Radix Albus Paeoniae Lactiflorae (*Bai Shao*).

If simultaneous blood vacuity is marked, replace *Bu Zhong Yi Qi Tang* etc. with *Gui Pi Tang Jia Wei* (Restore the Spleen Decoction with Added Flavors): Radix Astragali Membranacei (*Huang Qi*), 15g, Rhizoma Atractylodis Macrocephalae (*Bai Zhu*), 12g, Radix Codonopsitis Pilosulae (*Dang Shen*), Radix Angelicae Sinensis (*Dang Gui*), Arillus Euphoriae Longanae (*Long Yan Rou*), Semen Zizyphi Spinosae (*Suan Zao Ren*), Sclerotium Poriae Cocos (*Fu Ling*), Rhizoma Pinelliae Ternatae (*Ban Xia*), Pericarpium Citri Reticulatae (*Chen Pi*), Radix Polygalae Tenuifoliae (*Yuan Zhi*), and Radix Ledebouriellae Divaricatae (*Fang Feng*), 9g each, mix-fried Radix Glycyrrhizae (*Gan Cao*) and Radix Auklandiae Lappae (*Mu Xiang*), 6g, Fructus Zizyphi Jujubae (*Da Zao*), 5 pieces, and uncooked Rhizoma Zingiberis (*Sheng Jiang*), 3 slices.

If there is liver depression, lung-spleen qi vacuity, deep-lying phlegm, and stomach heat, replace *Bu Zhong Yi Qi Tang* etc. with *Xiao Chai Hu Tang Jia Wei* (Minor Bupleurum Decoction with Added Flavors): Radix Astragali Membranacei (*Huang Qi*), 15g, Rhizoma Atractylodis

Macrocephalae (*Bai Zhu*), 12g, Radix Bupleuri (*Chai Hu*), Rhizoma Pinelliae Ternatae (*Ban Xia*), Pericarpium Citri Reticulatae (*Chen Pi*), Sclerotium Poriae Cocos (*Fu Ling*), Radix Codonopsitis Pilosulae (*Dang Shen*), Radix Ledebouriellae Divaricatae (*Fang Feng*), and Radix Scutellariae Baicalensis (*Huang Qin*), 9g each, mix-fried Radix Glycyrrhizae (*Gan Cao*), 6g, uncooked Rhizoma Zingberis (*Sheng Jiang*), 3 slices, and Fructus Zizyphi Jujubae (*Da Zao*), 3 pieces. In this case, appetite will be normal or increased and fatigue, lack of strength, and coldness of the extremities are not usually pronounced. However, the tongue will be fat and the patient will frequently or easily catch cold.

If there is fall allergic rhinitis where summerheat has damaged the spleen qi, replace *Bu Zhong Yi Qi Tang* with *Huang Qi Ren Shen Tang Jia Wei* (Astragalus & Ginseng Decoction with Added Flavors): Radix Astragali Membranacei (*Huang Qi*), 15g, Tuber Ophiopogonis Japonici (*Mai Dong*), 12g, Rhizoma Atractylodis Macrocephalae (*Bai Zhu*), Rhizoma Atractylodis (*Cang Zhu*), Cortex Phellodendri (*Huang Bai*), Radix Angelicae Sinensis (*Dang Gui*), Radix Ledebouriellae Divaricatae (*Fang Feng*), and Fructus Schisandrae Chinensis (*Wu Wei Zi*), 9g each, mix-fried Radix Glycyrrhizae (*Gan Cao*) and Pericarpium Citri Reticulatae (*Chen Pi*), 6g each, Rhizoma Cimicifugae (*Sheng Ma*), 4.5g, and Massa Medica Fermentata (*Shen Qu*), 3g. If there is also marked liver depression qi stagnation, add 3-9 grams of Radix Bupleuri (*Chai Hu*). If there is marked worry and anxiety damaging the heart and spleen, add 6 grams each of Radix Auklandiae Lappae (*Mu Xiang*) and Fructus Amomi (*Sha Ren*).

ACUPUNCTURE & MOXIBUSTION: *Shang Xing* (GV 23), *Ying Xiang* (LI 20), *Fei Shu* (Bl 13), *He Gu* (LI 4), *Zu San Li* (St 36)

ANALYSIS OF FORMULA: Draining *Shang Xing* and *Ying Xiang* diffuses and frees the flow of the nose. Moxibustion should be used on *Shang Xing*. Supplementing *He Gu* and *Fei Shu* supplements the lungs and secures the exterior, while supplementing *Zu San Li* fortifies the spleen and supplements the qi. Since the spleen is the root of phlegm engenderment, supplementing *Zu San Li* also helps prevent the engenderment of phlegm. Moxibustion should also be used on *Fei Shu* and *Zu San Li*.

ADDITIONS & SUBTRACTIONS: If there is concomitant kidney qi vacuity, add *Qi Hai* (CV 6) and *Tai Xi* (Ki 3). If there is concomitant blood vacuity and/or blood stasis, add *San Yin Jiao* (Sp 6). If there is concomitant liver depression, add *Tai Chong* (Liv 3). For profuse phlegm, add *Feng Long* (St 40). One can also alternate *Shang Xing* with *Yin Tang* (M-HN-3).

3. KIDNEY QI VACUITY WITH LUNG LOSS OF WARMTH AND MOISTENING PATTERN

MAIN SYMPTOMS: Enduring, long-term clear nasal discharge, nasal itching, frequent sneezing, white, swollen nasal mucosa, aversion to wind and cold, especially in the upper back, chilled limbs, a pale facial complexion, devitalized essence spirit, low back and knee soreness and weakness, seminal emission, clear, long voidings of urine, nocturnal polyuria, a white tongue, and a deep, fine, weak pulse

NOTE: This pattern is most commonly seen in children whose kidneys have yet to mature. In most cases, kidney qi or yang vacuity complicates spleen vacuity. Therefore, this pattern is not that commonly met in its pure form in real-life patients.

TREATMENT PRINCIPLES: Warm the kidneys and supplement the lungs

RX: *Jin Gui Shen Qi Wan Jia Jian* (*Golden Cabinet* Kidney Qi Pills with Additions & Subtractions)

INGREDIENTS: Cooked Radix Rehmanniae (*Shu Di*) and Radix Dioscoreae Oppositae (*Shan Yao*), 12g each, Fructus Corni Officinalis (*Shan Zhu Yu*), Fructus Schisandrae Chinensis (*Wu Wei Zi*), and Flos Magnoliae Liliflorae (*Xin Yi Hua*), 9g each, Cortex Radicis Moutan (*Dan Pi*), Sclerotium Poriae Cocos (*Fu Ling*), Rhizoma Alismatis (*Ze Xie*), Radix Lateralis Praeparatus Aconiti Carmichaeli (*Fu Zi*), and Gecko (*Ge Jie*), 6g each, and Herba Asari Cum Radice (*Xi Xin*) and Cortex Cinnamomi Cassiae (*Rou Gui*), 3g each

ANALYSIS OF FORMULA: *Shu Di, Shan Yao, Shan Zhu Yu, Fu Ling, Dan Pi*, and *Ze Xie* are the six flavors of *Liu Wei Di Huang Wan* (Six Flavors Rehmannia Pills), a main Chinese medicinal formula for supplementing the kidneys and enriching yin. In this case, they nourish yin to supplement yang based on the sayings, "Yin and yang are mutually rooted," and, "Yang is engendered from yin." *Rou Gui, Fu Zi, Xi Xin*, and *Ge Jie* warm and supplement kidney yang. In addition, *Ge Jie* with *Wu Wei Zi* warms and supplements the lungs, while *Xi Xin* warms both the interior and the exterior as well as diffuses the lungs and frees the flow of the orifices. *Xin Yi Hua* helps *Xi Xin* to diffuse the nose and frees the flow of the orifices. *Wu Wei Zi* supplements both the lungs and kidneys, secure the exterior, and treats enduring sneezing.

ADDITIONS & SUBTRACTIONS: Please see pattern #2 above. If there is concomitant kidney yin and yang vacuity with vacuity heat, subtract *Fu Zi* and add 9 grams each of Rhizoma Anemarrhenae Asphodeloidis (*Zhi Mu*) and Cortex Phellodendri (*Huang Bai*).

ACUPUNCTURE & MOXIBUSTION: *Shang Xing* (GV 23), *Ying Xiang* (LI 20), *Fei Shu* (Bl 13), *Shen Shu* (Bl 23), *Tai Xi* (Ki 3)

ANALYSIS OF FORMULA: Draining *Shang Xing* and *Ying*

Xiang diffuses and frees the flow of the nose. Moxibustion should be used on *Shang Xing.* Supplementing *Shen Shu, Tai Xi,* and *Fei Shu* with moxibustion warms and supplements the kidneys and lungs.

ADDITIONS & SUBTRACTIONS: Please see pattern #2 above. If there is concomitant kidney yin and yang vacuity, omit moxibustion on *Shen Shu* and replace *Tai Xi* with *Fu Liu* (Ki 7).

REMARKS

1. During acute attacks, either use modified *Cang Er Zi San* alone or combine it with whatever formula addresses the patient's underlying disease mechanisms. However, in between attacks, the patient should take whatever formula is indicated for their habitual bodily vacuity and deep-lying phlegm. If the rhinitis is seasonal, begin supplementing the root six weeks to three months before the offending season. For instance, one can use modifications of *Huang Qi Ren Shen Tang* (Astragalus & Ginseng Decoction) for the prevention of fall season rhinitis. This formula is comprised of: Radix Astragali Membranacei (*Huang Qi*), 15g, Radix Codonopsitis Pilosulae (*Dang Shen*), 12g, Rhizoma Atractylodis Macrocephalae (*Bai Zhu*), Rhizoma Atractylodis (*Cang Zhu*), Tuber Ophiopogonis Japonici (*Mai Men Dong*), Cortex Phellodendri (*Huang Bai*), Radix Angelicae Sinensis (*Dang Gui*), Fructus Schisandrae Chinensis (*Wu Wei Zi*), and Pericarpium Citri Reticulatae (*Chen Pi*), 9g each, mix-fried Radix Glycyrrhizae (*Gan Cao*) and Massa Medica Fermentata (*Shen Qu*), 6g each, and Rhizoma Cimicifugae (*Sheng Ma*), 4.5g. In this case, summerheat and overconsumption of sweet foods and chilled liquids in the late summer damage the spleen and engender deep-lying phlegm rheum.

2. Appropriate Chinese dietary therapy is of utmost importance in this condition since a damaged spleen always plays a part in real-life Western patients. This means primarily avoidance of foods which damage the spleen as well as foods which strongly engender fluids and sticking to a clear, bland diet.

3. Most Chinese textbooks describe lung-spleen, spleen-kidney, and phlegm dampness patterns separately. However, phlegm dampness is the result of an underlying spleen qi vacuity, while kidney yang vacuity is always seen as an evolution of and in combination with spleen qi vacuity. Especially in this condition, we believe that listing the patterns separately in this way is not consonant with real-life practice.

4. Practitioners should note that there is no wind heat pattern of allergic rhinitis. The Western medical pathognomonic signs and symptoms of this condition include clear, watery nasal discharge. In a wind heat exterior pattern, there typically is yellow nasal mucus. A clear, white, watery nasal discharge, on the other hand, indicates cold rheum. If allergic rhinitis transforms into acute sinusitis, then there can be a yellow nasal discharge. However, that then is a different disease diagnosis.

3

ALZHEIMER'S DISEASE

Alzheimer's disease is a progressive, inexorable loss of cognitive function of unknown etiology associated with an excessive number of senile plaques in the cerebral cortex and subcortical gray matter which also contains beta-amyloid and neurofibrillary tangles consisting of tau protein. Approximately four million Americans are currently affected with this disease. The most common form of this disease mostly affects people over 60 years of age and its incidence increases with age. However, 2-7% of cases are earlier in onset. These early-onset cases are usually due to an inherited genetic mutation. A family history of Alzheimer's is present in 15-20% of all cases. The disease is twice as common in women as in men. It accounts for more than 65% of dementias in the elderly although vascular dementia and Alzheimer's disease coexist in approximately 15% of cases.

The clinical symptoms are divided into four stages of the progression of this disease. Its early stage is characterized by loss of recent memory, inability to learn and retain new information, language problems (especially word-finding), mood swings, and personality changes. Patients may have progressive difficulty performing daily activities and may become irritable and hostile due to this loss of control and memory. In the intermediate stage, patients become unable to learn and recall information. Memory of remote events is affected, although not totally lost, and patients may require assistance bathing, eating, dressing, and/or using the toilet. Behavioral disorganization is often characterized by wandering, agitation, hostility, uncooperativeness, or physical aggression. By this time, patients have lost all sense of time and place. Although they remain ambulatory, intermediate stage patients are at risk for falls or accidents due to confusion. In the severe stage, patients are unable to walk or perform any daily activity, and they are usually totally incontinent. Recent and remote memory is completely lost, and patients may even be unable to swallow and eat. Eventually, patients become mute. The end stage of Alzheimer's disease is coma and death, usually from infection masked by absence of febrile and leukocytic responses.

The Western medical diagnosis of Alzheimer's disease is usually based on the patient's history, physical examination, laboratory tests, and the exclusion of other causes of dementia. Basic tests include the Folstein Mini-mental Status Examination, CBC, electrolyte panel, Sequential Multiple Analyzer tests, thyroid function tests, folate and vitamin B_{12} levels, VDRL test, and urinanalysis. ECG and X-ray may be useful in some patients. In terms of Western medical treatment, some drugs that enhance cholinergic neurotransmission, such as donepezil, can temporarily improve memory during the early stages. Unfortunately, some of the drugs used to treat Alzheimer's disease, such as antipsychotics, can cause Parkinsonian movement disorder, while tricyclic antidepressants with anticholinergic side effects can cause constipation, urinary retention, glaucoma, and seizures. In addition, nonprescription antihistamines may worsen confusion. Antioxidants, such as vitamin E, estrogen therapy, and NSAIDs are currently under study. At this time, the cognitive decline of Alzheimer's disease is inevitable, but the rate of progression is unpredictable, with survival ranging from 2-20 years and an average of seven years.

CHINESE DISEASE CATEGORIZATION: Alzheimer's disease is categorized as *lao nian xing chi dai*, literally, senile feeble-mindedness but commonly translated as senile dementia, *wen chi*, civil madness, and *wu chi,* martial mania, in Chinese medicine. In the latter case, there is marked impetuosity, irritability, red face and eyes, restlessness, and agitated movement.

DISEASE CAUSES: Former heaven natural endowment insufficiency, aging, internal damage by the seven affects, and unregulated eating and drinking

DISEASE MECHANISMS: Due to former heaven natural endowment insufficiency and aging, there may be insufficient yin blood to transform essence and fill the sea of marrow or yang qi debility with loss of spiritual brightness. In either case, there may be decreased mental clarity and faulty memory. However, faulty or impaired memory and spirit abstraction may also be due to simple heart blood vacuity. If yin fails to control yang, liver yang may become hyperactive and ascend or heart fire may become hyperactive and exuberant. These mechanisms typically give rise to irritability, vexation and agitation, restlessness, and even hostility and aggression. Less pronounced irritability and taciturnity may be due to liver depression, with or without depressive heat. Faulty diet as well as heat stewing the juices may result in the engenderment of phlegm dampness which may mist the portals, causing mental confusion and aphasia. If yin and blood vacuity, fire heat, or phlegm give rise to internal stirring of liver wind, there may be convulsions and tremors. If there is liver depression qi stagnation, as there surely must be due to the frustration of this condition, this may give rise to blood stasis. Blood stasis may also be due to heart vacuity, liver blood vacuity, and phlegm obstruction as well as prolonged sitting and inactivity. Typically, several of these disease mechanisms combine in any given patient.

TREATMENT BASED ON PATTERN DISCRIMINATION:

1. LIVER DEPRESSION QI STAGNATION MIXED WITH PHLEGM & STASIS PATTERN

MAIN SYMPTOMS: Heart vexation, easy anger, depression, oppression, and emotional dysphoria, no desire to speak, bilateral rib-side distention and pain, a dark tongue with possible static macules and slimy fur, and a bowstring, slippery pulse

TREATMENT PRINCIPLES: Course the liver and rectify the qi, quicken the blood and dispel phlegm

RX: *Wu Shi Gan Yu Fang Jia Wei* (Master Wu's Liver Depression Formula with Added Flavors)

INGREDIENTS: Radix Ligustici Wallichii (*Chuan Xiong*) and Radix Salviae Miltiorrhizae (*Dan Shen*), 15g each, Semen Pruni Persicae (*Tao Ren*), Flos Carthami Tinctorii (*Hong Hua*), Radix Rubrus Paeoniae Lactiflorae (*Chi Shao*), and Rhizoma Cyperi Rotundi (*Xiang Fu*), 12g each, Rhizoma Pinelliae Ternatae (*Ban Xia*), Radix Bupleuri (*Chai Hu*), Pericarpium Citri Reticulatae (*Chen Pi*), Pericarpium Citri Reticulatae Viride (*Qing Pi*), and Rhizoma Acori Graminei (*Shi Chang Pu*), 9g each

ANALYSIS OF FORMULA: *Xiang Fu*, *Chai Hu*, and *Qing Pi* course the liver and resolve depression. *Chen Pi*, *Ban Xia*, and *Shi Chang Pu* dry dampness and transform phlegm. In addition, *Shi Chang Pu* opens the orifices and arouses the spirit. *Chuan Xiong*, *Dan Shen*, *Tao Ren*, *Hong Hua*, and *Chi Shao* quicken the blood and transform stasis.

ADDITIONS & SUBTRACTIONS: If there is depressive heat, add nine grams each of Fructus Gardeniae Jasminoidis (*Zhi Zi*) and Cortex Radicis Moutan (*Dan Pi*). If there is blood vacuity, add nine grams of Radix Angelicae Sinensis (*Dang Gui*) and replace Red Peony with Radix Albus Paeoniae Lactiflorae (*Bai Shao*). If there is spleen vacuity, add nine grams each of Rhizoma Atractylodis Macrocephalae (*Bai Zhu*) and Sclerotium Poriae Cocos (*Fu Ling*) and six grams of mix-fried Radix Glycyrrhizae (*Gan Cao*).

ACUPUNCTURE & MOXIBUSTION: *Bai Hui* (GV 20), *Si Shen Cong* (M-HN-1), *Tai Chong* (Liv 3), *San Yin Jiao* (Sp 6), *Feng Long* (St 40)

ANALYSIS OF FORMULA: Draining *Bai Hui* and *Si Shen Cong* opens the orifices, arouses the spirit, and boosts the intelligence. Draining *Tai Chong* courses the liver and resolves depression, *San Yin Jiao* quickens the blood and transforms stasis, while *Feng Long* dries dampness and transforms phlegm.

ADDITIONS & SUBTRACTIONS: For long-term treatment, alternate the above points with *Shen Ting* (GV 24), *Qian Ding* (GV 21), *Hou Ding* (GV 19), *Ge Shu* (Bl 17), *Gan Shu* (Bl 18), *Hun Men* (Bl 47), and *Pi Shu* (Bl 20). For depressive heat, replace *Tai Chong* with *Xing Jian* (Liv 2) and add *Xia Xi* (GB 43). For blood vacuity, add *Ge Shu* (Bl 17) and *Gan Shu* (Bl 18). For spleen vacuity, add *Zu San Li* (St 36). For bilateral rib-side distention and pain, add *Zhang Men* (Liv 13).

2. LIVER-KIDNEY YIN VACUITY MIXED WITH PHLEGM & STASIS PATTERN

MAIN SYMPTOMS: A relatively long disease course, dizziness, vertigo, numbness and tingling of the hands and feet, loss of intelligence and coordination, decreased memory power, lack of spirit in both eyes, a stagnant, torpid facial expression, malar flushing, night sweats, possible emaciation, dry, scaly skin, a predilection for abnormal anger, trembling or spasms and contractions, if severe, difficult, encumbered movement, possible hemilateral paralysis and aphasia, a dark red tongue with possible static macules and scanty fur, and a bowstring, fine, possibly rapid pulse

TREATMENT PRINCIPLES: Enrich and supplement the liver and kidneys, quicken the blood and dispel phlegm

RX: *Liu Wei Di Huang Wan Jia Jian* (Six Flavors Rehmannia Pills with Additions & Subtractions)

INGREDIENTS: Cooked Radix Rehmanniae (*Shu Di*) and

Sclerotium Poriae Cocos (*Fu Ling*), 15g each, Fructus Corni Officinalis (*Shan Zhu Yu*), Cortex Radicis Moutan (*Dan Pi*), Rhizoma Alismatis (*Ze Xie*), Radix Rubrus Paeoniae Lactiflorae (*Chi Shao*), Radix Albus Paeoniae Lactiflorae (*Bai Shao*), Radix Ligustici Wallichii (*Chuan Xiong*), and Flos Carthami Tinctorii (*Hong Hua*), 12g each, and Semen Pruni Persicae (*Tao Ren*), Radix Polygalae Tenuifoliae (*Yuan Zhi*), and Rhizoma Acori Graminei (*Shi Chang Pu*), 9g each

ANALYSIS OF FORMULA: *Shu Di* and *Shan Zhu Yu* enrich and supplement the liver and kidneys. *Bai Shao* nourishes liver blood and levels the liver. *Fu Ling, Ze Xie, Yuan Zhi*, and *Shi Chang Pu* seep dampness and transform phlegm. In addition, *Yuan Zhi* and *Shi Chang Pu* open the orifices and boost the intelligence, *Fu Ling* fortifies the spleen and calms the spirit, and *Ze Xie* downbears ministerial fire. *Dan Pi, Chi Shao, Chuan Xiong, Hong Hua*, and *Tao Ren* quicken the blood and transform stasis.

ADDITIONS & SUBTRACTIONS: If there is concomitant spleen vacuity, add nine grams each of Rhizoma Pinelliae Ternatae (*Ban Xia*) and Radix Dioscoreae Oppositae (*Shan Yao*) and six grams of Pericarpium Citri Reticulatae (*Chen Pi*). If there is vacuity heat/fire effulgence, add nine grams each of Rhizoma Anemarrhenae Aspheloidis (*Zhi Mu*) and Cortex Phellodendri (*Huang Bai*). If there is dizziness and vertigo, add 12 grams of Magnetitum (*Ci Shi*) and nine grams each of Rhizoma Gastrodiae Elatae (*Tian Ma*), Ramulus Uncariae Cum Uncis (*Gou Teng*), and Fructus Ligustri Lucidi (*Nu Zhen Zi*). If there is dry mouth and constipation, add nine grams each of Fructus Mori Albi (*Sang Shen*), Radix Trichosanthis Kirlowii (*Tian Hua Fen*), and Semen Biotae Orientalis (*Bai Zi Ren*). If there is vexation and agitation and a stiff tongue, add 12 grams each of Concha Margaritiferae (*Zhen Zhu Mu*) and Bulbus Lilii (*Bai He*). If there is hemiplegia or numbness of the hands and feet, add 15 grams each of Caulis Milletiae Seu Spatholobi (*Ji Xue Teng*) and Radix Salviae Miltiorrhizae (*Dan Shen*) and nine grams each of Radix Angelicae Sinensis (*Dang Gui*) and Gelatinum Corii Asini (*E Jiao*).

ACUPUNCTURE & MOXIBUSTION: *Gan Shu* (Bl 18), *Shen Shu* (Bl 23), *Zhi Shi* (Bl 52), *Si Shen Cong* (M-HN-1), *Bai Hui* (GV 20), *San Yin Jiao* (Sp 6), *Feng Long* (St 40)

ANALYSIS OF FORMULA: Supplementing *Gan Shu, Shen Shu*, and *Zhi Shi* enriches and supplements the liver and kidneys, fills the essence and boosts the intelligence. Supplementing *Si Shen Cong* and *Bai Hui* with moxibustion draws yin essence upward to fill the sea of marrow, opens the orifices, and boosts the intelligence. Draining *San Yin Jiao* quickens the blood and transforms stasis, while *Feng Long* dries dampness and transforms phlegm.

ADDITIONS & SUBTRACTIONS: If there is concomitant spleen vacuity, add *Zu San Li* (St 36). If there is yin vacuity-fire effulgence, add *Yong Quan* (Ki 1). If there is dizziness and vertigo, add *Feng Chi* (GB 20). If there is dry mouth and constipation, add *Zhao Hai* (Ki 6) and *Zhi Gou* (TB 6). For lack of spirit in both eyes, add *Yin Tang* (M-HN-3). For night sweats, add *Yin Xi* (Ht 6). For abnormal anger, add *Xing Jian* (Liv 2).

3. SPLEEN-KIDNEY YANG VACUITY MIXED WITH PHLEGM & STASIS PATTERN

MAIN SYMPTOMS: Slow movement, a torpid, dull affect, relatively scanty speech, if severe, aphasia, difficulty thinking, chaotic speech, decreased memory power, numbness of the limbs, loss of mental and physical sharpness and coordination, a pale but dark tongue with possible static macules and white, slimy fur, and a fine, slippery or fine, choppy pulse

TREATMENT PRINCIPLES: Warm the kidneys and supplement the spleen, dispel phlegm and transform stasis

RX: *Fu Zi Nan Xing Yu Jin Tang* (Aconite, Arisaema & Curcuma Decoction)

INGREDIENTS: Fructus Corni Officinalis (*Shan Zhu Yu*), Tuber Curcumae (*Yu Jin*), Radix Ligustici Wallichii (*Chuan Xiong*), Radix Rubrus Paeoniae Lactiflorae (*Chi Shao*), and Semen Pruni Persicae (*Tao Ren*), 12g each, Fructus Citri Aurantii (*Zhi Ke*), bile-processed Rhizoma Arisaematis (*Dan Nan Xing*), and Flos Carthami Tinctorii (*Hong Hua*), 9g each, and Cortex Cinnamomi Cassiae (*Rou Gui*) and blast-fried Radix Lateralis Praeparatus Aconiti Carmichaeli (*Fu Zi*), 6g each

ANALYSIS OF FORMULA: *Rou Gui, Shan Zhu Yu*, and *Fu Zi* warm and supplement the spleen and kidneys. Because memory and thought depend both on the warming and steaming of lifegate fire and the function of the spleen, these three medicinals also indirectly boost the intelligence. *Dan Nan Xing* and *Zhi Ke* move the qi and transform phlegm, and *Chuan Xiong, Chi Shao, Tao Ren*, and *Hong Hua* quicken the blood and transform stasis.

ADDITIONS & SUBTRACTIONS: If there is dizziness and tinnitus, add 12 grams of Ramulus Loranthi Seu Visci (*Sang Ji Sheng*) and nine grams each of Fructus Lycii Chinensis (*Gou Qi Zi*), Rhizoma Gastrodiae Elatae (*Tian Ma*), and Radix Dipsaci (*Xu Duan*). If there is marked fatigue and lack of strength, add 15 grams of Radix Astragali Membranacei (*Huang Qi*), nine grams each of Radix Codonopsitis Pilosulae (*Dang Shen*) and Rhizoma Atractylodis Macrocephalae (*Bai Zhu*), and six grams of mix-fried Radix Glycyrrhizae (*Gan Cao*).

ACUPUNCTURE & MOXIBUSTION: *Pi Shu* (Bl 20), *Shen*

Shu (Bl 23), *Zhi Shi* (Bl 52), *Si Shen Cong* (M-HN-1), *Bai Hui* (GV 20), *San Yin Jiao* (Sp 6), *Feng Long* (St 40)

ANALYSIS OF FORMULA: Supplementing *Pi Shu, Shen Shu,* and *Zhi Shi* with moxibustion warms and supplements the spleen and kidneys, fills the essence and boosts intelligence. Supplementing *Si Shen Cong* and *Bai Hui* with moxibustion draws the yang qi upward to the sea of marrow, opens the orifices, boosts the intelligence. Draining *San Yin Jiao* quickens the blood and transforms stasis, while *Feng Long* dries dampness and transforms phlegm.

ADDITIONS & SUBTRACTIONS: If there is dizziness, add *Feng Chi* (GB 20). If there is tinnitus, add *Ting Hui* (GB 2) and *Er Men* (TB 21). If there is marked fatigue and lack of strength, add *Zu San Li* (St 36). For lack of spirit in both eyes, add *Yin Tang* (M-HN-3). For anger, add *Xing Jian* (Liv 2).

4. HEART-SPLEEN DUAL VACUITY PATTERN

MAIN SYMPTOMS: Confused, chaotic thinking, a predilection to sorrow and a desire to cry, excessive stillness, scanty speech, slow movement, lack of involvement in the outside world, lassitude of the spirit, spontaneous perspiration, lack of strength, bodily emaciation, heart palpitations, susceptibility to fright, shortness of breath on slight exertion, torpid intake, lack of taste, an enlarged, pale tongue with thin fur, and a fine, weak pulse

TREATMENT PRINCIPLES: Supplement and boost the heart and spleen, quiet the spirit and stabilize the mind

RX: *Yang Xin Tang* (Nourish the Heart Decoction)

INGREDIENTS: Radix Panacis Ginseng (*Ren Shen*), Tuber Ophiopogonis Japonici (*Mai Men Dong*), and Semen Zizyphi Spinosae (*Suan Zao Ren*), 12g each, Radix Angelicae Sinensis (*Dang Gui*), uncooked Radix Rehmanniae (*Sheng Di*), cooked Radix Rehmanniae (*Shu Di*), and Sclerotium Poriae Cocos (*Fu Ling*), 9g each, Semen Biotae Orientalis (*Bai Zi Ren*) and Fructus Schisandrae Chinensis (*Wu Wei Zi*), 6g each, and mix-fried Radix Glycyrrhizae (*Gan Cao*), 3g

ANALYSIS OF FORMULA: *Ren Shen, Fu Ling,* and mix-fried *Gan Cao* fortify the spleen and supplement the qi, boost the intelligence and stabilize the mind. *Mai Men Dong, Suan Zao Ren, Dang Gui, Sheng Di, Shu Di, Bai Zi Ren,* and *Wu Wei Zi* together nourish yin blood and supplement the heart, quiet the spirit and stabilize the mind.

ADDITIONS & SUBTRACTIONS: If there is chaotic speech, add nine grams each of Rhizoma Acori Graminei (*Shi Chang Pu*), Dens Draconis (*Long Chi*), and Tuber Curcumae (*Yu Jin*). If there is dampness stagnating in the middle burner, delete *Dang Gui, Bai Zi Ren, Suan Zao Ren,* and *Wu Wei Zi* and add nine grams each of Herba Agastachis Seu Pogostemi (*Huo Xiang*), Herba Eupatorii Fortunei (*Pei Lan*), Rhizoma Acori Graminei (*Shi Chang Pu*), and Fructus Cardamomi (*Bai Dou Kou*). If the tongue is red and the pulse is rapid, add nine grams of Rhizoma Coptidis Chinensis (*Huang Lian*). If there is concomitant blood stasis, add nine grams of Radix Salviae Miltiorrhizae (*Dan Shen*) and three grams of Sucinum (*Hu Po*). If there is concomitant phlegm, add nine grams each of Rhizoma Acori Graminei (*Shi Chang Pu*), Radix Polygalae Tenuifoliae (*Yuan Zhi*), Rhizoma Pinelliae Ternatae (*Ban Xia*), and Pericarpium Citri Reticulatae (*Chen Pi*).

ACUPUNCTURE & MOXIBUSTION: *Xin Shu* (Bl 15), *Ge Shu* (Bl 17), *Pi Shu* (Bl 20), *Zhi Shi* (Bl 52), *Bai Hui* (GV 20), *Si Shen Cong* (M-HN-1)

ANALYSIS OF FORMULA: Supplementing *Xin Shu, Ge Shu,* and *Pi Shu* supplements and boosts the heart and spleen, quiets the spirit and stabilizes the mind. Supplementing *Zhi Shi* supplements the sea of marrow and boosts the intelligence. Supplementing *Bai Hui* and *Si Shen Cong* with moxibustion, draws the the qi and blood upward to the sea of marrow, opens the orifices and boosts the intelligence.

ADDITIONS & SUBTRACTIONS: For marked heart symptoms, such as heart palpitations, insomnia, and confused, chaotic thinking, add *Shen Men* (Ht 7). For concomitant blood stasis, add *San Yin Jiao* (Sp 6). For severe blood vacuity, also add *San Yin Jiao* (Sp 6). For phlegm, add *Feng Long* (St 40). For marked fatigue, lack of strength, or digestive symptoms, add *Zu San Li* (St 36). For a predilection to sorrow and a desire to cry, add *Yin Bai* (Sp 1). For susceptibility to fright, add *Da Ling* (Per 7).

5. ASCENDANT LIVER YANG HYPERACTIVITY PATTERN

MAIN SYMPTOMS: Headache, dizziness, red face and eyes, emotional vexation and agitation, restless stirring, a predilection to frenetic activity, scanty sleep, profuse dreams, a stiff tongue with slurred speech, numbness and tingling of the limbs, possible deviation of the mouth and eyes, hemiplegia, a red tongue with white or yellow fur, and a bowstring, slippery or bowstring, fine, and rapid pulse

NOTE: Some of the above symptoms suggest internal stirring of liver wind.

TREATMENT PRINCIPLES: Level the liver and subdue yang, arouse the spirit and open the orifices

RX: *Tian Ma Gou Teng Yin Jia Wei* (Gastrodia & Uncaria Drink with Added Flavors)

INGREDIENTS: Ramulus Loranthi Seu Visci (*Sang Ji Sheng*) and Semen Zizyphi Spinosae (*Suan Zao Ren*), 12g each,

Rhizoma Acori Graminei (*Shi Chang Pu*), Radix Albus Paeoniae Lactiflorae (*Bai Shao*), Fructus Lycii Chinensis (*Gou Qi Zi*), Rhizoma Gastrodiae Elatae (*Tian Ma*), Ramulus Uncariae Cum Uncis (*Gou Teng*), Cortex Eucommiae Ulmoidis (*Du Zhong*), Radix Cyathulae (*Chuan Niu Xi*), Caulis Polygoni Multiflori (*Ye Jiao Teng*), Radix Scutellariae Baicalensis (*Huang Qin*), and Herba Leonuri Heterophylli (*Yi Mu Cao*), 9g each, and Concha Haliotidis (*Shi Jue Ming*), Fructus Gardeniae Jasminoidis (*Zhi Zi*), and Sclerotium Poriae Cocos (*Fu Ling*), 6g each

ANALYSIS OF FORMULA: *Tian Ma, Bai Shao, Gou Teng,* and *Shi Jue Ming* level the liver and subdue yang. *Huang Qin* and *Zhi Zi* clear the liver and discharge fire. *Sang Ji Sheng, Bai Shao, Gou Qi,* and *Du Zhong* supplement the kidneys and enrich yin to control the yang. *Suan Zao Ren, Shi Chang Pu, Ye Jiao Teng,* and *Fu Ling* nourish the heart and quiet the spirit. *Shi Chang Pu* arouses the spirit and opens the orifices. *Chuan Niu Xi* and *Yi Mu Cao* quicken the blood and transform stasis.

ADDITIONS & SUBTRACTIONS: If there is constipation and reddish urine, add six grams of Radix Et Rhizoma Rhei (*Da Huang*) and nine grams of Lapis Chloriti Seu Micae (*Meng Shi*). If there is bilateral rib-side distention and pain, add nine grams of Pericarpium Citri Reticulatae Viride (*Qing Pi*) and 15 grams of Rhizoma Corydalis Yanhusuo (*Yan Hu Suo*). If there is agitation and restlessness, add 12 grams each of Concha Ostreae (*Mu Li*) and Os Draconis (*Long Gu*).

ACUPUNCTURE & MOXIBUSTION: *Bai Hui* (GV 20), *Si Shen Cong* (M-HN-1), *Feng Chi* (GB 20), *San Yin Jiao* (Sp 6), *Xuan Zhong* (GB 39)

ANALYSIS OF FORMULA: Draining *Bai Hui, Si Shen Cong,* and *Feng Chi* levels the liver and subdues yang, arouses the spirit and opens the orifices. Supplementing *San Yin Jiao* and draining *Xuan Zhong* nourishes yin and controls yang, supplements the liver and kidneys and levels the liver.

ADDITIONS & SUBTRACTIONS: If there is constipation, add *Zhao Hai* (Ki 6) and *Zhi Gou* (TB 6). If there is reddish urine, add *Yin Ling Quan* (Sp 9). If there is bilateral rib-side distention and pain, add *Tai Chong* (Liv 3). If there is agitation and restlessness, add *Da Ling* (Per 7). If there is a red face and eyes, emotional vexation and agitation, restless stirring, and a predilection for frenetic activity, add *Xing Jian* (Liv 2). If there is scanty sleep and profuse dreams, add *Da Ling* (Per 7).

6. HEART FIRE HYPERACTIVITY & EXUBERANCE PATTERN

MAIN SYMPTOMS: Headache, heart vexation, a red face and lips, scanty sleep, profuse dreams, chaotic, confused speech, laughing and crying without constancy, unregulated thinking and anxiety, a predilection to rash behavior, frequent, reddish urination, dry stools, a red tongue, especially the tip, with thin, yellow fur, and a bowstring, rapid pulse

TREATMENT PRINCIPLES: Clear the heart and drain fire, settle, still, and quiet the spirit

RX: *Xie Xin Tang* (Drain the Heart Decoction) & *Dao Chi San* (Abduct the Red Powder) with added flavors

INGREDIENTS: Uncooked Radix Rehmanniae (*Sheng Di*), 30g, Magnetitum (*Ci Shi*) and Radix Scrophulariae Ningpoensis (*Xuan Shen*), 15g each, Os Draconis (*Long Gu*), 12g, Radix Scutellariae Baicalensis (*Huang Qin*), Fructus Gardeniae Jasminoidis (*Zhi Zi*), Cortex Radicis Moutan (*Dan Pi*), and Tuber Curcumae (*Yu Jin*), 9g each, Radix Et Rhizoma Rhei (*Da Huang*), Caulis Akebiae (*Mu Tong*), and Herba Lophatheri Gracilis (*Dan Zhu Ye*), 6g each, and Rhizoma Coptidis Chinensis (*Huang Lian*) and Extremitas Radicis Glycyrrhizae (*Gan Cao Shao*), 3g each

ANALYSIS OF FORMULA: *Huang Lian, Huang Qin, Zhi Zi, Da Huang, Mu Tong,* and *Dan Zhu Ye* clear the heart and drain fire. *Ci Shi* and *Long Gu* heavily settle, still, and quiet the spirit. *Sheng Di* nourishes the yin blood of the heart and clears the heart. In addition, *Sheng Di* prevents damage to yin by the bitter flavor of the other medicinals. *Xuan Shen* clears vacuity heat. *Dan Pi* and *Yu Jin* quicken the blood and transform stasis. *Mu Tong, Dan Zhu Ye,* and *Gan Cao Shao* disinhibit dampness, clear the small intestine, and downbear heat through urination.

ADDITIONS & SUBTRACTIONS: If there is a dry mouth and throat, add 12 grams each of Tuber Ophiopogonis Japonici (*Mai Men Dong*), Tuber Asparagi Cochinensis (*Tian Men Dong*), and Bulbus Lilii (*Bai He*) and nine grams of Herba Dendrobii (*Shi Hu*). If there is insomnia and profuse dreams, add 12 grams each of Semen Zizyphi Spinosae (*Suan Zao Ren*) and Caulis Polygoni Multiflori (*Ye Jiao Teng*) and nine grams of Sclerotium Pararadicis Poriae Cocos (*Fu Shen*).

ACUPUNCTURE & MOXIBUSTION: *Tong Li* (Ht 5), *Da Ling* (Per 7), *Bai Hui* (GV 20), *Si Shen Cong* (M-HN-1)

ANALYSIS OF FORMULA: Draining *Tong Li* and *Da Ling* clears the heart and drains fire, settles and quiets the spirit. Draining *Bai Hui* and *Si Shen Cong* quiets the spirit and opens the orifices.

ADDITIONS & SUBTRACTIONS: For headache, add *Tou Wei* (St 8), *Tai Yang* (M-HN-9), *Yin Tang* (M-HN-3), and/or *Tong Tian* (Bl 7). For severe heart vexation, scanty sleep, and profuse dreams, bleed *Lao Gong* (Per 8) and *Shao Chong* (Ht 9). For a predilection to rash behavior, bleed *Lao Gong* (Per 8) and *Shao Chong* (Ht 9). For unregulated thinking and anxiety, bleed *Yin Bai* (Sp 1). For reddish urination, add *Zhong Ji* (CV 3). For a dry mouth and throat, add *Zhao Hai* (Ki 6).

7. DAMPNESS & PHLEGM MISTING THE ORIFICES PATTERN

MAIN SYMPTOMS: Heavy-headedness, a yellow, stagnant facial complexion, superficial edema, fatigue, lack of strength, profuse sleeping, phlegmy sounding respiration, a torpid affect, scanty speech or confused, chaotic speech, alternating sorrow and joy for no particular reason, no discrimination between good and bad, no care for human appearances, profuse phlegm drool from the mouth, ductal oppression, abdominal distention, if severe, lack of sensitivity, inability to manage one's activities by oneself, a pale, fat tongue with slimy, white fur, and a soggy, slippery pulse

TREATMENT PRINCIPLES: Fortify the spleen and transform phlegm, arouse the brain and open the orifices

RX: *Xi Xin Tang* (Cleanse the Heart Decoction)

INGREDIENTS: Radix Panacis Ginseng (*Ren Shen*), Semen Zizyphi Spinosae (*Suan Zao Ren*), and Sclerotium Pararadicis Poriae Cocos (*Fu Shen*), 12g each, Rhizoma Pinelliae Ternatae (*Ban Xia*), and Rhizoma Acori Graminei (*Shi Chang Pu*), 9g each, Pericarpium Citri Reticulatae (*Chen Pi*), Massa Medica Fermentata (*Shen Qu*), and mix-fried Radix Glycyrrhizae (*Gan Cao*), 6g each, and Radix Lateralis Praeparatus Aconiti Carmichaeli (*Fu Zi*), 3g

ANALYSIS OF FORMULA: *Ban Xia, Shi Chang Pu,* and *Chen Pi* transform phlegm, arouse the brain, and open the orifices. *Ren Shen, Fu Zi* and mix-fried *Gan Cao* warm and supplement the spleen to prevent further damp accumulation and phlegm engenderment. *Shen Qu* helps the transformation function of the spleen to prevent phlegm dampness. In addition, *Ren Shen* quiets the spirit and boosts the intelligence. *Suan Zao Ren* and *Fu Shen* nourish the heart, quiet the spirit, and boost the intelligence.

ADDITIONS & SUBTRACTIONS: If phlegm drool is profuse, add nine grams each of Bulbus Fritillariae Thunbergii (*Zhe Bei Mu*), Radix Polygalae Tenuifoliae (*Yuan Zhi*), and bile-processed Rhizoma Arisaematis (*Dan Nan Xing*). If there is abdominal distention and scanty intake, delete *Ren Shen, Fu Zi,* and *Suan Zao Ren* and add nine grams each of Herba Agastachis Seu Pogostemi (*Huo Xiang*), Herba Eupatorii Fortunei (*Pei Lan*), Cortex Magnoliae Officinalis (*Hou Po*), Semen Raphani Sativi (*Lai Fu Zi*), Fructus Citri Aurantii (*Zhi Ke*), and Radix Auklandiae Lappae (*Mu Xiang*).

ACUPUNCTURE & MOXIBUSTION: *Bai Hui* (GV 20), *Si Shen Cong* (M-HN-1), *Feng Chi* (GB 20), *Zu San Li* (St 36), *Yin Ling Quan* (Sp 9), *Feng Long* (St 40)

ANALYSIS OF FORMULA: Draining *Bai Hui, Si Shen Cong,* and *Feng Chi* clears the head, arouses the brain, and opens the orifices. Supplementing *Zu San Li* fortifies the spleen and boosts the qi to prevent new accumulation of phlegm. Draining *Yin Ling Quan* disinhibits dampness, while draining *Feng Long* transforms phlegm.

ADDITIONS & SUBTRACTIONS: If phlegm drool is profuse, add *Zhong Wan* (CV 12). If there is abdominal distention and scanty intake, add *Liang Men* (St 21) and *Zhong Wan* (CV 12). If there is marked fatigue and lack of strength, add *Zu San Li* (St 36). For excessive sleeping, add *San Jian* (LI 3). For scanty speech or confused, chaotic speech, add *Tong Li* (Ht 5). For alternating sorrow and joy for no particular reason, add *Shen Men* (Ht 7) and *Yin Bai* (Sp 1).

REMARKS

1. According to the famous Chinese medical geriatricist, Yan De-xin, blood stasis is the root cause or at least complicates most, if not all, cases of Alzheimer's disease. In *Aging & Blood Stasis,* Dr. Yan says:

> . . . through years of exploration, I have come to believe that the root of this disease is static blood obstructing the mansion of the clear spirit. Therefore, using the methods of quickening the blood and transforming stasis, I have gotten satisfactory therapeutic results, changing the stale point of view that this disease is irreversible.[1]

2. The Chinese language medical literature does not discriminate between Alzheimer's and other forms of senile dementia, such as vascular dementia. Therefore, although there is a relatively large body of literature on the Chinese medical treatment of senile dementia, it is hard to know exactly how many of the patients in the various studies did have a confirmed diagnosis of Alzheimer's disease. For more information on the Chinese medical treatment of senile dementia, please see Bob Flaws and James Lake's *Chinese Medical Psychiatry,* Blue Poppy Press, Boulder, CO, 2001.

ENDNOTES

[1] *Op. cit.,* trans. by Tang Guo-shun & Bob Flaws, Blue Poppy Press, Boulder, CO, 1995, p. 243

4

Amyotrophic Lateral Sclerosis

Amytrophic lateral sclerosis (ALS) is also know in the United States as Lou Gehrig's disease. It is not an autoimmune disease. Its Western medical etiology is currently unknown. ALS is a progressively degenerative motor neuron disease affecting the corticospinal tracts and anterior horn cells. Its symptoms depend on which part of the nervous system is affected. Onset is generally after 40 years of age, and its incidence is higher in males than females. Five to 10% of cases are familial.

The first symptoms of this condition are typically asymmetrical muscular weakness and atrophy usually manifesting distally. Forty percent of cases begin in the muscles of the hand. Cramps are common and may precede weakness. As the condition progresses, there are visible muscular fasciculations, spasticity, and hyperactive deep tendon reflexes. Dysarthria and dysphagia may also occur. Death usually occurs in 2-5 years with 20% of patients surviving five years. Western medicine has no specific treatment of this disease.

Chinese disease categorization: This condition is mainly categorized as *wei zheng*, wilting condition. However, its main symptoms are also Chinese disease categories in their own right. These include *shou zhi luan ji*, hypertonicity of the fingers of the hand, *zhen chan*, tremors, *shou chan*, tremors of the hands, and *ye ge*, dysphagia.

Disease causes: Damage by the seven affects, food and drink, alcohol, taxation fatigue, soaking in dampness, and living in a damp environment may all precipitate or aggravate this disease. In addition, former heaven natural endowment insufficiency and aging also play their parts.

Disease mechanisms: The three main viscera involved in this disease are the liver, kidneys, and spleen. Any of the above disease causing factors may result in detriment and damage of these three viscera. If the liver and kidneys are damaged, the sinews and bones will be deprived of proper nourishment. In addition, blood and yin vacuity may cause liver yang ascendant hyperactivity and engender internal stirring of liver wind. If the spleen is damaged, it may fail to engender and transform sufficient qi and blood, thus depriving the limbs of strength and nourishment and the muscles and flesh of filling and nourishment. Because spleen qi and kidney yang are mutually dependent and promoting, spleen qi vacuity may eventually result in kidney yang vacuity. Because blood and essence share a common source, long-standing blood vacuity may eventually evolve into yin essence vacuity. Because yin and yang are mutually rooted, kidney yin vacuity may result in kidney yang vacuity and *vice versa*. Further, because of visceral dysfunction, wind, damp, heat, stasis, or phlegm evils may be engendered. These evils may further damage the viscera of the liver, kidneys, and spleen as well as hinder and obstruct the flow of qi and blood to the body and limbs.

Treatment based on pattern discrimination:

1. Liver blood-kidney yin vacuity pattern

Main symptoms: Wilting, limpness, and lack of strength of the muscles and flesh which is most severe in the lower extremities, lower and upper back aching and limpness, emaciation of the muscles and flesh, tinnitus, dizziness, heart vexation, heat in the centers of the hands and feet, possible night sweats, seminal emission in men and menstrual irregularities in females, a red tongue with scanty fur, and a fine, rapid pulse. If, due to yin failing to control yang, liver yang becomes hyperactive and ascends resulting in internal stirring of liver wind, there will be pronounced muscular spasticity, spasms and contractures of the four limbs, a red tongue with scanty fur, and a bowstring, forceless pulse.

Treatment principles: Supplement and boost the liver

and kidneys, fill the essence and boost the marrow. If there is internal stirring of liver wind, also settle the liver and extinguish wind.

RX: *Hu Qian Wan* (Hidden Tiger Pills) & *Zuo Gui Wan* (Restore the Left [Kidney] Pills) with added flavors

INGREDIENTS: Cooked Radix Rehmanniae (*Shu Di*), 12g, Cortex Phellodendri (*Huang Bai*), Radix Albus Paeoniae Lactiflorae (*Bai Shao*), Herba Cynomorii Songarici (*Suo Yang*), Radix Dioscoreae Oppositae (*Shan Yao*), Fructus Lycii Chinensis (*Gou Qi Zi*), Fructus Corni Officinalis (*Shan Zhu Yu*), Radix Cyathulae (*Chuan Niu Xi*), Gelatinum Plastri Testudinis (*Gui Ban Jiao*), and Gelatinum Cornu Cervi (*Lu Jiao Jiao*), 9g each, and dry Rhizoma Zingiberis (*Gan Jiang*), 6g

ANALYSIS OF FORMULA: *Shu Di, Shan Yao, Gou Qi, Shan Zhu Yu,* and *Bai Shao* supplement and boost the liver and kidneys. *Lu Jiao Jiao* and *Gui Ban Jiao* enrich the yin and invigorate yang, nourish the blood, fill the essence, and boost the marrow. *Suo Yang* likewise invigorates yang and nourishes the blood, thus strengthening the sinews and bones and seeking yin within yang. *Huang Bai* clears vacuity heat. *Chuan Niu Xi* quickens the blood, strengthens the sinews and bones, and guides the others medicinals downward to the lower limbs. *Gan Jiang* warms yang and fortifies the spleen. In this formula, its purpose is to harmonize the spleen and stomach in order to protect them from the slimy, stagnating yin supplements on the one hand and the bitter, cold, heat-clearing ingredients on the other.

ADDITIONS & SUBTRACTIONS: For concomitant yang vacuity, add nine grams each of Herba Epimedii (*Yin Yang Huo*) and Cortex Radicis Acanthopanacis Gracilistylis (*Wu Jia Pi*). For concomitant qi vacuity, add 15 grams of Radix Astragali Membranacei (*Huang Qi*) and nine grams of Radix Codonopsitis Pilosulae (*Dang Shen*). For difficulty walking and severe lack of strength in the lower limbs, add 12 grams each of Cortex Radicis Acanthopanacis Gracilistylis (*Wu Jia Pi*) and Cortex Eucommiae Ulmoidis (*Du Zhong*) and replace *Chuan Niu Xi* with Radix Achyranthis Bidentatae (*Niu Xi*). For low back and knee soreness and limpness, add 12 grams each of Rhizoma Cibotii Barometsis (*Gou Ji*) and Cortex Eucommiae Ulmoidis (*Du Zhong*). For severe vacuity heat, add nine grams each of Rhizoma Alismatis (*Ze Xie*), Cortex Radicis Moutan (*Dan Pi*), and Rhizoma Anemarrhenae Asphodeloidis (*Zhi Mu*).

If there is liver wind stirring internally, replace *Hu Qian Wan* and *Zuo Gui Wan* with *Zhen Gan Xi Feng Tang Jia Wei* (Settle the Liver & Extinguish Wind Decoction with Added Flavors): Radix Achyranthis Bidentatae (*Niu Xi*) and Haemititum (*Dai Zhe Shi*), 30g each, Os Draconis (*Long Gu*), Concha Ostreae (*Mu Li*), Plastrum Testudinis (*Gui Ban*), Radix Scrophualriae Ningpoensis (*Xuan Shen*), Tuber Asparagi Cochinensis (*Tian Men Dong*), Radix Albus Paeoniae Lactiflorae (*Bai Shao*), and Rhizoma Gastrodiae Elatae (*Tian Ma*), 15g each, Ramulus Uncariae Cum Uncis (*Gou Teng*) and Flos Chrysanthemi Morifolii (*Ju Hua*), 12g each, Herba Artemisiae Capillaris (*Yin Chen Hao*) and Fructus Meliae Toosendan (*Chuan Lian Zi*), 9g each, Fructus Germinatus Hordei Vulgaris (*Mai Ya*), 6g, and Radix Glycyrrhizae (*Gan Cao*), 4.5g.

ACUPUNCTURE & MOXIBUSTION: *Shen Ting* (GV 24), *Bai Hui* (GV 20), *Feng Fu* (GV 16), *Da Zhui* (GV 14), *Ling Tai* (GV 10), *Ji Zhong* (GV 6), *Ming Men* (GV 4), *Chang Qiang* (GV 1), *Ge Shu* (Bl 17), *Gan Shu* (Bl 18), *Pi Shu* (Bl 20), *Shen Shu* (Bl 23)

ANAYLSIS OF FORMULA: Even supplementing-even draining *Shen Ting, Bai Hui, Feng Fu, Da Zhui, Ling Tai, Ji Zhong, Ming Men,* and *Chang Qiang* regulates the governing vessel and harmonizes yin and yang, opens the orifices and quiets the spirit, extinguishes wind, supports the righteous, and frees the flow of the network vessels. Supplementing *Ge Shu* and *Gan Shu* supplements and nourishes liver blood. Supplementing *Shen Shu* supplements the kidneys. Supplementing *Pi Shu* supplements the latter heaven to support and bolster the former heaven. In addition, the spleen is the root of qi and blood engenderment and transformation. Therefore, supplementing the spleen helps promote supplementation of the blood.

ADDITIONS & SUBTRACTIONS: For visual disturbances, add *Jing Ming* (Bl 1) or *Zan Zhu* (Bl 2) and *Tai Yang* (M-HN-9). For tremors or contractions in the limbs, add *Tai Chong* (Liv 3) and *He Gu* (LI 4). For dizziness, add *Feng Chi* (GB 20). For fatigue, add *Zu San Li* (St 36) and *Qi Hai* (CV 6). For atrophy, wilting, weakness, numbness, and/or insensitivity of the upper extremities, add *Jian Yu* (LI 15), *Bi Nao* (LI 14), *Qu Chi* (LI 11), *Shou San Li* (LI 10), *He Gu* (LI 4), and *Wai Guan* (TB 5). Select 2-3 points each treatment. For atrophy, wilting, weakness, numbness, and/or insensitivity of the lower extremities, add *Bi Guan* (St 31), *Fu Tu* (St 32), *Liang Qiu* (St 34), *Zu San Li* (St 36), *Shang Ju Xu* (St 37), and *Jie Xi* (St 41). Select 2-3 points each treatment. For weakness of the wrist, add *Yang Chi* (TB 4) and *Yang Xi* (LI 5). For weakness of the hand, add *He Gu* (LI 4) through to *Hou Xi* (SI 3) using the penetrating needle method. For weakness or numbness of the fingers, add *Ba Xie* (M-UE-22). For weakness of the knees, add *Wei Zhong* (Bl 40) and *Qu Quan* (Liv 8). For weakness of the feet or numbness of the toes, add *Ba Feng* (M-LE-8). For talipes equinus due to weakness of the sinew vessels of the foot yang ming, foot shao yang, and foot jue yin, use *Shang Ju Xu* (St 37), *Jie Xi* (St 41), *Qiu Xu* (GB 40), *Zhong Feng* (Liv 4), and *Yang Ling Quan* (GB 34). For talipes varus due to weakness of the sinew vessels of the foot tai yang and foot shao yang, add *Kun Lun* (Bl 60), *Shen Mai* (Bl 62), *Xuan Zhong* (GB 39), and *Qiu Xu* (GB 40). For talipes valgus due to weakness of the sinew vessels of the foot tai yin and foot shao yin, add *Gong Sun* (Sp 4), *San Yin Jiao* (Sp 6), *Tai Xi* (Ki 3), and *Zhao Hai* (Ki 6). For nausea or vomiting, add *Shang Wan* (CV 13) and *Nei Guan* (Per 6). For head distention, add *Tai Yang* (M-HN-9). For chest oppression, add *Nei Guan* (Per 6). For tinnitus, add *Ting Hui* (GB 2).

2. SPLEEN-KIDNEY YANG VACUITY PATTERN

MAIN SYMPTOMS: Muscle and flesh wilting, limpness, and lack of strength in the four limbs, shortness of breath, disinclination to speak, fear of cold, chilled limbs, a somber white facial complexion, torpid intake, loose stools, possible sweating, seminal emission or urinary incontinence, long, clear urination, lower limb puffy swelling, a pale red tongue which is also tender and fat with teeth-marks on its edges and white fur, and a deep, slow, forceless pulse

TREATMENT PRINCIPLES: Fortify the spleen and boost the qi, supplement the kidneys and invigorate yang

RX: *You Gui Wan* (Restore the Right [Kidney] Pills) & *Si Jun Zi Tang* (Four Gentlemen Decoction) with additions and subtractions

INGREDIENTS: Cooked Radix Rehmanniae (*Shu Di*) and Gelatinum Cornu Cervi (*Lu Jiao Jiao*), 12g each, Radix Lateralis Praeparatus Aconiti Carmichaeli (*Fu Zi*), Cortex Cinnamomi Cassiae (*Rou Gui*), Radix Dioscoreae Oppositae (*Shan Yao*), Fructus Corni Officinalis (*Shan Zhu Yu*), Fructus Lycii Chinensis (*Gou Qi Zi*), Semen Cuscutae Chinensis (*Tu Si Zi*), Cortex Eucommiae Ulmoidis (*Du Zhong*), Radix Angelicae Sinensis (*Dang Gui*), Radix Codonopsitis Pilosulae (*Dang Shen*), Rhizoma Atractylodis Macrocephalae (*Bai Zhu*), and Sclerotium Poriae Cocos (*Fu Ling*), 9g each, and mix-fried Radix Glycyrrhizae (*Gan Cao*), 6g

ANALYSIS OF FORMULA: *Shu Di, Shan Yao,* and *Shan Zhu Yu* are the three supplementing medicinals of *Liu Wei Di Huang Wan* (Six Flavors Rehmannia Pills), a basic formula for supplementing true yin. *Gou Qi Zi* and *Dang Gui* both nourish the blood and supplement the liver based on the sayings, "Blood and essence share a common source," and "The liver and kidneys share a common source." *Lu Jiao Jiao, Fu Zi, Rou Gui, Tu Si Zi,* and *Du Zhong,* warm and supplement the kidney yang. *Dang Shen, Shan Yao, Fu Ling, Bai Zhu,* and mix-fried *Gan Cao* fortify the spleen and boost the qi. In addition, *Lu Jiao Jiao* and *Shu Di* fill the essence and boost the marrow.

ADDITIONS & SUBTRACTIONS: For more severe fatigue, add 15 grams of Radix Astragali Membranacei (*Huang Qi*). For more extreme lack of strength, add 20-30 grams of Radix Astragali Membranacei (*Huang Qi*) and 12 grams of Cortex Radicis Acanthopanacis (*Wu Jia Pi*). For severe weakness and pain in the low back, add nine grams each of Radix Dipsaci (*Xu Duan*) and Radix Morindae Officinalis (*Ba Ji Tian*). For loose stools or diarrhea, add nine grams of Fructus Psoraleae Corylifoliae (*Bu Gu Zhi*) and six grams of Semen Myristicae Fragrantis (*Rou Dou Kou*). For frequent urination, urinary incontinence, or nocturia, add nine grams each of Fructus Alpiniae Oxyphyllae (*Yi Zhi Ren*), Fructus Rosae Laevigatae (*Jin Ying Zi*), and Fructus Rubi Chingii (*Fu Pen Zi*).

For predominant qi vacuity combined with blood vacuity, replace *You Gui Wan* & *Si Jun Zi Tang* with *Gui Pi Tang Jia Jian* (Return the Spleen Decoction with Additions & Subtractions): Radix Astragali Membranacei (*Huang Qi*), 60g, Radix Salviae Miltiorrhizae (*Dan Shen*) and Caulis Milletiae Seu Spatholobi (*Ji Xue Teng*), 30g each, Radix Codonopsitis Pilosulae (*Dang Shen*), Radix Angelicae Sinensis (*Dang Gui*), Radix Albus Paeoniae Lactiflorae (*Bai Shao*), Radix Rubrus Paeoniae Lactiflorae (*Chi Shao*), and Radix Dioscoreae Oppositae (*Shan Yao*), 15g each, Rhizoma Atractylodis Macrocephalae (*Bai Zhu*) and Sclerotium Poriae Cocos (*Fu Ling*), 9g each, and mix-fried Radix Glycyrrhizae (*Gan Cao*), 6g.

ACUPUNCTURE & MOXIBUSTION: *Shen Ting* (GV 24), *Bai Hui* (GV 20), *Feng Fu* (GV 16), *Da Zhui* (GV 14), *Ling Tai* (GV 10), *Ji Zhong* (GV 6), *Ming Men* (GV 4), *Chang Qiang* (GV 1), *Guan Yuan* (CV 4), *Pi Shu* (Bl 20), *Zu San Li* (St 36)

ANALYSIS OF FORMULA: Even supplementing-even draining *Shen Ting, Bai Hui, Feng Fu, Da Zhui, Ling Tai, Ji Zhong, Ming Men,* and *Chang Qiang* regulates the governing vessel and harmonizes yin and yang, opens the orifices and quiets the spirit, extinguishes wind, supports the righteous, and frees the flow of the network vessels. Supplementing *Guan Yuan* and *Shen Shu* with moxibustion supplements the kidneys and invigorates yang. Supplementing *Pi Shu* and *Zu San Li* with moxibustion warms and fortifies spleen yang.

ADDITIONS & SUBTRACTIONS: Please see pattern #1 above.

3. QI & YIN DUAL VACUITY PATTERN

MAIN SYMPTOMS: Wilting, limpness, and lack of strength of the four limbs, a dry mouth but no desire to drink, reduced food intake, loose or dry stools (depending on whether spleen qi or blood and yin vacuity is predominant), shortness of breath, disinclination to speak, dizziness, tinnitus, scanty sleep, impaired memory, low back and lower leg soreness and limpness, a red tongue with scanty fur, and a soggy, fine or fine and rapid pulse

TREATMENT PRINCIPLES: Boost the qi and nourish yin, bank and supplement the spleen and kidneys

RX: *Zuo Gui Wan Jia Wei* (Restore the Left [Kidney] Pills with Added Flavors)

INGREDIENTS: Radix Astragali Membranacei (*Huang Qi*), 15g, cooked Radix Rehmanniae (*Shu Di*), 12g, Radix Codonopsitis Pilosulae (*Dang Shen*), Radix Dioscoreae Oppositae (*Shan Yao*), Rhizoma Atractylodis Macrocephalae (*Bai Zhu*), Sclerotium Poriae Cocos (*Fu Ling*), Fructus Lycii Chinensis (*Gou Qi Zi*), Fructus Corni Officinalis (*Shan Zhu Yu*), Radix Achyranthis Bidentatae (*Niu Xi*), Semen Cuscuatae Chinensis (*Tu Si Zi*), Gelatinum Cornu Cervi (*Lu Jiao Jiao*), and Gelatinum Plastri Testudinis (*Gui Ban Jiao*), 9g each, and Radix Panacis Ginseng (*Ren Shen*), 6g

ANALYSIS OF FORMULA: *Shu Di, Gou Qi, Shan Zhu Yu,* and *Niu Xi* enrich the yin and supplement the kidneys. *Huang Qi, Dang Shen, Shan Yao, Bai Zhu, Fu Ling, Ren Shen,* and *Tu Si Zi* fortify the spleen and boost the qi. In addition *Tu Si Zi* supplements the kidneys and *Niu Xi* guides the other medicinals downward to the lower limbs. *Lu Jiao Jiao* and *Gui Ban Jiao* enrich yin and invigorate yang, nourish the blood, fill the essence, and boost the marrow.

ADDITIONS & SUBTRACTIONS: For severe low back and lower leg soreness and limpness, add nine grams each of Ramulus Loranthi Seu Visci (*Sang Ji Sheng*) and Cortex Eucommiae Ulmoidis (*Du Zhong*). For concomitant blood stasis, add 12 grams each of Radix Angelicae Sinensis (*Dang Gui*) and Radix Salviae Miltiorrhizae (*Dan Shen*). For insomnia and impaired memory, add 12 grams of Semen Zizyphi Spinosae (*Suan Zao Ren*) and 15 grams of Caulis Polygoni Multiflori (*Ye Jiao Teng*). For severe wilting, limpness, and lack of strength in the four limbs, add 12 grams each of Cortex Radicis Acanthopanacis Gracilistylis (*Wu Jia Pi*), Cortex Eucommiae Ulmoidis (*Du Zhong*), and Ramulus Loranthi Seu Visci (*Sang Ji Sheng*). For concomitant liver depression, add nine grams each of Radix Bupleuri (*Chai Hu*), Fructus Meliae Toosendan (*Chuan Lian Zi*), and Radix Albus Paeoniae Lactiflorae (*Bai Shao*).

ACUPUNCTURE & MOXIBUSTION: *Shen Ting* (GV 24), *Bai Hui* (GV 20), *Feng Fu* (GV 16), *Da Zhui* (GV 14), *Ling Tai* (GV 10), *Ji Zhong* (GV 6), *Ming Men* (GV 4), *Chang Qiang* (GV 1), *Pi Shu* (Bl 20), *Shen Shu* (Bl 23), *Zu San Li* (St 36), *Fu Liu* (Ki 7)

ANALYSIS OF FORMULA: Even supplementing-even draining *Shen Ting, Bai Hui, Feng Fu, Da Zhui, Ling Tai, Ji Zhong, Ming Men,* and *Chang Qiang* regulates the governing vessel and harmonizes yin and yang, opens the orifices and quiets the spirit, extinguishes wind, supports the righteous, and frees the flow of the network vessels. Supplementing *Pi Shu, Shen Shu, Zu San Li,* and *Fu Liu* fortifies the spleen and boosts the qi, supplements the kidneys and enriches yin.

ADDITIONS & SUBTRACTIONS: Please see pattern #1 above.

4. YIN & YANG DUAL VACUITY PATTERN

MAIN SYMPTOMS: Late stage disease, muscle and flesh falling and dropping, inability to function due to paralysis, fear of cold, chilled limbs, puffy face, swollen limbs, low, weak voice, dizziness, tinnitus, dry mouth and throat, tidal malar reddening, a somber white facial complexion, spontaneous perspiration and/or night sweats, seminal emission, urinary incontinence, possible heat in the centers of the hands and feet, a pale red tongue which may either be emaciated and small in size or fat with teeth-marks, scanty fur, and a deep, fine, forceless pulse

TREATMENT PRINCIPLES: Supplement both yin and yang

RX: *Jin Gui Shen Qi Wan Jia Wei* (*Golden Cabinet* Kidney Qi Pills with Added Flavors)

INGREDIENTS: Cooked Radix Rehmanniae (*Shu Di*), Plastrum Testudinis (*Gui Ban*), and Carapax Amydae Sinensis (*Bie Jia*), 12g each, Radix Dioscoreae Oppositae (*Shan Yao*), Fructus Corni Officinalis (*Shan Zhu Yu*), Sclerotium Poriae Cocos (*Fu Ling*), Radix Lateralis Praeparatus Aconiti Carmichaeli (*Fu Zi*), and Ramulus Cinnamomi Cassiae (*Gui Zhi*), 9g each, and Rhizoma Alismatis (*Ze Xie*) and Cortex Radicis Moutan (*Dan Pi*), 6g each

ANALYSIS OF FORMULA: *Shu Di, Shan Yao, Shan Zhu Yu, Dan Pi, Ze Xie,* and *Fu Ling* are the six flavors of *Liu Wei Di Huang Wan* (Six Flavors Rehmannia Pills), a basic formula for nourishing and supplementing liver blood and kidney yin. In this formula, they also nourish yin to supplement yang based on the sayings, "Yin and yang are mutually rooted," and "Yang is engendered from yin." When *Gui Ban* and *Bie Jia* are used together, they nourish yin and subdue yang, clear vacuity heat and strengthen the bones. *Fu Zi* and *Gui Zhi* warm and supplement kidney yang.

ADDITIONS & SUBTRACTIONS: Please see patterns #1, 2 & 3 above.

ACUPUNCTURE & MOXIBUSTION: *Shen Ting* (GV 24), *Bai Hui* (GV 20), *Feng Fu* (GV 16), *Da Zhui* (GV 14), *Ling Tai* (GV 10), *Ji Zhong* (GV 6), *Ming Men* (GV 4), *Chang Qiang* (GV 1), *Shen Shu* (Bl 23), *San Yin Jiao* (Sp 6), *Fu Liu* (Ki 7), *Guan Yuan* (CV 4)

ANALYSIS OF FORMULA: Even supplementing-even draining *Shen Ting, Bai Hui, Feng Fu, Da Zhui, Ling Tai, Ji Zhong, Ming Men,* and *Chang Qiang* regulates the governing vessel and harmonizes yin and yang, opens the orifices and quiets the spirit, extinguishes wind, supports the righteous, and frees the flow of the network vessels. Supplementing *Shen Shu* and *Fu Liu* supplements kidney yin. Supplementing *San Yin Jiao* supplements liver blood and kidney yin. Supplementing *Guan Yuan* with moxibustion supplements the kidneys and invigorates yang.

ADDITIONS & SUBTRACTIONS: Please see pattern #1 above.

5. DAMP HEAT DAMAGING THE SINEWS PATTERN

MAIN SYMPTOMS: Lower limb wilting, limpness, and lack of strength, slight swelling of the ankles and numbness of the feet, a predilection for chilled things and aversion to heat, body heaviness, a yellow facial complexion, chest and ductal glomus and fullness, sticky, stagnant, not crisp stools, red, astringent urination, a dark red tongue with slimy, yellow fur, and a soggy or slippery, rapid pulse

NOTE: In real-life Western patients, this pattern rarely presents as purely as the above description. Rather, damp heat often complicates any and all of these other patterns presented in this section and especially any patterns including spleen vacuity.

TREATMENT PRINCIPLES: Clear heat and disinhibit dampness

RX: *San Miao San Jia Wei* (Three Wonders Powder with Added Flavors)

INGREDIENTS: Cortex Phellodendri (*Huang Bai*), Rhizoma Atractylodis (*Cang Zhu*), Radix Achyranthis Bidentatae (*Niu Xi*), and Rhizoma Dioscoreae Hypoglaucae (*Bi Xie*), 9g each, and Rhizoma Acori Graminei (*Shi Chang Pu*), 6g

ANALYSIS OF FORMULA: When *Huang Bai*, *Cang Zhu*, *Bei Xie*, and *Shi Chang Pu* are used together, they clear heat and both dry and disinhibit dampness. *Niu Xi* guides the other medicinals downward toward the lower limbs, quickens the blood, and strengthens the sinews and bones.

ADDITIONS & SUBTRACTIONS: For concomitant spleen qi vacuity, add nine grams each of Rhizoma Atractylodis Macrocephalae (*Bai Zhu*), Sclerotium Poriae Cocos (*Fu Ling*), and Radix Codonopsitis Pilosulae (*Dang Shen*) and six grams of mix-fried Radix Glycyrrhizae (*Gan Cao*). For concomitant liver depression, add six grams each of Fructus Meliae Toosendan (*Chuan Lian Zi*), Tuber Curcumae (*Yu Jin*), and Radix Bupleuri (*Chai Hu*) and 12 grams of Radix Albus Paeoniae Lactiflorae (*Bai Shao*). For concomitant liver-kidney vacuity, add 15 grams of cooked Radix Rehmanniae (*Shu Di*) and nine grams of Cortex Radicis Acanthopanacis Gracilistylis (*Wu Jia Pi*). For severe damp heat, add six grams of Radix Scutellariae Baicalensis (*Huang Qin*) and nine grams each of Sclerotium Poriae Cocos (*Fu Ling*) and Rhizoma Alismatis (*Ze Xie*). If damp heat has damaged yin, add nine grams each of Radix Dioscoreae Oppositae (*Shan Yao*), Radix Glehniae Littoralis (*Sha Shen*), and Radix Trichosanthis Kirlowii (*Tian Hua Fen*).

ACUPUNCTURE & MOXIBUSTION: *Shen Ting* (GV 24), *Bai Hui* (GV 20), *Feng Fu* (GV 16), *Da Zhui* (GV 14), *Ling Tai* (GV 10), *Ji Zhong* (GV 6), *Ming Men* (GV 4), *Chang Qiang* (GV 1), *Zhong Wan* (CV 12), *Zhong Ji* (CV 3), *Yin Ling Quan* (Sp 9)

ANALYSIS OF FORMULA: Even supplementing-even draining *Shen Ting, Bai Hui, Feng Fu, Da Zhui, Ling Tai, Ji Zhong, Ming Men,* and *Chang Qiang* regulates the governing vessel and harmonizes yin and yang, opens the orifices and quiets the spirit, extinguishes wind, supports the righteous, and frees the flow of the network vessels. Draining *Zhong Wan, Zhong Ji,* and *Yin Ling Quan* clears heat and eliminates dampness.

ADDITIONS & SUBTRACTIONS: Please see pattern #1 above.

6. BLOOD STASIS OBSTRUCTING THE NETWORK VESSELS PATTERN

MAIN SYMPTOMS: Enduring wilting, atrophy and lack of strength of the muscles and flesh of the four limbs, non-pitting superficial edema of the four limbs, the affected area being greenish purple in color, dry skin, joint spasms and contractures, a dark pale or dark red, emaciated, small tongue with possible static macules or spots, and a fine, choppy, forceless pulse

NOTE: This pattern rarely presents in its pure form in this disease. However, it often complicates enduring conditions.

TREATMENT PRINCIPLES: Quicken the blood and free the flow of the network vessels

RX: *Xue Fu Zhu Yu Tang Jia Jian* (Blood Mansion Dispel Stasis Decoction with Additions & Subtractions)

INGREDIENTS: Semen Pruni Persicae (*Tao Ren*) and uncooked Radix Rehmanniae (*Sheng Di*), 12g each, Flos Carthami Tinctorii (*Hong Hua*), Radix Angelicae Sinensis (*Dang Gui*), Radix Rubrus Paeoniae Lactiflorae (*Chi Shao*), and Radix Cyathulae (*Chuan Niu Xi*), 9g each, Fructus Citri Aurantii (*Zhi Ke*), Radix Ligustici Wallichi (*Chuan Xiong*), Radix Bupleuri (*Chai Hu*), and Radix Platycodi Grandiflori (*Jie Geng*), 6g each, and Radix Glycyrrhizae (*Gan Cao*), 3g

ANALYSIS OF FORMULA: *Tao Ren, Hong Hua, Dang Gui, Chi Shao, Chuan Niu Xi,* and *Chuan Xiong* quicken the blood, transform stasis, and free the flow of the network vessels. *Sheng Di* both quickens and nourishes the blood. It is included in this formula because blood stasis causes blood vacuity and blood vacuity causes blood stasis. *Zhi Ke* and *Chai Hu* move the qi to help quicken the blood. This is based on the saying, "The qi moves the blood; when the qi moves, the blood moves." *Jie Geng* helps upbear clear yang, thus disinhibiting the qi mechanism and promoting the movement of qi and, therefore, blood. *Gan Cao* harmonizes all the other medicinals in this formula.

ADDITIONS & SUBTRACTIONS: For blood stasis with marked qi vacuity, replace *Xue Fu Zhu Yu Tang* with *Bu Yang Huan Wu Tang Jia Jian* (Supplement Yang & Restore the Five [Viscera] Decoction with Additions & Subtractions): Radix Astragali Membranacei (*Huang Qi*), 60g, Radix Ligustici Wallichii (*Chuan Xiong*) and Radix Salviae Miltiorrhizae (*Dan Shen*), 30g each, Radix Achyranthis Bidentatae (*Niu Xi*), Radix Rubrus Paeoniae Lactiflorae (*Chi Shao*), Radix Angelicae Sinensis (*Dang Gui*), Lumbricus (*Di Long*), and Radix Albus Paeoniae Lactiflorae (*Bai Shao*), 9g each, and Ramulus Cinnamomi Cassiae (*Gui Zhi*) and mix-fried Radix Glycyrrhizae (*Gan Cao*), 6g each.

ACUPUNCTURE & MOXIBUSTION: *Shen Ting* (GV 24), *Bai Hui* (GV 20), *Feng Fu* (GV 16), *Da Zhui* (GV 14), *Ling Tai* (GV 10), *Ji Zhong* (GV 6), *Ming Men* (GV 4), *Chang Qiang* (GV 1), *San Yin Jiao* (Sp 6), *He Gu* (LI 4)

ANALYSIS OF FORMULA: Even supplementing-even draining *Shen Ting, Bai Hui, Feng Fu, Da Zhui, Ling Tai, Ji Zhong, Ming Men,* and *Chang Qiang* regulates the governing vessel and harmonizes yin and yang, opens the orifices and quiets the spirit, extinguishes wind, supports the righteous, and frees the flow of the network vessels. Draining *San Yin Jiao* and *He Gu* quickens the blood and transforms stasis throughout the body.

ADDITIONS & SUBTRACTIONS: Please see pattern #1 above.

7. PHLEGM TURBIDITY CONGESTING & BLOCKING PATTERN

MAIN SYMPTOMS: Unclear speech, the sound of phlegm in the throat, coughing and vomiting white, sticky phlegm, chest and ductal glomus and fullness, nausea, a sticky, slimy feeling in the mouth, a dry mouth with no desire to drink, loose stools, a pale red tongue with slimy, white fur, and a soggy, moderate (*i.e.,* slightly slow) pulse

NOTE: The above pattern describes accumulation of phlegm turbidity due to spleen vacuity. Therefore, this pattern also does not typically present in such a pure form.

TREATMENT PRINCIPLES: Dry dampness and transform phlegm

RX: *Wen Dan Tang Jia Jian* (Warm the Gallbladder Decoction with Additions & Subtractions)

INGREDIENTS: Sclerotium Poriae Cocos (*Fu Ling*), 12g, Rhizoma Pinelliae Ternatae (*Ban Xia*), Caulis Bambusae In Taeniis (*Zhu Ru*), and Rhizoma Atractylodis (*Cang Zhu*), 9g each, Pericarpium Citri Reticulatae (*Chen Pi*), Fructus Immaturus Citri Aurantii (*Zhi Shi*), and Rhizoma Arisaematis (*Tian Nan Xing*), 6g each, and Radix Glycyrrhizae (*Gan Cao*), 3g

ANALYSIS OF FORMULA: *Ban Xia, Fu Ling, Zhu Ru,* and *Tian Nan Xing* transform phlegm and harmonize the stomach. *Chen Pi* and *Zhi Shi* move the qi to disperse the phlegm based on the saying, "To treat phlegm, first treat qi." *Fu Ling* seeps dampness, while *Ban Xia, Chen Pi,* and *Cang Zhu* dry dampness. *Fu Ling, Chen Pi,* and mix-fried *Gan Cao* fortify the spleen to prevent further phlegm engenderment. This is based on the saying, "The spleen is the root of phelgm engenderment."

ADDITIONS & SUBTRACTIONS: For concomitant spleen qi vacuity, add 12 grams each of Rhizoma Atractylodis Macrocephalae (*Bai Zhu*) and Radix Codonopsitis Pilosulae (*Dang Shen*). For concomitant liver depression, add nine grams each of Radix Bupleuri (*Chai Hu*) and Radix Albus Paeoniae Lactiflorae (*Bai Shao*). For concomitant kidney qi vacuity, add six grams of Radix Lateralis Praeparatus Aconiti Carmichaeli (*Fu Zi*) and 12 grams of Ramulus Cinnamomi Cassiae (*Gui Zhi*). For yellow phlegm, add six grams of Rhizoma Coptidis Chinensis (*Huang Lian*) and Radix Scutellariae Baicalensis (*Huang Qin*) and nine grams of Bulbus Fritillariae Thunbergii (*Zhe Bei Mu*).

ACUPUNCTURE & MOXIBUSTION: *Shen Ting* (GV 24), *Bai Hui* (GV 20), *Feng Fu* (GV 16), *Da Zhui* (GV 14), *Ling Tai* (GV 10), *Ji Zhong* (GV 6), *Ming Men* (GV 4), *Chang Qiang* (GV 1), *Yin Ling Quan* (Sp 9), *Feng Long* (St 40), *Zu San Li* (St 36)

ANALYSIS OF FORMULA: Even supplementing-even draining *Shen Ting, Bai Hui, Feng Fu, Da Zhui, Ling Tai, Ji Zhong, Ming Men,* and *Chang Qiang* regulates the governing vessel and harmonizes yin and yang, opens the orifices and quiets the spirit, extinguishes wind, supports the righteous, and frees the flow of the network vessels. Draining *Yin Ling Quan* and *Feng Long* transforms and eliminates phlegm and dampness. Supplementing *Zu San Li* supplements the spleen, and "The spleen is the root of phlegm engenderment."

ADDITIONS & SUBTRACTIONS: Please see pattern #1 above.

Remarks

1. Progressive spinal myoatrophy, *i.e.*, Aran-Duchenne muscular atrophy, is a variant to ALS in which anterior horn cells involvement outpaces corticospinal involvement and the condition is more benign. Onset can begin at any age, and survival of 25 or more years is possible. The Chinese disease causes and mechanisms and most of the patterns of this disease are the same as ALS. The patterns identified in the Chinese medical literature include: A) liver blood-kidney yin vacuity, B) spleen-kidney yang vacuity, C) blood stasis obstructing the network vessels, D) phlegm dampness obstucting the channels, and E) internal stirring of liver wind. Therefore, its treatment is essentially the same as ALS.

2. Although no Chinese source lists liver depression qi stagnation as a pattern of ALS, this disease mechanism will be present in every ALS sufferer. Thus, appropriate qi-rectifying medicinals will typically need to be added to all the above Chinese medicinal protocols.

3. Chinese medical treatment of this condition is primarily intended to slow its progression and to minimize suffering and disability.

4. Amyotrophic lateral sclerosis is a type of wilting condition according to Chinese medical disease categorization, and, in Chinese medicine, there is the famous ancient saying, "Treat wilting solely by choosing the yang ming." However, as the reader will note above, based on Wang Le-ting's extensive clinical experience treating wilting conditions, we prefer to emphasize Wang's saying, "To treat wilting, first choose the governing vessel." This contemporary teaching is based on the fact that the governing vessel is the sea of all yang vessels, governing the yang of the whole body. Since yang governs stirring or movement, all functional activities of the human body are governed by yang qi. In terms of the functional activities of the limbs are concerned, if yang qi is not able to ascend and be upborne or descend and extend, yin blood becomes depressed and blocked. In that case, the movement and transportation of the qi and blood are not easily and smoothly flowing, and the sinew vessels do not receive adequate nourishment. Therefore, there is wilting, weakness, and lack of use of the limbs.

5

Aplastic Anemia

Aplastic or hypoplastic anemia refers to anemia due to failure of the bone marrow to produce blood cells. If severe, it is considered a medical emergency and may (rarely) require immediate hospitalization. However, in most patients, AA is discovered during routine screenings. Fifty to 75% of all cases of true aplastic anemia are idiopathic. It is currently suspected that idiopathic aplastic anemia is an autoimmune disease. Recognized causes of aplastic anemia include chemicals, such as benzene, toluene, and DDT, radiation, and drugs, such as antibiotics, NSAIDs, anticonvulsants, and antineoplastics. Some cases are caused by viral infection, principally viral hepatitis, although Epstein Barr virus has also been implicated in a lesser number of cases. In addition, there seems to be a genetic predisposition to this disease. While some sources say that males are more prone to this disease than females, others say its incidence is equal between males and females. Its incidence is also said to increase with age.

The onset of aplastic anemia tends to be insidious, though it occasionally may be acute. The three main clinical characteristics of this disease are: 1) weakness and fatigue, 2) fever, and 3) petechiae and bleeding. General symptoms of anemia are usually severe, such as waxy pallor of the skin and mucous membranes. Chronic cases may show considerable brown skin pigmentation. Severe thrombocytopenia may occur with bleeding into the skin. However, thrombocytopenic purpura is dealt with separately in the following chapter. In terms of blood analysis, RBCs are normochromic-normocytic, WBC counts are equal to or less than 1500/mm^3. Platelets are often markedly reduced. Reticulocytes are decreased or absent, and aspirated bone marrow is acellular.

The Western medical treatment of aplastic anemia consists of intravenous infusion of immunosuppressive agents, such as equine antithymocyte globulin (ATG) and antilymphocyte globulin (ALG), over 4-6 hours for 10 consecutive days. This is effective in approximately 60% of patients. However, because ATG is a biologic product, allergic reactions and serum sickness may occur. Therefore, all patients receiving this therapy are given concomitant corticosteroids. Cyclosporine is as effective as ATG and has gotten a positive response in 50% of ATG failures. This has led to some physicians to prescribe joint ATG and cyclosporine therapy. Patients unresponsive to ATG or cyclosporine may respond to treatment with cytokines. Other medications in current use and under investigation include hemopoetic growth factors, colony stimulating factors, interleukin-3, and androgens. In severe cases of aplastic anemia, bone marrow transplantation from an identical twin or HLA-compatible sibling has proven successful, particularly in patients under 30 years of age. Because transfusions pose a risk to subsequent transplantation, blood products are used only when essential. When used, these consist of platelet transfusion. The risk of developing subsequent malignancy after treatment for aplastic anemia is 5.5 times greater than in healthy individuals.

Chinese disease categorization: The chronic form of this disease is traditionally classified as *xu lao*, vacuity taxation, *xue xu*, bood vacuity, *wang xue*, blood collapse, and *xu ku*, blood dessication. The acute form of this disease is traditionally classified as *xue zheng*, bleeding condition, *wen re*, warm heat, *ji lao*, acute taxation, and *re lao*, heat taxation.

Disease causes: Former heaven insufficiency, latter heaven lack of nourishment, external contraction of the six environmental excesses, unregulated eating and drinking, internal damage by the seven affects, enduring disease, and bedroom taxation

Disease mechanisms: The disease mechanisms of aplastic anemia are categorized as consisting of a root vacuity with branch repletions. Of these, the root vacuity is the more important. Another way of saying this is that there is a righteous vacuity with evil repletion. The disease is located in the three viscera of the liver, spleen, and kidneys. The foremost of these are the kidneys, and the second is the spleen. In terms of righteous vacuities, these may consist of qi and blood dual vacuity, liver-kidney yin vacuity, spleen-kidney yang vacuity, and yin and yang dual vacuity. As for evil repletions, these include heat toxins and blood stasis. Either one or more of these vacuities may lead to repletion, or repletion may lead to one or more of these vacuities. However, over time, vacuity and repletion become mixed.

In chronic aplastic anemia, the main disease mechanism is qi vacuity. The spleen is the latter heaven root of qi engenderment and transformation, while the kidneys are the former heaven root. Former or latter heaven causes may result in either of these two viscera not engendering the blood. However, because the spleen and kidneys support and bolster each other, disease of one may eventually reach the other. Because the blood and essence share a common source, enduring or severe blood vacuity may also evolve into a liver-kidney yin vacuity. In addition, because yin and yang are mutually rooted, either may eventually result in the other and hence yin and yang dual vacuity.

If qi is vacuous, there is fatigue and lack of strength as well as lack of warmth in the four extremities. In addition, vacuous qi may fail to contain the blood within its vessels. If blood is vacuous, there is pallor. If yin is vacuous, there is vacuity heat which may cause nose, subdermal, or gum bleeding. If yang is vacuous, there is even more pronounced cold, loose stools, and lower extremity edema.

In acute aplastic anemia, due to a righteous qi vacuity, heat toxins take advantage and enter. If these heat and fire evils blaze and become exuberant, they may cause high fever and vexatious thirst in the qi division and bleeding when they enter the blood division.

TREATMENT BASED ON PATTERN DISCRIMINATION:

1. ACUTE TAXATION WARM HEAT PATTERN

MAIN SYMPTOMS: Acute onset of disease, high fever or recurrent low-grade fever, sweating which does not decrease the fever, dizziness, shortness of breath, lack of strength, difficulty walking, a somber white facial complexion, oral thirst, vexation and agitation, dry throat, blood blisters in the mouth and on the tongue, heart palpitations, if severe, spirit clouding, confused speech, multiple sites of spontaneous ejection of blood, dry stools, reddish urine, a pale tongue with dry, yellow or black fur with lack of fluids, possible static spots or static macules on the tongue, and a fine, rapid or vacuous, large, forceless pulse

NOTE: This pattern describes acute aplastic anemia. It is also called marrow dessication heat exuberance pattern.

TREATMENT PRINCIPLES: Clear heat and resolve toxins, cool the blood and stop bleeding

RX: *Qing Ying Tang* (Clear the Constructive Decoction)

INGREDIENTS: Cornu Bubali (*Shui Niu Jiao*), 18g, uncooked Radix Rehmanniae (*Sheng Di*), 15g, Radix Scrophulariae Ningpoensis (*Xuan Shen*) and Tuber Ophiopogonis Japonici (*Mai Dong*), 12g each, Flos Lonicerae Japonicae (*Jin Yin Hua*) and Fructus Forsythiae Suspensae (*Lian Qiao*), 9g each, Folium Bambusae (*Zhu Ye*) and Radix Salviae Miltiorrhizae (*Dan Shen*), 6g each, and Rhizoma Coptidis Chinensis (*Huang Lian*), 3g

ANALYSIS OF FORMULA: *Shui Niu Jiao*, *Sheng Di*, *Xuan Shen*, and *Dan Shen* cool the blood and stop bleeding. *Mai Men Dong* and *Zhu Ye* clear heat, nourish yin, and engender fluids. *Jin Yin Hua*, *Lian Qiao*, *Xuan Shen*, and *Huang Lian* resolve toxins in the blood division or aspect.

ADDITIONS & SUBTRACTIONS: To replace *Shui Niu Jiao*, choose from among two or more of Cortex Phellodendri (*Huang Bai*), Radix Scutellariae Baicalensis (*Huang Qin*), Herba Taraxaci Mongolici Cum Radice (*Pu Gong Ying*), Herba Violae Yedoensitis Cum Radice (*Zi Hua Di Ding*), and Radix Isatidis Seu Baphicacanthi (*Ban Lan Geng*). For severe qi division fire, add 15 grams of Gypsum Fibrosum (*Shi Gao*). For severe depletion of yin fluids, add 12 grams of Radix Glehniae Littoralis (*Sha Shen*) and nine grams of Cortex Radicis Lycii Chinensis (*Di Gu Pi*). For tremors and convulsions, add 12 grams of Ramulus Uncariae Cum Uncis (*Gou Teng*) and nine grams of Lumbricus (*Di Long*). If bleeding due to heat is severe, add 30 grams of Rhizoma Imperatae Cylindricae (*Bai Mao Gen*) and 12 grams of Radix Rubiae Cordifoliae (*Qian Cao Gen*). For simultaneous bleeding due to blood heat and qi vacuity, add 30 grams of Herba Agrimoniae Pilosae (*Xian He Cao*), 15 grams of Radix Astragali Membranacei (*Huang Qi*), and six grams of Radix Panacis Ginseng (*Ren Shen*). For subdermal bleeding, add 15 grams of Radix Lithospermi Seu Arnebiae (*Zi Cao*) and nine grams each of Cortex Radicis Moutan (*Dan Pi*) and Radix Rubrus Paeoniae Lactiflorae (*Chi Shao*). To simultaneously supplement and nourish the blood, add 15 grams each of Radix Angelicae Sinensis (*Dang Gui*), cooked Radix Rehmanniae (*Shu Di*), and Radix Polygoni Multiflori (*He Shou Wu*).

For damp heat with jaundice, replace *Qing Ying Tang* with *Yin Zhi Hu Qin Tang* (Artemisia Capillaris, Gardenia, Polygonum Cuspidatum & Scutellaria Decoction): Herba Artemisiae Capillaris (*Yin Chen Hao*), 30g, Rhizoma Imperatae

Cyclindricae (*Bai Mao Gen*), Rhizoma Polygoni Cuspidati (*Hu Zhang*), Fructus Crategi (*Shan Zha*), and Fructus Germinatus Hordei Vulgaris (*Mai Ya*), 15g each, Tuber Curcumae (*Yu Jin*), 12g, and Fructus Gardeniae Jasminoidis (*Zhi Zi*), Radix Sctuellariae Baicalensis (*Huang Qin*), and Sclerotium Poriae Cocos (*Fu Ling*), 9g each. For nose and gum bleeding, add 15 grams of uncooked Radix Rehmanniae (*Sheng Di*) and nine grams of Cortex Radicis Moutan (*Dan Pi*). For constipation, add 6-9 grams of Radix Et Rhizoma Rhei (*Da Huang*). For vomiting, add nine grams of Rhizoma Pinelliae Ternatae (*Ban Xia*) and six grams of Pericarpium Citri Reticulatae (*Chen Pi*). For simultaneous food stagnation, add six grams each of Fructus Immaturus Citri Aurantii (*Zhi Shi*) and Massa Medica Fermentata (*Shen Qu*).

ACUPUNCTURE & MOXIBUSTION: *Wei Zhong* (Bl 40), *Shi Xuan* (M-UE-1), *Zhi Gou* (TB 6), *He Gu* (LI 4)

ANALYSIS OF FORMULA: In the acute stage, acupuncture is only a auxiliary therapy. Bleeding *Wei Zhong* and the *Shi Xuan* clears heat and cools the blood. Draining *Zhi Gou* and *He Gu* clears heat and resolves toxins in the three burners.

ADDITIONS & SUBTRACTIONS: For severe heat, add *Da Zhui* (GV 14) and *Qu Chi* (LI 11). For severe depletion of yin fluids, add *Fu Liu* (Ki 7). For tremors and convulsions, add *Tai Chong* (Liv 3) and *Feng Chi* (GB 20). If bleeding due to heat is severe, add *Ge Shu* (Bl 17), *San Yin Jiao* (Sp 6), and *Xi Men* (Per 4). For severe qi vacuity, add *San Yin Jiao* (Sp 6) and *Zu San Li* (St 36). For concomitant blood vacuity, add *Gao Huang Shu* (Bl 43). For constipation, add *Tian Shu* (St 25).

2. QI & BLOOD DUAL VACUITY PATTERN

MAIN SYMPTOMS: Slow, insidious onset, dizziness, blurred vision, heart palpitations, shortness of breath, fatigue, lack of strength, a somber white or sallow yellow facial complexion, a pale tongue with white fur, and a deep, fine pulse

TREATMENT PRINCIPLES: Boost the qi and nourish the blood

RX: *Ba Zhen Tang Jia Jian* (Eight Pearls Decoction with Additions & Subtractions)

INGREDIENTS: Radix Astragali Membranacei (*Huang Qi*), 18g, Radix Codonopsitis Pilosulae (*Dang Shen*), 15g, Radix Angelicae Sinensis (*Dang Gui*) and cooked Radix Rehmanniae (*Shu Di*), 12g each, Rhizoma Atractylodis Macrocephalae (*Bai Zhu*), Sclerotium Poriae Cocos (*Fu Ling*), Radix Albus Paeoniae Lactiflorae (*Bai Shao*), and Gelatinum Corii Asini (*E Jiao*), 9g each, and mix-fried Radix Glycyrrhizae (*Gan Cao*), 6g

ANALYSIS OF FORMULA: *Huang Qi*, *Dang Shen*, *Bai Zhu*, *Fu Ling*, and mix-fried *Gan Cao* fortify the spleen and boost the qi. In addition, *Huang Qi* with *Dang Gui* is an effective combination for supplementing the blood. *Dang Shen* supplements both the qi and the blood. *Dang Gui*, *Shu Di*, *Bai Shao*, and *E Jiao* nourish and harmonize the blood. In addition, *Dang Gui* quickens the blood without inducing bleeding so as to prevent or treat blood stasis. *E Jiao*, because of its fixed nature, stops bleeding.

ADDITIONS & SUBTRACTIONS: If there is bleeding, add 30 grams of Herba Agrimoniae Pilosae (*Xian He Cao*) and nine grams of carbonized Folium Artemisiae Argyii (*Ai Ye*). For fever, add 20 grams of Flos Lonicerae Japonicae (*Jin Yin Hua*) and nine grams each of Radix Bupleuri (*Chai Hu*) and Radix Scutellariae Baicalensis (*Huang Qin*). For marked blood vacuity, add three grams each of Cortex Cinnamomi Cassiae (*Rou Gui*) and Placenta Hominis (*Zi He Che*), both powdered and taken with the strained decoction.

ACUPUNCTURE & MOXIBUSTION: *San Yin Jiao* (Sp 6), *Tai Bai* (Sp 3), *Zu San Li* (St 36), *Ge Shu* (Bl 17), *Gao Huang Shu* (Bl 43)

ANALYSIS OF FORMULA: Supplementing *San Yin Jiao*, *Tai Bai*, and *Zu San Li* fortifies the spleen to boost the qi and nourish the blood. Supplementing *Ge Shu* and *Gao Huang Shu* supplements the blood and stops bleeding.

ADDITIONS & SUBTRACTIONS: If there is bleeding, add *Xue Hai* (Sp 10). For fever, add *He Gu* (LI 4) and *Wai Guan* (TB 5). If there is concomitant liver depression, add *Tai Chong* (Liv 3). For dizziness, add *Bai Hui* (GV 20) (moxa). For blurred vision, add *Gan Shu* (Bl 18) or *Guang Ming* (GB 37). For heart palpitations, add *Shen Men* (Ht 7).

3. SPLEEN-KIDNEY YANG VACUITY PATTERN

MAIN SYMPTOMS: A sallow, lusterless facial complexion, somber white lips and nails, shortness of breath, lack of strength in the four limbs, fatigue, a faint, weak voice, fear of cold, chilled limbs, low back and knee soreness and limpness, scanty intake, loose stools, lower extremity edema, clear, long, frequent urination, possible spontaneous perspiration, possible gum bleeding, subdermal bleeding, or uterine bleeding, a fat, pale tongue with teeth-marks on its edges, and a deep, fine pulse

NOTE: This pattern is seen in relatively light cases of chronic aplastic anemia or after the liver-kidney pattern has improved.

TREATMENT PRINCIPLES: Warm and supplement the spleen and kidneys

RX: *Si Jun Zi Tang* (Four Gentlemen Decoction) & *Zuo Gui Wan* (Restore the Left [Kidney] Pills) with additions and subtractions

INGREDIENTS: Radix Astragali Membranacei (*Huang Qi*) and Radix Codonopsitis Pilosulae (*Dang Shen*), 18g each, cooked Radix Rehmanniae (*Shu Di*), 15g, Rhizoma Atactylodis Macrocephalae (*Bai Zhu*) and Radix Dioscoreae Oppositae (*Shan Yao*), 12g each, Radix Angelicae Sinensis (*Dang Gui*), Fructus Psoraleae Corylifoliae (*Bu Gu Zhi*), Herba Epimedii (*Xian Ling Pi*), Radix Morindae Officinalis (*Ba Ji Tian*), and Gelatinum Cornu Cervi (*Lu Jiao Jiao*), 9g each, Pericarpium Citri Reticulatae (*Chen Pi*), 6g, and Cortex Cinnamomi Cassiae (*Rou Gui*), 3g

ANALYSIS OF FORMULA: *Huang Qi, Dang Shen, Bai Zhu,* and *Shan Yao* fortify the spleen and boost the qi. *Chen Pi* dries dampness, moves the qi, and helps the transformation function of the spleen. *Shu Di* and *Dang Gui* nourish kidney-liver yin essence from which to transform yang. *Bu Gu Zhi, Yin Yang Huo, Ba Ji Tian, Lu Jiao Jiao,* and *Rou Gui* warm and supplement kidney yang. In addition, *Lu Jiao Jiao* boosts the essence and stops bleeding.

ADDITIONS & SUBTRACTIONS: If there is concomitant upper respiratory infection, choose additions from among: Radix Platycodi Grandiflori (*Jie Geng*), Fructus Arctii Lappae (*Niu Bang Zi*), Semen Pruni Armeniacae (*Xing Ren*), Bulbus Fritillariae Thunbergii (*Zhe Bei Mu*), Radix Peucedani (*Qian Hu*), Herba Seu Flos Schizonepetae Tenuifoliae (*Jing Jie Sui*), Folium Lophatheri Gracilis (*Dan Zhu Ye*), Fructus Forsythiae Suspensae (*Lian Qiao*), and Flos Lonicerae Japonicae (*Jin Yin Hua*). If there are loose stools, add three grams of Fructus Evodiae Rutecarpae (*Wu Zhu Yu*) and nine grams of Semen Myristicae Fragrantis (*Rou Dou Kou*). If there is a faint, fine pulse, great sweating, and reversal counterflow of the four limbs, add six grams of Radix Lateralis Praeparatus Aconiti Carmichaeli (*Fu Zi*) and double the dose of *Rou Gui.* For marked kidney essence vacuity, add 15 grams of Fructus Lycii Chinensis (*Gou Qi* Zi) and three grams of Placenta Hominis (*Zi He Che*) powdered and taken with the strained decoction. For bleeding, add 15 grams each of Pollen Typhae (*Pu Huang*) and Herba Agrimoniae Pilosae (*Xian He Cao*) and increase the dosage of *Lu Jiao Jiao* up to 15g. For stomach and abdominal fullness and loose stools, add nine grams each of Fructus Amomi (*Sha Ren*) and Radix Auklandiae Lappae (*Mu Xiang*). For reduced appetite, add nine grams each of Massa Medica Fermentata (*Shen Qu*), Fructus Crataegi (*Shan Zha*), and Fructus Germinatus Hordei Vulgaris (*Mai Ya*). For edema, add 15 grams of Sclerotium Poriae Cocos (*Fu Ling*) and 12 grams of Rhizoma Alismatis (*Ze Xie*). For concomitant blood stasis, add 15 grams each of Pollen Typhae (*Pu Huang*) and Radix Salviae Miltiorrhizae (*Dan Shen*) and three grams of Radix Pseudoginseng (*San Qi*), powdered and taken with the strained decoction.

ACUPUNCTURE & MOXIBUSTION: *Pi Shu* (Bl 20), *Wei Shu* (Bl 21), *Shen Shu* (Bl 23), *Ming Men* (GV 4), *Da Zhui* (GV 14)

ANALYSIS OF FORMULA: Supplementing *Pi Shu, Wei Shu, Shen Shu, Ming Men,* and *Da Zhui* with moxibustion warms and supplements spleen and kidney yang.

ADDITIONS & SUBTRACTIONS: If there are loose stools, add *Yin Ling Quan* (Sp 9). If there is a faint, fine pulse, great sweating, and reversal counterflow of the four limbs, add *Guan Yuan* (CV 4) and *Qi Hai* (CV 6). For marked kidney essence vacuity, add *San Yin Jiao* (Sp 6). For bleeding, add *Ge Shu* (Bl 17) and *San Yin Jiao* (Sp 6). For stomach and abdominal fullness and loose stools, add *Nei Guan* (Per 6) and *Gong Sun* (Sp 4). For reduced appetite, add *Liang Men* (St 21). For edema, add *San Yin Jiao* (Sp 6) and *Yin Ling Quan* (Sp 9).

4. LIVER-KIDNEY YIN VACUITY PATTERN

MAIN SYMPTOMS: Pale lips and nails, a pale, lusterless facial complexion, bodily fatigue, lack of strength, headache, dizziness, tinnitus, heart vexation, heart palpitations, low-grade fever, night sweats, low back and knee soreness and limpness, blurred vision, dry eyes, dry throat, insomnia, profuse dreams, possible nosebleed, subdermal bleeding, and/or bleeding gums, in severe cases, hemafecia, hematemesis, or uterine bleeding, a pale red tongue with scanty or no fur, and a fine, rapid pulse

NOTE: This pattern mostly occurs in severe or acute aplastic anemia.

TREATMENT PRINCIPLES: Enrich and nourish the liver and kidneys

RX: *Da Bu Yuan Jian* (Greatly Supplementing the Source Decoction) & *Er Zhi Wan* (Two Ultimates Pills) with additions and subtractions

INGREDIENTS: Fructus Mori Albi (*Sang Shen*), 18g, Radix Codonopsitis Pilosulae (*Dang Shen*), cooked Radix Rehmanniae (*Shu Di*), uncooked Radix Rehmanniae (*Sheng Di*), Rhizoma Polygonati (*Huang Jing*), Fructus Lycii Chinensis (*Gou Qi Zi*), Herba Ecliptae Prostratae (*Han Lian Cao*), and Radix Polygoni Multiflori (*He Shou Wu*), 15g each, Fructus Corni Officinalis (*Shan Zhu Yu*), 12g, Radix Angelicae Sinensis (*Dang Gui*) and Fructus Ligustri Lucidi (*Nu Zhen Zi*), 9g each, and mix-fried Radix Glycyrrhizae (*Gan Cao*), 6g

ANALYSIS OF FORMULA: *Shu Di, Sheng Di, Sang Shen, Gou Qi, Han Lian Cao, He Shou Wu, Shan Zhu Yu, Nu Zhen Zi,* and *Dang Gui* together nourish liver blood and enrich kidney yin, fill the essence and boost the origin. *Dang Shen* and *Huang Jing* fortify the spleen and boost the qi, supplement the latter heaven to support the former heaven. *Gan Cao* harmonizes the other medicinals in this formula. In addition, *Sheng Di*, *Han Lian Cao*, and *Shan Zhu Yu* all stop bleeding.

ADDITIONS & SUBTRACTIONS: If there is fever, add 12 grams each of Herba Artemisiae Apiaceae (*Qing Hao*) and Cortex Radicis Lycii Chinensis (*Di Gu Pi*) and nine grams of Rhizoma Anemarrhenae Aspheloidis (*Zhi Mu*). For marked bleeding, add 12 grams of Radix Sanguisorbae (*Di Yu*) and nine grams each of Cacumen Biotae Orientalis (*Ce Bai Ye*) and Gelatinum Corii Asini (*E Jiao*). If concomitant qi vacuity is marked, add 15 grams of Radix Astragali Membranacei (*Huang Qi*) and nine grams of Radix Dioscoreae Oppositae (*Shan Yao*). For concomitant blood stasis, add 15 grams each of Pollen Typhae (*Pu Huang*), and Radix Salviae Miltiorrhizae (*Dan Shen*) and three grams of Radix Pseudoginseng (*San Qi*), powdered and taken with the strained decoction.

For qi and yin vacuity with concomitant heat toxins and blood stasis, replace *Da Bu Yuan Jian* and *Er Zhi Wan* with *Sheng Xue Tang San Hao* (Engender the Blood Decoction No. 3): Herba Oldenlandiae Diffusae Cum Radice (*Bai Hua She She Cao*), 40g, Rhizoma Polygoni Cuspidati (*Hu Zhang*), Radix Astragali Membranacei (*Huang Qi*), and Fructus Ligustri Lucidi (*Nu Zhen Zi*), 25g each, Fructus Lycii Chinensis (*Gou Qi Zi*), Rhizoma Polygonati (*Huang Jing*), Radix Angelicae Sinensis (*Dang Gui*), Radix Codonopsitis Pilosulae (*Dang Shen*), Radix Pseudostellariae (*Tai Zi Shen*), Radix Salviae Miltiorrhizae (*Dan Shen*), Caulis Polygoni Multiflori (*Ye Jiao Teng*), Fructus Corni Officinalis (*Shan Zhu Yu*), Rhizoma Atractylodis Macrocephalae (*Bai Zhu*), and Cortex Radicis Moutan (*Dan Pi*), 20g each, Gelatinum Corii Asini (*E Jiao*), Radix Polygoni Multiflori (*He Shou Wu*), Pericarpium Citri Reticulatae (*Chen Pi*), and cooked Radix Rehmanniae (*Shu Di*), 15g each, and Rhizoma Alismatis (*Ze Xie*), 9g.

ACUPUNCTURE & MOXIBUSTION: *San Yin Jiao* (Sp 6), *Tai Xi* (Ki 3), *Gan Shu* (Bl 18), *Shen Shu* (Bl 23)

ANALYSIS OF FORMULA: Supplementing *San Yin Jiao*, *Tai Xi*, *Gan Shu*, and *Shen Shu* together nourishes liver blood and enriches kidney yin, fills the essence, and boosts the origin.

ADDITIONS & SUBTRACTIONS: If there is fever, add *Da Zhui* (GV 14) and *Yin Xi* (Ht 6). For marked bleeding, add *Ge Shu* (Bl 17) and *Xue Hai* (Sp 10). If there is concomitant qi vacuity, add *Zu San Li* (St 36).

5. YIN & YANG DUAL VACUITY PATTERN

MAIN SYMPTOMS: A somber white facial complexion, dizziness, lack of strength, low back and lower leg soreness and limpness, seminal emission, decreased sexual desire, sometimes hot, sometimes chilled, spontaneous perspiration, night sweats, tinnitus, heart palpitations, a pale tongue with white or possibly scanty fur, and a deep, fine, forceless or deep, fine, rapid pulse depending on whether yin or yang vacuity is most severe

NOTE: This pattern mainly presents in chronic aplastic anemia or after liver-kidney pattern aplastic anemia has improved due to treatment.

TREATMENT PRINCIPLES: Supplement both yin and yang

RX: *Hei Long Bu Shen Zhu Yang Fang* (Black Dragon Supplement the Kidneys & Assist Yang Formula)

INGREDIENTS: Caulis Milletiae Seu Spatholobi (*Ji Xue Teng*), 15g, Radix Astragali Membranacei (*Huang Qi*), Radix Polygoni Multiflori (*He Shou Wu*), Radix Albus Paeoniae Lactiflorae (*Bai Shao*), and Fructus Lycii Chinensis (*Gou Qi Zi*), 12g each, Radix Angelicae Sinensis (*Dang Gui*), Tuber Asparagi Cocohinensis (*Tian Men Dong*), Tuber Ophiopogonis Japonici (*Mai Men Dong*), Herba Epimedii (*Xian Ling Pi*), Rhizoma Curculiginis Orchioidis (*Xian Mao*), Fructus Corni Officinalis (*Shan Zhu Yu*), and Semen Cuscutae Chinensis (*Tu Si Zi*), 9g each, Radix Lateralis Preparatus Aconiti Carmichaeli (*Fu Zi*), 6g, and Radix Rubrus Panacis Ginseng (*Hong Shen*), mix-fried Radix Glycyrrhizae (*Gan Cao*), and Cortex Cinnamomi Cassiae (*Rou Gui*), 3g each

ANALYSIS OF FORMULA: *He Shou Wu*, *Bai Shao*, *Gou Qi*, *Dang Gui*, *Tian Men Dong*, *Mai Men Dong*, and *Shan Zhu Yu* together nourish liver blood and enrich kidney yin, fill the essence and boost the origin. *Yin Yang Huo*, *Xian Mao*, *Shan Zhu Yu*, *Tu Si Zi*, *Fu Zi*, *Hong Shen*, and *Rou Gui* warm and supplement kidney yang. *Hong Shen*, *Huang Qi*, and mix-fried *Gan Cao* fortify the spleen, boost the qi, and supplement latter heaven to support former heaven. *Ji Xue Teng* nourishes and quickens the blood.

ADDITIONS & SUBTRACTIONS: If there are loose stools, add nine grams each of Radix Dioscoreae Oppositae (*Shan Yao*), Fructus Psoraleae Corylifoliae (*Bu Gu Zhi*), and Semen Myristicae Fragrantis (*Rou Dou Kou*). If the limbs are chilled at the same time as there is a sensation of burning heat within the heart and sores on the tongue, add 15 grams of Plastrum Testudinis (*Gui Ban*). For concomitant blood stasis, add 15 grams each of Pollen Typhae (*Pu Huang*) and Radix Salviae Miltiorrhizae (*Dan Shen*) and three grams of Radix Pseudoginseng (*San Qi*), powdered and taken with the strained decoction. Please, refer to patterns #3 and 4.

ACUPUNCTURE & MOXIBUSTION: *Gan Shu* (Bl 18), *Pi*

Shu (Bl 20), *Wei Shu* (Bl 21), *Shen Shu* (Bl 23), *San Yin Jiao* (Sp 6)

ANALYSIS OF FORMULA: *Gan Shu* supplements liver yin and blood. *Pi Shu* and *Wei Shu* fortify the spleen, boost the qi, and supplement latter heaven to support former heaven. *Shen Shu* supplements both kidney yin and yang. *San Yin Jiao* supplements former and latter heaven, the qi, blood, yin, essence, liver, spleen, and kidneys.

ADDITIONS & SUBTRACTIONS: For marked kidney yang vacuity, add *Ming Men* (GV 4). For marked kidney yin vacuity, add *Fu Liu* (Ki 7). For dizziness, add *Bai Hui* (GV 20). For lack of strength, add *Zu San Li* (St 36). For low back and lower leg soreness and limpness, add *Fu Liu* (Ki 7). For yin vacuity-fire effulgence, add *Zhao Hai* (Ki 6). For decreased sexual desire, add *Ming Men* (GV 4). For seminal emission, add *Zhi Shi* (Bl 52). For spontaneous perspiration, add *Da Zhui* (GV 14). For night sweats, add *Yin Xi* (Ht 6). For concomitant blood stasis or bleeding, add *Ge Shu* (Bl 17).

REMARKS

1. The first clinical symptom of anemia is fatigue, and fatigue is always a qi vacuity symptom. Therefore, it is important not to immediately confuse the Western idea of anemia as a blood disorder and deficiency with the Chinese medical concept of blood vacuity. There is only a pattern of blood vacuity when there is not only fatigue but marked facial and mucous membrane pallor. Qi vacuity typically complicates or is present in all other patterns of aplastic anemia whether or not the name of the pattern recognizes that fact.

6

Behçet's Syndrome

Behçet's syndrome is a chronic, relapsing, inflammatory disorder of unknown etiology that may involve the mucocutaneous, ocular, genital, articular, vascular, CNS, and GI systems. This syndrome generally begins in the 30s and occurs in twice as many men as women. Almost all patients with Behçet's syndrome have recurrent oral ulcers which are typically the first manifestation of this disease. Similar ulcers may appear on the penis and scrotum in men or on the vulva and vagina in women. Other symptoms develop in days to years. These may include eye pain, photophobia, blurred vision, blindness, skin papules, pustules, vesicles, and folliculitis, mild arthritis of the knees and other large joints, arterial aneurysms and thrombosis, and gastrointestinal manifestations ranging from nonspecific abdominal discomfort to regional enteritis resembling Crohn's disease.

Western medical diagnosis depends on the clinical manifestations since there are no specific, pathognomonic laboratory tests even though numerous immunologic abnormalities may be detected. Because this condition must be differentiated from RA, SLE, Crohn's disease, ulcerative colitis, ankylosing spondylitis, and herpes simplex infections, its diagnosis may require months, and there is no specific Western medical treatment for it in any case. Although topical corticosteriods are often used for temporary relief of eye and oral disease, neither topical nor internally administered corticosteroids alter the frequency of relapses. Immunosuppressive drugs have been used with some success in patients with severe disease. However, this syndrome is generally benign.

Chinese disease categorization: Behçet's syndrome is primarily categorized in Chinese medicine as *hu huo bing*, fox-like puzzling disease. "Fox puzzling" is first mentioned in Zhang Zhong-jing's *Jin Gui Yao Lue (Essentials of the Golden Cabinet)*:

> The disease of fox puzzling resembles damage due to cold. [The patient is] silent, desires to sleep but is not able to close their eyes, lying down and standing up restlessly. Sores in the throat are called puzzling, while sores on the yin are called fox-like. There is no desire to eat or drink, and [the patient] is averse to the odor of food. The face and eyes may be red, black, or white. If sores develop in the upper region of the body, there will be hoarseness.

Numerous signs and symptoms of Behçet's syndrome are also Chinese diseases in their own right. Oral sores are *kou gan*. Sores on the genitalia are *yin chuang*. Eye pain is *mu tong*, photophobia is *xiu ming*, and blurred vision is *hua yan*. Papules are *zhen*, vesicles are *shui pao*, and pustules and folliculitis commonly fall under the category of *yong* or welling abscesses. Arthritis is categorized as *bi*, impediment, thrombophlebitis usually is categorized as *tong zhong*, pain and swelling, and abdominal pain is *fu tong*.

Disease causes: External invasion of damp heat toxic qi, internal engenderment of damp evils which transform into heat, overeating acrid, hot, fatty, sweet foods, or retained toxins after a heat disease

Disease mechanisms: Due to any of the above causes, heat toxins may internally assault the liver, gallbladder, spleen, stomach, heart, or kidneys. Following the channels, these heat toxins may then travel to the mouth, eyes, and external yin, causing pathological changes in those areas. In the early stage of this disease, there is mostly spleen-stomach brewing of heat, liver-gallbladder damp heat, or damp heat pouring downward. Hence the condition during the early phase of this disease tends to be predominantly replete. When damp heat evils fall inward, they cause damage and detriment of the viscera. If they are emitted outward, they result in welling and flat abscesses. Thus, in the middle and later stages of this disease, there is mostly mixed vacuity and repletion. Damp heat remains the most important disease evil, but enduring damp heat may now have damaged the liver, spleen, and/or kidneys. Hence there may be liver-kidney yin vacuity, spleen-kidney yang vacuity, or qi and blood dual vacuity. Because of the inter-relationships between the qi, blood, and fluids and humors, there may also be blood stasis.

TREATMENT BASED ON PATTERN DISCRIMINATION:

1. SPLEEN-STOMACH BREWING HEAT PATTERN

MAIN SYMPTOMS: In the early stage of this disease, there are mouth, eye, and external genital sores of various sizes which are mostly painful. These are primarily located within the oral cavity. Diffuse, red-colored, macular lesions may be seen on the skin of the four limbs. There is oral thirst with a desire for chilled drinks, rapid hungering, clamoring stomach, possible addiction to alcohol, bad breath, swollen, painful gums, a red tongue with yellow fur, and a slippery, rapid pulse.

TREATMENT PRINCIPLES: Clear heat and disinhibit dampness using bitter and acrid to free the flow and downbear

RX: *Gan Cao Xie Xin Tang* (Licorice Drain the Heart Decoction)

INGREDIENTS: Mix-fried Radix Glycyrrhizae (*Gan Cao*), 15g, Radix Codonopsitis Pilosulae (*Dang Shen*), Rhizoma Pinelliae Ternatae (*Ban Xia*), and Radix Scutellariae Baicalensis (*Huang Qin*), 9g each, Fructus Zizyphi Jujubae (*Da Zao*), 3 pieces, dry Rhizoma Zingiberis (*Gan Jiang*), 6g, and Rhizoma Coptidis Chinensis (*Huang Lian*), 3g

ANALYSIS OF FORMULA: *Huang Qin* and *Huang Lian* clear heat and dry dampness. *Ban Xia* dries dampness and harmonizes the stomach. *Gan Jiang*, *Da Zao*, mix-fried *Gan Cao* and *Dang Shen* fortify the spleen to prevent damp accumulation.

ADDITIONS & SUBTRACTIONS: For constipation, add 3-6 grams of Radix Et Rhizoma Rhei (*Da Huang*). For sticky mouth and slimy tongue fur, add 30 grams of Herba Artemisiae Capillaris (*Yin Chen Hao*) and 15 grams of Talcum (*Hua Shi*). For external genital sores, add 30 grams of Rhizoma Smilacis Glabrae (*Tu Fu Ling*).

For more severe replete heat in the spleen-stomach, replace *Gan Cao Xie Xin Tang* with *Yu Nu Jian Jia Jian* (Jade Woman Decoction with Additions & Subtractions): Gypsum Fibrosum (*Shi Gao*) and Herba Artemisiae Capillaris (*Yin Chen Hao*), 30g each, uncooked Radix Rehmanniae (*Sheng Di*) and Rhizoma Anemarrhenae Asphodeloidis (*Zhi Mu*), 12g each, Herba Agastachis Seu Pogostemi (*Huo Xiang*), Cortex Radicis Moutan (*Dan Pi*), and Radix Cyathulae (*Chuan Niu Xi*), 9g each, and Rhizoma Coptidis Chinensis (*Huang Lian*), Rhizoma Cimicifugae (*Sheng Ma*), and Radix Glycyrrhizae (*Gan Cao*), 6g each.

ACUPUNCTURE & MOXIBUSTION: *Nei Ting* (St 44), *Zhong Wan* (CV 12), *He Gu* (LI 4), *Da Ling* (Per 7)

ANALYSIS OF FORMULA: Draining *Nei Ting*, *Zhong Wan*, and *He Gu* clears and discharges heat in the spleen and stomach. *Da Ling* is an empirical point for treating oral sores and bad breath.

ADDITIONS & SUBTRACTIONS: For eyes sores, add *Tai Yang* (M-HN-9), *Si Zhu Kong* (TB 23), *Tong Zi Liao* (GB 1), and *Zan Zhu* (Bl 2) (bleed). For external genital sores, add *Qu Gu* (CV 2) and *Li Gou* (Liv 5). For macular lesions on the skin, add *Ling Tai* (GV 10) and *Wei Zhong* (Bl 40). For constipation, add *Zhi Gou* (TB 6). For sticky mouth and slimy tongue fur, add *Yin Ling Quan* (Sp 9).

2. LIVER-GALLBLADDER DAMP HEAT PATTERN

MAIN SYMPTOMS: During acute episodes, there are oral, throat, and/or external genital sores and both eyes are red, burning hot, and painful. Sometimes there is yellow matter oozing from the corners of the eyes. In addition, there is generalized fever, heart vexation, chest fullness, rib-side pain, a bitter, sticky taste in the mouth, foul, fishy smelling, yellow vaginal discharge in females, testicular swelling and pain in males, a desire to sleep but insomnia or perturbed, restless sleep, constipation or uneasy defecation, possible joint pain, a red tongue with slimy, yellow fur, and a bowstring, rapid or slippery, rapid pulse.

TREATMENT PRINCIPLES: Clear heat and drain fire, dry dampness and resolve toxins

RX: *Long Dan Xie Gan Tang* (Gentiana Drain the Liver Decoction)

INGREDIENTS: Uncooked Radix Rehmanniae (*Sheng Di*) and Radix Scutellariae Baicalensis (*Huang Qin*), 12g each, Fructus Gardeniae Jasminoidis (*Zhi Zi*), Caulis Akebiae (*Mu Tong*), Radix Bupleuri (*Chai Hu*), and Extremitas Radicis Angelicae Sinensis (*Dang Gui Wei*), 9g each, Radix Gentianae Scabrae (*Long Dan Cao*), Rhizoma Alismatis (*Ze Xie*), and Semen Plantaginis (*Che Qian Zi*), 6g each, and Radix Glycyrrhizae (*Gan Cao*), 3g

ANALYSIS OF FORMULA: *Huang Qin*, *Zhi Zi*, and *Long Dan Cao* clear the liver and drain fire, dry dampness and resolve toxins. *Mu Tong*, *Ze Xie*, and *Che Qian Zi* clear and disinhibit dampness and heat. *Sheng Di* protects the yin of the liver from the bitter, drying nature of the other medicinals. *Chai*

Hu courses the liver and resolves depression. It prevents liver depression from transforming into heat. *Dang Gui Wei* quickens the blood and transforms stasis. *Gan Cao* harmonizes the other medicinals in this formula and protects the stomach from the bitter, drying medicinals in it.

Additions & subtractions: For fever, add 25 grams of Gypsum Fibrosum (*Shi Gao*) and 12 grams of Rhizoma Anemarrhenae Asphodeloidis (*Zhi Mu*). For edema in the lower limbs, add 12 grams each of Sclerotium Polypori Umbellati (*Zhu Ling*), Sclerotium Poriae Cocos (*Fu Ling*), and Semen Phaseoli Calcarati (*Chi Xiao Dou*). For skin pustules, vesicles, or folliculitis, add 12 grams each of Cortex Radicis Moutan (*Dan Pi*), Radix Rubrus Paeoniae Lactiflorae (*Chi Shao*), and Radix Lithospermi Seu Arnebiae (*Zi Cao*). For eye sores, add 12 grams each of Semen Cassiae Torae (*Jue Ming Zi*) and Semen Celosiae Argentae (*Qing Xiang Zi*). For external genital sores, add nine grams each of Spina Gleditschiae Chinensis (*Zao Jiao Ci*) and Cortex Phellodendri (*Huang Bai*) and 15 grams of Rhizoma Smilacis Glabrae (*Tu Fu Ling*). For pus anywhere in the body, add 15 grams each of Herba Taraxaci Mongolici Cum Radice (*Pu Gong Ying*) and Herba Scutellariae Barbatae (*Ban Zhi Lian*). For constipation, add 9-12 grams of Radix Et Rhizoma Rhei (*Da Huang*). For sore throat, add 15 grams of Radix Istadis Seu Baphicacanthi (*Ban Lan Gen*) and nine grams of Fructus Arctii Lappae (*Niu Bang Zi*).

Acupuncture & moxibustion: *Xing Jian* (Liv 2), *Yang Ling Quan* (GB 34), *Yin Ling Quan* (Sp 9), *Nei Ting* (St 44)

Analysis of formula: Draining *Xing Jian* and *Yang Ling Quan* clears the liver and drains fire, disinhibits dampness and resolves depression, while draining *Yin Ling Quan* and *Nei Ting* clears and disinhibits dampness and heat.

Additions & subtractions: For fever, add *Qu Chi* (LI 11). For edema in the lower limbs, add *Zhong Ji* (CV 3) and *San Yin Jiao* (Sp 6). For skin pustules, vesicles, or folliculitis, add *Ling Tai* (GV 10) and *Wei Zhong* (Bl 40). For eye sores, add *Tai Yang* (M-HN-9), *Si Zhu Kong* (TB 23), *Tong Zi Liao* (GB 1), and *Zan Zhu* (Bl 2) (bleed). For external genital sores, add *Qu Gu* (CV 2) and *Li Gou* (Liv 5). For constipation, add *Zhi Gou* (TB 6). For sore throat, add *Shao Shang* (Lu 11) (bleed), *Shang Yang* (LI 1) (bleed), and *Chi Ze* (Lu 5).

3. Damp heat pouring downward pattern

Main symptoms: During acute occurrences, there are relatively pronounced sores of various sizes in the genital region whose surfaces are covered in a yellowish white, thick, turbid matter or which exude pus. These are surrounded by redness and swelling and they are painful. These sores make movement difficult, and the lower abdomen is full and crampy. There may be a red-colored macular rash on the external genitalia or the two lower limbs. Sometimes this rash may be nodular or have a pussy head, in which case there is severe aching and pain. The urination is short and red or hot, astringent, strangurious, and painful. The tongue is red with yellow fur or only the fur at the root of the tongue may be yellow or yellow and slimy. The pulse is slippery and rapid.

Treatment principles: Clear heat, disinhibit dampness, and resolve toxins

Rx: *Huang Lian Jie Du Tang* (Coptis Resolve Toxins Decoction) & *Wu Wei Xiao Du Yin* (Five Flavors Disperse Toxins Drink)

Ingredients: Rhizoma Coptidis Chinensis (*Huang Lian*), Flos Lonicerae Japonicae (*Jin Yin Hua*), Flos Chrysanthemi Indici (*Ye Ju Hua*), Herba Violae Yedoensitis Cum Radice (*Zi Hua Di Ding*), Herba Taraxaci Mongolici Cum Radice (*Pu Gong Ying*), and Radix Scutellariae Baicalensis (*Huang Qin*), 12g each, and Cortex Phellodendri (*Huang Bai*), Fructus Gardeniae Jasminoidis (*Zhi Zi*), and Radix Semiaquilegiae (*Tian Kui Zi*), 9g each

Analysis of formula: *Huang Lian, Jin Yin Hua, Ye Ju Hua, Zi Hua Di Ding, Pu Gong Ying, Huang Qin, Huang Bai, Zhi Zi,* and *Tian Kui Zi* all clear heat and discharge fire, disinhibit or dry dampness, resolve toxins and disperse pus.

Additions & subtractions: Please see pattern #2 above.

Acupuncture & moxibustion: *Xing Jian* (Liv 2), *Yin Ling Quan* (Sp 9), *Nei Ting* (St 44), *Hui Yin* (CV 1), *Li Gou* (Liv 5), *Qu Gu* (CV 2)

Analysis of formula: Draining *Xing Jian* clears the liver and drains fire, disinhibits dampness and resolves depression. Draining *Yin Ling Quan* and *Nei Ting* clears and disinhibits dampness and heat. Draining *Hui Yin, Li Gou,* and *Qu Gu* clears and disinhibits damp heat in the liver channel and in the genital area.

Additions & subtractions: Same as above

4. Spleen vacuity mixed with dampness pattern

Main symptoms: Oral, eye, or genital sores which endure and do not close, pale colored lesions which are flat or concave in shape, lassitude of the spirit, lack of strength, devitalized eating and drinking, abdominal distention and discomfort, loose stools, long, clear urination, lack of warmth in the four limbs, possible low-grade fever, dizziness and/or a distended feeling of the head, a fat, pale tongue with teethmarks on its edges, and a fine, moderate (*i.e.*, slightly slow pulse)

TREATMENT PRINCIPLES: Fortify the spleen, boost the qi, and eliminate dampness

RX: *Bu Zhong Yi Qi Tang Jia Wei* (Supplement the Center & Boost the Qi Decoction with Added Flavors)

INGREDIENTS: Radix Astragali Membrancei (*Huang Qi*), 15g, Radix Codonopsitis Pilosulae (*Dang Shen*), 12g, Rhizoma Atractylodis Macrocephalae (*Bai Zhu*), Rhizoma Atractylodis (*Cang Zhu*), Herba Agastachis Seu Pogostemi (*Huo Xiang*) and Herba Eupatorei Fortunei (*Pei Lan*), 9g each, Radix Angelicae Sinensis (*Dang Gui*) and Pericarpium Citri Reticulatae (*Chen Pi*), 6g each, Rhizoma Cimicifugae (*Sheng Ma*), 4.5g, and Radix Bupleuri (*Chai Hu*) and mix-fried Radix Glycyrrhizae (*Gan Cao*), 3g each

ANALYSIS OF FORMULA: *Huang Qi, Dang Shen, Bai Zhu,* and mix-fried *Gan Cao* fortify the spleen and boost the qi, thus preventing further damp accumulation. *Bai Zhu, Cang Zhu, Huo Xiang, Pei Lan,* and *Chen Pi* arouse the spleen, dry dampness, and transform and downbear turbidity. *Dang Gui* harmonizes the blood, while *Chen Pi* rectifies the qi, and *Chai Hu* and *Sheng Ma* help *Huang Qi* upbear the clear.

ADDITIONS & SUBTRACTIONS: For undigested food in stools, reduced appetite, and nausea after meals, add 15 grams each of Endothelium Corneum Gigeriae Galli (*Ji Nei Jin*), Fructus Germinatus Hordei Vulgaris (*Mai Ya*), and Semen Coicis Lachryma-jobi (*Yi Yi Ren*). For phlegm, add nine grams each of Rhizoma Pinelliae Ternatae (*Ban Xia*) and Sclerotium Poriae Cocos (*Fu Ling*), and 15 grams of Fructus Trichosanthis Kirlowii (*Gua Lou*). For sores which endure and do not close, add nine grams of Semen Oroxyli Indici (*Mu Hu Die*) and 15 grams of Fructificatio Lasiospherae Seu Calvatiae (*Ma Bo*). For sliminess in the mouth and abdominal distention, add nine grams of Cortex Magnoliae Officinalis (*Hou Po*) and six grams of Semen Alpiniae Katsumadai (*Cao Dou Kou*).

ACUPUNCTURE & MOXIBUSTION: *Zu San Li* (St 36), *Tai Bai* (Sp 3), *Yin Ling Quan* (Sp 9)

ANALYSIS OF FORMULA: Supplementing *Zu San Li* and *Tai Bai* fortifies the spleen, boosts the qi, and prevents further dampness accumulation. Draining *Yin Ling Quan* eliminates dampness.

ADDITIONS & SUBTRACTIONS: For abdominal distention, add *Tian Shu* (St 25). For undigested food in the stools, reduced appetite, and nausea after meals, add *Liang Men* (St 21). For phlegm, add *Feng Long* (St 40). For severe spleen qi vacuity, add *Pi Shu* (Bl 20) and *Wei Shu* (Bl 21). For edema in the lower limbs, add *Zhong Ji* (CV 3) and *San Yin Jiao* (Sp 6). For eye sores, add *Tai Yang* (M-HN-9), *Si Zhu Kong* (TB 23), *Tong Zi Liao* (GB 1), and *Zan Zhu* (Bl 2) (bleed). For external genital sores, add *Qu Gu* (CV 2) and *Hui Yin* (CV 1). For sores in the oral cavity, add *Da Ling* (Per 7).

5. LIVER-KIDNEY YIN VACUITY PATTERN

MAIN SYMPTOMS: During the mid to latter stages of this disease or due to prolonged steroid use, there are oral and genital sores which endure without healing, are dark red, and are insidiously painful. Both eyes are dry and rough, the orbits of the eyes are dark, and the vision is not clear. There may also be photophobia. There is vexatious heat in the five hearts, insomnia, night sweats, low back and knee soreness and weakness, a red tongue with scanty fluids and thin fur or a red tip and no fur, and a fine, rapid pulse.

TREATMENT PRINCIPLES: Enrich and supplement the liver and kidneys assisted by clearing heat

RX: *Liu Wei Di Huang Wan* (Six Flavors Rehmannia Pills) & *Yi Guan Jian* (One Link Decoction)

INGREDIENTS: Cooked Radix Rehmanniae (*Shu Di*) and uncooked Radix Rehmanniae (*Sheng Di*), 12g each, Tuber Ophiopogonis Japonici (*Mai Dong*), Radix Glehniae Littoralis (*Sha Shen*), Radix Angelicae Sinensis (*Dang Gui*), Fructus Lycii Chinensis (*Gou Qi Zi*), Radix Dioscoreae Oppositae (*Shan Yao*), Fructus Corni Officinalis (*Shan Zhu Yu*), and Sclerotium Poriae Cocos (*Fu Ling*), 9g each, and Rhizoma Alismatis (*Ze Xie*), Fructus Meliae Toosendan (*Chuan Lian Zi*), and Cortex Radicis Moutan (*Dan Pi*), 6g each

ANALYSIS OF FORMULA: *Shu Di, Sheng Di, Mai Men Dong, Sha Shen, Dang Gui, Gou Qi, Shan Yao,* and *Shan Zhu Yu* together enrich and supplement the blood, yin, and essence of the liver and kidneys. *Ze Xie* disinhibits damp heat and downbears ministerial fire. *Fu Ling* seeps dampness and fortifies the spleen. *Dan Pi* cools the blood and clears the liver. *Chuan Lian Zi* courses and clears the liver while also eliminating damp heat. *Dang Gui* and *Dan Pi* quicken the blood and transform stasis.

ADDITIONS & SUBTRACTIONS: For tidal fever or enduring low-grade fever, add 12 grams each of Herba Artemisiae Apiacae (*Qing Hao*), Cortex Radicis Lycii Chinensis (*Di Gu Pi*), Radix Stellariae Dichotomae (*Yin Chai Hu*), and Rhizoma Picrorrhizae (*Hu Huang Lian*). For concomitant dampness, add 15 grams each of Rhizoma Smilacis Glabrae (*Tu Fu Ling*) and Rhizoma Dioscoreae Hypoglaucae (*Bei Xie*). For painful joints, add 12 grams each of Ramulus Lonicerae Japonicae (*Ren Dong Teng*), Caulis Trachelospermi Jasminoidis (*Luo Shi Teng*), and Radix Cyathulae (*Chuan Niu Xi*). For reduced appetite, add nine grams each of Pericarpium Citri Reticulatae (*Chen Pi*) and Fructus Crataegi (*Shan Zha*). For sore throat or mouth sores, add nine grams each of Radix Istadis Seu Baphicacanthi (*Ban Lan Gen*) and

Fructificatio Lasiospherae Seu Calvatiae (*Ma Bo*) and five grams of Rhizoma Coptidis Chinensis (*Huang Lian*). For red, rough, painful eyes, add 12 grams each of Flos Chrysanthemi Indici (*Ye Ju Hua*), Semen Celosiae Argentae (*Qing Xiang Zi*), and Semen Leonuri Heterophylli (*Chong Wei Zi*). For external genital sores, add 15 grams each of Rhizoma Smilacis Glabrae (*Tu Fu Ling*) and Herba Violae Yedoensitis Cum Radice (*Zi Hua Di Ding*). For insomnia, add 20 grams each of Semen Zizyphi Spinosae (*Suan Zao Ren*) and Caulis Polygoni Multiflori (*Ye Jiao Teng*). For scanty, dark urine, add 15 grams of Semen Plantaginis (*Che Qian Zi*). For concomitant kidney yang vacuity, add 12 grams each of Herba Epimedii (*Yin Yang Huo*) and Radix Morindae Officinalis (*Ba Ji Tian*). For nodular skin lesions, add nine grams each of Flos Carthami Tinctorii (*Hong Hua*), Radix Ligustici Wallichii (*Chuan Xiong*), and Radix Salviae Miltiorrhizae (*Dan Shen*).

ACUPUNCTURE & MOXIBUSTION: *San Yin Jiao* (Sp 6), *Tai Xi* (Ki 3), *Qu Gu* (CV 2), *Da Ling* (Per 7), *Tai Yang* (M-HN-9)

ANALYSIS OF FORMULA: Supplementing *San Yin Jiao* and *Tai Xi* enriches and supplements the blood, yin, and essence of the liver and kidneys. Draining *Qu Gu* clears heat and treats genital sores, draining *Da Ling* clears heat and treats oral sores, and draining *Tai Yang* clears heat and treats eye troubles.

ADDITIONS & SUBTRACTIONS: For tidal fever or enduring low-grade fever, add *Da Zhui* (GV 14), *Yin Xi* (Ht 6), and *Ran Gu* (Ki 2). For concomitant dampness, add *Yin Ling Quan* (Sp 9). For painful joints, add *Qu Chi* (LI 11), *Yin Ling Quan* (Sp 9), and *a shi* points. For reduced appetite, add *Liang Men* (St 21). For sore throat or mouth sores, add *Zhao Hai* (Ki 6). For red, rough, painful eyes, add *He Gu* (LI 4) and *Guang Ming* (GB 37). For external genital sores, add *Hui Yin* (CV 1). For insomnia, add *Bai Hui* (GV 20). For scanty, dark urine, add *Yin Ling Quan* (Sp 9). For concomitant kidney yang vacuity, add *Guan Yuan* (CV 4). For nodular skin lesions, add *Ling Tai* (GV 10) and *Wei Zhong* (Bl 40).

6. SPLEEN-KIDNEY YANG VACUITY PATTERN

MAIN SYMPTOMS: Enduring disease with repeated occurrences which are commonly precipitated by cold and chill in the fall, oral and genital sores which are not particularly painful or may be accompanied by chilly pain, sores which are pale red in color and tend to grow hollow, dry, rough, slightly painful eyes, a somber white facial complexion, dizziness, head distention, fatigue, torpid intake, loose stools, abdominal pain with a liking for warmth and pressure, lower and upper back aching and pain, aversion to cold, chilled limbs, easy lower limb and/or facial edema, a pale, watery, glossy tongue with thin, white fur, and a deep, fine or deep, slow, forceless pulse

TREATMENT PRINCIPLES: Warm and supplement the spleen and kidneys

RX: *Fu Zi Li Zhong Tang* (Aconite Rectify the Center Decoction) & *You Gui Yin* (Restore the Right [Kidney] Drink)

INGREDIENTS: Cooked Radix Rehmanniae (*Shu Di*) and Fructus Corni Officinalis (*Shan Zhu Yu*), 15g each, Rhizoma Atractylodis Macrocephalae (*Bai Zhu*), Fructus Lycii Chinensis (*Gou Qi Zi*), Radix Dioscoreae Oppositae (*Shan Yao*), Cortex Eucommiae Ulmoidis (*Du Zhong*), and Radix Lateralis Praeparatus Aconiti Carmichaeli (*Fu Zi*), 9g each, Radix Panacis Ginseng (*Ren Shen*) and dry Rhizoma Zingiberis (*Gan Jiang*), 6g each, and Cortex Cinnamomi Cassiae (*Rou Gui*) and mix-fried Radix Glycyrrhizae (*Gan Cao*), 3g each

ANALYSIS OF FORMULA: The combination of *Shu Di, Shan Zhu Yu, Gou Qi, Du Zhong, Fu Zi,* and *Rou Gui* warm and supplement kidney yang. *Bai Zhu, Shan Yao, Ren Shen,* mix-fried *Gan Cao,* and *Gan Jiang* together warm and supplement spleen yang.

ADDITIONS & SUBTRACTIONS: For sores which tend to grow hollow, add three grams of Cornu Cervi (*Lu Jiao*) (powdered and taken with the strained decoction). For frequent stools, add nine grams each of Semen Euryalis Ferocis (*Qian Shi*) and Pericarpium Punicae Granati (*Shi Liu Pi*). For blood and pus in the stools, add 12 grams each of Radix Pulsatillae Chinensis (*Bai Tou Weng*) and Radix Sanguisorbae Officinalis (*Di Yu*). For anemia, add 15 grams of Radix Astragali Membranacei (*Huang Qi*) and nine grams of Radix Angelicae Sinensis (*Dang Gui*). For leukopenia, add 12 grams each of Radix Astragali Membranacei (*Huang Qi*), Rhizoma Atractylodis Macrocephalae (*Bai Zhu*), and Fructus Psoraleae Corylifoliae (*Bu Gu Zhi*). For impotence and decreased sexual desire, add nine grams each of Rhizoma Curculiginis Orchioidis (*Xian Mao*) and Herba Epimedii (*Yin Yang Huo*). For eye disturbances, add nine grams each of Scapus Et Inflorescentia Eriocaulonis Buergeriani (*Gu Jing Cao*), Fructus Ligustri Lucidi (*Nu Zhen Zi*), and Semen Astragali Complanati (*Sha Yuan Zi*). For oral sores, add 15 grams each of Radix Pseudostellariae Heterophyllae (*Tai Zi Shen*) and Carapax Amydae Sinensis (*Bie Jia*). For genital sores, add three grams of Cornu Cervi (*Lu Jiao*) powdered and taken with the strained decoction. For edema in the lower limbs, add nine grams each of Cortex Radicis Acanthopanacis Gracilistylis (*Wu Jia Pi*) and Radix Stephaniae Tetrandrae (*Han Fang Ji*). For undigested food in stools and fifth watch or cockcrow diarrhea, add three grams of Fructus Evodiae Rutecarpae (*Wu Zhu Yu*) and nine grams of Semen Myristicae Fragrantis (*Rou Dou Kou*).

ACUPUNCTURE & MOXIBUSTION: *Zu San Li* (St 36), *Guan Yuan* (CV 4), *Ming Men* (GV 4), *Shen Shu* (Bl 23)

ANALYSIS OF FORMULA: Supplementing *Zu San Li* and *Guan Yuan* with moxibustion warms and supplements spleen yang. Supplementing *Ming Men* and *Shen Shu* with moxibustion warms and supplements kidney yang.

ADDITIONS & SUBTRACTIONS: For reduced appetite, add *Liang Men* (St 21). For sore throat or mouth sores, add *Zhao Hai* (Ki 6). For eye disturbances, add *Guang Ming* (GB 37). For external genital sores, add *Hui Yin* (CV 1). For frequent stools, add *Tian Shu* (St 25). For blood and pus in the stools, add *Xue Hai* (Sp 10) and *Shang Ju Xu* (St 37). For anemia, add *Gao Huang Shu* (Bl 43). For impotence and decreased sexual desire, add *Zhi Shi* (Bl 52). For edema in the lower limbs, add *Yin Ling Quan* (Sp 9) and *Shui Fen* (CV 9). For undigested food in stools and fifth watch diarrhea, add *Liang Men* (St 21) and *Yin Ling Quan* (Sp 9).

7. QI & BLOOD DUAL VACUITY MIXED WITH STASIS PATTERN

MAIN SYMPTOMS: Enduring disease which does not heal with repeated occurrences, oral and genital sores which will not heal and which are either not painful or piercingly painful (depending on whether vacuity or stasis is predominant), dark-colored sores, especially their borders, decreased visual acuity, nodular skin lesions which are either pale red or purple-red in color, possible hematuria or hemafecia, a somber white facial complexion, scanty qi, disinclination to speak, heart palpitations, fearful throbbing, dizziness, lack of strength, a pale tongue with thin fur and possible static macules or spots, and a fine, choppy pulse

NOTE: In actual fact, blood stasis may complicate any of the above patterns associated with enduring disease mechanisms.

TREATMENT PRINCIPLES: Boost the qi and supplement the blood, transform stasis and free the flow of the network vessels

RX: *Ba Zhen Tang* (Eight Pearls Decoction) & *Xue Fu Zhu Yu Tang* (Blood Mansion Dispel Stasis Decoction)

INGREDIENTS: Cooked Radix Rehmanniae (*Shu Di*) and uncooked Radix Rehmanniae (*Sheng Di*), 12g each, Radix Codonopsitis Pilosulae (*Dang Shen*), Rhizoma Atractylodis Macrocephalae (*Bai Zhu*), Sclerotium Poriae Cocos (*Fu Ling*), Semen Pruni Persicae (*Tao Ren*), Flos Carthami Tinctorii (*Hong Hua*), Radix Cyathulae (*Chuan Niu Xi*), Radix Angelicae Sinensis (*Dang Gui*), Radix Albus Paeoniae Lactiflorae (*Bai Shao*), and Radix Rubrus Paeoniae Lactiflorae (*Chi Shao*), 9g each, Fructus Citri Aurantii (*Zhi Ke*), Radix Platycodi Grandiflori (*Jie Geng*), Radix Ligustici Wallichii (*Chuan Xiong*), and Radix Bupleuri (*Chai Hu*), 6g each, and mix-fried Radix Glycyrrhizae (*Gan Cao*), 3g

ANALYSIS OF FORMULA: *Shu Di*, *Sheng Di*, *Bai Shao*, and *Dang Gui* nourish the blood to fill the vessels and thus prevent further blood stasis. *Dang Shen*, *Bai Zhu*, *Fu Ling*, and mix-fried *Gan Cao* boost the qi to move the qi and quicken the blood. *Zhi Ke* and *Chai Hu* move and rectify the qi to quicken the blood. *Jie Geng* upbears clear yang to also help move the qi and, thus, promote the movement of blood. *Tao Ren*, *Hong Hua*, *Chuan Niu Xi*, *Dang Gui*, *Chi Shao*, and *Chuan Xiong* all quicken the blood and transform stasis.

ADDITIONS & SUBTRACTIONS: For bleeding, add 12 grams each of Pollen Typhae (*Pu Huang*) and Nodus Rhizomatis Nelumbinis Nuciferae (*Ou Jie*). For decreased visual acuity, add 15 grams each of Fructus Lycii Chinensis (*Gou Qi Zi*) and Fructus Ligustri Lucidi (*Nu Zhen Zi*).

For a blood stasis due to yang qi vacuity, replace *Ba Zhen Tang* and *Xue Fu Zhu Yu Tang* with Radix Lateralis Praeparatus Aconiti Carmichaeli (*Fu Zi*), Rhizoma Pinelliae Ternatae (*Ban Xia*), Radix Codonopsitis Pilosulae (*Dang Shen*), Rhizoma Atractylodis Macrocephalae (*Bai Zhu*), Sclerotium Poriae Cocos (*Fu Ling*), Rhizoma Sparganii (*San Leng*), Rhizoma Curcumae Zedoariae (*E Zhu*), Extremitas Radicis Angelicae Sinensis (*Dang Gui Wei*), Radix Rubrus Paeoniae Lactiflorae (*Chi Shao*), Flos Carthami Tinctorii (*Hong Hua*), and Ramulus Cinnamomi Cassiae (*Gui Zhi*), 9g each, and mix-fried Radix Glycyrrhizae (*Gan Cao*), 6g.

ACUPUNCTURE & MOXIBUSTION: *Zu San Li* (St 36), *San Yin Jiao* (Sp 6), *Ge Shu* (Bl 17), *Pi Shu* (Bl 20)

ANALYSIS OF FORMULA: Supplementing *Zu San Li* and *Pi Shu* fortifies the spleen, boosts the qi, and, therefore, nourishes the blood. Draining *San Yin Jiao* and *Ge Shu* quickens the blood and transforms stasis.

ADDITIONS & SUBTRACTIONS: For sore throat or mouth sores, add *Da Ling* (Per 7). For eye disturbances, add *He Gu* (LI 4) and *Guang Ming* (GB 37). For external genital sores, add *Qu Gu* (CV 2) and *Hui Yin* (CV 1). For blood and pus in the stools, add *Xue Hai* (Sp 10) and *Shang Ju Xu* (St 37). For anemia, add *Gao Huang Shu* (Bl 43). For reduced appetite, add *Liang Men* (St 21).

REMARKS

1. As with most chronic, enduring conditions, liver depression qi stagnation typically plays a part in this disease even though no Chinese sources suggest a liver qi pattern of this disease.

2. Treatment by corticosteroids may first cause yin vacuity and later cause yin and yang vacuity, while prolonged or excessive treatment with antibiotics or bitter, cold Chinese

medicinals may cause damage to the spleen qi and, eventually, to kidney yang. In that case, Chinese medicinals prescribed based on the patient's total constellation of patterns while on the Western medications may alleviate the side effects of those Western medicines as well as achieve a better therapeutic effect eventually leading to a reduction in dose or discontinuation of use of those Westerns medicines.

3. This condition is more common in Asia than in the West.

7

Benign Prostatic Hypertrophy

Also called benign prostatic hyperplasia, this is a benign adenomatous hyperplasia of the periurethral prostate gland commonly seen in men over 50 years of age. In fact, one out of four men will eventually require treatment for BPH at some point in their life, and congestion and overgrowth of the prostate gland is virtually universal in men over the age of 60. This hyperplasia causes variable degrees of bladder outlet obstruction. Recent endocrine research has discovered that the male hormone dihydrotestosterone (DHT) is involved in the development of BPH, with levels of DHT increasing with age. Bladder outlet obstruction symptoms include progressive urinary frequency, urgency, and nocturia due to incomplete emptying and rapid refilling of the bladder. Hesitancy and intermittency with decreased size and force of the urinary stream occur. Sensations of incomplete emptying, terminal dribbling, almost continuous overflow incontinence, and complete urinary retention may ensue. Episodes of acute complete urinary retention may follow prolonged attempts to retain urine, immobolization, exposure to cold, anesthetic agents, anticholinergic and sympathomimetic drugs, and ingestion of alcohol. Prolonged urinary retention, whether partial or complete, may cause progressive renal failure and azotemia.

The Western medical diagnosis of BPH is based on the signs and symptoms and a rectal digital exam. Other tests include catheterization after voiding to measure residual urine and cystoscopy to estimate gland size. When BPH is complicated by secondary chronic bacterial prostatitis, antibiotics may be used to treat bacterial infection. Catheter drainage, whether urethral or suprapubic, may be used to treat acute urinary retention. Although new drugs (finasteride, Proscar) have shown some success in shrinking enlarged prostates, till recently, surgery (transurethral resection of the prostate) has been the definitive treatment. There are approximately 400,000 surgical operations each year in the U.S. for this condition. Though the prognosis after surgery is usually excellent, 18% of men experience complications, such as infection, bleeding, incontinence, and impotence.

Chinese disease categorization: Benign prostratic hypertrophy falls under several different categories in Chinese medicine depending on each patient's main clinical symptoms. Nocutria is called *ye niao* or *ye niao zeng duo zheng*. Urinary obstruction is referred to as *niao bi*, urinary impediment, and *long bi*, dribbling urinary block. If there is marked urinary urgency and polyuria, this is referred to as *lin zheng*, strangury condition.

Disease causes: Aging, enduring disease, internal damage by the seven affects, and unregulated eating and drinking

Disease mechanisms: This condition is associated with three main disease mechanisms. First, there may be spleen and/or kidney vacuity. It is the qi which moves the excess fluids outside the body as well as keeps righteous fluids inside the body. Therefore, either spleen or kidney qi vacuity may cause lack of force to discharge the urine and/or leakage and incontinence. Spleen and kidney vacuity in older middle-aged and elderly patients are the result of a lifetime accumulation of damages and detriments. Secondly, there may be something blocking the yin orifice. This may be either or any combination of qi stagnation, blood stasis, or phlegm obstruction. And third, damp heat may cause urinary urgency, frequency, burning, and pain.

Because the lungs also play a role in water metabolism in the body, there is one other disease mechanism which may play a part in this condition. If phlegm heat obstructs the diffusing and downbearing of the lungs, the lungs may lose control over the water passageways. In that case, fluids will not flow to and be discharged from the bladder. This disease mechanism helps explain why the symptoms of BPH often become aggravated during a cold or flu or in those with bronchial asthma.

TREATMENT BASED ON PATTERN DISCRIMINATION:

1. QI MECHANISM OBSTRUCTION & STAGNATION, PHLEGM CONGELATION & BLOOD STASIS PATTERN

MAIN SYMPTOMS: Perineal area pain and discomfort which may radiate to the lower abdomen and tops of the thighs, inhibited urination, urination with a thin or cleft stream, the necessity of urinating several times to empty the bladder or incomplete urination, dribbling urination, lower abdominal distention, fullness, and discomfort, a dark tongue with possible static macules or spots, and a slippery, bowstring, choppy pulse

TREATMENT PRINCIPLES: Move the qi and quicken the blood, transform phlegm and scatter nodulation

RX: *Ju He Wan* (Orange Seed Pills)

INGREDIENTS: Semen Citri Reticulatae (*Ju He*), Fructus Meliae Toosendan (*Chuan Lian Zi*), and Rhizoma Corydalis Yanhusuo (*Yan Hu Suo*), 15g each, Semen Pruni Persicae (*Tao Ren*), Herba Sargassii (*Hai Zao*), Thallus Algae (*Kun Bu*), and Herba Laminariae Japonicae (*Hai Dai*), 12g each, Radix Auklandiae Lappae (*Mu Xiang*), Caulis Akebiae (*Mu Tong*), and Cortex Magnoliae Officinalis (*Hou Po*), 9g each, and Fructus Immaturus Citri Aurantii (*Zhi Shi*) and Cortex Cinnamomi Cassiae (*Rou Gui*), 6g each

ANALYSIS OF FORMULA: *Ju He, Chuan Lian Zi, Mu Xiang, Hou Po*, and *Zhi Shi* move the qi, eliminate distention, and stop pain. *Yan Hu Suo* and *Tao Ren* quicken the blood and transform stasis, free the network vessels and stop pain. *Ju He, Hai Zao, Hai Dai,* and *Kun Bu* transform phlegm, soften the hard, and scatter nodulation. *Rou Gui* warms and strengthens the qi transformation of the bladder, especially its function of moving the excess fluids outside the body. *Mu Tong* disinhibits urination.

ADDITIONS & SUBTRACTIONS: For severe blood stasis, add nine grams each of Rhizoma Curcumae Zedoariae (*E Zhu*) and Rhizoma Sparganii (*San Leng*). For concomitant damp heat, delete Cinnamon and add nine grams each of Semen Plantaginis (*Che Qian Zi*), Rhizoma Alismatis (*Ze Xie*), and Rhizoma Smilacis Glabrae (*Tu Fu Ling*). If heat is more pronounced, add nine grams each of Radix Scutellariae Baicalensis (*Huang Qin*), Cortex Phellodendri (*Haung Bai*), and Radix Gentianae Scabrae (*Long Dan Cao*). If cold is marked, increase the dose of *Rou Gui* to nine grams and add three grams of Fructus Evodiae Rutecarpae (*Wu Zhu Yu*) and nine grams of Fructus Foeniculi Vulgaris (*Xiao Hui Xiang*). If there is concomitant qi vacuity, add 15 grams of Radix Astragali Membranacei (*Huang Qi*). For concomitant chronic bacterial prostatitis, add 12 grams each of Herba Taraxaci Mongolici Cum Radice (*Pu Gong Ying*), Herba Patriniae Heterophyllae Cum Radice (*Bai Jiang Cao*), and Fructus Forsythiae Suspensae (*Lian Qiao*). For hematuria, add 15 grams each of Herba Cephalanoploris Segeti (*Xiao Ji*), Rhizoma Imperatae Cylindricae (*Bai Mao Gen*), and Pollen Typhae (*Pu Huang*). For kidney vacuity, add nine grams each of Fructus Lycii Chinensis (*Gou Qi Zi*), Radix Dipsaci (*Xu Duan*), and Semen Cuscutae Chinensis (*Tu Si Zi*).

ACUPUNCTURE & MOXIBUSTION: *He Gu* (LI 4), *San Yin Jiao* (Sp 6), *Guan Yuan* (CV 4), *Zhong Ji* (CV 3), *Hui Yin* (CV 1)

ANALYSIS OF FORMULA: Draining *He Gu* and *San Yin Jiao* moves the qi and quickens the blood throughout the whole body. Their action is focused in the lower burner, bladder, and external genitals by their combination with *Guan Yuan* and *Zhong Ji*, which free the flow of the chong mai, ren mai, and bladder channels and disinhibit urine. With even supplementing-even draining method, *Hui Yin* frees the network vessels in the perineal area, eliminates distention, and stops pain.

ADDITIONS & SUBTRACTIONS: For severe blood stasis, add *Xue Hai* (Sp 10) and *Qu Quan* (Liv 8). For concomitant damp heat, add *Yin Ling Quan* (Sp 9). If heat is more pronounced, add *Nei Ting* (St 44) and *Xing Jian* (Liv 2). If cold is marked, add indirect moxibustion to *Hui Yin, Zhong Ji,* and *Guan Yuan.* For hematuria, add *Xue Hai* (Sp 10). For stabbing pain in the genitals, add *Da Dun* (Liv 1). For stabbing, or piercing pain during urination, add *Shui Dao* (St 28) and *Zhi Bian* (Bl 54). For difficult urination, add *Yin Ling Quan* (Sp 9) and *Zhi Bian* (Bl 54). For lower abdominal, groin region, and genital distention and pain, add *Qu Quan* (Liv 8). For concomitant kidney yin vacuity, add *Fu Liu* (Ki 7). For concomitant kidney yang vacuity, add *Tai Xi* (Ki 3). For concomitant qi vacuity, add *Tai Bai* (Sp 3). For constipation or dry stools, add *Zhi Gou* (TB 6).

2. LIVER DEPRESSION & PHLEGM NODULATION PATTERN

MAIN SYMPTOMS: Urinary stangury and obstruction which is worsened by emotional stress or upset, lower abdominal distention, irritability, easy anger, insomnia, possible flatulence, a normal or slightly dark tongue with white, slimy fur, and a bowstring, slippery pulse

TREATMENT PRINCIPLES: Course the liver and rectify the qi, transform phlegm and scatter nodulation

RX: *Shu Gan San Jie Fang* (Course the Liver & Scatter Nodulation Formula)

INGREDIENTS: Radix Salviae Miltiorrhizae (*Dan Shen*), Spica Prunellae Vulgaris (*Xia Ku Cao*), and Radix Scrophulariae Ningpoensis (*Xuan Shen*), 15g each, Concha Ostreae (*Mu Li*) and Pumice (*Hai Fu Shi*), 12g each, and Radix Bupleuri (*Chai Hu*), Radix Rubrus Paeoniae Lactiflorae (*Chi Shao*), Radix Angelicae Sinensis (*Dang Gui*), Radix Achyranthis Bidentatae (*Niu Xi*), Thallus Algae (*Kun Bu*), Herba Saragassii (*Hai Zao*), and Bulbus Fritillariae Thunbergii (*Zhe Bei Mu*), 9g each

ANALYSIS OF FORMULA: *Chai Hu* courses the liver and resolves depression. *Xia Ku Cao, Xuan Shen, Mu Li, Hai Fu Shi, Kun Bu, Hai Zao,* and *Zhe Bei Mu* soften the hard and scatter the nodulation. In addition, *Xia Ku Cao* clears the liver, *Mu Li* quiets the ethereal soul, and *Hai Fu Shi, Kun Bu, Hai Zao,* and *Zhe Bei Mu* transform phlegm. *Dan Shen, Chi Shao, Dang Gui,* and *Niu Xi* quicken the blood and transform stasis.

ADDITIONS & SUBTRACTIONS: For severe liver depression, add nine grams each of Rhizoma Cyperi Rotundi (*Xiang Fu*), Radix Albus Paeoniae Lactiflorae (*Bai Shao*), and Fructus Meliae Toosendan (*Chuan Lian Zi*). For inhibited urination which gets worse with emotional disturbance, such as anger, frustration, or depression, add 12 grams each of Semen Zizyphi Spinosae (*Suan Zao Ren*), Cortex Albizziae Julibrissinis (*He Huan Pi*), and Caulis Polygoni Multiflori (*Ye Jiao Teng*). Please also refer to the additions and subtractions of pattern #1.

ACUPUNCTURE & MOXIBUSTION: *Tai Chong* (Liv 3), *Qu Quan* (Liv 8), *San Yin Jiao* (Sp 6), *Zhong Ji* (CV 3), *Hui Yin* (CV 1)

ANALYSIS OF FORMULA: Draining *Tai Chong* and *Qu Quan* courses the liver and resolves depression, drains the liver channel and eliminates distention and pain. Draining *San Yin Jiao* quickens the blood and disinhibits urination. Draining *Zhong Ji* and *Hui Yin* disinhibits urination and frees the flow of the network vessels in the bladder and perineal area, eliminates distention and stops pain.

ADDITIONS & SUBTRACTIONS: Please see pattern #1 above.

3. DAMP HEAT, STASIS & STAGNATION PATTERN

MAIN SYMPTOMS: Numerous, frequent, short, and choppy urinations, urinary urgency, urinary pain, a constant feeling of the need to urinate, turbid, cloudy or yellow urine, possible nocturia, urination with a thin stream, dribbling urination, in severe cases, urinary stoppage with lower abdominal fullness and distention, lower abdominal and perineal distention and pain, dry, bound stools, a possible bitter taste in the mouth, a purple tongue with slimy, yellow fur, and a bowstring, slippery, rapid pulse

TREATMENT PRINCIPLES: Clear heat and disinhibit dampness, quicken the blood and free the flow of the network vessels

RX: *Yan Shi Qian Lie Xian Fang* (Master Yan's Prostate Formula)

INGREDIENTS: Radix Salviae Miltiorrhizae (*Dan Shen*), 15g, Rhizoma Anemarrhenae Aspheloidis (*Zhi Mu*), Cortex Phellodendri (*Huang Bai*), Semen Plantaginis (*Che Qian Zi*), Semen Pruni Persicae (*Tao Ren*), Rhizoma Cimicifugae (*Sheng Ma*), Rhizoma Dioscoreae Hypogalucae (*Bi Xie*), Herba Dianthi (*Qu Mai*), Talcum (*Hua Shi*), Fructus Gardeniae Jasminoidis (*Zhi Zi*), Semen Vaccariae Segetalis (*Wang Bu Liu Xing*), and Rhizoma Polygoni Cuspidati (*Hu Zhang*), 9g each, Radix Et Rhizoma Rhei (*Da Huang*), 6g, Caulis Akebiae (*Mu Tong*), 4.5g, and Radix Tenuis Glycyrrhizae (*Gan Cao Shao*), 3g

ANALYSIS OF FORMULA: *Che Qian Zi, Bei Xie, Qu Mai, Hua Shi, Hu Zhang, Shu Da Huang, Mu Tong,* and *Gan Cao Shao* together clear and disinhibit dampness and heat in the lower burner. *Zhi Mu* and *Sheng Ma* clear heat, while *Huang Bai* and *Zhi Zi* dry dampness and resolve toxins. *Wang Bu Liu Xing, Dan Shen, Tao Ren, Qu Mai,* and *Da Huang* quicken the blood, transform stasis, and free the flow of the network vessels.

ADDITIONS & SUBTRACTIONS: For hardness of the prostate gland, add 12 grams of Carapax Amydae Sinensis (*Bie Jia*) and nine grams of Squama Manitis Pentadactylis (*Chuan Shan Jia*). For dry mouth, add 12 grams of Radix Trichosanthis Kirlowii (*Tian Hua Fen*). If damp heat has damaged yin, add nine grams of Gelatinum Corii Asini (*E Jiao*). For hematuria, add 15 grams each of Herba Cephalanoploris Segeti (*Xiao Ji*), Rhizoma Imperatae Cylindricae (*Bai Mao Gen*), and Pollen Typhae (*Pu Huang*). For spasmodic pain, add 15 grams of Radix Albus Paeoniae Lactiflorae (*Bai Shao*) and nine grams of Rhizoma Acori Graminei (*Shi Chang Pu*) and increase the dosage of *Gan Cao Shao* up to nine grams. For concomitant chronic bacterial prostatitis, add 12 grams each of Herba Taraxaci Mongolici Cum Radice (*Pu Gong Ying*), Herba Patriniae Heterophyllae Cum Radice (*Bai Jiang Cao*), and Fructus Forsythiae Suspensae (*Lian Qiao*). For turbid or milky white urine, add 12 grams each of Sclerotium Poriae Cocos (*Fu Ling*) and Rhizoma Acori Graminei (*Shi Chang Pu*). For a damp, itchy scrotum, add nine grams each of Radix Sophorae Flavescentis (*Ku Shen*) and Fructus Kochiae Scopariae (*Di Fu Zi*). For nausea and stomach and abdominal distention, add nine grams each of Rhizoma Pinelliae Ternatae (*Ban Xia*) and Pericarpium Citri Reticulatae (*Chen Pi*). For concomitant spleen qi vacuity, add 15 grams each of Radix Astragali Membranacei (*Huang Qi*) and nine grams each of Radix Codonopsitis Pilosulae (*Dang Shen*), Rhizoma Atractylodis Macrocephalae (*Bai Zhu*), and Sclerotium Poriae Cocos (*Fu*

Ling). For concomitant qi stagnation, add 15 grams of Fructus Meliae Toosendan (*Chuan Lian Zi*) and nine grams of Radix Bupleuri (*Chai Hu*).

ACUPUNCTURE & MOXIBUSTION: *Zhong Ji* (CV 3), *Hui Yin* (CV 1), *Yin Ling Quan* (Sp 9), *San Yin Jiao* (Sp 6), *Zhi Bian* (Bl 54)

ANALYSIS OF FORMULA: Draining *Zhong Ji*, *Hui Yin*, and *Yin Ling Quan* clears heat and disinhibits dampness in the lower burner. *San Yin Jiao* and *Zhi Bian* quicken the blood and disinhibit urination, free the flow of the network vessels and stop pain. Needle *Zhi Bian* with deep insertion in the direction of *Gui Lai* (St 29) or *Shui Dao* (St 28).

ADDITIONS & SUBTRACTIONS: If damp heat has damaged yin with a dry mouth, add *Fu Liu* (Ki 7). For hematuria, add *Xue Hai* (Sp 10). For spasmodic pain, add *He Gu* (LI 4) and *Tai Chong* (Liv 3). For pain in the genitals, add *Da Dun* (Liv 1). For an itchy, damp scrotum, add *Li Gou* (Liv 5). For nausea and stomach and abdominal distention, add *Zhong Wan* (CV 12) and *Tian Shu* (St 25). For concomitant qi stagnation, add *Tai Chong* (Liv 3) and *Qu Quan* (Liv 8). For pain and distention in the lower abdomen, add *Gui Lai* (St 29) and *Qu Quan* (Liv 8). For concomitant spleen qi vacuity, add *Tai Bai* (Sp 3). For constipation or dry stools, add *Zhi Gou* (TB 6). For insomnia and restlessness, add *Tong Li* (Ht 5).

4. SPLEEN-KIDNEY YANG VACUITY PATTERN

MAIN SYMPTOMS: Urinary frequency, urgency, incontinence, and terminal dribbling, forceless urination with a thin stream, nocturia, clear or turbid, white urine, a possibly cool scrotum, cold extremities, especially the feet, fatigue, low back and knee soreness and limpness, loose stools or constipation, possible impotence or decreased sexual desire, a pale, fat tongue with thin, white fur, and a fine, weak pulse

TREATMENT PRINCIPLES: Fortify the spleen and supplement the qi, supplement the kidneys and invigorate yang

RX: *Huang Qi Fu Pen Tang* (Astragalus & Rubus Decoction)

INGREDIENTS: Radix Astragali Membranacei (*Huang Qi*), Radix Codonopsitis Pilosulae (*Dang Shen*), Radix Dioscoreae Oppositae (*Shan Yao*), Radix Dipsaci (*Xu Duan*), Ramulus Loranthi Seu Visci (*Sang Ji Sheng*), Sclerotium Poriae Cocos (*Fu Ling*), Radix Linderae Strychnifoliae (*Wu Yao*), and Fructus Rubi Chingii (*Fu Pen Zi*), 15g each, and Rhizoma Alismatis (*Ze Xie*) and Cortex Radicis Moutan (*Dan Pi*), 9g each

ANALYSIS OF FORMULA: *Huang Qi*, *Dang Shen*, *Shan Yao*, and *Fu Ling* fortify the spleen and boost the qi. *Shan Yao*, *Xu Duan*, *Sang Ji Sheng*, and *Fu Pen Zi* supplement the kidneys and invigorate yang. *Fu Ling* and *Ze Xie* disinhibit dampness and abduct turbidity, while *Fu Pen Zi* and *Shan Yao* secure the kidneys and restrain the essence. *Dan Pi* quickens the blood and transforms the stasis.

ADDITIONS & SUBTRACTIONS: For more severe cold, add nine grams each of Cortex Cinnamomi Cassiae (*Rou Gui*) and Radix Lateralis Praeparatus Aconiti Carmichaeli (*Fu Zi*). For more serious blood stasis, add 15 grams of Radix Salviae Miltiorrhizae (*Dan Shen*) and nine grams of Semen Vaccariae Segetalis (*Wang Bu Liu Xing*). If the central qi has fallen downward, add 4.5 grams of Rhizoma Cimcifugae (*Sheng Ma*). For severe enlargement of the prostate which is, nevertheless still soft, add 12 grams each of Herba Sargassii (*Hai Zao*), Thallus Algae (*Kun Bu*), and Concha Ostreae (*Mu Li*). For severe enlargement and hardening of the prostate, add 12 grams of Rhizoma Curcumae Zedoariae (*E Zhu*) and three grams of Hirudo Seu Whitmania (*Shui Zhi*), powdered and taken with the strained decoction. For concomitant damp heat, add nine grams each of Rhizoma Anemarrhenae Asphodeloidis (*Zhi Mu*) and Cortex Phellodendri (*Huang Bai*).

An alternative treatment is *Bu Shen Li Niao Tang* (Supplement the Kidneys & Disinhibit Urine Decoction): Radix Astragali Membranacei (*Huang Qi*), 30g, Radix Codonopsitis Pilosulae (*Dang Shen*), Herba Cistanchis Deserticolae (*Rou Cong Rong*), Rhizoma Alismatis (*Ze Xie*), and Semen Plantaginis (*Che Qian Zi*), 15g each, Sclerotium Poriae Cocos (*Fu Ling*), Semen Pruni Persicae (*Tao Ren*), and Flos Carthami Tinctorii (*Hong Hua*), 12g each, Squama Manitis Pentadactylis (*Chuan Shan Jia*) and Semen Vaccariae Segetalis (*Wang Bu Liu Xing*), 9g each, and Cortex Cinnamomi Cassiae (*Rou Gui*), 3g.

ACUPUNCTURE & MOXIBUSTION: *Hui Yin* (CV 1), *Guan Yuan* (CV 4), *San Yin Jiao* (Sp 6), *Shen Shu* (Bl 23)

ANALYSIS OF FORMULA: Supplementing *Hui Yin* with moxibustion supplements vacuity, harmonizes the network vessels, and secures the kidneys. Supplementing *Guan Yuan* and *Shen Shu* with moxibustion warms the lower origin and secures the kidneys. Supplementing *San Yin Jiao* supplements the spleen and kidneys, transforms dampness, divides the clear, and stops pain.

ADDITIONS & SUBTRACTIONS: For terminal dribbling which will not stop and nocturia, add *Zhi Shi* (Bl 52). For severe kidney yang vacuity, add *Ming Men* (GV 4). For low back pain, add *Fu Liu* (Ki 7). For fatigue and lassitude of the spirit, add *Tai Bai* (Sp 3). For decreased sexual desire or impotence, add *Ming Men* (GV 4). For loose stools, add *Gong Sun* (Sp 4). For concomitant damp heat, drain *Yin Ling Quan* (Sp 9). For more serious blood stasis, add *Xue Hai* (Sp 10).

5. Yin vacuity-fire effulgence pattern

Main symptoms: Frequent, scanty, inhibited urination, and terminal dribbling which is worse with taxation, yellow urine, low back pain, dizziness, tinnitus, impotence, seminal emission, insomnia, night sweats, vexatious heat in the five hearts, possible feverish sensation in the afternoon, constipation, red tongue with scanty fluids, and a fine, rapid, forceless pulse

Treatment principles: Enrich the yin and downbear fire

Rx: *Zhi Bai Di Huang Wan Jia Jian* (Anemarrhena & Phellodendron Rehmannia Pills with Additions & Subtractions)

Ingredients: Uncooked Radix Rehmanniae (*Sheng Di*), Tuber Asparagi Cochinensis (*Tian Men Dong*), Rhizoma Alismatis (*Ze Xie*), Sclerotium Poriae Cocos (*Fu Ling*), Cortex Phellodendri (*Huang Bai*), Rhizoma Anemarrhenae Asphodeloidis (*Zhi Mu*), and Rhizoma Dioscoreae Hypoglaucae (*Bei Xie*), 12g each, Cortex Radicis Moutan (*Dan Pi*), Radix Dioscoreae Oppositae (*Shan Yao*), Spica Prunellae Vulgaris (*Xia Ku Cao*), Bulbus Shancigu (*Shan Ci Gu*), and Squama Manitis Pentadactylis (*Chuan Shan Jia*), 9g each, Succinum (*Hu Po*), 1.5g (powdered and taken with the strained decoction), and Cortex Cinnamomi Cassiae (*Rou Gui*), 1g (powdered and taken with the strained decoction)

Analysis of formula: *Sheng Di*, *Shan Yao*, and *Tian Men Dong* enrich the yin, boost the essence, and supplement the kidneys. *Ze Xie*, *Huang Bai*, and *Zhi Mu* downbear ministerial fire. *Ze Xie*, *Bei Xie*, and *Fu Ling* clear and disinhibit dampness and heat in the lower burner. *Xia Ku Cao* and *Shan Ci Gu* soften the hard and scatter nodulation, while *Dan Pi* and *Chuan Shan Jia* quicken the blood and transform stasis. *Hu Po* quickens the blood and quiets the spirit, disinhibits dampness and stops pain. *Rou Gui* in a small dosage returns fire to its lower origin and strengthens the qi transformation of the bladder.

Additions & subtractions: For difficult urination and a burning sensation, add 15 grams of Semen Plantaginis (*Che Qian Zi*). For concomitant qi vacuity, add 15 grams of Radix Astragali Membranacei (*Huang Qi*) and nine grams of Radix Codonopsitis Pilosulae (*Dang Shen*). For severe stabbing pain, add nine grams of Eupolyphaga Seu Opisthoplatia (*Tu Bie Chong*). For concomitant kidney yang vacuity, add 12 grams each of Herba Epimedii (*Yin Yang Huo*) and Radix Morindae Officinalis (*Ba Ji Tian*). For frequent nocturia, add 12 grams each of Fructus Rosae Laevigatae (*Jin Ying Zi*), Semen Euryalis Ferocis (*Qian Shi*), and Fructus Schisandrae Chinensis (*Wu Wei Zi*). For restlessness and insomnia, add 12 grams each of Radix Polygalae Tenuifoliae (*Yuan Zhi*), Rhizoma Acori Graminei (*Shi Chang Pu*), and Sclerotium Pararadicis Poriae Cocos (*Fu Shen*).

Acupuncture & moxibustion: *Hui Yin* (CV 1), *Guan Yuan* (CV 4), *San Yin Jiao* (Sp 6), *Shen Shu* (Bl 23), *Fu Liu* (Ki 7)

Analysis of formula: With even supplementing-even draining technique, *Hui Yin* harmonizes the network vessels and secures the kidneys. Supplementing *Guan Yuan* and *Shen Shu* supplements the kidneys and secures and astringes. In addition, needling *Guan Yuan* leads ministerial fire back downward to its lower source. Supplementing *San Yin Jiao* supplements the spleen and kidneys, transforms dampness, divides the clear from turbid, and stops pain. Supplementing *Fu Liu*, the metal-mother point of the kidney channel, supplements the kidneys and enriches yin.

Additions & subtractions: Please see pattern #4 above.

6. Central qi downward falling pattern

Main symptoms: Frequent, scanty, forceless, inhibited urination, sometimes a desire to urinate but without success, fatigue, lassitude of the spirit, lack of strength, reduced appetite, shortness of breath, a weak voice, sagging and distention in the lower abdomen and perineal area, loose stools, a sallow facial complexion, a pale, fat tongue, and a fine, weak pulse

Treatment principles: Boost the qi, upbear yang, and raise the fallen

Rx: *Bu Zhong Yi Qi Tang Jia Wei* (Supplement the Center & Boost the Qi Decoction with Additions & Subtractions)

Ingredients: Radix Astragali Membranacei (*Huang Qi*), 20g, Radix Codonopsitis Pilosulae (*Dang Shen*), 15g, Rhizoma Atractylodis Macrocephalae (*Bai Zhu*), Sclerotium Poriae Cocos (*Fu Ling*), and Rhizoma Dioscoreae Hypoglaucae (*Bei Xie*), 9g each, and Radix Angelicae Sinensis (*Dang Gui*), Ramulus Cinnamomi Cassiae (*Gui Zhi*), Pericarpium Citri Reticulatae (*Chen Pi*), Rhizoma Cimicifugae (*Sheng Ma*), Radix Bupleuri (*Chai Hu*), Radix Platycodi Grandiflori (*Jie Geng*), and mix-fried Radix Glycyrrhizae (*Gan Cao*), 6g each

Analysis of formula: *Huang Qi*, *Dang Shen*, *Bai Zhu*, and mix-fried *Gan Cao* fortify the spleen and boost the qi. *Jie Geng*, *Chai Hu*, and *Sheng Ma* upbear yang qi. *Dang Gui* harmonizes the blood, while *Chen Pi* rectifies the qi. *Fu Ling* and *Bei Xie* disinhibit urination.

Additions & subtractions: For inhibited urination or

desire to urinate but no success, add nine grams each of Semen Plantaginis (*Che Qian Zi*) and Sclerotium Polypori Umbellati (*Zhu Ling*). For dribbling urination, add nine grams each of Fructus Alpiniae Oxyphyllae (*Yi Zhi Ren*), Semen Euryalis Ferocis (*Qian Shi*), and Semen Cuscutae Chinensis (*Tu Si Zi*). For severe enlargement of the prostate but which is still soft, add 12 grams each of Herba Sargassii (*Hai Zao*), Thallus Algae (*Kun Bu*), and Concha Ostreae (*Mu Li*). For severe enlargement but which is hard, add 12 grams of Rhizoma Curcumae Zedoariae (*E Zhu*) and three grams of Hirudo Seu Whitmania (*Shui Zhi*), powdered and taken with the strained decoction. For concomitant damp heat, add nine grams each of Radix Sophorae Flavescentis (*Ku Shen*) and Cortex Phellodendri (*Huang Bai*).

ACUPUNCTURE & MOXIBUSTION: *Hui Yin* (CV 1), *Guan Yuan* (CV 4), *Qi Hai* (CV 6), *Bai Hui* (GV 20), *Zu San Li* (St 36), *San Yin Jiao* (Sp 6)

ANALYSIS OF FORMULA: Supplementing *Guan Yuan*, *Qi Hai*, and *Bai Hui* with moxibustion boosts the qi and upbears the clear. Supplementing *Zu San Li* and *San Yin Jiao* fortifies the spleen, boosts the qi, and upbears the clear. Moxaing *Hui Yin* harmonizes the network vessels and supplements vacuity.

ADDITIONS & SUBTRACTIONS: For inhibited urination or desire to urinate but no success, add *Yin Ling Quan* (Sp 9). For dribbling urination, add *Zhi Shi* (Bl 52). For concomitant damp heat, add *Yin Ling Quan* (Sp 9) and *Nei Ting* (St 44). For sagging pain in the genitals, add *Da Dun* (Liv 1) with moxibustion. For distention and pain in the lower abdomen, groin, and genitals, add *Qu Quan* (Liv 8). For food stagnation, add *Liang Men* (St 21). For concomitant kidney qi vacuity, add *Tai Xi* (Ki 3). For concomitant, kidney yin vacuity, add *Fu Liu* (Ki 7). For heart-spleen dual vacuity, add *Shen Men* (Ht 7). For severe qi vacuity, add *Tai Bai* (Sp 3).

7. QI & YIN DUAL VACUITY PATTERN

MAIN SYMPTOMS: Urinary frequency, urgency, and dribbling which is worse with taxation, forceless urination with a thin stream, fatigue, lassitude of the spirit, lack of strength, dizziness, tinnitus, low back and knee soreness and limpness, vexatious heat in the five hearts, malar flushing, a dry mouth and throat, a fat, red tongue with scanty fluids or fur or a centerline crack, and a soggy and rapid or fine, rapid pulse

TREATMENT PRINCIPLES: Fortify the spleen and boost the qi, enrich yin and drain heat

RX: *Bu Zhong Yi Qi Tang* (Supplement the Center & Boost the Qi Decoction) & *Liu Wei Di Huang Wan* (Six Flavors Rehmannia Pills) with additions and subtractions

INGREDIENTS: Radix Astragali Membranacei (*Huang Qi*), 15g, cooked Radix Rehmanniae (*Shu Di*), 12g, Radix Dioscoreae Oppositae (*Shan Yao*), Sclerotium Poriae Cocos (*Fu Ling*), Rhizoma Atractylodis Macrocephalae (*Bai Zhu*), Radix Codonopsitis Pilosulae (*Dang Shen*), Radix Angelicae Sinensis (*Dang Gui*), and Fructus Corni Officinalis (*Shan Zhu Yu*), 9g each, Rhizoma Alismatis (*Ze Xie*), Cortex Radicis Moutan (*Dan Pi*), mix-fried Radix Glycyrrhizae (*Gan Cao*), and Rhizoma Cimicifugae (*Sheng Ma*), 6g each, and Pericarpium Citri Reticulatae (*Chen Pi*), 4.5g

ANALYSIS OF FORMULA: *Huang Qi*, *Shan Yao*, *Bai Zhu*, *Fu Ling*, and *Dang Shen* fortify the spleen and boost the qi. In addition, *Huang Qi*, *Bai Zhu*, and *Fu Ling* disinhibit urination, while *Shan Yao* secures the essence. *Shu Di*, *Shan Yao*, and *Shan Zhu Yu* together enrich yin and supplement the kidneys. *Dang Gui* nourishes liver blood and quickens the blood. *Dan Pi* cools and quickens the blood. *Chen Pi* dries dampness and rectifies the qi. *Ze Xie* disinhibits urination, and *Sheng Ma* clears heat and upbears the central qi.

ADDITIONS & SUBTRACTIONS: If there is marked blood stasis, add 15 grams each of Radix Salviae Miltiorrhizae (*Dan Shen*) and Semen Vaccariae Segetalis (*Wang Bu Liu Xing*). If there is phlegm nodulation, increase the *Chen Pi* to nine grams and add 15 grams each of Spica Prunellae Vulgaris (*Xiao Ku Cao*), Radix Scrophulariae Ningpoensis (*Xuan Shen*), and Semen Citri Reticulatae (*Ju He*), 12 grams of Concha Ostreae (*Mu Li*), and nine grams each of Thallus Algae (*Kun Bu*), Herba Sargassii (*Hai Zao*), Bulbus Fritillariae Thunbergii (*Zhe Bei Mu*), and Rhizoma Pinelliae Ternatae (*Ban Xia*). If there is low back pain, add nine grams each of Radix Achyranthis Bidentatae (*Niu Xi*), Ramulus Loranthi Seu Visci (*Sang Ji Sheng*), and Cortex Eucommiae Ulmoidis (*Du Zhong*). If there is more pronounced qi stagnation, add 15 grams of Fructus Meliae Toosendan (*Chuan Lian Zi*) and nine grams of Radix Auklandiae Lappae (*Mu Xiang*). For marked effulgent fire, add nine grams each of Rhizoma Anemarrhenae Asphodeloidis (*Zhi Mu*) and Cortex Phellodendri (*Huang Bai*). For dry mouth, add 12 grams of Radix Trichosanthis Kirlowii (*Tian Hua Fen*).

ACUPUNCTURE & MOXIBUSTION: *Hui Yin* (CV 1), *Guan Yuan* (CV 4), *Zu San Li* (St 36), *Fu Liu* (Ki 7), *Shen Shu* (Bl 23)

ANALYSIS OF FORMULA: With even supplementing-even draining method, *Hui Yin* supplements vacuity, harmonizes the network vessels, and secures kidneys. *Guan Yuan* supplements both the spleen and kidneys. Supplementing *Zu San Li* fortifies the spleen and boosts the qi. Supplementing *Shen Shu* and *Fu Liu* enriches yin and supplements the kidneys.

ADDITIONS & SUBTRACTIONS: Please see patterns #4, 5 and 6 above.

8. Lung loss of control & discipline pattern

Main symptoms: Uneasy urination which drips and drops but does not flow freely, lower abdominal distention and pain, a dry throat with a desire to drink, vexation and oppression within the chest, uneasy respiration, possible cough and/or phlegm panting, a red tongue with thin, yellow fur, and a slippery rapid pulse

Treatment principles: Clear and discharge lung heat, move the qi and disinhibit water

Rx: *Huang Qin Qing Fei Yin Jia Wei* (Scutellaria Clear the Lungs Drink with Added Flavors)

Ingredients: Uncooked Radix Rehmanniae (*Sheng Di*), 20g, Radix Trichosanthis Kirlowii (*Tian Hua Fen*), 15g, Radix Scutellariae Baicalensis (*Huang Qin*), Fructus Gardeniae Jasminoidis (*Zhi Zi*), Cortex Radicis Mori Albi (*Sang Bai Pi*), Sclerotium Rubrum Poriae Cocos (*Chi Fu Ling*), Semen Pruni Armeniacae (*Xing Ren*), and Radix Platycodi Grandiflori (*Jie Geng*), 9g each, and Radix Glycyrrhizae (*Gan Cao*), 6g

Analysis of formula: *Huang Qin, Zhi Zi, Sang Bai Pi, Tian Hua Fen, Gan Cao,* and *Jie Geng* all clear and discharge lung heat. *Jie Geng* also rectifies the qi and loosens the chest, thus promoting the lungs' diffusing and downbearing. *Sheng Di* nourishes yin and prevents heat from damaging lung yin. *Chi Fu Ling* and *Sang Bai Pi* disinhibit water.

Additions & subtractions: If there is heart fire effulgence with severe heart vexation, add nine grams of Folium Bambusae (*Zhu Ye*) and six grams of Rhizoma Coptidis Chinensis (*Huang Lian*). If there is concomitant lung yin insufficiency, add 12 grams each of Radix Glehniae Littoralis (*Sha Shen*) and Tuber Ophiopogonis Japonici (*Mai Men Dong*). If the stools are not free-flowing, add six grams of uncooked Radix Et Rhizoma Rhei (*Da Huang*).

For less lung heat and more urinary disorder, an alternative treatment is *Pi Pa Ye Qing Fei Tang* (Eriobotrya Clear the Lungs Decoction): Folium Eriobotryae Japonicae (*Pi Pa Ye*), Semen Pruni Armeniacae (*Xing Ren*), Spora Lygodii Japonici (*Hai Jin Sha*), Excrementum Bombicis Batryticati (*Can Sha*), Semen Plantaginis (*Che Qian Zi*), Rhizoma Alismatis (*Ze Xie*), and Sclerotium Polypori Umbellati (*Zhu Ling*), 9g each, Caulis Akebiae (*Mu Tong*), and Resina Olibani (*Ru Xiang*), 6g each, and Radix Platycodi Grandiflori (*Jie Geng*), 4.5g.

Acupuncture & moxibustion: *Chi Ze* (Lu 5), *He Gu* (LI 4), *Zhong Ji* (CV 3), *San Yin Jiao* (Sp 6), *Yin Ling Quan* (Sp 9)

Analysis of formula: Draining *Chi Ze* and *He Gu* clears and discharges lung heat and opens the upper. Draining *Zhong Ji, San Yin Jiao,* and *Yin Ling Quan* clears heat, disinhibits dampness, and flushes the lower.

Additions & subtractions: If there is heart fire effulgence with severe heart vexation, add *Tong Li* (Ht 5). If there is concomitant lung yin insufficiency, add *Fei Shu* (Bl 13) and *Gao Huang Shu* (Bl 43). If the stools are not free-flowing, add *Zhi Gou* (TB 6).

Remarks

1. Most cases of BPH consist of some combination of spleen qi vacuity, kidney yin or yang vacuity, qi stagnation, blood stasis, and phlegm nodulation. In addition, there may be damp heat in patients with habitual bodily yang exuberance combined with spleen vacuity and a faulty diet. The following modification of *Bu Zhong Yi Qi Tang* (Supplement the Center & Boost the Qi Decoction) is an example of a complex formula for the treatment of a complex combination of spleen vacuity, liver depression, kidney yin and yang vacuity, phlegm nodulation, blood stasis, and damp heat: Herba Patriniae Heterophyllae Cum Radice (*Bai Jiang Cao*) and Herba Artemisiae Capillaris (*Yin Chen Hao*), 25g each, Radix Astragali Membranacei (*Huang Qi*), 18g, Bulbus Fritillariae Thunbergii (*Zhe Bei Mu*), Spica Prunellae Vulgaris (*Xia Gu Cao*), and Radix Scrophulariae Ningpoensis (*Xuan Shen*), 15g each, cooked Radix Rehmanniae (*Shu Di*) and Sclerotium Poriae Cocos (*Fu Ling*), 12g each, Radix Codonopsitis Pilosulae (*Dang Shen*), Radix Dioscoreae Oppositae (*Shan Yao*), Rhizoma Atractylodis Macrocephalae (*Bai Zhu*), Herba Epimedii (*Xian Ling Pi*), Radix Angelicae Sinensis (*Dang Gui*), Semen Citri Reticulatae (*Ju He*), and Pericarpium Citri Reticulatae (*Chen Pi*), 9g each and mix-fried Radix Glycyrrhizae (*Gan Cao*), and Rhizoma Cimicifugae (*Sheng Ma*), 4.5g.

2. Whenever damp heat complicates BPH, a clear bland diet is extremely important.

3. Although some Western sources encourage frequent ejaculation as a way of discharging congestion in the prostate, Chinese medical theory usually suggests against ejaculation in prostate conditions. Clinically, it is our experience that ejaculation may worsen the symptoms of BPH when the patient's pattern includes, as it so often does, an element of either kidney yin or yang vacuity.

4. Daily self-massage of the perineum can be very helpful in reducing prostate enlargement. However, the key to success with self-massage is regularity and persistence, since it usually takes several weeks to notice significant change.

5. BPH is relapsing in nature. During acute exacerbations,

use decocted medicinals in large doses. During remissions, use appropriate combinations of Chinese medicinal ready-made pills and concentrate on diet and lifestyle.

6. In the West, transurethral resection of the prostate (TURP) is considered the definitive treatment of this condition. However, after this procedure, 5-10% of patients experience problems with sexual function and/or urinary incontinence. In the case of postsurgical urinary incontinence, research in China has shown the following protocol to be 92.2% effective, with a 60% cure rate:[1] *Bu Zhong Yi Qi Tang Jia Wei* (Supplement the Center & Boost the Qi Decoction with Added Flavors): Radix Codonopsitis Pilosulae (*Dang Shen*), 15g, Radix Astragali Membranacei (*Huang Qi*), 20g, Rhizoma Atractylodis Macrocephalae (*Bai Zhu*), 9g, Radix Angelicae Sinensis (*Dang Gui*), 9g, Pericarpium Citri Reticulatae (*Chen Pi*), 12g, Rhizoma Cimicifugae (*Sheng Ma*), 3g, Radix Bupleuri (*Chai Hu*), 6g, Sclerotium Poriae Cocos (*Fu Ling*), 15g, Fructus Alpiniae Oxyphyllae (*Yi Zhi Ren*), 12g, Rhizoma Dioscoreae Hypoglaucae (*Bi Xie*), 1g, and Radix Glycyrrhizae (*Gan Cao*), 6g. If there is accompanying qi vacuity and lassitude of the spirit, increase *Huang Qi* up to 30g and replace *Dang Shen* with eight grams of Radix Rubrus Panacis Ginseng (*Hong Shen*). If there is yang qi vacuity weakness, add 12 grams of Herba Epimedii (*Xian Ling Pi*). If there is accompanying damp heat, remove *Dang Shen* and add 30-60 grams of Herba Artemisiae Capillaris (*Yin Chen Hao*) and six grams of Cortex Phellodendri (*Huang Bai*).

7. Digital rectal examination should be a routine part of the physical examination of all men over 50 years of age.

ENDNOTES

[1] Li Zhi-qiang & Yang Jun, "The Treatment of 40 Cases of Postsurgical Prostatic Hypertrophy Urinary Incontinence with *Bu Zhong Yi Qi Tang Jia Wei*," *He Nan Zhong Yi (Henan Chinese Medicine)*, #6, 2000, p. 29

8

Bronchial Asthma

Bronchial asthma is a typically episodic and remittent obstructive lung disorder characterized by narrowing of the large and small airways due to spasm of the smooth muscles of the bronchi, edema, inflammation of the bronchial mucosa, and production of tenacious mucus. A great deal of bronchial asthma is allergic in nature. Patients diagnosed as suffering from asthma differ greatly in the frequency and severity of their symptoms. In some patients, asthmatic attacks are infrequent, of short duration, and mild in their severity. Between these attacks, patients may be completely asymptomatic. Other patients may suffer from mild coughing and wheezing much of the time, punctuated by severe exacerbations following exposure to known allergens, viral infections, exercise, or nonspecific irritants. Psychoemotional stress may also either precipitate attacks or aggravate their severity. During acute attacks, there is tight-sounding, generally unproductive coughing, dyspnea, tachypnea, tightness and/or pressure in the chest, and wheezing. If dyspnea is severe, patients may not be able to breathe lying down and may experience great anxiety. In life-threatening attacks, there may be rapid, shallow, ineffectual breathing, cyanosis, lethargy, and confusion premonitory to respiratory failure. As the attack subsides, adult patients, but not young children, may expectorate tenacious, thick, sticky phlegm.

The Western medical diagnosis of asthma is based on the presence of wheezing, a family history, a personal history of episodic wheezing and dyspnea, often beginning in childhood or early adulthood, and a family or personal history of allergies. If diagnosis from the above is difficult or complicated by other factors, especially in patients whose wheezing and dyspnea begin after age 50, chest x-rays, blood cell examination, pulmonary function tests, and allergic skin testing may all be used to confirm the diagnosis. The Western medical treatment of asthma is mostly drug-based, and a wide range of medications may be prescribed based on the severity and staging of the disease. These medications include orally administered and inhaled prescriptions. The main classes of Western drugs used in the treatment of asthma are 1) beta-adrenergic agents, such as epinephrine, ephedrine, isoproterenol, and theophylline to relax the smooth muscles of the bronchi and bronchioles, 2) corticosteroids to inhibit allergic reactions, 3) anticholinergic agents to block the cholinergic pathways that cause airway obstruction, and 4) cromolyn sodium used prophylatcially to reduce airway hyper-reactivity. During severe attacks, patients may also be treated with oxygen to reduce hypoxia and with fluids and electrolytes to prevent or treat dehydration. When viral respiratory tract infections become complicated by secondary bacterial infections, antibiotics, such as ampicillin, erthromycin, or tetracycline, may be given. Unfortunately, all of the above medications have side effects, and satisfactory asthma control in adults may be difficult to achieve.

Chinese disease categorization: In Chinese medicine, bronchial asthma is referred to as *chuan zheng*, panting condition, *chuan ke*, panting and coughing, *chuan cu*, hasty panting, *xiao zheng*, wheezing condition, and *xiao chuan*, wheezing and panting.

Disease causes: External contraction of the six environmental excesses, internal damage by the seven affects, faulty diet, iatrogenesis, immaturity and aging

Disease mechanisms: The disease mechanisms of asthma are essentially the same as those of allergic rhinitis. There is typically a spleen qi vacuity resulting in A) defensive qi not securing and B) engenderment of phlegm dampness. Defensive qi not securing allows easy entry of external evils which hinder and obstruct the lung qi's diffusion and downbearing. When external evils mix with accumulated deep-lying phlegm in the lungs, impairment of the lungs' depurating and downbearing becomes even more severe. If enduring phlegm and dampness or severe qi stagnation leads to transformation of heat, phlegm dampness may be brewed into phlegm heat. Enduring non-diffusion and stagnation of the qi and obstruction by phlegm dampness may lead to concomitant blood stasis. Former heaven natural endowment insufficiency, latter heaven immaturity, enduring disease, or aging may lead to yin and/or yang vacuity. Especially in children and the elderly, kidney qi vacuity may fail to grasp the qi downborne by the lungs. Thus the three main viscera involved in asthma are the lungs, spleen, and kidneys. However, since the lungs and liver together govern the flow of qi throughout the body, most cases of asthma are also complicated by liver depression qi stagnation. This is because the lungs' downbearing and depurating works hand in hand with the liver's coursing and discharging. If the lungs do not downbear and depurate, this may lead to or aggravate liver depression, while liver depression leading to upward counterflow of qi and/or depressive heat may cause or aggravate loss of the lungs' depuration and downbearing.

TREATMENT BASED ON PATTERN DISCRIMINATION:

1. WIND COLD ASSAILING THE LUNGS PATTERN

MAIN SYMPTOMS: Acute or initial stage of asthma, panting with rales in the throat which usually occurs when exposed to cold, worse panting when lying flat, chest and diaphragmatic fullness and oppression, white, sticky or clear, watery, foamy phlegm, possible coughing, possible cold upper back, a green-blue, dull, stagnant facial complexion, no thirst or thirst with a liking for hot drinks, possible slight effusion of heat (*i.e.*, fever), aversion to cold, headache, itchy throat, sneezing, a runny nose, body aches or itching especially at the beginning of the acute stage, white, glossy tongue fur, and a floating, tight or bowstring pulse

TREATMENT PRINCIPLES: Dispel wind and scatter cold, diffuse the lungs, level panting, and transform phlegm

RX: *Ma Huang Tang* (Ephedra Decoction)

INGREDIENTS: Semen Pruni Armeniacae (*Xing Ren*), 12g, Herba Ephedrae (*Ma Huang*), 9g, Ramulus Cinnamomi Cassiae (*Gui Zhi*), 6g, and mix-fried Radix Glycyrrhizae (*Gan Cao*), 3g

ANALYSIS OF FORMULA: Within this formula, *Ma Huang* resolves the exterior and diffuses the lungs, stops coughing and levels panting. *Gui Zhi* resolves the exterior and scatters cold. When combined with *Ma Huang*, *Gui Zhi* strengthens *Ma Huang's* function of promoting diaphoresis. *Xing Ren* frees the flow of the lung qi and transforms phlegm, stops wheezing and loosens the chest, while mix-fried *Gan Cao* harmonizes the other medicinals in this formula and moderates *Ma Huang's* strongly diaphoretic action.

ADDITIONS & SUBTRACTIONS: For severe hasty panting, add nine grams each of Fructus Perillae Frutescentis (*Zi Su Zi*) and Radix Peucedani (*Qian Hu*). For chest oppression, add nine grams each of Radix Platycodi Grandiflori (*Jie Geng*) and Fructus Citri Aurantii (*Zhi Ke*).

For wind cold with disharmony between the constructive and defensive accompanied by hasty panting not stabilized after sweating, fever, aversion to cold, sweating, and a floating, moderate (*i.e.*, slightly slow) pulse, replace *Ma Huang Tang* with *Gui Zhi Jia Hou Po Xing Ren Tang* (Cinnamon Twig Plus Magnolia & Armeniaca Decoction): Ramulus Cinnamomi Cassiae (*Gui Zhi*), Radix Albus Paeoniae Lactiflorae (*Bai Shao*), Semen Pruni Armeniacae (*Xing Ren*), and Cortex Magnoliae Officinalis (*Hou Po*), 9g each, mix-fried Radix Glycyrrhizae (*Gan Cao*), 6g, uncooked Rhizoma Zingiberis (*Sheng Jiang*), 3 slices, and Fructus Zizyphi Jujubae (*Da Zao*), 5 pieces.

For profuse phlegm, replace *Ma Huang Tang* with modified *Xiao Qing Long Tang* (Minor Blue-green Dragon Decoction): uncooked Herba Ephedrae (*Ma Huang*), Rhizoma Pinelliae Terantae (*Ban Xia*), and Ramulus Cinnamomi Cassiae (*Gui Zhi*), Semen Pruni Armeniacae (*Xing Ren*), and Fructus Perillae Frutescentis (*Su Zi*), 9g each, Radix Albus Paeoniae Lactiflorae (*Bai Shao*), mix-fried Radix Glycyrrhizae (*Gan Cao*), and dry Rhizoma Zingiberis (*Gan Jiang*), 6g each, and Herba Asari Cum Radice (*Xi Xin*) and Fructus Schisandrae Chinensis (*Wu Wei Zi*), 3g each.

ACUPUNCTURE & MOXIBUSTION: *Da Zhui* (GV 14), *Feng Men* (Bl 12), *Fei Shu* (Bl 13), *Lie Que* (Lu 7), *Tian Tu* (CV 22)

ANALYSIS OF FORMULA: Draining *Da Zhui*, *Feng Men*, *Fei Shu*, and *Lie Que* dispels wind and scatters cold, diffuses the lungs and levels panting. Draining *Tian Tu* diffuses the lungs and transforms phlegm, strongly downbears the qi and levels panting.

ADDITIONS & SUBTRACTIONS: For severe panting, add *Ding Chuan* (M-BW-1). For headache, nasal congestion, and runny nose, add *Ying Tang* (M-HN-3) and *Yin Xiang* (LI 20). For effusion of heat (*i.e.*, fever), add *He Gu* (LI 4). For simultaneous effusion of heat and aversion to cold, add *Wai Guan* (TB 5). For profuse phlegm, add *Zhong Wan* (CV 12), *Feng Long* (St 40), and *Zu San Li* (St 36). For severe coughing, add *Chi Ze* (Lu 5). For chest oppression, add *Dan Zhong* (CV 17) and *Nei Guan* (Per 6). In children, especially with underlying food stagnation, bleed *Si Feng* (M-UE-9).

ADJUNCTIVE THERAPY: To help level panting and stop wheezing, grind Radix Lateralis Praeparatus Aconiti Carmichaeli (*Fu Zi*), 10%, Ramulus Cinnamomi Cassiae (*Gui Zhi*), 20%,

Semen Sinapis Albae (*Bai Jie Zi*), 10%, Herba Asari Cum Radice (*Xi Xin*), 20%, dry Rhizoma Zingiberis (*Gan Jiang*), 20%, and Pericarpium Zanthoxyli Bungeani (*Chuan Jiao*), 20%, into fine powder. Add fresh ginger juice and make into medicinal discs 2cm in diameter. Place one disc each on *Fei Shu* (Bl 13), *Gao Huang* (Bl 43), and *Dan Zhong* (CV 17) each night before bed, keeping them on with adhesive tape. Remove in the morning on arising.

2. WIND HEAT INVADING THE LUNGS PATTERN

SYMPTOMS: An acute episode of wheezing and panting, possible itching throat and/or sneezing, difficulty breathing, vexation and oppression, flaring nostrils, gaping mouth, raised shoulders, coughing of thick, yellow phlegm which is difficult to expectorate, possible effusion of heat (*i.e.*, fever), sweating, aversion to wind, thirst, pain in the chest, thin, white or thin, yellow tongue fur, and a floating, rapid pulse

TREATMENT PRINCIPLES: Clear heat and resolve the exterior, diffuse the lungs, level panting, and transform phlegm

RX: *Ma Xing Shi Gan Tang Jia Wei* (Ephedra, Armeniaca, Gypsum & Licorice Decoction with Added Flavors)

INGREDIENTS: Uncooked Gypsum Fibrosum (*Shi Gao*), 30g, Pericarpium Trichosanthis Kirlowii (*Gua Lou Pi*), 12g, Semen Pruni Armeniacae (*Xing Ren*), Radix Scutellariae Baicalensis (*Huang Qin*), and Fructus Forsythiae Suspensae (*Lian Qiao*), 9g each, and Herba Ephedrae (*Ma Huang*), Radix Glycyrrhizae (*Gan Cao*), and Radix Platycodi Grandiflori (*Jie Geng*), 6g each

ANALYSIS OF FORMULA: *Shi Gao* resolves the muscles, clears heat, drains lung heat, and, in combination with *Ma Huang,* resolves the exterior and levels panting due to wind heat. In addition, *Ma Huang* levels panting and stops cough. *Gua Lou Pi* diffuses the lungs and disperses phlegm, while *Xing Ren* downbears the qi and transforms phlegm. Both these medicinals also level panting and stop cough. *Jie Geng* diffuses the lungs and leads the other medicinals to the chest and lungs. *Lian Qiao* and *Huang Qin* clear the lungs.

ADDITIONS & SUBTRACTIONS: For severe contraction of external wind heat with aversion to wind and fever, add nine grams of Folium Mori Albi (*Sang Ye*), six grams of Herba Menthae Haplocalysis (*Bo He*), and 15 grams of Flos Lonicerae Japonicae (*Jin Yin Hua*). For profuse phlegm and severe hasty panting, add nine grams each of Semen Lepidii Seu Descurainiae (*Ting Li Zi*) and Rhizoma Belamcandae Chinensis (*She Gan*) and six grams each of Bulbus Fritillariae Thunbergii (*Zhe Bei Mu*) and Lumbricus (*Di Long*). For severe lung heat, add nine grams of Cortex Radicis Mori Albi (*Sang Bai Pi*). For constipation, add 3-9 grams of Radix Et Rhizoma Rhei (*Da Huang*).

For dryness and heat damaging the lungs with fever, aversion to cold, hasty panting, difficult expectoration of scanty, thick, sticky phlegm, phlegm containing blood, or dry coughing, pain in the chest, dry nose and throat, itchy sore throat, constipation, a red tongue tip with dry, yellow fur, and a floating, rapid pulse, replace *Ma Xing Shi Gan Tang* with *Sang Xing Tang Jia Jian* (Morus & Armeniaca Decoction with Additions & Subtractions): Folium Mori Albi (*Sang Ye*), Semen Pruni Armeniacae (*Xing Ren*), Radix Adenophorae Strictae (*Nan Sha Shen*), warm Semen Praeparatus Sojae (*Dan Dou Chi*), stir-fried Fructus Gardeniae Jasminoidis (*Zhi Zi*), Folium Eriobotryae Japonicae (*Pi Pa Ye*), and Fructus Aristolochiae (*Ma Dou Ling*), 9g each, and Bulbus Fritillariae Cirrhosae (*Chuan Bei Mu*) and Rhizoma Polygonati Odorati (*Yu Zhu*), 6g each. For malodorous, green phlegm, add Herba Houttuyniae Cordatae Cum Radice (*Yu Xing Cao*), 18g, and Rhizoma Phragmitis Communis (*Lu Gen*), 9g.

ACUPUNCTURE & MOXIBUSTION: *Da Zhui* (GV 14), *He Gu* (LI 4), *Fei Shu* (Bl 13), *Chi Ze* (Lu 5), *Tian Tu* (CV 22)

ANALYSIS OF FORMULA: Draining *Da Zhui* and *He Gu* resolves the exterior and clears heat. Draining *Fei Shu* drains the lungs and diffuses the qi, while draining *Chi Ze* clears and drains lung heat. Together, these points resolve the exterior and clear heat, diffuse the lungs and level panting. Draining *Tian Tu* diffuses the lungs and transforms phlegm, strongly downbears the qi and levels panting.

ADDITIONS & SUBTRACTIONS: For severe panting with flaring nostrils, gaping mouth, and raised shoulders when breathing, add *Ding Chuan* (M-BW-1) and *Fu Tu* (LI 18). For headache, nasal congestion, and runny nose, add *Ying Tang* (M-HN-3) and *Yin Xiang* (LI 20). For effusion of heat (*i.e.,* fever), add *Qu Chi* (LI 11). For simultaneous effusion of heat and aversion to cold, add *Wai Guan* (TB 5). For bloody phlegm, add *Kong Zui* (Lu 6). For profuse phlegm, add *Zhong Wan* (CV 12), *Feng Long* (St 40), and *Zu San Li* (St 36). For severe coughing, add *Yu Ji* (Lu 10). For chest oppression, add *Dan Zhong* (CV 17) and *Nei Guan* (Per 6). For constipation, add *Zhi Gou* (TB 6) and *Tian Shu* (St 25). In children, especially with underlying food stagnation, bleed *Si Feng* (M-UE-9).

3. EXTERIOR COLD COUPLED WITH INTERIOR HEAT PATTERN

MAIN SYMPTOMS: An acute episode of wheezing and panting, chest oppression, effusion of heat (*i.e.*, fever), aversion to cold, body aches, headache, vexatious thirst, difficult expectoration of thick phlegm or profuse, yellow phlegm, yellow and white tongue fur, and a floating, rapid pulse

TREATMENT PRINCIPLES: Diffuse the lungs and clear heat, transform phlegm and stabilize panting

Rx: *Ding Chuan Tang* (Stabilize Panting Decoction)

Ingredients: Herba Ephedrae (*Ma Huang*), Semen Pruni Armeniacae (*Xing Ren*), Flos Tussilaginis Farfarae (*Kuan Dong Hua*), Rhizoma Pinelliae Ternatae (*Ban Xia*), Semen Ginkgonis Bilobae (*Bai Guo*), Cortex Radicis Mori Albi (*Sang Bai Pi*), and Radix Scutellariae Baicalensis (*Huang Qin*), 9g each, Semen Pruni Armeniacae (*Xing Ren*) and Fructus Perillae Frutescentis (*Zi Su Zi*), 6g each, and Radix Glycyrrhizae (*Gan Cao*), 3g

Analysis of formula: *Ma Huang* resolves the exterior and scatters cold, while *Huang Qin* clears interior heat. Both enter the lungs. The former diffuses; the latter drains. *Xing Ren, Kuan Dong Hua,* and *Zi Su Zi* transform phlegm, downbear the qi, and level panting. *Ban Xia* transforms phlegm and downbears the qi. *Sang Bai Pi* helps *Huang Qin* clear the lungs and also levels panting. *Bai Guo* constrains the lung qi and levels painting.

Additions & subtractions: For profuse yellow phlegm and severe hasty panting, add nine grams each of Semen Lepidii Seu Descurainiae (*Ting Li Zi*) and Rhizoma Belamcandae Chinensis (*She Gan*) and six grams of Bulbus Fritillariae Thunbergii (*Zhe Bei Mu*). For clear, watery phlegm, add six grams of dry Rhizoma Zingiberis (*Gan Jiang*) and three grams of Herba Asari Cum Radice (*Xi Xin*). For severe exterior cold, add nine grams of Folium Perillae Frutescentis (*Zi Su Ye*) and six grams of Ramulus Cinnamomi Cassiae (*Gui Zhi*). For thirst, add nine grams of Rhizoma Phragmitis Communis (*Lu Gen*). For constipation, add six grams of Radix Et Rhizoma Rhei (*Da Huang*). For interior heat, add 20 grams of Gypsum Fibrosum (*Shi Gao*), nine grams of Folium Eriobotryae Japonicae (*Pi Pa Ye*) and three grams of Lumbricus (*Di Long*) (powdered and taken with the strained decoction). For severe panting and wheezing, add three grams of Lumbricus (*Di Long*), (powdered and taken with the strained decoction) and nine grams each of Semen Lepidii Seu Descurainiae (*Ting Li Zi*) and Cortex Magnoliae Officinalis (*Hou Po*). For contraction of external wind heat with aversion to wind and effusion of heat, add nine grams each of Semen Praeparatus Sojae (*Dan Dou Chi*) and Herba Menthae Haplocalysis (*Bo He*) and 15 grams of Flos Lonicerae Japonicae (*Jin Yin Hua*). For profuse phlegm, add nine grams each of Radix Platycodi Grandiflori (*Jie Geng*) and bile-processed Rhizoma Arisaematis (*Dan Nan Xing*).

Acupuncture & moxibustion: *Da Zhui* (GV 14), *Feng Men* (Bl 12), *Fei Shu* (Bl 13), *Nei Ting* (St 44), *He Gu* (LI 4), *Tian Tu* (CV 22)

Analysis of formula: Draining *Da Zhui, Feng Men,* and *Fei Shu* dispels wind and scatters cold, diffuses the lungs and levels panting. Draining *He Gu* and *Nei Ting* together clears the lungs and drains the interior. Draining *Tian Tu* diffuses the lungs and transforms phlegm, strongly downbears the qi and levels panting.

Additions & subtractions: For severe panting, add *Ding Chuan* (M-BW-1) and/or *Fu Tu* (LI 18). For severe lung heat, add *Yu Ji* (Lu 10). For headache, nasal congestion, and itchy, runny nose, add *Ying Tang* (M-HN-3) and *Yin Xiang* (LI 20). For effusion of heat (*i.e.*, fever), add *Qu Chi* (LI 11). For simultaneous effusion of heat and aversion to cold, add *Wai Guan* (TB 5). For profuse phlegm, add *Zhong Wan* (CV 12), *Feng Long* (St 40), and *Zu San Li* (St 36). For severe coughing, add *Chi Ze* (Lu 5). For chest oppression, add *Dan Zhong* (CV 17) and *Nei Guan* (Per 6). In children, especially with underlying food stagnation, bleed *Si Feng* (M-UE-9).

4. Phlegm turbidity obstructing the lungs pattern

Main symptoms: Wheezing and panting with difficulty breathing, a gurgling sound of phlegm, coughing with difficult to expectorate profuse, thick, white phlegm, chest oppression and a suffocating feeling, possible nausea and torpid intake, slimy, white tongue fur, and a slippery pulse

Treatment principles: Transform phlegm, downbear the qi, and stop panting

Rx: *Er Chen Tang* (Two Aged [Ingredients] Decoction) & *San Zi Yang Xin Tang* (Three Seeds Nourish the New Decoction) with additions and subtractions

Ingredients: Rhizoma Pinelliae Ternatae (*Ban Xia*), Pericarpium Citri Reticulatae (*Chen Pi*), Sclerotium Poriae Cocos (*Fu Ling*), Fructus Perillae Frutescentis (*Su Zi*), Semen Sinapis Albae (*Bai Jie Zi*), Semen Raphani Sativi (*Lai Fu Zi*), Cortex Magnoliae Officinalis (*Hou Po*), and Semen Pruni Armeniacae (*Xing Ren*), 9g each, mix-fried Radix Glycyrrhizae (*Gan Cao*), 6g, and Fructus Pruni Mume (*Wu Mei*), 1 piece

Analysis of formula: *Bai Jie Zi* warms the lungs and disinhibits the qi, disinhibits the diaphragm and transforms phlegm. *Zi Su Zi* downbears the qi and transforms phlegm, stops cough and levels panting. *Lai Fu Zi* moves the qi and expels phlegm. When these three medicinals are used together, they comprise *San Zi Yang Xin Tang.* This is a basic formula for treating asthma due to phlegm accumulation in the lungs. Nevertheless, this formula is relatively weak for transforming phlegm and downbearing the qi. Thus, we add *Ban Xia, Fu Ling, Chen Pi,* and mix-fried *Gan Cao,* the main ingredients of *Er Chen Tang.* This is a basic formula for treating phlegm dampness. To this foundation are added *Xing Ren* to transform phlegm, diffuse the lungs, and level panting, *Hou Po* to move and downbear the qi and level panting, and *Wu Mei* to constrain the lung qi to level panting.

ADDITIONS & SUBTRACTIONS: For profuse phlegm, add nine grams each of processed Rhizoma Arisaematis (*Tian Nan Xing*) and Flos Inulae Racemosae (*Xuan Fu Hua*). For cold phlegm or spleen yang vacuity, add six grams of dry Rhizoma Zingiberis (*Gan Jiang*) and three grams of Herba Asari Cum Radice (*Xi Xin*). For phlegm dampness transforming into phlegm heat, add nine grams each of Radix Scutellariae Baicalensis (*Huang Qin*) and Pericarpium Trichosanthis Kirlowii (*Gua Lou Pi*) and six grams of bile-processed Rhizoma Arisaematis (*Dan Nan Xing*). For severe qi vacuity with reduced food intake, abdominal distention, and fatigue, add 15 grams of Rhizoma Atractylodis Macrocephalae (*Bai Zhu*) and nine grams of Radix Codonopsitis Pilosulae (*Dang Shen*). For damp turbidity in the center with a slimy, bland taste in the mouth, reduced food intake, nausea, abdominal distention, and loose stools, add nine grams of Rhizoma Atractylodis (*Cang Zhu*) and three grams of Fructus Amomi (*Sha Ren*). For thick, white phlegm which is difficult to expectorate, add nine grams of Radix Platycodi Grandiflori (*Jie Geng*), Fructus Citri Aurantii (*Zhi Ke*), and Fructus Trichosanthis Kirlowii (*Gua Lou*). For severe panting and wheezing, add nine grams each of Radix Asteris Tatarici (*Zi Wan*) and Flos Tussilaginis Farfarae (*Kuan Dong Hua*) and three grams of Lumbricus (*Di Long*), powdered and taken with the strained decoction. For concomitant kidney yang vacuity, combine with *Shen Qi Wan* (Kidney Qi Pills, a Chinese ready-made medicine) or eventually add 12 grams of Fructus Psoraleae Corylifoliae (*Bu Gu Zhi*), nine grams of Fructus Schisandrae Chinensis (*Wu Wei Zi*), and three grams of Lignum Aquilariae Agallochae (*Chen Xiang*), powdered and taken with the strained decoction. For concomitant lung yin vacuity, add nine grams each of Radix Adenophorae Strictae (*Nan Sha Shen*), Bulbus Lilii (*Bai He*), and Tuber Ophiopogonis Japonici (*Mai Men Dong*). For concomitant kidney yin vacuity, combine with *Liu Wei Di Huang Wan* (Six Flavors Rehmannia Pills, a Chinese ready-made medicine) or eventually add 12 grams each of cooked Radix Rehmanniae (*Shu Di*) and Fructus Schisandrae Chinensis (*Wu Wei Zi*).

ACUPUNCTURE & MOXIBUSTION: *Da Zhui* (GV 14), *Fei Shu* (Bl 13), *Zu San Li* (St 36), *Feng Long* (St 40), *Nei Guan* (Per 6), *Tian Tu* (CV 22)

ANALYSIS OF FORMULA: Draining *Da Zhui* and *Fei Shu* diffuses the lungs and disperses phlegm, downbears the qi and levels panting. Supplementing *Zu San Li* fortifies the spleen and prevents damp accumulation and, thus, the engenderment of new phlegm. Draining *Feng Long* eliminates dampness and transforms already engendered phlegm. One treats the root of phlegm engenderment, *i.e.*, the spleen, while the other treats the branch, the phlegm. Draining *Nei Guan* guides the action of the last two points to the chest and then helps the first two points to disperse phlegm and loosen the chest. Draining *Tian Tu* diffuses the lungs and transforms phlegm, strongly downbears the qi and levels panting.

ADDITIONS & SUBTRACTIONS: See patterns #1, 2 and 3 above.

5. PHLEGM HEAT CONGESTING IN THE LUNGS PATTERN

MAIN SYMPTOMS: Wheezing and panting, hoarse panting with loud rales in the throat which often occur when exposed to heat, coughing of thick, sticky, yellow phlegm, difficulty breathing, possible flaring nostrils, possible fever, heart vexation, disquieted spirit, thirst with a liking for chilled drinks, a dry throat, a red facial complexion, dark-colored urine, constipation, a red tongue with slimy, yellow fur, and a slippery, rapid pulse

NOTE: The difference between this pattern and the wind heat pattern above is that here there is internally engendered depressive and yang ming heat and no particular exterior signs or symptoms.

TREATMENT PRINCIPLES: Clear heat and transform phlegm, downbear the qi and stop panting

RX: *Sang Bai Pi Tang Jia Jian* (Cortex Mori Decoction with Additions & Subtractions)

INGREDIENTS: Cortex Radicis Mori Albi (*Sang Bai Pi*), Rhizoma Pinelliae Ternatae (*Ban Xia*), Fructus Perillae Frutescentis (Zi *Su Zi*), Semen Pruni Armeniacae (*Xing Ren*), Bulbus Fritillariae Thunbergii (*Zhe Bei Mu*), Radix Scutellariae Baicalensis (*Huang Qin*), Fructus Gardeniae Jasminoidis (*Zhi Zi*), and Semen Lepidii Seu Descurainiae (*Ting Li Zi*), 9g each, and Radix Glycyrrhizae (*Gan Cao*), 6g

ANALYSIS OF FORMULA: *Sang Bai Pi*, *Zhi Zi*, and *Huang Qin* clear the lungs and drain heat. In addition, *Sang Bai Pi* levels panting. *Ban Xia* and *Zhe Bei Mu* transform phlegm heat. *Zi Su Zi* and *Xing Ren* transform phlegm, while *Ting Li Zi* flushes phlegm accumulation in the lungs. In addition, *Ting Li Zi* drains the lungs and stabilizes panting, while *Zi Su Zi* and *Xing Ren* diffuse and downbear the lung qi and level panting. *Gan Cao* harmonizes all the other medicinals in the formula.

ADDITIONS & SUBTRACTIONS: For severe hasty panting, add nine grams of Rhizoma Belamcandae Chinensis (*She Gan*) and six grams of Herba Ephedrae (*Ma Huang*). For fever, add 20 grams of Gypsum Fibrosum (*Shi Gao*) and nine grams of Rhizoma Anemarrhenae Asphodeloidis (*Zhi Mu*). For profuse phlegm, add nine grams of Pericarpium Trichosanthis Kirlowii (*Gua Lou Pi*) and six grams of Radix Platycodi Grandiflori (*Jie Geng*). For blood-streaked phlegm, malodorous phlegm, and chest pain, add nine grams each of Herba Houttuyniae Cordatae Cum Radice (*Yu Xing Cao*), Semen Benincasae Hispidae (*Dong Gua Zi*), and Rhizoma Phragmitis Communis (*Lu Gen*). For heat damaging the network vessels in the lungs with coughing of blood or hacking of blood, add three grams each of Rhizoma Bletillae Striatae (*Bai Ji*) and Radix Pseudoginseng (*San Qi*). For constipation, add six grams of Radix Et Rhizoma Rhei (*Da Huang*) and nine grams of Semen Trichosanthis Kirlowii (*Gua Lou Ren*). For sticky phlegm which is difficult to expectorate, add nine grams of Radix Platycodi Grandiflori (*Jie Geng*) and Semen Benincasae Hispidae (*Dong Gua Zi*) and six grams of Fructus Citri Aurantii (*Zhi Ke*). For severe panting and wheezing, add three grams each of Lumbricus (*Di Long*) and Bombyx Batryticatus (*Jiang Can*), both powdered and taken with the strained decoction. For severe lung yin damage due to heat, subtract *Ban Xia* and *Huang Qin* and add nine grams each of Bulbus Fritillariae Cirrhosae (*Chuan Bei Mu*), Fructus Trichosanthis Kirlowii (*Gua Lou*), Tuber Ophiopogonis Japonici (*Mai Men Dong*), and Bulbus Lilii (*Bai He*) and three grams of Lumbricus (*Di Long*), powdered and taken with the strained decoction. For severe heat accumulation with phlegm heat transforming into fire accompanied by high fever, a red facial complexion, sweating, thirst with a liking for chilled drinks, and a surging pulse, add *Bai Hu Tang* (White Tiger Decoction), *i.e.*, 30 grams of uncooked Gypsum Fibrosum (*Shi Gao*), nine grams of uncooked Rhizoma Anemarrhenae Asphodeloidis (*Zhi Mu*), and six grams each of Radix Glycyrrhizae (*Gan Cao*), and Semen Oryzae Sativae (*Geng Mi*) as well as nine grams of Rhizoma Phragmitis Communis (*Lu Gen*).

ACUPUNCTURE & MOXIBUSTION: *Da Zhui* (GV 14), *Fei Shu* (Bl 13), *Zu San Li* (St 36), *Feng Long* (St 40), *Yu Ji* (Lu 10), *Tian Tu* (CV 22)

ANALYSIS OF FORMULA: Draining *Da Zhui* and *Fei Shu* clears the lungs and drains heat, disperses phlegm, downbears the qi, and levels panting. Supplementing *Zu San Li* fortifies the spleen and prevents damp accumulation and, thus, the engenderment of new phlegm. Draining *Feng Long* eliminates dampness and transforms already engendered phlegm. Draining *Yu Ji* clears and disperses phlegm heat, downbears the qi and stabilizes panting. Draining *Tian Tu* diffuses the lungs and transforms phlegm, strongly downbears the qi and levels panting.

ADDITIONS & SUBTRACTIONS: Please see pattern #2 above.

6. PHLEGM & QI DEPRESSION & BINDING PATTERN

MAIN SYMPTOMS: Sudden onset of wheezing and panting, chest oppression, a possible feeling of something stuck in the throat which can neither be spit up nor swallowed down, chest and rib-side distention and pain, emotional depression, impatience and irritability, insomnia, heart palpitations, thin, white tongue fur, and a bowstring pulse

NOTE: In most real-life cases of asthma, liver depression complicates other patterns. It does not typically cause asthma by itself.

TREATMENT PRINCIPLES: Transform phlegm and resolve the depression, downbear the qi and stabilize panting

RX: *Wu Mo Yin Zi* (Five Grindings Drink) & *Er Chen Tang* (Two Aged [Ingredients] Decoction) with additions and subtractions

INGREDIENTS: Rhizoma Pinelliae Ternatae (*Ban Xia*), Sclerotium Poriae Cocos (*Fu Ling*), and Semen Arecae Catechu (*Bing Lang*), 9g each, Radix Auklandiae Lappae (*Mu Xiang*), Lignum Aquilariae Agallochae (*Chen Xiang*), Fructus Immaturus Citri Aurantii (*Zhi Shi*), Radix Bupleuri (*Chai Hu*), Pericarpium Citri Reticulatae (*Chen Pi*), and Radix Albus Paeoniae Lactiflorae (*Bai Shao*), 6g each, and Radix Glycyrrhizae (*Gan Cao*), 3g

ANALYSIS OF FORMULA: Within this formula, *Bing Lang, Mu Xiang, Chen Xiang, Zhi Shi, Chai Hu*, and *Chen Pi* all move and rectify the qi, thus loosening the chest and downbearing counterflow. *Ban Xia* transforms phlegm at the same time as it downbears counterflow, while *Fu Ling* fortifies the spleen and seeps dampness, thus aiding in the elimination of phlegm dampness. These two ingredients are aided by *Chen Pi* which also eliminates dampness, transforms phlegm, and downbears counterflow. *Bai Shao* nourishes liver blood to enable the liver to regain control over coursing and discharge, while *Gan Cao* harmonizes all the medicinals in this formula.

ADDITIONS & SUBTRACTIONS: For chest pain, oppression, and distention, add nine grams each of Rhizoma Cyperi Rotundi (*Xiang Fu*) and Flos Inulae Racemosae (*Xuan Fu Hua*). For heart palpitations and insomnia, add nine grams each of Bulbus Lilii (*Bai He*), Flos Albizziae Julibrissinis (*He Huan Hua*), Semen Zizyphi Spinosae (*Suan Zao Ren*), and Radix Polygalae Tenuifoliae (*Yuan Zhi*). For severe plum-pit qi and/or severe hasty panting, add nine grams of Cortex Magnoliae Officinalis (*Hou Po*) and six grams of Folium Perillae Frutescentis (*Zi Su Ye*).

For enduring depression transforming fire, replace *Wu Mo Yin Zi* and *Er Chen Tang* with *Dan Zhi Xiao Yao San Jia Wei* (Moutan & Gardenia Rambling Powder with Added Flavors): Radix Angelicae Sinensis (*Dang Gui*), Radix Albus Paeoniae Lactiflorae (*Bai Shao*), Radix Ligustici Wallichii (*Chuan Xiong*), Tuber Curcumae (*Yu Jin*), Rhizoma Cyperi Rotundi (*Xiang Fu*), and Cortex Radicis

Moutan (*Dan Pi*), 9g each, Radix Bupleuri (*Chai Hu*), Fructus Gardeniae Jasminoidis, and Sclerotium Poriae Cocos (*Fu Ling*), 6g each, mix-fried Radix Glycyrrhizae (*Gan Cao*) and Herba Menthae Haplocalycis (*Bo He*), 3g each, and uncooked Rhizoma Zingiberis (*Sheng Jiang*), 2 slices.

Acupuncture & moxibustion: *Da Zhui* (GV 14), *Fei Shu* (Bl 13), *Zu San Li* (St 36), *Feng Long* (St 40), *Nei Guan* (Per 6), *Tai Chong* (Liv 3)

Analysis of formula: Draining *Da Zhui* and *Fei Shu* diffuses the lungs and disperses phlegm, downbears the qi and level panting. Supplementing *Zu San Li* fortifies the spleen and prevents damp accumulation and, thus, the engenderment of new phlegm. Draining *Feng Long* eliminates dampness and transforms already engendered phlegm. Draining *Nei Guan* guides the action of the last two points to the chest and then helps the first two points disperse phlegm and loosen the chest. In addition, it also helps *Tai Chong*, which should also be drained, to course the liver and resolve the depression.

Additions & subtractions: Please see patterns #1, 2, and 3 above.

7. Lung qi & yin dual vacuity pattern

Main symptoms: Wheezing and panting, shortness of breath which gets worse on exertion, a weak voice and/or disinclination to speak, aversion to wind, spontaneous perspiration, susceptibility to catching cold, fatigue, a dry mouth and throat, malar flushing in the afternoon, reduced sleep, heart vexation, a pale tongue with red tip, and a soggy or vacuous and weak pulse. The wheezing and panting in this pattern often appear and worsen due to changes in the weather. The acute stage tends to occur during the fall and winter when the climate turns cooler and drier or in the spring in those with an allergic constitution. The remission stage is in the summer.

Note: Although no signs and symptoms of phlegm are included in the above list, there will be deep-lying or hidden phlegm in all cases of asthma, and phlegm is taken into account in the Chinese medicinal formula suggested below. This pattern is commonly seen in those with enduring disease, those living in dry climates, the elderly, and as an iatrogenic complication to prolonged use of beta-adrenergic agents and corticosteriods.

Treatment principles: Supplement the lungs, nourish yin, and stabilize panting

Rx: *Bu Fei Tang Jia Jian* (Supplement the Lungs Decoction with Additions & Subtractions)

Ingredients: Radix Astragali Membranacei (*Huang Qi*), 12g, Radix Codonopsis Pilosulae (*Dang Shen*), Fructus Schisandrae Chinensis (*Wu Wei Zi*), Radix Asteris Tatarici (*Zi Wan*), Cortex Radicis Mori Albi (*Sang Bai Pi*), Tuber Ophiopogonis Japonici (*Mai Men Dong*), and Radix Adenophorae Strictae (*Nan Sha Shen*), 9g each, and cooked Radix Rehmanniae (*Shu Di*), 6g

Analysis of formula: *Huang Qi* and *Dang Shen* both fortify the spleen and boost the qi. *Wu Wei Zi*, *Mai Men Dong*, and *Shu Di* all supplement yin. *Wu Wei Zi* also constrains the lung qi, while *Mai Men Dong* also clears heat and transforms phlegm. *Zi Wan* stops coughing, and *Sang Bai Pi* clears the lungs.

Additions & subtractions: For predominant lung qi vacuity, add nine grams of Radix Dioscoreae Oppositae (*Shan Yao*) and 1.5 grams of powdered Gecko (*Ge Jie*). For predominant lung yin vacuity, add nine grams of Bulbus Lilii (*Bai He*) and six grams of Rhizoma Polygonati Odorati (*Yu Zhu*). For severe hasty panting, add nine grams each of Fructus Terminaliae Chebulae (*He Zi*) and Semen Ginkgonis Bilobae (*Bai Guo*). For susceptibility to common cold, add six grams of Radix Ledebouriellae Divaricatae (*Fang Feng*) and nine grams of Rhizoma Atractylodis Macrocephalae (*Bai Zhu*). For phlegm dampness obstructing the lungs manifesting as coughing of white phlegm, add nine grams each of Rhizoma Pinelliae Ternatae (*Ban Xia*) and Sclerotium Poriae Cocos (*Fu Ling*) and six grams of Pericarpium Citri Reticulatae (*Chen Pi*). For coughing, add nine grams each of Semen Pruni Armeniacae (*Xing Ren*) and Fructus Perillae Frutescentis (*Su Zi*). For concomitant spleen qi vacuity with reduced appetite, abdominal fullness, and loose stools, add nine grams each of Radix Codonopsitis Pilosulae (*Dang Shen*) and Rhizoma Atractylodis Macrocephalae (*Bai Zhu*).

Acupuncture & moxibustion: *Da Zhui* (GV 14), *Fei Shu* (Bl 13), *Tai Yuan* (Lu 9), *He Gu* (LI 4), *Fu Liu* (Ki 7)

Analysis of formula: *Da Zhui* is the intersection point of all the yang channels, *Fei Shu* is the back transport point of the lungs, *Tai Yuan* is the source point of the lungs, and *He Gu* is one of the master or ruling points of the qi, exterior, and lungs. When these four points are used together with supplementing technique, they supplement the lungs and boost the qi, secure the exterior and level panting. Supplementing *Fu Liu,* the metal-mother point on the kidney channel, nourishes not only the kidneys but also the yin of the entire body. *Fei Shu* and *Tai Yuan* then guide the yin-supplementing action of *Fu Liu* to the lungs.

Note: Acupuncture's ability to supplement yin is limited.

Additions & subtractions: For severe qi vacuity, add *Zu San Li* (St 36). For phlegm, add *Feng Long* (St 40) and *Zu*

San Li (St 36). For severe panting, add *Ding Chuan* (M-BW-1) and/or *Fu Tu* (LI 18). For chest oppression, add *Dan Zhong* (CV 17) and *Nei Guan* (Per 6). In children, especially with underlying food stagnation, bleed *Si Feng* (M-UE-9).

8. LUNG-KIDNEY YIN VACUITY PATTERN

MAIN SYMPTOMS: Wheezing and panting which gets worse on exertion, difficult expectoration of scanty, sticky phlegm, a dry mouth and throat, tidal heat, night sweats, vexatious heat in the five hearts, low back and knee soreness and limpness, tinnitus, a red tongue with scanty fur and fluids, and a thin, rapid pulse

NOTE: This pattern is commonly seen in those with enduring disease, those living in dry climates, the elderly, and as an iatrogenic complication to prolonged use of beta-adrenergic agents and corticosteriods.

TREATMENT PRINCIPLES: Nourish yin and foster essence, supplement the lungs and kidneys

RX: *Du Qi Wan Jia Jian* (Capital Qi Pills with Additions & Subtractions)

INGREDIENTS: Cooked Radix Rehmanniae (*Shu Di*), 24g, Fructus Schisandrae Chinensis (*Wu Wei Zi*), 18g, Fructus Corni Officinalis (*Shan Zhu Yu*), 12g, Radix Dioscoreae Oppositae (*Shan Yao*), Sclerotium Poriae Cocos (*Fu Ling*), Bulbus Lilii (*Bai He*), and Tuber Ophiopogonis Japonici (*Mai Dong*), 9g each, Rhizoma Alismatis (*Ze Xie*) and Cortex Radicis Moutan (*Dan Pi*), 6g each, and Lignum Aquilariae Agallochae (*Chen Xiang*), 3g (powdered and taken with the strained decoction)

ANALYSIS OF FORMULA: *Shu Di, Shan Yao, Shan Zhu Yu, Fu Ling, Dan Pi*, and *Ze Xie* are the six flavors of *Liu Wei Di Huang Wan* (Six Flavors Rehmannia Pills) which enrich liver-kidney yin. *Wu Wei Zi* engenders fluids, constrains the lung qi, and helps stabilize panting. *Mai Men Dong* and *Bai He* nourish lung yin.

ADDITIONS & SUBTRACTIONS: For scanty phlegm which is difficult to expectorate, add nine grams each of Bulbus Fritillariae Cirrhosae (*Chuan Bei Mu*), Semen Pruni Armeniacae (*Xing Ren*), and Fructus Perillae Frutescentis (*Su Zi*). For concomitant spleen vacuity, add 15 grams of Radix Astragali Membranacei (*Huang Qi*) and nine grams of Radix Codonopsitis Pilosulae (*Dang Shen*).

ACUPUNCTURE & MOXIBUSTION: *Da Zhui* (GV 14), *Fei Shu* (Bl 13), *Tai Yuan* (Lu 9), *Tai Xi* (Ki 3)

ANALYSIS OF FORMULA: When needled together with supplementing technique, *Da Zhui, Fei Shu*, and *Tai Yuan* supplement the lungs and level panting, while supplementing *Tai Xi* supplements lung and kidney yin and promotes qi absorption.

ADDITIONS & SUBTRACTIONS: For concomitant spleen vacuity, add *Zu San Li* (St 36). For phlegm, add *Feng Long* (St 40) and *Zu San Li* (St 36). For severe panting, add *Ding Chuan* (M-BW-1) and/or *Fu Tu* (LI 18). For chest oppression, add *Dan Zhong* (CV 17) and *Nei Guan* (Per 6). In children, especially with underlying food stagnation, bleed *Si Feng* (M-UE-9).

9. LUNG-SPLEEN QI VACUITY

MAIN SYMPTOMS: Wheezing and panting and shortness of breath which get worse on exertion, coughing of clear, watery phlegm, a pale facial complexion, a weak voice or disinclination to speak, aversion to wind, spontaneous perspiration, susceptibility to catching cold, fatigue, a pale, fat tongue with teeth-marks on its edges and white fur, and a weak or soggy pulse. When spleen qi vacuity is dominant, wheezing and panting appear and worsen with dietary irregularities and especially excessive consumption of uncooked, chilled foods, iced drinks, sweet or fatty foods, dairy products, fish, shrimp, or other sea foods. When lung qi vacuity is dominant, wheezing and panting appear and worsen due to changes in the weather. In addition, there is a susceptibility to catching cold, frequent sneezing, or runny nose. The former is a pattern of food allergy; the second is a respiratory allergy.

NOTE: This pattern is commonly seen in infants and children whose spleen's are inherently immature. It may also be due to faulty diet as well as over-use or prolonged use of antibiotics. In addition, women are especially prone to spleen vacuity due to menstruation, gestation, and lactation. Further, both men and women tend to become spleen vacuous and weak with aging.

TREATMENT PRINCIPLES: Fortify the spleen and supplement the lungs, transform phlegm and stop panting

RX: *Liu Jun Zi Tang* (Six Gentlemen Decoction) & *Yu Ping Feng San* (Jade Windscreen Powder) with added flavors

INGREDIENTS: Rhizoma Atractylodis Macrocephalae (*Bai Zhu*) and Radix Astragali Membranacei (*Huang Qi*), 12g each, Radix Codonopsitis Pilosulae (*Dang Shen*), Sclerotium Poriae Cocos (*Fu Ling*), lime-processed Rhizoma Pinelliae Ternatae (*Ban Xia*), and Flos Inulae Racemosae (*Xuan Fu Hua*), 9g each, and mix-fried Radix Glycyrrhizae (*Gan Cao*), Pericarpium Citri Reticulatae (*Chen Pi*), and Radix Ledebouriellae Divaricatae (*Fang Feng*), 6g each

ANALYSIS OF FORMULA: *Bai Zhu, Huang Qi, Fu Ling, Dang*

Shen, and mix-fried *Gan Cao* fortify the spleen and supplement the lungs, boost the qi and secure the exterior. *Ban Xia*, *Fu Ling*, *Chen Pi*, and *Xuan Fu Hua* eliminate dampness, move the qi, and transform phlegm. In addition, *Xuan Fu Hua* downbears the qi and stabilizes panting. *Fang Feng* gently out-thrusts any wind evils.

ADDITIONS & SUBTRACTIONS: For vacuity cold of the lungs with aversion to cold and profuse white, watery phlegm, add 6 grams of dry Rhizoma Zingiberis (*Gan Jiang*) and 3 grams of Herba Asari Cum Radice (*Xi Xin*). For spleen yang vacuity with a cold body, diarrhea, etc., add 6 grams each of dry Rhizoma Zingiberis (*Gan Jiang*) and stir-fried Ramulus Cinnamomi Cassiae (*Gui Zhi*). For severe hasty panting, add 9 grams each of Fructus Schisandrae Chinensis (*Wu Wei Zi*) and Fructus Terminaliae Chebulae (*He Zi*). For severe spleen qi vacuity with diarrhea, add 9 grams of Semen Nelumbinis Nuciferae (*Lian Zi*) and Radix Dioscoreae Oppositae (*Shan Yao*). For concomitant food stagnation with no thought for eating and indigestion, add 9 grams of Cortex Magnoliae Officinalis (*Hou Po*). For nausea or vomiting, add 9 grams of Flos Inulae Racemosae (*Xuan Fu Hua*) and 3 slices of uncooked Rhizoma Zingiberis (*Sheng Jiang*). For damp turbidity in the center with a slimy, bland taste in the mouth, reduced food intake, nausea, abdominal distention, and loose stools, add 9 grams of Cortex Magnoliae Officinalis (*Hou Po*) and 6 grams of Rhizoma Atractylodis (*Cang Zhu*).

ACUPUNCTURE & MOXIBUSTION: *Da Zhui* (GV 14), *Fei Shu* (Bl 13), *Zu San Li* (St 36), *Feng Long* (St 40)

ANALYSIS OF FORMULA: Supplementing *Da Zhui* boosts the qi, secures the exterior, and levels panting. *Fei Shu* supplements and warms the lungs, disperses phlegm, downbears the qi, and levels panting. *Zu San Li* fortifies the spleen and prevents damp accumulation, thus, preventing the engenderment of new phlegm. *Feng Long* eliminates dampness and transforms phlegm.

ADDITIONS & SUBTRACTIONS: Please see patterns #1, 2, and 3 above.

10. KIDNEYS NOT ABSORBING THE QI PATTERN

MAIN SYMPTOMS: Enduring wheezing and panting, shortness of breath, more difficulty inhaling than exhaling, worsening on exertion, low back and knee soreness and limpness, a possibly blue-green facial complexion (if complicated by blood stasis), chilled limbs, a pale tongue with white fur, and a deep, fine pulse

NOTE: This pattern is most often seen in the young whose kidneys are inherently immature, in the elderly, and in the chronically ill. In the later case, "Enduring illness reaches the kidneys." As described above, this pattern is mainly a kidney qi vacuity pattern. Children with this pattern typically also suffer from enuresis.

TREATMENT PRINCIPLES: Supplement the kidneys to absorb the qi

RX: *Ren Shen Hu Tao Ren Tang Jia Wei* (Ginseng & Walnut Decoction with Added Flavors)

INGREDIENTS: Fructus Schisandrae Chinensis (*Wu Wei Zi*), 12g, Semen Juglandis Regiae (*Hu Tao Ren*) and Fructus Psoraleae Corylifoliae (*Bu Gu Zhi*), 9g each, Radix Panacis Ginseng (*Ren Shen*), 6g, Lignum Aquilariae Agallochae (*Chen Xiang*) and Placenta Hominis (*Zi He Che*), 3g each, Gecko (*Ge Jie*), 1.5g, uncooked Rhizoma Zingiberis (*Sheng Jiang*), 2 slices

ANALYSIS OF FORMULA: *Zi He Che* supplements the kidneys and boosts the essence, thus promoting qi absorption. *Ren Shen* supplements the latter heaven to support the former heaven. *Hu Tao Ren* and *Ge Jie* supplement lungs and kidneys and stabilize panting. *Bu Gu Zhi* supplements the kidneys, while *Chen Xiang* scatters cold and moves the qi. Both these two medicinals also promote the qi absorption and level panting. *Wu Wei Zi* supplements the lungs and kidneys and constrains the lung qi. *Sheng Jiang* aides the qi transformation.

ADDITIONS & SUBTRACTIONS: For kidney yang vacuity with enduring hasty panting, shortness of breath, more exhalation than inhalation, worsening on exertion, aversion to cold, night-time urination, sweating, lassitude of the spirit, low back and knee soreness and limpness, chilled limbs, a pale tongue with white fur, and a deep, fine, forceless pulse, replace *Ren Shen Hu Tao Ren Tang* with *Shen Qi Wan Jia Wei* (Kidney Qi Pills with Added Flavors): cooked Radix Rehmanniae (*Shu Di*), 15g, Radix Dioscoreae Oppositae (*Shan Yao*), Fructus Corni Officinalis (*Shan Zhu Yu*), and Fructus Psoraleae Corylifoliae (*Bu Gu Zhi*), 9g each, Rhizoma Alismatis (*Ze Xie*), Radix Lateralis Praeparatus Aconiti Carmichaeli (*Fu Zi*), and Sclerotium Poriae Cocos (*Fu Ling*), 6g each, and Cortex Radicis Moutan (*Dan Pi*), Cortex Cinnamomi Cassiae (*Rou Gui*), and Lignum Aquilariae Agallochae (*Chen Xiang*), 3g each.

For kidney yang vacuity with phlegm accumulation, panting more on exhalation than inhalation, shortness of breath, coughing with profuse, white phlegm, chest and diaphragm oppression and fullness, low backache, chilled limbs, frequent urination, slimy, white tongue fur, and a deep, fine or soggy, slippery, forceless pulse, replace *Ren Shen Hu Tao Ren Tang* with *Su Zi Jiang Qi Tang* (Perilla Seed Downbear the Qi Decoction): Fructus Perillae Frutescentis (*Zi Su Zi*), Fructus Psoraleae Corylifoliae (*Bu Gu Zhi*), and lime-processed

Rhizoma Pinelliae Ternatae (*Ban Xia*), 9g each, Radix Angelicae Sinensis (*Dang Gui*), mix-fried Radix Glycyrrhizae (*Gan Cao*), Radix Peucedani (*Qian Hu*), Cortex Magnoliae Officinalis (*Hou Po*), Sclerotium Poriae Cocos (*Fu Ling*), and Pericarpium Citri Reticulatae (*Chen Pi*), 6g each, and Cortex Cinnamomi Cassiae (*Rou Gui*), 3g.

NOTE: In this latter formula, *Dang Gui* is not used to nourish the blood but to downbear the qi. This function of this medicinal is not very well known but is real and effective.

ACUPUNCTURE & MOXIBUSTION: *Da Zhui* (GV 14), *Shen Shu* (Bl 23), *Qi Hai* (CV 6), *Tai Xi* (Ki 3). Use supplementing method and moxibustion at *Da Zhui, Shen Shu*, and *Qi Hai.*

ANALYSIS OF FORMULA: Supplementing *Da Zhui* strengthens the yang of the entire body, secures the exterior, downbears the qi, and levels panting. *Shen Shu* and *Tai Xi* warm and supplement kidney yang, promote qi absorption, and level panting. *Qi Hai* warms the cinnabar field and secures the kidneys, leads the qi back to its lower origin, and stabilizes the panting.

ADDITIONS & SUBTRACTIONS: For concomitant spleen vacuity, add *Zu San Li* (St 36). For phlegm, add *Feng Long* (St 40) and *Zu San Li* (St 36). For severe panting, add *Ding Chuan* (M-BW-1) and/or *Fu Tu* (LI 18). For chest oppression, add *Dan Zhong* (CV 17) and *Nei Guan* (Per 6). In children, especially with underlying food stagnation, bleed *Si Feng* (M-UE-9).

11. YANG VACUITY COUPLED WITH WATER FLOODING PATTERN

MAIN SYMPTOMS: Wheezing, panting, and rapid breathing, inability to lie flat, heart palpitations, fear of cold, low back pain, chilled limbs, scanty urination, edema, a pale, fat tongue with white, glossy fur, and a deep, fine pulse

NOTE: This pattern mostly describes asthma associated with cardiopulmonary disease. This is a potentially fatal pattern requiring emergency medical care. Patients with this pattern not under the care of an MD should be referred to one.

TREATMENT PRINCIPLES: Warm yang, disinhibit water, and stabilize panting

RX: *Zhen Wu Tang Jia Wei* (True Warrior Decoction with Added Flavors)

INGREDIENTS: Radix Astragali Membranacei (*Huang Qi*), 12g, Rhizoma Atractylodis Macrocephalae (*Bai Zhu*), Sclerotium Poriae Cocos (*Fu Ling*), Radix Stephaniae Tetrandrae (*Han Fang Ji*), and Semen Lepidii Seu Descurainiae (*Ting Li Zi*), 9g each, Radix Lateralis Praeparatus Aconiti Carmichaeli (*Fu Zi*), Radix Albus Paeoniae Lactiflorae (*Bai Shao*), Ramulus Cinnamomi Cassiae (*Gui Zhi*), and mix-fried Radix Glycyrrhizae (*Gan Cao*), 6g each, uncooked Rhizoma Zingiberis (*Sheng Jiang*), 2 slices

ANALYSIS OF FORMULA: *Fu Zi, Sheng Jiang*, and *Gui Zhi* warm yang and scatter the cold. In addition, *Gui Zhi* promotes the qi transformation of the bladder. *Huang Qi, Bai Zhu, Fu Ling*, and *Gui Zhi* disinhibit dampness and transform water. *Ting Li Zi,* with the help of *Han Fang Ji,* drains water accumulation in the lungs and also stabilizes panting. Since blood is the mother of the qi, *Bai Shao* is used to harmonize the blood to regulate qi. Also, in combination with *Gui Zhi*, it harmonizes the constructive and defensive. *Gan Cao* harmonizes all the other medicinals in the formula.

ADDITIONS & SUBTRACTIONS: For severe heart palpitations and cyanotic face, lips, and nails, add nine grams of Radix Salviae Miltiorrhizae (*Dan Shen*) and three grams of Radix Pseudoginseng (*San Qi*). For severe edema, add nine grams each of Sclerotium Polypori Umbellati (*Zhu Ling*) and Rhizoma Alismatis (*Ze Xie*). For severe hasty panting, add nine grams of Cortex Magnoliae Officinalis (*Hou Po*) and six grams of Herba Ephedrae (*Ma Huang*).

ACUPUNCTURE & MOXIBUSTION: *Xin Shu* (Bl 15), *Ju Que* (CV 14), *Nei Guan* (Per 6), *Dan Zhong* (CV 17)

ANALYSIS OF FORMULA: Moxaing *Xin Shu* and *Ju Que* warms heart yang and frees the flow of the network vessels of the heart, moves the qi and quickens the blood. Draining *Nei Guan* and *Dan Zhong* rectifies the ancestral (or gathering) qi and loosens the chest, disinhibits water in the lungs and stabilizes panting.

REMARKS

1. The treatment of asthma with Chinese medicine is typically divided into two phases, the acute attack phase and the remittent, asymptomatic phase. During the acute phase, it is assumed that there are unseen wind evils provoking the attack mixed with deep-lying or hidden phlegm. This is especially so in allergic asthma. Then, depending on the patient's signs and symptoms, their pattern is divided into cold wheezing and panting or hot wheezing and panting (corresponding to the wind cold and wind heat patterns above). During the remittent phase, treatment is directed at the lungs, spleen, and kidneys as well as the liver. Most patients with asthma have a liver-spleen disharmony. Because of this disharmony, phlegm and dampness are engendered internally as well as transformative heat. Enduring heat and aging may lead to yin vacuity, while enduring spleen vacuity and aging may lead to yang vacuity. And enduring qi stagnation

and phlegm damp depression may lead to blood stasis. Therefore, during the remittent phase, treatment should mainly course the liver and rectify the qi, fortify the spleen and boost the qi, transform phlegm and eliminate dampness. If there is concomitant heat, clear heat as and where appropriate. If there is concomitant yin vacuity, nourish and enrich yin. If there is concomitant yang vacuity, warm and invigorate yang. If there is blood stasis, quicken the blood and transform stasis.

Although the main emphasis in treating acute episodes of asthma is on draining evils and diffusing the lungs, if there is an exterior repletion with an interior vacuity, one must supplement and drain at the same time. If one does not supplement as well as drain in such cases, the righteous qi will not be strong enough to expel or dispel the evil qi. Therefore, the evils will remain lodged within the body waiting to be stirred up or mix with other externally invading or internally engendered evils. Such simultaneous supplementing and draining will not supplement repletion as long as there are simultaneously coexisting replete evils and a righteous qi vacuity.

2. In modern Chinese medicine, many respiratory specialists add wind-extinguishing, network vessel quickening worm and insect medicinals to formulas for the treatment of acute asthma. This is based on the assumption that, "Enduring disease enters the network vessels." However, from a Western pharmacodynamic point of view, these medicinals are also spasmolytic, and asthma is associated with spasm of the large and small air passageways. These worm and insect medicinals include Buthus Martensis (*Quan Xie*), Scolopendra Subspinipes (*Wu Gong*), Lumbricus (*Di Long*), Bombyx Batryticatus (*Jiang Can*), and Periostracum Cicadae (*Chan Tui*). The first two of these are somewhat toxic and should not be used for prolonged periods of time. When these worm or insect medicinals are added to asthma formulas, they are used when there is wheezing and panting, not during remission stages.

3. Although no Chinese textbooks with which we are aware list a food stagnation pattern of asthma *per se*, food stagnation may aggravate or precipitate asthmatic attacks, especially in little children. Therefore, for wheezing and panting worsened by food intake due to food accumulation accompanied by abdominal distention, reduced food intake, nausea, bad breath, putrid belching, diarrhea with foul-smelling stools, thick, slimy, possibly yellow tongue fur, and a slippery pulse, we should disperse food and abduct stagnation, transform phlegm, and stop panting. To accomplish these purposes, one may combine the Chinese ready-made medicine *Bao He Wan* (Preserve Harmony Pills) with other appropriate formulas discussed above.

4. Because of the relationship between the lungs and large intestine, if an acute attack of asthma is accompanied by constipation, epigastric and abdominal glomus and fullness, and abdominal pain that refuses pressure, we should free the flow of the stools no matter what else we do. One way to do that is to first prescribe *Da Cheng Qi Tang* (Major Order the Qi Decoction): Cortex Magnoliae Officinalis (*Hou Po*), 6-15g, uncooked Radix Et Rhizoma Rhei (*Da Huang*) and Fructus Immaturus Citri Aurantii (*Zhi Shi*), 6-12g each, and Mirabilitum (*Mang Xiao*), 3-9g. One can also add some or all of these medicinals to other appropriate formulas discussed above.

5. In China, various treatments are used during the remission stage so as the lessen or prevent future acute occurrences. The most commonly used and convenient ones are as follows:

a. Summer moxibustion: During the summer, apply 3-5 cones of moxa indirectly on sliced uncooked ginger to *Fei Shu* (Bl 13), *Gao Huang* (Bl 43), *Da Zhui* (GV 14), *Pi Shu* (Bl 20), and *Shen Shu* (Bl 23) until the skin becomes red at each point. Do this once per day, with 10 times equaling one course of treatment. Do one such course each month for three months before the asthma season, *i.e.*, the fall/winter, begins.

b. Do sliding cupping along *Fei Shu* (Bl 13) to *Gao Huang* (Bl 43) until the skin becomes dark red. Do this once a week, with four times equaling one course of treatment. Do this two months before the asthma season begins.

c. Suppurative moxibustion: This treatment is usually applied in mid-summer, once per year. The points moxaed include *Fei Shu* (Bl 13), *Gao Huang* (Bl 43), *Da Zhui* (GV 14), *Feng Men* (Bl 12), and *Zu San Li* (St 36). Local anesthesia may be given before the direct moxibustion. After moxibustion, make sure the burnt areas do not become infected. Although this technique is reputed to be very effective, for a variety of legal and personal reasons, it is difficult to do direct moxibustion on Western patients. This is a pity since heavy, rice-sized direct moxibustion or suppurative moxibustion is often the most effective Chinese medical treatment for many diseases.

d. Preventive Chinese medicinal formula: Two to three weeks before the beginning of the usual onset of the acute stage of asthma, the patient should use the appropriate Chinese medicinal formula from the remission stage according to their constitution, *i.e.*, lung, spleen, or kidney vacuity, along with the inclusion of Chinese medicinals that diffuse the lungs and downbear the qi, level panting and stop wheezing, such as Cortex Magnoliae Officinalis (*Hou Po*), Semen Pruni Armeniacae (*Xing Ren*), Semen Lepidii Seu Descurainiae (*Ting Li Zi*), Herba Ephedrae (*Ma Huang*), Semen Ginkgonis Bilobae (*Bai Guo*), and Fructus Schisandrae Chinensis (*Wu Wei Zi*).

6. Both patients and practitioners alike should keep in mind

that asthma is a serious disease and is difficult to treat even for the best Chinese doctors. Typically, it requires a long course of persistent treatment.

7. Both asthma and emphysema are chronic obstructive pulmonary diseases (COPD) in Western medicine. In Chinese medicine, emphysema is called *fei zhong*, lung swelling. When emphysema is due to cigarette smoking (more than 20 cigarettes per day for more than 20 years), its main symptoms are cough developing in the early 40s or 50s and exertional dyspnea developing in the 50s to mid 60s. Since emphysema's main clinical symptoms are panting and coughing, its Chinese medical pattern discrimination and treatment are similar to those of bronchial asthma. The three main patterns of this condition are lung qi depletion and vacuity, lung-kidney qi vacuity, and lung qi not securing. For lung qi depletion and vacuity, consider using *Bu Fei Tang* (Supplement the Lungs Decoction): Radix Astragali Membranacei (*Huang Qi*), 15g, cooked Radix Rehmanniae (*Shu Di*), 12g, Cortex Radicis Mori Albi (*Sang Bai Pi*), Fructus Schisandrae Chinensis (*Wu Wei Zi*), and Radix Asteris Tatarici (*Zi Wan*), 9g each, and Radix Panacis Ginseng (*Ren Shen*), 6g. If there is concomitant kidney qi, add 9 grams each of Lignum Aquilariae Agallochae (*Chen Xiang*), Cortex Cinnamomi Cassiae (*Rou Gui*), and Semen Julgandis Regiae (*Hu Tao Ren*). If there is a tendency to kidney yang vacuity, also add 6 grams of Radix Lateralis Praeparatus Aconiti Carmichaeli (*Fu Zi*).

For lung qi not securing, consider using *Jiu Xian San* (Nine Immortals Powder): Gelatinum Corii Asini (*E Jiao*), 12g, Flos Tussilaginis Farfarae (*Kuan Dong Hua*), Cortex Radicis Mori Albi (*Sang Bai Pi*), Fructus Schisandrae Chinensis (*Wu Wei Zi*), Fructus Pruni Mume (*Wu Mei*), Bulbus Fritillariae Cirrhosae (*Chuan Bei Mu*), and Pericarpium Papaveris Somniferi (*Ying Su Ke*), 9g each, and Radix Panacis Ginseng (*Ren Shen*) and Radix Platycodi Grandiflori (*Jie Geng*), 6g each.

In individual patients, one may also have to modify either of the above two formulas for concomitant phlegm rheum, blood stasis, and/or qi stagnation.

8. Herba Ephedrae (*Ma Huang*) must always be used with caution and only for a short period of time. This medicinal can cause psychiatric disturbances, including hallucinations, as well as increase the blood pressure and cause cardiac arrhythmia. This medicinal should not be used in case of either spontaneous perspiration or night sweats, and it is contraindicated in qi and/or yin vacuity patterns.

9

Carpal Tunnel Syndrome

Carpal tunnel syndrome (CTS) describes the symptoms when the median nerve traveling through the tunnel of the wrist bones is compressed by the tendons which also run through the carpal tunnel. Although CTS may be the result of a single acute traumatic event, this syndrome is the most common of the cumulative trauma disorders resulting from repetitive motions of modest force. Carpal tunnel syndrome affects as many as 15% of workers in high risk industries, such as electronic parts assemblers, musicians, keyboarders, and dental hygienists. Other factors associated with the development besides repetitive wrist movements are diabetes mellitus, RA, thyroid disease, and pregnancy. In 1994 in the U.S. alone, 849,000 new problem visits were made to physicians in office-based practice because of CTS. Approximately 260,000 carpal tunnel release operations are performed each year, and 47% of these are considered work-related. In addition, carpal tunnel syndrome results in the highest median number of days of work lost (30 days) among all major work-related injury or illness categories, with almost half (47.5%) resulting in 31 days or more of work loss.

Carpal tunnel syndrome is perceived at first as an uncomfortable feeling in the hand frequently associated with tingling. This paresthesia becomes more and more frequent as the condition progresses and may sometimes become continuous. These uncomfortable sensations associated with CTS tend to occur more frequently at night and during sleep and may wake patients from their sleep. The classic CTS comment is, "I wake in the middle of the night with my hands tingling and have to shake them to make them stop." Other early symptoms of CTS include inability to manipulate objects, weakness, hypoesthesia, and wrist pain which may, but only rarely, migrate into the upper arm or even the shoulder region. Eventually tingling is replaced by numbness which is frequently described as if one were wearing a rubber glove. Numbness and tingling are distributed in the areas served by the median nerve – the thumb, index, and middle fingers. As the disease progresses, lack of co-ordination turns into severe, debilitating weakness, especially in the motion of opposing the thumb to the rest of the hand. Such debilitating weakness is commonly associated with muscular wasting of the thenar eminence.

The definitive Western medical diagnosis of CTS consists of an electromyograph (EMG) of the wrist showing compression of the median nerve. EMGs are capable of detecting over 90% of all CTS cases. The Western medical treatment of CTS is divided into nonsurgical and surgical treatments. The first and foremost nonsurgical treatment consists of rest of the wrist, wearing a wrist-splint, and various anti-inflammatory medicines, including steroid injections into the wrist. Specialized exercises may help alleviate early symptoms of carpal tunnel syndrome. Such specialized exercises include both stretching and strengthening exercises. In addition, oral administration of vitamin B_6 has shown wide-spread evidence of alleviating the symptoms of CTS. The standard surgical treatment for CTS is the carpal tunnel release which has as much as a 90% success rate. After surgery, office workers can be back on the job in as little as one week. Carpenters and athletes may be incapacitated for 4-6 weeks.

Chinese disease categorization: Carpal tunnel syndrome is categorized as *shou zhi ma mu*, hand and finger tingling and numbness. Wrist pain is categorized as *bi zheng*, impediment condition, in general and as *wan tong*, wrist pain in particular.

Disease causes: Overwork taxation, traumatic injury, enduring disease, and pregnancy

Disease mechanisms: Numbness and tingling are primarily due to malnourishment of the sinews and vessels. This malnourishment may be either due to qi and especially blood insufficiency due to overwork taxation, habitual bodily weakness, enduring disease, and/or pregnancy. Pain in the wrist is mainly due to blood stasis, but may be complicated by wind cold damp evils having taken advantage of righteous vacuity to enter and lodge in the channels and vessels of the wrist joint causing impediment. Blood stasis may be due to either or both repetitive micro-trauma or blood vacuity not nourishing the vessels. Because the blood returns for storage to the liver during rest and sleep at night, numbness and tingling tend to be worse at night.

TREATMENT BASED ON PATTERN DISCRIMINATION:

1. BLOOD VACUITY NOT NOURISHING THE SINEWS & VESSELS PATTERN

MAIN SYMPTOMS: Tingling and/or numbness of the fingers of one or both hands which tend to be thin in form and pale in color accompanied by possible pale lips and nails, a pale white or sallow yellow facial complexion, night-blindness, brittle nails, dry skin, dizziness, heart palpitations, a pale tongue, and a fine pulse

TREATMENT PRINCIPLES: Nourish the blood and harmonize the constructive

RX: *Si Wu Tang Jia Wei* (Four Materials Decoction with Added Flavors)

INGREDIENTS: Cooked Radix Rehmanniae (*Shu Di*) and Caulis Milletiae Seu Spatholobi (*Ji Xue Teng*), 15g each, Radix Angelicae Sinensis (*Dang Gui*) and Radix Albus Paeoniae Lactiflorae (*Bai Shao*), 12g each, and Radix Ligustici Wallichii (*Chuan Xiong*), and Radix Salviae Miltiorrhizae (*Dan Shen*), 9g each

ANALYSIS OF FORMULA: *Shu Di, Dang Gui, Bai Shao*, and *Ji Xue Teng* all nourish the blood. In addition, *Dang Gui, Ji Xue Teng, Dan Shen*, and *Chuan Xiong* all quicken the blood and dispel stasis. *Ji Xue Teng* also treats wind damp impediment pain as well as numbness in the extremities. *Bai Shao* also relieves or relaxes spasms.

ADDITIONS & SUBTRACTIONS: If there is concomitant qi vacuity, add 15 grams of Radix Astragali Membranacei (*Huang Qi*) and nine grams of Radix Codonopsitis Pilosulae (*Dang Shen*). If there is concomitant yang vacuity as evidenced by cold, purplish fingertips, add six grams of Radix Lateralis Praeparatus Aconiti Carmichaeli (*Fu Zi*) and three grams of Herba Asari Cum Radice (*Xi Xin*).

ACUPUNCTURE & MOXIBUSTION: Needle the *Ba Xie* (M-UE-22), *Da Ling* (Per 7), *Ge Shu* (Bl 17), *Gan Shu* (Bl 18), *Pi Shu* (Bl 20)

ANALYSIS OF FORMULA: Supplementing *Ge Shu, Gan Shu*, and *Pi Shu* supplements the qi and nourishes the blood. Using even supplementing-even draining technique at *Ba Xie* and *Da Ling* frees the flow of qi and blood and harmonizes the network vessels in the local area.

ADDITIONS & SUBTRACTIONS: For heart palpitations and insomnia, add *Xin Shu* (Bl 15) and *Shen Men* (Ht 7). For dizziness and vertigo, add *Bai Hui* (GV 20). For more pronounced blood stasis, add *Qu Chi* (LI 11) and *Xue Hai* (Sp 10). For fatigue and lassitude of the spirit, add *Zu San Li* (St 36).

2. QI STAGNATION & BLOOD STASIS PATTERN

MAIN SYMPTOMS: Wrist pain which is relatively severe, fixed in location, and is worse at night. Possible systemic symptoms may include a dark, purple tongue with static macules or spots and a bowstring, choppy pulse.

TREATMENT PRINCIPLES: Quicken the blood and dispel stasis, free the flow of the network vessels and stop pain

RX: *Shen Tong Zhu Yu Tang Jia Jian* (Body Pain Dispel Stasis Decoction with Additions & Subtractions)

INGREDIENTS: Semen Pruni Persicae (*Tao Ren*), Flos Carthami Tinctorii (*Hong Hua*), Radix Angelicae Sinensis (*Dang Gui*), and Radix Ligustici Wallichii (*Chuan Xiong*), 9g each, Radix Et Rhizoma Notopterygii (*Qiang Huo*), Lumbricus (*Di Long*), Resina Myrrhae (*Mo Yao*), Feces Trogopterori Seu Pteromi (*Wu Ling Zhi*), and Radix Glycyrrhizae (*Gan Cao*), 6g each, and Rhizoma Cyperi Rotundi (*Xiang Fu*), 3g

ANALYSIS OF FORMULA: *Tao Ren, Hong Hua, Dang Gui, Chuan Xiong, Wu Ling Zhi*, and *Mo Yao* all quicken the blood and dispel stasis. *Dang Gui* also nourishes the blood, while *Mo Yao* also frees the flow of the network vessels and stops pain. *Di Long* enters the network vessels and tracks down wind. *Qiang Huo* guides all the other medicinals to the upper extremities and frees the flow of impediment. *Xiang Fu* moves the qi to move the blood, and *Gan Cao* harmonizes all the other medicinals in the formula.

ADDITIONS & SUBTRACTIONS: For fatigue and weakness of the limbs, add 15 grams of Radix Astragali Membranacei (*Huang Qi*) and nine grams of Radix Codonopsitis Pilosulae (*Dang Shen*), and replace uncooked *Gan Cao* with six grams of mix-fried *Gan Cao*.

ACUPUNCTURE & MOXIBUSTION: *Xue Hai* (Sp 10), *Da Ling* (Per 7), *Yang Chi* (TB 4), *Ba Xie* (M-UE-22)

ANALYSIS OF FORMULA: Draining *Xue Hai* quickens the blood and dispels stasis. Draining *Da Ling, Yang Chi*, and *Ba*

Xie frees the flow of the network vessels in the affected area and stops pain.

ADDITIONS & SUBTRACTIONS: If the pain migrates into the upper arm or even the shoulder region, add *Wai Guan* (TB 5). For severe tingling and pain in the palm, add *Lao Gong* (Per 8). For weakness in the hand, add *He Gu* (LI 4). For cervical vertebrae disease, add *Jia Ji* (M-BW-35) of the sixth cervical vertebra and/or *Da Zhui* (GV 14).

3. WIND DAMP IMPEDIMENT PATTERN

MAIN SYMPTOMS: Wrist pain that comes and goes or migrates up the arm, numbness and heaviness in the hand and fingers, somewhat inhibited finger joints, worse pain or impediment on exposure to cold or during damp, rainy weather, a pale tongue with slimy, white fur, and a possibly soggy, bowstring pulse

TREATMENT PRINCIPLES: Dispel wind and eliminate dampness, supplement the qi and nourish the blood

RX: For predominant wind impediment, *Fang Feng Tang Jia Jian* (Ledebouriella Decoction with Additions & Subtractions)

INGREDIENTS: Radix Ledebouriellae Divaricatae (*Fang Feng*), 12g, Sclerotium Poriae Cocos (*Fu Ling*), Fasciculus Vascularis Luffae Cylindricae (*Si Gua Luo*), Radix Gentianae Macrocphyllae (*Qin Jiao*), Radix Puerariae (*Ge Gen*), Ramulus Mori Albi (*Sang Zhi*), and Radix Et Rhizoma Notopterygii (*Qiang Huo*), 9g each, and Ramulus Cinnamomi Cassiae (*Gui Zhi*) and Lumbricus (*Di Long*), 6g

ANALYSIS OF FORMULA: *Fang Feng, Jin Qiao, Ge Gen, Sang Zhi,* and *Qiang Huo* all dispel wind and eliminate dampness in the treatment of impediment conditions. Most of these medicinals have a tropism for the upper body and extremities. *Si Gua Luo* and *Di Long* quicken the network vessels, while *Gui Zhi* warms the channels and scatters cold. *Fu Ling* seeps dampness and fortifies the spleen. *Gan Cao* harmonizes all the other medicinals in this formula.

For predominant cold impediment, *Wu Tou Tang Jia Jian* (Aconite Decoction with Additions & Subtractions)

INGREDIENTS: Radix Astragali Membranacei (*Huang Qi*), 12g, Ramulus Mori Albi (*Sang Zhi*), Radix Albus Paeoniae Lactiflorae (*Bai Shao*), Radix Et Rhizoma Notopterygii (*Qiang Huo*), and Fasciculus Vascularis Luffae Cylindricae (*Si Gua Luo*), 9g each, Ramulus Cinnamomi Cassiae (*Gui Zhi*) and Radix Aconiti Carmichaeli (*Chuan Wu*), 6g each, and Radix Glycyrrhizae (*Gan Cao*), 3g

ANALYSIS OF FORMULA: *Sang Zhi* and *Qiang Huo* treat wind damp impediment pain. *Gui Zhi* and *Chuan Wu* strongly warm the channels and scatter cold. *Huang Qi* boosts the qi, while *Bai Shao* nourishes the blood and relaxes tension or cramping. *Si Gua Luo* quickens the network vessels, and *Gan Cao* harmonizes all the other medicinals.

For predominant dampness impediment, *Qiang Huo Sheng Shi Tang Jia Jian* (Notopterygium Overcome Dampness Decoction with Additions & Subtractions)

INGREDIENTS: Radix Et Rhizoma Notopterygii (*Qiang Huo*), Radix Angelicae Pubescentis (*Du Huo*), Ramulus Cinnamomi Cassiae (*Gui Zhi*), and Ramulus Mori Albi (*Sang Zhi*), 9g each, Radix Et Rhizoma Ligustici Chinensis (*Gao Ben*), Radix Ledebouriellae Divaricatae (*Fang Feng*), Radix Ligustici Wallichii (*Chuan Xiong*), Radix Clematidis Chinensis (*Wei Ling Xian*), and Rhizoma Atractylodis (*Cang Zhu*), 6g each, and Radix Glycyrrhizae (*Gan Cao*), 3g

ANALYSIS OF FORMULA: *Qiang Huo, Du Huo, Sang Zhi, Fang Feng, Wei Ling Xian,* and *Cang Zhu* all treat wind damp impediment pain. *Cang Zhu* also strongly dries dampness. *Gao Ben* dispels wind and stops pain, especially in the upper body. *Chuan Xiong* quickens the blood and transforms stasis, while *Gui Zhi* warms the channels and scatters cold. *Gan Cao* once again harmonizes all the other medicinals in this formula.

ACUPUNCTURE & MOXIBUSTION: *Ba Xie* (M-UE-22), *Da Ling* (Per 7), *He Gu* (LI 4), *Hou Xi* (SI 3), *Zu San Li* (St 36)

ANALYSIS OF FORMULA: Draining *He Gu* and *Hou Xi* dispels wind and eliminates dampness from the upper extremities. When combined with draining *Ba Xie* and *Da Ling,* they also free the flow of the network vessels in the affected area. Supplementing *Zu San Li* supplements the spleen, the latter heaven root of qi and blood engenderment and transformation.

ADDITIONS & SUBTRACTIONS: For predominant cold, add warm needle technique to the local points. For inhibited movement of the fingers, add *Yang Chi* (TB 4). For pain radiating up the forearm, add *Wai Guan* (TB 5).

REMARKS

1. When treating CTS with acupuncture, it is usual to needle directly into the carpal tunnel at *Da Ling* (Per 7). Use strong stimulation and do not retain the needle. In some cases, needling *Nei Guan* (Per 6) and *Lao Gong* (Per 8) may achieve an even better effect.

2. Most patients with CTS also have liver depression qi stagnation, if not before, then as a sequela to the frustration of not being able to work or play. Depending on how promi-

nent this liver depression is, one may choose to modify such formulas as *Xiao Chai Hu Tang* (Minor Bupleurum Decoction) or *Xiao Yao San* (Rambling Powder) with blood-nourishing, blood-quickening, and/or wind damp treating medicinals. In other words, for best results, take the bodily constitution as the root and modify a guiding formula for that constitution for the disease mechanisms specifically associated with CTS.

3. Cessation of activities aggravating CTS, at least long enough for the condition to heal, are a prerequisite for its successful Chinese medical treatment. Often recurrences of this condition can be prevented either by ergonomically more efficient tools and appliances or kinesiological re-education and counseling. Therefore, patients with work or sports-related CTS should be referred to a physiatrist, occupational therapist, kinesiologist, etc.

4. External applications of Chinese herbal liniments, ointments, or fomentations may help speed recovery. In that case, one should use a liniment, ointment, or fomentation whose main medicinals match the patient's pattern. Such external treatments are more effective for qi stagnation and blood stasis and wind damp impediment patterns of CTS and are not as effective for blood vacuity not nourishing the sinews and vessels. Heat therapy with a TDP lamp may help all patterns of CTS.

10

CELIAC DISEASE

Celiac disease, also called sprue, is an autoimmune digestive disease that damages the villi of the small intestine and interferes with the absorption of nutrients from food. People with this disorder cannot tolerate the gluten found in wheat, barley, rye, and possibly oats. When people with this condition eat foods containing gluten, their immune system responds by attacking the villi of the small intestine. When the villi are attacked, they first become inflamed. Later they shrivel up, flatten out, and may even disappear. Without functioning villi, the body cannot absorb food properly.

Celiac is a genetic disease which is more common in those of European descent than in Asians and Africans. Its incidence may be as high as one in 250-300 in those of European descent. In Europe, more people are screened for celiac disease. For instance, celiac disease is so common in Italy that all children are routinely screened for it. Therefore, this diagnosis is more common in Europe than in North America. However, random blood sampling suggests that its incidence is just as high on both continents. Because this condition's symptoms are so diverse, its diagnosis in the U.S. is often missed unless accompanied by its classic manifestations of diarrhea and weight loss. Although genetics predispose a person to sprue, genetics alone do not explain the incidence of this disease. Surveys suggest that only one out of every ten close relatives of a person with this disease will also develop it. Therefore, there must be other cofactors involved.

Celiac disease may affect those of any age. However, sometimes it is triggered by surgery, pregnancy, childbirth, viral infection, or severe emotional stress. Its symptoms include recurring abdominal distention and pain, chronic diarrhea, weight loss, pale, foul-smelling stools, unexplained anemia, flatulence, joint and bone pain, muscle cramps, behavior changes, fatigue, possible seizures, tingling and numbness due to peripheral neuropathy, pale-colored sores inside the mouth, painful skin rash (*i.e.*, dermatitis herpetiformis), tooth discoloration, and delayed menstruation, hypomenorrhea, or amenorrhea due to excessive weight loss.

The Western medical diagnosis of sprue is based on the detection of certain gluten antibodies in the blood, such as antigliadin, anti-endomysium, and antireticulin. This diagnosis is confirmed by a tissue biopsy of the small intestine. The Western medical treatment of this condition consists of a strict, life-time gluten-free diet. Healing typically occurs 3-6 months after initiation of such a diet. However, it may take two years or so in older adults. Complications of celiac disease include lymphoma and adenocarcinoma, osteoporosis, miscarriage and congenital malformation, short stature, and seizures. Patients with celiac disease tend to also suffer from other autoimmune diseases. These include Hashimoto's thyroiditis, SLE, RA, Sjögren's Syndrome, liver disease, insulin-dependant diabetes mellitus (IDDM), and collagen vascular disease.

CHINESE DISEASE CATEGORIZATION: This disease is mostly categorized as *xie tong*, painful diarrhea, *xing ti xiao shou*, bodily emaciation and whittling, and *lei ruo*, emaciation and weakness. Muscle joint pain is usually categorized as some kind of *bi* or impediment. Flatulence is *xia qi*, descending qi, fatigue is *pi juan*, numbness and tingling are *ma mu*, oral sores are *kou chuang*, herpes-like sores are *chuang yang*, sores and open sores, delayed menstruation is *yu jing hou qi*, menstruation behind schedule, hypomenorrhea is *yue jing guo shao*, excessively scanty menstruation, and amenorrhea is *jing bi* or *bi jing*, blocked menstruation.

DISEASE CAUSES & MECHANISMS: The disease causes and mechanisms of sprue are the same as those of irritable bowel above, with liver-spleen disharmony being the core mechanisms of this condition. However, in the case of serious, symptomatic sprue with chronic diarrhea and weight loss, spleen vacuity and damp heat are more prominent. The spleen controls the muscles and flesh and the spleen controls the four limbs. If, for any reason, the spleen becomes vacuous and weak, it may fail to engender and transform the qi and blood which then fail to nourish and construct the muscles and flesh. If blood vacuity endures, it may evolve into yin vacuity, thus giving rise to a qi and yin dual vacuity. Pale-colored stools are usually a sign of spleen vacuity, while foul-smelling stools suggest dampness and heat.

TREATMENT BASED ON PATTERN DISCRIMINATION:

1. LIVER-SPLEEN DISHARMONY WITH INTERNAL BREWING OF DAMP HEAT PATTERN

MAIN SYMPTOMS: Enduring diarrhea with pale-colored, foul-smelling stools which may be the color of mustard and/or explosive, possible burning around the anus after defecation, abdominal distention and/or painful diarrhea, possible pale-colored mouth sores, fatigue, lack of strength, emaciation, a pale but possibly dark, fat, swollen tongue with white or yellow, slimy fur, and a slippery, bowstring, possibly rapid pulse

TREATMENT PRINCIPLES: Harmonize the liver and spleen, clear heat, eliminate dampness, and stop diarrhea

RX: *Ban Xia Xie Xin Tang Jia Wei* (Pinelliae Drain the Heart Decoction with Added Flavors)

INGREDIENTS: Radix Scutellariae Baicalensis (*Huang Qin*), 12g, Radix Bupleuri (*Chai Hu*), Radix Codonopsitis Pilosulae (*Dang Shen*), and Rhizoma Pinelliae Ternatae (*Ban Xia*), 9g each, mix-fried Radix Glycyrrhizae (*Gan Cao*) and dry Rhizoma Zingiberis (*Gan Jiang*), 6g each, Rhizoma Coptidis Chinensis (*Huang Lian*), 3g, and Fructus Zizyphi Jujubae (*Da Zao*), 3 pieces

ANALYSIS OF FORMULA: *Chai Hu* courses the liver and resolves the depression. *Dang Shen*, *Da Zao*, and mix-fried *Gan Cao* supplement the center and boost the qi. *Ban Xia* harmonizes the stomach. Together, these medicinals harmonize the liver and spleen. *Gan Jiang* warms the spleen and stops diarrhea. *Huang Qin* and *Huang Lian* clear heat, dry dampness, and stop diarrhea.

ADDITIONS & SUBTRACTIONS: If there is marked fatigue and enduring diarrhea, add 15 grams of Radix Astragali Membranacei (*Huang Qi*) and 4.5 grams of Rhizoma Cimicifugae (*Sheng Ma*). If dampness is pronounced, add nine grams each of Rhizoma Atractylodis Macrocephalae (*Bai Zhu*) and Sclerotium Poriae Cocos (*Fu Ling*). If enduring heat has damaged yin fluids, add 12 grams of Tuber Ophiopogonis Japonici (*Mai Dong*) and nine grams of Radix Puerariae (*Ge Gen*). If chilled limbs are pronounced, add nine grams of Ramulus Cinnamomi Cassiae (*Gui Zhi*). If there is painful diarrhea, add 18 grams of Radix Albus Paeoniae Lactiflorae (*Bai Shao*). If there are heart palpitations and worry and anxiety due to spleen vacuity reaching the heart, increase mix-fried Licorice to 18 grams and Red Dates to 10 pieces. If there are no signs of chilling or cold, replace *Gan Jiang* with three slices of uncooked Rhizoma Zingiberis (*Sheng Jiang*).

ACUPUNCTURE & MOXIBUSTION: *Zu San Li* (St 36), *Tian Shu* (St 25), *Xia Wan* (CV 10), *Jian Li* (CV 11), *Tai Chong* (Liv 3)

ANALYSIS OF FORMULA: Draining *Tai Chong* courses the liver and resolves depression. Supplementing *Zu San Li* fortifies the spleen and boosts the qi. Together, these two points harmonize the liver and spleen. With even supplementing-even draining method, *Tian Shu*, *Xia Wan*, and *Jian Li* harmonize the stomach and intestines, eliminate dampness, and stop diarrhea.

ADDITIONS & SUBTRACTIONS: For pale-colored stools and cold limbs, add *Shen Que* (CV 8). For foul-smelling stools and yellow, slimy tongue fur, add *Nei Ting* (St 44). For severe spleen vacuity, add *Tai Bai* (Sp 3). For severe liver depression, add *Nei Guan* (Per 6). For mouth sores, add *Da Ling* (Per 7). For food stagnation, add *Liang Men* (St 21). For abdominal distention, add *Zhong Wan* (CV 12).

2. QI & YIN VACUITY WITH INTERNAL BREWING OF DAMP HEAT PATTERN

MAIN SYMPTOMS: Enduring diarrhea or loose stools, fatigue, lack of strength, bodily emaciation, numbness and tingling, a pale face with possible malar flushing, cold hands and feet with possible vexatious heat in the five hearts, dizziness, tinnitus, heart palpitations, insomnia, night sweats, mouth and/or tongue sores, dry mouth and throat, scanty, delayed, or blocked menstruation in females, a tender, red or fat, pale tongue with a red tip and scanty fur, and a soggy, possibly rapid pulse

TREATMENT PRINCIPLES: Boost the qi and nourish yin, clear heat, eliminate dampness, and stop diarrhea

RX: *Gan Lu Yin Jia Wei* (Sweet Dew Drink with Added Flavors)

INGREDIENTS: Uncooked Radix Rehmanniae (*Sheng Di*) and Tuber Ophiopogonis Japonici (*Mai Dong*), 12 each, Fructus Schisandrae Chinensis (*Wu Wei Zi*), Radix Trichosanthis Kirlowii (*Tian Hua Fen*), Sclerotium Poriae Cocos (*Fu Ling*), Radix Puerariae (*Ge Gen*), Radix Dioscoreae Oppositae (*Shan Yao*), Semen Dolichoris Lablab (*Bai Bian Dou*), and Rhizoma Anemarrhenae Aspheloidis

(*Zhi Mu*), 9g each, and mix-fried Radix Glycyrrhizae (*Gan Cao*), Radix Panacis Ginseng (*Ren Shen*), and Fructus Citri Aurantii (*Zhi Ke*), 6g each

ANALYSIS OF FORMULA: *Ren Shen, Fu Ling, Shan Yao, Bai Bian Dou,* and mix-fried *Gan Cao* fortify the spleen and boost the qi. *Sheng Di, Mai Men Dong, Wu Wei Zi,* and *Zhi Mu* nourish yin. *Tian Hua Fen, Zhi Mu,* and *Ge Gen* engender fluids. In addition, *Ge Gen* stops diarrhea and *Zhi Mu* drains fire. *Fu Ling* eliminates dampness, and *Zhi Ke* moves the qi.

ADDITIONS & SUBTRACTIONS: For upper burner fire, add nine grams of Fructus Gardeniae Jasminoidis (*Zhi Zi*) and Plumula Nelumbinis Nuciferae (*Lian Xin*) and six grams of Radix Platycodi Grandiflori (*Jie Geng*). For middle burner fire, add 20 grams of Gypsum Fibrosum (*Shi Gao*), and three grams of Rhizoma Coptidis Chinensis (*Huang Lian*). And for lower burner fire, add nine grams of Cortex Phellodendri (*Huang Bai*). For more severe yin vacuity, add 12 grams of Tuber Asparagi Cochinensis (*Tian Men Dong*). For numbness and tingling, add nine grams of Bombyx Batryticatus (*Jiang Can*). For reduced appetite and abdominal distention after taking the above decoction, add six grams of Fructus Amomi (*Sha Ren*) and 15 grams of Fructus Germinatus Hordei Vulgaris (*Mai Ya*).

ACUPUNCTURE & MOXIBUSTION: *Zu San Li* (St 36), *Tian Shu* (St 25), *Xia Wan* (CV 10), *Jian Li* (CV 11), *Fu Liu* (Ki 7)

ANALYSIS OF FORMULA: Supplementing *Fu Liu* nourishes yin and engenders fluids. Supplementing *Zu San Li* fortifies the spleen and boosts the qi. Together, these two points support the righteous or correct qi. When needled with even supplementing-even draining method, *Tian Shu, Xia Wan,* and *Jian Li* harmonize the stomach and intestines, eliminate dampness, and stop diarrhea.

ADDITIONS & SUBTRACTIONS: For pale-colored stools and cold limbs, add *Shen Que* (CV 8). For foul-smelling stools and yellow, slimy tongue fur, add *Nei Ting* (St 44). For severe yin vacuity, add *San Yin Jiao* (Sp 6) and *Wei Shu* (Bl 21). For severe spleen vacuity, add *Tai Bai* (Sp 3). For concomitant liver depression, add *Nei Guan* (Per 6). For mouth sores, add *Da Ling* (Per 7). For food stagnation, add *Liang Men* (St 21). For abdominal distention, add *Zhong Wan* (CV 12).

REMARKS

1. Chinese medical treatment is not a substitute for a gluten-free diet. Rice should become the main grain eaten by patients with celiac disease, and the diet should generally conform to a Chinese medical clear, bland diet. Although such a gluten-free diet will itself heal most cases of sprue, Chinese medical treatment typically quickens the relief of accompanying symptoms without side effects.

2. For mouth sores, one can spray powdered Cortex Phellodendri (*Huang Bai*) or the Chinese ready-made medicine *Xi Gua Shuang* (Watermelon Frost) directly on the sores or rinse the mouth with a decoction of Phellodendron.

3. For the treatment of delayed menstruation, excessively scanty menstruation, or amenorrhea, see Bob Flaws's *A Handbook of Menstrual Diseases in Chinese Medicine* also published by Blue Poppy Press.

4. For numbness and tingling due to peripheral neuropathy, also see the chapter on peripheral neuropathy below.

11

Cerebral Vascular Disease

Cerebral vascular disease is also referred to as cerebrovascular accident (CVA) and, more colloquially, as stroke. It is the most common cause of neurologic disability in Western countries. Cerebral vascular disease is a generic term covering several different cerebrovascular diseases. These are cerebral insufficiency, cerebral infarction, cerebral hemorrhage, and cerebral arteriovenous malformation. However, all of these diseases result in nerve damage in a specific region of the brain due to acute, non-traumatic obstruction to the blood flow. The main clinical manifestations of both ischemic stroke and cerebral hemorrhage are sudden onset, obstruction of consciousness, and hemiplegia. The exact signs and symptoms of cerebrovascular disease depend upon the area of the brain affected and not necessarily on the involved artery. Predisposing factors to stroke include hypertension, atherosclerosis, heart disease, diabetes mellitus, and polycythemia. Attacks are most common in the middle-aged and elderly. Preceding attacks, there may be transient numbness of the limbs, fatigue, and aphasia. Attacks often occur during sleep when blood flow is slower.

The Western medical diagnosis of stroke is usually made clinically based on the patient's signs and symptoms, age (50 years or over), and a history of hypertension, diabetes, or atherosclerosis. Diagnosis may be aided or confirmed by x-ray or CT scan. However, laboratory findings are nonspecific. Angiography is sometimes used to determine the site of arterial occlusion, especially when surgery is contemplated. The Western medical treatment of this condition mainly revolves around its prevention by treating the disease conditions which predispose one to stroke. After a CVA has occurred, immediate treatment focuses on keeping the patient alive. Once the patient has stabilized, the emphasis shifts to rehabilitation through physical therapy and nursing aftercare for disabled patients. During the early days of either evolving or completed stroke, neither progression nor ultimate outcome can be predicted. Approximately 35% of patients die in the hospital with the mortality rate increasing with age. Any deficits remaining after six months are likely to be permanent.

Chinese disease categorization: This disease is categorized as *zhong feng*, wind stroke, *zu zhong*, death stroke, *da jue*, great reversal, *bo jue*, slight reversal, *ban shen bu sui*, hemiplegia, *pian ku*, one-sided withering, and *ya fei*, muteness, in Chinese medicine.

Disease causes: Habitual bodily exuberance and/or vacuity due to age, internal damage by the seven affects, drinking too much alcohol and/or overeating fatty, sweet, thick-flavored foods, bedroom taxation (*i.e.*, excessive sexual activity), or taxation fatigue.

Disease mechanisms: Due to habitual bodily yang exuberance, depressive heat stirring ministerial fire and damaging yin, or yin vacuity due to aging, liver yang may become hyperactive and ascend above. Yang is nothing other than qi, and it is qi which moves the blood and body fluids. Therefore, when yang becomes hyperactive and counterflows upward, it may draft along with it blood and phlegm dampness. If phlegm and dampness block the heart orifices, there may be loss of consciousness, aphasia, and the sound of phlegm in the throat. If phlegm blocks the channels and vessels, there may be hemiplegia. Hyperactive yang may also give rise to internally engendered wind. When this wind moves frenetically, it may cause spasms and contractures, tic and tremors. Because of evil heat, phlegm obstruction, blood stasis, and chaotic qi flow affecting the qi mechanism, the viscera and bowels lose their normal function, resulting in inability to engender and transform the qi and blood. During the acute stage of this disease, the condition is potentially life-threatening, manifesting the symptoms of internal blockage and external desertion. During the post-stroke recovery stage, qi vacuity and blood stasis are the principal disease mechanisms.

TREATMENT BASED ON PATTERN DISCRIMINATION:

1. BLOCKAGE PATTERN

MAIN SYMPTOMS: The patient suddenly falls down in a faint, unconscious of human affairs. The teeth are tightly closed. The mouth is silent and not open. The two hands are tightly clenched. There is constipation and urinary retention. The limbs are stiff. Clinically, stroke may be divided into yang blockage and yin blockage. In yang blockage, there is a combination of wind, fire, phlegm, and heat blocking and obstructing the clear orifices. The face is red and the body is hot. There is forceful breathing, bad breath, vexation, worry, and restlessness. The tongue fur is yellow and slimy, and the pulse is bowstring, slippery, and rapid. In yin blockage, there is a combination of internal wind, phlegm, and dampness clouding and blocking the clear orifices. The face is white, while the lips are dark. The patient lies still and is not vexed. The four limbs are not warm. Phlegm drool congests and is exuberant. The tongue fur in this case is white and slimy, and the pulse is deep, slippery, and moderate (*i.e.*, slightly slow).

TREATMENT PRINCIPLES: For yang blockage, clear the liver and track down wind, open the orifices and transform stasis

RX: *Han Shui Long Chi Tang* (Calcitum & Dragon's Teeth Decoction)

INGREDIENTS: Calcitum (*Han Shui Shi*) and Dens Draconis (*Long Chi*), 30g each, Ramulus Uncariae Cum Uncis (*Gou Teng*), 15g, Rhizoma Acori Graminei (*Chang Pu*), 12g, Radix Et Rhizoma Rhei (*Da Huang*), Concretio Silicea Bambusae (*Tian Zhu Huang*), and Radix Scutellariae Baicalensis (*Huang Qin*), 9g each, Herba Menthae Haplocalycis (*Bo He*), 4.5g, Rhizoma Coptidis Chinensis (*Chuan Lian*), 3g, powdered Cornu Antelopis Saigae Tataricae (*Ling Yang Jiao*), 1.5g, and *An Gong Niu Huang Wan* (Quiet the Palace Bezoar Pills, a Chinese ready-made medicine), 1 bolus (dissolved and taken with the other decocted medicinals)

ANALYSIS OF FORMULA: *An Gong Niu Huang Wan* clears heat and resolves toxins, opens the orifices and quiets the spirit. It is a basic formula for yang blockage, treating the acute stage of stroke. *Han Shui Shi* is very cold. It clears heat and discharges fire. When *Da Huang*, *Huang Qin*, and *Huang Lian* are used together, they discharge fire from each of the three burners. *Long Chi*, *Gou Teng*, and *Ling Yang Jiao* settle the liver and extinguish wind, *Shi Chang Pu* and *Tian Zhu Huang* transform phlegm and open the orifices, and *Bo He* courses and clears the liver.

ADDITIONS & SUBTRACTIONS: This is an emergency treatment that is typically not modified since it is primarily aimed at treating the branch.

ACUPUNCTURE & MOXIBUSTION: *Bai Hui* (GV 20), *Si Shen Cong* (M-HN-1), *Shui Gou* (GV 26), *Cheng Jiang* (CV 24), *Feng Chi* (GB 20), *He Gu* (LI 4), *Lao Gong* (Per 8), *Tai Chong* (Liv 3), *Yong Quan* (Ki 1).

ANALYSIS OF FORMULA: Bleeding *Bai Hui* and *Si Shen Cong* clears the brain, arouses the spirit, and opens the orifices. Needling the remaining points with draining method clears the heart and discharges heat, quiets the spirit and opens the orifices.

ADDITIONS & SUBTRACTIONS: For severe heat, bleed the 12 well points on the hands and feet.

For yin blockage, break up phlegm and track down wind, open the orifices and transform stasis

RX: Unnamed protocol by Yan De-xin

INGREDIENTS: *Su He Xiang Wan* (Styrax Pills, a Chinese ready-made medicine), 1 bolus, taken orally dissolved in warm water. Wait a bit and then use the following formula: Flos Carthami Tinctorii (*Hong Hua*), Semen Pruni Persicae (*Tao Ren*), Rhizoma Acori Graminei (*Chang Pu*), Radix Ligustici Wallichii (*Chuan Xiong*), Radix Rubrus Paeoniae Lactiflorae (*Chi Shao*), Rhizoma Pinelliae Ternatae (*Ban Xia*), Tuber Curcumae (*Yu Jin*), Fructus Immaturus Citri Aurantii (*Zhi Shi*), and Rhizoma Arisaematis (*Nan Xing*), 9g each, Ramulus Cinnamomi Cassiae (*Gui Zhi*), 6g, Fasciculus Vascularis Citri Reticulatae (*Ju Luo*), 4.5g.

ANALYSIS OF FORMULA: *Su He Xiang Wan* warms, frees, and opens the orifices, moves the qi, and transforms turbidity. It is a basic formula for yin blockage, treating the acute stage of stroke. *Hong Hua*, *Tao Ren*, *Chuan Xiong*, *Chi Shao*, and *Yu Jin* all quicken the blood and transform stasis. *Shi Chang Pu* and *Yu Jin* open the orifices. *Tian Nan Xing*, *Shi Chang Pu*, and *Ban Xia* transform phlegm. *Zhi Shi* moves the qi to help quicken the blood and to help disperse the phlegm. *Gui Zhi* and *Ju Luo* warm and free the flow of the channels and network vessels.

ADDITIONS & SUBTRACTIONS: This is an emergency treatment that is typically not modified since it is primarily aimed at treating the branch.

ACUPUNCTURE & MOXIBUSTION: The same points as for yang blockage above but without bleeding *Bai Hui* and *Si Shen Cong*.

2. DESERTION PATTERN

MAIN SYMPTOMS: If blockage pattern is not rescued with force or if the condition of the disease deteriorates, it will develop into desertion pattern. The manifestations of this pattern are blockage of the eyes, open mouth, snoring, faint breathing, hands spread open, chilled limbs, sweat like oil, urinary incontinence, a slack, lolling tongue, and a faint pulse tending to expiry.

TREATMENT PRINCIPLES: Boost the qi and quicken the blood, return yang and stem yin

RX: *Li Zhong Wan* (Rectify the Center Pills) & *Sheng Mai San* (Added Flavors Engender the Pulse Powder) with added flavors

INGREDIENTS: Radix Lateralis Praeparatus Aconiti Carmichaeli (*Fu Zi*), Rhizoma Atractylodis Macrocephalae (*Bai Zhu*), Semen Pruni Persicae (*Tao Ren*), Flos Carthami Tinctorii (*Hong Hua*), Radix Panacis Ginseng (*Ren Shen*), Tuber Ophiopogonis Japonicae (*Mai Dong*), and Fructus Schizandrae Chinensis (*Wu Wei Zi*), 9g each, and mix-fried Radix Glycyrrhizae (*Gan Cao*) and dry Rhizoma Zingiberis (*Gan Jiang*), 3g each

ANALYSIS OF FORMULA: *Ren Shen*, mix-fried *Gan Cao*, and *Bai Zhu* boost the qi and stem desertion. *Fu Zi* and *Gan Jiang* return and rescue yang. *Mai Men Dong* and *Wu Wei Zi* engender fluids and rescue yin. *Tao Ren* and *Hong Hua* quicken the blood and transform stasis.

ACUPUNCTURE & MOXIBUSTION: *Shen Que* (CV 8), *Qi Hai* (CV 6), *Guan Yuan* (CV 4), *Bai Hui* (GV 20), *Nei Guan* (Per 6), *Zu San Li* (St 36), *Yong Quan* (Ki 1)

ANALYSIS OF FORMULA: Repeated indirect moxa over salt and ginger at *Shen Que* and over ginger at *Qi Hai* and *Guan Yuan* boosts the qi, rescues yang, and stems counterflow. Supplementing *Zu San Li* fortifies the spleen and boosts the qi as well as rectifies and regulates the channel qi of the entire body. Draining the remaining points opens the orifices, quiets the spirit, and downbears counterflow.

3. HEMIPLEGIA

MAIN SYMPTOMS: Movement of the limbs on one side of the body is not able to be consciously controlled. In mild cases, there is numbness. In severe cases, there is complete loss of sensitivity. The body and limbs are paralyzed and weak. The tongue is purple and dark, and the tongue fur is white and slimy. The pulse is slippery, moderate (*i.e.*, slightly slow), and forceless.

TREATMENT PRINCIPLES: Boost the qi and transform stasis, extinguish wind and free the flow of channels and vessels

RX: *Bu Yang Huan Wu Tang Jia Jian* (Supplement Yang & Restore the Five [Viscera] Decoction with Additions & Subtractions)

INGREDIENTS: Radix Astragali Membranacei (*Huang Qi*) and Radix Salviae Miltiorrhizae (*Dan Shen*), 30g each, Radix Achyranthis Bidentatae (*Niu Xi*), 15g, Radix Ligustici Wallichii (*Chuan Xiong*), Radix Rubrus Paeoniae Lactiflorae (*Chi Shao*), Radix Angelicae Sinensis (*Dang Gui*), and Lumbricus (*Di Long*), 12g each, and Ramulus Cinnamomi Cassiae (*Gui Zhi*), Semen Pruni Persicae (*Tao Ren*), and Flos Carthami Tinctorii (*Hong Hua*), 9g each

ANALYSIS OF FORMULA: Uncooked *Huang Qi* enters the exterior and the channels where it strongly boosts the qi to help quicken the blood. *Dan Shen, Niu Xi, Chuan Xiong, Chi Shao, Dang Gui, Tao Ren,* and *Hong Hua* quicken the blood and transform stasis. In addition, *Niu Xi* nourishes the liver and kidneys, the sinews and bones and *Dang Gui* (especially when combined with *Huang Qi*) nourishes the blood to fill the vessels. *Di Long* and *Gui Zhi* free the flow of network vessels. At the same time, *Di Long* extinguishes wind.

ADDITIONS & SUBTRACTIONS: For severe blood stasis, add six grams of Eupolyphaga Seu Ophisthoplatia (*Zhe Chong*) and 1.5 grams of Hirudo (*Shu Zhi*). For marked qi vacuity, add 15 grams of Radix Codonopsitis Pilosulae (*Dang Shen*). If cold is pronounced, add six grams of Radix Lateralis Praeparatus Aconiti Carmichaeli (*Fu Zi*). If there is profuse phlegm, add nine grams each of Rhizoma Pinelliae Ternatae (*Ban Xia*) and Concretio Silicea Bambusae (*Tian Zhu Huang*). For aphasia, add nine grams each of Rhizoma Acori Graminei (*Shi Chang Pu*) and Radix Polygalae Tenuifoliae (*Yuan Zhi*). For deviated eye and mouth, add nine grams each of Bombyx Batryticatus (*Jiang Can*), and nine grams each of Rhizoma Typhonii Gigantei (*Bai Fu Zi*), and Buthus Martensis (*Quan Xie*). If there is constipation, add nine grams of Semen Cannabis Sativae (*Huo Ma Ren*). For paralysis of mainly the lower extremities, add 15 grams each of Radix Polygoni Multiflori (*He Shou Wu*), cooked Radix Rehmanniae (*Shu Di*), and Ramulus Loranthi Seu Visci (*Sang Ji Sheng*).

ACUPUNCTURE & MOXIBUSTION: *Bai Hui* (GV 20), *Feng Fu* (GV 16), *He Gu* (LI 4), *San Yin Jiao* (Sp 6)

ANALYSIS OF FORMULA: According to the *Ling Shu (Spiritual Pivot), Feng Fu* and *Bai Hui* govern the flow of qi and blood in the sea of marrow. When drained, they transform stasis, extinguish wind, and transform phlegm in the head. Supplementing *He Gu* boosts the qi, while supplementing *San Yin Jiao* nourishes the blood. Together, they harmonize yin and yang and help free the flow of the network vessels.

ADDITIONS & SUBTRACTIONS: For concomitant kidney vacuity, add *Tai Xi* (Ki 3) and/or *Shen Shu* (Bl 23). For spasmodic or tense hemiplegia, add *Tai Chong* (Liv 3), draining *He Gu* as well. For hemiplegia of the upper limbs, select 3-5 points from *Jian Yu* (LI 15), *Bi Nao* (LI 14), *Qu Chi* (LI 11), *Shou San Li* (LI 10), and *Wai Guan* (TB 5). For hemiplegia of the lower limbs, select 4-6 points from *Bi Guan* (St 31), *Fu Tu* (St 32), *Zu San Li* (St 36), *Jie Xi* (St 41), *Huan Tiao* (GB 30), *Feng Shi* (GB 31), *Yang Ling Quan* (GB 34), and *Xuan Zhong* (GB 39). For contraction of the arm, add *Nei Guan* (Per 6), *Jian Shi* (Per 5), and *Chi Ze* (Lu 5). For difficult flexion of the wrist, add *Yang Chi* (TB 4). For difficulty moving the thumb, add *Yang Xi* (LI 5). For swelling or numbness of the fingers, add *Ba Xie* (M-UE-22). For contraction or difficult flexion of the knee, add *Wei Zhong* (Bl 40) and *Qu Quan* (Liv 8). For swelling or numbness of the toes, add *Ba Feng* (M-LE-8). If the leg and foot twist to the inside, add *Gong Sun* (Sp 4), *San Yin Jiao* (Sp 6), *Tai Xi* (Ki 3), and *Zhao Hai* (Ki 6). If the leg and foot twist to the outside, add *Xuan Zhong* (GB 39), *Qiu Xu* (GB 40), *Kun Lun* (Bl 60), and *Shen Mai* (Bl 62). If the foot bends downward, add *Jie Xi* (St 41), *Shang Ju Xu* (St 37), *Qiu Xu* (GB 40), and *Zhong Feng* (Liv 4).

4. Speech obstructed & rough

MAIN SYMPTOMS: The tongue does not move freely. Speech is not clear. Drool flows by itself. The tongue is mostly wry and deviated. The tongue fur is thin and slimy. The pulse is slippery and moderate (*i.e.*, slightly slow).

TREATMENT PRINCIPLES: Break the phlegm and disinhibit the orifices, quicken the blood and transform stasis

RX: *Dan Er Chong Tang* (Salvia Two Worms Decoction)

INGREDIENTS: Radix Salviae Miltiorrhizae (*Dan Shen*), 15g, Fructus Trichosanthis Kirlowii (*Quan Gua Lou*), 12g, Rhizoma Typhonii Gigantei (*Bai Fu Zi*), bile-processed Rhizoma Arisaematis (*Dan Nan Xing*), Fructus Immaturus Citri Aurantii (*Zhi Shi*), Concretio Silicea Bambusae (*Tian Zhu Huang*), Rhizoma Acori Graminei (*Shi Chang Pu*), Radix Polygalae Tenuifoliae (*Yuan Zhi*), Radix Ligustici Wallichii (*Chuan Xiong*), and Flos Carthami Tinctorii (*Hong Hua*), 9g each, Rhizoma Gastrodiae Elatae (*Tian Ma*), 4.5g, Hirudo (*Shui Zhi*), 3g, and Buthus Martensis (*Quan Xie*), 1.5g

ANALYSIS OF FORMULA: *Bai Fu Zi, Quan Gua Lou, Dan Nan Xing, Tian Zhu Huang, Shi Chang Pu,* and *Yuan Zhi* all break phlegm and disinhibit the orifices. In addition, *Bai Fu Zi* and *Tian Zhu Huang* extinguish wind, treat wind stroke, and have a marked tropism for the face, mouth, and head, *Yuan Zhi* and *Shi Chang Pu* also open the orifices. *Zhi Shi* moves the qi to help quicken the blood and disperse phlegm. *Dan Shen, Chuan Xiong, Hong Hua,* and *Shui Zhi* break the blood and transform stasis. *Tian Ma* and *Quan Xie* extinguish wind, help transform phlegm, and free the flow of the network vessels.

ADDITIONS & SUBTRACTIONS: For concomitant qi vacuity, add 15 grams of Radix Astragali Membranacei (*Huang Qi*) and 12 grams of Radix Codonopsitis Pilosulae (*Dang Shen*). For concomitant blood vacuity, add 12 grams each of Radix Angelicae Sinensis (*Dang Gui*) and Radix Albus Paeoniae Lactiflorae (*Bai Shao*). For nausea and vomiting of drool, subtract *Dan Nan Xing* and add nine grams each of Rhizoma Pinelliae Ternatae (*Ban Xia*) and uncooked Rhizoma Zingiberis (*Sheng Jiang*).

ACUPUNCTURE & MOXIBUSTION: *Bai Hui* (GV 20), *Feng Fu* (GV 16), *He Gu* (LI 4), *San Yin Jiao* (Sp 6), *Liang Quan* (CV 23), *Tong Li* (Ht 5)

ANALYSIS OF FORMULA: For an analysis of *Bai Hui, Feng Fu, He Gu,* and *San Yin Jiao,* please see the preceding pattern. *Tong Li* is the network point of the heart, and the heart governs speech. Therefore, needling it frees the heart qi, opens the orifices, and eases the speech. *Liang Quan* is located on the conception vessel at the level of the throat, just below the tongue. Needling it frees the flow of the network vessels of the throat and tongue and harmonizes the qi and blood flow locally. Together, these two points treat aphasia due to wind stroke.

ADDITIONS & SUBTRACTIONS: Please see the preceding pattern. One can also alternate *Feng Fu* and *Tong Li* with *Ya Men* (GV 15). For deviated mouth, add *Di Cang* (St 4), *Cheng Jiang* (CV 24), and *Shui Gou* (GV 26).

REMARKS

1. The above discussion of cerebrovascular disease is based on Yan De-xin's discussion of this condition in *Aging & Blood Stasis.* Dr. Yan believes that blood stasis plays a part in all strokes. Therefore, blood stasis medicinals are found in all of the above formulas. Dr. Yan cautions his readers not to become confused between modern Western and traditional Chinese medicines. Even in hemorrhagic stroke, one should still use blood-quickening, stasis-transforming medicinals based on Chinese theories. As Dr. Yan points out, "where there is hemorrhage, there must be stasis." This is because the blood only flows freely when it remains within its vessels. If blood extravasates due to hemorrhage, then such extravasation must, *ipso facto,* result in blood stasis. Only when this stasis is transformed and dispelled can the function of the spirit brilliance be restored.

2. The sooner treatment is initiated after a stroke with acupuncture and Chinese medicinals, the less permanent sequelae there usually are.

3. For the blockage pattern of stroke, another first aid acupuncture treatment is to bleed *Yu Ye* and *Jin Jin* (M-HN-

20). To do this, clamp the tongue between two chopsticks in order to prevent the patient from retracting it at the moment of puncture.

4. For more information specifically on the acupuncture treatment of stroke and hemiplegia, see Wu & Han's *Golden Needle Wang Le-ting* also published by Blue Poppy Press.

5. Some Chinese doctors prefer to use head or so-called scalp acupuncture for the treatment of stroke. For information on that acupuncture specialty, please see any of the various books on this subject available in English.

6. Ultimately, in Chinese medicine just as in Western medicine, the best treatment for cerebral vascular accident is prevention. This means treating hypertension, atherosclerosis, heart disease, and diabetes mellitus. When liver repletion patterns are accompanied by constipation, freeing the flow of the bowels is also important for preventing stroke according to Chinese medicine.

12

CERVICAL SPONDYLOSIS

Cervical spondylosis refers to chronic degenerative changes in both the intervertebral discs and anuli in the region of the neck as well as the formation of bony osteophytes, all of which may narrow the cervical canal causing spinal stenosis which may result in progressive myelopathy. For instance, osteophytes may develop on the vertebral bodies adjacent to the areas of motion at the intervertebral disks or the ligamentum flavum may undergo hypertrophy and buckling. If such pathological changes compress the spinal cord, certain motor and sensory deficits may result. This is then referred to as myelopathy. Symptoms of cervical spondylosis include headaches, especially occipital headaches, tinnitus, and progressive neck pain. Another symptom of cervical spondylosis is Lhermitte's sign. This refers to a sudden electrical sensation down the neck and back triggered by flexing the neck. Although myelopathy due to spondylosis has no single pathognomonic sign or symptom, the most common combination of symptoms in patients with this condition are weakness and clumsiness of the hands, paresthesias in the hand, and gait disturbances. Leg weakness leading to gait disturbances usually first manifests as a feeling of heaviness in the legs and noticeable difficulty in walking usual distances and up stairs. There may also be loss of balance, stiffness, and unsteadiness. A "myelopathic gait" may appear which is a sort of shuffle with disruption in smooth, rhythmic function. As the myelopathy progresses, sphincter and sexual function may also be compromised. Bowel and bladder dysfunction occur in 15-18% of patients.[1]

Cervical spondylosis is most commonly seen in the elderly.[2] Some degree of spondylotic change is seen in 25-50% of the adult population over 50 years of age and in 75% of those over 75 years old. However, myelopathy occurs in only 5-10% of patients with symptomatic spondylosis.[3] Risks include old neck injury which may have occurred several years prior to the onset of present symptoms. However, this disorder also occurs commonly in older people who have no history of neck injury. Cervical spondylosis is thought to result from normal changes in vertebral anatomy due to aging.

Physical examination findings of cervical spondylitic myelopathy (CSM) vary widely depending on the level and degree of cord compression. In general, lower motor neuron findings are seen at the level of the lesion, while upper level motor neuron findings are seen below the level of the lesion, for instance hyporeflexia in the upper extremities and hyporeflexia in the lower extremities. Another feature of CSM is that it involves the axial skeleton and does not affect the head and face. Definitive diagnosis of this condition is by x-ray, CT scan, myelogram, MRI, and somatosensory evoked potentials (SSEPs).

Occasionally, this condition improves or stabilizes on its own. However, unlike cervical disc herniation, most patients do not improve with nonsurgical treatment due to the progressive degenerative nature of spondylotic disease. Conservative Western medical treatment includes a soft collar to restrict neck movement causing pain and physical therapy to strengthen the neck muscles. Intermittent neck traction may be recommended instead of, or in addition to, a cervical collar. For severe cases, hospitalization with complete bed rest and traction for 1-2 weeks may be necessary. Analgesics and/or muscle relaxants may help to reduce pain. If the signs and symptoms of cervical myelopathy are progressive, surgical options include anterior or posterior decompression. In some cases, the entire vertebral body may be removed (corpectomy) between adjacent levels of spondylosis or even several bodies may be removed. A bony graft is then placed for fusion and plates and screws are used to reinforce long grafts. Improvement postsurgery in neck and arm pain due to radiculopathy is approximately 90%, while improvement in leg weakness due to myelopathy occurs in 60-80% of cases. Serious neurologic complications from surgery, including permanent disability, is rare, around 2%.

Factors negatively impacting the degree of improvement from surgery include age greater than 50, duration of symptoms for more than 12 months, and involvement of multiple levels. Patients who are poor surgical candidates or who are treated nonsurgically for some other reason should be followed closely for worsening myelopathy.

CHINESE DISEASE CATEGORIZATION: Depending on its signs and symptoms, this disease is categorized variously as *bi zheng*, impediment condition, *wei zheng*, wilting condition, *tou tong*, headache, *yun zhen*, dizziness, *jing qiang*, stiff neck, *jing jin ji*, neck sinew cramping or tension, and *jing jian tong*, neck and shoulder pain.

DISEASE CAUSES: External invasion by wind, cold, damp evils, faulty diet, enduring taxation detriment, and vacuity due to aging

DISEASE MECHANISMS: If externally invading wind, cold, and/or damp evils invade and cause impediment to the free flow of the channel and vessel qi and blood, this will usually result in pain and lack or restriction of movement. Often such evils take advantage of bodily weakness in the elderly, in which case the interstices are hollow and vacuous and the qi and blood are scanty and weak. Damp evils may also be internally engendered, commonly due to spleen vacuity and faulty diet. If dampness endures, it may transform into phlegm. If phlegm and dampness spill over into the region of the neck and shoulders, they may block the free flow of qi and blood there, resulting in aching and pain. In addition, habitual bodily vacuity due to aging may also result in lack of moistening and nourishment of the sinews and bones, thus leading to aching, pain, and insensitivity. Habitual bodily vacuity resulting in neck pain, stiffness, and numbness, is usually characterized as liver blood-kidney yin vacuity. Further, long-term microtrauma to the neck may result in taxation detriment to the cervical muscles and joints. If any of these disease mechanisms endure and do not heal, they may give rise to qi stagnation and blood stasis which then complicate these other disease mechanisms.

TREATMENT BASED ON PATTERN DISCRIMINATION:

1. WIND COLD IMPEDIMENT & OBSTRUCTION PATTERN

MAIN SYMPTOMS: Head, neck, shoulder, and upper back aching and pain, fixed neck pain, tender points on the neck, a possible palpable cord-like feeling in the neck, stiff neck, inhibited movement, soreness, pain, and numbness of the four limbs, possible weakness and heaviness of the upper limbs and also heavy-headedness, a liking for heat and an aversion to cold, a pale tongue with thin, white fur, and a floating, moderate (*i.e.*, slightly slow) or tight pulse

TREATMENT PRINCIPLES: Dispel wind and scatter cold, free the flow of the network vessels and diffuse impediment

RX: *Gui Zhi Jia Ge Gen Tang Jia Jian* (Cinnamon Twig Plus Pueraria Decoction with Additions & Subtractions)

INGREDIENTS: Radix Puerariae (*Ge Gen*), 15g, Ramulus Cinnamomi Cassiae (*Gui Zhi*), Radix Albus Paeoniae Lactiflorae (*Bai Shao*), Radix Angelicae Sinensis (*Dang Gui*), Radix Ligustici Wallichii (*Chuan Xiong*), Rhizoma Atractylodis (*Cang Zhu*), Fructus Chaenomelis Lagenariae (*Mu Gua*), 9g each, Radix Glycyrrhizae (*Gan Cao*), 6g, Radix Pseudoginseng (*San Qi*), 3g, uncooked Rhizoma Zingiberis (*Sheng Jiang*), 3 slices, and Fructus Zizyphi Jujubae (*Da Zao*), 3 pieces

ANALYSIS OF FORMULA: *Ge Gen, Gui Zhi, Chuan Xiong* and *Cang Zhu* dispel wind. *Ge Gen* effuses the exterior and resolves the muscle, especially treating muscular pain in the upper back and the back of the neck. Therefore, it is a key medicinal for this condition. *Gui Zhi* scatters cold and, with *Bai Shao,* harmonizes the defensive and constructive to prevent further invasion of evils in the exterior. In addition, *Bai Shao* relaxes cramping, thus helping *Ge Gen* stop pain in the neck. *Chuan Xiong* and *Cang Zhu* dispel wind dampness and treat impediment pain, especially in the upper part of the body. *Dang Gui, Chuan Xiong* and *San Qi* free the flow of the network vessels, transform stasis, and stop pain. *Dang Gui* and *Bai Shao* also nourish the blood to fill the vessels to avoid penetration of cold into the channels of the neck. *Mu Gua* eliminates dampness, frees the flow of impediment, relaxes cramping, and soothes the sinews. When combined with *Ge Gen,* it relaxes tension in the neck. *Da Zao, Sheng Jiang* and *Gan Cao* are the other standard ingredients of *Gui Zhi Tang* (Cinnamon Twig Decoction) which help *Gui Zhi* and *Bai Shao* dispel wind, scatter cold, and harmonize the defensive and constructive.

ADDITIONS & SUBTRACTIONS: For inhibited movement, add nine grams each of Herba Lycopodii (*Shen Jin Cao*) and Caulis Trachelospermi Jasminoidis (*Luo Shi Teng*). For severe fixed pain, add six grams each of Resina Olibani (*Ru Xiang*) and Resina Myrrhae (*Mo Yao*).

For preponderant damp impediment with a bag-over-the-head sensation, heavy, aching limbs, painful joints, and chest oppression, replace *Gui Zhi Jia Ge Gen Tang Jia Jian* with *Qiang Huo Sheng Shi Tang Jia Wei* (Notopterygium Overcome Dampness Decoction with Added Flavors): Radix Puerariae (*Ge Gen*), 12g, Radix Et Rhizoma Notopterygii (*Qiang Huo*), Radix Angelicae Pubescentis (*Du Huo*), and Ramulus Cinnamomi Cassiae (*Gui Zhi*), 9g each, Radix Et Rhizoma Ligustici Chinensis (*Gao Ben*), Radix Ledebouriellae Divaricatae (*Fang Feng*), Radix Ligustici Wallichii (*Chuan Xiong*), Radix Clematidis Chinensis (*Wei

Ling Xian), and Rhizoma Atractylodis (*Cang Zhu*), 6g each, and Radix Glycyrrhizae (*Gan Cao*), 3g.

For preponderant cold impediment with severe aversion to cold, a cold sensation in the back of the neck, and worsening of pain with cold, replace *Gui Zhi Jia Ge Gen Tang Jia Jian* with *Wu Tou Tang Jia Wei* (Aconite Decoction with Added Flavors): Radix Puerariae (*Ge Gen*), 12g, Radix Et Rhizoma Notopterygii (*Qiang Huo*), Radix Albus Paeoniae Lactiflorae (*Bai Shao*), and uncooked Radix Astragali Membranacei (*Huang Qi*), 9g each, Radix Aconiti Carmichaeli (*Chuan Wu*) (decocted at least 30 minutes before adding the other medicinals), Herba Ephedrae (*Ma Huang*), and Ramulus Cinnamomi Cassiae (*Gui Zhi*), 6g each, and Herba Asari Cum Radice (*Xi Xin*) and Radix Glycyrrhizae (*Gan Cao*), 3g each.

For preponderant wind impediment with migratory pain and aversion to wind, replace *Gui Zhi Jia Ge Gen Tang Jia Jian* with *Fang Feng Tang Jia Jian* (Ledebouriella Decoction with Additions & Subtractions): Radix Ledebouriellae Divaricatae (*Fang Feng*) and Radix Puerariae (*Ge Gen*), 12g each, Radix Gentianae Macrophyllae (*Qin Jiao*), Radix Clematidis Chinensis (*Wei Ling Xian*), and Radix Et Rhizoma Notopterygii (*Qiang Huo*), 9g each, Sclerotium Poriae Cocos (*Fu Ling*), Radix Angelicae Sinensis (*Dang Gui*), and Ramulus Cinnamomi Cassiae (*Gui Zhi*), 6g each, and Herba Ephedrae (*Ma Huang*), 3g.

ACUPUNCTURE & MOXIBUSTION: *Hou Xi* (SI 3), *Feng Chi* (GB 20), *Da Zhui* (GV 14), *Lie Que* (Lu 7)

ANALYSIS OF FORMULA: *Hou Xi* is the meeting point of the governing vessel which penetrates the cervical vertebrae. It is one of the best points for treating neck stiffness and/or pain when needled with draining technique. Draining *Lie Que*, *Da Zhui*, and *Feng Chi* dispels wind and scatters cold. In addition, *Lie Que* is the master or ruling point of the head and neck area, *Da Zhui* is the intersection point of the six yang channels and the governing vessel, while *Feng Chi* is the intersection point of the gallbladder and triple burner channels and the yang qiao mai and yang wei mai. Therefore, when all these points are needled together, they free the flow of the channels to stop pain in the affected area.

ADDITIONS & SUBTRACTIONS: If wind damp is predominant, subtract *Lie Que* and *Da Zhui* and add *Yin Ling Quan* (Sp 9) and *Da Zhu* (Bl 11). For neck pain along the distribution of the foot tai yang channel, subtract *Feng Chi* while adding *Tian Zhu* (Bl 10) and *Kun Lun* (Bl 60). If the pain is along the hand yang ming channel, add *Shou San Li* (LI 10). If located along the hand tai yang channel, add *Tian Zong* (SI 11) and *Qu Yuan* (SI 13). If located along the course of the hand shao yang channel, add *Tian Liao* (TB 15) and/or *Tian You* (TB 16) and replace *Lie Que* with *Zhong Zhu* (TB 3). If located along the governing vessel, add *Ya Men* (GV 15) and *Feng Fu* (GV 16). For pain causing avoidance of backward bending of the neck, add *Chen Jiang* (CV 24). For pain causing avoidance of forward bending of the head, add *Shui Gou* (GV 26). For pain that involves the shoulders, add *Tian Liao* (TB 15) and *Jian Yu* (LI 15) or the "three shoulder needles," *i.e.*, *Jian Yu* (LI 15), *Jian Liao* (TB 14), and *Jian Zhen* (SI 9). For pain which simultaneously involves the neck, the trapezius muscle, and the scapula, one can use the following strategy: First, needle the "five heavens," *i.e.*, *Tian Zhu* (Bl 10), *Tian You* (TB 16), *Tian Jing* (GB 21), *Tian Liao* (TB 15) and *Tian Zong* (SI 11), locally. Secondly, choose 1-3 distant points depending on the location of the pain. If the pain is located on the governing vessel, choose *Hou Xi* (SI 3) or *Chang Jiang* (GV 1). If on the bladder channel, use *Kun Lun* (Bl 60) or *Shen Mai* (Bl 62). If it is on the gallbladder channel, choose *Qiu Xu* (GB 40) or *Xuan Zhong* (GB 39). If it is on the small intestine channel, needle *Hou Xi* (SI 3) or *Yang Lao* (SI 6). If it is on the triple burner channel, use *Zhong Zhu* (TB 3) or *Zhi Gou* (TB 6). This seemingly simple strategy achieves good results for this kind of pain.

2. PHLEGM & DAMPNESS OBSTRUCTING THE NETWORK VESSELS PATTERN

MAIN SYMPTOMS: Head, neck, shoulder, and upper back aching and pain, dizziness and vertigo, heavy-headedness, bodily heaviness, lack of strength, nausea, chest and ductal fullness and oppression, a pale tongue with white, possibly slimy fur, and a bowstring, slippery pulse

NOTE: This pattern does not commonly present in this pure form, but internally phlegm and dampness often complicate other patterns of this condition.

TREATMENT PRINCIPLES: Transform phlegm and dispel dampness, quicken the blood and free the flow of the network vessels

RX: *Fu Ling Wan Jia Jian* (Poria Pills with Additions & Subtractions)

INGREDIENTS: Sclerotium Poriae Cocos (*Fu Ling*), Pericarpium Citri Reticulatae (*Chen Pi*), Lumbricus (*Di Long*), 12g each, bile-processed Rhizoma Arisaematis (*Dan Nan Xing*), Rhizoma Pinelliae Ternatae (*Ban Xia*), Semen Sinapis Albae (*Bai Jie Zi*), Fructus Schisandrae Chinensis (*Wu Wei Zi*), 10g each, Radix Platycodi Grandiflori (*Jie Geng*), 6g, and Radix Pseudoginseng (*San Qi*), 3g

ANALYSIS OF FORMULA: *Fu Ling*, *Chen Pi*, and *Ban Xia* are the three ruling ingredients in *Er Chen Tang* (Two Aged [Ingredients] Decoction) for transforming phlegm and dispelling dampness. *Bai Jie Zi* scatters cold and disperses phlegm as well as stops pain. *Dan Nan Xing* disperses phlegm and frees the flow of the channels and vessels. *Di Long* frees the flow of the network vessels and resolves tetany. *Wu Wei Zi* secures the exterior to prevent simultaneous invasion by external evils, while *San Qi* quickens the blood and dispels stasis. *Jie Geng* guides the other medicinals to the upper body at the same time as it transforms phlegm.

ADDITIONS & SUBTRACTIONS: For concomitant wind cold damp impediment, add nine grams each of Ramulus Cinnamomi Cassiae (*Gui Zhi*) and Radix Et Rhizoma Notopterygii (*Qiang Huo*). For dizziness, add 12 grams each of Rhizoma Gastrodiae Elatae (*Tian Ma*) and Rhizoma Atractylodis Macrocephalae (*Bai Zhu*). For chest impediment, add nine grams each of Radix Salviae Miltiorrhizae (*Dan Shen*), Bulbus Allii (*Xie Bai*), and Pericarpium Trichosanthis Kirlowii (*Gua Lou Pi*).

For phlegm heat intruding into the tai yang, replace *Fu Ling Wan Jia Wei* with *Er Chen Tang Jia Wei* (Two Aged [Ingredients] Decoction with Added Flavors): Rhizoma Pinelliae Ternatae (*Ban Xia*) and Radix Scutellariae Baicalensis (*Huang Qin*), 12g each, Sclerotium Poriae Cocos (*Fu Ling*), Pericarpium Citri Reticulatae (*Chen Pi*), Flos Carthami Tinctorii (*Hong Hua*), and Radix Et Rhizoma Notopterygii (*Qiang Huo*), 9g each, Radix Glycyrrhizae (*Gan Cao*), 6g, and uncooked Rhizoma Zingiberis (*Sheng Jiang*), 2 slices.

ACUPUNCTURE & MOXIBUSTION: *Hou Xi* (SI 3), *Feng Chi* (GB 20), *Da Zhui* (GV 14), *Yin Ling Quan* (Sp 9), *Feng Long* (St 40)

ANALYSIS OF FORMULA: Draining *Hou Xi*, *Feng Chi*, and *Da Zhui* frees the flow of the channels and vessels in the affected area and stops pain. *Yin Ling Quan* is the master point for disinhibiting dampness, while *Feng Long* is the master point for transforming phlegm. Therefore, when these two points are used together with draining technique, they form a key combination for treating dampness and phlegm.

ADDITIONS & SUBTRACTIONS: Please see pattern #1 above.

3. QI STAGNATION & BLOOD STASIS PATTERN

MAIN SYMPTOMS: Head, neck, shoulder, and upper back aching, pain, and numbness, lancinating pain, pain which is fixed in location and which is worse at night but better during the day, pressure pain, possible numbness which is also worse at night, spasms and tension or cramping of the four limbs, vexation and agitation, a dry mouth, a dark purple tongue or possible static macules or spots, and a bowstring, choppy pulse

NOTE: This pattern rarely presents in its pure form but often complicates other patterns of this condition.

TREATMENT PRINCIPLES: Quicken the blood and transform stasis, free the flow of the network vessels and stop pain

Rx: *Tao Hong Yin Jia Jian* (Persica & Carthamus Drink with Additions & Subtractions)

INGREDIENTS: Semen Pruni Persicae (*Tao Ren*), Flos Carthami Tinctorii (*Hong Hua*), Radix Ligustici Wallichii (*Chuan Xiong*), Radix Angelicae Sinensis (*Dang Gui*), Feces Trogopterori Seu Pteromi (*Wu Ling Zhi*), Fructus Immaturus Citri Aurantii (*Zhi Shi*), Rhizoma Corydalis Yanhusuo (*Yan Hu Suo*), and Radix Clematidis Chinensis (*Wei Ling Xian*), 9g each

ANALYSIS OF FORMULA: *Tao Ren*, *Hong Hua*, *Chuan Xiong*, *Dang Gui*, *Wu Ling Zhi*, and *Yan Hu Suo* quicken the blood and transform stasis, free the flow of the network vessels and stop pain. *Hong Hua* and *Chuan Xiong* work especially in the upper part of the body. *Chuan Xiong*, *Zhi Shi*, and *Yan Hu Suo* move the qi to quicken the blood and stop pain. *Wei Ling Xian* and *Chuan Xiong* dispel wind dampness and treat impediment pain.

ADDITIONS & SUBTRACTIONS: If there are symptoms of cold, add nine grams of Ramulus Cinnamomi Cassiae (*Gui Zhi*) and three grams each of processed Radix Aconiti Carmichaeli (*Chuan Wu Tou*) and Herba Asari Cum Radice (*Xi Xin*). For heat symptoms, add 12 grams of Herba Patriniae Heterophyllae Cum Radice (*Bai Jiang Cao*) and Cortex Radicis Moutan (*Dan Pi*). For concomitant qi vacuity, add 18 grams of Radix Astragali Membranacei (*Huang Qi*). For concomitant blood vacuity, add 12 grams of Radix Albus Paeoniae Lactiflorae (*Bai Shao*). For liver-kidney vacuity, add 12 grams of Cortex Radicis Acanthopanacis (*Wu Jia Pi*) and nine grams each of Ramulus Loranthi Seu Visci (*Sang Ji Sheng*) and Rhizoma Drynariae (*Gu Sui Bu*).

If qi stagnation and blood stasis are complicated by qi vacuity and wind, replace *Tao Hong Yin* with *Yi Qi Huo Xue San Feng Tang* (Boost the Qi, Quicken the Blood & Scatter Wind Decoction): Radix Puerariae (*Ge Gen*) and Radix Albus Paeoniae Lactiflorae (*Bai Shao*), 18g each, Radix Astragali Membranacei (*Huang Qi*), 15g, uncooked Radix Rehmanniae (*Sheng Di*) and Squama Manitis Pentadactylis (*Chuan Shan Jia*), 12g each, and Radix Codonopsitis Pilosulae (*Dang Shen*), Radix Salviae Miltiorrhizae (*Dan Shen*), Semen Pruni Persicae (*Tao Ren*), Flos Carthami Tinctorii (*Hong Hua*), Rhizoma Cyperi Rotundi (*Xiang Fu*), Lumbricus (*Di Long*), Eupolyphaga Seu Ophisthoplatia (*Zhe Chong*), and Radix Clematidis Chinensis (*Wei Ling Xian*), 9g each.

ACUPUNCTURE & MOXIBUSTION: *Hou Xi* (SI 3), *Shen Mai* (Bl 62), *He Gu* (LI 4), *San Yin Jiao* (Sp 6), *a shi* points

ANALYSIS OF FORMULA: *Hou Xi* is the meeting point of the governing vessel which penetrates the cervical vertebrae. *Shen Mai* is the meeting point of yang qiao mai. Together, they form a traditional combination for freeing the flow of the governing vessel and bladder channel to stop pain in the neck when needled with draining technique. Draining *He Gu* moves qi, while draining *San Yin Jiao* quickens the blood. Together, these two points form a special combination to treat qi stagnation and blood stasis in the whole body. Draining the *a shi* points frees the flow of the network vessels and stops pain in the local area.

ADDITIONS & SUBTRACTIONS: Please see pattern #1 above.

4. QI & BLOOD VACUITY PLUS BLOOD STASIS PATTERN

MAIN SYMPTOMS: Head and neck pain with inhibited movement, weakness of the neck and the four limbs especially the upper extremities, numbness of the shoulder and arms, general fatigue, insomnia, profuse dreams, spontaneous perspiration or night sweats, dizziness, heart palpitations, shortness of breath, a pale facial complexion, menstrual irregularities, a pale tongue with thin, white fur, and a fine, weak pulse

TREATMENT PRINCIPLES: Supplement the qi and nourish the blood, free the flow of the network vessels and move the impediment

RX: *Huang Qi Gui Zhi Wu Wu Tang Jia Wei* (Astragalus & Cinnamon Twig Five Materials Decoction with Added Flavors)

INGREDIENTS: Radix Astragali Membranacei (*Huang Qi*) 18g, Caulis Milletiae Seu Spatholobi (*Ji Xue Teng*), 15g, Radix Rubrus Paeoniae Lactiflorae (*Chi Shao*) and Radix Albus Paeoniae Lactiflorae (*Bai Shao*), 12g each, Ramulus Cinnamomi Cassiae (*Gui Zhi*) and Radix Puerariae (*Ge Gen*), 9g each, uncooked Rhizoma Zingiberis (*Sheng Jiang*), 6g, Fructus Zizyphi Jujubae (*Da Zao*), 4 pieces

ANALYSIS OF FORMULA: Within this formula, *Huang Qi* supplements the qi and *Ji Xue Teng* nourishes the blood. *Huang Qi* is aided by *Sheng Jiang* and *Da Zao*, while *Ji Xue Teng* is aided by *Bai Shao* and *Da Zao*. *Ji Xue Teng* and *Chi Sao* quicken the blood and dispel stasis. *Bai Shao* and *Ge Gen* relax cramping and tension specifically in the upper back and back of the neck. *Gui Zhi* quickens the blood in the upper part of the body and also promotes *Huang Qi's* supplementation of the qi.

ADDITIONS & SUBTRACTIONS: For concomitant wind damp impediment, add nine grams each of Radix Clematidis Chinensis (*Wei Ling Xian*) and Radix Et Rhizoma Notopterygii (*Qiang Huo*). For concomitant blood stasis, add nine grams each of Lumbricus (*Di Long*) and Flos Carthami Tinctorii (*Hong Hua*) and six grams of Resina Olibani (*Ru Xiang*). For concomitant kidney vacuity, add nine grams each of Cortex Radicis Acanthopanacis Gracilistylis (*Wu Jia Pi*), Herba Epimedii (*Yin Yang Huo*), and Rhizoma Cibotii Barometsis (*Gou Ji*).

ACUPUNCTURE & MOXIBUSTION: *Zu San Li* (St 36), *Da Zhui* (GV 14), *Ge Shu* (Bl 17), *Gan Shu* (Bl 18), *Pi Shu* (Bl 20), *San Yin Jiao* (Sp 6), *He Gu* (LI 4)

ANALYSIS OF FORMULA: Supplementing *Zu San Li* supplements the spleen, the latter heaven root of qi and blood engenderment and transformation. *Da Zhui* is a meeting point of all the yang channels. Supplementing it raises yang qi in the body and especially to the head and neck region. *Ge Shu* is the meeting point of the blood, and *Gan Shu* is the transport point of the liver, the viscus which stores the blood. When used together, these two points are called the "four flowers." Supplementing them supplements the blood. *Pi Shu* is the back transport point of the spleen. Supplementing it fortifies the spleen and boosts the qi, especially when needled together with *Zu San Li*. When needled with even supplementing-even draining technique, *San Yin Jiao* both supplements the spleen and quickens the blood, while *He Gu* governs the qi of the upper body.

ADDITIONS & SUBTRACTIONS: Please see pattern #1 above.

5. LIVER-KIDNEY YIN DEBILITY PATTERN

MAIN SYMPTOMS: Neck, shoulder, and upper back aching and pain, possible distended pain in the head, numbness and lack of strength of the four limbs, low back and knee soreness and limpness, dizziness, blurred vision, tidal redness, night sweats, dry mouth and throat, a red tongue with scanty fur, and a fine, rapid pulse

TREATMENT PRINCIPLES: Supplement and nourish the liver and kidneys, quicken the blood and free the flow of the network vessels

RX: *Hu Qian Wan Jia Jian* (Hidden Tiger Pills with Additions & Subtractions)

INGREDIENTS: Radix Achyranthis Bidentatae (*Niu Xi*), cooked Radix Rehmanniae (*Shu Di*), and Radix Salviae Miltiorrhizae (*Dan Shen*), 12g each, and Radix Angelicae Sinensis (*Dang Gui*), Radix Albus Paeoniae Lactiflorae (*Bai Shao*), Herba Cynomorii Songarici (*Suo Yang*), Rhizoma

Anemarrhenae Aspheloidis (*Zhi Mu*), Cortex Phellodendri (*Huang Bai*), Plastrum Testudinis (*Gui Ban*), Semen Cuscutae Chinensis (*Tu Si Zi*), and Caulis Milletiae Seu Spatholobi (*Ji Xue Teng*), 9g each

ANALYSIS OF FORMULA: Withing this formula, *Niu Xi*, *Shu Di*, and *Gui Ban* enrich kidney yin, and, because liver and kidneys share a common source, *Dang Gui* and *Bai Shao* nourish liver blood. *Suo Yang* and *Tu Si Zi* supplement kidney yang because yin and yang are mutually rooted. In addition, *Suo Yang*, *Niu Xi* and *Gui Ban* reinforce or strengthen the sinews and bones. *Dang Gui* with *Ji Xue Teng* and *Dan Shen* quickens the blood and transforms the stasis due to vacuity. These three medicinals also stop pain. *Zhi Mu* and *Huang Bai* clear vacuity heat and downbear ministerial fire.

ADDITIONS & SUBTRACTIONS: If there is yin and yang vacuity with concomitant cold feet, decreased sexual desire, and loose stools as well as blood stasis, replace *Hu Qian Wan* with *He Shi Jing Zhui Bing Fang* (Master He's Cervical Vertebrae Disease Formula): cooked Radix Rehmanniae (*Shu Di*), uncooked Pollen Typhae (*Pu Huang*), Radix Drynariae (*Gu Sui Bu*), and Caulis Milletiae Seu Spatholobi (*Ji Xue Teng*), 15g each, Herba Pyrolae (*Lu Ti Cao*), 12g, Radix Salviae Miltiorrhizae (*Dan Shen*), Ramulus Mori Albi (*Sang Zhi*), Fructus Germinatus Hordei Vulgaris (*Mai Ya*), Herba Cistanchis Deserticolae (*Rou Cong Rong*), and Extremitas Radicis Angelicae Sinensis (*Dang Gui Wei*), 9g each, and Scolopendra Subspinipes (*Wu Gong*), 6g.

For vertigo, dizziness, and blurred vision, add 12 grams each of Rhizoma Gastrodiae Elatae (*Tian Ma*) and Ramulus Uncariae Cum Uncis (*Gou Teng*). For concomitant wind damp impediment, add nine grams each of Radix Clematidis Chinensis (*Wei Ling Xian*), Radix Puerariae (*Ge Gen*), and Herba Siegesbeckiae (*Xi Xian Cao*). For blood vacuity, add nine grams of Gelatinum Corii Asini (*E Jiao*). For osteoporosis, subtract *Suo Yang* and *Tu Si Zi* and add nine grams of Rhizoma Drynariae (*Gu Sui Bu*), Radix Dipsaci (*Xu Duan*), and Cortex Radicis Acanthopanacis Gracilistylis (*Wu Jia Pi*).

ACUPUNCTURE & MOXIBUSTION: *Tai Xi* (Ki 3), *Da Zhu* (Bl 11), *Xuan Zhong* (GB 39)

ANALYSIS OF FORMULA: The kidneys store the essence, the essence engenders the marrow, and the marrow nourishes the bones. If the kidneys are strong, the essence is abundant, the marrow is prosperous, and then the bones are firm. Therefore, if there is weakness of the bones, one should supplement the kidneys, boost the marrow, and strengthen the bones. *Tai Xi* is the source point of the kidney channel. Supplementing it supplements both yin and yang of the kidneys and also the former heaven essence. *Xuan Zhong* is the meeting point of the marrow. Supplementing it, therefore, boosts the marrow. *Da Zhu* is the meeting point of the bones. Supplementing it reinforces the bones. This is a key combination for bone diseases due to kidney vacuity.

ADDITIONS & SUBTRACTIONS: Please see pattern #1 above.

REMARKS

1. Though osteoporosis is a main cause of spondylosis in our (P.S.) clinic, the severity of the osteoporosis is not proportional to the degree of pain. In other words, slight osteoporosis can give rise to severe pain, and severe osteoporosis can manifest only slight pain. Therefore, pain, which is the main clinical symptom of this disease, should be the reference point for its Chinese diagnosis and treatment, not the degree of osteoporosis.

2. Spondylosis with bony osteophytes and stenosis of the cervical canal is very often due to qi and blood or liver-kidney vacuity which then allows the penetration of external evils or results in qi stagnation and blood stasis. In such cases, one should drain and supplement at the same time.

3. When spondylosis causes severe narrowing of the cervical canal, it may result in pain and stiffness of the neck with dizziness, vertigo, nausea, vomiting, tinnitus, and blurred vision. In that case, the following formula is suitable for extinguishing wind and transforming phlegm, quickening the blood and stopping pain: *Ding Xuan Tang* (Calm Vertigo Decoction): Radix Salviae Miltiorrhizae (*Dan Shen*), 30g, Radix Albus Paeoniae Lactiflorae (*Bai Shao*) and Caulis Polygoni Multiflori (*Ye Jiao Teng*), 24g each, Ramulus Uncariae Cum Uncis (*Gou Teng*), 20g, Sclerotium Poriae Cocos (*Fu Ling*), 15g, Rhizoma Gastrodiae Elatae (*Tian Ma*), Rhizoma Pinelliae Ternatae (*Ban Xia*), and Bombyx Batryticatus (*Jiang Can*), 9g each, Buthus Martensis (*Quan Xie*), 6g. One to two months of treatment are typically necessary.

4. There are many new Chinese medicinal formulas for spondylosis. Looking at their composition, one can draw the following conclusions: Herba Pyrolae (*Lu Ti Cao*) and Radix Puerariae (*Ge Gen*), 15-30g each, seem to be two empirically specific medicinals for treating cervical spondylosis. The former treats the bones, while the latter treats the sinews. Radix Albus Paeoniae Lactiflorae (*Bai Shao*) and Fructus Chaenomelis Lagenariae (*Mu Gua*), 15-30g each, are commonly used for muscle tension and spasm. Rhizoma Drynariae (*Gu Sui Bu*) and Cornu Cervi (*Lu Jiao*) seem to be the main Chinese medicinals for osteoporosis or bone impediment, while Radix Clematidis Chinensis (*Wei Ling Xian*) and Radix Et Rhizoma Notopterygii (*Qiang Huo*) are most often used for wind damp impediment. Lumbricus (*Di Long*) and Caulis Milletiae Seu Spatholobi (*Ji Xue Teng*) are commonly used for inhibited movement, and Radix Salviae

Miltiorrhizae (*Dan Shen*), Radix Ligustici Wallichii (*Chuan Xiong*), Buthus Martensis (*Quan Xie*), and Scolopendra Subspinipes (*Wu Gong*) are commonly used for pain.

5. Some Chinese acupuncturist use the single point *Yin Gu* (Ki 10) or *Cheng Shan Xia* (N-LE-43, 2 *cun* under *Cheng Shan,* Bl 57) for cervical spondylosis with reported success.

ENDNOTES

[1] Clark, C.R., "CSM: History and Physical Findings," *Spine*, #13, 1988, p. 847-849

[2] Ben Eliyahu, David, "Cervical Myelopathy and Spinal Stenosis," www.chrioweb.com/archives/16/18/04.html

[3] "Spinal Diseases & Disorders: Cervical Stenosis," http://neurosun.medsch.ucla.edu/Diagnoses/Spinal/SpinalDis_2.html

13

CHOLECYSTITIS/CHOLELITHIASIS

Cholecystitis means inflammation of the gallbladder, while cholelithiasis means stones within the gallbladder and bile duct. Modern methods of imaging have now shown that gallstones obstructing the bile duct are the most common cause of cholecystitis. Therefore, we are discussing these two related conditions under a single heading. The symptoms of acute cholecystitis are severe, acute, colicky pain localized in the upper right quadrant which often radiates around to the lower right scapula. This pain is typically accompanied by nausea and vomiting. Approximately, 75% of patients have experienced these symptoms one or more times before. Typical episodes improve in 2-3 days and resolve within a week. Risk factors include being obese, female, and over 40 years of age, the so-called three F's of gallbladder disease.

The Western medical diagnosis of this disease is based on the patient's presenting signs and symptoms, their history, and either hepatobiliary scintigraphy or ultrasound. The Western medical treatment of this condition consists mainly of fasting, rehydration with IV fluids and electrolytes, and the prescription of antacids and anticholingerics. Antibiotics may be prescribed if cholecystitis is complicated by infection. Cholecystectomy is routinely used for the management of acute cholecystitis and is considered the treatment of choice by many MDs. Noninvasive methods of lithotripsy, such as those using sonic pulses, are only sometimes used.

CHINESE DISEASE CATEGORIZATION: Cholecystitis and cholelithiasis are mainly categorized as *xie tong*, rib-side pain, *fu tong*, abdominal pain, and *huang dan*, jaundice. Accompanying nausea and vomiting are categorized as *e xin* and *ou tu* respectively.

DISEASE CAUSES: Unregulated eating and drinking, internal damage by the seven affects, aging, and worms

DISEASE MECHANISMS: Over-eating oily, slimy foods may damage the spleen and engender dampness internally. If evil dampness transform heat, dampness and heat may bind, forming damp heat which then obstructs the free flow of qi and blood and the qi mechanism. Inhibited flow of the qi and blood results in rib-side and abdominal pain, while inhibition of the qi mechanism results in nausea and vomiting. It is also possible for damp heat brewing and binding to engender or transform worms which also inhibit both the flow of qi and blood and the qi mechanism with the same results. If dampness and heat spill over from the center into the skin, jaundice may appear.

On the other hand, unfulfilled desires and anger may both damage the liver which then loses control over coursing and discharge. Qi stagnation results in rib-side and abdominal pain. If the liver assails the stomach, the stomach qi may become disharmonious, thus leading to nausea and vomiting. If liver depression endures for a long time, it may transform into depressive heat. If qi stagnation endures, it may engender blood stasis, since the qi moves the blood, and, if, the qi stops, the blood stops. If the liver invades the spleen, the spleen typically becomes vacuous and weak and loses its control over movement and transformation. Therefore, there may be food stagnation and/or damp accumulation. If internally engendered dampness due to spleen vacuity combines with depressive heat due to liver depression, this may also give rise to damp heat obstructing the center.

If either internally engendered or dietarily caused damp heat brews internally, it may produce heat toxins burning and blazing. Because enduring damp heat damages and consumes both the qi and yin, qi and yin vacuity symptoms may be seen, especially in older patients.

TREATMENT BASED ON PATTERN DISCRIMINATION:

1. LIVER-GALLBLADDER DEPRESSION & STAGNATION PATTERN

MAIN SYMPTOMS: Insidious right-sided rib-side pain or distention and pain possibly radiating to the upper back and right shoulder, chest and ductal oppression, nausea, vomiting, aversion to oily, slimy food, reduced appetite, belching, possible slight fever, a dry mouth with a bitter taste, emotional tension, easy anger, irregular bowel movements, a possibly red tongue with thin, white or thin, yellow tongue fur, and a bowstring pulse

NOTE: This pattern may manifest either during acute episodes or in the remission period after the expulsion of stones.

TREATMENT PRINCIPLES: Course the liver and rectify the qi, disinhibit the gallbladder and expel stones

RX: *Da Chai Hu Tang Jia Jian* (Major Bupleurum Decoction with Additions & Subtractions)

INGREDIENTS: Tuber Curcumae (*Yu Jin*), Radix Albus Paeoniae Lactiflorae (*Bai Shao*), and Spora Lygodii Japonici (*Hai Jin Sha*), 15g each, Radix Bupleuri (*Chai Hu*), Radix Scutellariae Baicalensis (*Huang Qin*), Endothelium Corneum Gigeriae Galli (*Ji Nei Jin*), Fructus Citri Aurantii (*Zhi Ke*), and Radix Auklandiae Lappae (*Mu Xiang*), 9g each, Radix Et Rhizoma Rhei (*Da Huang*) and uncooked Radix Glycyrrhizae (*Gan Cao*), 6g each

ANALYSIS OF FORMULA: *Chai Hu*, *Bai Shao*, and *Yu Jin* course the liver and rectify the qi, resolve depression and stop pain. *Huang Qin* and *Da Huang* clear and disinhibit dampness and heat and discharge the liver. *Hai Jin Sha* disinhibits the gallbladder and expels stones. *Ji Nei Jin* transforms hardness and disperses stones. *Mu Xiang* and *Zhi Ke* move the qi to stop pain, and *Gan Cao* harmonizes the other medicinals in the formula. In addition, when combined with *Bai Shao*, it relaxes urgency (*i.e.*, cramping) and stops pain.

ADDITIONS & SUBTRACTIONS: If there is devitalized eating and drinking, add nine grams each of Fructus Germinatus Hordei Vulgaris (*Mai Ya*), Fructus Crataegi (*Shan Zha*), and Massa Medica Fermentata (*Shen Qu*). If spleen vacuity is marked, add nine grams each of Radix Codonopsitis Pilosulae (*Dang Shen*), Rhizoma Atractylodis Macrocephalae (*Bai Zhu*), and Sclerotium Poriae Cocos (*Fu Ling*) and change uncooked *Gan Cao* to mix-fried *Gan Cao*. For simultaneous phlegm dampness, add nine grams each of Rhizoma Pinelliae Ternatae (*Ban Xia*), Sclerotium Poriae Cocos (*Fu Ling*), and Pericarpium Citri Reticulatae (*Chen Pi*). If there is no constipation, delete *Da Huang*. If there is more marked constipation, add six grams of Mirabilitum (*Mang Xiao*). If there is more marked heat, add 30 grams of Flos Lonicerae Japonicae (*Jin Yin Hua*) and 15 grams of Fructus Forsythiae Suspensae (*Lian Qiao*). If there is concomitant blood stasis, add 15 grams of Radix Salviae Miltiorrhizae (*Dan Shen*) and nine grams each of Radix Rubrus Paeoniae Lactiflorae (*Chi Shao*) and Cortex Radicis Moutan (*Dan Pi*). For nausea and vomiting, add nine grams each of Caulis Bambusae In Taeniis (*Zhu Ru*) and Rhizoma Pinelliae Ternatae (*Ban Xia*).

ACUPUNCTURE & MOXIBUSTION: *Ri Yue* (GB 24) (right side), *Yang Ling Quan* (GB 34), *Zhi Gou* (TB 6), *Dan Shu* (Bl 19), *Dan Nang Xue* (M-LE-23)

ANALYSIS OF FORMULA: *Ri Yue* is the alarm point of the gallbladder, and *Yang Ling Quan* is the uniting point of the gallbladder channel. *Dan Shu* is the back transport point of the gallbladder, and *Zhi Gou* is the fire point on the triple burner channel. *Dan Nang Xue* is an empirical point for the treatment of cholecystitis and cholelithiasis. When all these points are used together, they course the liver and resolve the depression, disinhibit the gallbladder, expel stones, and stop pain. Use draining method on all points. Do not needle *Dan Nang Xue* if it is not painful. For cholelithiasis, one can use electroacupuncture on all points except *Zhi Gou*.

ADDITIONS & SUBTRACTIONS: For severe pain, add *He Gu* (LI 4) and *Qi Men* (Liv 14). For jaundice, add *Zhi Yang* (GV 9). For abdominal distention and pain, add *Zu San Li* (St 36). For nausea and vomiting, add *Nei Guan* (Per 6). For fever and chills, add *Qu Chi* (LI 11) and *He Gu* (LI 4).

2. DAMP HEAT INTERNALLY BREWING PATTERN

MAIN SYMPTOMS: Severe right-sided rib-side distention and pain, ductal and abdominal distention and fullness, palpable pain in the gallbladder area and pain when pressed, palpation pain at *Tian Zong* (SI 11) and *Dan Nang Xue* (M-LE-23), torpid intake, nausea, vomiting, dry mouth with a bitter taste, thirst with no desire to drink, fear of cold and emission of heat or cold and heat mixed together, jaundice, dry stools, yellow urine, slimy, yellow tongue fur, however, if heat is heavy, there may be dry, yellow fur, and a bowstring, slippery, rapid pulse

NOTE: This pattern mostly manifests in relatively severe acute attacks or when cholecystitis is complicated by infection.

TREATMENT PRINCIPLES: Clear heat and disinhibit dampness, disinhibit the gallbladder and expel stones, free the flow on the interior and attack and precipitate

RX: If heat is greater than dampness, *Yin Chen Hao Tang* (Artemisia Capillaris Decoction) & *Long Dan Xie Gan Tang*

(Gentiana Drain the Liver Decoction) with additions and subtractions

INGREDIENTS: Herba Artemisiae Capillaris (*Yin Chen Hao*) and Flos Lonicerae Japonicae (*Jin Yin Hua*), 30g each, Radix Scutellariae Baicalensis (*Huang Qin*), Radix Bupleuri (*Chai Hu*), Tuber Curcumae (*Yu Jin*), Spora Lygodii Japonici (*Hai Jin Sha*), and Fructus Forsythiae Suspensae (*Lian Qiao*), 15g each, Radix Gentianae Scabrae (*Long Dan Cao*) and Fructus Gardeniae Jasminoidis (*Zhi Zi*), 12g each, Radix Et Rhizoma Rhei (*Da Huang*), Fructus Immaturus Citri Aurantii (*Zhi Shi*), Radix Auklandiae Lappae (*Mu Xiang*), Endothelium Corneum Gigeriae Galli (*Ji Nei Jin*), and Radix Glycyrrhizae (*Gan Cao*), 9g each

ANALYSIS OF FORMULA: *Yin Chen Hao, Huang Qin, Long Dan Cao, Zhi Zi,* and *Da Huang* all clear heat, eliminate dampness, and disinhibit the gallbladder. *Jin Yin Hua, Lian Qiao, Huang Qin,* and *Zhi Zi* clear heat and resolve toxins. *Da Huang* attacks and precipitates in order to discharge damp heat and heat toxins through the stool. *Yu Jin* and *Chai Hu* course the liver and resolve the depression. With *Mu Xiang* and *Zhi Shi,* they also move the qi and stop pain. *Hai Jin Sha* and *Ji Nei Jin,* with the help of *Yu Jin, Chai Hu, Mu Xiang* and *Zhi Shi,* disinhibit the gallbladder and expel stones.

ADDITIONS & SUBTRACTIONS: If there is high fever, add 30 grams each of uncooked Gypsum Fibrosum (*Shi Gao*) and Radix Isatidis Seu Baphicacanthi (*Ban Lan Gen*). For nausea and vomiting, add nine grams each of Caulis Bambusae In Taeniis (*Zhu Ru*) and Rhizoma Pinelliae Ternatae (*Ban Xia*). For devitalized eating and drinking, add nine grams each of Fructus Germinatus Hordei Vulgaris (*Mai Ya*), Fructus Crataegi (*Shan Zha*), and Massa Medica Fermentata (*Shen Qu*). If there is concomitant blood stasis, add 15 grams each of Radix Salviae Miltiorrhizae (*Dan Shen*) and uncooked Radix Rehmanniae (*Sheng Di*) and nine grams of Extremitas Radicis Angelicae Sinensis (*Dang Gui Wei*). If dampness is greater than heat, delete *Long Dan Cao, Jin Yin Hua,* and *Lian Qiao* and add *San Ren Tang* (Three Seeds Decoction): Semen Coicis Lachryma-jobi (*Yi Yi Ren*) and Talcum (*Hua Shi*), 15g each, Semen Pruni Armeniacae (*Xing Ren*), 12g, Rhizoma Pinelliae Ternatae (*Ban Xia*), 9g, Fructus Caradmomi (*Bai Dou Kou*), Cortex Magnoliae Officinalis (*Hou Po*), Folium Bambusae (*Zhu Ye*), and Medulla Tetrapanacis Papyriferi (*Tong Cao*), 6g each. If there is no constipation, delete *Da Huang.* If there is jaundice, add 25 grams of Herba Lysimachiae Seu Desmodii (*Jin Qian Cao*). If stones obstruct the bile duct, add 30 grams each of Radix Clematidis Chinensis (*Wei Ling Xian*) and Herba Lysimachiae Seu Desmodii (*Jin Qian Cao*).

ACUPUNCTURE & MOXIBUSTION: Same as above. However, for this pattern acupuncture should always be used in conjunction with Chinese medicinals.

ADDITIONS & SUBTRACTIONS: Same as above.

3. HEAT TOXINS BURNING & BLAZING PATTERN

MAIN SYMPTOMS: Severe right-sided upper abdominal pain, glomus lumps below the rib-side, abdominal area hardness and fullness refusing pressure, severe jaundice, scanty, reddish urine, constipation, spirit clouding, deranged speech, a crimson tongue with dry, yellow or yellowish black fur, and a bowstring, rapid or fine, rapid pulse. If extremely severe, there may be reversal chilling of the four extremities, great sweating dribbling and dripping, listlessness of the essence spirit, and a faint pulse on the verge of expiry or a deep, fine, forceless pulse.

NOTE: This pattern is mostly seen in acute purulent, obstructive bile duct inflammation.

TREATMENT PRINCIPLES: Clear the constructive, cool the blood, and resolve toxins, free the flow and precipitate and expel stones, support the righteous and dispel evils, secure yang and stem desertion

RX: *Xi Jiao Di Huang Tang Jia Jian* (Rhinoceros Horn & Rehmannia Decoction with Additions & Subtractions)

INGREDIENTS: Cornu Bubali (*Shui Niu Jiao*), 30-60g, uncooked Radix Rehmanniae (*Sheng Di*) and Rhizoma Smilacis Glabrae (*Tu Fu Ling*), 30g each, Herba Artemisiae Capillaris (*Yin Chen Hao*) and Radix Scrophulariae Ningpoensis (*Xuan Shen*), 20g each, Flos Chrysanthemi Indici (*Ye Ju Hua*), 15g, Cortex Radicis Moutan (*Dan Pi*), Rhizoma Coptidis Chinensis (*Huang Lian*), uncooked Radix Et Rhizoma Rhei (*Da Huang*), Fructus Gardeniae Jasminoidis (*Zhi Zi*), uncooked Radix Glycyrrhizae (*Gan Cao*), and Rhizoma Cimicifugae (*Sheng Ma*), 9g each

ANALYSIS OF FORMULA: *Shui Niu Jiao, Sheng Di, Xuan Shen,* and *Dan Pi* clear the constructive and cool the blood. *Tu Fu Ling, Xuan Shen, Ye Ju Hua, Huang Lian, Zhi Zi, Sheng Ma,* and *Da Huang* clear heat and resolve toxins, while *Tu Fu Ling, Yin Chen Hao, Huang Lian, Zhi Zi,* and *Da Huang* clear heat and disinhibit dampness.

ADDITIONS & SUBTRACTIONS: If there is clouded spirit and deranged speech, add *An Gong Niu Huang Wan* (Quiet the Palace Bezoar Pills, a Chinese ready-made medicine), one pill two times per day. If urination is frequent, scanty, and reddish in color, add 30 grams each of Rhizoma Imperatae Cylindricae (*Bai Mao Gen*) and Herba Verbenae (*Ma Bian Cao*).

If there is yang desertion, replace *Xi Jiao Di Huang Tang Jia Jian* with *Shen Fu Tang* (Ginseng & Aconite Decoction) and *Sheng Mai San* (Engender the Pulse Powder): Radix Panacis

Ginseng (*Ren Shen*), 15g, Radix Lateralis Praeparatus Aconiti Carmichaeli (*Fu Zi*) and Tuber Ophiopogonis Japonici (*Mai Dong*), 12g each, and Fructus Schisandrae Chinensis (*Wu Wei Zi*), 9g.

ACUPUNCTURE & MOXIBUSTION: For this acute emergency condition, acupuncture can help for pain but should be combined with Chinese medicinals and/or Western medicine. For the selection of points, please see pattern #1 above with its additions and subtractions.

4. QI & BLOOD DUAL VACUITY, PHLEGM & TURBIDITY MUTUALLY BINDING PATTERN

MAIN SYMPTOMS: Yellowing of the eyes and body which is sometimes worse and sometimes better, dizziness and vertigo, a shiny, greenish blue facial complexion, fatigue, lassitude of the spirit, lack of strength, disinclination to speak, scanty qi, rib-side distention, fullness, oppression, and discomfort or insidious pain which comes and goes, accumulation lumps below the rib-side if severe, reduced food intake, a pale but dark tongue with possible static macules or spots, engorged, distended, tortuous sublingual veins, and a bowstring, fine or bowstring, choppy pulse

NOTE: Although the name of this pattern does not mention blood stasis, static blood is a part of its disease mechanisms.

TREATMENT PRINCIPLES: Fortify the spleen and dispel dampness, rectify the qi and harmonize the blood

RX: *Si Jun Zi Tang* (Four Gentlemen Decoction) & *Ge Xia Zhu Yu Tang* (Below the Diaphragm Dispel Stasis Decoction) with additions and subtractions:

INGREDIENTS: Radix Scutellariae Barbatae (*Ban Zhi Lian*), Radix Codonopsitis Pilosulae (*Dang Shen*), and Sclerotium Poriae Cocos (*Fu Ling*), 15g each, Rhizoma Atractylodis Macrocephalae (*Bai Zhu*), Semen Pruni Persicae (*Tao Ren*), Radix Angelicae Sinensis (*Dang Gui*), Radix Bupleuri (*Chai Hu*), Herba Artemisiae Capillaris (*Yin Chen Hao*), Rhizoma Cyperi Rotundi (*Xiang Fu*), and Rhizoma Corydalis Yanhusuo (*Yan Hu Suo*), 9g each, Flos Carthami Tinctorii (*Hong Hua*) and Cortex Radicis Moutan (*Dan Pi*), 6g each, Radix Glycyrrhizae (*Gan Cao*), 3g

ANALYSIS OF FORMULA: *Dang Shen*, *Fu Ling*, and *Bai Zhu* supplement the spleen, the latter heaven root of qi and blood engenderment and transformation. *Yin Chen Hao* clears heat and eliminates dampness, especially in the liver-gallbladder, while *Ban Zhi Lian* clears heat and resolves toxins at the same time as it quickens the blood. *Chai Hu* and *Xiang Fu* move the qi, while *Tao Ren*, *Hong Hua*, and *Dan Pi* quicken the blood. *Yan Hu Suo* quickens the blood and stops pain. *Gan Cao* harmonizes all the other medicinals in the formula.

ADDITIONS & SUBTRACTIONS: If there are loose stools or diarrhea, delete *Dan Pi* and add nine grams each of Rhizoma Atractylodis (*Cang Zhu*) and Radix Astragali Membranacei (*Huang Qi*). If there are accumulation lumps below the rib-side and pain, add 15 grams each of Carapax Amydae Sinensis (*Bei Jia*) and Radix Salviae Miltiorrhizae (*Dan Shen*).

ACUPUNCTURE & MOXIBUSTION: *Ri Yue* (GB 24) (right side), *Dan Shu* (Bl 19), *Tai Chong* (Liv 3), *Zu San Li* (St 36)

ANALYSIS OF FORMULA: Supplementing *Zu San Li* fortifies the spleen and disinhibits dampness. Supplementing *Tai Chong* nourishes liver blood. Together, these two points form a special combination for the treatment of jaundice and cholecystitis. *Ri Yue* is the alarm point of the gallbladder, while *Dan Shu* is its back transport point, both of which have a direct connection with the gallbladder not mediated by the channels and network vessels. Therefore, they are very effective for disinhibiting the gallbladder, expelling stones, and stopping pain in the gallbladder.

ADDITIONS & SUBTRACTIONS: If a stone in the bile duct is suspected, add *Dan Nang Xue* (M-LE-23) and/or *Yang Ling Quan* (GB 34). If there are concretion lumps below the rib-side, add *Qi Men* (Liv 14) and *Yang Ling Quan* (GB 34). For severe jaundice, add *Zhi Yang* (GV 9). For abdominal distention and pain, add *Zhong Wan* (CV 12). For nausea and vomiting, add *Nei Guan* (Per 6).

5. QI & YIN INSUFFICIENCY PATTERN

MAIN SYMPTOMS: Insidious rib-side pain accompanied by marked fatigue, lack of strength, torpid intake, and abdominal distention after meals in patients typically over 40 years of age, dry mouth with a bitter taste, constipation, a fat, swollen tongue with teeth-marks on its edges, a red tip, cracks in its center, and scanty or peeled fur, and a fine, bowstring, rapid pulse

NOTE: Although the name of this pattern does not say so, there is lingering damp heat evils which have damaged and consumed the qi and yin.

TREATMENT PRINCIPLES: Supplement yin and boost the qi, clear heat and eliminate dampness, move the qi

RX: *Yi Qi Ruan Gan Tang* (Boost the Qi & Soften the Liver Decoction)

INGREDIENTS: Radix Astragali Membranacei (*Huang Qi*), 30g, uncooked Radix Rehmanniae (*Sheng Di*), Fructus Lycii Chinensis (*Gou Qi Zi*), Radix Albus Paeoniae Lactiflorae (*Bai Shao*), Fructus Corni Officinalis (*Shan Zhu Yu*), Herba Artemisiae Capillaris (*Yin Chen Hao*), Fructus Crateagi

(*Shan Zha*), and Rhizoma Polygoni Cuspidati (*Hu Zhang*), 12g each, processed Radix Et Rhizoma Rhei (*Da Huang*), 9g, Pericarpium Citri Reticulatae (*Chen Pi*), Pericarpium Citri Reticulatae Viride (*Qing Pi*), and mix-fried Radix Glycyrrhizae (*Gan Cao*), 6g each

ANALYSIS OF FORMULA: *Huang Qi* and mix-fried *Gan Cao* supplement the center and boost the qi. *Sheng Di, Gou Qi, Bai Shao,* and *Shan Zhu Yu* enrich yin and nourish liver blood. *Qing Pi* and *Chen Pi* rectify the qi of the spleen and liver. *Yin Chen Hao, Hu Zhang,* and *Da Huang* clear heat and disinhibit dampness. *Shan Zha* disperses food and especially treats stagnation due to meaty, oily, fatty foods which tend to generate damp heat in the liver-gallbladder.

ADDITIONS & SUBTRACTIONS: If rib-side pain is severe, add 12 grams each of Tuber Curcumae (*Yu Jin*) and Rhizoma Corydalis Yanhusuo (*Yan Hu Suo*). If there are simultaneous heat signs, add nine grams each of Fructus Gardeniae Jasminoidis (*Zhi Zi*) and Radix Scutellariae Baicalensis (*Huang Qin*). If there are concomitant damp evils, add 20 grams of Semen Coicis Lachryma-jobi (*Yi Yi Ren*) and 12 grams of Sclerotium Poriae Cocos (*Fu Ling*). If abdominal distention is marked, add nine grams each of Fructus Citri Sacrodactylis (*Fo Shou*) and Pericarpium Arecae Catechu (*Da Fu Pi*). If the stools are dry and bound, replace processed *Da Huang* with uncooked *Da Huang*. If there are loose stools, subtract *Da Huang* and add nine grams of Rhizoma Atractylodis Macrocephalae (*Bai Zhu*).

If there is liver blood-kidney yin vacuity with qi stagnation but without qi vacuity, replace *Yi Qi Ruan Gan Tang* with *Yi Guan Jian Jia Wei* (One Link Decoction with Added Flavors): Fructus Meliae Toosendan (*Chuan Lian Zi*), 15g, Radix Glehniae Littoralis (*Sha Shen*), Tuber Ophiopogonis Japonici (*Mai Men Dong*), uncooked Radix Rehmanniae (*Sheng Di*), Fructus Lycii Chinensis (*Gou Qi*), Herba Artemisiae Capillaris (*Yin Chen Hao*), and Herba Lysimachiae Seu Desmodii (*Jin Qian Cao*), 12g each, and Radix Angelicae Sinensis (*Dang Gui*), 9g.

ACUPUNCTURE & MOXIBUSTION: *Ge Shu* (Bl 17), *Gan Shu* (Bl 18), *Pi Shu* (Bl 20), *Ri Yue* (GB 24), *Yang Ling Quan* (GB 34)

ANALYSIS OF FORMULA: Needling *Ge Shu, Gan Shu,* and *Pi Shu* together fortifies the spleen and supplements the qi, nourishes the blood, enriches yin, and emolliates the liver. Draining *Ri Yue* and *Yang Ling Quan* clears heat and eliminates dampness, moves the qi and disinhibits the gallbladder.

ADDITIONS & SUBTRACTIONS: For a severe yin vacuity, add *Fu Liu* (Ki 7). For a severe qi vacuity, add *Zu San Li* (St 36). If stones are suspected in the bile duct, add *Dan Nang Xue* (M-LE-23). For yellow eyes or skin, add *Zhi Yang* (GV 9) and *Zu San Li* (St 36). For abdominal distention and pain, add *Zhong Wan* (CV 12). For nausea and vomiting, add *Nei Guan* (Per 6).

6. ROUNDWORM REVERSAL PATTERN

MAIN SYMPTOMS: Intermittent attack of stomach ductal and rib-side pain, chest oppression, irritability, vexatious heat, vomiting after eating and/or vomiting of roundworms, cold hands and feet, a red tongue with peeled, slimy, white fur, and a deep, slippery, bowstring or deep, fine, and bowstring pulse

TREATMENT PRINCIPLES: Warm the viscera and clear heat, drain evils and quiet roundworms

RX: *Wu Mei Wan Jia Wei* (Mume Pills with Added Flavors)

INGREDIENTS: Fructus Pruni Mume (*Wu Mei*), 15g, Rhizoma Coptidis Chinensis (*Huang Lian*), Cortex Phellodendri (*Huang Bai*), dry Rhizoma Zingiberis (*Gan Jiang*), Radix Angelicae Sinensis (*Dang Gui*), Cortex Radicis Meliae Azardachis (*Ku Lian Gen Pi*), Semen Arecae Catechu (*Bing Lang*), and Radix Panacis Ginseng (*Ren Shen*), 9g each, Ramulus Cinnamomi Cassiae (*Gui Zhi*), Radix Lateralis Praeparatus Aconiti Carmichaeli (*Fu Zi*), and Fructus Quisqualis Indicae (*Shi Jun Pi*), 6g each, Herba Asari Cum Radice (*Xi Xin*) and Fructus Zanthoxyli Bungeani (*Chuan Jiao*), 3g each

ANALYSIS OF FORMULA: *Wu Mei* quiets roundworms, while *Ku Lian Gen Pi, Bing Lang, Shi Jun Pi,* and *Chuan Jiao* kill worms and stop pain. *Huang Lian* and *Huang Bai* clear heat and dry dampness, while *Gan Jiang, Gui Zhi, Fu Zi, Xi Xin,* and *Chuan Jiao* warm the viscera and stop pain. *Dang Gui* nourishes the blood, and *Ren Shen* supplements the qi.

ADDITIONS & SUBTRACTIONS: If there are no cold symptoms, delete *Fu Zi* and *Gui Zhi*. If the righteous qi is not yet vacuous, delete *Ren Shen* and *Dang Gui*. For severe abdominal pain, add 15 grams each of Fructus Meliae Toosendan (*Chuan Lian Zi*) and Rhizoma Corydalis Yanhusuo (*Yan Hu Suo*) and nine grams each of Tuber Curcumae (*Yu Jin*) and Radix Auklandiae Lappae (*Mu Xiang*). For constipation, add nine grams of Fructus Immaturus Citri Aurantii (*Zhi Shi*).

ACUPUNCTURE & MOXIBUSTION: *Ying Xiang* (LI 20) through to *Di Cang* (St 4), *Shang Wan* (CV 13), *Dan Shu* (Bl 19), *Zhong Wan* (CV 12), *Yang Ling Quan* (GB 34)

ANALYSIS OF FORMULA: *Ying Xiang* needled through to *Di Cang* is a special combination to kill roundworms. *Shang Wan* plus *Dan Shu* and *Zhong Wan* plus *Yang Ling Quan* are also empirical combinations for treating roundworms in the bile duct. They harmonize the center and disinhibit the gallbladder, relax urgency and stop pain. All these points should be needled with draining method, and acupuncture should be combined with Chinese medicinals.

ADDITIONS & SUBTRACTIONS: For nausea, add *Nei Guan* (Per 6). For severe pain, use electroacupuncture on all points except *Ying Xiang*. For fatigue and loose stools, add *Zu San Li* (St 36) and *Pi Shu* (Bl 20). For children, prick *Si Feng* (M-UE-9).

REMARKS

1. During acute attacks, patients should be treated with both acupuncture and internally administered Chinese medicinals. Typically such medicinals are prescribed in relatively high doses in order to achieve as quick pain relief as possible. In between attacks, most patients suffer from a liver-spleen disharmony. During periods of remission, patients should be encouraged to take low doses of Chinese medicinals on a daily basis in either desiccated powdered extract or pill form. An alternative is to take higher doses in decoction for 21 days every three months. Since almost all cholecystitis is due to gallstones, preventive formulas taken during periods of remission should usually include stone-expelling medicinals, such as Endothelium Corneum Gigeriae Galli (*Ji Nei Jin*). When combined with correct diet, this condition is very amenable to Chinese medical treatment.

For liver-spleen disharmony during remissions, use *Xiao Yao San Jia Jian* (Moutan & Gardenia Rambling Powder with Additions & Subtractions): Radix Angelicae Sinensis (*Dang Gui*), Radix Albus Paeoniae Lactiflorae (*Bai Shao*), Tuber Curcumae (*Yu Jin*), Rhizoma Cyperi Rotundi (*Xiang Fu*), 9g each, Rhizoma Atractylodis Macrocephalae (*Bai Zhu*), Sclerotium Poriae Cocos (*Fu Ling*), Radix Bupleuri (*Chai Hu*), Radix Auklandiae Lappae (*Mu Xiang*), mix-fried Radix Glycyrrhizae (*Gan Cao*), 6g each. If liver-spleen disharmony is complicated by damp or depressive heat, add 15 grams of Herba Artemisiae Capillaris (*Yin Chen Hao*) and nine grams each of Cortex Radicis Moutan (*Dan Pi*) and Fructus Gardeniae Jasminoidis (*Zhi Zi*). If qi stagnation has resulted in blood stasis with piercing, fixed pain in the rib-side, add nine grams of Pollen Typhae (*Pu Huang*), Feces Trogopterori Seu Pteromi (*Wu Ling Zhi*), Rhizoma Curcumae Longae (*Jiang Huang*) and Rhizoma Corydalis Yanhusuo (*Yan Hu Suo*). If stones are suspected or present, add nine grams of Endothelium Corneum Gigeriae Galli (*Ji Nei Jin*), Herba Lysimachiae Seu Desmodii (*Jin Qian Cao*), and Radix Clematidis Chinensis (*Wei Ling Xian*).

In the case of chronic cholecystitis, if there is predominantly spleen vacuity in a liver-spleen disharmony with depressive heat and, therefore, a yin fire scenario, consider using *Sheng Yang Yi Wei Tang* (Upbear Yang & Boost the Stomach Decoction): Radix Codonopsitis Pilosulae (*Dang Shen*), Radix Astragali Membranacei (*Huang Qi*), Rhizoma Atractylodis Macrocephalae (*Bai Zhu*), Sclerotium Poriae Cocos (*Fu Ling*), Rhizoma Alismatis (*Ze Xie*), and Radix Albus Paeoniae Lactiflorae (*Bai Shao*), 9g each, Rhizoma Coptidis Chinensis (*Huang Lian*), 2g, Rhizoma Pinelliae Ternatae (*Ban Xia*), Radix Et Rhizoma Notopterygii (*Qiang Huo*), and Radix Angelicae Pubescentis (*Du Huo*), 6g each, Pericarpium Citri Reticulatae (*Chen Pi*), Radix Ledebouriellae Divaricatae (*Fang Feng*), and Radix Bupleuri (*Chai Hu*), 5g each, and mix-fried Radix Glycyrrhizae (*Gan Cao*), 3g.

2. Women are more prone to this condition than men because women are more prone to spleen vacuity and, therefore, liver depression than men. This condition typically occurs around 40 years of age because spleen vacuity becomes pronounced, especially in women, around that age. In addition, people who are obese usually have a habitual spleen vacuity with dampness and phlegm obstructing the flow of qi and blood. This then explains the three F's – fat, female, and forty. Therefore, a liver-spleen disharmony is typically at the root of this condition complicated by damp heat and/or blood stasis.

3. In most Western patients, there will be a complex combination of vacuity and repletion patterns. The presence of stones should be assumed as should at least some element of smoldering damp heat. Typically, there will be pronounced qi stagnation. If the condition has endured, there may also be blood stasis.

4. Diet is extremely important in the treatment of cholecystitis and cholelithiasis. This mainly means a clear, bland diet, taking care to stay away from sugars and sweets as well as oily, fatty foods. In addition, patients need to get adequate exercise. When acute episodes are precipitated by emotional stress, daily exercise and deep relaxation need to go hand in hand as well as trying to change one's lifestyle in order to reduce stress.

5. In case of acute cholelithiasis, there is a famous modern protocol called "general offensive" which is commonly used in Chinese medical hospitals in China. This protocol is a combination of a Chinese medicinal formula, acupuncture, and Western drug therapy. Because this type of protocol aims to expel stones, it is important to know if the stone is small enough to pass through the bile duct so as to avoid obstruction and a worsening of the patient's condition. Usually, large stones in the gallbladder stay "cold and calm." Therefore, it is unnecessary to try to expel these. In this case, the preventive formulas above are sufficient to "keep the dragon in its den."

6. Chinese medicinals which regulate the gallbladder and treat cholecystitis are: Radix Clematidis Chinensis (*Wei Ling Xian*), Radix Et Rhizoma Rhei (*Da Huang*), Herba

Lysimachiae Seu Desmodii (*Jin Qian Cao*), Herba Artemisiae Capillaris (*Yin Chen Hao*), Semen Vaccariae Segetalis (*Wang Bu Liu Xing*), Radix Et Rhizoma Polygoni Cuspidati (*Hu Zhang*), Tuber Curcumae (*Yu Jin*), and Rhizoma Curcumae Longae (*Jiang Huang*).

Chinese medicinals which expel stones from the gallbladder are: Herba Lysimachiae Seu Desmodii (*Jin Qian Cao*), Rhizoma Curcumae Longae (*Jiang Huang*), Tuber Curcumae (*Yu Jin*), Endothelium Corneum Gigeriae Galli (*Ji Nei Jin*), Semen Vaccariae Segetalis (*Wang Bu Liu Xing*), Radix Clematidis Chinensis (*Wei Ling Xian*), and Radix Et Rhizoma Rhei (*Da Huang*).

Chinese medicinals which treat roundworms in the bile duct are: Fructus Pruni Mume (*Wu Mei*), Cortex Radicis Meliae Azardachis (*Ku Lian Gen Pi*), Semen Arecae Catechu (*Bing Lang*), Caulis Sargentodoxae (*Hong Teng*), Semen Crotonis Tiglii (*Ba Dou*).

7. Pressure pain at *Dan Nang Xue* (M-LE-23) helps confirm the cholecystitis and cholelithiasis. This point should only be used in treatment when it is painful. The location of *Dan Nang Xue* is not fixed. It can be anywhere 0.5-3 *cun* below *Yang Ling Quan* (GB 34). Therefore, palpatory examination should be careful.

Other effective points for cholecystitis and cholelithiasis include: *Yang Ling Quan* (GB 34), *Zhi Gou* (TB 6), *Nei Guan* (Per 6), *Dan Shu* (Bl 19), *Qiu Xu* (GB 40), and *Ri Yue* (GB 24). Empirically effective combinations include: *Yang Ling Quan* (GB 34) + *Zhi Gou* (TB 6); *Yang Ling Quan* (GB 34) + *Dan Nang Xue* (M-LE-23); *Yang Ling Quan* (GB 34) + *Nei Guan* (Per 6); *Nei Guan* (Per 6) + *Qiu Xu* (GB 40); *Qiu Xu* (GB 40) + *Zhao Hai* (Ki 6); *Ri Yue* (GB 24) + *Qi Men* (Liv 14); *Yang Ling Quan* (GB 34) + *Tai Chong* (Liv 3); *Yang Ling Quan* (GB 34) + *Zu San Li* (St 36); and *Zu San Li* (St 36) + *Tai Chong* (Liv 3).

8. Many Chinese acupuncturists use electroacupuncture when treating acute cholelithiasis in order to stop the pain and expel the stones.

14

CHRONIC ACTIVE HEPATITIS

Chronic active hepatitis is also referred to as hepatitis C. It is due to contraction of the hepatitis virus transmitted either via blood, sex, or perinatally. This condition accounts for 60-70% of chronic hepatitis and 30% of liver cirrhosis in the United States. It also accounts for 8,000-10,000 deaths per year in the U.S. Approximately four million Americans or 1.8% of the population are infected with this virus. Although one may remain asymptomatic for years after contracting this virus, 20% of patients develop cirrhosis within 10-20 years. The clinical symptoms of this condition are fatigue, mild upper right quadrant discomfort or tenderness, nausea, poor appetite, diarrhea, muscle-joint pain, and possible vascular spiders or palmar erythema. The symptoms of cirrhosis of the liver are enlarged liver and/or spleen, jaundice, muscle wasting, ascites, and swollen ankles. Extrahepatic complications include skin rashes, kidney disease, glomerulonephritis, and peripheral neuropathy. Many patients with this disease also test positive for rheumatoid factor or suffer from Sjögren's syndrome, fibromylagia syndrome, or lichen planus.

The Western medical diagnosis of this disease is based on the detection of anti-HCV antibodies by enzyme immunoassay (EIA). Liver biopsy is then used to stage the disease. There are currently two main treatment regimes for this condition. The first is called monotherapy and consists of administration of alpha-interferon. Alpha-interferon, however, has multiple neuropsychiatric side effects. The second is called combination therpay and consists of administration of interferon and ribavirin. Liver transplants are done in severe cases.

CHINESE DISEASE CATEGORIZATION: Chronic active hepatitis is mainly categorized as *pi juan*, fatigue, *xie tong*, rib-side pain, *e xin*, nausea, *na dai*, torpid intake, *xie xie*, diarrhea, and *bi zheng*, impediment condition. Cirrhosis of the liver is categorized as *zheng jia*, concretions and conglomerations, *huang dan*, jaundice, *xiao xue*, dispersion and whittling, *i.e.*, emaciation, and *zu zhong*, foot swelling.

DISEASE CAUSES: External contraction of perverse qi, unregulated eating and drinking, internal damage by the seven affects, and aging

DISEASE MECHANISMS: *Li qi* or perverse qi refers to contagious evil qi which can cause serious, potentially life-threatening disease. In this case, the perverse qi associated with chronic active hepatitis should be described as a hidden or deep-lying warm evil that is damp and hot in nature and lodges in the blood division. This deep-lying warm evil damages the blood and consumes the qi at the same time as it obstructs the free flow of qi and blood. It is activated or aggravated by any other damp heat in the body. The two main causes of enduring, internally engendered damp heat are faulty diet and emotional stress. Over-eating of spicy, hot foods, sweet, fatty, thick-flavored foods, and alcohol may damage the spleen, thus engendering dampness, at the same time as they brew and transform heat. However, damp heat may also be due to emotional stress causing liver depression. In this case, enduring depression transforms heat as well as assails the spleen. Spleen vacuity then engenders dampness which binds with depressive heat to become damp heat. When faulty diet is combined with emotional stress, the recipe for damp heat becomes all the more assured. In addition, the spleen becomes vacuous and weak with age and, therefore, so does the righteous qi. If the righteous qi becomes too weak to keep hidden evils under control, then these hidden evils become active and further damage the righteous.

Damp heat evils not only obstruct the free flow of qi and blood, but heat may consume yin, blood, and fluids, thus resulting in yin and/or blood vacuity. Damp heat may engender phlegm and result in stasis. If damp heat transforms into fire and brews toxins, it may harass the constructive and the blood. And if damp heat evils so damage the spleen qi, spleen disease may reach the kidneys, thus resulting in a spleen qi-kidney yang vacuity. However, in all these cases, it is damp heat evils that sit at the center of these disease mechanisms. Because there is a typically a combination of damp heat, liver depression, and spleen vacuity at least in cases of chronic active hepatitis, the disease mechanisms of this condition may also be described as yin fire. Because damp evils typically predominate over heat, symptoms of heat may be minimal and the condition may simmer for years. Thus there is frequently a long course of few symptoms until accumulated damage to the righteous qi and viscera and bowels becomes severe.

Treatment based on pattern discrimination:

1. Liver depression qi stagnation pattern

Main symptoms: Stomach ductal and/or rib-side distention and pain, chest oppression, a tendency to sigh, irritability, burping and belching, premenstrual syndrome and/or menstrual irregularities in females, a normal or dark tongue with thin, white fur, and a bowstring pulse

Note: This pattern rarely presents in Westerners in this simple, discrete form. However, liver depression complicates essentially all chronic hepatitis.

Treatment principles: Course the liver and resolve depression, move the qi and stop pain

Rx: *Chai Hu Shu Gan San* (Bupleurum Course the Liver Powder)

Ingredients: Radix Bupleuri (*Chai Hu*), 12g, Radix Albus Paeoniae Lactiflorae (*Bai Shao*), and Rhizoma Cyperi Rotundi (*Xiang Fu*), 9g each, Fructus Citri Aurantii (*Zhi Ke*) and Radix Ligustici Wallichii (*Chuan Xiong*), 6g each, and Radix Glycyrrhizae (*Gan Cao*), 3g

Analysis of formula: *Chai Hu*, *Xiang Fu*, and *Zhi Ke* course the liver and resolve depression, move the qi and stop pain. *Bai Shao* nourishes the blood to harmonize the liver and prevent further qi depression. *Chuan Xiong* quickens the blood to prevent liver stasis due to qi stagnation. It also stops pain.

Additions & subtractions: If there is abdominal pain, add 15 grams of Rhizoma Corydalis Yanhusuo (*Yan Hu Suo*) and 12 grams of Fructus Meliae Toosendan (*Chuan Lian Zi*). If there is abdominal distention, add nine grams each of Cortex Magnoliae Officinalis (*Hou Po*) and Radix Auklandiae Lappae (*Mu Xiang*). If liver depression transforms heat, add nine grams of Radix Scutellariae Baicalensis (*Huang Qin*) and three grams of Rhizoma Coptidis Chinensis (*Huang Lian*). If depressive heat has entered the blood division, add nine grams each of Fructus Gardeniae Jasminoidis (*Zhi Zi*) and Cortex Radicis Moutan (*Dan Pi*). If liver qi assails the stomach, delete the uncooked *Gan Cao* and add nine grams of Folium Perillae Frutescentis (*Zi Su Ye*) and six grams each of Pericarpium Citri Reticulatae (*Chen Pi*) and mix-fried Radix Glycyrrhizae (*Gan Cao*). If there is lack of appetite due to food stagnation, add nine grams each of Massa Medica Fermentata (*Shen Qu*) and Fructus Germinatus Hordei Vulgaris (*Mai Ya*).

Acupuncture & moxibustion: *Gan Shu* (Bl 18), *Dan Shu* (Bl 19), *Tai Chong* (Liv 3), *Yang Ling Quan* (GB 34)

Analysis of formula: *Gan Shu* is the back transport point of the liver, while *Dan Shu* is the back transport point of the gallbladder. *Tai Chong* is the source point of the liver channel, and *Yang Ling Quan* is the uniting point of the gallbladder channel. Together, these points course the liver and resolve depression, move the qi and stop pain when drained. All are key points in the treatment of hepatitis.

Additions & subtractions: If there is upper abdominal distention or pain, add *Zhong Wan* (CV 12). If there is abdominal distention or pain at the level of the waist, add *Tian Shu* (St 25). If liver depression transforms heat, replace *Tai Chong* with *Xing Jian* (Liv 2). If liver qi assails the stomach with vomiting, nausea, and/or belching, add *Nei Guan* (Per 6) and *Shang Wan* (CV 13). If there is lack of appetite due to food stagnation, add *Liang Men* (St 21).

2. Liver-spleen disharmony pattern

Main symptoms: Chest, breast, stomach venter, and rib-side distention and pain, irritability, frequent sighing, possible emotional tension or depression, fatigue, lack of strength, cold hands and feet, possible torpid intake, premenstrual syndrome and/or menstrual irregularities in females, a bland taste in the mouth, loose stools, a swollen, fat tongue which may be pale and/or dark with thin, white fur, and a bowstring, fine pulse

Note: In a liver-spleen disharmony, liver depression may manifest only by irritability and a bowstring pulse with some menstrual irregularity in females.

Treatment principles: Course the liver and rectify the qi, fortify the spleen and boost the qi

Rx: *Xiao Yao San* (Rambling Powder)

Ingredients: Radix Bupleuri (*Chai Hu*), Radix Angelicae Sinensis (*Dang Gui*), Radix Albus Paeoniae Lactiflorae (*Bai Shao*), Rhizoma Atractylodis Macrocephalae (*Bai Zhu*), and Sclerotium Poriae Cocos (*Fu Ling*), 9g each, mix-fried Radix Glycyrrhizae (*Gan Cao*) and Herba Menthae Haplocalycis (*Bo He*), 6g each, and uncooked Rhizoma Zingiberis (*Sheng Jiang*), 2 slices

ANALYSIS OF FORMULA: *Chai Hu* and *Bo He* course the liver and rectify the qi. *Bai Shao* and *Dang Gui* nourish the blood, harmonizing and emolliating the liver. *Bai Zhu, Fu Ling,* and mix-fried *Gan Cao* fortify the spleen and supplement the qi. *Sheng Jiang* harmonizes the other medicinals in the formula, aids in moving the qi, and benefits the spleen by helping transform dampness.

ADDITIONS & SUBTRACTIONS: For marked qi vacuity causing serious fatigue, add up to 60 grams of Radix Astragali Membranacei (*Huang Qi*). For more pronounced qi stagnation, add nine grams each of Rhizoma Cyperi Rotundi (*Xiang Fu*), Radix Auklandiae Lappae (*Mu Xiang*), and Radix Meliae Toosendan (*Chuan Lian Zi*). For more pronounced spleen vacuity with fatigue, add 15 grams of Radix Astragali Membranacei (*Huang Qi*) and nine grams of Radix Codonopsitis Pilosulae (*Dang Shen*). For phlegm dampness, add nine grams of Rhizoma Pinelliae Ternatae (*Ban Xia*) and six grams of Pericarpium Citri Reticulatae (*Chen Pi*). For liver depression transforming heat, add nine grams each of Fructus Gardeniae Jasminoidis (*Zhi Zi*) and Cortex Radicis Moutan (*Dan Pi*). For concomitant blood vacuity, add 12 grams of cooked Radix Rehmanniae (*Shu Di*) and nine grams of Radix Polygoni Multiflori (*He Shou Wu*). For concomitant blood stasis, add nine grams each of Radix Ligustici Wallichii (*Chuan Xiong*), Semen Pruni Persicae (*Tao Ren*), and Flos Carthami Tinctorii (*Hong Hua*). If there are cold hands and feet, add nine grams of Ramulus Cinnamomi Cassiae (*Gui Zhi*).

If there is liver-spleen disharmony diarrhea, replace *Xiao Yao San* with *Tong Xie Yao Fang* (Painful Diarrhea Essential Formula): Rhizoma Atractylodis Macrocephalae (*Bai Zhu*), Radix Albus Paeoniae Lactiflorae (*Bai Shao*), and Radix Ledebouriellae Divaricatae (*Fang Feng*), 9g each, Pericarpium Citri Reticulatae (*Chen Pi*), 6g. If spleen vacuity and dampness are more severe, combine this with *Shen Ling Bai Zhu San* (Ginseng, Poria & Atractylodes Powder), *i.e.*, add Semen Coicis Lachryma-jobi (*Yi Yi Ren*), 20g, Semen Nelumbinis Nuciferae (*Lian Zi*) and Radix Dioscoreae Oppositae (*Shan Yao*), 15g each, Sclerotium Poriae Cocos (*Fu Ling*) and Semen Dolichoris Lablab (*Bai Bian Dou*), 12g each, and Radix Panacis Ginseng (*Ren Shen*), Fructus Cardamomi (*Bai Dou Kou*), Radix Platycodi (*Jie Geng*), and mix-fried Radix Glycyrrhizae (*Gan Cao*), 6g each. If there is marked rib-side and flank distention and pain, add nine grams each of Tuber Curcumae (*Yu Jin*) and Fructus Meliae Toosendan (*Chuan Lian Zi*). If there is severe abdominal distention, add nine grams each of Cortex Magnoliae Officinalis (*Hou Po*) and Pericarpium Arecae Catechu (*Da Fu Pi*). If there is shortness of breath and lack of strength, add 15 grams of Radix Astragali Membranacei (*Huang Qi*) and nine grams of Radix Codonopsitis Pilosulae (*Dang Shen*). If there are cold hands and feet, add nine grams of Ramulus Cinnamomi Cassiae (*Gui Zhi*).

ACUPUNCTURE & MOXIBUSTION: *Gan Shu* (Bl 18), *Zu San Li* (St 36), *Tai Chong* (Liv 3), *Yang Ling Quan* (GB 34)

ANALYSIS OF FORMULA: *Gan Shu* is the back transport point of the liver and *Tai Chong* is the source point of the liver channel. *Yang Ling Quan* is the uniting point of the gallbladder channel. Together, these points course the liver and resolve depression, move the qi and stop pain. *Zu San Li* is the uniting point of the stomach. It fortifies the spleen and boosts the qi, harmonizes the stomach and disinhibits dampness. The first three points should be needled with draining method, while the last one is needled with supplementing method. All are key points for the treatment of hepatitis.

ADDITIONS & SUBTRACTIONS: For more pronounced qi stagnation, add *Nei Guan* (Per 6). For more pronounced spleen vacuity with fatigue, add *Pi Shu* (Bl 20) and *Wei Shu* (Bl 21). For phlegm dampness, add *Feng Long* (St 40). For liver depression transforming heat, replace *Tai Chong* with *Xing Jian* (Liv 2). For concomitant blood vacuity, add *San Yin Jiao* (Sp 6) and *Ge Shu* (Bl 17). For concomitant blood stasis, add *San Yin Jiao* (Sp 6) and *Ge Shu* (Bl 17). If there is abdominal distention or pain, add *Zhong Wan* (CV 12). If there is abdominal distention or pain at the level of the waist, add *Tian Shu* (St 25). If liver qi assails the stomach with vomiting, nausea, and/or belching, add *Nei Guan* (Per 6) and *Shang Wan* (CV 13). If there is lack of appetite due to food stagnation, add *Liang Men* (St 21).

3. SPLEEN-STOMACH DAMP HEAT PATTERN

MAIN SYMPTOMS: Abdominal distention, torpid intake, nausea, a sticky, slimy, unclean feeling in the mouth, dizziness, fatigue, lack of strength, possible mouth sores, loose stools or diarrhea, pale but bright yellow stools, foul-smelling stools, possible anal burning after defecation, a possibly red, fat, enlarged tongue with slimy, white or slimy, yellow fur, and a slippery, soggy, rapid pulse

NOTE: Although Chinese sources give this pattern for chronic active hepatitis, in real-life practice there is typically fatigue. Therefore, there is usually also marked spleen qi vacuity.

TREATMENT PRINCIPLES: Clear and transform dampness and heat, rectify the spleen and harmonize the stomach

RX: *Huo Po Ban Ling Tang Jia Jian* (Agastaches, Magnolia, Pinellia & Poria Decoction with Additions & Subtractions)

INGREDIENTS: Herba Agastachis Seu Pogostemi (*Huo Xiang*), 15g, Rhizoma Pinelliae Ternatae (*Ban Xia*) and Sclerotium Poriae Cocos (*Fu Ling*), 12g each, Cortex Magnoliae Officinalis (*Hou Po*) and Folium Perillae Frutescentis (*Zi Su Ye*), 9g each, and Fructus Cardamomi

(*Bai Dou Kou*) and Rhizoma Coptidis Chinensis (*Huang Lian*), 6g each

ANALYSIS OF FORMULA: *Huo Xiang, Hou Po*, and *Bai Dou Kou* transform dampness, while *Huang Lian* clears the heat. Together, they clear and transform dampness and heat. In addition, *Huo Xiang* treats the sticky, slimy, unclean feeling in the mouth. *Fu Ling* seeps dampness, while *Zi Su Ye* and *Ban Xia* harmonize the stomach and stop vomiting.

ADDITIONS & SUBTRACTIONS: For spleen vacuity with heavy dampness, add 18 grams of Semen Coicis Lachryma-jobi (*Yi Yi Ren*) and nine grams each of Radix Codonopsitis Pilosulae (*Dang Shen*), Rhizoma Atractylodis Macrocephalae (*Bai Zhu*), and Rhizoma Atractylodis (*Cang Zhu*). If heat is more pronounced, add nine grams each of Radix Scutellariae Baicalensis (*Huang Qin*) and Fructus Gardeniae Jasminoidis (*Zhi Zi*). If heat has damaged yin, add 12 grams of Tuber Ophiopogonis Japonici (*Mai Men Dong*) and nine grams of Herba Dendrobii (*Shi Hu*). For scanty, reddish yellow urine, add 15 grams of Semen Plantaginis (*Che Qian Zi*). For nausea and vomiting, add nine grams each of Caulis Bambusae In Taeniis (*Zhu Ru*) and Pericarpium Citri Reticulatae (*Chen Pi*).

ACUPUNCTURE & MOXIBUSTION: *Zu San Li* (St 36), *Yin Ling Quan* (Sp 9), *Nei Ting* (St 44), *Yang Ling Quan* (GB 34)

ANALYSIS OF FORMULA: Supplementing *Zu San Li* fortifies the spleen and boosts the qi, harmonizes the stomach and disinhibits dampness. Draining *Nei Ting* clears heat from the spleen and stomach. Draining *Yin Ling Quan* and *Yang Ling Quan* clear and disinhibit damp heat.

ADDITIONS & SUBTRACTIONS: For more pronounced spleen vacuity with fatigue, add *Pi Shu* (Bl 20) and *Wei Shu* (Bl 21). For concomitant liver depression, add *Tai Chong* (Liv 3). For concomitant blood vacuity and/or blood stasis, add *San Yin Jiao* (Sp 6) and *Ge Shu* (Bl 17). If there is abdominal distention or pain, add *Zhong Wan* (CV 12). If there is abdominal distention or pain at the level of the waist, add *Tian Shu* (St 25). For vomiting, nausea, and/or belching, add *Nei Guan* (Per 6) and *Shang Wan* (CV 13). If there is lack of appetite due to food stagnation, add *Liang Men* (St 21).

4. LIVER-GALLBLADDER DAMP HEAT PATTERN

MAIN SYMPTOMS: Rib-side pain, low-grade fever or alternating fever and chills, red eyes, headache, a bitter taste in the mouth, torpid intake, aversion to greasy, fatty foods, nausea, vomiting, reddish yellow urine, possible jaundice, a red tongue with slimy, yellow fur, and a bowstring, slippery, rapid pulse

TREATMENT PRINCIPLES: Course the liver and disinhibit the gallbladder, clear heat and eliminate dampness

RX: *Long Dan Xie Gan Tang Jia Jian* (Gentiana Drain the Liver Decoction with Additions & Subtractions)

INGREDIENTS: Talcum (*Hua Shi*), 18g, uncooked Radix Rehmanniae (*Sheng Di*) and Radix Scutellariae Baicalensis (*Huang Qin*), 12g each, Fructus Gardeniae Jasminoidis (*Zhi Zi*), Rhizoma Alismatis (*Ze Xie*), Semen Plantaginis (*Che Qian Zi*), Caulis Akebiae (*Mu Tong*), and Radix Bupleuri (*Chai Hu*), 9g each, Radix Gentianae Scabrae (*Long Dan Cao*), Pulvis Indigonis (*Qing Dai*), and Extremitas Radicis Angelicae Sinensis (*Dang Gui Wei*), 6g each, and Radix Glycyrrhizae (*Gan Cao*), 3g

ANALYSIS OF FORMULA: *Hua Shi, Ze Xie, Mu Tong*, and *Che Qian Zi* disinhibit damp heat through urination. *Zhi Zi, Huang Qin*, and *Long Dan Cao* clear the liver and dry dampness. *Qing Dai* clears the liver and discharges fire. *Sheng Di* nourishes liver yin. It also protects yin from the dry nature of the majority of the medicinals in this formula. *Chai Hu* courses the liver to prevent further liver depression transforming into heat. *Dang Gui Wei* quickens the blood and prevents blood stasis due to heat, while *Gan Cao* harmonizes the other medicinals in this formula.

ADDITIONS & SUBTRACTIONS: If heat has transformed into fire, add 3-6g of Radix Et Rhizoma Rhei (*Da Huang*). If heat has damaged yin, add 12 grams each of Tuber Ophiopogonis Japonici (*Mai Men Dong*) and Tuber Asparagi Cochinensis (*Tian Men Dong*). If there is accompanying jaundice, add 30 grams of Herba Artemisiae Capillaris (*Yin Chen Hao*). For nausea and vomiting, add nine grams of Caulis Bambusae In Taeniis (*Zhu Ru*) and Pericarpium Citri Reticulatae (*Chen Pi*). For aversion to greasy, fatty foods or undigested food in the stools, add 15 grams of Fructus Crataegi (*Shan Zha*) and nine grams each of Fructus Germinatus Hordei Vulgaris (*Mai Ya*) and Massa Medica Fermentata (*Shen Qu*).

ACUPUNCTURE & MOXIBUSTION: *Gan Shu* (Bl 18), *Dan Shu* (Bl 19), *Tai Chong* (Liv 3), *Yang Ling Quan* (GB 34)

ANALYSIS OF FORMULA: *Gan Shu* is the back transport point of the liver, while *Dan Shu* is the back transport point of the gallbladder. *Tai Chong* is the source point of the liver channel, and *Yang Ling Quan* is the uniting point of the gallbladder channel. Together, these points course the liver and disinhibit the gallbladder, clear heat and eliminate dampness. All these points should be needled with draining method. All are key points for the treatment of hepatitis.

ADDITIONS & SUBTRACTIONS: For bodily weakness and fatigue, add *Zu San Li* (St 36). For jaundice, add *Qiu Xu* (GB 40) and *Zhi Yang* (GV 9). For abdominal distention or pain, add *Zhong Wan* (CV 12). For abdominal distention or pain at the level of the waist, add *Tian Shu* (St 25). For vomiting, nausea, and/or belching, add *Nei Guan* (Per 6) and *Shang*

Wan (CV 13). For aversion to greasy, fatty foods, or lack of appetite due to food stagnation, add *Hua Rou Men* (St 24).

5. DAMP HEAT TRANSFORMING INTO FIRE & BREWING TOXINS PATTERN

MAIN SYMPTOMS: Rib-side pain, abdominal distention, glomus, and fullness, a bitter taste in the mouth, bad breath, dry tongue and parched lips, possible red eyes, headache, vexation and agitation, easy anger, insomnia, susceptibility to fright, red, turbid urination, loose stools with a foul odor, a red tongue with slimy, yellow, filthy fur, and a surging, slippery, rapid pulse

NOTE: Fire may either flare upward to harass the heart spirit, congest and obstruct the middle burner, or force its way downward. Depending on where the fire is located, various of the above signs and symptoms may manifest. It is also possible for fire to be present in all three burners simultaneously.

TREATMENT PRINCIPLES: Clear heat and resolve toxins, course the liver and disinhibit the gallbladder

RX: *Yin Chen Hao Tang Jia Wei* (Artemisia Capillaris Decoction with Added Flavors)

INGREDIENTS: Rhizoma Polygoni Bistortae (*Quan Shen*), Herba Oldenlandiae Diffusae (*Bai Hua She She Cao*), and Rhizoma Guanchong (*Guan Zhong*), 15g each, Herba Artemisiae Capillaris (*Yin Chen Hao*), 12g, Fructus Gardeniae Jasminoidis (*Zhi Zi*), Radix Lithospermi Seu Arnebiae (*Zi Cao*), Rhizoma Smilacis Glabrae (*Tu Fu Ling*), and Rhizoma Cimicifugae (*Sheng Ma*), 9g each, Radix Et Rhizoma Rhei (*Da Huang*), 3-6g, and uncooked Radix Glycyrrhizae (*Gan Cao*), 3g

ANALYSIS OF FORMULA: *Da Huang, Zhi Zi, Quan Shen, Bai Hua She She Cao,* and *Tu Fu Ling* all clear heat, disinhibit or dry dampness, and resolve toxins. *Yin Chen Hao* clears heat, eliminates dampness, and disinhibits the gallbladder. *Guan Zhong* and *Sheng Ma* also clear heat and resolve toxins. *Zi Cao* cools and quickens the blood, clears the heat and resolves toxins, and *Gan Cao* harmonizes the other medicinals in this formula.

ADDITIONS & SUBTRACTIONS: If rib-side pain is marked, add 15 grams each of Rhizoma Corydalis Yanhusuo (*Yan Hu Suo*) and Fructus Meliae Toosendan (*Chuan Lian Zi*). If fire is damaging and consuming yin fluids, add 12 grams each of Radix Glehniae Littoralis (*Sha Shen*) and Tuber Ophiopogonis Japonici (*Mai Men Dong*). If there is insomnia and susceptibility to fright, add 15 grams each of Caulis Polygoni Multiflori (*Ye Jiao Teng*) and Cortex Albizziae Julibrissinis (*He Huan Pi*). If there is abdominal distention, glomus, and fullness, add nine grams each of Tuber Curcumae (*Yu Jin*), Cortex Magnoliae Officinalis (*Hou Po*), and Radix Auklandiae Lappae (*Mu Xiang*). If there is red, turbid urine, add 12 grams each of Rhizoma Alismatis (*Ze Xie*) and Semen Plantaginis (*Che Qian Zi*). If there are foul-smelling loose stools, add nine grams of Radix Scutellariae Baicalensis (*Huang Qin*).

ACUPUNCTURE & MOXIBUSTION: Same as pattern #4 above but add *Qiu Xu* (GB 40) to clear the liver and disinhibit the gallbladder.

ADDITIONS & SUBTRACTIONS: Same as pattern #4 above. For insomnia or susceptibility to fright, add *Da Ling* (Per 7). For vexation and agitation, add *Shen Ting* (GV 24). For easy anger, add *Xing Jian* (Liv 2).

6. DAMP HEAT HARASSING THE CONSTRUCTIVE & BLOOD PATTERN

MAIN SYMPTOMS: The above signs and symptoms plus spontaneous ejection of blood, *i.e.,* epistaxis, bleeding gums, subdermal bleeding, or erysipelas

NOTE: This pattern describes a late stage complication or crisis of chronic hepatitis.

TREATMENT PRINCIPLES: Disinhibit dampness and clear heat, clear the constructive and cool the blood

RX: *Yin Chen Hao Tang* (Artemisia Capillaris Decoction), *Xi Jiao Di Huang San* (Rhinoceros Horn & Rehmannia Powder) & *Yin Hua Jie Du Tang* (Lonicera Resolve Toxins Decoction) with additions and subtractions

INGREDIENTS: Cornu Bubali (*Shui Niu Jiao*), 30g, Radix Et Rhizoma Rhei (*Da Huang*), 18g, Flos Lonicerae Japonicae (*Jin Yin Hua*), Herba Violae Yedoensitis Cum Radice (*Zi Hua Di Ding*), and Spica Prunellae Vulgaris (*Xia Ku Cao*), 15g each, Cortex Radicis Moutan (*Dan Pi*), Radix Rubrus Paeoniae Lactiflorae (*Chi Shao*), Fructus Gardeniae Jasminoidis (*Zhi Zi*), and Herba Artemisiae Capillaris (*Yin Chen Hao*), 9g each, and Rhizoma Coptidis Chinensis (*Huang Lian*), 6g

ANALYSIS OF FORMULA: *Da Huang, Xia Ku Cao, Zhi Zi,* and *Huang Lian* clear heat, disinhibit or dry dampness, and resolve toxins. In addition, *Huang Lian* clears the heart and *Da Huang* stops bleeding. *Yin Chen Hao* clears heat, eliminates dampness, and disinhibits the gallbladder. *Shui Niu Jiao, Dan Pi,* and *Chi Shao* cool the constructive and blood and stop bleeding. *Zi Hua Di Ding* and *Jin Yin Hua* clear heat and resolve toxins.

ADDITIONS & SUBTRACTIONS: Please see pattern #5 above. For nosebleeding, add 12 grams each of Herba

Patriniae Heterophyllae Cum Radice (*Bai Jiang Cao*) and Cacumen Biotae Orientalis (*Ce Bai Ye*). For hematuria, add 12 grams each of Herba Seu Radix Cirsii Japonici (*Da Ji*), Herba Cephalanoploris Segeti (*Xiao Ji*), and Cacumen Biotae Orientalis (*Ce Bai Ye*). For vomiting of blood or bleeding gums, add 12-15 grams each of Rhizoma Imperatae Cylindricae (*Bai Mao Gen*) and Cacumen Biotae Orientalis (*Ce Bai Ye*).

ACUPUNCTURE & MOXIBUSTION: *Gan Shu* (Bl 18), *Dan Shu* (Bl 19), *Yang Ling Quan* (GB 34), *Xia Xi* (GB 43), *Ge Shu* (Bl 17)

ANALYSIS OF FORMULA: Draining *Gan Shu*, *Dan Shu*, *Yang Ling Quan*, and *Xia Xi* together clears the liver and discharges fire, eliminates dampness and disinhibits the gallbladder. *Ge Shu* is the meeting point of the blood. Draining it cools the constructive and blood and stops bleeding.

ADDITIONS & SUBTRACTIONS: For nosebleeding, add *Xi Men* (Per 4). For hematuria, add *San Yin Jiao* (Sp 6). For vomiting of blood, add *Nei Ting* (St 44) and *Xi Men* (Per 4). For bleeding gums, add *He Gu* (LI 4) and *Nei Ting* (St 44).

7. PHLEGM NODULATION PATTERN

MAIN SYMPTOMS: Profuse phlegm, plum pit qi, chest and abdominal glomus and fullness, fatigue, lack of strength, lassitude of the spirit, torpid intake, possible nausea and vomiting, a tendency to loose stools, mucus in the stools, subdermal nodulations or accumulation lumps below the rib-side, slimy tongue fur, and a slippery bowstring or soggy, bowstring pulse

NOTE: In this case damp heat has both damaged the spleen qi and brewed fluids into phlegm.

TREATMENT PRINCIPLES: Fortify the spleen and transform phlegm, scatter nodulation and disperse accumulation

RX: *Liu Jun Zi Tang Jia Jian* (Four Gentlemen Decoction with Additions & Subtractions)

INGREDIENTS: Radix Astragali Membranacei (*Huang Qi*), Semen Citri Reticulatae (*Ju He*), and Spica Prunellae Vulgaris (*Xia Ku Cao*), 15g, Bulbus Fritillariae Thunbergii (*Zhe Bei Mu*), Concha Ostreae (*Mu Li*), and Herba Sargassii (*Hai Zao*), 12g each, Radix Codonopsitis Pilosulae (*Dang Shen*), Rhizoma Atractylodis Macrocephalae (*Bai Zhu*), Sclerotium Poriae Cocos (*Fu Ling*), Rhizoma Pinelliae Ternatae (*Ban Xia*), Endothelium Corneum Gigeriae Galli (*Ji Nei Jin*), and scorched Fructus Crataegi (*Shan Zha*), 9g each, and Pericarpium Citri Reticulatae (*Chen Pi*), 6g

ANALYSIS OF FORMULA: *Huang Qi*, *Dang Shen*, *Bai Zhu*, and *Fu Ling* fortify the spleen and supplement the qi, thus treating the root and preventing further engenderment of phlegm. *Zhe Bei Mu*, *Ban Xia*, *Fu Ling*, and *Chen Pi* transform phlegm. In addition, *Ban Xia* and *Zhe Bei Mu* soften the hard and scatter nodulation, as do *Xia Ku Cao*, *Ju He*, *Mu Li*, and *Hai Zao*. *Ji Nei Jin* and *Shan Zha* abduct stagnation and disperse accumulation.

ADDITIONS & SUBTRACTIONS: For severe qi vacuity, add 15 grams of Fructus Schisandrae Chinensis (*Wu Wei Zi*) and nine grams of Fructificatio Ganodermae Lucidi (*Ling Zhi*). For concomitant blood vacuity, add nine grams each of Radix Angelicae Sinensis (*Dang Gui*) and Fructus Lycii Chinensis (*Gou Qi Zi*). For phlegm heat, add six grams each of Radix Scutellariae Baicalensis (*Huang Qin*) and Rhizoma Coptidis Chinensis (*Huang Lian*). For concomitant liver depression, add nine grams each of Radix Bupleuri (*Chai Hu*) and Radix Albus Paeoniae Lactiflorae (*Bai Shao*). For accumulation lumps below the rib-side, add 12 grams each of Rhizoma Sparganii (*San Leng*), Rhizoma Curcumae Zedoariae (*E Zhu*), and Radix Salviae Miltiorrhizae (*Dan Shen*).

ACUPUNCTURE & MOXIBUSTION: *Zhang Men* (Liv 13), *Zu San Li* (St 36), *Yin Ling Quan* (Sp 9), *Feng Long* (St 40)

ANALYSIS OF FORMULA: Supplementing *Zu San Li* fortifies the spleen and boosts the qi. *Yin Ling Quan* is a key point for eliminating dampness, while *Feng Long* is the main point for transforming phlegm. When needled with draining method, they transform phlegm and disperse accumulation. When *Zhang Men* is also drained, it rectifies the qi and disperses accumulation lumps below the rib-side. However, in case of hepatomegaly, care should be taken when needling this point.

ADDITIONS & SUBTRACTIONS: In case of damp heat, add *Yang Ling Quan* (GB 34). If there is food stagnation, add *Liang Men* (St 21). If there are accumulation lumps below the rib-side, add *Qi Men* (Liv 14), *Ge Shu* (Bl 17), and *San Yin Jiao* (Sp 6). If there is nausea and vomiting add *Nei Guan* (Per 6). For stomach and abdominal fullness, add *Zhong Wan* (CV 12), and for severe qi vacuity, add *Tai Bai* (Sp 3).

8. BLOOD STASIS OBSTRUCTING THE NETWORK VESSELS PATTERN

MAIN SYMPTOMS: Lancinating pain below the rib-side, pain which is worse at night, accumulation lumps below the rib-side, a dark, stagnant facial complexion with dark, purplish lips, head, neck, and chest region red spots and red threads, possible spider nevi and/or palmar eythema, a dark, purplish tongue or static macules or spots, and a bowstring, choppy pulse

NOTE: Blood stasis may complicate any pattern of chronic

active hepatitis and especially when there is either fibrosis or cirrhosis of the liver.

TREATMENT PRINCIPLES: Quicken the blood and transform stasis, free the flow of the network vessels and disperse accumulations

RX: *Ge Xia Zhu Yu Tang Jia Jian* (Below the Diaphragm Dispel Stasis Decoction with Additions & Subtractions)

INGREDIENTS: Rhizoma Corydalis Yanhuso (*Yan Hu Suo*) and Radix Salviae Miltiorrhizae, 15g each, Radix Angelicae Sinensis (*Dang Gui*), Radix Ligustici Wallichii (*Chuan Xiong*), Semen Pruni Persicae (*Tao Ren*), Flos Carthami Tinctorii (*Hong Hua*), Feces Trogopterori Seu Pteromi (*Wu Ling Zhi*), Radix Rubrus Paeoniae Lactiflorae (*Chi Shao*), Cortex Radicis Moutan (*Dan Pi*), and Rhizoma Cyperi Rotundi (*Xiang Fu*), 9g each, Fructus Citri Aurantii (*Zhi Ke*), 6g, and Radix Glycyrrhizae (*Gan Cao*), 3g

ANALYSIS OF FORMULA: *Yan Hu Suo, Dan Shen, Dang Gui, Chuan Xiong, Tao Ren, Hong Hua, Wu Ling Zhi, Chi Shao,* and *Dan Pi* all quicken the blood and transform stasis. *Yan Hu Suo, Chuan Xiong, Zhi Ke,* and *Xiang Fu* move the qi to quicken the blood, while *Dan Shen* and *Dang Gui* also nourish the blood.

ADDITIONS & SUBTRACTIONS: If there are accumulation lumps below the rib-side and the righteous qi is not yet debilitated, add 15g of Carapax Amydae Sinensis (*Bei Jia*) and nine grams each of Rhizoma Sparganii (*San Leng*) and Rhizoma Curcumae Zedoariae (*E Zhu*). If there is heat stasis, add nine grams each of Fructus Gardeniae Jasminoidis (*Zhi Zi*) and Radix Scutellariae Baicalensis (*Huang Qin*). If there is concomitant qi vacuity, add 15 grams of Radix Astragali Membranacei (*Huang Qi*) and nine grams each of Radix Codonopsitis Pilosulae (*Dang Shen*) and Sclerotium Poriae Cocos (*Fu Ling*). If qi stagnation is more pronounced, add nine grams each of Pericarpium Citri Reticulatae Viride (*Qing Pi*) and Radix Linderae Strychnifoliae (*Wu Yao*). If there is chest oppression and fullness, add nine grams each of Tuber Curcumae (*Yu Jin*) and Flos Inulae Racemosae (*Xuan Fu Hua*). If phlegm and stasis have bound together, add 12 grams each of Bulbus Fritillariae Thunbergii (*Zhe Bei Mu*), Semen Trichosanthis Kirlowii (*Gua Lou Ren*), and Radix Trichosanthis Kirlowii (*Tian Hua Fen*), nine grams each of Radix Platycodi Grandiflori (*Jie Geng*) and Sclerotium Poriae Cocos (*Fu Ling*), and six grams of Pericarpium Citri Reticulatae (*Chen Pi*).

If there is a qi and blood dual vacuity with blood stasis, replace *Ge Xia Zhu Yu Tang Jia Jian* with *Ba Zhen Tang* (Eight Pearls Decoction) and *Hua Ji Wan* (Transform Accumulation Pills) with additions and subtractions: cooked Radix Rehmanniae (*Shu Di*), 12g, Radix Codonopsitis Pilosulae (*Dang Shen*), Rhizoma Atractylodis Macrocephalae (*Bai Zhu*), Sclerotium Poriae Cocos (*Fu Ling*), Radix Angelicae Sinensis (*Dang Gui*), Radix Albus Paeoniae Lactiflorae (*Bai Shao*), Radix Ligustici Wallichii (*Chuan Xiong*), Rhizoma Sparganii (*San Leng*), Rhizoma Curcumae Zedoariae (*E Zhu*), Semen Pruni Persicae (*Tao Ren*), Rhizoma Cyperi Rotundi (*Xiang Fu*), and Fructus Crataegi (*Shan Zha*), 9g each and mix-fried Radix Glycyrrhizae (*Gan Cao*), Semen Raphani Sativi (*Lai Fu Zi*), and Massa Medica Fermentata (*Shen Qu*), 6g each. If there is concomitant damp or depressive heat, add nine grams of Fructus Gardeniae Jasminoidis (*Zhi Zi*) and three grams of Rhizoma Coptidis Chinensis (*Huang Lian*). If phlegm accumulation is severe, add nine grams each of Rhizoma Pinelliae Ternatae (*Ban Xia*) and Bulbus Fritillariae Thunbergii (*Zhe Bei Mu*). If there is spleen-kidney yang vacuity, add *Shen Qi Wan* (Kidney Qi Pills, a Chinese ready-made medicine). If righteous vacuity is severe, reduce the doses of the attacking medicinals and increase the doses of the supporting medicinals.

ACUPUNCTURE & MOXIBUSTION: *Gan Shu* (Bl 18), *Dan Shu* (Bl 19), *Ge Shu* (Bl 17), *Zhang Men* (Liv 13)

ANALYSIS OF FORMULA: Draining *Gan Shu, Dan Shu,* and *Ge Shu* quickens the blood and transforms stasis, especially liver blood and stasis. Draining *Zhang Men* frees the flow of the network vessels and disperses accumulations in the rib-side.

ADDITIONS & SUBTRACTIONS: For marked concomitant liver depression, add *Tai Chong* (Liv 3). For pain in the rib-side, add *Zhi Gou* (TB 6). For severe blood stasis, add *He Gu* (LI 4) and *San Yin Jiao* (Sp 6). For concomitant blood vacuity, add *San Yin Jiao* (Sp 6). For concomitant qi vacuity, add *Zu San Li* (St 36).

9. LIVER-KIDNEY YIN VACUITY PATTERN

MAIN SYMPTOMS: Insidious right-sided rib-side pain, low back and knee soreness and limpness, dry mouth and parched throat, vexatious heat in the five hearts, possible insomnia with profuse dreams, emaciation, possible low-grade fever in the afternoons, dizziness, tinnitus, bilateral dry, rough eyes, a red tongue with scanty fur, and a bowstring, fine, and/or rapid pulse

TREATMENT PRINCIPLES: Nourish the liver and enrich the kidneys

RX: *Yi Guan Jian* (One Link Decoction)

INGREDIENTS: Uncooked Radix Rehmanniae (*Sheng Di*), 15g, Radix Glehniae Littoralis (*Sha Shen*) and Tuber Ophiopogonis Japonici (*Mai Dong*), 12g each, Radix Angelicae Sinensis (*Dang Gui*) and Fructus Lycii Chinensis

(*Gou Qi Zi*), 9g each, and Fructus Meliae Toosendan (*Chuan Lian Zi*), 6g

ANALYSIS OF FORMULA: *Sheng Di* and *Gou Qi Zi* nourish liver blood and kidney yin. *Sha Shen* and *Mai Men Dong* nourish yin and engender fluids. *Dang Gui* and *Gou Qi Zi* nourish liver blood. *Chuan Lian Zi* courses the liver and resolves depression without plundering yin.

ADDITIONS & SUBTRACTIONS: If there is lingering damp heat, add 15grams of Rhizoma Imperatae Cylindricae (*Bai Mao Gen*) and nine grams of Herba Artemisiae Capillaris (*Yin Chen Hao*). If there is vexatious heat in the heart and sleep is poor, add 12 grams of Semen Zizyphi Spinosae (*Suan Zao Ren*) and nine grams of Fructus Gardeniae Jasminoidis (*Zhi Zi*). If there is a bitter taste in the mouth, add three grams of Rhizoma Coptidis Chinensis (*Huang Lian*). If there is dizziness, add nine grams each of Rhizoma Polygonati (*Huang Jing*), Flos Chrysanthemi Morifolii (*Ju Hua*), and Ramulus Uncariae Cum Uncis (*Gou Teng*). If qi stagnation is marked, add nine grams each of Fructus Citri Sacrodactylis (*Fo Shou*), Folium Citri Reticulatae (*Ju Ye*), and Flos Rosae Rugosae (*Mei Gui Hua*). If there is blurred or dim vision, add 12 grams each of Fructus Ligustri Lucidi (*Nu Zhen Zi*) and Semen Cassiae Torae (*Cao Jue Ming*). If there is constipation, add 12 grams of Semen Trichosanthis Kirlowii (*Gua Lou Ren*). If there is concomitant phlegm, add 12 grams of Bulbus Fritillariae Thunbergii (*Zhe Bei Mu*). If there are below the rib-side accumulation lumps, add 12 grams each of Carapax Amydae Sinensis (*Bei Jia*) and Radix Salviae Miltiorrhizae (*Dan Shen*). If there is vexatious heat and thirst, add 12 grams of Gypsum Fibrosum (*Shi Gao*) and nine grams of Rhizoma Anemarrhenae Aspheloidis (*Zhi Mu*). If there is severe abdominal pain, add 18 grams of Radix Albus Paeoniae Lactiflorae (*Bai Shao*) and six grams of mix-fried Radix Glycyrrhizae (*Gan Cao*). If there is concomitant spleen qi vacuity, add 15 grams of Radix Astragali Membrancei (*Huang Qi*) and nine grams each of Radix Panacis Quinquefolii (*Xi Yang Shen*), Radix Pseudostellariae (*Tai Zi Shen*), and/or Radix Dioscoreae Oppositae (*Shan Yao*).

ACUPUNCTURE & MOXIBUSTION: *Gan Shu* (Bl 18), *Shen Shu* (Bl 23), *San Yin Jiao* (Sp 6), *Tai Chong* (Liv 3)

ANALYSIS OF FORMULA: *Gan Shu* is the back transport point of the liver. Supplementing it nourishes liver blood. *Shen Shu* is the back transport point of the kidneys. Supplementing it enriches kidney yin. *San Yin Jiao* is the meeting point of the three yin. Supplementing it nourishes the blood and yin, the liver and kidneys. *Tai Chong* is the source point of the liver channel. Draining it courses the liver, recedes jaundice, and prevents liver depression.

ADDITIONS & SUBTRACTIONS: If there is lingering damp heat, add *Qiu Xu* (GB 40). If there is a bitter taste in the mouth, add *Xia Xi* (GB 43). If there is dizziness, add *Feng Chi* (GB 20). If there is blurred or dim vision, add *Guang Ming* (GB 37). If there is constipation, add *Zhi Gou* (TB 6). If there is concomitant phlegm, add *Feng Long* (St 40). If there are accumulation lumps below the rib-side, add *Zhang Men* (Liv 13) and/or *Qi Men* (Liv 14). If there is severe abdominal pain, add *Tian Shu* (St 25). If there is concomitant spleen qi vacuity, add *Zu San Li* (St 36).

10. SPLEEN-KIDNEY YANG VACUITY PATTERN

MAIN SYMPTOMS: Abdominal distention and ductal glomus, loose stools, possible cockcrow diarrhea, undigested food in the stools, fatigue, weakness of the limbs, lack of warmth in the four extremities, a lusterless facial complexion, low back and knee chilly pain, lower extremity edema, reduced food intake, a pale, fat tongue with teeth-prints on its edges, and a deep, fine, forceless pulse

TREATMENT PRINCIPLES: Fortify the spleen and supplement the kidneys, invigorate yang and eliminate dampness

RX: *Li Zhong Wan* (Rectify the Center Pills) & *Si Shen Wan* (Four Spirits Pills)

INGREDIENTS: Radix Panacis Ginseng (*Ren Shen*), Rhizoma Atractylodis Macrocephalae (*Bai Zhu*), dry Rhizoma Zingiberis (*Gan Jiang*), Fructus Psoraleae Corylifoliae (*Bu Gu Zhi*), Fructus Schisandrae Chinensis (*Wu Wei Zi*), and Semen Myristicae Fragrantis (*Rou Dou Kou*), 9g each , mix-fried Radix Glycyrrhizae (*Gan Cao*), 6g, and Fructus Evodiae Rutecarpae (*Wu Zhu Yu*), 3g

ANALYSIS OF FORMULA: *Ren Shen*, *Bai Zhu*, and mix-fried *Gan Cao* fortify the spleen and boost the qi. *Gan Jiang*, *Rou Dou Kou*, and *Wu Zhu Yu* warm the spleen and scatter cold. *Bu Gu Zhi* and *Wu Wei Zi* warm and supplement the kidneys.

ADDITIONS & SUBTRACTIONS: If qi vacuity is severe with enduring diarrhea, add 15 grams of Radix Astragali Membranacei (*Huang Qi*), six grams of Pericarpium Citri Reticulatae (*Chen Pi*), 4.5 grams of Rhizoma Cimicifugae (*Sheng Ma*), and three grams of Radix Bupleuri (*Chai Hu*). If yang qi is severely debilitated with yin cold exuberant internally, add six grams of Radix Lateralis Praeparatus Aconiti Carmichaeli (*Fu Zi*). If there is low back and knee soreness and limpness, add nine grams of Radix Dipsaci (*Xu Duan*) and Rhizoma Cibotii Barometsis (*Gou Ji*). If there is scanty urination and edema, add nine grams each of Ramulus Cinnamomi Cassiae (*Gui Zhi*), Rhizoma Alismatis (*Ze Xie*), and Semen Plantaginis (*Che Qian Zi*). For pain in the liver area, add nine grams each of Radix Rubrus Paeoniae Lactiflorae (*Chi Shao*), Radix Salviae Miltiorrhizae (*Dan Shen*), and Radix Bupleuri (*Chai Hu*). For severe kidney yang vacuity, add 12 grams of cooked Radix Rehmanniae (*Shu Di*), nine grams each of Radix Dioscoreae Oppositae (*Shan Yao*) and Fructus Corni Officinalis (*Shan Zhu Yu*), and six grams each of Fructus Amomi (*Sha Ren*) and Radix Lateralis Praeparatus Aconiti Carmichaeli (*Fu Zi*).

ACUPUNCTURE & MOXIBUSTION: *Ming Men* (GV 4), *Guan Yuan* (CV 4), *Qi Hai* (CV 6), *Zu San Li* (St 36)

ANALYSIS OF FORMULA: Supplementing *Ming Men, Guan Yuan, Qi Hai,* and *Zu San Li* with moxibustion fortifies the spleen and supplements the kidneys, invigorates yang and eliminates dampness.

ADDITIONS & SUBTRACTIONS: For severe spleen vacuity, add *Pi Shu* (Bl 20). For severe kidney vacuity, add *Shen Shu* (Bl 23). For diarrhea, add *Tian Shu* (St 25). For low back and knee soreness and limpness, add *Gong Sun* (Sp 4) and *Fu Liu* (Ki 7).

11. COLD DAMPNESS BREWING INTERNALLY PATTERN

MAIN SYMPTOMS: Right-sided rib-side pain and distention, abdominal fullness, yin jaundice, aversion to cold, chilled limbs, no thirst and a tasteless feeling in the mouth, torpid intake, loose stools, fatigue, lack of strength, lassitude of the spirit, edema, ascites, a pale or sallow facial complexion, a pale, fat tongue with teeth-marks on its edges and white, slimy fur, and a soggy, moderate (*i.e.*, slightly slow) pulse

TREATMENT PRINCIPLES: Fortify the spleen and warm yang, transform dampness and recede jaundice

RX: *Yin Chen Zhu Fu Tang Jia Wei* (Artemisia Capillaris, Atractylodes & Aconite Decoction with Added Flavors)

INGREDIENTS: Rhizoma Atractylodis Macrocephalae (*Bai Zhu*), Sclerotium Poriae Cocos (*Fu Ling*), Herba Artemisiae Capillaris (*Yin Chen Hao*), and Rhizoma Alismatis (*Ze Xie*), 9g each, and Cortex Cinnamomi Cassiae (*Rou Gui*), Radix Lateralis Praeparatus Aconiti Carmichaeli (*Fu Zi*), dry Rhizoma Zingiberis (*Gan Jiang*), and mix-fried Radix Glycyrrhizae (*Gan Cao*), 6g each

ANALYSIS OF FORMULA: *Bai Zhu, Fu Ling,* and mix-fried *Gan Cao* fortify the spleen and supplement the qi. *Gan Jiang, Fu Zi,* and *Rou Gui* warm the spleen and scatter the cold, thus helping to transform cold dampness. *Bai Zhu* dries dampness, *Fu Ling* and *Ze Xie* seep dampness, and *Yin Chen Hao* disinhibits dampness. In addition, *Yin Chen Hao* treats yin jaundice.

ADDITIONS & SUBTRACTIONS: If there is abdominal distention and thick tongue fur, add nine grams each of Rhizoma Atractylodis (*Cang Zhu*), Cortex Magnoliae Officinalis (*Hou Po*), and Pericarpium Arecae Catechu (*Bing Lang*). For diarrhea or watery stools, add nine grams each of Fructus Amomi (*Sha Ren*), Herba Agastachis Seu Pogostemi (*Huo Xiang*), and Rhizoma Atractylodis (*Cang Zhu*). For severe jaundice, increase the dosage of *Bai Zhu* up to 15 grams and that of *Yin Chen Hao* up to 25 grams.

ACUPUNCTURE & MOXIBUSTION: *Zu San Li* (St 36), *Zhong Wan* (CV 12), *Yin Ling Quan* (Sp 9), *Tai Chong* (Liv 3), *Zhang Men* (Liv 13)

ANALYSIS OF FORMULA: *Zhong Wan, Yin Ling Quan,* and *Zu San Li* fortify the spleen, warm yang, and transform dampness. *Zhang Men* rectifies the qi and disperses accumulations in the rib-side. *Tai Chong* recedes jaundice. All these points should be drained except *Zu San Li.* Also moxa *Zu San Li* and *Zhong Wan.*

ADDITIONS & SUBTRACTIONS: For marked fatigue and lack of strength, add *Tai Bai* (Sp 3). For severe jaundice, add *Gan Shu* (Bl 18) and *Pi Shu* (Bl 20). For upper abdominal distention, add *Shang Wan* (CV 13). For abdominal distention at the level of the waist, add *Tian Shu* (St 25). For nausea and vomiting, add *Nei Guan* (Per 6). For diarrhea, add *Shen Que* (CV 8).

REMARKS

1. Ultimately, no matter what the disease, one should always treat the patient's personal pattern or combination of patterns. Although Western MDs say that chronic active hepatitis may be asymptomatic, patients with this condition are never asymptomatic from the point of view of Chinese medicine. In other words, every person with chronic active hepatitis does display one or more patterns, remembering that a Chinese pattern is made up of a combination of signs and symptoms, tongue signs, and pulse signs. These signs and symptoms may not have anything to do with hepatitis from a Western medical point of view. For instance, women with liver depression qi stagnation, typically have menstrual and premenstrual symptoms. Men will at least be irritable or easily frustrated. Therefore, it is extremely important to do a complete intake using the four examinations. Even if there is nothing other than an enlarged tongue with a red right edge and slimy tongue fur plus a bowstring, slippery pulse, this does add up to a Chinese medical pattern.

At the very least, there is usually a liver-stomach and/or liver-spleen disharmony. The above are the most commonly seen patterns in chronic active hepatitis. However, they merely give some general guidelines to pattern discrimination and treatment. Individual treatment plans will usually be a combination of several of the above elements.

2. It has recently been reported from Japan that several patients on interferon therapy have died due to liver failure while simultaneously taking *Xiao Chai Hu Tang* (Minor Bupleurum Decoction). As of this writing, the exact pharmacodynamics have not been determined. Some synergism between interferon and Radix Bupleuri (*Chai Hu*) is suspected. However, it may also be that *Xiao Chai Hu Tang* was misprescribed to these patients. Until this issue has been cleared up, we advise not prescribing Bupleurum with interferon.

3. Although a combination of enduring damp heat evils and aging often damage and consume the spleen qi resulting in spleen vacuity with cold dampness and even spleen-kidney yang vacuity, care should be taken when using interior-warming medicinals such as Radix Lateralis Praeparatus Aconiti Carmichael (*Fu Zi*), Cortex Cinnamomi Cassiae (*Rou Gui*), and dry Rhizoma Zingiberis (*Gan Jiang*). These intensely hot medicinals can aggravate any lingering heat evils in the body. Therefore, practitioners should monitor their patients carefully. If symptoms of evil heat become apparent, either these medicinals should be deleted, their dose should be reduced, or they should be combined with appropriate heat-clearing medicinals.

4. The righteous qi of patients waiting for liver transplant surgery is usually vacuous and weak. In such cases, supplementing the righteous helps reduce blood loss during surgery and helps guarantee a successful outcome. Postsurgery, patients are extremely debilitated and also typically require strong supplementation of the qi and blood. Other postsurgical symptoms should be dealt with on a case by case basis determined by their personal pattern discrimination.

5. According to both the Chinese literature and our own clinical experience, chronic active hepatitis can be treated successfully with Chinese medicine as evidenced by positive changes in such markers as transaminase, SGPT, and SGOT. However, patients must eat a proper diet, live a regular lifestyle, and take Chinese medicines for at least 12-24 months continuously. After liver enzymes are stabilized, preventive therapy can be given for 20 days every three months.

6. Although Chinese medical treatment should always be based on each patient's personal pattern discrimination, modern laboratory research has shown that the following Chinese medicinals can achieve the following effects:

Regulating transaminase: Fructus Schisandrae Chinensis (*Wu Wei Zi*), Radix Istadis Seu Baphicacanthi (*Ban Lan Gen*), Herba Artemisiae Capillaris (*Yin Chen Hao*), Radix Rubrus Paeoniae Lactiflorae (*Chi Shao*), Concretio Silicea Bambusae (*Tian Zhu Huang*), Radix Glycyrrhizae (*Gan Cao*), Herba Sedi Sarmentosi (*Chui Pen Cao*), Radix Angelicae Sinensis (*Dang Gui*), Herba Patriniae Heterophyllae Cum Radice (*Bai Jiang Cao*), Radix Et Rhizoma Polygoni Cuspidati (*Hu Zhang*), Rhizoma Coptidis Chinensis (*Huang Lian*), Cortex Phellodendri (*Huang Bai*), Radix Gentianae Scabrae (*Long Dan Cao*), Sclerotium Poriae Cocos (*Fu Ling*), Rhizoma Cimicifugae (*Sheng Ma*), Radix Puerariae (*Ge Gen*), and Fructificatio Ganodermae Lucidi (*Ling Zhi*)

Lowering SGPT & SGOT: Fructus Schisandrae Chinensis (*Wu Wei Zi*), Radix Angelicae Sinensis (*Dang Gui*), Radix Gentianae Scabrae (*Long Dan Cao*), Herba Patriniae Heterophyllae Cum Radice (*Bai Jiang Cao*), Radix Glycyrrhizae (*Gan Cao*), Radix Istadis Seu Baphicacanthi (*Ban Lan Gen*), Fructus Forsythiae Suspensae (*Lian Qiao*), Radix Salviae Miltiorrhizae (*Dan Shen*), Fructificatio Ganodermae Lucidi (*Ling Zhi*), Endothelium Corneum Gigeriae Galli (*Ji Nei Jin*), and Radix Bupleuri (*Chai Hu*)

Protecting liver function and promoting the regeneration of liver cells: Radix Angelicae Sinensis (*Dang Gui*), uncooked Radix Rehmanniae (*Sheng Di*), Radix Salviae Miltiorrhizae (*Dan Shen*), Fructus Lycii Chinensis (*Gou Qi*), Rhizoma Atractylodis Macrocephalae (*Bai Zhu*), Radix Astragali Membranacei (*Huang Qi*), Radix Codonopsitis Pilosulae (*Dang Shen*), Fructus Zizyphi Jujubae (*Da Zao*), Radix Glycyrrhizae (*Gan Cao*), Rhizoma Polygonati (*Huang Jing*), Fructificatio Ganodermae Lucidi (*Ling Zhi*), Radix Bupleuri (*Chai Hu*), Herba Artemisiae Capillaris (*Yin Chen Hao*), Radix Et Rhizoma Polygoni Cuspidati (*Hu Zhang*), Rhizoma Alismatis (*Ze Xie*), Herba Patriniae Heterophyllae Cum Radice (*Bai Jiang Cao*), and Fructus Forsythiae Suspensae (*Lian Qiao*)

Treating liver fibrosis: Rhizoma Sparganii (*San Leng*), Rhizoma Curcumae Zedoariae (*E Zhu*), Squama Manitis Pentadactylis (*Chuan Shan Jia*), Carapax Amydae Sinensis (*Bie Jia*), Fructus Crataegi (*Shan Zha*), Radix Salviae Miltiorrhizae (*Dan Shen*), Radix Bupleuri (*Chai Hu*), and Radix Glycyrrhizae (*Gan Cao*)

Treating hepatomegaly (due to hepatitis): Radix Salviae Miltiorrhizae (*Dan Shen*), Rhizoma Sparganii (*San Leng*), Rhizoma Curcumae Zedoariae (*E Zhu*), Carapax Amydae Sinensis (*Bie Jia*), Squama Manitis Pentadactylis (*Chuan Shan Jia*), Radix Albus Paeoniae Lactiflorae (*Bai Shao*), Tuber Curcumae (*Yu Jin*), Fructus Meliae Toosendan (*Chuan Lian Zi*), Spica Prunellae Vulgaris (*Xia Ku Cao*), Radix Bupleuri (*Chai Hu*), and Herba Verbenae (*Ma Bian Cao*)

Chinese medicinals which treat steatosis of the liver: Fructus Crataegi (*Shan Zha*), Concha Haliotidis (*Shi Jue Ming*), and Fructificatio Ganodermae Lucidi (*Ling Zhi*)

15

CHRONIC FATIGUE IMMUNE DEFICIENCY SYNDROME

Chronic fatigue immune deficiency syndrome (CFIDS) is currently used in the United States to describe a disabling and poorly understood multisystem illness. This syndrome is also called chronic fatigue syndrome (CFS) and, colloquially, "yuppie flu" in the U.S. and myalgic encephalomyelitis (ME) or post-viral fatigue in the United Kingdom, Canada, Australia, and New Zealand. This is a constellation of neurological, neuromuscular, and immunological abnormalities combined with cognitive impairments, disabling fatigue, and recurrent bouts of flu-like illness which can be either short and mild or prolonged and extremely debilitating. While its etiology is unknown, viral infection is strongly suspected, with 85% of sufferers experiencing an initial acute onset of flu-like symptoms, such as mild fever, sore throat, tender lymph nodes, and chills, accompanied by extreme fatigue after minimal exertion. This is then followed by such chronic manifestations as myalgia, migrating arthralgias (but no joint swelling or pain), sleep disorders, headaches, hypo- or hypersensitivities, cognitive disorders, such as spatial disorientation and short-term memory loss, disabling fatigue and malaise, depression, anxiety, irritability, and confusion, fluctuations in weight, and abdominal pain, nausea, and vomiting. Other complaints include muscle fatigue, worsening PMS, blurred vision, tachycardia, paresthesias, dry eyes, dry mouth, cough, night sweats, skin rashes, and decreased sexual desire. While the incidence of the above symptoms vary from patient to patient, the incidence of severe, disabling fatigue is 100%. In addition, patients with this condition often have a history of multiple allergies. Early studies indicated that this disease affected a predominance of women. However, recent studies suggest this may not be the case. Most patients are between 25-40 years of age.

In terms of Western medical diagnosis, there are no absolute clinical indicators or laboratory tests confirming this diagnosis. It is diagnosed mainly by the patient's presenting symptoms and history and by ruling out all other conditions with similar constellations of signs and symptoms, such as SLE, RA, and FMS. Some sources lump CFIDS and FMS together. However, we believe that there are differences between these two conditions. For instance, FMS sufferers experience a much higher and more significant incidence of myalgias and arthralgias. In addition, CFIDS sufferers suffer from more recurrent flu-like symptoms, often "catching cold" with every in-coming low pressure system. In all probability, FMS is the more common condition and CFIDS is the rarer condition. It has been estimated that 75% of those patients diagnosed with FMS actually have CFIDS.

There is no specific Western medical treatment for CFIDS. Its current treatment is based on the management of its symptoms. For sleep disturbances, tricyclic antidepressants, serotonin-uptake inhibitors, and benzodiazepine and clonazepam are the drugs of choice. For headaches, NSAIDs are recommended for tension headaches and calcium channel blockers are prescribed for migraines. Muscle-relaxants, such as Flexeril, NSAIDs, and clonazepam are used for arthralgias and myalgias. H-2 blockers such as Zantac are prescribed for gastro-intestinal symptoms. Candidiasis is treated with ketoconazole (Nizoral) and fluconazole (Diflucan). Fatigue is treated with buproprion (Wellbutrin) and intramuscular injections of vitamin B_{12} and/or gamma globulin. For depression, antidepressants such as fluoxetine (Prozac) are prescribed. In addition, various immunomodulating and antiviral agents are sometimes prescribed experimentally.

CHINESE DISEASE CATEGORIZATION: The main, over-riding complaint of this condition is fatigue. Therefore, it is categorized as *xu lao*, vacuity taxation, in Chinese medicine. As with FMS above, each of its major accompanying symptoms is also typically its own traditional disease in Chinese medicine. For instance, swollen, tender cervical lymphnodes are categorized as *luo li,* scrofula, while low-grade fever is *fa re*, literally "emission of heat."

DISEASE CAUSES: External contraction of the six environmental excesses, internal damage by the seven affects, unregulated eating and drinking, iatrogenesis, and aging

DISEASE MECHANISMS: In our experience, the core disease mechanisms at work in CFIDS are a liver-spleen disharmony. Liver depression qi stagnation may be due to unfulfilled desires or anger damaging the liver. However, it may also be due to insufficient blood nourishing the liver or insufficient yang warming and steaming the liver. Spleen vacuity is due to either faulty diet, excessive taxation, excessive thinking and especially worry and anxiety, too little physical exercise, overuse of bitter, cold medicinals, including Western antibiotics, living in a damp, hot environment, and liver wood assailing spleen earth. If the liver becomes depressed, the qi and, therefore, blood and body fluids all will not flow smoothly and easily as they should. Liver qi symptoms include chest, breast, rib-side, and abdominal oppression, distention, fullness, and pain, emotional depression, irritability, headaches, PMS, and dysmenorrhea. Spleen qi vacuity symptoms include fatigue, lack of strength and/or warmth in the extremities, poor appetite, and loose stools. Damp accumulation symptoms include edema, abnormal vaginal discharge, damp skin lesions, and damp impediment. If dampness congeals into phlegm, there may be phlegm nodulation, phlegm in the lungs, or phlegm harassing and disquieting the heart spirit. Blood stasis may result in painful menstruation or any fixed location pain in the body.

Based on this core disease mechanism of liver-spleen disharmony, numerous other disease mechanisms may also be engendered. Since the defensive qi issues from the middle burner, spleen qi vacuity leads to defensive qi not securing with easy invasion of external evils. If spleen vacuity fails to transform and engender sufficient new blood, there will be heart and/or liver blood vacuity. If blood vacuity endures, it may give rise to yin vacuity, internal stirring of wind, worsening of liver depression, or blood stasis. If spleen vacuity endures, it may eventually reach the kidneys, damaging yang. In that case, there will be a spleen-kidney yang vacuity and vacuity cold which may constrict and congeal the blood, hence also causing blood stasis. In addition, if both the spleen and kidney yang are vacuous and weak, water metabolism must be even more negatively affected. If liver depression worsens or endures, qi depression may transform heat. This may give rise to liver fire flaming upward or ascendant liver yang hyperactivity. Heat in the liver may mutually engender heat in the stomach, spleen, heart, lungs, bladder, and/or blood. If heat endures it will damage and consume yin fluids. Further, when heat flares upward, it harasses the spirit and the clear orifices above. According to Li Dong-yuan, when heat flares upward from the lower burner, it also consumes and damages the spleen qi. If dampness due to spleen vacuity and faulty diet unites with or engenders depressive heat, damp heat may pour downward, to the bladder, uterus, and lower limbs. It may also spill over into the space between the muscles and the skin. Damp heat pouring downward may damage liver and kidney yin at the same time as it stirs ministerial fire to flare upward. All of the signs and symptoms of CFIDS are due to some combination of these inter-related disease mechanisms.

Because CFIDS and fibromyalgia syndrome are so similar in clinical manifestations, the causes and disease mechanisms of these disorders are essentially the same. However, in CFIDS, there is typically a definite initial wind heat external invasion, and retained or deep-lying warm evils are suspected thereafter. In addition, any arthralgias and myalgias present in CFIDS tend to manifest more as wind damp cold impediment and malnourishment of the sinews and vessels as opposed to wind damp heat impediment patterns. Under "Treatment based on pattern discrimination" below, we only discuss those patterns which are unique to this condition. Therefore, the reader should also refer to the patterns and their treatments under fibromyalgia syndrome for a fuller range of possible presenting patterns.

TREATMENT BASED ON PATTERN DISCRIMINATION:

1. INTERIOR VACUITY-EXTERIOR REPLETION PATTERN

MAIN SYMPTOMS: Acute onset of sore, swollen throat, fever, sweating or no sweating, muscle aches, fatigue, lack of strength, torpid intake, a pale, fat tongue with teeth-marks on its edges and yellow and white fur, and a floating, fine, bowstring, slightly rapid pulse

NOTE: In our experience, all patients who develop CFIDS have an underlying habitual bodily vacuity which allows wind heat evils to lodge in the body and become deep-lying. Therefore, simply resolving the exterior and clearing heat is not clinically adequate or even standard professional Chinese medicine.

TREATMENT PRINCIPLES: Dispel wind and clear heat while supporting the righteous

RX: *Xiao Chai Hu Tang Jia Wei* (Minor Bupleurum Decoction with Added Flavors)

INGREDIENTS: Radix Isatidis Seu Baphicacanthi (*Ban Lan Gen*) and Radix Scrophualariae Ningpoensis (*Xuan Shen*), 15g each, Radix Arctii Lappae (*Niu Bang Zi*) and Radix Scutellariae Baicalensis (*Huang Qin*), Radix Bupleuri (*Chai Hu*), Radix Codonopsitis Pilosulae (*Dang Shen*), and Rhizoma Pinelliae Ternatae (*Ban Xia*), 9g each, mix-fried Radix Glycyrrhizae (*Gan Cao*), 6g, uncooked Rhizoma

Zingberis (*Sheng Jiang*), 2 slices, and Fructus Zizyphi Jujubae (*Da Zao*), 2 pieces

ANALYSIS OF FORMULA: *Chai Hu, Niu Bang Zi,* and *Sheng Jiang* together dispel wind from the exterior. *Chai Hu, Ban Xia,* and *Huang Qin* together resolve and harmonize the shao yang and drain evils lodged in the body which have become deep-lying. *Ban Lan Gen* and *Xuan Shen* clear heat, resolve toxins, and disinhibit the throat. *Dang Shen, Da Zao,* mix-fried *Gan Cao,* and *Dang Shen* boost the qi and support the righteous. In addition, *Dang Shen* supplements without retaining evils inside the body as do many supplementing medicinals.

ADDITIONS & SUBTRACTIONS: If there is marked swelling of the lymphnodes, add 15 grams each of Bulbus Fritillariae Thunbergii (*Zhe Bei Mu*) and Spica Prunellae Vulgaris (*Xia Ku Cao*). If there is blood vacuity or the patient "catches cold" at each menstruation, add 12 grams of cooked Radix Rehmanniae (*Shu Di*) and nine grams each of Radix Angelicae Sinensis (*Dang Gui*), Radix Albus Paeoniae Lactiflorae (*Bai Shao*), and Radix Ligustici Wallichii (*Chuan Xiong*). If there is nasal congestion, add nine grams each of Radix Angelicae Dahuricae (*Bai Zhi*) and Herba Menthae Haplocalycis (*Bo He*). If there is marked muscle-joint pain, add nine grams each of Radix Et Rhizoma Notopterygii (*Qiang Huo*) and Radix Ledebouriellae Divaricatae (*Fang Feng*) and 15 grams of Radix Puerariae (*Ge Gen*). If there is high fever and thirst, add 20 grams of Gypsum Fibrosum (*Shi Gao*) and 12 grams of Rhizoma Anemarrhenae Aspheloidis (*Zhi Mu*).

ACUPUNCTURE & MOXIBUSTION: *He Gu* (LI 4), *Da Zhui* (GV 14), *Feng Men* (Bl 12), *Zu San Li* (St 36)

ANALYSIS OF FORMULA: Draining *He Gu, Da Zhui,* and *Feng Men* dispels wind and clears heat. Supplementing *Zu San Li* boosts the qi and supports the righteous.

ADDITIONS & SUBTRACTIONS: If there is marked swelling of the lymphnodes, add *Que Pen* (St 12) and *Nao Hui* (TB 13). If there is blood vacuity or the patient "catches cold" at each menstruation, add *San Yin Jiao* (Sp 6). If there is nasal congestion, add *Yin Tang* (M-HN-3). If there is marked muscle-joint pain, add *Qu Chi* (LI 11) and *Yin Ling Quan* (Sp 9). If there is high fever and thirst, add *Wai Guan* (TB 5) and *Qu Chi* (LI 11).

2. TAXATION MALARIA PATTERN

MAIN SYMPTOMS: Taxation malaria-like disorders are characterized by chronic extreme fatigue and recurrent low-grade fevers due to a combination of qi and yin vacuities with vacuity heat harassing internally and liver depression qi stagnation. The signs and symptoms of spleen qi vacuity include: fatigue, especially after eating, abdominal bloating after eating, a tendency to loose stools but possibly constipation, cold hands and feet, lack of strength in the four extremities, dizziness when standing up, easy bruising, easy contraction of colds and flus, a swollen tongue with teeth-marks on its edges, and a fine pulse which is often soggy or soft in the right bar position. The signs and symptoms of liver blood-kidney yin vacuity with vacuity heat include: night sweats, hot flashes, vexatious heat in the five hearts, tinnitus, dizziness, thirst or a dry mouth but little or no desire to drink, recurrent, dry, sore throat, especially in the evening and upon waking, malar and/or auricular flushing in the afternoon or early evening, stiffness of the sinews, numbness and/or tingling of the extremities, matitudinal insomnia, a pale red tongue or a pale tongue with red tip and scanty tongue fur, and a fine, rapid or possibly floating, surging pulse. The signs and symptoms of liver depression include: premenstrual or menstrual lower abdominal distention, lower abdominal cramping, premenstrual breast distention and pain, irritability, emotional depression, and a bowstring pulse.

NOTE: In our experience, this pattern describes a common one in Westerners with CFIDS. In Chinese medicine, malaria does not just mean an infection by *Plasmodium faciliparum.* It includes any disease characterized by shortly spaced remittent episodes, and there are several kinds of malaria-like diseases in Chinese medicine, taxation malaria being one of them. We have chosen to use this pattern name to emphasize the probable existence of hidden warm evils in this condition.

TREATMENT PRINCIPLES: Supplement vacuity and check malaria, course the liver and rectify the qi

RX: *Bu Zhong Yi Qi Tang Jia Wei* (Supplement the Center & Boost the Qi Decoction with Added Flavors)

INGREDIENTS: Radix Astragali Membranacei (*Huang Qi*) and processed Radix Polygoni Multiflori (*He Shou Wu*), 15g each, Radix Achyranthis Bidentatae (*Niu Xi*), 12g, Radix Codonopsitis Pilosulae (*Dang Shen*), Rhizoma Atractylodis Macrocephalae (*Bai Zhu*), Rhizoma Anemarrhenae Aspheloidis (*Zhi Mu*), Fructus Pruni Mume (*Wu Mei*), and Fructus Amomi Tsao-kuo (*Cao Guo*), 9g each, mix-fried Radix Glycyrrhizae (*Gan Cao*), Radix Angelicae Sinensis (*Dang Gui*), and Pericarpium Citri Reticulatae (*Chen Pi*), 6g each, Rhizoma Cimicifugae (*Sheng Ma*), 4.5g, and Radix Bupleuri (*Chai Hu*), 1-3g

ANALYSIS OF FORMULA: *Huang Qi, Dang Shen,* mix-fried *Gan Cao,* and *Bai Zhu* all fortify the spleen and boost the qi. *Huang Qi* and *Bai Zhu* particularly supplement and secure the defensive qi. *Chai Hu* and *Sheng Ma* upbear yang and disinhibit the qi mechanism. Rectification of the qi is also aided by *Chen Pi*'s harmonizing of the stomach and downbearing of turbidity. Because *Chai Hu* and *Sheng Ma* both also resolve the exterior, these two ingredients in small doses can out-thrust any lingering exterior evils as well as exteriorize evils hidden or latent in the blood division. *Dang Gui* and *He Shou Wu* both nourish and supplement the blood. Nourishment of liver blood indirectly promotes the liver's function of coursing and discharging. *Dang Gui* also quickens the blood, while *He Shou Wu* has some ability to quiet the spirit. The combination of *Dang Gui, He Shou Wu* and *Niu Xi* supplements yin and nourishes the sinews. *Niu Xi* also leads the blood and, therefore, ministerial fire back downward to its lower source, especially when combined with *Zhi Mu* which enriches yin and clears vacuity heat. *Wu Mei* engenders fluids, kills parasites, astringes the lung and large intestine qi, and, according to Ye Tian-shi, restrains or controls liver repletion. *Cao Guo* strongly dries dampness, stops malarial disorders, and rectifies the qi. The combination of *Cao Guo, Zhi Mu,* and *Chai Hu* is a recognized anti-*nue* combination recommended by Bensky & Gamble. Likewise, Wiseman & Feng recommend the combination of *He Shou Wu, Niu Xi,* and *Wu Mei* for taxation *nue*, while the Qing dynasty writer, Xin Fuzhong, recommends the combination of *Wu Mei* and *Cao Guo* for taxation *nue*.[1]

ADDITIONS & SUBTRACTIONS: For severe fatigue, increase the dosage of *Dang Shen* up to 20 grams and *Huang Qi* up to 30 grams. For fatigue and/or abdominal bloating after eating, add nine grams of Rhizoma Acori Graminei (*Shi Chang Pu*) and Radix Auklandiae Lappae (*Mu Xiang*). For easy contraction of colds and flus, add nine grams of Radix Ledebouriellae Divaricatae (*Fang Feng*). For night sweats, add nine grams each of Cortex Phellodendri (*Huang Bai*) and Fructus Schisandrae Chinensis (*Wu Wei Zi*). For hot flashes and vexatious heat in the five hearts, add nine grams each of Cortex Phellodendri (*Huang Bai*) and Cortex Radicis Lycii Chinensis (*Di Gu Pi*). For thirst or a dry mouth but little or no desire to drink, add nine grams of Tuber Ophiopogonis Japonici (*Mai Men Dong*). For recurrent, dry, sore throat, especially in the evening, add 12 grams of Radix Scrophulariae Ningpoensis (*Xuan Shen*) and one gram of Cortex Cinnamomi Cassiae (*Rou Gui*). For stiffness of the sinews and numbness and/or tingling of the extremities, add 20 grams of Caulis Milletiae Seu Spatholobi (*Ji Xue Teng*). For matitudinal insomnia, add 12 grams each of Semen Zizyphi Spinosae (*Suan Zao Ren*), Cortex Albizziae Julibrissinis (*He Huan Pi*), and Semen Biotae Orientalis (*Bai Zi Ren*). For premenstrual or menstrual lower abdominal distention, lower abdominal cramping, premenstrual breast distention and pain, irritability, and emotional depression, add nine grams each of Rhizoma Cyperi Rotundi (*Xiang Fu*), Radix Ligustici Wallichii (*Chuan Xiong*), and Radix Albus Paeoniae Lactiflorae (*Bai Shao*).

ACUPUNCTURE & MOXIBUSTION: *Jian Shi* (Per 5), *Da Zhui* (GV 14), *He Gu* (LI 4), *Zu San Li* (St 36), *Fu Liu* (Ki 7)
ANALYSIS OF FORMULA: *Jian Shi* is a key point for treating malaria. When drained, it also courses the liver and rectifies the qi. *Da Zhui* is the intersection point of all the yang channels. It is also a main point for treating malaria. When needled with the supplementing method, it supplements vacuity. Supplementing *He Gu* supplements the exterior, while supplementing *Zu San Li* supplements the interior. *Fu Liu* enriches yin, supplements the liver and kidneys, and supports the righteous.

ADDITIONS & SUBTRACTIONS: For severe fatigue, add *Pi Shu* (Bl 20) and *Wei Shu* (Bl 21). For marked liver depression, add *Tai Chong* (Liv 3). For marked liver-kidney yin vacuity, add *Gan Shu* (Bl 18) and *Shen Shu* (Bl 23). For fatigue and/or abdominal bloating after eating, add *Tai Bai* (Sp 3) and *Yin Ling Quan* (Sp 9). For night sweats, hot flashes, and vexatious heat in the five hearts, add *Yin Xi* (Ht 6). For recurrent, dry, sore throat, especially in the evening, add *Zhao Hai* (Ki 6) and *Lie Que* (Lu 7). For stiffness of the sinews and numbness and/or tingling of the extremities, add *Wai Guan* (TB 5) and *Cheng Shan* (Bl 57). For matitudinal insomnia, add *Shen Men* (Ht 7) and *Shen Ting* (GV 24). For premenstrual or menstrual lower abdominal distention, lower abdominal cramping, premenstrual breast distention and pain, irritability, and emotional depression, add *Gui Lai* (St 29) and *Tai Chong* (Liv 3) and replace *Fu Liu* with *San Yin Jiao* (Sp 6).

3. HEART MALNOURISHMENT WITH LIVER DEPRESSION PATTERN

MAIN SYMPTOMS: A long period of extreme fatigue, a wan affect, emotional depression, insomnia, impaired memory, occasional desire to sigh, shortness of breath, a faint, weak voice or disinclination to speak, heart palpitations or fluster, no thought of eating or drinking, lack of strength, flabby muscles, possible muscle-joint soreness and pain, a fat, pale red tongue with white fur, and a fine, bowstring pulse

NOTE: This pattern has also been called liver qi vacuity. However, we believe that name is a misnomer for a liver-spleen disharmony where spleen vacuity resulting in heart qi and blood vacuity are more pronounced than liver depression.

TREATMENT PRINCIPLES: Supplement the heart qi and blood by fortifying the spleen and boosting the qi, course the liver and resolve depression, quiet the spirit

RX: *Bu Gan Yi Qi Tang* (Supplement the Liver & Boost the Qi Decoction)

INGREDIENTS: Radix Astragali Membranacei (*Huang Qi*),

Herba Agrimoniae Pilosae (*Xian He Cao*), and Bulbus Lilii (*Bai He*), 30g each, Radix Rubrus Panacis Ginseng (*Hong Shen*), Fructus Corni Officinalis (*Shan Zhu Yu*), Radix Bupleuri (*Chai Hu*), Fructus Citri Aurantii (*Zhi Ke*), Pericarpium Citri Reticulatae (*Chen Pi*), and Radix Angelicae Sinensis (*Dang Gui*), 9g each, and Rhizoma Atractylodis Macrocephalae (*Bai Zhu*) and Radix Albus Paeoniae Lactiflorae (*Bai Shao*), 12g each

ANALYSIS OF FORMULA: Within this formula, *Huang Qi, Xian He Cao, Hong Shen,* and *Bai Zhu* all supplement the spleen and boost the qi. *Chai Hu, Zhi Ke,* and *Chen Pi* course the liver and rectify the qi. *Dang Gui* and *Bai Shao* supplement the blood, thus nourishing the heart spirit above as well as harmonizing and emolliating the liver below. *Bai He* nourishes heart blood and yin and thus quiets the spirit. *Shan Zhu Yu* is an astringing medicinal, but it also supplements liver blood and kidney qi. Hence, it is sometimes also said to fill the essence and invigorate yang. Since the former and latter heavens are mutually rooted, its inclusion in this formula helps make the formula more harmonious and holistic.

ADDITIONS & SUBTRACTIONS: If there is a tendency toward heat, add 3-6 grams of Rhizoma Coptidis Chinensis (*Huang Lian*) and nine grams of Radix Scutellariae Baicalensis (*Huang Qin*). If there is concomitant yang vacuity, add nine grams each of Herba Epimedii (*Xian Ling Pi*) and Rhizoma Curculiginis Orchioidis (*Xian Mao*). If there is torpid intake, add nine grams each of Massa Medica Fermentata (*Shen Qu*), Fructus Crataegi (*Shan Zha*), and Fructus Germinatus Hordei Vulgaris (*Mai Ya*). If there is insomnia and heart palpitations, add nine grams of Radix Sophorae Flavescentis (*Ku Shen*) and 12-15 grams of stir-fried Semen Zizyphi Spinosae (*Suan Zao Ren*). If there is concomitant dampness, add 12 grams of Sclerotium Poriae Cocos (*Fu Ling*) and nine grams of Rhizoma Pinelliae Ternatae (*Ban Xia*), at least as a beginning. If there is yin vacuity, add 9-12 grams of Fructus Lycii Chinensis (*Gou Qi Zi*), Fructus Ligustri Lucidi (*Nu Zhen Zi*), Fructus Schisandrae Chinensis (*Wu Wei Zi*), and/or processed Radix Polygoni Multiflori (*He Shou Wu*). If there is vacuity heat, add 9-12 grams of Rhizoma Anemarrhenae Aspheloidis (*Zhi Mu*) and Cortex Phellodendri (*Huang Bai*). If there is blood stasis, add nine grams of Radix Rubrus Paeoniae Lactiflorae (*Chi Shao*), Radix Salviae Miltiorrhizae (*Dan Shen*), Cortex Radicis Moutan (*Dan Pi*), and/or Herba Leonuri Heterophylli (*Yi Mu Cao*). If there are lingering wind evils in the exterior, add nine grams of Radix Ledebouriellae Divaricatae (*Fang Feng*), while for warm evils hidden or deeply lying in the blood, consider adding 9-15 grams of Radix Lithospermi Seu Arnebiae (*Zi Cao*), Flos Lonicerae Japonicae (*Jin Yin Hua*), Fructus Forsythiae Suspensae (*Lian Qiao*), Herba Taraxaci Mongolici Cum Radice (*Pu Gong Ying*), and/or Radix Isatidis Seu Baphicacanthi (*Ban Lan Gen*).

ACUPUNCTURE & MOXIBUSTION: *Xin Shu* (Bl 15), *Dan Zhong* (CV 17), *Shen Men* (Ht 7), *Zu San Li* (St 36), *San Yin Jiao* (Sp 6), *Tai Chong* (Liv 3)

ANALYSIS OF FORMULA: Using supplementing technique on *Xin Shu, Dan Zhong,* and *Shen Men* supplements the heart and quiets the spirit. Supplementing *Zu San Li* and *San Yin Jiao* fortifies the spleen and supplements the qi. Draining *Tai Chong* courses the liver and rectifies the qi.

ADDITIONS & SUBTRACTIONS: For marked liver depression qi stagnation, add *He Gu* (LI 4). If there is rib-side distention, add *Qi Men* (Liv 14) and/or *Zhang Men* (Liv 13). If there is heat harassing the heart, add *Da Ling* (Per 7). If there is liver depression/depressive heat, replace *Tai Chong* with *Xing Jian* (Liv 2). If there is stomach heat, add *Nei Ting* (St 44). If there are heart palpitations, add *Nei Guan* (Per 6) and/or *Jian Shi* (Per 5). If there are night sweats, add *Yin Xi* (Ht 6). If there are loose stools or diarrhea due to spleen vacuity, add *Pi Shu* (Bl 20) and *Wei Shu* (Bl 21). If there is muscle-joint soreness and pain, add *Yang Ling Quan* (GB 34) and *Ge Shu* (Bl 17) as well as local points near the affected area. If there is concomitant kidney yang vacuity, add moxibustion at *Shen Shu* (Bl 23) and *Ming Men* (GV 4).

REMARKS

1. Most patients with CFIDS have a history of one or more allergies, hypoglycemia, and candidiasis. Therefore, Chinese dietary therapy is extremely important. This means eating a hypoallergenic, yeast-free, clear, bland diet.

2. Although patients with CFIDS suffer from severe, debilitating disease, they should, nevertheless, try to get some physical exercise. The amount of exercise needs to be carefully regulated, however, so that the net result is more energy and feeling of dynamic well-being as opposed to further exhaustion and fatigue. The right amount of exercise for a particular patient can usually be arrived at by trial and error and usually needs to be constantly adjusted. It is very important to realize the spleen-fortifying, liver-coursing, depression-resolving, and dampness-overcoming effects of exercise.

[1] The idea that many cases of CFIDS manifest qi and yin vacuities with vacuity heat and liver depression is corroborated by Yin Heng-ze in *Shang Hai Zhong Yi Yao Za Zhi (The Shanghai Journal of Chinese Medicine & Medicinals)*, #3, 1999, p. 19-20.

16

Chronic Glomerulonephritis

Chronic glomerulonephritis, also called chronic nephritic-proteinuric syndrome and slowly progressive glomerular disease, is a progressive deteriorating condition of the kidneys associated with a number of other diseases of different etiologies, including, for instance systemic lupus erythmatosus. However, each of these other diseases results in diffuse sclerosis of the glomeruli damaging kidney function. This disease or syndrome is, in fact, the most common cause of chronic kidney failure leading to end stage renal disease (ESRD). In its early stages, typically lasting for years, it is frequently asymptomatic, although urinanalysis is abnormal with RBCs, WBCs, and protein in the urine. During this stage, there is also often hypertension. As the disease progresses, there is edema in the lower extremities and persistent high blood pressure which is often recalcitrant to treatment. Signs of kidney failure or uremia are noted when there is severe loss of kidney function.

The Western medical diagnosis of glomerulonephritis in its early stage depends entirely on urinanalysis. Often this condition is diagnosed during routine physical examinations including blood analysis in otherwise asymptomatic patients. Certain blood tests which show inflammation in the kidneys can also show how much kidney function has been lost. Often it is necessary to do a kidney biopsy to determine the exact diagnosis and determine short- and long-term prognosis. In terms of Western medical treatment, this consists of treating the hypertension and restricting sodium intake. In addition, dietary phosphate and protein reduction and the administration of ACE inhibitors may slow the deterioration. However, as of this writing, no Western medical therapy has been proven to prevent progression of this condition.

Chinese disease categorization: Once this condition becomes symptomatic, it is categorized in Chinese medicine as *shui zhong*, water swelling, *yao tong*, low back pain, *xu lao*, vacuity taxation, and *xue niao*, hematuria.

Disease causes: Enduring disease and debility and decline due to aging

Disease mechanisms: According to Zhang Jie-bin in his *Jing Yue Quan Shu (The Complete Writings of Jing-yue)*, "Water swelling is associated with disease of the lungs, spleen, and kidneys. . . with its root being located in the kidneys." The lungs, spleen, and kidneys are the three viscera which control water fluids in the body. The lungs control the water passageways. It is the downward diffusion of the lung qi which moves water fluids downward through the body for eventual discharge from the bladder. The spleen governs the movement and transformation of water, and the kidneys govern the water of the entire body. If any or all of these three viscera fail to do their duty *vis à vis* water metabolism, edema may result. The ways in which the lungs, spleen, and kidneys may be damaged are legion. However, most chronic diseases result in spleen qi vacuity which eventually reaches the kidneys or in yin vacuity which also reaches the kidneys. In addition, the qi moves fluids throughout the body. Therefore, liver depression qi stagnation may result in accumulation of dampness. Further, blood and fluids flow together. Hence, anything that causes blood stasis may also give rise to damp accumulation, while damp accumulation may likewise engender blood stasis.

Treatment based on pattern discrimination:

1. Stasis & heat struggling & binding pattern

Main symptoms: Water swelling of the cheeks of the face and the four limbs which, when pressed, easily rebound, aversion to cold, fever, headache, dizziness, a dry mouth, a bitter taste in the mouth, eczema, ceaseless itching, scanty, hot, reddish yellow urine, a purple red tongue with slimy, yellow fur, and a bowstring, slippery, rapid pulse

NOTE: This pattern describes glomerulonephritis due to an infection that has reached the kidneys and become chronic. While the name of this pattern and its Chinese medicinal treatment below imply blood stasis, there are none of the common blood stasis signs or symptom listed above except for the purple tongue. However, itching can be a symptom of stasis, and stasis may also be assumed due to A) the presence of heat toxins and B) the chronic nature of this condition.

TREATMENT PRINCIPLES: Clear heat and resolve toxins, quicken the blood and disinhibit water

RX: *Long Kui She Mei Yi Mi Tang* (Solanum Negrum, Duchnesea & Coix Decoction)

INGREDIENTS: Herba Solani Nigri (*Long Kui*), Herba Duchneseae Indicae (*She Mei*), Semen Coicis Lachryma-jobi (*Yi Yi Ren*), Herba Leonuri Heterophylli (*Yi Mu Cao*), and Herba Solani Lyrati (*Shu Yang Quan*), 30g each, Cortex Phellodendri (*Huang Bai*), Rhizoma Atractylodis (*Cang Zhu*), Cortex Radicis Moutan (*Dan Pi*), uncooked Pollen Typhae (*Pu Huang*), Radix Salviae Miltiorrhizae (*Dan Shen*), Herba Lycopi Lucidi (*Ze Lan*), and Sclerotium Poriae Cocos (*Fu Ling*), 9g each, and Bombyx Batryticatus (*Jiang Can*), 4.5g

ANALYSIS OF FORMULA: *Long Kui* clears heat and resolves toxins, quickens the blood and disperses swelling, while *Shu Yang Quan* clears heat and resolves toxins, disinhibits dampness and dispels wind. *Huang Bai* clears heat and dries dampness. *Dan Pi* and *Dan Shen* cool and quicken the blood. *She Mei* also clears heat and cools the blood. However, it also resolves toxins and disperses swelling. *Cang Zhu*, *Fu Ling*, and *Yi Yi Ren* dry and seep dampness. *Yi Mu Cao*, *Pu Huang*, and *Ze Lan* quicken the blood and disinhibit dampness, and *Jiang Can* clears heat, dispels wind, and stops itching.

ADDITIONS & SUBTRACTIONS: For concomitant righteous qi vacuity, add 45 grams of Radix Astragali Membranacei (*Huang Qi*) and 15 grams each of Radix Codonopsitis Pilosulae (*Dang Shen*) and Rhizoma Atractylodis Macrocephalae (*Bai Zhu*).

ACUPUNCTURE & MOXIBUSTION: *He Gu* (LI 4), *San Yin Jiao* (Sp 6), *Yin Ling Quan* (Sp 9), *Xue Hai* (Sp 10), *Zhong Ji* (CV 3)

ANALYSIS OF FORMULA: Draining *San Yin Jiao, Yin Ling Quan*, and *Zhong Ji* clears heat and eliminates dampness, disperses swelling and disinhibits urination. Draining *San Yin Jiao, Xue Hai*, and *He Gu* quickens the blood and dispels stasis. *He Gu* also clears heat and frees the flow in the exterior.

ADDITIONS & SUBTRACTIONS: For marked blood stasis, add *Ge Shu* (Bl 17). For marked aversion to cold and fever, add *Wai Guan* (TB 5). For headache and dizziness, add *Feng Chi* (GB 20). For a dry mouth with a bitter taste, add *Qiu Xu* (GB 40). For eczema and ceaseless itching, add *Qu Chi* (LI 11). For scanty, hot, reddish yellow urine, add *Pang Guang Shu* (Bl 28) and *Tong Li* (Ht 5).

2. FLOODING OF WIND & WATER PATTERN

MAIN SYMPTOMS: Puffy eyelids initially leading to generalized edema, recent onset, rapidly developing edema which is most pronounced in the face, a bright, shiny facial complexion, possible fever and chills, generalized aching and pain, inhibited urination, a normal tongue or a somewhat red tongue with either thin, white or thin, yellow fur, and a floating, tight or floating, rapid pulse

NOTE: This pattern describes external contraction of evils and an exterior pattern. In real-life patients, this pattern typically only complicates other patterns in which the righteous qi is already damaged and external evils are taking advantage of vacuity to invade and enter the body. Therefore, although the edema may be sudden, the patient has probably had albuminuria and hypertension for some time.

TREATMENT PRINCIPLES: Course wind and resolve the exterior, seep dampness and disperse swelling

RX: *Ma Huang Lian Qiao Chi Xiao Dou Tang Jia Jian* (Ephedra, Forsythia & Aduki Bean Decoction with Additions & Subtractions)

INGREDIENTS: Semen Phaseoli Calcarati (*Chi Xiao Dou*), 30g, Sclerotium Poriae Cocos (*Fu Ling*) and Rhizoma Alismatis (*Ze Xie*), 24g each, Fructus Forsythiae Suspensae (*Lian Qiao*), 15g, honey mix-fried Herba Ephedrae (*Ma Huang*), Rhizoma Atractylodis Macrocephalae (*Bai Zhu*), and Radix Stephaniae Tetrandrae (*Fan Ji*), 12g each, uncooked Rhizoma Zingiberis (*Sheng Jiang*), 3 slices, and Fructus Zizyphi Jujubae (*Da Zao*), 3 pieces

ANALYSIS OF FORMULA: *Ma Huang* and *Sheng Jiang* course wind and resolve the exterior. In addition, *Ma Huang* disinhibits the urination. *Chi Xiao Dou*, *Ze Xie*, *Fu Ling*, *Bai Zhu*, and *Han Fang Ji* disinhibit water and disperse swelling, and *Lian Qiao* clears heat and resolves toxins. *Da Zao* harmonizes the other medicinals in this formula.

ADDITIONS & SUBTRACTIONS: If wind heat is pronounced with marked sore throat, add 30 grams of uncooked Gypsum Fibrosum (*Shi Gao*), 15 grams each of

Flos Lonicerae Japonicae (*Jin Yin Hua*), Rhizoma Phragmitis Communis (*Lu Gen*), and Radix Isatidis Seu Baphicacanthi (*Ban Lan Gen*), and six grams of Radix Platycodi Grandiflori (*Jie Geng*). If wind cold is marked with aversion to cold and a floating, tight pulse, delete *Lian Qiao* and add nine grams each of Folium Perillae Frutescentis (*Zi Su Ye*) and Radix Ledebouriellae Divaricatae (*Fang Feng*) and six grams each of Ramulus Cinnamomi Cassiae (*Gui Zhi*) and Herba Lemnae Seu Spirodelae (*Fu Ping*). If cough is severe, add nine grams each of Radix Peucedani (*Qian Hu*) and Semen Pruni Armeniacae (*Xing Ren*).

ACUPUNCTURE & MOXIBUSTION: *Lie Que* (Lu 7), *He Gu* (LI 4), *Fei Shu* (Bl 13), *Yin Ling Quan* (Sp 9), *Zhong Ji* (CV 3)

ANALYSIS OF FORMULA: Draining *Lie Que*, *Fei Shu*, and *He Gu* clears heat and resolves toxins, diffuses the lungs and disinhibits water, especially in the face and upper part of the body. Draining *Yin Ling Quan* and *Zhong Ji* eliminates dampness, disinhibits urination, and treats the edema.

ADDITIONS & SUBTRACTIONS: If wind heat is pronounced with marked sore throat, add *Wai Guan* (TB 5) and *Qu Chi* (LI 11). If wind cold is marked, add *Feng Chi* (GB 20) with moxibustion. If cough is severe, add *Chi Ze* (Lu 5) or *Feng Men* (Bl 12).

3. LUNG-KIDNEY QI VACUITY PATTERN

MAIN SYMPTOMS: Facial edema, swollen limbs, a yellow facial complexion, scanty urination, scanty qi, lack of strength, easy catching of cold, lower and upper back soreness and pain, a pale tongue with white, moist fur and teethmarks on its edges, and a fine, weak pulse

TREATMENT PRINCIPLES: Boost the lungs and enrich the kidneys

RX: *Yu Ping Feng San Jia Wei* (Jade Windscreen Powder with Added Flavors)

INGREDIENTS: Semen Plantaginis (*Che Qian Zi*) and Epicarpium Benincasae Hispidae (*Dong Gua Pi*), 30g each, uncooked Radix Astragali Membranacei (*Huang Qi*), Radix Codonopsitis Pilosulae (*Dang Shen*), Sclerotium Poriae Cocos (*Fu Ling*), Sclerotium Polypori Umbellati (*Zhu Ling*), Rhizoma Alismatis (*Ze Xie*), Radix Achyranthis Bidentatae (*Niu Xi*), and Ramulus Loranthi Seu Visci (*Sang Ji Sheng*), 15g each, Rhizoma Atractylodis Macrocephalae (*Bai Zhu*) and Radix Ledebouriellae Divaricatae (*Fang Feng*), 9g each, and Ramulus Cinnamomi Cassiae (*Gui Zhi*), Fructus Amomi (*Sha Ren*), and Fructus Cardamomi (*Bai Dou Kou*), 6g each

ANALYSIS OF FORMULA: *Huang Qi*, *Dang Shen*, and *Bai Zhu* supplement the qi and secure the exterior, while *Gui Zhi* and *Fang Feng* gently out-thrust any lingering exterior evils. In addition, *Huang Qi* and *Bai Zhu* disinhibit the urination. *Che Qian Zi*, *Dong Gua Pi*, *Fu Ling*, *Zhu Ling*, and *Ze Xie* disinhibit dampness and disperse swelling, while *Niu Xi* and *Sang Ji Sheng* supplement the kidneys. *Sha Ren* and *Bai Dou Kou* warm the spleen and dry dampness.

ADDITIONS & SUBTRACTIONS: If there is aversion to cold with fever and cough, add six grams of Herba Ephedrae (*Ma Huang*), 20 grams of Gypsum Fibrosum (*Shi Gao*), and three grams of uncooked Rhizoma Zingiberis (*Sheng Jiang*). For fever with a sore, swollen throat, subtract *Gui Zhi*, *Sha Ren*, and *Bai Dou Kou* and add 12 grams each of Fructus Forsythiae Suspensae (*Lian Qiao*), Flos Lonicerae Japonicae (*Jin Yin Hua*), and Radix Sophorae Subprostratae (*Shan Dou Gen*). For severe edema, add 15 grams each of Semen Plantaginis (*Che Qian Zi*) and Pericarpium Arecae Catechu (*Da Fu Pi*). For hematuria, add 15 grams of Herba Cephalanoploris Segeti (*Xiao Ji*). For concomitant blood stasis, add 12 grams each of Herba Lycopi Lucidi (*Ze Lan*) and Herba Leonuri Heterophylli (*Yi Mu Cao*).

For lung-spleen qi vacuity, without severe kidney qi vacuity, use *Yu Ping Feng San Jia Wei* (Jade Windscreen Powder with Added Flavors): Radix Astragali Membranacei (*Huang Qi*) and Sclerotium Poriae Cocos (*Fu Ling*), 15-30g each, Radix Dioscoreae Oppositae (*Shan Yao*), 15g, Rhizoma Atractylodis Macrocephalae (*Bai Zhu*), 12g, Radix Codonopsitis Pilosulae (*Dang Shen*) and Semen Nelumbinis Nuciferae (*Lian Zi*), 9g each, and Radix Ledebouriellae Divaricatae (*Fang Feng*), 6g. If there is severe edema and/or scanty urine, add 9-12 grams each of Semen Plantaginis (*Che Qian Zi*), Rhizoma Alismatis (*Ze Xie*), and Sclerotium Polypori Umbellati (*Zhu Ling*). For reduced appetite, add nine grams each of Endothelium Corneum Gigeriae Galli (*Ji Nei Jin*) and Fructus Germinatus Hordei Vulgaris (*Mai Ya*). For more marked kidney vacuity, add nine grams each of Radix Achyranthis Bidentatae (*Niu Xi*) and Ramulus Loranthi Seu Visci (*Sang Ji Sheng*).

ACUPUNCTURE & MOXIBUSTION: *Shen Shu* (Bl 23), *Jing Gu* (Bl 64), *He Gu* (LI 4), *Zu San Li* (St 36), *Zhong Ji* (CV 3)

ANALYSIS OF FORMULA: *Shen Shu* and *Jing Gu* are an empirical formula for the treatment of glomerulonephritis. When needled with even supplementing-even draining method, they supplement the kidneys and disinhibit water. Supplementing *He Gu* and *Zu San Li* supplements the lungs, secures the exterior, and disinhibits dampness. Draining *Zhong Ji* disinhibits water and disperses swelling.

ADDITIONS & SUBTRACTIONS: If there is aversion to cold with fever and cough, add *Lie Que* (Lu 7), *Fei Shu* (Bl 13), and temporarily drain *He Gu* (LI 4). For fever with a sore, swollen throat, add *Wai Guan* (TB 5) and *Qu Chi* (LI 11) and temporarily drain *He Gu* (LI 4). For severe edema, add *Shui Dao* (St 28) and *Shui Fen* (CV 9). For hematuria, add *Xue Hai* (Sp 10). For concomitant blood stasis, add *San Yin Jiao* (Sp 6). For severe qi vacuity, add *Tai Bai* (Sp 3) and *Guan Yuan* (CV 4). For easy catching of cold, add *Da Zhui* (GV 14) with moxibustion. For lung-spleen qi vacuity without severe kidney qi vacuity, subtract *Shen Shu* and *Jing Gu* and add *San Yin Jiao* (Sp 6) and *Tai Bai* (Sp 3).

4. Spleen-kidney yang vacuity pattern

Main symptoms: Marked superficial edema which tends to be worse in the lower half of the body, pitting edema, clear, scanty urination, a bright, white or dark facial complexion, fear of cold, chilled limbs, lower and upper back soreness or neck soreness and lower leg limpness, heel pain, lassitude of the spirit, torpid intake, possible loose stools, decreased sexual function or menstrual irregularity, a tender, fat, pale tongue with teeth-marks on its edges, and a deep, fine or deep, slow, forceless pulse

Treatment principles: Warm and supplement the spleen and kidneys, seep water and disperse swelling

Rx: If spleen yang vacuity is more pronounced, use *Shi Pi Yin Jia Jian* (Replete the Spleen Drink with Additions & Subtractions)

Ingredients: Semen Plantaginis (*Che Qian Zi*) and Epicarpium Benincasae Hispidae (*Dong Gua Pi*), 30g each, Sclerotium Poriae Cocos (*Fu Ling*) and Semen Phaseoli Calcarati (*Chi Xiao Dou*), 15g each, Rhizoma Atractylodis Macrocephalae (*Bai Zhu*), Cortex Magnoliae Officinalis (*Hou Po*), Pericarpium Arecae Catechu (*Da Fu Pi*), Radix Auklandiae Lappae (*Mu Xiang*), Radix Lateralis Praeparatus Aconiti Carmichaeli (*Fu Zi*), Fructus Amomi (*Sha Ren*), and Fructus Cardamomi (*Bai Dou Kou*), 9g each, and Fructus Amomi Tsao-ko (*Cao Guo*) and dried Rhizoma Zingiberis (*Gan Jiang*), 6g each

Analysis of formula: *Bai Zhu, Fu Ling, Fu Zi, Sha Ren, Bai Dou Kou, Cao Guo,* and *Gan Jiang* together supplement and warm the spleen, dry and/or seep dampness. *Che Qian Zi, Dong Gua Pi, Fu Ling, Chi Xiao Dou,* and *Da Fu Pi* seep dampness and disperse swelling. *Hou Po* and *Mu Xiang* combined with *Sha Ren* and *Bai Dou Kou* move the qi and arouse the spleen.

Additions & subtractions: If fatigue and lack of strength are marked, add 15 grams of Radix Astragali Membranacei (*Huang Qi*) and nine grams of Radix Codonopsitis Pilosulae (*Dang Shen*). For more marked kidney vacuity, add nine grams each of Radix Achyranthis Bidentatae (*Niu Xi*), Ramulus Loranthi Seu Visci (*Sang Ji Sheng*), and Herba Epimedii (*Yin Yang Huo*). For nausea, add 12 grams each of Rhizoma Pinelliae Ternatae (*Ban Xia*) and Pericarpium Citri Reticulatae (*Chen Pi*). For abdominal fullness after eating, borborygmus, flatulence, and edema which is worse in the abdominal region, add nine grams each of Semen Arecae Catechu (*Bing Lang*) and Fructus Immaturus Citri Aurantii (*Zhi Shi*). For concomitant blood stasis, add 12 grams each of Herba Lycopi Lucidi (*Ze Lan*) and Herba Leonuri Heterophylli (*Yi Mu Cao*).

For spleen vacuity with damp encumbrance but without kidney vacuity, replace *Shi Pi Yin Jia Jian* with *Shen Ling Bai Zhu San Jia Jian* (Ginseng, Poria & Atractylodes Powder with Additions & Subtractions): Radix Astragali Membranacei (*Huang Qi*) and Herba Leonuri Heterophylli (*Yi Mu Cao*), 30g each, Radix Dioscoreae Oppositae (*Shan Yao*) and Semen Coicis Lachryma-jobi (*Yi Yi Ren*), 20g each, Radix Codonopsitis Pilosulae (*Dang Shen*), Rhizoma Atractylodis Macrocephalae (*Bai Zhu*), Sclerotium Poriae Cocos (*Fu Ling*), Rhizoma Alismatis (*Ze Xie*), and Radix Stephaniae Tetrandrae (*Han Fang Ji*), 15g each, and Pericarpium Arecae Catechu (*Da Fu Pi*), 9g. For severe albuminuria, increase the dosage of *Huang Qi* up to 45 grams and add nine grams each of Semen Phaseoli Calcarati (*Chi Xiao Dou*) and Periostracum Cicadae (*Chan Tui*). For edema primarily in the upper body, add nine grams each of Herba Ephedrae (*Ma Huang*) and Folium Perillae Frutescentis (*Zi Su Ye*). For edema mainly in the lower part of the body, add nine grams of Semen Plantaginis (*Che Qian Zi*) and six grams of Semen Zanthoxyli Bungeani (*Jiao Mu*). For severe damp encumbrance, add nine grams each of Rhizoma Atractylodis (*Cang Zhu*) and Cortex Magnoliae Officinalis (*Hou Po*).

If there is damp heat with skin sores, replace *Shi Pi Yin Jia Jian* with *Wei Ling Tang Jia Wei* (Stomach Poria Decoction with Added Flavors): Semen Coicis Lachryma-jobi (*Yi Yi Ren*), 30g, Rhizoma Alismatis (*Ze Xie*), Semen Plantaginis (*Che Qian Zi*), and Sclerotium Poriae Cocos (*Fu Ling*), 20g each, Pericarpium Arecae Catechu (*Da Fu Pi*), Flos Lonicerae Japonicae (*Jin Yin Hua*), Fructus Forsythiae Suspensae (*Lian Qiao*), Radix Sophorae Flavescentis (*Ku Shen*), and Herba Taraxaci Mongolici Cum Radice (*Pu Gong Ying*), 15g each, Rhizoma Atractylodis Macrocephalae (*Bai Zhu*) and Rhizoma Atractylodis (*Cang Zhu*), 12g each, uncooked Cortex Rhizomatis Zingiberis (*Sheng Jiang Pi*) and Pericarpium Citri Reticulatae (*Chen Pi*), 6g each, and Radix Glycyrrhizae (*Gan Cao*), 3g. If there is concomitant constipation and dark urine, add 6-9 grams of Radix Et Rhizoma Rhei (*Da Huang*).

Acupuncture & moxibustion: *Zu San Li* (St 36), *San Yin Jiao* (Sp 6), *Yin Ling Quan* (Sp 9), *Guan Yuan* (CV 4)

Analysis of formula: Supplementing *Zu San Li, Guan*

Yuan, and *San Yin Jiao* with moxibustion warms and supplements mainly the spleen but also the kidneys. Draining *San Yin Jiao* and *Yin Ling Quan* disinhibits water and disperses swelling.

ADDITIONS & SUBTRACTIONS: If fatigue and lack of strength are marked, add *Tai Bai* (Sp 3). For nausea, add *Zhong Wan* (CV 12). For abdominal fullness after eating, borborygmus, flatulence, and edema predominantly in the abdomen, add *Nei Guan* (Per 6) and *Gong Sun* (Sp 4). For severe edema in the abdomen, also add *Shui Fen* (CV 9). For concomitant blood stasis, add *Ge Shu* (Bl 17). For severe edema in the limbs, add *Shui Dao* (St 28).

If kidney yang vacuity is more pronounced, use *Shen Qi Tang Jia Wei* (Kidney Qi Decoction with Added Flavors)

INGREDIENTS: Rhizoma Dioscoreae Hypoglaucae (*Bei Xie*) and Semen Plantaginis (*Che Qian Zi*), 30g each, uncooked Radix Rehmanniae (*Sheng Di*), Sclerotium Poriae Cocos (*Fu Ling*), Rhizoma Alismatis (*Ze Xie*), Radix Achyranthis Bidentatae (*Niu Xi*), Herba Epimedii (*Xiang Ling Pi*), and Ramulus Loranthi Seu Visci (*Sang Ji Sheng*), 15g each, Radix Dioscoreae Oppositae (*Shan Yao*), Fructus Corni Officinalis (*Shan Zhu Yu*), Cortex Radicis Moutan (*Dan Pi*), Radix Lateralis Praeparatus Aconiti Carmichaeli (*Fu Zi*), Fructus Amomi (*Sha Ren*), and Fructus Cardamomi (*Bai Dou Kou*), 9g each, Ramulus Cinnamomi Cassiae (*Gui Zhi*), 6g

ANALYSIS OF FORMULA: *Sheng Di, Niu Xi,* and *Sang Ji Sheng* enrich yin to engender yang. *Shan Yao, Yin Yang Huo, Shan Zhu Yu, Fu Zi,* and *Gui Zhi* supplement the kidneys and warm and invigorate yang. In addition, *Shan Yao* supplements the spleen and *Gui Zhi* frees the flow of yang and transforms the qi of the bladder. *Sha Ren* and *Bai Dou Kou* warm the spleen and dry dampness. *Bei Xie, Che Qian Zi, Ze Xie,* and *Fu Ling* disinhibit water and disperse swelling.

ADDITIONS & SUBTRACTIONS: If yang disease has reached yin, subtract *Yin Yang Huo* and add 12 grams each of Fructus Lycii Chinensis (*Gou Qi Zi*) and Tuber Asparagi Cochinensis (*Tian Men Dong*). For concomitant blood stasis, add 12 grams each of Herba Lycopi Lucidi (*Ze Lan*) and Herba Leonuri Heterophylli (*Yi Mu Cao*). For severe aversion to cold and low back pain with a cold sensation, add nine grams each of Radix Morindae Officinalis (*Ba Ji Tian*) and Rhizoma Curculiginis Orchioidis (*Xian Mao*). For heart palpitation and hasty panting, add 12 grams each of Semen Lepidii Seu Descurainiae (*Ting Li Zi*), Cortex Radicis Mori Albi (*Sang Bai Pi*), Herba Lycopi Lucidi (*Ze Lan*), and Radix Stephaniae Tetrandrae (*Han Fang Ji*). For hematuria, add 12 grams of Rhizoma Imperatae Cylindricae (*Bai Mao Gen*). If edema disappears but protein in the urine continues, add nine grams each of Fructus Rosae Laevigatae (*Jin Ying Zi*) and Fructus Alpiniae Oxyphyllae (*Yi Zhi Ren*).

For strangury taxation due to spleen-kidney yang vacuity without edema but with dizziness, low back and knee soreness and limpness, aversion to cold, turbid urine, reduced appetite, lack of strength, a sallow or dark facial complexion, a pale tongue, and a thin, weak pulse, replace *Shen Qi Tang Jia Wei* with *Liu Wei Di Huang Tang Jia Jian* (Six Flavors Rehmannia Decoction with Additions & Subtractions): Radix Astragali Membranacei (*Huang Qi*), 30g, cooked Radix Rehmanniae (*Shu Di*), Semen Cuscutae Chinensis (*Tu Si Zi*), and Terra Falva Ustae (*Fu Long Gan*), 15g each, Radix Dioscoreae Oppositae (*Shan Yao*), Fructus Psoraleae Corylifoliae (*Bu Gu Zhi*), Semen Euryalis Ferocis (*Qian Shi*), and Radix Codonopsitis Pilosulae (*Dang Shen*), 12g each, and Fructus Corni Officinalis (*Shan Zhu Yu*), Fructus Rosae Laevigatae (*Jin Ying Zi*), Rhizoma Atractylodis Macrocephalae (*Bai Zhu*), and Sclerotium Poriae Cocos (*Fu Ling*), 9g each. For marked kidney yang vacuity, add one gram each of Cornu Cervi (*Lu Jiao*) and Cortex Cinnamomi Cassiae (*Rou Gui*), powdered and taken with the strained decoction. For concomitant kidney yin vacuity, subtract *Bu Gu Zhi* and add 15 grams of Plastrum Testudinis (*Gui Ban*) and nine grams of Cortex Phellodendri (*Huang Bai*). For numerous red blood cells in the urine due to concomitant blood stasis, add nine grams each of Flos Carthami Tinctorii (*Hong Hua*), Herba Leonuri Heterophylli (*Yi Mu Cao*), and Herba Lycopi Lucidi (*Ze Lan*) and three grams of Radix Pseudoginseng (*San Qi*), powdered and taken with the strained decoction.

ACUPUNCTURE & MOXIBUSTION: *Shen Shu* (Bl 23), *San Yin Jiao* (Sp 6), *Guan Yuan* (CV 4), *Yin Ling Quan* (Sp 9)

ANALYSIS OF FORMULA: Supplementing *Shen Shu, Guan Yuan,* and *San Yin Jiao* with moxibustion, supplements and warms mainly the kidneys but also the spleen. Draining *San Yin Jiao* and *Yin Ling Quan* disinhibits water and disperses swelling.

ADDITIONS & SUBTRACTIONS: If yang disease has reached yin, add *Fu Liu* (Ki 7). For severe edema, especially below the waist, severe aversion to cold, and low back pain with a cold sensation, add *Ming Men* (GV 4) with moxibustion. If, in addition, there is hematuria, add *Xue Chou* (extra point located just above the spinous process of L2) with moxibustion. For heart palpitation and hasty panting, add *Nei Guan* (Per 6), *Liang Quan* (CV 23), and *Lie Que* (Lu 7). For severe edema in the limbs, add *Shui Dao* (St 28). If there is severe edema in the abdomen, add *Shui Fen* (CV 9).

5. QI VACUITY & BLOOD STASIS PATTERN

MAIN SYMPTOMS: Water swelling in the cheeks, face, and feet which is aggravated by over-taxation, bodily form vacuous and debilitated, fatigue, weakness of the four limbs, a sallow yellow complexion, devitalized appetite, epigastric and abdominal distention and falling, inhibited urination and defecation or possible diarrhea, a fat tongue with static macules or spots and thin, slimy fur, and a bowstring, choppy pulse

TREATMENT PRINCIPLES: Boost the qi and move water, quicken the blood and transform stasis

RX: *Yi Qi Shen Shi Tang Jia Wei* (Boost the Qi & Seep Dampness Decoction with Added Flavors)

INGREDIENTS: Radix Astragali Membranacei (*Huang Qi*) and Herba Leonuri Heterophylli (*Yi Mu Cao*), 30g each, Radix Codonopsitis Pilosulae (*Dang Shen*), Rhizoma Atractylodis (*Cang Zhu*), Rhizoma Atractylodis Macrocephalae (*Bai Zhu*), Radix Stephaniae Tetrandrae (*Han Fang Ji*), Sclerotium Polypori Umbellati (*Zhu Ling*), Sclerotium Poriae Cocos (*Fu Ling*), Rhizoma Alismatis (*Ze Xie*), Radix Ligustici Wallichii (*Chuan Xiong*), and Semen Pruni Persicae (*Tao Ren*), 9g each, and Ramulus Cinnamomi Cassiae (*Gui Zhi*) and Pericarpium Citri Reticulatae (*Chen Pi*), 6g each

ANALYSIS OF FORMULA: *Huang Qi, Dang Shen, Bai Zhu,* and *Fu Ling* fortify the spleen and boost the qi. In addition, *Huang Qi* and *Bai Zhu* disinhibit water. *Chen Pi* and *Cang Zhu* dry dampness, while *Zhu Ling, Fu Ling, Han Fang Ji,* and *Ze Xie* disinhibit water and disperse swelling. *Gui Zhi* warms yang and transforms the qi of the bladder to help disinhibit urination. *Chuan Xiong, Yi Mu Cao,* and *Tao Ren* quicken the blood and transform stasis.

ADDITIONS & SUBTRACTIONS: For marked blood stasis, add nine grams each of Flos Carthami Tinctorii (*Hong Hua*) and Herba Lycopi Lucidi (*Ze Lan*). For concomitant kidney vacuity, add 12 grams each of Radix Achyranthis Bidentatae (*Niu Xi*) and Ramulus Loranthi Seu Visci (*Sang Ji Sheng*). For yang vacuity, add nine grams of Herba Epimedii (*Yin Yang Huo*). For yin vacuity, add 12 grams of cooked Radix Rehmanniae (*Shu Di*).

ACUPUNCTURE & MOXIBUSTION: *Zu San Li* (St 36), *Shen Shu* (Bl 23), *Ge Shu* (Bl 17), *San Yin Jiao* (Sp 6), *Yin Ling Quan* (Sp 9)

ANALYSIS OF FORMULA: Supplementing *Zu San Li, Shen Shu,* and *San Yin Jiao* fortifies and supplements the spleen and the kidneys and boosts the qi. Draining *San Yin Jiao* and *Yin Ling Quan* disinhibits water and disperses swelling. Draining *Ge Shu* and *San Yin Jiao* quickens the blood and transforms stasis.

ADDITIONS & SUBTRACTIONS: For marked blood stasis, add *Xue Hai* (Sp 10) and *Xue Chou* (extra point located just above the spinous process of L2) with moxibustion. For concomitant kidney yang vacuity, add *Guan Yuan* (CV 4). For concomitant kidney yin vacuity, add *Fu Liu* (Ki 7). If fatigue and lack of strength are marked, add *Tai Bai* (Sp 3). For abdominal fullness after eating, borborygmus, flatulence, and edema predominantly in the abdomen, add *Nei Guan* (Per 6) and *Gong Sun* (Sp 4). For severe edema in the abdomen, also add *Shui Fen* (CV 9). For severe edema in the limbs, add *Shui Dao* (St 28). Please also refer to pattern #4 above.

6. YANG VACUITY & BLOOD STASIS PATTERN

MAIN SYMPTOMS: Facial and bodily superficial edema, especially below the waist, pressure causing the skin to be like mud (*i.e.*, pitting edema), a somber, dark complexion, fear of cold, lassitude of the spirit, fatigue, counterflow chilling of the four limbs, heart palpitations, shortness of breath, bluish purple lips and nails, low back soreness, heaviness, aching, and pain, inhibited urination, a pale, purple, and fat tongue with slimy, white fur, and a deep, choppy, forceless pulse

TREATMENT PRINCIPLES: Warm the kidneys and supplement yang, boost the qi and quicken the blood

RX: *Wen Shen Shen Shi Hua Yu Tang* (Warm the Kidneys, Seep Dampness & Transform Stasis Decoction)

INGREDIENTS: Herba Leonuri Heterophylli (*Yi Mu Cao*), 30g, Rhizoma Alismatis (*Ze Xie*), 15g, Radix Astragali Membranacei (*Huang Qi*), 12g, Cornu Cervi (*Lu Jiao Pian*), Radix Morindae Officinalis (*Ba Ji Tian*), Cortex Eucommiae Ulmoidis (*Du Zhong*), Sclerotium Polypori Umbellati (*Zhu Ling*), Sclerotium Poriae Cocos (*Fu Ling*), Radix Rubrus Paeoniae Lactiflorae (*Chi Shao*), and Semen Pruni Persicae (*Tao Ren*), 9g each, Radix Ligustici Wallichii (*Chuan Xiong*) and Radix Lateralis Praeparatus Aconiti Carmichaeli (*Fu Zi*), 6g each, and Cortex Cinnamomi Cassiae (*Rou Gui*), 3g

ANALYSIS OF FORMULA: *Lu Jiao, Ba Ji Tian, Du Zhong, Fu Zi,* and *Rou Gui* warm and invigorate kidney yang. *Huang Qi* and *Fu Ling* fortify the spleen and boost the qi. *Yi Mu Cao, Chi Shao, Tao Ren,* and *Chuan Xiong* quicken the blood and transform stasis. *Yi Mu Cao, Ze Xie, Zhu Ling,* and *Fu Ling* disinhibit water and disperse swelling.

ADDITIONS & SUBTRACTIONS: Please see pattern #4 above.

ACUPUNCTURE & MOXIBUSTION: *Shen Shu* (Bl 23), *Ge Shu* (Bl 17), *Pi Shu* (Bl 20), *Ming Men* (GV 4), *Fu Liu* (Ki 7)

ANALYSIS OF FORMULA: Supplementing *Shen Shu, Ming Men,* and *Fu Liu* with moxibustion warms and invigorates kidney yang. In addition, *Fu Liu* disinhibits water. Draining *Ge Shu* quickens the blood and transforms stasis.

Supplementing *Pi Shu* fortifies the spleen and boosts the qi. ADDITIONS & SUBTRACTIONS: Please see patterns #4 & 5 above.

7. LIVER-KIDNEY YIN VACUITY PATTERN

MAIN SYMPTOMS: Possible slight edema of the eyelids, face, and lower limbs, eyes dark, rough, and dry or cloudy vision, dizziness, tinnitus, vexatious heat in the five hearts, a dry mouth and parched throat, lower and upper back soreness and pain, urinary incontinence, possible menstrual irregularity, possible restless sleep, a red tongue with scanty fur, and a bowstring, rapid, or fine, bowstring, rapid pulse

TREATMENT PRINCIPLES: Enrich and nourish the liver and kidneys, clear heat and subdue yang

RX: *Liu Wei Di Huang Tang* (Six Flavors Rehmannia Decoction) & *Jian Ling Tang* (Fortify the Roof-tiles Decoction) with additions and subtractions

INGREDIENTS: Uncooked Concha Ostreae (*Mu Li*) and Os Draconis (*Long Gu*), 30g each, uncooked Radix Rehmanniae (*Sheng Di*), Radix Achyranthis Bidentatae (*Niu Xi*), Radix Albus Paeoniae Lactiflorae (*Bai Shao*), Flos Chrysanthemi Morifolii (*Ju Hua*), Ramulus Loranthi Seu Visci (*Sang Ji Sheng*), and Sclerotium Poriae Cocos (*Fu Ling*), 15g each, and Fructus Corni Officinalis (*Shan Zhu Yu*), Cortex Radicis Moutan (*Dan Pi*), Radix Dioscoreae Oppositae (*Shan Yao*), Fructus Lycii Chinensis (*Gou Qi Zi*), Rhizoma Anemarrhenae Aspheloidis (*Zhi Mu*), and Cortex Phellodendri (*Huang Bai*), 9g each

ANALYSIS OF FORMULA: *Sheng Di, Sang Ji Sheng, Shan Zhu Yu, Shan Yao, Niu Xi,* and *Gou Qi Zi* together enrich and nourish the liver and kidneys. *Mu Li, Long Gu, Ju Hua, Bai Shao,* and *Niu Xi* level the liver and subdue yang. In addition, *Ju Hua* with *Gou Qi Zi* brighten the eyes. *Huang Bai* and *Zhi Mu* clear vacuity heat. *Dan Pi* cools and quickens the blood.

ADDITIONS & SUBTRACTIONS: For inhibited, rough urination, add 15 grams each of Rhizoma Imperatae Cylindricae (*Bai Mao Gen*) and Semen Plantaginis (*Che Qian Zi*). For edema, add 12 grams each of Radix Stephaniae Tetrandrae (*Han Fang Ji*) and Semen Plantaginis (*Che Qian Zi*). For severe dizziness and tinnitus, add 12 grams each of Ramulus Uncariae Cum Uncis (*Gou Teng*) and Rhizoma Gastrodiae Elatae (*Tian Ma*). For painful throat, add 15 grams each of Radix Scrophulariae Ningpoensis (*Xuan Shen*) and Tuber Ophiopogonis Japonici (*Mai Men Dong*). For insomnia and heart palpitations, add 20 grams each of Semen Zizyphi Spinosae (*Suan Zao Ren*) and Caulis Polygoni Multiflori (*Ye Jiao Teng*). For concomitant liver fire, add nine grams each of Spica Prunellae Vulgaris (*Xia Ku Cao*) and Fructus Gardeniae Jasminoidis (*Zhi Zi*). For blood stasis, add 12 grams each of Herba Lycopi Lucidi (*Ze Lan*) and Herba Leonuri Heterophylli (*Yi Mu Cao*). For severe high blood pressure, add 30 grams each of Semen Celosiae Argentae (*Qing Xiang Zi*) and Herba Leonuri Heterophylli (*Yi Mu Cao*).

For liver-kidney yin vacuity with damp heat and blood stasis, replace *Liu Wei Di Huang Tang* and *Jian Ling Tang* with *Zi Shen Tang* (Enrich the Kidneys Decoction): Rhizoma Imperatae Cylindricae (*Bai Mao Gen*), 30g, uncooked Radix Rehmanniae (*Sheng Di*), Radix Achyranthis Bidentatae (*Niu Xi*), Radix Rubrus Paeoniae Lactiflorae (*Chi Shao*), and Herba Leonuri Heterophylli (*Yi Mu Cao*), 15g each, Radix Angelicae Sinensis (*Dang Gui*), Radix Ligustici Wallichii (*Chuan Xiong*), Fructus Ligustri Lucidi (*Nu Zhen Zi*), Herba Ecliptae Prostratae (*Han Lian Cao*), Fructus Rosae Laevigatae (*Jin Ying Zi*), Semen Euryalis Ferocis (*Qian Shi*), Rhizoma Atractylodis (*Cang Zhu*), and Cortex Phellodendri (*Huang Bai*), 9g each.

ACUPUNCTURE & MOXIBUSTION: *Shen Shu* (Bl 23), *Jing Gu* (Bl 64), *Gan Shu* (Bl 18), *Fu Liu* (Ki 7)

ANALYSIS OF FORMULA: *Shen Shu* and *Jing Gu* are an empirical combination for treating enduring glomerulonephritis. *Gan Shu* and *Fu Liu* further enrich and nourish the liver and kidneys and subdue yang. All these points should be supplemented.

ADDITIONS & SUBTRACTIONS: For inhibited, rough urination, add *Zhong Ji* (CV 3). For edema, add *Zhong Ji* (CV 3) and *Shui Dao* (St 28). For severe dizziness and tinnitus, add *Feng Chi* (GB 20) and *Yi Feng* (TB 17). For painful throat, add *Zhao Hai* (Ki 6). For insomnia and heart palpitations, add *Shen Men* (Ht 7). For concomitant liver fire, add *Xing Jian* (Liv 2). For blood stasis, add *San Yin Jiao* (Sp 6). For severe high blood pressure, add *Qu Chi* (LI 11) and *Zu San Li* (St 36).

8. QI & YIN DUAL VACUITY PATTERN

MAIN SYMPTOMS: A lusterless facial complexion, scanty qi, lack of strength, possible easy catching of cold, afternoon low-grade fever or heat in the hands, feet, and heart, a dry mouth and parched throat or enduring sore throat, a reddish tongue with scanty fur, and a fine and/or weak pulse

TREATMENT PRINCIPLES: Boost the qi and nourish yin, clear heat and seep dampness

RX: *Shen Qi Di Huang Tang Jia Wei* (Ginseng & Astragalus Rehmannia Decoction with Added Flavors)

INGREDIENTS: Herba Verbenae Officinalis (*Ma Bian Cao*)

and Caulis Lonicerae Japonicae (*Ren Dong Teng*), 30g each, Radix Pseudostellariae (*Tai Zi Shen*), uncooked Radix Astragali Membranacei (*Huang Qi*), Sclerotium Poriae Cocos (*Fu Ling*), and Rhizoma Alismatis (*Ze Xie*), 15g each, and uncooked Radix Rehmanniae (*Sheng Di*), Fructus Corni Officinalis (*Shan Zhu Yu*), Radix Dioscoreae Oppositae (*Shan Yao*), Cortex Radicis Moutan (*Dan Pi*), Fructus Ligustri Lucidi (*Nu Zhen Zi*), and Herba Ecliptae Prostratae (*Han Lian Cao*), 9g each

ANALYSIS OF FORMULA: *Tai Zi Shen, Huang Qi, Fu Ling,* and *Shan Yao* fortify the spleen and boost the qi. In addition, *Tai Zi Shen* engenders fluids, *Fu Ling* seeps dampness, *Huang Qi* disinhibits water, and *Shan Yao* supplements the kidneys. *Sheng Di, Nu Zhen Zi, Han Lian Cao,* and *Shan Zhu Yu* supplement the kidneys and enrich yin. *Ze Xie* disinhibits water, while *Dan Pi* transforms stasis. *Ma Bian Cao* and *Ren Dong Teng* clear heat and resolve toxins, leading ministerial fire back down to its lower source via urination.

ADDITIONS & SUBTRACTIONS: For low back pain, add nine grams each of Radix Achyranthis Bidentatae (*Niu Xi*) and Radix Dipsaci (*Xu Duan*). For dry mouth and parched throat or enduring sore throat and afternoon low-grade fever, add nine grams each of Tuber Ophiopogonis Japonici (*Mai Men Dong*), Cortex Phellodendri (*Huang Bai*), and Rhizoma Anemarrhenae Asphodeloidis (*Zhi Mu*). For reduced appetite and abdominal fullness especially after eating, add nine grams each of Radix Auklandiae Lappae (*Mu Xiang*) and Fructus Amomi (*Sha Ren*). For constipation, add nine grams each of Radix Scrophulariae Ningpoensis (*Xuan Shen*) and Semen Biotae Orientalis (*Bai Zi Ren*).

ACUPUNCTURE & MOXIBUSTION: *Shen Shu* (Bl 23), *Pi Shu* (Bl 20), *Zu San Li* (St 36), *Fu Liu* (Ki 7)

ANALYSIS OF FORMULA: Supplementing *Shen Shu, Pi Shu, Zu San Li,* and *Fu Liu* together fortifies and supplements the spleen and kidneys, boosts the qi, nourishes yin, and seeps dampness.

ADDITIONS & SUBTRACTIONS: For low back pain, add *Tai Xi* (Ki 3). For dry mouth and parched throat or enduring sore throat and afternoon low-grade fever, add *Zhao Hai* (Ki 6) and *Yin Xi* (Ht 6). For reduced appetite and abdominal fullness, especially after eating, add *Nei Guan* (Per 6) and *Gong Sun* (Sp 4). For constipation, add *Zhi Gou* (TB 6).

9. DAMP HEAT INHIBITING THE THREE BURNERS PATTERN

MAIN SYMPTOMS: Puffy eyelids or generalized edema, short, rough urination, chest oppression, nausea, reduced food intake, bodily heaviness, sores on the skin, slimy, yellow tongue fur, and a slippery, rapid or soggy pulse

TREATMENT PRINCIPLES: Clear heat and disinhibit dampness, free the flow of and disinhibit the three burners

RX: *San Ren Tang Jia Jian* (Three Seeds Decoction with Additions & Subtractions)

INGREDIENTS: Talcum (*Hua Shi*), 15-30g, uncooked Semen Coicis Lachryma-jobi (*Yi Yi Ren*), 20g, Semen Pruni Armeniacae (*Xing Ren*), Cortex Magnoliae Officinalis (*Hou Po*), ginger stir-fried Rhizoma Pinelliae Ternatae (*Ban Xia*), and Herba Lophatheri Gracilis (*Dan Zhu Ye*), 9g each, and Fructus Cardamomi (*Bai Dou Kou*) and Medulla Tetrapanacis Papyriferi (*Tong Cao*), 6g each

ANALYSIS OF FORMULA: *Hua Shi, Yi Yi Ren, Dan Zhu Ye,* and *Tong Cao* clear heat and disinhibit dampness. *Ban Xia, Hou Po,* and *Bai Dou Kou* transform and dry dampness. In addition, *Ban Xia* harmonizes the stomach and stops vomiting. *Xing Ren* and *Ban Xia* free the flow of and disinhibit the upper burner, *Hou Po* and *Bai Dou Kou* free and disinhibit the middle burner, and *Hua Shi, Yi Yi Ren, Dan Zhu Ye,* and *Tong Cao* free and disinhibit the lower burner.

ADDITIONS & SUBTRACTIONS: If diffusion and downbearing is also impaired with inhibition of the water passageways, add 30g of Semen Phaseoli Calcarati (*Chi Xiao Dou*) and 12g each of Fructus Forsythiae Suspensae (*Lian Qiao*) and honey mix-fried Herba Ephedrae (*Ma Huang*). If there are skin sores due to heat toxins, add 15g each of Flos Lonicerae Japonicae (*Jin Yin Hua*), Rhizoma Smilacis Glabrae (*Tu Fu Ling*), Herba Taraxaci Mongolici Cum Radice (*Pu Gong Ying*), and Herba Violae Yedoensitis Cum Radice (*Zi Hua Di Ding*). If defecation is inhibited, add 12g each of Semen Pruni Persicae (*Tao Ren*) and Semen Pruni (*Yu Li Ren*). If there is concomitant hematuria, add 12g each of Herba Cephalanoploris Segeti (*Xiao Ji*), uncooked Radix Rehmanniae (*Sheng Di*), Radix Rubiae Cordifoliae (*Qian Cao*), and Rhizoma Imperatae Cylindricae (*Bai Mao Gen*).

ACUPUNCTURE & MOXIBUSTION: *He Gu* (LI 4), *Nei Ting* (St 44), *Zhi Gou* (TB 6), *Yin Ling Quan* (Sp 9), *Zhong Ji* (CV 3)

ANALYSIS OF FORMULA: Draining *Yin Ling Quan* and *Zhong Ji* clears heat and eliminates dampness, disinhibits water and treats the edema, while draining *Nei Ting, He Gu,* and *Zhi Gou* clears heat and resolves toxins, frees the flow of and disinhibits the three burners.

ADDITIONS & SUBTRACTIONS: If diffusion and downbearing is also impaired with inhibition of the water passageway, add *Wai Guan* (TB 5), *Qu Chi* (LI 11), and *Shui Dao* (St 28). If there are skin sores due to heat toxins, add *Ling Tai* (GV 10),

Wei Zhong (Bl 40), *Xue Hai* (Sp 10), and *Qu Chi* (LI 11). If defecation is inhibited, add *Zhi Gou* (TB 6). If there is hematuria, add *San Yin Jiao* (Sp 6) and *Ran Gu* (Ki 2).

10. Blood stasis pattern

MAIN SYMPTOMS: Enduring disease which does not heal, a dark facial complexion, blackness around the eyes, dryness and darkness of the lower lobe of the ear, dry skin, liver spots on the hands, possible hematuria, a dark purplish tongue and/or possible static spots or macules on the tongue, and a deep or deep and choppy pulse

TREATMENT PRINCIPLES: Quicken the blood and transform stasis

RX: *Xue Fu Zhu Yu Tang Jia Jian* (Blood Mansion Dispel Stasis Decoction with Additions & Subtractions)

INGREDIENTS: Uncooked Radix Rehmanniae (*Sheng Di*), 9-30g, Radix Rubrus Paeoniae Lactiflorae (*Chi Shao*), 12g, Semen Pruni Persicae (*Tao Ren*), Flos Carthami Tinctorii (*Hong Hua*), Fructus Citri Aurantii (*Zhi Ke*), Radix Cyathulae (*Chuan Niu Xi*), and Radix Angelicae Sinensis (*Dang Gui*), 9g each, and Radix Bupleuri (*Chai Hu*), Radix Platycodi Grandiflori (*Jie Geng*), and Radix Ligustici Wallichii (*Chuan Xiong*), 6g each

ANALYSIS OF FORMULA: *Tao Ren*, *Hong Hua*, *Chi Shao*, *Chuan Xiong*, and *Dang Gui* quicken the blood and transform stasis. *Jie Geng* moves qi in the upper burner, *Chai Hu* moves qi in the middle burner, while *Zhi Ke* moves qi in the lower burner, and, if the qi moves, the blood moves. *Sheng Di* and *Dang Gui* also nourish the blood.

ADDITIONS & SUBTRACTIONS: If there is concomitant qi vacuity with fatigue, add 18 grams of Radix Astragali Membranacei (*Huang Qi*) and 12 grams of Radix Pseudostellariae Heterophyllae (*Tai Zi Shen*). For qi stagnation with abdominal and/or rib-side distention and pain, add 12 grams each of Rhizoma Cyperi Rotundi (*Xiang Fu*), Tuber Curcumae (*Yu Jin*), and Pericarpium Arecae Catechu (*Da Fu Pi*). For edema, add nine grams each of Radix Stephaniae Tetrandrae (*Han Fang Ji*), Rhizoma Alismatis (*Ze Xie*), Sclerotium Polypori Umbellati (*Zhu Ling*), and Herba Lycopi Lucidi (*Ze Lan*). For concomitant phlegm heat with nausea, chest and stomach fullness and oppression, a bitter taste in the mouth, and a sticky feeling in the mouth, add 3-6 grams of Rhizoma Coptidis Chinensis (*Huang Lian*) and 6-9 grams each of Pericarpium Citri Reticulatae (*Chen Pi*), Rhizoma Pinelliae Ternatae (*Ban Xia*), and Caulis Bambusae In Taeniis (*Zhu Ru*).

ACUPUNCTURE & MOXIBUSTION: *San Yin Jiao* (Sp 6), *He Gu* (LI 4), *Ge Shu* (Bl 17), *Xue Hai* (Sp 10), *Zhong Ji* (CV 3)

ANALYSIS OF FORMULA: Draining *San Yin Jiao* and *He Gu* quickens the blood in the whole of the body by moving the qi. Draining *Ge Shu* quickens the blood in the upper burner, while draining *Xue Hai* quickens the blood in the lower burner. Draining *Zhong Ji*, the bladder front *mu* or alarm point, clears and disinhibits the lower burner.

ADDITIONS & SUBTRACTIONS: If there is concomitant qi vacuity with fatigue, add *Zu San Li* (St 36) and *Tai Bai* (Sp 3). For qi stagnation with abdominal and/or rib-side distention and pain, add *Tian Shu* (St 25) and *Qi Men* (Liv 14). For edema, add *Yin Ling Quan* (Sp 9) and *Shui Dao* (St 28). For concomitant phlegm heat with nausea, chest and stomach fullness and oppression, a bitter taste and a sticky feeling in the mouth, add *Zhong Wan* (CV 12) and *Feng Long* (St 40).

Remarks

1. In Chinese medicine, chronic nephritis can also generally be referred to as a water and qi disease (*shui qi bing*). This is because damp, turbid substances obstruct and stagnate the qi mechanism. Thus the qi transformation cannot reach all the regions of the body and the kidneys lose their control over the body's water fluids, resulting in water swelling or edema. However, in chronic glomerulonephritis, edema does not have to be present, and many patients are asymptomatic for the first several years. For instance, edema is not necessarily present in patterns #3, 4, 5, and 6 and only may be present in patterns #7 and 8.

2. Because this disease is usually the result of long-term, enduring disease and tends to present most often in older patients, blood stasis typically plays a part in its disease mechanisms. Therefore, most formulas for this condition include or should be modified by the addition of blood-quickening, stasis-dispelling medicinals. Yan De-xin, author of *Aging & Blood Stasis,* believes that virtually all chronic nephritis in the elderly involves blood stasis, and that quickening the blood and dispelling stasis is essential to achieve a good treatment effect. In terms of blood-quickening medicinals, at the beginning of this disease, Dr. Yan says one should consider using Herba Lycopi Lucidi (*Ze Lan*) and Herba Leonuri Heterophylli (*Yi Mu Cao*) to transform blood into water. In the middle stage, Dr. Yan says to use uncooked Pollen Typhae (*Pu Huang*) and Hirudo (*Shui Zhi*) to transform stasis and free the flow of the network vessels.

3. If there is concomitant liver depression qi stagnation, add appropriate qi-rectifying or exterior-resolving medicinals to any of the above formulas.

4. Several Chinese medicinals contain nephrotoxic con-

stituents, such as aristolochic acid. Therefore, the following medicinals should not be used in patients that suffer glomerulonephritis or chronic renal failure: uncooked Fructus Xanthii Sibirici (*Cang Er Zi*), Fructus Bruceae Javanicae (*Ya Dan Zi*), Radix Dichroae Febrifugae (*Chang Shan*), uncooked Semen Ginkgonis Bilobae (*Bai Guo*), Semen Strychnotis (*Ma Qian Zi*), Mylabris (*Ban Mao*), Herba Asari Cum Radice (*Xi Xin*), uncooked Rhizoma Pinelliae Ternatae (*Ban Xia*), Herba Tripterygii Wilfordii (*Lei Gong Teng*), and Realgar (*Xiong Huang*).

5. Herba Leonuri Heterophylli (*Yi Mu Cao*), 25g per day, and Fructus Crataegi (*Shan Zha*), 50-90g per day, are especially useful in the treatment of glomerulonephritis complicated by hypertension, while fresh Herba Plantaginis (*Che Qian Cao*) and Rhizoma Imperatae Cylindricae (*Bai Mao Gen*), 30g each per day, plus Stylus Zeae Maydis (*Yu Mi Xu*), 60g per day, are especially effective for albuminuria. Radix Astragali Membranacei (*Huang Qi*) is also one of the best medicinals to treat chronic glomerulonephritis and relieve albuminuria.

6. According to Dr. Wan Ge, the most common pattern of chronic glomerulonephritis is spleen-kidney yin and yang vacuity with blood stasis.

17

CHRONIC PANCREATITIS

Chronic pancreatitis refers to chronic inflammation of the pancreas. In the United States, the most common cause of this condition is alcoholism. The main symptom of chronic pancreatitis is severe epigastric pain which may last for hours or even days. This pain may radiate straight through to the back in 50% of patients. The pain usually develops suddenly and reaches maximal intensity within minutes. Its quality is steady and boring, and it is not relieved by pressure or changes in position. However, coughing, deep breathing, or vigorous movement may accentuate this pain. Most patients also experience nausea and vomiting to the point of dry heaves. While chronic pancreatitis is usually characterized by recurrent attacks of symptoms identical to acute pancreatitis, some few patients may not experience any pain. Other symptoms include diarrhea, anorexia, emaciation, jaundice, and abdominal lumps.

The Western medical diagnosis of this condition is made by first ruling out all other causes of severe paroxysmal epigastric pain. It is then confirmed by x-ray, ultrasound, CT scan, and/or endoscopic retrograde cholangiopancreatography. In addition, tests of pancreatic function assess endocrine and exocrine function. The Western medical treatment of chronic pancreatitis begins with abstinence from alcohol. Episodes similar to acute pancreatitis are treated in the same way as that disease, *i.e.*, primarily by fasting and infusion of IV fluids. The Western medical treatment of chronic pancreatic pain is frequently unsatisfactory. Antacid and H_2 receptor blockers are often administered as well as narcotics to relieve pain. However, often increasing amounts of narcotics are required, and there is the very real danger of the patient becoming addicted to these. Surgery is sometimes resorted to for pain relief in cases of pancreatic pseudocyst or other causes of compression of the pancreatic duct. Unfortunately, such surgery is effective in relieving pain in only 40-70% of cases. Chronic pancreatitis often coexists with diabetes mellitus. In that case, oral hypoglycemics are rarely effective, while insulin must only be used cautiously since the pathophysiology of pancreatitis means that the hypoglycemic effects of insulin are unopposed.

CHINESE DISEASE CATEGORIZATION: Based on this condition's main clinical symptoms, it is mainly categorized in Chinese medicine as *fu tong*, abdominal pain, *xie tong*, rib-side pain, *xie xie*, diarrhea, *huang dan*, jaundice, *na dai*, torpid intake, *xiao xue*, emaciation (literally, dispersion and whittling), and *zheng jia*, concretions and conglomerations. In addition, nausea is *e xin* and vomiting is *ou tu*.

DISEASE CAUSES: Unregulated eating and drinking, internal damage by the seven affects, roundworms internally harassing, and habitual bodily vacuity weakness

DISEASE MECHANISMS: Over-eating fatty, sweet, thick-flavored foods or drinking too much alcohol may result in damage and detriment to the spleen and stomach, further resulting in the internal engenderment of accumulation and stagnation. If this endures, it may brew dampness and transform heat. In that case, dampness and heat and food and drink may mutually bind in the center, obstructing and stagnating the qi mechanism and causing loss of normalcy in upbearing and downbearing. This then results in epigastric pain, nausea, vomiting, torpid intake, diarrhea, emaciation, and jaundice. It is also possible that, due to eating unclean foods, dampness and heat brew worms. If roundworms obstruct the intestines, there will be pain, nausea, vomiting, torpid intake, diarrhea, and jaundice.

Either unfulfilled desires or anger may damage the liver, while worry and anxiety damage the spleen. If the liver is damaged, coursing and discharge will lose their normalcy. If the spleen is damaged, movement and transformation will lose their normalcy. If this endures for days, qi stagnation may result in pain, while inhibition of upbearing and downbearing result in nausea, vomiting, torpid intake, diarrhea, emaciation, and jaundice.

Commonly, there is a combination of both faulty diet and habitual emotional stress. In that case, there is a tendency to liver repletion and spleen vacuity. In addition, if qi stagnation endures, it may give rise to blood stasis, and blood stasis may result in severe, fixed, boring pain and concretions and conglomerations. If depressive and/or damp heat lingers and endures, heat evils will damage and consume yin fluids, thus giving rise to concomitant yin vacuity.

TREATMENT BASED ON PATTERN DISCRIMINATION:

1. LIVER DEPRESSION QI STAGNATION PATTERN

MAIN SYMPTOMS: Upper abdominal and/or rib-side distention and pain or insidious pain that comes and goes and is not fixed or stable. If severe, the pain may radiate to the chest, upper back, shoulder, and upper arm. There may also be accompanying chest oppression, burping and belching, possible dry heaves, reduced appetite, frequent sighing, etc. Acute attacks are associated with emotional disturbance. The tongue is normal or darkish in color with thin, white fur, while the pulse is bowstring and fine or deep and fine.

TREATMENT PRINCIPLES: Course the liver, rectify the qi, and stop pain

RX: *Chai Hu Shu Gan San Jia Wei* (Bupleurum Course the Liver Powder with Added Flavors)

INGREDIENTS: Rhizoma Corydalis Yanhusuo (*Yan Hu Suo*), 15g, Radix Bupleuri (*Chai Hu*) and Fructus Meliae Toosendan (*Chuan Lian Zi*), 12g, Rhizoma Cyperi Rotundi (*Xiang Fu*), Fructus Citri Sacrodactylis (*Fo Shou*), Flos Rosae Rugosae (*Mei Gui Hua*), Radix Albus Paeoniae Lactiflorae (*Bai Shao*) and Fructus Citri Aurantii (*Zhi Ke*), 9g each, Radix Ligustici Wallichii (*Chuan Xiong*), 6g, and Radix Glycyrrhizae (*Gan Cao*), 3g

ANALYSIS OF FORMULA: *Chai Hu, Chuan Lian Zi, Xiang Fu, Fo Shou, Mei Gui Hua*, and *Zhi Ke* course the liver, rectify the qi, and stop pain. *Yan Hu Suo* and *Chuan Xiong* move the qi, quicken the blood, and stop pain. *Bai Shao* nourishes the blood and emolliates the liver to prevent liver depression. *Gan Cao* harmonizes the other medicinals.

ADDITIONS & SUBTRACTIONS: If liver depression has transformed heat, add nine grams of Radix Scutellariae Baicalensis (*Huang Qin*) and 4.5 grams of Rhizoma Coptidis Chinensis (*Huang Lian*). For nausea and vomiting due to heat, add nine grams each of Caulis Bambusae In Taeniis (*Zhu Ru*) and Rhizoma Pinelliae Ternatae (*Ban Xia*) and six grams of Pericarpium Citri Reticulatae (*Chen Pi*). If spleen vacuity is marked, add nine grams each of Radix Codonopsitis Pilosulae (*Dang Shen*), Rhizoma Atractylodis Macrocephalae (*Bai Zhu*), and Sclerotium Poriae Cocos (*Fu Ling*) and replace uncooked *Gan Cao* with mix-fried *Gan Cao*. If there is concomitant blood stasis, add 15 grams of Radix Salviae Miltiorrhizae (*Dan Shen*) and nine grams of Radix Angelicae Sinensis (*Dang Gui*). If heat has damaged stomach fluids, add 12 grams of Tuber Ophiopogonis Japonici (*Mai Men Dong*). If there is severe rib-side distention and pain, add nine grams of Pericarpium Citri Reticulatae Viride (*Qing Pi*). For constipation, add 6-12 grams of Radix Et Rhizoma Rhei (*Da Huang*). For stomach and abdominal fullness, add nine grams each of Cortex Magnoliae Officinalis (*Hou Po*) and Radix Auklandiae Lappae (*Mu Xiang*).

For liver depression which has transformed heat with food stagnation, replace *Chai Hu Shu Gan San Jia Wei* with *Qing Yi Tang Jia Wei* (Clear the Pancreas Decoction with Added Flavors): Radix Albus Paeoniae Lactiflorae (*Bai Shao*), 15g, Fructus Crataegi (*Shan Zha*) and Massa Medica Fermentata (*Shen Qu*), 12g each, Radix Bupleuri (*Chai Hu*), Radix Scutellariae Baicalensis (*Huang Qin*), Radix Auklandiae Lappae (*Mu Xiang*), Rhizoma Corydalis Yanhusuo (*Yan Hu Suo*), and Cortex Magnoliae Officinalis (*Hou Po*), 6g each, Rhizoma Picrorrhizae (*Hu Huang Lian*), 3g. If there is concomitant constipation, add 3-12 grams of Radix Et Rhizoma Rhei (*Da Huang*).

ACUPUNCTURE & MOXIBUSTION: *Qi Men* (Liv 14), *Zhang Men* (Liv 13), *Zhi Gou* (TB 6), *Nei Guan* (Per 6)

ANALYSIS OF FORMULA: Draining *Qi Men, Zhang Men, Zhi Gou*, and *Nei Guan* courses the liver and resolves depression, rectifies the qi and stops pain.

ADDITIONS & SUBTRACTIONS: If liver depression has transformed heat, add *Xing Jian* (Liv 2) and replace *Nei Guan* with *Yang Ling Quan* (GB 34). For nausea and vomiting add *Zhong Wan* (CV 12). If spleen vacuity is marked, add *Zu San Li* (St 36). If there is concomitant blood stasis, add *Ge Shu* (Bl 17) and *San Yin Jiao* (Sp 6). If there is food stagnation, add *Liang Men* (St 21). For constipation, add *Zhao Hai* (Ki 6). For stomach and abdominal fullness, add *Zhong Wan* (CV 12).

2. QI STAGNATION AND BLOOD STASIS PATTERN

MAIN SYMPTOMS: Ductal and rib-side lancinating pain or distention and pain which is fixed in location and worse at night, bodily emaciation, scaly skin, a dark, lusterless facial complexion, brittle, ridged fingernails, abdominal lumps and concretions, especially below the rib-side, menstrual irregularities, a dark, purplish tongue or possible static macules or spots, distended, engorged, tortuous sublingual veins, and a fine, bowstring, choppy pulse

TREATMENT PRINCIPLES: Rectify the qi and quicken the blood, transform stasis and soften the hard

RX: *Ge Xia Zhu Yu Tang* (Below the Diaphragm Dispel Stasis Decoction)

INGREDIENTS: Radix Angelicae Sinensis (*Dang Gui*), Radix Ligustici Wallichii (*Chuan Xiong*), Semen Pruni Persicae (*Tao Ren*), Flos Carthami Tinctorii (*Hong Hua*), Feces Trogopterori Seu Pteromi (*Wu Ling Zhi*), Radix Rubrus Paeoniae Lactiflorae (*Chi Shao*), Cortex Radicis Moutan (*Dan Pi*), and Rhizoma Cyperi Rotundi (*Xiang Fu*), 9g each, Rhizoma Corydalis Yanhusuo (*Yan Hu Suo*) and Fructus Citri Aurantii (*Zhi Ke*), 6g each, and Radix Glycyrrhizae (*Gan Cao*), 3g

ANALYSIS OF FORMULA: *Dang Gui, Chuan Xiong, Tao Ren, Hong Hua, Wu Ling Zhi, Chi Shao, Dan Pi,* and *Yan Hu Suo* quicken the blood, transform stasis, and stop pain. *Yan Hu Suo, Chuan Xiong, Xiang Fu,* and *Zhi Ke* rectify the qi and stop pain. *Dang Gui* also nourishes the blood, while *Dan Pi* and *Chi Shao* cool the blood. *Gan Cao* harmonizes the other medicinals in this formula.

ADDITIONS & SUBTRACTIONS: For reduced appetite with undigested food in the stools, add 12 grams each of Rhizoma Atractylodis Macrocephalae (*Bai Zhu*), Fructus Crataegi (*Shan Zha*), Massa Medica Fermentata (*Shen Qu*), and Fructus Germinatus Hordei Vulgaris (*Mai Ya*). For lumps below the rib-side, add 30 grams of Caulis Sargentodoxae (*Hong Teng*) and 12 grams each of Rhizoma Sparganii (*San Leng*) and Rhizoma Curcumae Zedoariae (*E Zhu*). For marked liver depression, add 15 grams of Radix Albus Paeoniae Lactiflorae (*Bai Shao*) and nine grams of Radix Bupleuri (*Chai Hu*). For severe pain, add nine grams each of Fructus Meliae Toosendan (*Chuan Lian Zi*) and Radix Auklandiae Lappae (*Mu Xiang*). For blood stasis with replete heat in the spleen and stomach with constipation, dry stools, dry mouth, and severe abdominal distention, subtract *Chuan Xiong* and *Hong Hua*, and add 6-15 grams of Radix Et Rhizoma Rhei (*Da Huang*), 15 grams of Radix Albus Paeoniae Lactiflorae (*Bai Shao*), and nine grams each of Radix Scutellariae Baicalensis (*Huang Qin*) and Radix Bupleuri (*Chai Hu*).

ACUPUNCTURE & MOXIBUSTION: *Qi Men* (Liv 14), *Zhang Men* (Liv 13), *Zhi Gou* (TB 6), *Nei Guan* (Per 6), *San Yin Jiao* (Sp 6)

ANALYSIS OF FORMULA: Draining *Qi Men* and *Zhang Men* rectifies the qi, resolves depression, and stops pain locally in the region of the upper abdomen and rib-side. Draining *Zhi Gou* moves the qi in the three burners and especially below the rib-side. Draining *Nei Guan* quickens the blood, transforms stasis, and stops pain, especially in the rib-side, diaphragm, and chest. Draining *San Yin Jiao* cools and quickens the blood and transforms stasis in the whole body.

ADDITIONS & SUBTRACTIONS: If there is severe blood stasis, add *Ge Shu* (Bl 17) and *He Gu* (LI 4). If qi stagnation has transformed heat, add *Xing Jian* (Liv 2) and replace *Nei Guan* with *Yang Ling Quan* (GB 34). For nausea and vomiting, add *Zhong Wan* (CV 12). If spleen vacuity is marked, add *Zu San Li* (St 36). If there is food stagnation, add *Liang Men* (St 21). For constipation, add *Zhao Hai* (Ki 6) and *Tian Shu* (St 25). For stomach and abdominal fullness, add *Zhong Wan* (CV 12).

3. LIVER-GALLBLADDER (SPLEEN-STOMACH) DAMP HEAT PATTERN

MAIN SYMPTOMS: This pattern is mostly seen in chronic pancreatitis where there are acute attacks accompanied by chest oppression, torpid intake, aversion to fatty, oily foods, abdominal distention and pain, rib-side pain, possible fever, a yellowish body and eyes, possible nausea and vomiting, a dry mouth with a bitter taste, yellow urine, dry, bound stools or diarrhea which is yellow or brown in color and foul-smelling, possible jaundice, slimy, yellow tongue fur, and a bowstring, slippery, rapid pulse

TREATMENT PRINCIPLES: Clear heat and disinhibit dampness assisted by freeing the flow and descending

RX: *Da Chai Hu Tang* (Major Bupleurum Decoction)

INGREDIENTS: Radix Bupleuri (*Chai Hu*) and Radix Scutellariae Baicalensis (*Huang Qin*), 12g each, Fructus Immaturus Citri Aurantii (*Zhi Shi*), Rhizoma Pinelliae Ternatae (*Ban Xia*), and Radix Albus Paeoniae Lactiflorae (*Bai Shao*), 9g each, Radix Et Rhizoma Rhei (*Da Huang*), 6g, uncooked Rhizoma Zingiberis (*Sheng Jiang*), 3 slices, and Fructus Zizyphi Jujubae (*Da Zao*), 3 pieces

ANALYSIS OF FORMULA: *Chai Hu* and *Bai Shao* course the liver, rectify the qi, and stop pain. *Huang Qin* and *Da Huang* clear heat and dry and disinhibit dampness. *Zhi Shi* and *Da Huang* free the flow and descend. *Ban Xia* and *Sheng Jiang* harmonize the stomach and stop vomiting. *Da Zao* harmonizes the other medicinals in this formula.

ADDITIONS & SUBTRACTIONS: If there is jaundice, add 15 grams of Herba Artemisiae Capillaris (*Yin Chen Hao*) and nine grams each of Fructus Gardeniae Jasminoidis (*Zhi Zi*) and Cortex Phellodendri (*Huang Bai*). If jaundice is severe, increase the dosage of Herba Artemisiae Capillaris (*Yin Chen Hao*) up to 60 grams. If there is constipation, add six grams of Mirabilitum (*Mang Xiao*). If there is vomiting, add nine grams of Caulis Bambusae In Taeniis (*Zhu Ru*), six grams of Fructus Evodiae Rutecarpae (*Wu Zhu Yu*), and three grams of Rhizoma Coptidis Chinensis (*Huang Lian*). For severe abdominal pain, add 15 grams of Rhizoma Corydalis Yanhusuo (*Yan Hu Suo*), 12 grams of Fructus Meliae Toosendan (*Chuan Lian Zi*), and nine grams of Rhizoma Cyperi Rotundi (*Xiang Fu*). If there is severe rib-side pain and distention, add nine grams each of Tuber Curcumae (*Yu Jin*), Fructus Meliae Toosendan (*Chuan Lian Zi*), and Pericarpium Citri Reticulatae Viride (*Qing Pi*). For nausea with aversion to food, add 12 grams of Caulis Bambusae In Taeniis (*Zhu Ru*), nine grams each of Endothelium Corneum Gigeriae Galli (*Ji Nei Jin*) and Fructus Crataegi (*Shan Zha*), and three grams of Rhizoma Coptidis Chinensis (*Huang Lian*).

ACUPUNCTURE & MOXIBUSTION: *Qi Men* (Liv 14), *Zhang Men* (Liv 13), *Zhi Gou* (TB 6), *Yang Ling Quan* (GB 34), *Yin Ling Quan* (Sp 9)

ANALYSIS OF FORMULA: Draining *Qi Men* and *Zhang Men* rectifies the qi, resolves depression, and stops pain locally. Draining *Zhi Gou* moves the qi and clears heat in the three burners, stops pain in the rib-side, and frees the flow and descends. Draining *Nei Guan* rectifies the qi, quickens the blood, and stops pain, especially in the rib-side, diaphragm, and chest. Draining *Yang Ling Quan* clears heat and disinhibits dampness, especially in the liver-gallbladder. Draining *Yin Ling Quan* clears heat and disinhibits dampness, especially in the spleen-stomach.

ADDITIONS & SUBTRACTIONS: If there is jaundice, add *Gan Shu* (Bl 18) and *Zhi Yang* (GV 9). If there is blood stasis, add *Ge Shu* (Bl 17) and *San Yin Jiao* (Sp 6). If qi stagnation has transformed heat, add *Xing Jian* (Liv 2). For nausea and vomiting add *Zhong Wan* (CV 12). If there is concomitant spleen vacuity, add *Zu San Li* (St 36). If there is food stagnation, add *Liang Men* (St 21). For constipation, add *Zhao Hai* (Ki 6) and *Tian Shu* (St 25). For stomach and abdominal fullness, add *Zhong Wan* (CV 12).

4. SPLEEN VACUITY WITH DAMP ENCUMBRANCE PATTERN

MAIN SYMPTOMS: Damp evils obstructing the middle burner and the qi mechanism with chest and venter glomus and stagnation, distention and oppression after eating, reduced food intake, torpid intake, possible diarrhea or loose stools if dampness is overwhelming, possible dizziness if dampness prevents the clear yang from being upborne, possible lack of strength in the four extremities if dampness obstructs the channels and network vessels, slimy, white tongue fur, and a soggy, moderate (*i.e.*, slightly slow) pulse

TREATMENT PRINCIPLES: Fortify the spleen and dry dampness, move the qi and harmonize the stomach

RX: *Ping Wei San Jia Wei* (Level the Stomach Powder with Added Flavors)

INGREDIENTS: Rhizoma Atractylodis (*Cang Zhu*), Rhizoma Atractylodis Macrocephalae (*Bai Zhu*), and Sclerotium Poriae Cocos (*Fu Ling*), 15g each, Radix Codonopsitis Pilosulae (*Dang Shen*), 12g, Cortex Magnoliae Officinalis (*Hou Po*), 9g, Radix Glycyrrhizae (*Gan Cao*), 6g

ANALYSIS OF FORMULA: *Cang Zhu* dries dampness and fortifies the spleen, while *Bai Zhu* fortifies the spleen and dries dampness. When both *Zhu* are used together, they strongly dry dampness. *Fu Ling* seeps dampness and fortifies the spleen. *Dang Shen* fortifies the spleen and supplements the qi. *Hou Po* moves the qi, transforms dampness, and eliminates stagnation. *Gan Cao* aids in the fortification of the spleen and supplementation of the qi at the same time as protecting the stomach qi.

ADDITIONS & SUBTRACTIONS: If there is a liver-spleen disharmony, replace *Ping Wei San Jia Wei* with *Xiao Yao San* (Rambling Powder): Radix Bupleuri (*Chai Hu*), Rhizoma Atractylodis Macrocephalae (*Bai Zhu*), Sclerotium Poriae Cocos (*Fu Ling*), and Radix Albus Paeoniae Lactiflorae (*Bai Shao*), 9g each, mix-fried Radix Glycyrrhizae (*Gan Cao*), Herba Menthae Haplocalycis (*Bo He*), and Radix Angelicae Sinensis (*Dang Gui*), 6g each, and uncooked Rhizoma Zingiberis (*Sheng Jiang*), 2 slices.

If there is qi and blood vacuity, replace *Ping Wei San Jia Wei* with *Gui Pi Tang Jia Jian* (Return the Spleen Decoction with Additions & Subtractions): Radix Astragali Membranacei (*Huang Qi*), Radix Albus Paeoniae Lactiflorae (*Bai Shao*), and Semen Zizyphi Spinosae (*Suan Zao Ren*), 12g each, Radix Codonopsitis Pilosulae (*Dang Shen*), Radix Salviae Miltiorrhizae (*Dan Shen*), Arillus Euphoriae Longanae (*Long Yan Rou*), Rhizoma Atractylodis Macrocephalae (*Bai Zhu*), Radix Bupleuri (*Chai Hu*), and Radix Auklandiae Lappae (*Mu Xiang*), 9g each, Radix Angelicae Sinensis (*Dang Gui*) and mix-fried Radix Glycyrrhizae (*Gan Cao*), 6g each, Fructus Zizyphi Jujubae (*Da Zao*), 3 pieces, and uncooked Rhizoma Zingiberis (*Sheng Jiang*), 2 slices.

If there is spleen-stomach vacuity cold, with stomach and abdominal pain which gets better with warmth, reduced appetite, nausea, vomiting, loose stools, undigested food in stools, emaciation, cold form, cold limbs, replace *Ping Wei San Jia Wei* with *Si Jun Zi Tang Jia Wei* (Four Gentlemen Decoction with Added Flavors): Rhizoma Atractylodis Macrocephalae (*Bai Zhu*), Sclerotium Poriae Cocos (*Fu Ling*), Radix Dioscoreae Oppositae (*Shan Yao*), 12g each, Radix Codonopsitis Pilosulae (*Dang Shen*), mix-fried Radix

Glycyrrhizae (*Gan Cao*), Radix Auklandiae Lappae (*Mu Xiang*), and Fructus Terminaliae Chebulae (*He Zi*), 9g each, and dry Rhizoma Zingiberis (*Gan Jiang*), Semen Myristicae Fragrantis (*Rou Dou Kou*), and Fructus Amomi (*Sha Ren*), 6g each. Without aversion to cold and cold limbs, subtract *Gan Jiang*. For concomitant food stagnation, add nine grams each of Fructus Crataegi (*Shan Zha*), Massa Medica Fermentata (*Shen Qu*), and Fructus Germinatus Hordei Vulgaris (*Mai Ya*).

If there is spleen-kidney yang vacuity, replace *Ping Wei San Jia Wei* with *Jin Gui Shen Qi Wan* (*Golden Cabinet* Kidney Qi Pills) & *Si Shen Wan* (Four Spirits Pills): cooked Radix Rehmanniae (*Shu Di*), 20-30g, Radix Dioscoreae Oppositae (*Shan Yao*), Fructus Corni Officinalis (*Shan Zhu Yu*), Fructus Psoraleae Corylifoliae (*Bu Gu Zhi*), and Sclerotium Poriae Cocos (*Fu Ling*), 12g each, Cortex Radicis Moutan (*Dan Pi*), Rhizoma Alismatis (*Ze Xie*), Fructus Schisandrae Chinensis (*Wu Wei Zi*), Fructus Myristicae Fragrantis (*Rou Dou Kou*), and Radix Lateralis Praeparatus Aconiti Carmichaeli (*Fu Zi*), 9g each, Fructus Evoidae Rutecarpae (*Wu Zhu Yu*) and Cortex Cinnamomi Cassiae (*Rou Gui*), 6g each, Fructus Zizyphi Jujubae (*Da Zao*), 3 pieces, and uncooked Rhizoma Zingiberis (*Sheng Jiang*), 2 slices.

If there is qi and yin dual vacuity, replace *Ping Wei San Jia Wei* with *Shen Ling Bai Zhu San Jia Jian* (Ginseng, Poriae & Atractylodes Powder with Additions & Subtractions): Semen Coicis Lachryma-jobi (*Yi Yi Ren*), 20g, Dolichoris Lablab (*Bai Bian Dou*), Radix Dioscoreae Oppositae (*Shan Yao*), and Semen Nelumbinis Nuciferae (*Lian Zi*), 15g each, Radix Codonopsitis Pilosulae (*Dang Shen*) and Sclerotium Poriae Cocos (*Fu Ling*), 12g each, Rhizoma Atractylodis Macrocephalae (*Bai Zhu*), Radix Bupleuri (*Chai Hu*), Radix Albus Paeoniae Lactiflorae (*Bai Shao*), Radix Auklandiae Lappae (*Mu Xiang*), and Radix Platycodi Grandiflori (*Jie Geng*), 9g each, mix-fried Radix Glycyrrhizae (*Gan Cao*), 6g, and Fructus Cardamomi (*Bai Dou Kou*), 3g.

If qi and yin vacuity are complicated by fire effulgence, one can use the following unnamed Chinese medicinal formula: Radix Dioscoreae Oppositae (*Shan Yao*) and Radix Astragali Membranacei (*Huang Qi*), 20g each, Gypsum Fibrosum (*Shi Gao*) and Rhizoma Anemarrhenae Asphodeloidis (*Zhi Mu*), 15g each, Tuber Ophiopogonis Japonici (*Mai Men Dong*), Radix Scrophulariae Ningpoensis (*Xuan Shen*), and uncooked Radix Rehmanniae (*Sheng Di*), 9g each, and Radix Panacis Ginseng (*Ren Shen*) and Radix Et Rhizoma Rhei (*Da Huang*), 6g each. If there is no constipation, subtract *Da Huang*. For severe constipation, add nine grams of Mirabilitum (*Mang Xiao*). For emaciation, add 15 grams each of Rhizoma Atractylodis Macrocephalae (*Bai Zhu*) and Rhizoma Polygonati (*Huang Jing*). For severe thirst, add 15 grams each of Radix Trichosanthis Kirlowii (*Tian Hua Fen*), Rhizoma Polygonati Odorati (*Yu Zhu*), and Radix Puerariae (*Ge Gen*). For frequent, profuse urination, add nine grams each of Fructus Lycii Chinensis (*Gou Qi Zi*), Fructus Pruni Mume (*Wu Mei*), and Fructus Rosae Laevigatae (*Jin Ying Zi*).

ACUPUNCTURE & MOXIBUSTION: *Shang Wan* (CV 13), *Zhong Wan* (CV 12), *Xia Wan* (CV 10), *Qi Hai* (CV 6), *Tian Shu* (St 25), *Nei Guan* (Per 6), *Zu San Li* (St 36)

ANALYSIS OF FORMULA: Draining *Shang Wan*, *Zhong Wan*, and *Xia Wan* disinhibits the qi mechanism and regulates and rectifies upbearing and downbearing. Draining *Tian Shu* and *Qi Hai* regulates and rectifies the qi of the lower burner in general and intestines in particular. Supplementing *Zu San Li* supplements the spleen and boosts the qi on the one hand and regulates and rectifies the qi of the yang ming on the other. *Nei Guan* is a point on the hand jue yin. Draining it courses the liver and rectifies the qi, harmonizes the stomach and downbears counterflow.

ADDITIONS & SUBTRACTIONS: For symptoms of cold, add moxibustion on *Zu San Li*, *Zhong Wan*, *Qi Hai*, and *Tian Shu*. For a liver-spleen disharmony, subtract *Zhong Wan* and *Xia Wan* and add *Zhang Men* (Liv 13). For concomitant food stagnation, replace *Shang Wan* and *Qi Hai* with *Liang Men* (St 21) and *Xuan Ji* (CV 21).

5. FOOD STAGNATION PATTERN

MAIN SYMPTOMS: Ductal and abdominal distention and pain, bad breath, putrid belching, no desire to eat or drink, rotten egg smelling diarrhea, decreased pain after defecation, uncrisp defecation (meaning that it may be either or both sticky and difficult), thick, slimy, turbid tongue fur, and a bowstring, slippery pulse

NOTE: This pattern only really complicates other of the above patterns.

TREATMENT PRINCIPLES: Disperse food and abduct stagnation

RX: *Bao He Wan Jia Jian* (Protect Harmony Pills with Additions & Subtractions)

INGREDIENTS: Fructus Crataegi (*Shan Zha*), 12g, Massa Medica Fermentata (*Shen Qu*), Semen Raphani Sativi (*Lai Fu Zi*), Rhizoma Pinelliae Ternatae (*Ban Xia*), Sclerotium Poriae Cocos (*Fu Ling*), Fructus Immaturus Citri Aurantii (*Zhi Shi*), and Cortex Magnoliae Officinalis (*Hou Po*), 9g each, and Pericarpium Citri Reticulatae (*Chen Pi*), 6g

ANALYSIS OF FORMULA: *Shan Zha* and *Shen Qu* disperse food and abduct stagnation. *Lai Fu Zi* and *Chen Pi* disperse food and move the qi. *Zhi Shi* moves the qi and breaks accumulation, while *Hou Po* moves the qi and transforms dampness. *Fu Ling* fortifies the spleen and disinhibits dampness, and *Ban Xia* harmonizes the stomach and dries dampness.

ADDITIONS & SUBTRACTIONS: For constipation, add 6-9 grams of Radix Et Rhizoma Rhei (*Da Huang*). For heat symptoms, add nine grams of Radix Scutellariae Baicalensis (*Huang Qin*) and three grams of Rhizoma Coptidis Chinensis (*Huang Lian*). For cold symptoms, add six grams of dry Rhizoma Zingiberis (*Gan Jiang*) and nine grams of Rhizoma Atractylodis Macrocephalae (*Bai Zhu*). For concomitant spleen qi vacuity, add 15 grams of Rhizoma Atractylodis Macrocephalae (*Bai Zhu*). For severe distention and pain below the rib-side, add 15 grams each of Radix Bupleuri (*Chai Hu*) and Tuber Curcumae (*Yu Jin*).

ACUPUNCTURE & MOXIBUSTION: *Zhong Wan* (CV 12), *Xia Wan* (CV 10), *Tian Shu* (St 25), *Nei Guan* (Per 6), *Zu San Li* (St 36), *Liang Men* (St 21), *Xuan Ji* (CV 21)

ANALYSIS OF FORMULA: Please see pattern #4 above. Draining *Liang Men* and *Xuan Ji* disperses food and abducts stagnation.

ADDITIONS & SUBTRACTIONS: Please see pattern #4 above.

REMARKS

1. Most cases of chronic pancreatitis manifest spleen vacuity with qi stagnation and blood stasis. Another way of stating this is a liver-spleen disharmony with blood stasis. Then, depending on the constitution of the patient, these are complicated by heat (*i.e.*, damp heat) and/or food stagnation or, in the case of diabetes mellitus, yin vacuity.

2. Chinese medicinal and acupuncture therapy are secondary to a correct diet, abstinence from alcohol, and stress reduction. Without these three as a basis, Chinese medicinals and acupuncture cannot be expected to achieve their full effects in the treatment of this condition.

18

CHRONIC PROSTATITIS

Chronic prostatitis refers to chronic inflammation of the prostate gland. It is divided into two types: bacterial and nonbacterial. In chronic bacterial prostatitis, there is relapsing urinary tract infection due to the same pathogen as found in the prostatic secretions. Most patients experience low back and perineal pain, urinary urgency and frequency, and painful urination. Diagnosis is based on history, presenting signs and symptoms, and cultures taken from the urethra, bladder, and prostatic secretions. The symptoms of nonbacterial prostatitis are similar to those of bacterial prostatitis. However, no pathogenic bacteria can be cultured and there is rarely a history of urinary tract infection. Nonbacterial prostatitis is far more common than the bacterial form. Its etiology is unknown, and it does not respond to antimicrobial therapy. Hot sitz baths and anticholinergic drugs may provide some symptomatic relief, and periodic prostate massage helps improve symptoms in some patients.

CHINESE DISEASE CATEGORIZATION: Chronic prostatitis is categorized as *qi lin*, qi strangury, or *tong lin*, painful strangury, when characterized by pain and distention. It is categorized as *lao lin*, taxation strangury, when it is associated with fatigue, and it is categorized as *re lin*, heat strangury, when it is accompanied by burning urination.

DISEASE CAUSES: Enduring disease, internal damage by the seven affects, unregulated eating and drinking, taxation fatigue, and aging

DISEASE MECHANISMS: Faulty diet may give rise to dampness and heat pouring downward. When these accumulate in the bladder, they hinder and obstruct the bladder's qi mechanism. This results in painful urination, choppy, rough urination, frequent, urgent urination, and burning urination. Due to unfulfilled desires, the liver may be damaged and fail to control coursing and discharge. In that case, the bladder qi mechanism may become inhibited, thus giving rise to difficulty urinating, painful urination, and incomplete urination. If damp heat and/or qi stagnation endure, they may give rise to blood stasis which even further inhibits the bladder's qi mechanism. Hence there is more serious and enduring urinary difficulty and more severe, localized, sharp, and/or stabbing pain. Due to enduring damp heat or to over-taxation, faulty diet, and too much thinking and worrying, the spleen qi may become vacuous and weak. Also due to enduring damp heat or to aging, the kidney qi may be consumed. In either or both cases, there will be insufficient qi to move fluids out of the bladder and insufficient qi to hold fluids within the bladder. Thus there is hesitant, difficult urination and terminal dribbling. Kidney qi vacuity may be associated with either kidney yin or kidney yang vacuity or both.

TREATMENT BASED ON PATTERN DISCRIMINATION:

1. DAMP HEAT STASIS & STAGNATION PATTERN

MAIN SYMPTOMS: Recurrent bouts of urinary pain, frequency, and urgency, pain in the genitals radiating to the groin, lower abdomen, and perineum, scanty, yellow or turbid urine, possible constipation or dry stools or, more rarely, uneasy defecation of loose stools with a burning sensation in the anus, effort to defecate causing a milky white, turbid discharge from the urethra, possible dryness, bitterness, and/or sliminess in the mouth, restlessness, possible itchy and/or damp scrotum, possible fever, aversion to cold, and body pains when severe, headache, a red tongue with slimy, thick, yellow fur, and a slippery, bowstring, rapid or soggy, rapid pulse

TREATMENT PRINCIPLES: Clear heat and eliminate dampness, quicken the blood and transform stasis

RX: *Huang Bai Jiang Cao Tang* (Phellodendron & Patrinia Decoction)

INGREDIENTS: Semen Vaccariae Segetalis (*Wang Bu Liu Xing*), Cortex Phellodendri (*Huang Bai*), Herba Patriniae Heterophyllae Cum Radice (*Bai Jiang Cao*), and Herba Taraxaci Mongolici Cum Radice (*Pu Gong Ying*), 15g each, Rhizoma Corydalis Yanhusuo (*Yan Hu Suo*) and Radix Rubrus Paeoniae Lactiflorae (*Chi Shao*), 12g each, Cortex Radicis Moutan (*Dan Pi*), Squama Manitis Pentadactylis (*Chuan Shan Jia*), and Spina Gleditschiae Chinensis (*Zao Jiao Ci*), 9g each, Radix Auklandiae Lappae (*Mu Xiang*), 6g, and Radix Glycyrrhizae (*Gan Cao*), 3g

ANALYSIS OF FORMULA: *Huang Bai* clears heat and dries dampness, especially in the lower burner. *Pu Gong Ying* and *Bai Jiang Cao* clear heat and resolve toxins. In addition, *Bai Jiang Cao* transforms stasis and stops pain. *Zao Jiao Ci* quickens the blood, disperses swelling, and expels pus. *Wang Bu Liu Xing, Yan Hu Suo, Chi Shao, Dan Pi,* and *Chuan Shan Jia* quicken the blood, transform stasis, and stop pain. In addition, *Chuan Shan Jia* disperses swelling and expels pus. *Mu Xiang* moves the qi and stops pain, and *Gan Cao* harmonizes the other medicinals in the formula.

ADDITIONS & SUBTRACTIONS: For concomitant spleen qi vacuity, add 15 grams each of Radix Astragali Membranacei (*Huang Qi*) and 9 grams each of Radix Codonopsitis Pilosulae (*Dang Shen*), Rhizoma Atractylodis Macrocephalae (*Bai Zhu*), and Sclerotium Poriae Cocos (*Fu Ling*). If there is more pronounced qi stagnation, add 15 grams of Fructus Meliae Toosendan (*Chuan Lian Zi*) and 9 grams of Radix Bupleuri (*Chai Hu*). For marked damp heat with scanty, burning, urgent, frequent, painful urination or simply difficult urination, add 12 grams each of Semen Plantaginis (*Che Qian Zi*), Rhizoma Dioscoreae Hypoglaucae (*Bei Xie*), and Herba Dianthi (*Qu Mai*). For bacterial type, add 15 grams of Flos Lonicerae Japonicae (*Jin Yin Hua*), and nine grams of Radix Et Rhizoma Polygoni Cuspidati (*Hu Zhang*). For turbid or milky white urine, add 12 grams each of Sclerotium Poriae Cocos (*Fu Ling*) and Rhizoma Acori Graminei (*Shi Chang Pu*). For a thick, turbid discharge dripping from the urethra, add 12 grams each of Rhizoma Smilacis Glabrae (*Tu Fu Ling*), Rhizoma Acori Graminei (*Shi Chang Pu*), and Semen Coicis Lachryma-jobi (*Yi Yi Ren*). For constipation or dry stools, add 6-9 grams of Radix Et Rhizoma Rhei (*Da Huang*). For dry mouth, add 12 grams of Radix Trichosanthis Kirlowii (*Tian Hua Fen*). For damp and itchy scrotum, add nine grams each of Radix Sophorae Flavescentis (*Ku Shen*) and Fructus Kochiae Scopariae (*Di Fu Zi*). For nausea and stomach and abdominal distention, add nine grams each of Rhizoma Pinelliae Ternatae (*Ban Xia*) and Pericarpium Citri Reticulatae (*Chen Pi*). For severe distention and pain in the *Hui Yin* (CV 1) area, add 15 grams each of Semen Litchi Sinensis (*Li Zhi He*) and Semen Citri Reticulatae (*Ju He*) and nine grams of Fructus Meliae Toosendan (*Chuan Lian Zi*). For fever, add nine grams of Rhizoma Coptidis Chinensis (*Huang Lian*) and 30 grams of Herba Taraxaci Mongolici Cum Radice (*Pu Gong Ying*). For bloody urine, add nine grams each of Herba Seu Radix Cirsii Japonici (*Da Ji*) and Herba Cephalanoploris Segeti (*Xiao Ji*) and 20 grams each of uncooked Radix Rehmanniae (*Sheng Di*) and Rhizoma Imperatae Cylindricae (*Bai Mao Gen*). For insomnia and restlessness, add 12 grams each of Rhizoma Acori Graminei (*Shi Chang Pu*), Sclerotium Pararadicis Poriae Cocos (*Fu Shen*), and Radix Polygalae Tenuifoliae (*Yuan Zhi*).

If enduring damp heat has damaged yin and there is stasis and stagnation, replace *Huang Bai Jiang Cao Tang* with *Xuan Shen Sheng Di Tang* (Scrophularia & Uncooked Rehmannia Decoction): Radix Scrophulariae Ningpoensis (*Xuan Shen*) and uncooked Radix Rehmanniae (*Sheng Di*), 15g each, Radix Lithospermi Seu Arnebiae (*Zi Cao*), Herba Violae Yedoensitis Cum Radice (*Zi Hua Di Ding*), and Semen Plantaginis (*Che Qian Zi*), 12g each, Gelatinum Corii Asini (*E Jiao*), Cortex Phellodendri (*Huang Bai*), Resina Olibani (*Ru Xiang*), Resina Myrrhae (*Mo Yao*), and Herba Leonuri Heterophylli (*Yi Mu Cao*), 9g each. If there is qi vacuity with fatigue and lack of strength, add 15 grams of Radix Astragali Membranacei (*Huang Qi*) and nine grams of Radix Codonopsitis Pilosulae (*Dang Shen*). If there is concomitant yang vacuity, add 6-9 grams each of Radix Lateralis Praeparatus Aconiti Carmichaeli (*Fu Zi*) and Cortex Cinnamomi Cassiae (*Rou Gui*). If there is constipation, add six grams of Radix Et Rhizoma Rhei (*Da Huang*). If there is lower abdominal distention, add nine grams each of Fructus Meliae Toosendan (*Chuan Lian Zi*) and Radix Linderae Strychnifoliae (*Wu Yao*).

ACUPUNCTURE & MOXIBUSTION: *Qu Gu* (CV 2), *Hui Yin* (CV 1), *Yin Ling Quan* (Sp 9), *Zhi Bian* (Bl 54)

ANALYSIS OF FORMULA: Draining *Qu Gu, Hui Yin,* and *Yin Ling Quan* clears heat and disinhibits dampness in the lower burner. *Zhi Bian* quickens the blood and disinhibits dampness, frees the flow of the network vessels and stops pain. Needle *Zhi Bian* with deep insertion in the direction of *Gui Lai* (St 29) or *Shui Dao* (St 28).

ADDITIONS & SUBTRACTIONS: For pain in the genitals, add *Da Dun* (Liv 1). For itchy, damp scrotum, add *Li Gou* (Liv 5). For severe distention in the *Hui Yin* (CV 1) area, add *Zhong Liao* (Bl 33) and *Hui Yang* (Bl 35). For pain and distention in the lower abdomen, add *Gui Lai* (St 29). For concomitant spleen qi vacuity, add *Tai Bai* (Sp 3) and *San Yin Jiao* (Sp 6). For marked damp heat with scanty, burning, urgent, frequent, painful urination or simply difficult urination, add *San Yin Jiao* (Sp 6) and *Zhi Bian* (Bl 54). For turbid or milky white urine, add *San Yin Jiao* (Sp 6). For constipation or dry stools, add *Zhi Gou* (TB 6). For dry mouth, add *Fu Liu* (Ki 7). For nausea and stomach and abdominal distention, add *Zhong Wan* (CV 12) and *Tian Shu* (St 25). For fever, add *He Gu* (LI 4), *Wai Guan* (TB 5), and *Qu Chi* (LI 11). For bloody urine, add *Xue Hai* (Sp 10). For insomnia and restlessness, add *Tong Li* (Ht 5).

2. QI STAGNATION & BLOOD STASIS PATTERN

MAIN SYMPTOMS: Enduring disease which does not heal, marked, possibly lancinating perineal area pain, pain radiating to the testes, penis, lower abdomen, or low back, dark circles around the eyes, possible penile indurations, urinary dribbling, rough, astringent, painful urination, painful sexual intercourse and especially ejaculation, possible spermaturia or hematuria, a hard prostate or possible nodulations on the prostate on rectal examination, possible mental-emotional depression, irritability, insomnia, restlessness, a dark, purplish tongue or possible static macules or spots, and a bowstring, choppy pulse

TREATMENT PRINCIPLES: Quicken the blood and dispel stasis, move the qi and stop pain

RX: *Huo Xue San Yu Tang* (Quicken the Blood & Scatter Stasis Decoction)

INGREDIENTS: Radix Salviae Miltiorrhizae (*Dan Shen*), 15g, Herba Lycopi Lucidi (*Ze Lan*), Radix Rubrus Paeoniae Lactiflorae (*Chi Shao*), Semen Pruni Persicae (*Tao Ren*), Radix Ligustici Wallichii (*Chuan Xiong*), Lignum Sappan (*Su Mu*), Cortex Radicis Moutan (*Dan Pi*), and Semen Arecae Catechu (*Bing Lang*), 9g each, and Fructus Citri Aurantii (*Zhi Ke*), 6g

ANALYSIS OF FORMULA: *Dan Shen, Ze Lan, Chi Shao, Tao Ren, Chuan Xiong, Su Mu,* and *Dan Pi* quicken the blood, transform and stop stasis. *Bing Lang* and *Zhi Ke* move the qi and stop pain, especially in the lower burner.

ADDITIONS & SUBTRACTIONS: If there is constipation, add nine grams of Fructus Trichosanthis Kirlowii (*Gua Lou*) and six grams of Radix Et Rhizoma Rhei (*Da Huang*). For stabbing pain, add three grams of Radix Pseudoginseng (*San Qi*). For stabbing, piercing pain on urination, add three grams of Succinum (*Hu Po*), powdered and taken with the strained decoction. For bacterial prostatitis, add 12 grams each of Herba Patriniae Heterophyllae Cum Radice (*Bai Jiang Cao*), Caulis Sargentodoxae (*Hong Teng*), and Herba Taraxaci Mongolici Cum Radice (*Pu Gong Ying*). For lower abdomen, groin, or genital distention and pain, add nine grams each of Radix Bupleuri (*Chai Hu*) and Rhizoma Cyperi Rotundi (*Xiang Fu*). For white, milky drops discharged from the urethra, add nine grams each of Rhizoma Acori Graminei (*Shi Chang Pu*), Sclerotium Poriae Cocos (*Fu Ling*), and Rhizoma Dioscoreae Hypoglaucae (*Bei Xie*). For nodulations on the prostate, add 12 grams each of Ramulus Cinnamomi Cassiae (*Gui Zhi*), Sclerotium Poriae Cocos (*Fu Ling*), and Rhizoma Curcumae Zedoariae (*E Zhu*) and one gram of Hirudo Seu Whitmania (*Shui Zhi*), powdered and taken with the strained decoction. For distention and pain in the scrotum with an enlarged prostate, add 12 grams each of Semen Citri Reticulatae (*Ju He*), Semen Litchi Sinensis (*Li Zhi He*), and Fructus Meliae Toosendan (*Chuan Lian Zi*). For mental depression, irritability, and insomnia, add nine grams each of Radix Bupleuri (*Chai Hu*) and Radix Albus Paeoniae Lactiflorae (*Bai Shao*) and 20 grams each of Cortex Albizziae Julibrissinis (*He Huan Pi*) and Caulis Polygoni Multiflori (*Ye Jiao Teng*). For spermaturia or hematuria, add 15 grams each of Pollen Typhae (*Pu Huang*) and Feces Trogopterori Seu Pteromi (*Wu Ling Zhi*). For a cold sensation in the lower abdomen and/or scrotal area, add nine grams each of Radix Linderae Strychnifoliae (*Wu Yao*) and Fructus Foeniculi Vulgaris (*Xiao Hui Xiang*). For a burning sensation in the lower abdomen and/or scrotal area, add nine grams each of Cortex Phellodendri (*Huang Bai*) and Radix Sophorae Flavescentis (*Ku Shen*). For difficult urination, add 30 grams of Herba Leonuri Heterophylli (*Yi Mu Cao*). For concomitant kidney yin vacuity, add nine grams each of Fructus Ligustri Lucidi (*Nu Zhen Zi*), Fructus Lycii Chinensis (*Gou Qi Zi*), and Herba Ecliptae Prostratae (*Han Lian Cao*). For concomitant kidney yang vacuity, add nine grams each of Herba Epimedii (*Yin Yang Huo*), Semen Cuscutae Chinensis (*Tu Si Zi*), and Radix Morindae Officinalis (*Ba Ji Tian*). For concomitant qi vacuity, add 15 grams of Radix Astragali Membranacei (*Huang Qi*) and nine grams of Radix Codonopsitis Pilosulae (*Dang Shen*).

If there is cold congealing in the blood vessels with pain and cool sensation in the perineum, scrotum, and lower abdomen, frequent, urgent painful, dribbling urination, a milky white discharge from the urethra, aversion to cold, normal or loose stools, a pale, purple tongue with thin, white fur, and a bowstring, rough pulse, replace *Huo Xue San Yu Tang* with *Gui Zhi Fu Ling Wan Jia Wei* (Cinnamon & Poria Pills with Added Flavors): Ramulus Cinnamomi Cassiae (*Gui Zhi*), Radix Albus Paeoniae Lactiflorae (*Bai Shao*), Fructus Foeniculi Vulgaris (*Xiao Hui Xiang*), Radix Linderae Strychnifoliae (*Wu Yao*), and Semen Litchi Sinensis (*Li Zhi He*), 12g each, Sclerotium Poriae Cocos (*Fu Ling*), Radix Rubrus Paeoniae Lactiflorae (*Chi Shao*), Cortex Radicis Moutan (*Dan Pi*), and Semen Pruni Persicae (*Tao Ren*), 9g each, uncooked Rhizoma Zingiberis (*Sheng Jiang*) and mix-fried Radix Glycyrrhizae (*Zhi Gan Cao*), 6g each, and Radix Lateralis Praeparatus Aconiti Carmichaeli (*Fu Zi*), 3g.

ACUPUNCTURE & MOXIBUSTION: *Qu Gu* (CV 2), *Hui Yin* (CV 1), *Xue Hai* (Sp 10), *San Yin Jiao* (Sp 6), *Zhi Bian* (Bl 54)

ANALYSIS OF FORMULA: Draining *Qu Gu* and *Hui Yin* disinhibits dampness, frees the flow of the network vessels in the lower burner, and stops pain. Draining *Zhi Bian* in combination with *San Yin Jiao* and *Xue Hai* disinhibits dampness and quickens the blood, transforms stasis, frees the flow of the network vessels, and stops pain. Needle *Zhi Bian* with deep insertion in the direction of *Gui Lai* (St 29) or *Shui Dao* (St 28). In addition, *San Yin Jiao* and *Xue Hai* cool the blood and stop bleeding.

ADDITIONS & SUBTRACTIONS: For stabbing pain in the genitals, add *Da Dun* (Liv 1). For stabbing, piercing pain on urination, add *Shui Dao* (St 28). For lower abdominal, groin, and genital distention and pain, add *Qu Quan* (Liv 8). For severe distention in the perineal area, add *Zhong Liao* (Bl 33) and *Hui Yang* (Bl 35). For nodulations on the prostate gland, add *Zhong Liao* (Bl 33) and *Hui Yang* (Bl 35). For mental depression, irritability, and insomnia, add *Zhong Feng* (Liv 4), *Da Dun* (Liv 1), and *Tong Li* (Ht 5). For spermaturia or hematuria, add *Da Dun* (Liv 1) with moxibustion. For a cold sensation in the lower abdomen and/or scrotal area, add *Guan Yuan* (CV 4) with moxibustion. For a burning sensation in the lower abdomen and/or scrotal area, add *Da Dun* (Liv 1) and *Li Dui* (St 45) (bleed). For difficult urination, add *Yin Ling Quan* (Sp 9). For concomitant, kidney yin vacuity, add *Fu Liu* (Ki 7). For concomitant kidney yang vacuity, add *Tai Xi* (Ki 3). For concomitant qi vacuity, add *Tai Bai* (Sp 3). For constipation or dry stools, add *Zhi Gou* (TB 6).

3. SPLEEN QI VACUITY PATTERN

MAIN SYMPTOMS: Enduring disease, terminal dribbling which is worse with fatigue, frequent, urgent urination, a desire to urinate but without success, white deposits in the urine, possible long, clear urination, possible slight hematuria, sagging pain in the perineal area, fatigue, lassitude of the spirit, lack of strength, a lusterless facial complexion, a pale, fat tongue, and a fine, soft pulse

NOTE: This pattern rarely appears in its simple, discrete form. However, it often complicates many, if not all, the other patterns in this chapter.

TREATMENT PRINCIPLES: Supplement the center and boost the qi

RX: *Bu Zhong Yi Qi Tang* (Supplement the Center & Boost the Qi Decoction)

INGREDIENTS: Radix Astragali Membranacei (*Huang Qi*), 18g, Radix Codonopsitis Pilosulae (*Dang Shen*), 12g, Rhizoma Atractylodis Macrocephalae (*Bai Zhu*), 9g, Radix Angelicae Sinensis (*Dang Gui*), Pericarpium Citri Reticulatae (*Chen Pi*), and mix-fried Radix Glycyrrhizae (*Gan Cao*), 6g each, Rhizoma Cimicifugae (*Sheng Ma*), 4.5g, and Radix Bupleuri (*Chai Hu*), 3g

ANALYSIS OF FORMULA: *Huang Qi*, *Dang Shen*, *Bai Zhu* and mix-fried *Gan Cao* fortify the spleen and boost the qi. *Chai Hu* and *Sheng Ma* upbear yang and raise the fallen. *Dang Gui* harmonizes the blood, while *Chen Pi* rectifies the qi.

ADDITIONS & SUBTRACTIONS: For dribbling urination, add nine grams each of Fructus Alpiniae Oxyphyllae (*Yi Zhi Ren*), Semen Euryalis Ferocis (*Qian Shi*), and Semen Cuscutae Chinensis (*Tu Si Zi*). For difficult urination, add nine grams each of Sclerotium Poriae Cocos (*Fu Ling*) and Sclerotium Polypori Umbellati (*Zhu Ling*).

ACUPUNCTURE & MOXIBUSTION: *Hui Yin* (CV 1), *Guan Yuan* (CV 4), *Qi Hai* (CV 6), *Bai Hui* (GV 20), *Zu San Li* (St 36), *San Yin Jiao* (Sp 6)

ANALYSIS OF FORMULA: Supplementing *Guan Yuan*, *Qi Hai*, and *Bai Hui* with moxibustion boosts the qi and upbears the clear. Supplementing *Zu San Li* and *San Yin Jiao* fortifies the spleen, boosts the qi, and upbears the clear. Moxaing *Hui Yin* harmonizes the network vessels and supplements vacuity.

ADDITIONS & SUBTRACTIONS: For sagging pain in the genitals, add *Da Dun* (Liv 1) with moxibustion. For lower abdominal, groin and genital distention and pain, add *Qu Quan* (Liv 8). For hematuria, add *Da Dun* (Liv 1) with moxibustion. For frequent urination, add *Zhong Ji* (CV 3) with supplementing method. For difficult urination, add *Yin Ling Quan* (Sp 9). For susceptibility to common cold, add *He Gu* (LI 4) and *Da Zhui* (GV 14). For food stagnation, add *Liang Men* (St 21). For concomitant kidney qi vacuity, add *Tai Xi* (Ki 3). For concomitant kidney yin vacuity, add *Fu Liu* (Ki 7). For heart-spleen dual vacuity, add *Shen Men* (Ht 7). For severe qi vacuity, add *Tai Bai* (Sp 3).

4. KIDNEY YIN VACUITY PATTERN

MAIN SYMPTOMS: Discharge of a clear, thin fluid from the urethra, frequent but scanty urination, dribbling urination which is worse with taxation, frequent nocturia, yellow urine, low back pain, dizziness, tinnitus, impotence, seminal emission, insomnia, night sweats, vexatious heat in the five hearts, possible feverish sensation or low-grade fever in the afternoon, constipation, a red tongue with scanty fluids, and a fine, rapid pulse

TREATMENT PRINCIPLES: Enrich yin and supplement the kidneys, disinhibit dampness and abduct the turbid

RX: *Liu Wei Di Huang Wan* (Six Flavors Rehmannia Decoction) & *Er Zhi Wan* (Two Ultimates Pills) plus added flavors

INGREDIENTS: Uncooked Radix Rehmanniae (*Sheng Di*),

cooked Radix Rehmanniae (*Shu Di*), Radix Dioscoreae Oppositae (*Shan Yao*), Sclerotium Poriae Cocos (*Fu Ling*), and Rhizoma Alismatis (*Ze Xie*), 15g each, and Fructus Corni Officinalis (*Shan Zhu Yu*), Cortex Radicis Moutan (*Dan Pi*), Fructus Ligustri Lucidi (*Nu Zhen Zi*), Herba Ecliptae Prostratae (*Han Lian Cao*), Rhizoma Smilacis Glabrae (*Tu Fu Ling*), and Rhizoma Dioscoreae Hypoglaucae (*Bei Xie*), 9g each

ANALYSIS OF FORMULA: *Sheng Di, Shu Di, Shan Yao, Shan Zhu Yu, Nu Zhen Zi*, and *Han Lian Cao* together enrich yin, boost the essence, and supplement the kidneys. In addition, *Shan Yao* and *Shan Zhu Yu* astringe the essence. *Dan Pi* cools and quickens the blood. *Ze Xie, Fu Ling, Tu Fu Ling*, and *Bei Xie* clear and disinhibit dampness and heat in the lower burner and abduct the turbid.

ADDITIONS & SUBTRACTIONS: For frequent nocturia and seminal emission, add 12 grams each of Fructus Rosae Laevigatae (*Jin Ying Zi*), Semen Euryalis Ferocis (*Qian Shi*), and Fructus Schisandrae Chinensis (*Wu Wei Zi*). For concomitant qi vacuity, add 15 grams of Radix Astragali Membranacei (*Huang Qi*) and nine grams of Rhizoma Atractylodis Macrocephalae (*Bai Zhu*). For nodules on the prostate gland, add 12 grams each of Semen Litchi Sinensis (*Li Zhi He*), Semen Citri Reticulatae (*Ju He*), and Endothelium Corneum Gigeriae Galli (*Ji Nei Jin*). For concomitant kidney yang vacuity, add 1 one gram of Cortex Cinnamomi Cassiae (*Rou Gui*) and 12 grams each of Herba Epimedii (*Yin Yang Huo*) and Radix Morindae Officinalis (*Ba Ji Tian*). For difficult urination with a burning sensation, add 15 grams of Semen Plantaginis (*Che Qian Zi*). For restlessness and insomnia, add 12 grams each of Radix Polygalae Tenuifoliae (*Yuan Zhi*), Rhizoma Acori Graminei (*Shi Chang Pu*), and Sclerotium Pararadicis Poriae Cocos (*Fu Shen*).

If there is yin vacuity fire effulgence with the same symptoms as above but with increased sexual desire, easy erection, hyperactive sexuality but with absence of ejaculation or ejaculation stopping suddenly during coitus, slight distention and pain in the scrotum and perinenal area which is better after ejaculation, frequent, urgent, painful urination, seminal emission while dreaming, and a dry mouth and throat, replace *Liu Wei Di Huang Wan* (Six Flavors Rehmannia Decoction) plus *Er Zhi Wan* (Two Ultimates Pills) with *Zhi Bai Di Huang Wan* (Anemarrhena & Phellodendron Rehmannia Pills) plus *Bei Xie Fen Qing Yin* (Dioscorea Hypoglauca Divide the Clear Drink) with additions and subtractions: uncooked Radix Rehmanniae (*Sheng Di*), Rhizoma Alismatis (*Ze Xie*), Sclerotium Poriae Cocos (*Fu Ling*), Cortex Radicis Moutan (*Dan Pi*), Radix Dioscoreae Oppositae (*Shan Yao*), Fructus Corni Officinalis (*Shan Zhu Yu*), Radix Salviae Miltiorrhizae (*Dan Shen*), Plumula Nelumbinis Nuciferae (*Lian Xin*), and Semen Plantaginis (*Che Qian Zi*), 15g each, Cortex Phellodendri (*Huang Bai*), Rhizoma Anemarrhenae Asphodeloidis (*Zhi Mu*), and Rhizoma Dioscoreae Hypoglaucae (*Bei Xie*), 12g each, and Rhizoma Acori Graminei (*Shi Chang Pu*) and Rhizoma Atractylodis Macrocephalae (*Bai Zhu*), 9g each.

ACUPUNCTURE & MOXIBUSTION: *Hui Yin* (CV 1), *Qu Gu* (CV 2), *Fu Liu* (Ki 7), *Shen Shu* (Bl 23), *Hui Yang* (Bl 35)

ANALYSIS OF FORMULA: Using even supplementing-even draining on *Hui Yin* and *Qu Gu* clears and disinhibits dampness and heat, abducts the turbid, and harmonizes the network vessels. Supplementing *Fu Liu* and *Shen Shu* enriches yin and secures the kidneys. *Hui Yang* with the even supplementing-even draining method transforms dampness, divides the clear, and stops pain. *Hui Yang* should be needled deeply, 2-3 cun, to induce a qi sensation in the affected area.

ADDITIONS & SUBTRACTIONS: Please see patterns #1 and 2 above.

5. QI & YIN VACUITY PATTERN

MAIN SYMPTOMS: Enduring low back and sacral soreness and pain, perineal pain, testicular sagging and distention, symptoms worse with fatigue, dizziness, insomnia, heart palpitations, a red tongue with scanty fur, and a fine, bowstring, rapid pulse

NOTE: Although the name of this pattern does not say so, there is persistent damp heat consuming qi and yin complicated by an element of blood stasis.

TREATMENT PRINCIPLES: Fortify the spleen and boost the qi, enrich yin and drain heat

RX: *Shen Ling Liu Huang Tang* (Ginseng & Poria Six Yellows Decoction)

INGREDIENTS: Radix Astragali Membranacei (*Huang Qi*) and uncooked Radix Rehmanniae (*Sheng Di*), 30g each, Radix Codonopsitis Pilosulae (*Dang Shen*), Sclerotium Poriae Cocos (*Fu Ling*), Rhizoma Polygonati (*Huang Jing*), and Semen Plantaginis (*Che Qian Zi*), 15g each, Radix Achyranthi Bidentatae (*Niu Xi*), 12g, and Rhizoma Coptidis Chinensis (*Huang Lian*), Cortex Phellodendri (*Huang Bai*), and Pollen Typhae (*Pu Huang*), 9g each

ANALYSIS OF FORMULA: *Dang Shen, Fu Ling, Huang Qi*, and *Huang Jing* fortify the spleen and boost the qi. In addition, *Huang Qi* and *Fu Ling* with *Che Qian Zi* disinhibit dampness. *Sheng Di* and *Niu Xi* enrich yin and supplement the kidneys. *Huang Bai* and *Huang Lian* clear and disinhibit dampness and heat, especially in the lower burner. *Niu Xi* and *Pu Huang* quicken the blood and transform stasis.

ADDITIONS & SUBTRACTIONS: Please see patterns # 1, 2, and 3 above.

ACUPUNCTURE & MOXIBUSTION: *Zhi Bian* (Bl 54), *San Yin Jiao* (Sp 6), *Zu San Li* (St 36), *Fu Liu* (Ki 7), *Hui Yin* (CV 1)

ANALYSIS OF FORMULA: Draining *Hui Yin, Zhi Bian,* and *San Yin Jiao* clears and disinhibits dampness and heat, quickens the blood, frees the flow of the network vessels, and stops pain in the lower burner. Supplementing *Zu San Li* with moxibustion fortifies the spleen and boosts the qi, while supplementing *Fu Liu* enriches yin and supplements the kidneys.

ADDITIONS & SUBTRACTIONS: Please see patterns #1, 2, and 3 above.

6. KIDNEY YANG VACUITY WITH DAMP TURBIDITY PATTERN

MAIN SYMPTOMS: Enduring insidious perineal pain, white deposits in the urine, nocturia, possible spermaturia, decreased sexual desire or impotence, possible sterility, low back pain, fear of cold, terminal dribbling which will not stop, a sticky, whitish discharge at the end of urination, fatigue, lassitude of the spirit, a somber white facial complexion, puffy edema of the lower extremities, loose stools, a pale, fat tongue with white, moist fur, and a deep, slow, forceless pulse

TREATMENT PRINCIPLES: Supplement the kidneys and warm yang, transform dampness and divide the clear

RX: *Shen Qi Wan Jia Wei* (Kidney Qi Pills with Added Flavors) & *Bei Xie Fen Qing Yin* (Dioscorea Hypoglauca Divide the Clear Drink)

INGREDIENTS: Cooked Radix Rehmanniae (*Shu Di*) and Fructus Alpiniae Oxyphyllae (*Yi Zhi Ren*), 15g each, Rhizoma Dioscoreae Hypoglaucae (*Bei Xie*), 12g, Radix Dioscoreae Oppositae (*Shan Yao*), Fructus Corni Officinalis (*Shan Zhu Yu*), Sclerotium Poriae Cocos (*Fu Ling*), Cortex Radicis Moutan (*Dan Pi*), Rhizoma Alismatis (*Ze Xie*), Rhizoma Acori Graminei (*Shi Chang Pu*), Radix Linderae Strychnifoliae (*Wu Yao*), and Radix Lateralis Praeparatus Aconiti Carmichaeli (*Fu Zi*), 9g each, and Cortex Cinnamomi Cassiae (*Rou Gui*), 6g

ANALYSIS OF FORMULA: *Shu Di* supplements the kidneys, boosts the essence, and enrichs yin to engender yang. *Yi Zhi Ren, Shan Yao, Shan Zhu Yu, Wu Yao, Fu Zi,* and *Rou Gui* supplement the kidneys and warm the lower source, secure the kidneys and divide the clear. *Bei Xie, Fu Ling, Ze Xie,* and *Shi Chang Pu* disinhibit, dry, and seep dampness and downbear the turbid to divide the clear. *Dan Pi* quickens the blood and transforms stasis.

ADDITIONS & SUBTRACTIONS: For severe terminal dribbling, nocturia, long, clear, urination, and a whitish discharge at the end of urination, subtract *Rou Gui* and add nine grams each of Herba Epimedii (*Yin Yang Huo*), Semen Astragali Complanati (*Sha Yuan Zi*), Semen Euryalis Ferocis (*Qian Shi*), and Semen Cuscutae Chinensis (*Tu Si Zi*). For decreased sexual desire or impotence, add nine grams each of Herba Epimedii (*Yin Yang Huo*) and Herba Cistanchis Deserticolae (*Rou Cong Rong*). For lower abdominal, perineal, and/or scrotal distention and pain, add nine grams each of Fructus Meliae Toosendan (*Chuan Lian Zi*), Semen Citri Reticulatae (*Ju He*), and Semen Litchi Sinensis (*Li Zhi He*). For low back pain, add 12 grams of Cortex Eucommiae Ulmoidis (*Du Zhong*). For concomitant qi vacuity, add 15 grams of Radix Astragali Membranacei (*Huang Qi*) and nine grams of Rhizoma Atractylodis Macrocephalae (*Bai Zhu*). For a sagging, distended feeling in the perineal area and scrotum due to concomitant central qi downward fall, besides the previous two additions, add six grams each of Fructus Citri Aurantii (*Zhi Ke*), Rhizoma Cimicifugae (*Sheng Ma*), and Radix Bupleuri (*Chai Hu*). For white blood cells in the prostatic fluid, add 12 grams each of Herba Taraxaci Mongolici Cum Radice (*Pu Gong Ying*) and Herba Patriniae Heterophyllae Cum Radice (*Bai Jiang Cao*). For red blood cells in the prostatic fluid or in the sperm, add 12 grams each of Fructus Ligustri Lucidi (*Nu Zhen Zi*) and Herba Ecliptae Prostratae (*Han Lian Cao*) and nine grams of Gelatinum Corii Asini (*E Jiao*).

ACUPUNCTURE & MOXIBUSTION: *Hui Yin* (CV 1), *Guan Yuan* (CV 4), *Shen Shu* (Bl 23), *Hui Yang* (Bl 35)

ANALYSIS OF FORMULA: Moxaing *Hui Yin* supplements vacuity, harmonizes the network vessels, and secures the kidneys. Supplementing *Guan Yuan* and *Shen Shu* with moxibustion warms the lower source and secures the kidneys. *Hui Yang* with the even supplementing-even draining method transforms dampness, divides the clear, and stops pain. *Hui Yang* should be needle deeply, 2-3 cun, to induce a qi sensation in the affected area.

ADDITIONS & SUBTRACTIONS: For terminal dribbling which will not stop and nocturia, add *Zhi Shi* (Bl 52). For severe kidney yang vacuity, add *Ming Men* (GV 4). For low back pain, add *Fu Liu* (Ki 7). For fatigue and lassitude of the spirit, add *San Yin Jiao* (Sp 6). For decreased sexual desire or impotence, add *Ming Men* (GV 4). For loose stools, add *Gong Sun* (Sp 4).

REMARKS

1. Most Western cases of chronic prostatitis involve at least some element of damp heat. When there is a history of urinary tract infection, this damp heat may have been an externally invading damp heat or at least a totally replete damp

heat. However, if damp heat lingers and endures, it damages the spleen and consumes yin. Therefore, chronic prostatitis is commonly complicated by qi and yin vacuity. Because lingering damp heat obstructs the free flow of qi, it is also typically complicated by stasis and stagnation.

2. Although the Chinese literature contains case histories of yang vacuity chronic prostatitis, we have never seen this pattern in its pure form in this disease. However, because of the inter-relationship between yin and yang, qi and yin vacuity may be complicated by an element of yang vacuity.

3. Because damp heat plays a part in so many patient's chronic prostatitis, dietary therapy is extremely important for the long-term management of this condition. Basically, this means a clear, bland diet.

4. Daily perineal self-massage can be very beneficial in the treatment of chronic prostatitis. In order for such self-massage to be effective, it must be done regularly over a relatively long period of time.

5. There are several special point combinations which should be considered when treating chronic prostatitis:

Ci Liao (Bl 32) and *Zhong Ji* (CV 3). Both points should be needled in direction of the genitals to induce a qi sensation in the affected area.

Zhi Bian (Bl 54) and *San Yin Jiao* (Sp 6). *Zhi Bian* should be needled deeply in direction of *Gui Lai* (St 29) to induce a qi sensation in the affected area.

Hui Yang (Bl 35) and *Shen Shu* (Bl 23). *Hui Yang* should be needled deeply, 2-3 cun, to induce a qi sensation in the affected area.

Hui Yang (Bl 35) and *Guan Yuan* (CV 4). *Hui Yang* should be needled deeply, 2-3 cun, and *Guan Yuan* should be needled in direction of the genitals so as to induce a qi sensation in the affected area.

Jing Gu (Bl 64) and *Da Zhong* (Ki 4). Both points should be needled with even supplementing-even draining method.

However, the key point for treating this disease is still *Hui Yin* (CV 1). This should be needled deeply 2-3 cun or treated with indirect moxibustion depending on the condition. In addition, there is a new extra channel point, *Qian Lie Yan Xue* (prostatitis point), which is located midway between *Hui Yin* and the anus. This point should be needled 1.5-2 cun deep.

6. There are many new Chinese medicinal formulas for the treatment of chronic prostatitis. The following two formulas are for the types of complex pattern presentations common in our practice:

Fu Fang Di Hu Tang (Compound Lumbricus & Polygonum Cuspidatum Decoction) treats qi vacuity, damp heat, and blood stasis: Radix Astragali Membranacei (*Huang Qi*), 30g, Lumbricus (*Di Long*), Radix Et Rhizoma Polygoni Cuspidati (*Hu Zhang*), Semen Raphani Sativi (*Lai Fu Zi*), and Squama Manitis Pentadactylis (*Chuan Shan Jia*), 20g each, Caulis Akebiae (*Mu Tong*) and Semen Plantaginis (*Che Qian Zi*), 15g each, and Radix Glycyrrhizae (*Gan Cao*), 9g

Qing Hua Tang (Clear & Transform Decoction) treats yin vacuity, damp heat, and blood stasis: cooked Radix Rehmanniae (*Shu Di*) and uncooked Radix Rehmanniae (*Sheng Di*), 30g each, Cortex Phellodendri (*Huang Bai*) and Radix Salviae Miltiorrhizae (*Dan Shen*), 15g each, Semen Plantaginis (*Che Qian Zi*), Rhizoma Dioscoreae Hypoglaucae (*Bei Xie*), and Fructus Alpiniae Oxyphyllae (*Yi Zhi Ren*), 9g each, and cooked Radix Et Rhizoma Rhei (*Da Huang*), 5g

7. Simple popular formulas include:

A. Powdered Radix Pseudoginseng (*San Qi*), 3g twice daily, for stabbing pain in chronic prostatitis
B. Powdered Succinum (*Hu Po*), 1.5g twice daily, for burning, difficult, painful urination
C. Powdered uncooked Radix Glycyrrhizae (*Gan Cao*), 20-40g daily, taken with warm water

8. Long-term use of Caulis Akebiae (*Mu Tong*) is forbidden due to the possibility of aristocloch acid induced nephrotoxicity.

9. According Wang Qi, a Chinese authority in male disease (*nan ke*), the key Chinese medicinals for treating chronic prostatitis are the following:

For disinhibiting water and seeping dampness: Semen Plantaginis (*Che Qian Zi*), Herba Polygoni Avicularis (*Bian Xu*), Rhizoma Dioscoreae Hypoglaucae (*Bei Xie*), Talcum (*Hua Shi*), Caulis Akebiae (*Mu Tong*), Sclerotium Poriae Cocos (*Fu Ling*), Herba Dianthi (*Qu Mai*), Medulla Junci Effusi (*Deng Xin Cao*), Rhizoma Alismatis (*Ze Xie*), Medulla Tetrapanacis Papyriferi (*Tong Cao*), Folium Pyrrosiae (*Shi Wei*), Semen Coicis Lachryma-jobi (*Yi Yi Ren*), Succinum (*Hu Po*), and Sclerotium Polypori Umbellati (*Zhu Ling*)

For clearing heat and resolving toxins: Herba Taraxaci Mongolici Cum Radice (*Pu Gong Ying*), Herba Patriniae Heterophyllae Cum Radice (*Bai Jiang Cao*), Herba Portulacae Oleraceae (*Ma Chi Xian*), Herba Houttuyniae Cordatae Cum Radice (*Yu Xing Cao*), Rhizoma Smilacis Glabrae (*Tu Fu Ling*), Radix Et Rhizoma Polygoni Cuspidati

(*Hu Zhang*), Flos Lonicerae Japonicae (*Jin Yin Hua*), Fructus Forsythiae Suspensae (*Lian Qiao*), Fructus Gardeniae Jasminoidis (*Zhi Zi*), Herba Oldenlandiae Diffusae Cum Radice (*Bai Hua She She Cao*), Herba Scutellariae Barbatae (*Ban Zhi Lian*), and Radix Scrophulariae Ningpoensis (*Xuan Shen*)

For clearing heat and drying dampness: Cortex Phellodendri (*Huang Bai*), Radix Gentianae Scabrae (*Long Dan Cao*), Radix Sophorae Flavescentis (*Ku Shen*), and Radix Scutellariae Baicalensis (*Huang Qin*)

For clearing heat and cooling the blood: Radix Rubrus Paeoniae Lactiflorae (*Chi Shao*), Cortex Radicis Moutan (*Dan Pi*), and uncooked Radix Rehmanniae (*Sheng Di*)

For quickening the blood and transforming stasis: Radix Salviae Miltiorrhizae (*Dan Shen*), Radix Cyathulae (*Chuan Niu Xi*), Herba Lycopi Lucidi (*Ze Lan*), Semen Vaccariae Segetalis (*Wang Bu Liu Xing*), Pollen Typhae (*Pu Huang*), Rhizoma Corydalis Yanhusuo (*Yan Hu Suo*), Squama Manitis Pentadactylis (*Chuan Shan Jia*), Semen Pruni Persicae (*Tao Ren*), Flos Carthami Tinctorii (*Hong Hua*), Rhizoma Curcumae Zedoariae (*E Zhu*), Resina Olibani (*Ru Xiang*), Resina Myrrhae (*Mo Yao*), and Spina Gleditschiae Chinensis (*Zao Jiao Ci*)

For rectifying the qi: Fructus Meliae Toosendan (*Chuan Lian Zi*), Fructus Citri Aurantii (*Zhi Ke*), Radix Linderae Strychnifoliae (*Wu Yao*), Radix Bupleuri (*Chai Hu*), Semen Citri Reticulatae (*Ju He*), Pericarpium Citri Reticulatae Viride (*Qing Pi*), Rhizoma Cyperi Rotundi (*Xiang Fu*), and Semen Litchi Sinensis (*Li Zhi He*)

For softening the hard and scattering nodulation: Bulbus Fritillariae Thunbergii (*Zhe Bei Mu*), Concha Ostreae (*Mu Li*), Herba Sargassii (*Hai Zao*), and Thallus Algae (*Kun Bu*)

For astringing and securing: Fructus Alpiniae Oxyphyllae (*Yi Zhi Ren*), Ootheca Mantidis (*Sang Piao Xiao*), Os Draconis (*Long Gu*), Fructus Corni Officinalis (*Shan Zhu Yu*), Fructus Rubi Chingii (*Fu Pen Zi*), Fructus Rosae Laevigatae (*Jin Ying Zi*), and Semen Euryalis Ferocis (*Qian Shi*)

For supplementing yang: Herba Epimedii (*Yin Yang Huo*), Semen Cuscutae Chinensis (*Tu Si Zi*), Radix Morindae Officinalis (*Ba Ji Tian*), Herba Cistanchis Deserticolae (*Rou Cong Rong*), and Semen Astragali Complanati (*Sha Yuan Zi*)

For supplementing yin: Uncooked Radix Rehmanniae (*Sheng Di*), Fructus Lycii Chinensis (*Gou Qi*), Fructus Ligustri Lucidi (*Nu Zhen Zi*), Herba Ecliptae Prostratae (*Han Lian Cao*), Herba Dendrobii (*Shi Hu*), Tuber Ophiopogonis Japonici (*Mai Men Dong*), Tuber Asparagi Cochinensis (*Tian Men Dong*), and Gelatinum Plastri Testudinis (*Gui Ban Jiao*)

For supplementing the qi: Radix Panacis Ginseng (*Ren Shen*), Radix Codonopsitis Pilosulae (*Dang Shen*), Radix Pseustellariae Heterophyllae (*Tai Zi Shen*), Radix Astragali Membranacei (*Huang Qi*), Radix Dioscoreae Oppositae (*Shan Yao*), Radix Glycyrrhizae (*Gan Cao*), and Rhizoma Polygonati (*Huang Jing*)

Other commonly used medicinals: Radix Pseudoginseng (*San Qi*), Rhizoma Acori Graminei (*Shi Chang Pu*), Rhizoma Anemarrhenae Asphodeloidis (*Zhi Mu*), Radix Et Rhizoma Rhei (*Da Huang*), Lumbricus (*Di Long*), Fructus Foeniculi Vulgaris (*Xiao Hui Xiang*), and Herba Cephalanoplos Segeti (*Xiao Ji*)

19

Chronic Renal Failure

Also called uremia and end stage renal disease (ESRD), chronic renal failure (CRF) may evolve from chronic glomerulonephritis or any other major cause of renal dysfunction. This clinical condition results from chronic derangement and insufficiency of renal excretory and regulatory function. Its most common causes are diabetic nephropathy and hypertensive nephroangiosclerosis. Patients with mild to moderate renal insufficiency may only have vague symptoms accompanied by marked nocturia. The first symptoms of uremia are usually lassitude, extreme fatigue even after a good night's sleep, decreased mental acuity, difficulty sleeping, itching and dry skin. Neuromuscular features include coarse muscular twitches, peripheral neuropathies, muscle cramps, and convulsions which tend to worsen at night. Other symptoms include anorexia, nausea, vomiting, stomatitis, and an unpleasant taste in the mouth. In case of chronic uremia, there is usually generalized tissue wasting due to malnutrition. In advanced CRF, GI ulceration and bleeding are common. Hypertension is present in more than 80% of patients with advanced CRF.

Chronic renal failure should be suspected when serum creatinine concentration is more than 1.5-2mg/dL. The definitive Western medical diagnostic tool for CRF is renal biopsy. However, this is contraindicated when ultrasonography shows that the kidneys are small and fibrotic. Usually moderate acidosis and anemia are also characteristic. The Western medical treatment of this condition primarily revolves around treatment of the primary disease, such as diabetes or hypertension. In particular, ACE inhibitors and angiotensin receptor blockers are used to decrease the rate of decline in cases of diabetic nephropathy. Other factors, such as heart disease and infections, should also be treated specifically. Maintaining proper fluid and electrolyte levels are an important aspect of management. Chronic metabolic acidosis is usually treated with sodium bicarbonate. The tendency to bleeding is lessened by RBC, platelet, or cryoprecipitate infusions. Pruritus may respond to ultraviolet phototherapy. If uremia results from a progressive and untreatable disorder and conventional therapy is no longer effective, dialysis and transplantation are required. The prognosis of this condition depends on the nature of the underlying disorder and superimposed complications.

Chinese disease categorization: Inhibition of urination is called *guan* or block, while vomiting is called *ge*, repulsion. Therefore, this condition is most commonly categorized as *guan ge*, block and repulsion, based on its main, end stage clinical manifestations. Fatigue is called *pi ji*, lack of strength is called *shi li*, anorexia is *na dai*, torpid intake, insomnia is *shi mian*, and pruritus is simply *yang*, itching.

Disease causes: Enduring disease and bodily vacuity due to aging, possible contraction of external evils

Disease mechanisms: This disease is mainly caused by yang vacuity and yin congelation. Due to congestion and exuberance of stasis and turbidity, the triple burner qi transformation loses its normalcy. The clear qi is not able to rise and be upborne, while turbid qi is not able to obtain precipitation and be downborne. Damp depression may give rise to damp heat. If damp heat binds with blood stasis, there will be stasis heat. If enduring heat damages yin, there will be qi and yin or yin and yang vacuities. Thus, the root of this condition is vacuity, while its branch is repletion.

Treatment based on pattern discrimination:

Vacuity detriment stage:

1. Qi & yin vacuity pattern

Main symptoms: A lusterless, sallow yellow facial complexion, fatigue, generalized lack of strength, shortness of breath on movement, low back and knee soreness and limpness, torpid intake, a dry and/or sticky mouth, no or little desire to drink water, the taste of urine in the mouth, dry, bound stools, scanty, yellow urine during the day but long, clear urination at night, hand, foot, and heart heat, a pale tongue with teeth-marks on its edges, and a deep, fine pulse

TREATMENT PRINCIPLES: Fortify the spleen and boost the qi, supplement the kidneys and nourish yin

RX: *Shen Qi Di Huang Tang Jia Wei* (Ginseng, Astragalus & Rehmannia Decoction with Added Flavors)

INGREDIENTS: Radix Codonopsitis Pilosulae (*Dang Shen*), Radix Astragali Membranacei (*Huang Qi*), uncooked Radix Rehmanniae (*Sheng Di*), Sclerotium Poriae Cocos (*Fu Ling*), and Rhizoma Alismatis (*Ze Xie*), 15-30g each, Fructus Corni Officinalis (*Shan Zhu Yu*), Radix Dioscoreae Oppositae (*Shan Yao*), Cortex Radicis Moutan (*Dan Pi*), and Pericarpium Citri Reticulatae (*Chen Pi*), 9g each, and Fructus Amomi (*Sha Ren*) and Caulis Bambusae In Taeniis (*Zhu Ru*), 6g each

ANALYSIS OF FORMULA: *Dang Shen, Huang Qi, Fu Ling,* and *Shan Yao* fortify the spleen, boost the qi, and upbear the clear. *Ze Xie* and *Fu Ling* disinhibit water and downbear the turbid. *Sha Ren* and *Chen Pi* warm and fortify the spleen, dry dampness and move the qi. In addition, *Huang Qi* disinhibits the urination. *Sheng Di, Shan Yao,* and *Shan Zhu Yu* supplement the kidneys and enrich yin. *Dan Pi* cools and quickens the blood. *Zhu Ru* clears and harmonizes the stomach.

ADDITIONS & SUBTRACTIONS: For more marked yin vacuity, add 12 grams each of Radix Achyranthis Bidentatae (*Niu Xi*) and Fructus Lycii Chinensis (*Gou Qi Zi*). For concomitant kidney yang vacuity, add one gram each of Cornu Cervi (*Lu Jiao*) and Cortex Cinnamomi Cassiae (*Rou Gui*), powdered and taken with the strained decoction. For concomitant lung yin vacuity, add 12 grams each of Tuber Ophiopogonis Japonici (*Mai Men Dong*), Radix Scrophulariae Ningpoensis (*Xuan Shen*), and Radix Platycodi Grandiflori (*Jie Geng*). For heart palpitations and insomnia, add 12 grams each of Tuber Ophiopogonis Japonici (*Mai Men Dong*), Semen Zizyphi Spinosae (*Suan Zao Ren*), and Fructus Schisandrae Chinensis (*Wu Wei Zi*). For low back pain, add nine grams each of Cortex Eucommiae Ulmoidis (*Du Zhong*) and Radix Morindae Officinalis (*Ba Ji Tian*).

ACUPUNCTURE & MOXIBUSTION: *Shen Shu* (Bl 23), *Pi Shu* (Bl 20), *Zu San Li* (St 36), *Fu Liu* (Ki 7)

ANALYSIS OF FORMULA: Supplementing *Shen Shu, Pi Shu, Zu San Li,* and *Fu Liu* fortifies and supplements the spleen and kidneys, boosts the qi, nourishes yin, and seeps dampness.

ADDITIONS & SUBTRACTIONS: For low back pain, add *Tai Xi* (Ki 3). For dry mouth and parched throat or enduring sore throat and afternoon low-grade fever, add *Zhao Hai* (Ki 6) and *Yin Xi* (Ht 6). For reduced appetite and abdominal fullness, especially after eating, add *Nei Guan* (Per 6) and *Gong Sun* (Sp 4). For constipation, add *Zhi Gou* (TB 6).

2. LIVER-KIDNEY YIN VACUITY PATTERN

MAIN SYMPTOMS: A sallow yellow facial complexion, bodily fatigue, lack of strength, dry, rough eyes, dry skin, a bitter taste in the mouth, dry throat, thirst with a desire for chilled drinks, an odor of urine in the mouth, vexatious heat in the five hearts, insomnia, profuse dreams, low back and knee soreness and limpness, dry, bound stools, scanty reddish yellow urine, if severe, headache, dizziness, tinnitus, and vexation and agitation, a pale, emaciated tongue with scanty or thin, yellow fur, and a bowstring, fine pulse

TREATMENT PRINCIPLES: Enrich and nourish the liver and kidneys

RX: *Zhi Bai Di Huang Tang Jia Wei* (Anemarrhena & Phellodendron Rehmannia Decoction with Added Flavors)

INGREDIENTS: Uncooked Radix Rehmanniae (*Sheng Di*), Sclerotium Poriae Cocos (*Fu Ling*), Rhizoma Alismatis (*Ze Xie*), and Radix Salviae Miltiorrhizae (*Dan Shen*), 30g each, Cortex Radicis Moutan (*Dan Pi*), 12g, Rhizoma Anemarrhenae Aspheloidis (*Zhi Mu*), Cortex Phellodendri (*Huang Bai*), Fructus Corni Officinalis (*Shan Zhu Yu*), Radix Dioscoreae Oppositae (*Shan Yao*), Tuber Ophiopogonis Japonici (*Mai Dong*), and Tuber Asparagi Cochinensis (*Tian Men Dong*), 9g each, and processed Radix Et Rhizoma Rhei (*Da Huang*), 6-15g

ANALYSIS OF FORMULA: *Sheng Di, Shan Zhu Yu, Shan Yao, Mai Men Dong,* and *Tian Men Dong* supplement the liver and kidneys and enrich yin. *Ze Xie* and *Fu Ling* disinhibit water and downbear the turbid. *Dan Shen* and *Dan Pi* quicken the blood and transform stasis. *Zhi Mu* and *Huang Bai* clear vacuity heat. *Da Huang* frees the flow of the stools.

ADDITIONS & SUBTRACTIONS: If there is no constipation, subtract *Da Huang*. For mild, transient constipation subtract *Da Huang* and add nine grams of Radix Angelicae Sinensis (*Dang Gui*). For edema, add 12 grams of Semen Plantaginis (*Che Qian Zi*) and 15 grams of Herba Plantaginis (*Che Qian Cao*). For fatigue and cold limbs, add one gram of Cortex Cinnamomi Cassiae (*Rou Gui*) and 15 grams of Semen Cuscutae Chinensis (*Tu Si Zi*). For marked yin blood vacuity, add 12 grams each of Radix Polygoni Multiflori (*He Shou Wu*) and Fructus Lycii Chinensis (*Gou Qi Zi*). For dizziness, headache, and stiffness of the neck and back, add 12 grams each of Rhizoma Gastrodiae Elatae (*Tian Ma*) and Radix Puerariae (*Ge Gen*) and 18 grams of Caulis Milletiae Seu Spatholobi (*Ji Xue Teng*).

Acupuncture & moxibustion: *Shen Shu* (Bl 23), *Jing Gu* (Bl 64), *Gan Shu* (Bl 18), *Fu Liu* (Ki 7)

Analysis of formula: *Shen Shu* and *Jing Gu* are an empirical combination for treating enduring glomerulonephritis. *Gan Shu* and *Fu Liu* further enrich and nourish the liver and kidneys and subdue yang. All these points should be supplemented.

Additions & subtractions: For inhibited, rough urination, add *Zhong Ji* (CV 3). For edema, add *Zhong Ji* (CV 3) and *Shui Dao* (St 28). For severe dizziness and tinnitus, add *Feng Chi* (GB 20) and *Yi Feng* (TB 17). For painful throat, add *Zhao Hai* (Ki 6). For insomnia and heart palpitations, add *Shen Men* (Ht 7). For concomitant liver fire, add *Xing Jian* (Liv 2). For blood stasis, add *San Yin Jiao* (Sp 6). For severe high blood pressure, add *Qu Chi* (LI 11) and *Zu San Li* (St 36).

3. Spleen-kidney qi vacuity pattern

Main symptoms: A lusterless facial complexion, scanty qi, lack of strength, torpid intake, abdominal distention, a tendency to loose stools, a sticky feeling and bland taste in the mouth and either no thirst or thirst but no desire to drink, low back and knee soreness and pain, lack of warmth in the hands and feet, frequent, numerous night-time urinations, a pale tongue with teeth-marks on its edges, and a deep, weak pulse

Treatment principles: Fortify the spleen and supplement the kidneys

Rx: *Bao Yuan Tang Jia Wei* (Protect the Source Decoction with Added Flavors)

Ingredients: Sclerotium Poriae Cocos (*Fu Ling*), 30g, Radix Codonopsitis Pilosulae (*Dang Shen*), Radix Astragali Membranacei (*Huang Qi*), Ramulus Loranthi Seu Visci (*Sang Ji Sheng*), and Cortex Eucommiae Ulmoidis (*Du Zhong*), 15g each, Rhizoma Atractylodis Macrocephalae (*Bai Zhu*), Fructus Amomi (*Sha Ren*), and Pericarpium Citri Reticulatae (*Chen Pi*), 9g each, and Cortex Cinnamomi Cassiae (*Rou Gui*) and mix-fried Radix Glycyrrhizae (*Gan Cao*), 3g each

Analysis of formula: *Huang Qi, Dang Shen, Fu Ling, Bai Zhu*, and mix-fried *Gan Cao* fortify the spleen and boost the qi. In addition, *Fu Ling, Huang Qi*, and *Bai Zhu* disinhibit water. *Sha Ren* and *Chen Pi* warm and fortify the spleen, dry dampness and move the qi. *Sang Ji Sheng, Du Zhong*, and *Rou Gui* together supplement the kidney qi. In addition, *Rou Gui* warms yang and transforms the qi.

Additions & subtractions: For edema, add 15 grams of Semen Plantaginis (*Che Qian Zi*) and 12 grams of Sclerotium Polypori Umbellati (*Zhu Ling*). For damp accumulation, add 12 grams each of Cortex Magnoliae Officinalis (*Hou Po*) and Fructus Amomi (*Sha Ren*). Please also refer to pattern #4 below.

For a spleen-kidney qi vacuity plus water stasis binding with edema mainly below the waist, fatigue, cold limbs, low back and knee soreness and pain, loose stools, scanty urine, a dark facial complexion, purple lips and nails, menstrual irregularities in women, a fat, purple tongue with possible static macules or spots and thin, slimy fur, and a deep, choppy pulse, replace *Bao Yuan Tang Jia Wei* with *Shi Pi Yin* (Replete the Spleen Drink) plus *Xue Fu Zhu Yu Tang* (Blood Mansion Dispel Stasis Decoction) with additions and subtractions: Radix Salviae Miltiorrhizae (*Dan Shen*), 15g, Tuber Curcumae (*Yu Jin*), Cortex Radicis Moutan (*Dan Pi*), Herba Lycopi Lucidi (*Ze Lan*), Radix Achyranthis Bidentatae (*Niu Xi*), Radix Angelicae Sinensis (*Dang Gui*), Herba Leonuri Heterophylli (*Yi Mu Cao*), Sclerotium Poriae Cocos (*Fu Ling*), Sclerotium Polypori Umbellati (*Zhu Ling*), Cortex Magnoliae Officinalis (*Hou Po*), Rhizoma Atractylodis Macrocephalae (*Bai Zhu*), and Pericarpium Arecae Catechu (*Da Fu Pi*), 12g each, and Radix Auklandiae Lappae (*Mu Xiang*), 6g.

For a simple spleen qi vacuity without apparent kidney vacuity symptoms, replace *Bao Yuan Tang Jia Wei* with *Liu Jun Zi Tang Jia Wei* (Six Gentlemen Decoction with Added Flavors): Radix Astragali Membranacei (*Huang Qi*) and Radix Codonopsitis Pilosulae (*Dang Shen*), 15g each, Sclerotium Poriae Cocos (*Fu Ling*), 15-30g, Rhizoma Atractylodis Macrocephalae (*Bai Zhu*), Pericarpium Citri Reticulatae (*Chen Pi*), and Rhizoma Pinelliae Ternatae (*Ban Xia*), 9g each, and mix-fried Radix Glycyrrhizae (*Gan Cao*), 6g. For enduring diarrhea, add six grams each of Radix Bupleuri (*Chai Hu*) and Rhizoma Cimicifugae (*Sheng Ma*). For the odor of urine in the mouth, add nine grams each of Excrementum Bombicis Batryticati (*Can Sha)* and Rhizoma Smilacis Glabrae (*Tu Fu Ling*). For reduced appetite, add nine grams each of Fructus Germinatus Hordei Vulgaris (*Mai Ya*), Fructus Crataegi (*Shan Zha*), and Endothelium Corneum Gigeriae Galli (*Ji Nei Jin*).

For spleen-kidney qi vacuity with marked blood vacuity, use *Ren Shen Yang Rong Tang Jia Jian* (Ginseng Nourish the Constructive Decoction with Additions & Subtractions): Radix Astragali Membranacei (*Huang Qi*), 30g, cooked

Radix Rehmanniae (*Shu Di*), Radix Angelicae Sinensis (*Dang Gui*), Radix Albus Paeoniae Lactiflorae (*Bai Shao*), Radix Codonopsitis Pilosulae (*Dang Shen*), Rhizoma Atractylodis Macrocephalae (*Bai Zhu*), Sclerotium Poriae Cocos (*Fu Ling*), Fructus Schisandrae Chinensis (*Wu Wei Zi*), Radix Achyranthis Bidentatae (*Niu Xi*), and Rhizoma Polygonati (*Huang Jing*), 9g each, and Cortex Cinnamomi Cassiae (*Rou Gui*), 1g.

ACUPUNCTURE & MOXIBUSTION: *Shen Shu* (Bl 23), *San Yin Jiao* (Sp 6), *Guan Yuan* (CV 4), *Yin Ling Quan* (Sp 9)

ANALYSIS OF FORMULA: Supplementing *Shen Shu* and *Guan Yuan* with moxibustion supplements and warms the kidneys. Even supplementing-even draining *San Yin Jiao* supplements the spleen at the same time as it disinhibits water and disperses swelling, especially when combined with draining *Yin Ling Quan*.

ADDITIONS & SUBTRACTIONS: If yang disease has reached yin, add *Fu Liu* (Ki 7). For severe edema, especially below the waist, severe aversion to cold, and low back pain with a cold sensation, add *Ming Men* (GV 4) with moxibustion. If, in addition, there is hematuria, add *Xue Chou* (extra point located just above the spinous process of L2) with moxibustion. For heart palpitation and hasty panting, add *Nei Guan* (Per 6), *Liang Quan* (CV 23), and *Lie Que* (Lu 7). For severe edema in the limbs, add *Shui Dao* (St 28). If there is severe edema in the abdomen, add *Shui Fen* (CV 9).

4. SPLEEN-KIDNEY YANG VACUITY PATTERN

MAIN SYMPTOMS: A somber white or bright white facial complexion, lassitude of the spirit, lack of strength, torpid intake, loose stools, a sticky feeling and bland taste in the mouth with no thirst, low back and knee soreness and pain, chilly pain in the lumbar region, or fear of cold and chilled extremities, possible edema, frequent, numerous night-time urination which is long and clear or scanty urination, a pale, tender, fat tongue with marked teeth-marks on its edges, and a deep, weak pulse

TREATMENT PRINCIPLES: Warm and supplement the spleen and kidneys

RX: *Zhen Wu Tang Jia Wei* (True Warrior Decoction with Added Flavors)

INGREDIENTS: Sclerotium Poriae Cocos (*Fu Ling*), 30g, Radix Codonopsitis Pilosulae (*Dang Shen*), 15g, and Radix Lateralis Praeparatus Aconiti Carmichaeli (*Fu Zi*), Rhizoma Atractylodis Macrocephalae (*Bai Zhu*), Radix Albus Paeoniae Lactiflorae (*Bai Shao*), dry Rhizoma Zingiberis (*Gan Jiang*), Ramulus Cinnamomi Cassiae (*Gui Zhi*), and Fructus Amomi (*Sha Ren*), 9g each

ANALYSIS OF FORMULA: *Dang Shen*, *Fu Ling*, *Bai Zhu*, *Gan Jiang*, and *Sha Ren* together warm and fortify the spleen. In addition, *Fu Ling* and *Bai Zhu*, disinhibit water. *Fu Zi* and *Gui Zhi* warm and supplement kidney yang. *Bai Shao* nourishes the blood and protects yin from the warm and drying nature of the other medicinals in this formula.

ADDITIONS & SUBTRACTIONS: For marked kidney yang vacuity, add nine grams each of Radix Morindae Officinalis (*Ba Ji Tian*), Herba Epimedii (*Yin Yang Huo*), and Herba Cistanchis Deserticolae (*Rou Cong Rong*). For low back pain, add nine grams each of Cortex Eucommiae Ulmoidis (*Du Zhong*) and Radix Dipsaci (*Xu Duan*). For diarrhea, add 12 grams each of Fructus Psoraleae Corylifoliae (*Bu Gu Zhi*), Fructus Schisandrae Chinensis (*Wu Wei Zi*), and Semen Myristicae Fragrantis (*Rou Dou Kou*) and five grams of Fructus Evodiae Rutecarpae (*Wu Zhu Yu*). For edema, add 15 grams each of Semen Plantaginis (*Che Qian Zi*) and Pericarpium Arecae Catechu (*Da Fu Pi*) and 12 grams each of Sclerotium Polypori Umbellati (*Zhu Ling*) and Semen Zanthoxyli Bungeani (*Jiao Mu*). For damp accumulation, add 12 grams each of Herba Agastachis Seu Pogostemi (*Huo Xiang*) and Pericarpium Citri Reticulatae (*Chen Pi*). For frequent urination at night, add nine grams each of Fructus Alpiniae Oxyphyllae (*Yi Zhi Ren*) and Semen Cuscutae Chinensis (*Tu Si Zi*).

ACUPUNCTURE & MOXIBUSTION: Same as pattern #3 above.

5. YIN & YANG DUAL VACUITY PATTERN

MAIN SYMPTOMS: Extreme lack of strength, fear of cold, chilled limbs, hand, foot, and heart heat, a dry mouth with desire to drink but not drinking a lot of water, a taste of urine in the mouth, low back and knee soreness and pain, no thought for eating food, a tendency to loose stools with yellow-red urine or dry, bound stools with long, clear urination, a pale, fat tongue with teeth-marks on its edges, and a deep, fine, or deep, weak pulse

TREATMENT PRINCIPLES: Supplement both yin and yang

RX: *Jin Gui Shen Qi Wan Jia Jian* (*Golden Cabinet* Kidney Qi Pills with Additions & Subtractions)

INGREDIENTS: Sclerotium Poriae Cocos (*Fu Ling*), 30g, Rhizoma Alismatis (*Ze Xie*), 15g, Radix Lateralis Praeparatus Aconiti Carmichaeli (*Fu Zi*), uncooked Radix Rehmanniae (*Sheng Di*), Fructus Corni Officinalis (*Shan Zhu Yu*), Rhizoma Atractylodis Macrocephalae (*Bai Zhu*), and Radix Achyranthis Bidentatae (*Niu Xi*), 9g each, and Cortex Cinnamomi Cassiae (*Rou Gui*) and Cortex Radicis Moutan (*Dan Pi*), 6g each

ANALYSIS OF FORMULA: *Sheng Di*, *Shan Yao*, *Niu Xi*, and

Shan Zhu Yu supplement the kidneys and enrich yin. *Fu Zi, Shan Zhu Yu,* and *Rou Gui* warm and supplement kidney yang. *Fu Ling, Ze Xie,* and *Bai Zhu,* fortify the spleen and disinhibit dampness. *Dan Pi* quickens the blood and transforms stasis.

ADDITIONS & SUBTRACTIONS: Please see patterns #1, 2, and 4 above.

ACUPUNCTURE & MOXIBUSTION: *Shen Shu* (Bl 23), *San Yin Jiao* (Sp 6), *Fu Liu* (Ki 7), *Tai Xi* (Ki 3)

ANALYSIS OF FORMULA: Supplementing *Shen Shu, San Yin Jiao, Fu Liu,* and *Tai Xi* supplements both yin and yang. In addition, *San Yin Jiao* fortifies the spleen and disinhibits water.

ADDITIONS & SUBTRACTIONS: For marked kidney yang vacuity, add *Ming Men* (GV 4) with moxibustion. For dry mouth and parched throat or enduring sore throat and afternoon low-grade fever, add *Zhao Hai* (Ki 6) and *Yin Xi* (Ht 6). For reduced appetite and abdominal fullness, especially after eating, add *Nei Guan* (Per 6) and *Gong Sun* (Sp 4). For constipation, add *Zhi Gou* (TB 6).

BLOCK & REPULSION STAGE:

1. SPLEEN-KIDNEY YANG VACUITY PATTERN

MAIN SYMPTOMS: A bright white or dark, stagnant facial complexion, lack of warmth in the four limbs, low back and knee soreness and weakness, legs and feet aching and painful, superficial edema which is more marked below the waist, nausea, vomiting, no thought for food or drink, scanty urination or even anuria (however, urination may, in some cases, be clear, long, and frothy). The pulse is deep and fine. The tongue fur is thin and slimy like white jade.

TREATMENT PRINCIPLES: Warm the spleen and boost the kidneys, quicken the blood and transform stasis

RX: *Yi Qi Jian Pi Fu Zheng Tang* (Boost the Qi, Fortify the Spleen & Support the Righteous Decoction)

INGREDIENTS: Radix Astragali Membranacei (*Huang Qi*), Radix Salviae Miltiorrhizae (*Dan Shen*), and Sclerotium Poriae Cocos (*Fu Ling*), 30g each, Herba Epimedii (*Xian Ling Pi*), 20g, Radix Codonopsitis Pilosulae (*Dang Shen*), Rhizoma Atractylodis Macrocephalae (*Bai Zhu*), Radix Albus Paeoniae Lactiflorae (*Bai Shao*), and Fructus Forsythiae Suspensae (*Lian Qiao*), 15g each, Radix Angelicae Sinensis (*Dang Gui*), Rhizoma Pinelliae Ternatae (*Ban Xia*), Pericarpium Citri Reticulatae (*Chen Pi*), and Rhizoma Curculiginis Orchioidis (*Xian Mao*), 12g each, and Endoethelium Corneum Gigeriae Galli (*Ji Nei Jin*), 9g

ANALYSIS OF FORMULA: *Huang Qi, Dang Shen, Fu Ling, Ji Nei Jin,* and *Bai Zhu* fortify the spleen and boost the qi. In addition, *Huang Qi, Fu Ling,* and *Bai Zhu* disinhibit water and seep dampness. *Ban Xia* and *Chen Pi* dry dampness, harmonize the stomach, and stop vomiting. *Yin Yang Huo* and *Xian Mao* warm and supplement kidney yang. *Bai Shao* and *Dang Gui* nourish the blood and protect yin from the dry, warm nature of the other medicinals. *Dan Shen* and *Dang Gui* quicken the blood and transform stasis without further damaging it. *Ji Nei Jin* improves the spleen's transporting function at the same time as it secures the essence and stops excessive urination. *Lian Qiao* clears depressive heat.

ADDITIONS & SUBTRACTIONS: For nausea and vomiting, add 30 grams of uncooked Rhizoma Zingiberis (*Sheng Jiang*) and nine grams of Caulis Bambusae In Taeniis (*Zhu Ru*). For marked torpid intake, add nine grams each of scorched Fructus Crataegi (*Shan Zha*), stir-fried Fructus Germinatus Hordei Vulgaris (*Mai Ya*), Massa Medica Fermentata (*Shen Qu*), and Fructus Amomi (*Sha Ren*). For pronounced edema, add 15 grams each of Semen Plantaginis (*Che Qian Zi*), Sclerotium Polypori Umbellati (*Zhu Ling*), and Pericarpium Arecae Catechu (*Da Fu Pi*). For marked abdominal distention, add 15 grams of Pericarpium Arecae Catechu (*Da Fu Pi*) and nine grams of Radix Auklandiae Lappae (*Mu Xiang*). If tending to cold, add 12 grams of dry Rhizoma Zingiberis (*Gan Jiang*) and six grams of Cortex Cinnamomi Cassiae (*Rou Gui*). If anemia is marked, add 15 grams of Radix Polygoni Multiflori (*He Shou Wu*). If there is itching of the skin, add 30 grams of Cortex Radicis Dictamni Dasycarpi (*Bai Xian Pi*) and 15 grams of Herba Taraxaci Mongolici Cum Radice (*Pu Gong Ying*).

In the terminal stage when there is block and repulsion due to even more severe yin congelation (*i.e.*, vacuity cold and blood stasis), replace *Yi Qi Jian Pi Fu Zheng Tang* with *Wen Pi Tang Jia Wei* (Warm the Spleen Decoction with Added Flavors): Radix Angelicae Sinensis (*Dang Gui*), Radix Lateralis Praeparatus Aconiti Carmichaeli (*Fu Zi*), Radix Et Rhizoma Rhei (*Da Huang*), Lignum Sappan (*Su Mu*), Flos Carthami Tinctorii (*Hong Hua*), and Semen Pruni Persicae (*Tao Ren*) 9g each, Radix Panacis Ginseng (*Ren Shen*) and Mirabilitum (*Mang Xiao*), 6g each, Radix Glycyrrhizae (*Gan Cao*), 3g, and dry Rhizoma Zingiberis (*Gan Jiang*), 2.4g.

ACUPUNCTURE & MOXIBUSTION: *Shen Shu* (Bl 23), *Pi Shu* (Bl 20), *Guan Yuan* (CV 4), *San Yin Jiao* (Sp 6), *Yin Ling Quan* (Sp 9)

ANALYSIS OF FORMULA: Supplementing *Shen Shu, Pi Shu,* and *Guan Yuan* with moxibustion warms the spleen and boosts the kidneys. In addition, *Guan Yuan* disinhibits water. Draining *San Yin Jiao* and *Yin Ling Quan* disinhibits water and disperses swelling. *San Yin Jiao* also quickens the blood and transforms stasis.

ADDITIONS & SUBTRACTIONS: For nausea and vomiting, add *Nei Guan* (Per 6) and *Gong Sun* (Sp 4). For marked torpid intake, add *Liang Men* (St 21). For pronounced edema, add *Shui Dao* (St 28) and *Shui Fen* (CV 9). For marked abdominal distention, add *Tian Shu* (St 25). If tending to cold, add *Ming Men* (GV 4) with moxibustion. If anemia is marked, add *Gao Huang Shu* (Bl 43). If there is itching of the skin, add *Qu Chi* (LI 11) and *Xue Hai* (Sp 10).

2. TURBIDITY FLOODING THE TRIPLE BURNER PATTERN

MAIN SYMPTOMS: A lusterless facial complexion, nausea, vomiting, lack of appetite, abdominal distention, a slimy mouth and sweet taste, inhibited defecation, heaviness of the four limbs, a fat, pale tongue with teeth-marks on its edges, and a deep, fine pulse

TREATMENT PRINCIPLES: Warm yang and assist transportation, harmonize the stomach and discharge turbidity

RX: *Niao Du Er Hao Fang* (No. 2 Uremia Formula)

INGREDIENTS: Rhizoma Pinelliae Ternatae (*Ban Xia*), Haematitum (*Dai Zhe Shi*), Folium Eupatorii Chinensis (*Liu Yue Xue*), and Semen Glycinis Hispidae (*Hei Da Dou*), 30g each, Flos Inulae Racemosae (*Xuan Fu Hua*) and Sclerotium Poriae Cocos (*Fu Ling*), 9g each, Cortex Magnoliae Officinalis (*Hou Po*), 6g, uncooked Rhizoma Zingiberis (*Sheng Jiang*), 5 slices, ginger-processed Rhizoma Coptidis Chinensis (*Chuan Lian*), 3g, and Fructus Evodiae Rutecarpae (*Wu Zhu Yu*), 2.4g

ANALYSIS OF FORMULA: *Ban Xia, Hou Po, Fu Ling, Liu Yue Xue*, and *Sheng Jiang* dry dampness and discharge turbidity, harmonize the stomach and stop vomiting. *Dai Zhe Shi* and *Xuan Fu Hua* downbear counterflow and stop vomiting. Based on the saying, "A small amount of bitter harmonizes the stomach," a small amount of *Huang Lian* harmonizes the stomach and stops vomiting. In addition, its cold nature prevents stagnation from transforming into heat. *Wu Zhu Yu* warms yang and stops vomiting, while *Hei Da Dou* nourishes yin blood and prevents its damage by the other ingredients in this formula at the same time as it seeps dampness and disinhibits urination.

ADDITIONS & SUBTRACTIONS: If edema is more pronounced, especially in the lower extremities, and there are coughing and panting, heart palpitations, and inability to lie down, and nausea and vomiting are less, replace *Niao Du Er Hao Fang* with *Dao Shui Fu Ling Tang Jia Jian* (Abduct Water Poria Decoction with Additions & Subtractions): Sclerotium Poriae Cocos (*Fu Ling*), Rhizoma Alismatis (*Ze Xie*), Semen Plantaginis (*Che Qian Zi*), Pericarpium Arecae Catechu (*Da Fu Pi*), and Cortex Radicis Mori Albi (*Sang Bai Pi*), 30g each, and Rhizoma Atractylodis Macrocephalae (*Bai Zhu*), Semen Arecae Catechu (*Bing Lang*), Fructus Chaenomelis Lagenariae (*Mu Gua*), Pericarpium Citri Reticulatae (*Chen Pi*), and Radix Achyranthis Bidentatae (*Niu Xi*), 9g each.

ACUPUNCTURE & MOXIBUSTION: *Nei Guan* (Per 6), *Gong Sun* (Sp 4), *Yin Ling Quan* (Sp 9), *Shang Wan* (CV 13)

ANALYSIS OF FORMULA: Draining *Nei Guan* and *Gong Sun* is a traditional treatment for moving the qi and promoting transportation, harmonizing the stomach and stopping vomiting. Draining *Yin Ling Quan* also assists transportation, discharges turbidity, and disinhibits dampness, while draining and moxibustion at *Shang Wan* warms yang and assists transportation, discharges turbidity and stops vomiting.

ADDITIONS & SUBTRACTIONS: If edema is more pronounced, especially in the lower extremities, and there are coughing and panting, heart palpitations, and inability to lie down, and nausea and vomiting are less, replace *Shang Wan* with *Dan Zhong* (CV 17) and *Shui Fen* (CV 9). For constipation, add *Zhi Gou* (TB 6).

3. DAMP HEAT OBSTRUCTING THE MIDDLE PATTERN

MAIN SYMPTOMS: Nausea, vomiting, a bitter taste and sticky feeling in the mouth, and odor of urine in the mouth, torpid intake, abdominal distention, dry, bound or loose stools and diarrhea, yellow urine, fatigue, lack of strength, a pale red tongue with slimy, white or slimy, yellow fur, and a bowstring, slippery pulse

TREATMENT PRINCIPLES: Clear heat and transform dampness, harmonize the center and stop vomiting

RX: *Huang Lian Wen Dan Tang Jia Jian* (Coptis Warm the Gallbladder Decoction with Additions & Subtractions)

INGREDIENTS: Sclerotium Poriae Cocos (*Fu Ling*), 30g, Rhizoma Pinelliae Ternatae (*Ban Xia*), Pericarpium Citri Reticulatae (*Chen Pi*), Fructus Citri Aurantii (*Zhi Ke*), and uncooked Rhizoma Zingiberis (*Sheng Jiang*), 9g each, Rhizoma Coptidis Chinensis (*Huang Lian*) and Caulis Bambusae In Taeniis (*Zhu Ru*), 6g each, and processed Radix Et Rhizoma Rhei (*Da Huang*), 3-9g

ANALYSIS OF FORMULA: *Huang Lian* and *Zhu Ru* clear heat and dry dampness, harmonize the stomach and stop vomiting. *Ban Xia, Fu Ling*, and *Sheng Jiang* dry dampness and discharge turbidity, harmonize the stomach and stop vomiting. *Zhi Ke* and *Da Huang* clear heat and free the flow of the stools, thus discharging heat and turbidity via defecation.

ADDITIONS & SUBTRACTIONS: For diarrhea, subtract *Da Huang*. For edema, add 15 grams each of Semen Plantaginis (*Che Qian Zi*) and Sclerotium Polypori Umbellati (*Zhu Ling*). For spirit mind abstraction, add 12 grams each of Rhizoma Acori Graminei (*Shi Chang Pu*) and Tuber Curcumae (*Yu Jin*).

ACUPUNCTURE & MOXIBUSTION: *Nei Guan* (Per 6), *Gong Sun* (Sp 4), *Shang Wan* (CV 13), *Zhong Wan* (CV 12), *Xia Wan* (CV 10), *Nei Ting* (St 44)

ANALYSIS OF FORMULA: Draining *Nei Guan* and *Gong Sun* harmonizes the stomach, downbears counterflow, and stops vomiting. Draining *Shang Wan*, *Zhong Wan*, and *Xia Wan* transforms dampness, harmonizes the center, and stops vomiting, while draining *Nei Ting* clears heat in the middle burner.

4. LIVER WIND INTERNALLY STIRRING PATTERN

MAIN SYMPTOMS: Urinary blockage, trembling fingers, headache, red, swollen gums, oral ulcers, itching, in severe cases, spirit darkness (*i.e.*, syncope), tremors, agitation, worry, and restlessness, a dry, crimson tongue with scorched yellow fur, a curled upward or trembling tongue, and a fine, weak, rapid pulse

NOTE: In this case, liver wind is engendered by yin vacuity/vacuity heat in turn caused by damp depression transforming heat and enduring heat damaging yin.

TREATMENT PRINCIPLES: Subdue yang and track down wind, quicken the blood and transform stasis

RX: *Niao Du San Hao Fang* (No. 3 Uremia Formula)

INGREDIENTS: Herba Portulacae Oleraceae (*Ma Chi Xian*), 30g, Carapax Amydae Sinensis (*Bie Jia*), Plastrum Testudinis (*Gui Ban*), Ramulus Uncariae Cum Uncis (*Shuang Gou*), uncooked Radix Rehmanniae (*Sheng Di*), and Radix Scrophulariae Ningpoensis (*Xuan Shen*), 15g each, and Herba Dendrobii (*Shi Hu*), Radix Et Rhizoma Rhei (*Da Huang*), Sclerotium Pararadicis Poriae Cocos (*Fu Shen*), Tuber Ophiopogonis Japonicae (*Mai Men Dong*), Semen Plantaginis (*Che Qian Zi*), and Radix Achyranthis Bidentatae (*Niu Xi*), 9g each

ANALYSIS OF FORMULA: *Bei Jia* and *Gui Ban* enrich yin and subdue yang. *Gou Teng* clears the liver, subdues yang, and extinguishes the wind. *Sheng Di*, *Shi Hu*, *Mai Men Dong*, and *Niu Xi* enrich liver-kidney yin to check yang. In addition, *Sheng Di* and *Niu Xi* quicken the blood and transform stasis. *Ma Chi Xian* clears heat and resolves toxins, draining the heart and thus treating oral ulcers. *Xuan Shen* nourishes yin and drains fire, clears heat and resolves toxins. *Da Huang* likewise clears heat while discharging turbidity through the stools. *Fu Shen* quiets the spirit at the same time as it seeps dampness, and *Che Qian Zi* disinhibits urination.

ADDITIONS & SUBTRACTIONS: For dry, rough eyes, add 12 grams each of Flos Chrysanthemi Morifolii (*Ju Hua*) and Fructus Lycii Chinensis (*Gou Qi Zi*). For severe headache and dizziness, add 12 grams each of Rhizoma Gastrodiae Elatae (*Tian Ma*) and Radix Puerariae (*Ge Gen*). For restlessness, insomnia, and easy anger, add nine grams each of Fructus Gardeniae Jasminoidis (*Zhi Zi*) and Cortex Radicis Moutan (*Dan Pi*) and 15 grams of Caulis Polygoni Multiflori (*Ye Jiao Teng*). For concomitant blood stasis, add 15 grams each of Herba Lycopi Lucidi (*Ze Lan*) and Herba Leonuri Heterophylli (*Yi Mu Cao*). For reduced appetite and abdominal fullness, add six grams of Fructus Amomi (*Sha Ren*) and 12 grams each of Pericarpium Citri Reticulatae (*Chen Pi*) and Endothelium Corneum Gigeriae Galli (*Ji Nei Jin*). For loose stools, add 12 grams each of Radix Codonopsitis Pilosulae (*Dang Shen*) and Rhizoma Atractylodis Macrocephalae (*Bai Zhu*).

ACUPUNCTURE & MOXIBUSTION: *Shen Shu* (Bl 23), *San Yin Jiao* (Sp 6), *Zhong Ji* (CV 3), *He Gu* (LI 4), *Tai Chong* (Liv 3), *Feng Chi* (GB 20)

ANALYSIS OF FORMULA: *Shen Shu* and *San Yin Jiao* enrich liver-kidney yin to check yang. *San Yin Jiao* and *Zhong Ji* clear damp heat and disinhibit urine. *He Gu* and *Tai Chong*, the so-called four bars or gates, regulate and rectify the qi of the entire body, thus resolving depression which might transform into heat and fan wind. *Feng Chi* and *He Gu* extinguish wind. In addition, *He Gu* and *San Yin Jiao* quicken the blood and transform stasis. Supplement *Shen Shu*, even supplement-even drain *San Yin Jiao*, and simply drain the other points.

ADDITIONS & SUBTRACTIONS: For dry, rough eyes, add *Guang Ming* (GB 37). For severe headache and dizziness, add *Bai Hui* (GV 20). For restlessness, insomnia, and easy anger, add *Xing Jian* (Liv 2) and *Da Ling* (Per 7). For concomitant blood stasis, add *Xue Hai* (Sp 10). For reduced appetite and abdominal fullness, add *Nei Guan* (Per 6) and *Gong Sun* (Sp 4). For loose stools, add *Zu San Li* (St 36).

REMARKS

1. For uremia, Yan De-xin commonly uses 30 grams each of Folium Eupatorii Chinensis (*Liu Yue Xue*) and uncooked Radix Et Rhizoma Rhei (*Da Huang*). These are decocted in water down to 150ml of liquid and used as a retention enema, one time per day, in order to discharge turbidity through the intestinal tract. According to Dr. Yan, this treatment helps reduce retention of blood urea nitrogen (BUN) and creatinine.

However, this is a strongly attacking treatment liable to produce strong diarrhea. Therefore, it should be used with care or modified for use in those who are vacuous and weak.

Another enema formula for uremia consists of 15- 30 grams of calcined Concha Ostreae (*Mu Li*), 20 grams of Fructus Forsythiae Suspensae (*Lian Qiao*), and 15 grams of Radix Et Rhizoma Rhei (*Da Huang*). Do once every other day for 14 days with a week's rest between courses.

Yet another Chinese medicinal enema is *Jun Kun Tang* (Army & Feminine Decoction). Here "army" refers to *Da Huang* which is also called *Jun* and "feminine" refers to *Yi Mu Cao* which is also called *Kun Cao.* Ingredients: Radix Et Rhizoma Rhei (*Da Huang*), 40g, Herba Leonuri Heterophylli (*Yi Mu Cao*), 30g, Concha Ostreae (*Mu Li*), 30g, and Radix Lateralis Praeparatus Aconiti Carmichaeli (*Fu Zi*), 15g. Put the medicinals in 500ml of water and decoct until reduced to 200ml. Retain the resulting warm (but not hot) liquid for 20-30 minutes each time. Do one enema per day for 20 days. Then stop for five days before resuming another 20 day course. If there is concomitant yang vacuity, add 3 grams of Cortex Cinnamomi Cassiae (*Rou Gui*). If there is yin vacuity, subtract *Fu Zi.* If there is high blood pressure, subtract *Fu Zi* and add 12 grams each of Radix Rubrus Paeoniae Lactiflorae (*Chi Shao*) and Flos Immaturus Sophorae Japonicae (*Huai Hua Mi*). For bloody stools, add 15 grams of Radix Sanguisorbae Officinalis (*Di Yu*). If there are white blood cells in the urine, add 30 grams each of Herba Taraxaci Mongolici Cum Radice (*Pu Gong Ying*) and Cortex Phellodendri (*Huang Bai*).

2. During remission, decoct 60 grams of Rhizoma Atractylodis Macrocephalae (*Bai Zhu*) with rice soup and take one time per day. Since the core mechanism of this condition is spleen(-kidney) vacuity, this treatment can lengthen the period of remission according to Dr. Yan.

3. If stasis heat damages liver-kidney yin and blood heat moves frenetically while the spirit brightness is depressed, then the condition will become very critical.

4. According to recent research, Radix Et Rhizoma Rhei (*Da Huang*), Cordyceps Sinensis (*Dong Chong Xia Cao*), Radix Polygoni Multiflori (*He Shou Wu*), Radix Astragali Membranacei (*Huang Qi*), and Radix Salviae Miltiorrhizae (*Dan Shen*) are particularly good medicinals for treating chronic renal failure.

5. As with chronic glomerulonephritis, one should avoid prescribing any medicinals that are nephrotoxic to patients with chronic renal failure. Please see chronic glomerulonephritis for a list of some of the most commonly used Chinese medicinals which may be toxic to the kidneys.

20

CHRONIC SINUSITIS

Sinusitis is an inflammation of the mucus membranes that line the sinus cavities. This inflammation may be either acute or chronic and causes the mucus glands in the sinuses to secret more mucus. In fact, so much mucus may be secreted and the tissue may become so swollen that the sinuses become obstructed, thus preventing drainage. In that case, there will be nasal congestion, anosmia, and head and face pain in the areas of the sinuses. In addition, there may be postnasal drip, cough, sore throat, and thick, yellow or green nasal mucus. Acute sinusitis is usually due to secondary bacterial infection subsequent to either a viral upper respiratory tract infection or allergic rhinitis. While chronic sinusitis may be asymptomatic, it is usually associated with pain in the head, face, or neck, runny nose and/or postnasal drip, a cough which is worse at night, anorexia, and a general feeling of malaise which may last from several weeks to several months. Chronic sinusitis may be due to incomplete or ineffective treatment of acute sinusitis or repeated attacks of acute sinusitis. However, it is often not associated with infection and may also be caused by allergies, changes in temperature and air pressure and airborne irritants, such as smoke. Over-use of decongestant nasal sprays, smoking, and swimming and diving increase the risk of developing sinusitis. Systemic factors include ciliary dyskinesia syndrome, cystic fibrosis, and immunoglobulin deficiency. Complications of sinusitis include orbital or periorbital cellulitis or edema, cavernous sinus thrombosis, optic neuritis, epidural or subdural abscesses, and meningitis.

The Western medical diagnosis of chronic sinusitis is mostly based on the patient's presenting signs and symptoms and history. Some clinicians will confirm their diagnosis via x-rays which show thickening of the membrane lining and clouding due to accumulation of fluid in the sinuses. Neck X-rays are used to rule out enlarged adenoids. If the history and symptoms are suggestive of sinusitis but X-rays are negative, CT scan may be used. Nasal endoscopy may also be used to diagnose chronic sinusitis. The Western medical treatment of sinusitis includes saline solution nasal washes, antibiotics in case of bacterial infection, corticosteroid nasal spray, decongestants, antihistamines, NSAIDs, and occasionally surgery to remove diseased tissue and restore sinus drainage. The indications for surgery include failure of medical management for more than three months, anatomical obstruction, complications, and intense pain.

CHINESE DISEASE CATEGORIZATION: Both acute and chronic sinusitis are mainly categorized as *bi yuan*, deep source nasal congestion. Deep source nasal congestion refers to persistent nasal congestion with turbid snivel. Other names include *nao lou*, brain leakage, *nao beng*, brain flooding, *nao xie*, brain drainage, *nao shen*, brain seepage, and *kong nao sha*, brain cavity sand. Postnasal drip is categorized as *mei he qi*, plum pit qi. Cough is *ke sou*. Headache is *tou tong*, while face pain is *mian tong*. Sore throat is *yan hou tong*, and anorexia is *na dai*, torpid intake.

DISEASE CAUSES: External contraction of evil qi, retained evils, unregulated eating and drinking, taxation fatigue, internal damage by the seven affects, and habitual bodily vacuity due to immaturity or aging

DISEASE MECHANISMS: Due to bodily vacuity, the defensive exterior may be insecure. In this case, wind evils may repeatedly enter the body and assail the lungs, lodging in the nasal passageways, the orifice of the lungs. If these wind evils transform heat, evil heat will brew body fluids, engendering phlegm and damaging the lungs' depurative downbearing, thus causing sneezing, nasal congestion, and cough. If external evils are not completely eliminated either by the body's righteous qi or medical treatment, they may be retained and become depressed in the areas of the body corresponding to the lungs. However, it is also possible for over-eating spicy, hot, fatty, sweet, thick-flavored foods or drinking alcohol to engender dampness and heat in the body. Damp may congeal into phlegm, while heat may draft this phlegm upward to lodge in the orifices of the lungs. Typically, this damp heat is associated with spleen vacuity. However, it may also be associated with depressive heat in the liver due to emotional stress and frustration. If depressive counterflows upward, it may lodge in the lungs, the florid canopy, brewing and stewing lung fluids into phlegm. Because phlegm is a yin depression which obstructs the flow of qi, enduring phlegm obstruction is often complicated by blood stasis.

The above scenarios of chronic sinusitis all involve some kind of evil heat. However, chronic sinusitis may also be associated with vacuity cold. If, for any reason, the spleen becomes vacuous and weak, it may lose control over movement and transformation. In that case, fluids may gather and collect, transforming into dampness. If dampness endures, it may congeal into phlegm. The lungs are the child of the spleen. Therefore, if the spleen qi becomes vacuous and weak, so must the lungs. In that case, the lungs may not be able to diffuse and downbear and hence fluids accumulate and spill over into the clear orifice of the nose. This results in white, watery nasal discharge and nasal congestion. In addition, spleen vacuity leads to anorexia, fatigue, lack of strength, and general malaise.

TREATMENT BASED ON PATTERN DISCRIMINATION:

1. LUNG CHANNEL WIND HEAT PATTERN

MAIN SYMPTOMS: Runny nose with profuse thick yellowish white phlegm, episodic nasal congestion, decreased sense of smell, swollen, red nasal membranes, frontal or maxillary aching and pain, possible aversion to cold, cough with profuse phlegm, headache, a dry mouth with a desire to drink, a possibly red tongue with thin, white fur, and a floating, rapid or floating, slippery, and rapid pulse

TREATMENT PRINCIPLES: Course wind and clear heat, penetratingly and aromatically free the flow of the orifices

RX: *Cang Er Zi San Jia Wei* (Xanthium Powder with Added Flavors)

INGREDIENTS: Flos Chrysanthemi Morifolii (*Ju Hua*), Radix Puerariae (*Ge Gen*) and Fructus Forsythiae Suspensae (*Lian Qiao*), 12g each, Fructus Xanthii Sibirici (*Cang Er Zi*), Flos Magnoliae Liliflorae (*Xin Yi*), and Radix Angelicae Dahuricae (*Bai Zhi*), 9g each, and Herba Menthae Haplocalycis (*Bo He*), 6g

ANALYSIS OF FORMULA: *Ju Hua*, *Ge Gen*, and *Bo He* dispel wind heat. *Lian Qiao* clears heat and resolves toxins. *Cang Er Zi*, *Xin Yi Hua*, and *Bai Zhi* course wind, diffuse the lungs, disinhibit and free the flow of the orifices of the nose.

ADDITIONS & SUBTRACTIONS: For severe lung heat with foul-smelling, green nasal discharge, add 18 grams of Herba Houttuyniae Cordatae Cum Radice (*Yu Xing Cao*) and nine grams of Radix Scutellariae Baicalensis (*Huang Qin*). These two medicinals can be alternated with 15 grams of Herba Taraxaci Mongolici Cum Radice (*Pu Gong Ying*) and Herba Patriniae Heterophyllae Cum Radice (*Bai Jiang Cao*). For cough with profuse phlegm, add nine grams each of Radix Platycodi Grandiflori (*Jie Geng*) and Semen Pruni Armeniacae (*Xing Ren*). For headache at the vertex, add 12 grams of Radix Et Rhizoma Ligustici Chinensis (*Gao Ben*). For frontal headache or supraorbital bone pain, add 12 grams of Fructus Viticis (*Man Jing Zi*) and increase the dosage of *Bai Zhi* up to 15 grams. For pain in the *Tai Yang* (M-HN-9) area, add nine grams of Radix Bupleuri (*Chai Hu*). For occipital headache, increase the dosage of *Ge Gen* up to 18 grams. For severe nasal congestion, add 18 grams of Herba Houttuyniae Cordatae Cum Radice (*Yu Xing Cao*) and nine grams of Herba Agastachis Seu Pogostemi (*Huo Xiang*).

ACUPUNCTURE & MOXIBUSTION: *He Gu* (LI 4), *Qu Chi* (LI 11), *Ying Xiang* (LI 20), *Chi Ze* (Lu 5). Use draining technique.

ANALYSIS OF FORMULA: Frontal or maxillary sinusitis involves the yang ming channel. Therefore, draining *He Gu* and *Qu Chi* are used to clear heat from the yang ming. At the same time, they course wind and clear heat. In addition, *He Gu* is the master or ruling point of the face. Therefore, it can treat any pain or disease in the orifices of the head. Draining *Ying Xiang*, the final point of the large intestine channel, disinhibits and frees the flow of the orifices of the nose, while draining *Chi Ze* diffuses and clears the lungs, and helps the other points dispel heat from the lung channel.

ADDITIONS & SUBTRACTIONS: For severe lung heat, add *Yu Ji* (Lu 10) and bleed *Chi Ze* (Lu 5). For local pain in the sinus cavities area, needle perpendicularly every painful *a shi* point in the center of the pain. For pain in the maxilla, add *Si Bai* (St 2). For severe runny nose, add *Shang Xing* (GV 23). For cough with profuse phlegm, add *Lie Que* (Lu 7). For supraorbital bone pain, add *Zan Zhu* (Bl 2), *Yin Tang* (M-HN-3), and eventually *Yu Yao* (M-HN-6). For pain in the temples, add *Tai Yang* (M-HN-9). For headache in the occiput, add *Feng Chi* (GB 20). For severe nasal congestion, add *Yin Tang* (M-HN-3).

2. GALLBLADDER BOWEL DEPRESSIVE HEAT PATTERN

MAIN SYMPTOMS: Runny nose with profuse, thick, foul-smelling, sticky, yellow or yellow-green, turbid, purulent phlegm, possible filaments of blood in the phlegm, nasal congestion, anosmia, very red, swollen, and distended nasal membranes, severe headache, frontal headache, orbital or supraorbital bone pain, possible bilateral temple headache, maxillary bone pain, generalized fever, a dry throat and bitter taste in the mouth, tinnitus, deafness, dizziness, insomnia, red eyes, a red tongue with yellow fur, and a bowstring, rapid pulse

NOTE: This pattern is also sometimes called lung channel depressive heat pattern. The name gallbladder bowel depressive heat pattern emphasizes that depressive heat has been engendered in the liver but has shifted to the paired yang channel, the gallbladder, where it has followed the channel upward to the head. In either case, the heat is being transformed in the liver due to depression and then counterflowing upward. In its full-blown form, this pattern describes an acute crisis of otherwise chronic sinusitis.

TREATMENT PRINCIPLES: Clear and discharge gallbladder heat, disinhibit dampness and free the flow of the orifices

RX: *Long Dan Bi Yuan Fang* (Gentiana Deep Source Nasal Congestion Formula)

INGREDIENTS: Semen Coicis Lachryma-jobi (*Yi Yi Ren*), 20g, Radix Scutellariae Baicalensis (*Huang Qin*), Herba Houttuyniae Cordatae Cum Radice (*Yu Xing Cao*), Spica Prunellae Vulgaris (*Xia Ku Cao*), Flos Chrysanthemi Morifolii (*Ju Hua*), Radix Angelicae Dahuricae (*Bai Zhi*), Fructus Xanthii Sibirici (*Cang Er Zi*), Radix Platycodi Grandiflori (*Jie Geng*), Semen Plantaginis (*Che Qian Zi*), and Herba Agastachis Seu Pogostemi (*Huo Xiang*), 9g each, and Radix Gentianae Scabrae (*Long Dan Cao*), 6g

ANALYSIS OF FORMULA: *Long Dan Cao*, *Huang Qin*, *Ju Hua*, and *Xia Ku Cao* strongly clear and discharge gallbladder heat. *Yi Yi Ren* and *Che Qian Zi* disinhibit dampness and guide heat downward via urination. *Huang Qin*, *Yu Xing Cao*, and *Jie Geng* diffuse and clear the lungs. *Bai Zhi*, *Cang Er Zi*, and *Huo Xiang* free the flow of the orifices. In addition, *Huang Qin* and *Yu Xing Cao* resolve toxins, especially in the lungs, while *Bai Zhi* stops pain in the face, especially in the large intestine and stomach channel. *Huo Xiang* is an empirical medicinal for treating nasal discharge, and *Jie Geng* is a messenger which leads the other medicinals into the lungs and the upper part of the body.

ADDITIONS & SUBTRACTIONS: If depressive heat has endured and damaged qi and yin, replace *Long Dan Bi Yuan Fang* with *Xin Yi Qing Fei Yin* (Flos Magnoliae Clear the Lungs Drink) and *Cang Er Zi San* (Xanthium Powder): uncooked Gypsum Fibrosum (*Shi Gao*), 30g, Radix Astragali Membranacei (*Huang Qi*) and Radix Angelicae Dahuricae (*Bai Zhi*), 18g each, Folium Eriobotryae Japonicae (*Pi Pa Ye*), Fructus Gardeniae Jasminoidis (*Zhi Zi*), Tuber Ophiopogonis Japonici (*Mai Men Dong*), and Bulbus Lilii (*Bai He*), 15g each, Rhizoma Anemarrhenae Aspheloidis (*Zhi Mu*), Rhizoma Cimicifugae (*Sheng Ma*), Herba Menthae Haplocalycis (*Bo He*), and Fructus Xanthii Sibirici (*Cang Er Zi*), 9g each, and Radix Glycyrrhizae (*Gan Cao*), 6g.

If there is a liver-spleen disharmony with depressive heat and phlegm, replace *Long Dan Bi Yuan Fang* with *Xiao Chai Hu Tang* (Minor Bupleurum Decoction) and *Cang Er Zi San* (Xanthium Powder) with added flavors: Radix Angelicae Dahuricae (*Bai Zhi*), 15g, Radix Scutellariae Baicalensis (*Huang Qin*), 12g, Radix Bupleuri (*Chai Hu*), Radix Codonopsitis Pilosulae (*Dang Shen*), Rhizoma Pinelliae Ternatae (*Ban Xia*), Fructus Xanthii Sibirici (*Cang Er Zi*), Flos Magnoliae Liliflorae (*Xin Yi*), and Herba Menthae Haplocalycis (*Bo He*), 9g each, Rhizoma Acori Graminei (*Shi Chang Pu*) and mix-fried Radix Glycyrrhizae (*Gan Cao*), 6g each, uncooked Rhizoma Zingiberis (*Sheng Jiang*), 2 slices, and Fructus Zizyphi Jujubae (*Da Zao*), 3 pieces. For profuse purulent greenish yellow phlegm, add 15 grams each of Flos Lonicerae Japonicae (*Jin Yin Hua*), Herba Houttuyniae Cordatae Cum Radice (*Yu Xing Cao*), and Herba Centipedae (*E Bu Shi Cao*).

ACUPUNCTURE & MOXIBUSTION: *Ying Xiang* (LI 20), *Shang Xing* (GV 23), *Xuan Zhong* (GB 39), *Feng Chi* (GB 20)

ANALYSIS OF FORMULA: Draining *Ying Xiang* and *Shang Xing* disinhibits and frees the flow of the orifices of the nose and stops pain. In Chinese medicine, sinusitis is variously called *nao lou*, brain leakage, *nao beng*, brain flooding, *nao xie*, brain drainage, *nao shen*, brain seepage, and *kong nao sha*, brain cavity. *Xuan Zhong* is the meeting point of the brain. Draining it drains heat from the gallbladder channel and clears liver fire. Therefore, it treats deep source nasal congestion due to gallbladder bowel depressive heat. *Feng Chi* is a local point which, when drained, clears the head and helps *Xuan Zhong* clear liver-gallbladder heat.

ADDITIONS & SUBTRACTIONS: For severe lung heat, add *He Gu* (LI 4) and *Chi Ze* (Lu 5). For emission of heat or fever, add *He Gu* (LI 4) and *Qu Chi* (LI 11). For local pain in the sinus cavities area, add *He Gu* (LI 4) and needle perpendicularly every painful *a shi* point in the center of the pain. For pain in the maxilla, add *He Gu* (LI 4) and *Si Bai* (St 2). For severe runny nose, add *Yin Tang* (M-HN-3). For cough with profuse phlegm, add *Chi Ze* (Lu 5). For supraorbital bone pain, add *Zan Zhu* (Bl 2), *Yin Tang* (M-HN-3), and eventually *Yu Yao* (M-HN-6). For pain in the temples, add *Tai Yang* (M-HN-9). For headache at the vertex, add *Bai Hui* (GV 20). For severe nasal congestion, add *Yin Tang* (M-HN-3).

3. Spleen channel damp heat pattern

Main symptoms: Runny nose with profuse, yellow, turbid phlegm, a prolonged, sluggish, trickling flow, relatively severe nasal congestion, anosmia, red, swollen nasal membranes, possible severe headache or heavy-headedness, distention, and discomfort, heavy body and encumbered limbs, devitalized eating and drinking, venter and abdominal distention and fullness, yellow urine, a red tongue with slimy, yellow fur, and a slippery, rapid or soggy pulse

Treatment principles: Clear the spleen and drain heat, disinhibit dampness and dispel turbidity

Rx: *Huang Qin Hua Shi Tang* (Scutellaria & Talcum Decoction)

Ingredients: Pericarpium Arecae Catechu (*Da Fu Pi*), 20g, Sclerotium Poriae Cocos (*Fu Ling*), Sclerotium Polypori Umbellati (*Zhu Ling*), and Radix Scutellariae Baicalensis (*Huang Qin*), 15g each, Fructus Cardamomi (*Bai Dou Kou*), 12g, Talcum (*Hua Shi*), 9g, and Medulla Tetrapanacis Papyriferi (*Tong Cao*), 6g

Analysis of formula: *Da Fu Pi* loosens the center, moves the qi, and treats damp accumulation with qi stagnation. It also moves water and disperses swelling. *Bai Dou Kou* moves the qi, warms the center, disperses food, and treats damp turbid accumulation in the center. *Fu Ling* and *Zhu Ling* disinhibit dampness and dispel turbidity, while *Fu Ling* fortifies the spleen. These four medicinals prevent further damp turbid obstruction in the center which might transform into heat. *Huang Qin, Hua Shi,* and *Tong Cao* clear the spleen and disinhibit dampness. In addition, *Huang Qin* clears heat in the upper burner and lungs.

Additions & subtractions: For severe nasal congestion with very swollen nasal membranes, add nine grams each of Herba Agastachis Seu Pogostemi (*Huo Xiang*), Rhizoma Acori Graminei (*Shi Chang Pu*), and Fructus Xanthii Sibirici (*Cang Er Zi*). For foul-smelling, green nasal discharge or very profuse yellow discharge, add 18 grams of Herba Houttuyniae Cordatae Cum Radice (*Yu Xing Cao*) and nine grams of Fructus Gardeniae Jasminoidis (*Zhi Zi*). These two medicinals can be alternated with 15 grams each of Herba Taraxaci Mongolici Cum Radice (*Pu Gong Ying*) and Herba Patriniae Heterophyllae Cum Radice (*Bai Jiang Cao*). For marked spleen vacuity, add 15 grams of Rhizoma Atractylodis Macrocephalae (*Bai Zhu*) and nine grams of Radix Codonopsitis Pilosulae (*Dang Shen*). For abdominal distention, especially after meals, add nine grams each of Cortex Magnoliae Officinalis (*Hou Po*) and Rhizoma Atractylodis Macrocephalae (*Bai Zhu*). For cough with profuse phlegm, add nine grams each of Radix Platycodi Grandiflori (*Jie Geng*) and Pericarpium Trichosanthis Kirlowii (*Gua Lou Pi*). For headache at the vertex, add 12 grams of Radix Et Rhizoma Ligustici Chinensis (*Gao Ben*). For frontal headache or supraorbital bone pain, add 12 grams each of Fructus Viticis (*Man Jing Zi*) and Radix Angelicae Dahuricae (*Bai Zhi*). For pain in the *Tai Yang* (M-HN-9) area, add nine grams of Radix Bupleuri (*Chai Hu*). For occipital headache, add 12 grams of Radix Puerariae (*Ge Gen*). For heavy body and encumbered limbs, add nine grams each of Rhizoma Alismatis (*Ze Xie*), Rhizoma Acori Graminei (*Shi Chang Pu*), and Rhizoma Atractylodis (*Cang Zhu*). For severe damp heat, add 15 grams of Herba Artemisiae Capillaris (*Yin Chen Hao*) and three grams of Rhizoma Coptidis Chinensis (*Huang Lian*).

Acupuncture & moxibustion: *He Gu* (LI 4), *Nei Ting* (St 44), *Zhong Wan* (CV 12), *Ying Xiang* (LI 20), *Shang Xing* (GV 23)

Analysis of formula: Draining *He Gu, Nei Ting,* and *Zhong Wan* clears heat from the spleen and drains heat from the center, disinhibits dampness and dispels turbidity. In addition, *He Gu* is the master or ruling point of the face which treats any disease in the orifices of the head. It is a key point for nose problems. Draining *Ying Xiang* and *Shang Xing* disinhibits and frees the flow of the orifices of the nose.

Additions & subtractions: For local pain in the sinus cavities area, needle perpendicularly every painful *a shi* point in the center of the pain. For pain in the maxilla, add *Si Bai* (St 2). For severe runny nose, add *Yin Tang* (M-HN-3). For marked spleen vacuity, add *Zu San Li* (St 36). For cough with profuse phlegm, add *Lie Que* (Lu 7). For supraorbital bone pain, add *Zan Zhu* (Bl 2), *Yin Tang* (M-HN-3), and eventually *Yu Yao* (M-HN-6). For pain in the temples, add *Tai Yang* (M-HN-9). For occipital headache, add *Feng Chi* (GB 20). For severe nasal congestion, add *Yin Tang* (M-HN-3).

4. Lung qi vacuity cold pattern

Main symptoms: Runny nose with profuse, sticky, white phlegm, anosmia or decreased sense of smell, nasal congestion which may be either slight or severe, swollen, distended, pale red nasal membranes, worsening of symptoms on exposure to wind and chill, easy contraction of wind evils, heavy-headedness, dizziness, spontaneous perspiration, shortness of breath, lack of strength, disinclination to speak, weak voice, cough with thin, watery phlegm, a pale tongue with thin, white fur, and a moderate (*i.e.*, slightly slow), weak pulse

Treatment principles: Warm and supplement the lung qi, course and scatter wind cold

Rx: *Wen Fei Zhi Liu Dan* (Warm the Lungs & Stop Running Elixir) & *Cang Er Zi San* (Xanthium Powder)

INGREDIENTS: Radix Angelicae Dahuricae (*Bai Zhi*), 18g, Herba Seu Flos Schizonepetae Tenuifoliae (*Jing Jie*), 12g, Fructus Xanthii Sibirici (*Cang Er Zi*), Flos Magnoliae Liliflorae (*Xin Yi*), Herba Menthae Haplocalycis (*Bo He*), mix-fried Radix Glycyrrhizae (*Gan Cao*), Fructus Terminaliae Chebulae (*He Zi*), Radix Platycodi Grandiflori (*Jie Geng*), Otolith Pseudosciaenae (*Yu Nao Shi*), and Radix Panacis Ginseng (*Ren Shen*), 9g each, and Herba Asari Cum Radice (*Xi Xin*), 3g

ANALYSIS OF FORMULA: *Ren Shen* and mix-fried *Gan Cao* supplement the lungs. *He Zi* constrains the lung qi to avoid further loss of the lung qi. *Yu Nao Shi, Cang Er Zi, Xi Xin, Xin Yi Hua,* and *Bai Zhi* free the flow of the nasal orifices and prevent wind cold invasion. *Jing Jie, Xi Xin,* and *Bo He* also prevent wind cold.

NOTE: *Yu Nao Shi* is a very effective medicinal for chronic sinusitis. However, it is not easy to find in Western countries. It can be replaced by Herba Agastachis Seu Pogostemi (*Huo Xiang*) though this latter medicinal is not as strong acting.

ADDITIONS & SUBTRACTIONS: For concomitant spleen vacuity, add 12 grams each of Radix Codonopsitis Pilosulae (*Dang Shen*) and Radix Astragali Membranacei (*Huang Qi*). For frequent and easy contraction of wind evils, add *Yu Ping Feng San* (Jade Wind-screen Powder): Radix Astragali Membranacei (*Huang Qi*), 15g, Rhizoma Atractylodis Macrocephalae (*Bai Zhu*), 12g, and Radix Ledebouriellae Divaricatae (*Fang Feng*), 6g. For enduring cough with profuse phlegm, add nine grams each of Radix Asteris Tatarici (*Zi Wan*), Semen Pruni Armeniacae (*Xing Ren*), and Fructus Schisandrae Chinensis (*Wu Wei Zi*). For headache, heavy-headedness, or dizziness, add nine grams each of Radix Angelicae Dahuricae (*Bai Zhi*), Radix Ligustici Wallichii (*Chuan Xiong*), and Rhizoma Acori Graminei (*Shi Chang Pu*). For severe nasal congestion, add nine grams each of Rhizoma Acori Graminei (*Shi Chang Pu*) and Herba Agastachis Seu Pogostemi (*Huo Xiang*). For white nasal discharge alternating with yellow discharge, add six grams of Radix Scutellariae Baicalensis (*Huang Qin*) and 12 grams of Herba Houttuyniae Cordatae Cum Radice (*Yu Xing Cao*).

ACUPUNCTURE & MOXIBUSTION: *Feng Men* (Bl 12), *Fei Shu* (Bl 13), *He Gu* (LI 4), *Ying Xiang* (LI 20), *Shang Xing* (GV 23)

ANALYSIS OF FORMULA: Supplementing *Feng Me* and *Fei Shu* with moxibustion warms and supplements the lungs and prevents contraction of wind cold. Even supplementing-even draining *He Gu* courses and scatters wind cold and secures the exterior to also help avoid further wind damage. Draining *Ying Xiang* and *Shang Xing* disinhibits and frees the flow of the orifices of the nose.

ADDITIONS & SUBTRACTIONS: For marked lung vacuity, add *Tai Yuan* (Lu 9). For concomitant spleen vacuity, add *Zu San Li* (St 36). For frequent and easy contraction of wind evils, add *Da Zhui* (GV 14). For local pain in the sinus cavities area, needle perpendicularly every painful *a shi* point in the center of the pain. For pain in the maxilla, add *Si Bai* (St 2). For severe runny nose, add *Yin Tang* (M-HN-3). For severe congestion, add *Yin Tang* (M-HN-3). For cough with profuse phlegm, add *Lie Que* (Lu 7). For supra-orbital bone pain, add *Zan Zhu* (Bl 2), *Yin Tang* (M-HN-3), and eventually *Yu Yao* (M-HN-6). For pain in the temples, add *Tai Yang* (M-HN-9). For occipital headache, add *Feng Chi* (GB 20).

5. SPLEEN QI VACUITY WEAKNESS PATTERN

MAIN SYMPTOMS: Runny nose with profuse thick, white or thick, yellow phlegm, anosmia, relatively severe nasal congestion, pale red nasal membranes with severe swelling and distention, heavy-headedness, dizziness, bodily fatigue, a weak constitution, lack of strength, reduced food intake, abdominal distention, especially after meals, a somber white or sallow yellow facial complexion, loose stools, a pale tongue with thin, white fur, and a moderate (*i.e.*, slightly slow), weak pulse

NOTE: This pattern and the preceding one often combine.

TREATMENT PRINCIPLES: Fortify the spleen and boost the qi, clear and disinhibit dampness and turbidity

RX: *Shen Ling Bai Zhu San Jia Jian* (Ginseng, Poria & Atractylodes Powder with Additions & Subtractions)

INGREDIENTS: Radix Astragali Membranacei (*Huang Qi*) and Radix Codonopsitis Pilosulae (*Dang Shen*), 20g each, Rhizoma Atractylodis Macrocephalae (*Bai Zhu*), Sclerotium Poriae Cocos (*Fu Ling*), Semen Coicis Lachryma-jobi (*Yi Yi Ren*), and Radix Dioscoreae Oppositae (*Shan Yao*), 15g each, Rhizoma Alismatis (*Ze Xie*), 12g, mix-fried Radix Glycyrrhizae (*Gan Cao*), Semen Dolichoris Lablab (*Bai Bian Dou*), and Semen Nelumbinis Nuciferae (*Lian Zi*), 9g each, Fructus Amomi (*Sha Ren*), Radix Platycodi Grandiflori (*Jie Geng*), and Pericarpium Citri Reticulatae (*Chen Pi*), 6g each, and Fructus Zizyphi Jujubae (*Da Zao*), 3 pieces

ANALYSIS OF FORMULA: *Huang Qi, Dang Shen, Bai Zhu, Fu Ling, Shan Yao, Bai Bian Dou,* mix-fried *Gan Cao,* and *Da Zao* all fortify the spleen and boost the qi. They treat the root of the disease. *Fu Ling, Yi Yi Ren,* and *Ze Xie* percolate or seep dampness, and dampness is the spleen's worst enemy. *Sha Ren* and *Chen Pi* move the qi and thus move dampness as well as dry dampness. *Jie Geng,* the messenger within this formula, leads the other medicinals to the lungs and its related orifice, *i.e.*, the nose.

ADDITIONS & SUBTRACTIONS: For severe nasal congestion, add nine grams each of Fructus Xanthii Sibirici (*Cang Er Zi*) and Herba Agastachis Seu Pogostemi (*Huo Xiang*) and three grams of Herba Asari Cum Radice (*Xi Xin*). For clear, watery nasal discharge, add six grams of dry Rhizoma Zingiberis (*Gan Jiang*) and three grams of Herba Asari Cum Radice (*Xi Xin*). For white discharge alternating with yellow discharge, add six grams of Radix Scutellariae Baicalensis (*Huang Qin*) and 12 grams of Herba Houttuyniae Cordatae Cum Radice (*Yu Xing Cao*). For frequent and easy contraction of wind evils, add six grams each of Herba Schizonepetae Tenuifoliae (*Jing Jie*) and Radix Ledebouriellae Divaricatae (*Fang Feng*). For enduring cough with profuse phlegm, add nine grams each of Radix Asteris Tatarici (*Zi Wan*), Semen Pruni Armeniacae (*Xing Ren*), and Fructus Schisandrae Chinensis (*Wu Wei Zi*). For headache, heavy-headedness, or dizziness, add nine grams each of Radix Angelicae Dahuricae (*Bai Zhi*), Radix Ligustici Wallichii (*Chuan Xiong*), and Rhizoma Acori Graminei (*Shi Chang Pu*).

ACUPUNCTURE & MOXIBUSTION: *Zu San Li* (St 36), *He Gu* (LI 4), *Yin Ling Quan* (Sp 9), *Ying Xiang* (LI 20), *Shang Xing* (GV 23)

ANALYSIS OF FORMULA: Supplementing *Zu San Li* fortifies the spleen and boosts the qi. Even supplementing-even draining *He Gu* supplements the qi and secures the exterior as well as drains any replete evils in the region of the head and face. *Yin Ling Quan* is a key point for dampness. Draining it disinhibits dampness and dispels turbidity. Draining *Ying Xiang* and *Shang Xing* disinhibits and frees the flow of the orifices of the nose.

ADDITIONS & SUBTRACTIONS: For frequent and easy contraction of wind evils, add *Da Zhui* (GV 14). For local pain in the sinus cavities area, needle perpendicularly every painful *a shi* point in the center of the pain. For pain in the maxilla, add *Si Bai* (St 2). For severe runny nose, add *Yin Tang* (M-HN-3). For severe nasal congestion, add *Yin Tang* (M-HN-3). For cough with profuse phlegm, add *Lie Que* (Lu 7). For supraorbital bone pain, add *Zan Zhu* (Bl 2), *Yin Tang* (M-HN-3), and eventually *Yu Yao* (M-HN-6). For pain in the temples, add *Tai Yang* (M-HN-9). For occipital headache, add *Feng Chi* (GB 20).

REMARKS

1. Most Western patients with chronic sinusitis have a combination of liver depression/depressive heat wafting up to accumulate in and damage the lungs plus spleen vacuity with phlegm and dampness. For instance, the following formula treats chronic sinusitis due to liver-spleen disharmony and lung vacuity with depressive heat and blood stasis: *Bi Shu Ling* (Nose Soothing Elixir): Herba Houttuyniae Cordatae Cum Radice (*Yu Xing Cao*) and Herba Taraxaci Mongolici Cum Radice (*Pu Gong Ying*), 15g each, Radix Bupleuri (*Chai Hu*) and Fructus Xanthii Sibirici (*Cang Er Zi*), 12g each, and Herba Agastachis Seu Pogostemi (*Huo Xiang*), Semen Coicis Lachryma-jobi (*Yi Yi Ren*), Radix Salviae Miltiorrhizae (*Dan Shen*), Radix Scutellariae Baicalensis (*Huang Qin*), Rhizoma Atractylodis Macrocephalae (*Bai Zhu*), Radix Astragali Membranacei (*Huang Qi*), and Ramulus Cinnamomi Cassiae (*Gui Zhi*), 9g each.

If there is chronic sinusitis with a liver-spleen disharmony and the spleen vacuity is predominant at the same time as there is clearly depressive heat counterflowing upward to steam and putrefy the nasal mucosa, this may be seen as a yin fire scenario. In that case, one may consider using *Bu Pi Wei Xie Yin Huo Sheng Yang Tang* (Supplement the Spleen & Stomach, Drain Yin Fire & Upbear Yang Decoction): Radix Bupleuri (*Chai Hu*), Radix Et Rhizoma Notopterygii (*Qiang Huo*), Rhizoma Cimicifugae (*Sheng Ma*), Radix Codonopsitis Pilosulae (*Dang Shen*), Radix Astragali Membranacei (*Huang Qi*), Rhizoma Atractylodis (*Cang Zhu*), and Fructus Xanthii Sibirici (*Cang Er Zi*), 9g each, Radix Scutellariae Baicalensis (*Huang Qin*), 6g, and Rhizoma Coptidis Chinensis (*Huang Lian*) and mix-fried Radix Glycyrrhizae (*Gan Cao*), 3g each.

2. If chronic sinusitis, head and face pain, and nasal obstruction endure for some time, any of the above patterns may become complicated by blood stasis. In that case, add nine grams each of Radix Rubrus Paeoniae Lactiflorae (*Chi Shao*) and Cortex Radicis Moutan (*Dan Pi*).

3. Because of the relationship of diet to spleen function and, therefore, the internal engenderment of dampness and phlegm and also because heat can be caused or aggravated by hot, spicy foods, diet is typically important in the overall Chinese medical treatment of chronic sinusitis. As with so many other chronic conditions, this means eating a clear, bland diet.

4. Chinese medicinal nose drops can be a useful adjunct to the treatment of this condition. The following is a simple recipe for nose drops: Dissolve small, equal amounts of Borax (*Peng Sha*) and Alumen (*Ming Fan*) plus a third amount of Borneol (*Bing Pian*) in a small amount of water. Store in a dropper bottle. Drip several drops of this solution into the affected nostril(s) 2-3 times per day.

5. Most effective new contemporary Chinese formulas to treat this condition use Fructus Xanthii Sibirici (*Cang Er Zi*). For instance, *Zhong Cang Ping Yuan Tang* (Heavy [Dosage of] Xanthum Level the Deep Source Decoction) treats the acute crisis of sinusitis. Because of the slight toxicity and heavy dosage of *Cang Er Zi*, this formula should only be used for a short period of time and with careful observation of the patient. This formula's ingredients are: Fructus Xanthii

Sibirici (*Cang Er Zi*), 30g, Fructus Forsythiae Suspensae (*Lian Qiao*), Radix Scrophulariae Ningpoensis (*Xuan Shen*), and Cortex Radicis Mori Albi (*Sang Bai Pi*), 20g each, Radix Platycodi Grandiflori (*Jie Geng*), 18g, Gypsum Fibrosum (*Shi Gao*), Cortex Radicis Moutan (*Dan Pi*), and Herba Agastachis Seu Pogostemi (*Huo Xiang*), 15g each, Radix Angelicae Dahuricae (*Bai Zhi*) and Flos Magnoliae Liliflorae (*Xin Yi Hua*), 12g each, Herba Schizonepetae Tenuifoliae (*Jing Jie*) and Radix Glycyrrhizae (*Gan Cao*), 9g each, and Herba Ephedrae (*Ma Huang*), 6g. Decoct each bag of medicinals three times, drinking the resulting medicinal decoction each time after meals. For emission of heat or fever and aversion to cold due to wind heat in the lung orifice, add nine grams each of Flos Lonicerae Japonicae (*Jin Yin Hua*) and Radix Scutellariae Baicalensis (*Huang Qin*). For irascibility and a bitter taste in the mouth due to liver fire, add nine grams each of Radix Gentianae Scabrae (*Long Dan Cao*) and Fructus Gardeniae Jasminoidis (*Zhi Zi*). For mouth sores, dry stools, and thirst due to stomach fire, add 3-6 grams each of Radix Et Rhizoma Rhei (*Da Huang*) and Mirabilitum (*Mang Xiao*).

21

Coronary Artery Disease

Coronary artery disease (CAD) is primarily due to atherosclerosis of the large and medium-sized arteries supplying the heart. The major complications of CAD are angina pectoris, myocardial infarction, arrhythmia, and sudden cardiac death. Atherosclerosis is the most common form of arteriosclerosis. Arteriosclerosis is a generic term for thickening and loss of elasticity of the arterial walls thus restricting and reducing blood flow through those arteries. Risk factors for arteriosclerosis include hypertension, elevated serum lipids, cigarette smoking, diabetes mellitus, obesity, and the male sex. From ages 25-34, the death rate from CAD in white males is 1 per 10,000. From age 55-64, it is nearly 1 per 100. Between the ages of 35-44, the death rate from CAD among white males is 6.1 times greater than that for women. In non-whites, for some unknown reason, the sex difference in death rates from CAD is less apparent.

The discomfort of angina pectoris is highly variable. It is most commonly felt beneath the sternum as a vague, barely troublesome ache. However, it may rapidly become a severe, intense precordial crushing sensation. Pain may radiate to the left shoulder and down the inside of the left arm possibly reaching the fingers. This pain may also radiate straight through to the upper back. In addition, it sometimes radiates to the throat, jaws, teeth, and even occasionally down the right arm. Angina pectoris is characteristically triggered by physical activity and usually lasts only a few minutes, subsiding with rest. It is even more easily triggered by exercise following a meal and is also exaggerated by exposure to cold. In some patients, angina may occur at night when resting or asleep. Attacks may vary in frequency from several per day to occasional attacks separated by asymptomatic intervals of weeks, months, or even years. Since the symptoms of angina are usually constant for a given individual, any change or worsening in the pattern of these symptoms should be viewed as serious.

The Western medical diagnosis of CAD is based on the patient's symptoms, if any, plus palpation of the precordium, listening to the heart sounds via stethoscope, ischemic ECG changes, exercise tolerance tests, coronary arteriography, and radionuclide studies. Western medical treatment of CAD consists of diet and exercise plus prophylatic and remedial use of nitrate vasodilators, such as nitroglycerin and amyl nitrate, beta-adrenergic agents, calcium blockers, antiplatelet drugs, such as aspirin, coronary arterial bypass surgery, and angioplasty. Prognosis is determined by age, extent of coronary disease, severity of symptoms, and ventricular function. For instance, men with CAD with angina but no history of myocardial infarction, normal blood pressure, and a normal resting ECG have an annual mortality rate of 1.4%, while men with CAD with systolic hypertension and an abnormal ECG have a 12% annual mortality rate.

Chinese disease categorization: In Chinese medicine, CAD is traditionally categorized as *xiong bi*, chest impediment, *xiong tong*, chest pain, *zhen xin tong*, true heart pain, and *jue xin tong*, reversal heart pain, *i.e.*, heart pain with chilled limbs.

Disease causes: Habitual bodily exuberance, external invasion by the six environmental excesses, internal damage by the seven affects, unregulated eating and drinking, unregulated stillness (*i.e.*, rest) and activity, and aging

Disease mechanisms: The elderly tend to be both qi and yin vacuous. The heart controls the blood. This means that the heart qi pushes the blood through its vessels. If qi vacuity reaches yang, heart yang may become devitalized. In addition, due to concomitant defensive yang vacuity, cold evils may be contracted. Thus yin cold may become exuberant in the temple of the chest. This then leads to yang qi losing its diffusion and cold congealing in the blood vessels. It is also possible that drinking alcohol and over-eating fatty, sweet, thick-flavored floods may cause detriment and damage to the spleen and stomach. Therefore, phlegm turbidity and fatty substances are engendered internally. This may also hinder and obstruct the movement and transportation of qi and blood. Further, due to emotional depression, qi may stagnate in the upper burner. Hence chest yang loses its spreading and out-thrusting, and the blood vessels are not harmonious. Rather, the blood vessels may become blocked and obstructed and the heart loses its nourishment. Therefore, there are chest pain, heart palpitations, and chilling of the extremities. If severe, this may even lead to reversal condition, *i.e.*, loss of consciousness, and death.

TREATMENT BASED ON PATTERN DISCRIMINATION:

1. CHEST YANG IMPEDIMENT & OBSTRUCTION PATTERN

MAIN SYMPTOMS: Heart pain which is often induced by cold, shortness of breath or a suffocating feeling, chest oppression, heart pain radiating to the upper back in severe cases, heart palpitations, slimy, white tongue fur, and a bowstring, slippery, regularly interrupted, or bound pulse

NOTE: This pattern is a combination of cold impediment, phlegm obstruction, qi stagnation, and blood stasis. The next three patterns each describe blood stasis, qi stagnation, and phlegm obstruction as more discrete entities (though even liver depression and phlegm obstruction are complicated by an element of blood stasis). However, in clinical practice, they are rarely seen in such simple forms.

TREATMENT PRINCIPLES: Loosen the chest and free the flow of yang, quicken the blood and transform stasis

RX: *Gua Lou Xie Bai Ban Xia Tang Jia Wei* (Trichosanthes, Allium & Pinellia Decoction with Added Flavors)

INGREDIENTS: Radix Salviae Miltiorrhizae (*Dan Shen*), 15g, Fructus Trichosanthis Kirlowii (*Gua Lou*), Bulbus Allii Macrostemi (*Xie Bai*), Radix Ligustici Wallichii (*Chuan Xiong*), Pollen Typhae (*Pu Huang*), Rhizoma Cyperi Rotundi (*Xiang Fu*), Rhizoma Pinelliae Ternatae (*Ban Xia*), and Flos Carthami Tinctorii (*Hong Hua*), 9g each, Ramulus Cinnamomi Cassiae (*Gui Zhi*), 4.5g, and powdered Sanguis Draconis (*Xue Jie*) and powdered Radix Pseudoginseng (*San Qi*), 1.5g each (swallowed in divided doses with the liquid decoction)

ANALYSIS OF FORMULA: This is a basic formula to treat CAD, especially due to a combination of cold impediment, phlegm obstruction, and qi stagnation. With modifications, *Gua Lou Xie Bai Ban Xia Tang* can be adapted to many conditions. *Ban Xia* transforms phlegm, while *Gua Lou* disperses it. At the same time, *Gua Lou* loosens the chest. *Xie Bai* and *Gui Zhi* free the flow of yang, warm and reinforce the heart yang, warm and free the flow of the channels and network vessels. *Xiang Fu* and *Chuan Xiong* move the qi and stop pain. *Xiang Fu* also courses the liver. *Chuan Xiong, Dan Shen, Pu Huang, Hong Hua, Xue Jie,* and *San Qi* all quicken the blood, dispel stasis, and stop heart pain. Also, *Dan Shen, Pu Huang,* and *San Qi* treat hyperlipoproteinemia, while *San Qi* and *Pu Huang* dispel blood stasis at the same time as stop bleeding, thus preventing infarct. Except for *Xiang Fu,* all the medicinals in this formula are empirically well-known for treating chest impediment and CAD. Remark: to loosen the chest and treat *xiong bi,* chest impediment, Pericarpium Trichosanthis Kirlowii (*Gua Lou Pi*) is better than Fructus Trichosanthis Kirlowii (*Gua Lou*).

ADDITIONS & SUBTRACTIONS: For severe cold impediment, add six grams of Radix Lateralis Praeparatus Aconiti Carmichaeli (*Fu Zi*) and nine grams of Herba Epimedii (*Yin Yang Huo*). For concomitant heart yang vacuity, add 15 grams of Radix Astragali Membranacei (*Huang Qi*) and three grams each of Herba Asari Cum Radice (*Xi Xin*) and Radix Lateralis Praeparatus Aconiti Carmichaeli (*Fu Zi*). For qi vacuity with fatigue, shortness of breath, and weakness of the limbs, add 15 grams of Radix Astragali Membranacei (*Huang Qi*) and nine grams of Radix Codonopsitis Pilosulae (*Dang Shen*). For severe chest oppression, add nine grams of Cortex Magnoliae Officinalis (*Hou Po*) and Fructus Citri Aurantii (*Zhi Ke*). For profuse phlegm, add nine grams of Radix Platycodi Grandiflori (*Jie Geng*). For severe heart pain, add 20 grams of Rhizoma Corydalis Yanhusuo (*Yan Hu Suo*).

ACUPUNCTURE & MOXIBUSTION: *Xin Shu* (Bl 15), *Ju Que* (CV 14), *Nei Guan* (Per 6), *Ge Shu* (Bl 17)

ANALYSIS OF FORMULA: *Xin Shu* is the back transport point of the heart, while *Ju Que* is the front *mu* or alarm point of the heart. This combination of back transport and front alarm points scatters cold and dispels phlegm, quickens the blood and moves the qi of the heart. *Ge Shu* is the meeting point of the blood. However, it regulates and rectifies both the qi and blood of the heart. *Nei Guan* is the network point of the pericardium. It is a main point for the treatment of heart disease. It frees the flow of the network vessels of the heart and regulates cardiac rhythm, reinforces the left ventricle of the heart and treats CAD. All points should be needled with the even supplementing-even draining method.

ADDITIONS & SUBTRACTIONS: If there is severe chest oppression, add *Dan Zhong* (CV 17). After 10 treatments, if the result is not satisfactory, alternate the preceding points with *Gong Sun* (Sp 4) and *Nei Guan* (Per 6). This famous combination of eight extraordinary vessel meeting points especially treats repletion pattern CAD when combined with *Dan Zhong* (CV 17). For cold hands or a cold sensation in the cardiac area, add moxibustion on *Xin Shu* (Bl 15), *Ju Que* (CV 14), and *Ge Shu* (Bl 17). If there is profuse phlegm or slimy tongue fur, add *Feng Long* (St 40). For concomitant qi vacuity, add *Zu San Li* (St 36). For concomitant ascendant liver yang hyperactivity with hypertension, add *Tai Chong* (Liv 3) and *Feng Chi* (GB 20).

2. Heart vessel stasis & obstruction pattern

Main symptoms: Piercing pain in the chest and heart which may radiate to the upper back, bilateral rib-side distention and fullness, heart palpitations, shortness of breath, heart vexation, restlessness, dark, purplish lips and facial complexion, a dark, purplish tongue or possible static macules or spots, purple, engorged, tortuous sublingual veins, and a bowstring, choppy, regularly interrupted, or bound pulse

Treatment principles: Move the qi and quicken the blood, transform stasis and free the flow of the network vessels

Rx: *Dan Shen Yin* (Salvia Drink) & *Tao Hong Si Wu Tang* (Persica & Carthamus Four Materials Decoction) with additions and subtractions

Ingredients: Radix Salviae Miltiorrhizae (*Dan Shen*) and Lignum Santali Albi (*Tan Xiang*), 15g each, Semen Pruni Persicae (*Tao Ren*), Flos Carthami Tinctorii (*Hong Hua*), Radix Bupleuri (*Chai Hu*), Radix Ligustici Wallichii (*Chuan Xiong*), Feces Trogopterori Seu Pteromi (*Wu Ling Zhi*), Pollen Typhae (*Pu Huang*), Radix Angelicae Sinensis (*Dang Gui*), Radix Rubrus Paeoniae Lactiflorae (*Chi Shao*), and Radix Albus Paeoniae Lactiflorae (*Bai Shao*), 9g each, and mix-fried Radix Glycyrrhizae (*Gan Cao*) and Ramulus Cinnamomi Cassiae (*Gui Zhi*), 4.5g each

Analysis of formula: *Dan Shen, Tao Ren, Hong Hua, Chuan Xiong, Wu Ling Zhi, Pu Huang, Dang Gui,* and *Chi Shao* all quicken the blood, transform stasis, and free the flow of the network vessels. In addition, *Wu Ling Zhi* and *Pu Huang* strongly stop heart pain and also prevent bleeding due to blood stasis, especially when combined with *Dan Shen.* Also, *Dan Shen, Pu Huang, Dang Gui,* and *Gan Cao* treat hyperlipoproteinemia, a main cause of CAD. *Chuan Xiong* and *Chai Hu* move the qi to quicken the blood. *Tan Xiang* also moves the qi and stops pain, especially chest pain. *Dang Gui* and *Bai Shao* nourish the blood to prevent further blood stasis. *Gui Zhi* warms and frees the flow of the blood vessels and invigorates heart yang to improve blood circulation. *Gan Cao* harmonizes the other medicinals in the formula and also supplements the heart qi to quicken the blood.

Additions & subtractions: If qi stagnation is more pronounced, add 12 grams of Fructus Meliae Toosendan (*Chuan Lian Zi*) and nine grams of Rhizoma Cyperi Rotundi (*Xiang Fu*). If blood stasis is even more severe, add nine grams each of Resina Olibani (*Ru Xiang*) and Resina Myrrhae (*Mo Yao*). If there is concomitant qi vacuity, add 15 grams of Radix Astragali Membranacei (*Huang Qi*) and nine grams of Radix Codonopsitis Pilosulae (*Dang Shen*). If there is blood vacuity, add 12 grams of cooked Radix Rehmanniae (*Shu Di*). If there is impaired memory and insomnia due to blood vacuity, add 20 grams of Caulis Polygoni Multiflori (*Ye Jiao Teng*) and 12 grams of Semen Biotae Orientalis (*Bai Zi Ren*). For severe chest oppression, add nine grams of Radix Platycodi Grandiflori (*Jie Geng*) and Fructus Citri Aurantii (*Zhi Ke*). If there is the risk of cardiac infarct, add nine grams of Bulbus Allii (*Xie Bai*) and three grams of Sanguis Draconis (*Xue Jie*) and Radix Pseudoginseng (*San Qi*), powdered and taken with the strained decoction.

Acupuncture & moxibustion: *Dan Zhong* (CV 17), *Ge Shu* (Bl 17), *Nei Guan* (Per 6), *Xi Men* (Per 4)

Analysis of formula: *Dan Zhong* is the meeting point of the qi, and *Ge Shu* is the meeting point of the blood. Together, they move the gathering or chest qi and quicken the heart blood, transform stasis and free the flow of the network vessels. *Nei Guan* is the network point of the pericardium. It frees the flow of the network vessels of the heart and regulates cardiac rhythm, reinforces the left ventricle of the heart and treats the CAD. *Xi Men* is the cleft point of the pericardium. The cleft point of yin channels are well-known for treating pain and acute diseases and for stopping bleeding. *Xi Men* treats heart pain and prevents infarct of the heart. All these points should be needled with draining method.

Additions & subtractions: If there are cold hands or a cold sensation in the cardiac area, add moxibustion on *Dan Zhong* and *Ge Shu.* If there is concomitant qi vacuity, add *Zu San Li* (St 36). If there is concomitant ascendant liver yang hyperactivity with hypertension, add *Tai Chong* (Liv 3) and *Feng Chi* (GB 20). If qi stagnation is more pronounced, add *He Gu* (LI 4). If blood stasis is even more severe, add *San Yin Jiao* (Sp 6). After 10 treatments, alternate *Nei Guan* and *Xi Men* with *Ling Dao* (Ht 4) and *Jian Shi* (Per 5) and *Dan Zhong* and *Ge Shu* with *Xin Shu* (Bl 15) and *Ju Que* (CV 14). If there is impaired memory and insomnia due to blood vacuity, add *Shen Men* (Ht 7). If there is hyperlipoproteinemia, add *Zu San Li* (St 36) or *Feng Long* (St 40).

3. Liver depression counterflow chilling pattern

Main symptoms: Dull heart pain accompanied by chest oppression which comes in waves and is caused or worsened by emotional stress, shortness of breath, emotional tension or depression, restlessness, possible frequent sighing, bilateral rib-side discomfort, cold hands as a reaction to stress, a normal or slightly dark tongue with thin, white fur, and a bowstring pulse

TREATMENT PRINCIPLES: Soothe the liver and rectify the qi, quicken the blood and transform stasis

Rx: *Si Ni San Jia Wei* (Four Counterflows Powder with Added Flavors)

INGREDIENTS: Radix Salviae Miltiorrhizae (*Dan Shen*), 15g, Tuber Curcumae (*Yu Jin*), 12g, Radix Bupleuri (*Chai Hu*), Fructus Immaturus Citri Aurantii (*Zhi Shi*), Radix Albus Paeoniae Lactiflorae (*Bai Shao*), Radix Ligustici Wallichii (*Chuan Xiong*), Rhizoma Cyperi Rotundi (*Xiang Fu*), 9g each, Radix Glycyrrhizae (*Gan Cao*), 4.5g, and Lignum Dalbergiae Odoriferae (*Jiang Xiang*), 1-2g (powdered and swallowed with the decocted liquid)

ANALYSIS OF FORMULA: *Chai Hu, Yu Jin, Zhi Shi,* and *Xiang Fu* soothe the liver and rectify the qi. *Bai Shao* nourishes the blood and emolliates the liver. *Dan Shen, Chuan Xiong,* and *Jiang Xiang* quicken the blood and transform stasis. In addition, *Dan Shen* and *Jiang Xiang* are a well-known empirical combination for treating CAD, while *Yu Jin, Gan Cao,* and *Dan Shen* treat hyperlipoproteinemia.

ADDITIONS & SUBTRACTIONS: If there is severe chest pain, add *Jing Ling Zi San* (Fructus Meliae Toosendan Powder): Rhizoma Corydalis Yanhusuo (*Yan Hu Suo*), 15g, and Fructus Meliae Toosendan (*Chuan Lian Zi*), 9g. If there is insomnia, add 15 grams each of Caulis Polygoni Multiflori (*Ye Jiao Teng*) and Semen Zizyphi Spinosae (*Suan Zao Ren*). If there is vomiting, add nine grams of Rhizoma Pinelliae Ternatae (*Ban Xia*) and six grams of uncooked Rhizoma Zingiberis (*Sheng Jiang*). For reduced food intake, add nine grams each of the three immortals, *i.e.,* Fructus Crataegi (*Shan Zha*), Massa Medica Fermentata (*Shen Qu*), and Fructus Germinatus Hordei Vulgaris (*Mai Ya*). For spleen qi vacuity, add nine grams each of Radix Codonopsitis Pilosulae (*Dang Shen*), Rhizoma Atractylodis Macrocephalae (*Bai Zhu*), and Sclerotium Poriae Cocos (*Fu Ling*). For liver depression transforming into heat, add nine grams each of Cortex Radicis Moutan (*Dan Pi*) and Fructus Gardeniae Jasminoidis (*Zhi Zi*). For blood vacuity, add nine grams of Radix Angelicae Sinensis (*Dang Gui*). For yang vacuity, add nine grams of Ramulus Cinnamomi Cassiae (*Gui Zhi*) and three grams of Herba Asari Cum Radice (*Xi Xin*).

ACUPUNCTURE & MOXIBUSTION: *Nei Guan* (Per 6), *Ju Que* (CV 14), *Ge Shu* (Bl 17), *Tai Chong* (Liv 3)

ANALYSIS OF FORMULA: *Tai Chong* and *Nei Guan* soothe the liver and rectify the qi. *Nei Guan* also frees the flow of the network vessels of the heart and treats CAD. *Ge Shu* is the meeting point of the blood. It is an important point for regulating the blood, it also regulates the qi of the chest, rib-side, and diaphragm areas. Further, combined with *Ju Que,* the alarm point of the heart, it quickens the blood and transforms stasis. All these points should be needled with even supplementing-even draining method.

ADDITIONS & SUBTRACTIONS: If there is persistent dull pain in the chest, add *Dan Zhong* (CV 17). For insomnia, add *Shen Men* (Ht 7). For occasional piercing chest pain, add *Ling Dao* (Ht 4) or *Qu Ze* (Per 3). If there is severe emotional tension or depression, add *Gan Shu* (Bl 18) and *Hun Men* (Bl 47). If there is concomitant qi vacuity, add *Zu San Li* (St 36). If there is concomitant ascendant liver yang hyperactivity with hypertension, add *Xuan Zhong* (GB 39) and *Feng Chi* (GB 20). If there is blood vacuity, add *Gan Shu* (Bl 18) and *Shen Men* (Ht 7). If liver depression transforming into heat, add *Xuan Zhong* (GB 39) and replace *Tai Chong* with *Xing Jian* (Liv 2).

4. PHLEGM TURBIDITY INTERNALLY OBSTRUCTING PATTERN

MAIN SYMPTOMS: Chest oppression or chest pain, a fat body, bodily heaviness, lack of strength, extremely profuse phlegm, a tendency to hypersomnia or somnolence, heavy-headedness, possible dizziness, heart palpitations, possible nausea and reduced food intake, a sticky, slimy feeling within the mouth, thick, slimy or filthy, turbid tongue fur, and a slippery, bowstring pulse

TREATMENT PRINCIPLES: Use fragrant, aromatic medicinals to transform turbidity, disinhibit phlegm, and dispel stasis

Rx: *Wen Dan Tang Jia Wei* (Warm the Gallbladder Decoction with Added Flavors)

INGREDIENTS: Fructus Trichosanthis Kirlowii (*Quan Gua Lou*), 21g, Radix Salviae Miltiorrhizae (*Dan Shen*), 15g, and Tuber Curcumae (*Yu Jin*), 12g, Rhizoma Pinelliae Ternatae (*Ban Xia*), Pericarpium Citri Reticulatae (*Chen Pi*), Sclerotium Poriae Cocos (*Fu Ling*), Caulis Bambusae In Taeniis (*Zhu Ru*), Fructus Citri Aurantii (*Zhi Ke*), and Fructus Cardamomi (*Bai Dou Kou*), 9g each

ANALYSIS OF FORMULA: *Ban Xia, Chen Pi,* and *Fu Ling,* the three main ingredients of *Er Chen Tang* (Two Aged [Ingredients] Decoction), with *Zhu Ru* dry dampness and transform phlegm, while *Quan Gua Lou* dispels phlegm accumulation in the chest. In addition, *Quan Gua Lou* is a main medicinal for treating chest impediment due to phlegm. Combined with *Zhi Ke* which moves the qi, it loosens the chest. *Bai Dou Kou* aromatically dries dampness and transforms turbidity. *Yu Jin, Chen Pi,* and *Zhi Ke* move the qi to dispel phlegm according to the saying, "To treat phlegm, first move the qi." *Dan Shen* quickens the blood and transforms stasis due to phlegm obstruction in the chest. Although none of these medicinals is a penetrating, aromatic orifice-opener, all are acrid, windy, moving, and scattering ingredients.

ADDITIONS & SUBTRACTIONS: If there is a bitter taste in the mouth, thirst, yellow tongue fur, and a red facial complexion due to phlegm heat, add six grams each of Rhizoma Coptidis Chinensis (*Huang Lian*), bile-processed Rhizoma Arisaematis (*Dan Nan Xing*) and Concretio Silicea Bambusae (*Tian Zhu Huang*). If there is aversion to cold, cold limbs, and clear phlegm, subtract *Zhu Ru* and add six grams of dry Rhizoma Zingiberis (*Gan Jiang*), nine grams of Bulbus Allii (*Xie Bai*), and three grams of Herba Asari Cum Radice (*Xi Xin*). If there is piercing pain in the chest, add nine grams of Radix Ligustici Wallichii (*Chuan Xiong*) and three grams each of Radix Pseudoginseng (*San Qi*) and Lignum Dalbergiae Odoriferae (*Jiang Xiang*), powdered and taken with the strained decoction. If there is constipation, add six grams of Radix Et Rhizoma Rhei (*Da Huang*). If there is diarrhea, poor appetite, and fatigue, add nine grams of Rhizoma Atractylodis Macrocephalae (*Bai Zhu*) and Radix Codonopsitis Pilosulae (*Dang Shen*) and 15 grams of Radix Astragali Membranacei (*Huang Qi*).

ACUPUNCTURE & MOXIBUSTION: *Nei Guan* (Per 6), *Dan Zhong* (CV 17), *Zu San Li* (St 36), *Feng Long* (St 40)

ANALYSIS OF FORMULA: Draining *Feng Long* transforms phlegm, while supplementing *Zu San Li* fortifies the spleen to prevent further phlegm engenderment. *Dan Zhong,* the meeting point of the qi, moves the gathering or chest qi, loosens the chest, and dispels phlegm accumulated in the chest. *Nei Guan* moves the qi and quickens the blood, transforms stasis and frees the flow of the network vessels of the heart. These two last points should be needled with even supplementing-even draining method.

ADDITIONS & SUBTRACTIONS: For piercing pain in the chest, add *Ling Dao* (Ht 4) or *Qu Ze* (Per 3). For phlegm heat, add *Nei Ting* (St 44) and *He Gu* (LI 4). For cold phlegm, add moxibustion on *Dan Zhong* and *Zu San Li.* For spleen qi vacuity, add *Tai Bai* (Sp 3). For severe bodily heaviness, add *Yin Ling Quan* (Sp 9). For heart palpitations, add *Shen Men* (Ht 7).

5. QI & YIN DUAL VACUITY PATTERN

MAIN SYMPTOMS: Insidious heart pain, generalized fatigue, lack of strength, shortness of breath, heart palpitations, chest oppression, spontaneous perspiration, a dry mouth with scanty fluids, dizziness, insomnia, a dry throat, a red tongue with scanty or no fur, and a fine, rapid or bound, regularly interrupted pulse depending on whether yin vacuity with vacuity heat or qi vacuity predominate

TREATMENT PRINCIPLES: Boost the qi and nourish yin assisted by quickening the blood

RX: *Sheng Mai San Jia Jian* (Engender the Pulse Powder with Additions & Subtractions)

INGREDIENTS: Semen Cassiae Torae (*Jue Ming Zi*) and Concha Margaritiferae (*Zhen Zhu Mu*), 30g each, Radix Pseudostellariae (*Tai Zi Shen*), Radix Astragali Membranacei (*Huang Qi*), and Radix Salviae Miltiorrhizae (*Dan Shen*), 15g each, Radix Puerariae (*Ge Gen*), Fructus Crataegi (*Shan Zha*), Radix Rubrus Paeoniae Lactiflorae (*Chi Shao*), and Tuber Ophiopogonis Japonici (*Mai Dong*), 9g each, Fructus Schizandrae Chinensis (*Wu Wei Zi*), 6g, and Rhizoma Gastrodiae Elatae (*Tian Ma*), 4.5g

ANALYSIS OF FORMULA: *Tai Zi Shen, Huang Qi,* and *Dang Shen* boost the qi. Also, *Tai Zi Shen* engenders fluids and nourishes yin, while *Dang Shen* and *Huang Qi* are well-known to regulate the blood pressure. *Ge Gen* and *Shan Zha* treat hyperlipoproteinemia and hypertension, two important causes of CAD. In addition, *Ge Gen* engenders fluids and *Shan Zha* disperses food and helps the transforming function of the spleen. *Mai Men Dong* and *Wu Wei Zi* engender fluids and nourish yin. With *Dang Shen,* they compose *Sheng Mai San* (Engender the Pulse Powder), a very effective formula for treating CAD due to qi and yin vacuity. *Jue Ming Zi, Zhen Zhu Mu,* and *Tian Ma* subdue ascendant yang due to yin vacuity. Also, *Jue Ming Zi* and *Tian Ma* treat hyperlipoproteinemia and hypertension. *Chi Shao,* with the help of *Shan Zha,* quickens the blood and transforms stasis due to qi vacuity.

ADDITIONS & SUBTRACTIONS: If there is ascendant liver yang hyperactivity with marked dizziness, add nine grams each of Fructus Lycii Chinensis (*Gou Qi Zi*) and Flos Chrysanthemi Morifolii (*Ju Hua*). If heart palpitations and insomnia are marked, add 30 grams of Caulis Polygoni Multiflori (*Ye Jiao Teng*) and 12 grams of Semen Zizyphi Spinosae (*Suan Zao Ren*). If there is severe dry mouth and throat with thirst, add 15 grams of Radix Glehniae Littoralis (*Sha Shen*) and 12 grams of Rhizoma Polygonati Odorati (*Yu Zhu*). If there is severe pain and chest oppression, add 15 grams of Radix Salviae Miltiorrhizae (*Dan Shen*) and three grams of Radix Pseudoginseng (*San Qi*), powdered and taken with the strained decoction.

If there is dual qi and blood vacuity of the heart with the same symptoms as above but without vacuity heat and dryness and with a pale facial complexion, white nails, lips and tongue, etc., replace *Sheng Mai San Jia Jian* with *Bu Xin Dan Jia Jian* (Supplement the Heart Elixir with Additions & Subtractions): Radix Albus Paeoniae Lactiflorae (*Bai Shao*), 20g, Radix Salviae Miltiorrhizae (*Dan Shen*), Radix Astragali Membranacei (*Huang Qi*), Sclerotium Poriae Cocos (*Fu Ling*), and Pericarpium Trichosanthis Kirlowii (*Gua Lou Pi*), 15g each, Radix Pseustellariae Heterophyllae (*Tai Zi Shen*), Pericarpium Citri Reticulatae (*Chen Pi*), Semen Zizyphi Spinosae (*Suan Zao Ren*), Radix Angelicae Sinensis (*Dang Gui*), Radix Polygalae Tenuifoliae (*Yuan Zhi*), Rhizoma Atractylodis Macrocephalae (*Bai Zhu*), and Fructus Citri

Aurantii (*Zhi Ke*), 9g each, and mix-fried Radix Glycyrrhizae (*Gan Cao*), 8g.

If there is heart yin and blood vacuity without qi vacuity, replace *Sheng Mai San Jia Jian* with *Tian Wang Bu Xin Dan Jia Jian* (Heavenly Emperor Supplement the Heart Elixir with Additions & Subtractions): uncooked Radix Rehmanniae (*Sheng Di*), 30g, Radix Salviae Miltiorrhizae (*Dan Shen*), 15g, Radix Scrophulariae Ningpoensis (*Xuan Shen*), Radix Angelicae Sinensis (*Dang Gui*), Tuber Ophiopogonis Japonici (*Mai Men Dong*), and Sclerotium Pararadicis Poriae Cocos (*Fu Shen*), 12g each, Semen Biotae Orientalis (*Bai Zi Ren*), Semen Zizyphi Spinosae (*Suan Zao Ren*), and Fructus Schisandrae Chinensis (*Wu Wei Zi*), 9g each, and Radix Pseustellariae Heterophyllae (*Tai Zi Shen*) and mix-fried Radix Glycyrrhizae (*Gan Cao*), 6g each, and Radix Polygalae Tenuifoliae (*Yuan Zhi*), 3g.

For liver-kidney yin vacuity with blood stasis and chest oppression, insomnia, and chest pain at night, replace *Sheng Mai San Jia Jian* with *Yang Yin Tong Bi Tang Jia Jian* (Nourish Yin & Free the Flow of Impediment Decoction with Additions & Subtractions): cooked Radix Rehmanniae (*Shu Di*), uncooked Radix Rehmanniae (*Sheng Di*), and Pericarpium Trichosanthis Kirlowii (*Gua Lou Pi*), 18g each, Tuber Ophiopogonis Japonici (*Mai Men Dong*), Fructus Schisandrae Chinensis (*Wu Wei Zi*), Fructus Ligustri Lucidi (*Nu Zhen Zi*), and Radix Codonopsitis Pilosulae (*Dang Shen*), 12g each, Semen Pruni Persicae (*Tao Ren*) and Rhizoma Corydalis Yanhusuo (*Yan Hu Suo*), 9g each, and Flos Carthami Tinctorii (*Hong Hua*), 6g. If there is arrhythmia and heart palpitations, add 9 grams of Gelatinum Corii Asini (*E Jiao*) and 20 grams of mix-fried Radix Glycyrrhizae (*Gan Cao*).

NOTE: If there is essential hypertension or the blood pressure rises after administration of this formula, the dosage of *Gan Cao* should be lowered to nine grams or less. The active substance in *Gan Cao* which tends to increase the blood pressure is mainly in the outer bark or skin of the root. Processing *Gan Cao* with honey seems to attenuate this side effect. *Gan Cao* is a key medicinal for treating arrhythmia, but the practitioner should take care in its use when there is simultaneous hypertension.

ACUPUNCTURE & MOXIBUSTION: *Xin Shu* (Bl 15), *Shen Men* (Ht 7), *Fu Liu* (Ki 7), *Zu San Li* (St 36), *Nei Guan* (Per 6)

ANALYSIS OF FORMULA: *Xin Shu* is the back transport point of the heart and *Shen Men* is the source point of the heart channel. Therefore, both points have a pronounced action on the heart. When supplemented together, they boost the qi and nourish the yin of the heart. Supplementing *Fu Liu* is added to more strongly engender fluids and nourish yin. Likewise, supplementing *Zu San Li* is added to more strongly boost the qi. Draining *Nei Guan* frees the flow of the network vessels of the heart and transforms stasis. This is because vacuity of the heart always leads to blood stasis.

ADDITIONS & SUBTRACTIONS: If there are night sweats, add *Yin Xi* (Ht 6). If there is severe chest oppression, add *Dan Zhong* (CV 17). If there are cold hands or a cold sensation in the cardiac area, add moxibustion on *Xin Shu*. For piercing pain in the chest, add *Ling Dao* (Ht 4) or *Qu Ze* (Per 3). If spleen qi vacuity is marked, add *Tai Bai* (Sp 3). If there is concomitant ascendant liver yang hyperactivity with hypertension, add *Xuan Zhong* (GB 39) and *Tai Chong* (Liv 3). If there is liver blood or yin vacuity, add *Gan Shu* (Bl 18).

6. YIN & YANG DUAL VACUITY PATTERN

MAIN SYMPTOMS: Heart palpitations and fearful throbbing, heart pain, shortness of breath, lassitude of the spirit, chest oppression which is worse at night and may awake the patient, a white facial complexion with malar flushing, fear of cold, exacerbation of heart pain when exposed to chill, lack of warmth in the four limbs alternating with vexatious heat in the five centers, dizziness and vertigo, low back and knee soreness and limpness, nocturnal polyuria, a pale tongue with a red or dark, purplish tip, and a deep, fine or bound, regularly interrupted.

NOTE: This pattern frequently complicates qi and yin vacuity, in which case there is a yin and yang vacuity. Here it is presented as a discreet pattern.

TREATMENT PRINCIPLES: Warm yang and nourish yin, supplement the kidneys and quicken the blood

RX: *Shen Qi Wan Jia Wei* (Kidney Qi Pills) & *Si Wu Tang* (Four Materials Decoction) with additions and subtractions

INGREDIENTS: Radix Rubrus Paeoniae Lactiflorae (*Chi Shao*) and uncooked Radix Rehmanniae (*Sheng Di*), 15g each, Fructus Corni Officinalis (*Yu Rou*), Radix Dioscoreae Oppositae (*Shan Yao*), Sclerotium Poriae Cocos (*Fu Ling*), Rhizoma Alismatis (*Ze Xie*), Cortex Radicis Moutan (*Dan Pi*), Radix Ligustici Wallichii (*Chuan Xiong*), and Radix Angelicae Sinensis (*Dang Gui*), 9g each, Radix Lateralis Praeparatus Aconiti Carmichaeli (*Fu Zi*), 6g, and Ramulus Cinnamomi Cassiae (*Gui Zhi*), 4.5g

ANALYSIS OF FORMULA: *Sheng Di, Shan Zhu Yu, Shan Yao, Fu Ling, Ze Xie*, and *Dan Pi* are the six ingredients of *Liu Wei Di Huang Wan* (Six Flavors Rehmannia Pills). This is a basic formula for enriching the true yin. By adding *Fu Zi* and *Gui Zhi*, both of which warm yang, this formula becomes *Shen Qi Wan* (Kidney Qi Pills) which supplements both kidney yin and yang. *Chi Shao, Chuan Xiong, Dang Gui*, and *Dan Pi* quicken the blood and transform stasis due to yin and yang vacuity. In addition, *Sheng Di* and *Dang Gui* nourish the blood, while *Shan Yao* and *Fu Ling* boost the qi. Further, *Dang Gui* and *Ze Xie* treat hyperlipoproteinemia, and *Dan Pi* and *Ze Xie* treat hypertension.

ADDITIONS & SUBTRACTIONS: If there is arrhythmia and heart palpitations, replace the preceding formula with *Zhi Gan Cao Tang Jia Jian* (Mix-fried Licorice Decoction with Additions & Subtractions): mix-fried Radix Glycyrrhizae (*Gan Cao*), Radix Codonopsitis Pilosulae (*Dang Shen*), uncooked Radix Rehmanniae (*Sheng Di*), and Radix Salviae Miltiorrhizae (*Dan Shen*), 15g each, Ramulus Cinnamomi Cassiae (*Gui Zhi*), Tuber Ophiopogonis Japonici (*Mai Men Dong*), Radix Angelicae Sinensis (*Dang Gui*), and Bulbus Allii (*Xie Bai*), 9g each, and Gelatinum Corii Asini (*E Jiao*) and Radix Lateralis Praeparatus Aconiti Carmichaeli (*Fu Zi*), 5g each. For predominant liver-kidney yin vacuity, subtract *Fu Zi* and add 12 grams of Radix Polygoni Multiflori (*He Shou Wu*) and Radix Salviae Miltiorrhizae (*Dan Shen*). If there is concomitant essential hypertension due to ascendant liver yang hyperactivity, add 15 grams each of Ramulus Uncariae Cum Uncis (*Gou Teng*) and Semen Cassiae Torae (*Jue Ming Zi*). For severe yang vacuity, add nine grams each of Bulbus Allii (*Xie Bai*) and Herba Epimedii (*Yin Yang Huo*) and three grams of Herba Asari Cum Radice (*Xi Xin*). If there is pirecing pain of the heart, add 12 grams each of Radix Salviae Miltiorrhizae (*Dan Shen*), Feces Trogopterori Seu Pteromi (*Wu Ling Zhi*), and Pollen Typhae (*Pu Huang*). For concomitant qi vacuity, add 15 grams of Radix Astragali Membranacei (*Huang Qi*) and six grams of Radix Panacis Ginseng (*Ren Shen*).

ACUPUNCTURE & MOXIBUSTION: Same as pattern #5 above with the addition of *Guan Yuan* (CV 4) and moxibustion on *Zu San Li* and *Xin Shu*

ANALYSIS OF FORMULA: *Guan Yuan* warms and supplements both heart and kidney yang.

ADDITIONS & SUBTRACTIONS: Please see pattern #5 above.

7. YANG VACUITY ON THE VERGE OF DESERTION PATTERN

MAIN SYMPTOMS: Heart pain, shortness of breath, great perspiration dribbling and dripping, reversal chilling of the four limbs, bluish purple nails, a somber white facial complexion, a dark tongue with white fur, and a deep, fine pulse on the verge of expiry

TREATMENT PRINCIPLES: Return yang and secure desertion, quicken the blood and stem counterflow

RX: *Shen Fu Long Mu Tang Jia Wei* (Ginseng, Aconite, Dragon Bone & Oyster Shell Decoction with Added Flavors)

INGREDIENTS: Os Draconis (*Long Gu*) and Concha Ostreae (*Mu Li*), 30g each, Radix Panacis Ginseng (*Ren Shen*), Radix Lateralis Praeparatus Aconiti Carmichaeli (*Fu Zi*), Radix Albus Paeoniae Lactiflorae (*Bai Shao*), Radix Ligustici Wallichii (*Chuan Xiong*), Flos Carthami Tinctorii (*Hong Hua*), Radix Rubrus Paeoniae Lactiflorae (*Chi Shao*), and Semen Pruni Persicae (*Tao Ren*), 9g each, and mix-fried Radix Glycyrrhizae (*Gan Cao*) and Ramulus Cinnamomi (*Gui Zhi*), 4.5g each

ANALYSIS OF FORMULA: *Ren Shen* strongly boosts the qi, and *Fu Zi* strongly returns yang. Together, they strongly secure desertion. *Bai Shao* secures yin and stops sweating. *Gui Zhi* helps warm and supplement heart and kidney yang. *Long Gu* and *Mu Li* astringe, secure, and stop sweating, thus helping *Ren Shen* and *Fu Zi* to secure desertion. *Chuan Xiong*, *Hong Hua*, *Tao Ren*, and *Chi Shao* quicken the blood, transform stasis, and stop pain. *Gan Cao* boosts the qi and harmonizes the other medicinals in this formula.

ADDITIONS & SUBTRACTIONS: For a mild case of yang desertion or for heart yang vacuity, use *Qi Fu Tang* (Astragalus & Aconite Decoction) plus *Sheng Mai San* (Engender the Pulse Powder) with additions and subtractions: Radix Astragali Membranacei (*Huang Qi*), 25g, Tuber Ophiopogonis Japonici (*Mai Men Dong*), Fructus Schisandrae Chinensis (*Wu Wei Zi*), Radix Salviae Miltiorrhizae (*Dan Shen*), and Ramulus Cinnamomi Cassiae (*Gui Zhi*), 12g each, Radix Panacis Ginseng (*Ren Shen*), Radix Lateralis Praeparatus Aconiti Carmichaeli (*Fu Zi*), and mix-fried Radix Glycyrrhizae (*Gan Cao*), 5g each, and Herba Asari Cum Radice (*Xi Xin*), 3g.

ACUPUNCTURE & MOXIBUSTION: *Nei Guan* (Per 6), *Xin Shu* (Bl 15), *Guan Yuan* (CV 4), *Qi Hai* (CV 6)

ANALYSIS OF FORMULA: Moxaing *Guan Yuan* and *Qi Hai* returns yang, secures desertion, and stems counterflow. Supplementing *Xin Shu* with moxibustion warms and supplements heart yang. Draining *Nei Guan* quickens the blood, transforms stasis, and frees the flow of the network vessels of the heart.

ADDITIONS & SUBTRACTIONS: Please see the preceding patterns.

8. YANG VACUITY, WATER FLOODING PATTERN

MAIN SYMPTOMS: Heart palpitation, panting, chest oppression, inability to lie down comfortably, aversion to cold, cold limbs, possible cold sweats, low back soreness, scanty urination, a pale, lusterless or bluish purple facial complexion, possible generalized edema or edema in the lower limbs or thoracic region, possible abdominal inflation, reduced food intake, abdominal distention, nausea, a pale tongue with teeth-marks on its edges and white fur, and a deep, thin, bound or regularly interrupted pulse

NOTE: This pattern is a combination of heart and kidney yang vacuity resulting in the non-transportation and transformation of water fluids and thus the accumulation of water rheum in the chest which then further obstructs chest yang.

TREATMENT PRINCIPLES: Warm yang and disinhibit water

RX: *Zhen Wu Tang Jia Jian* (True Warrior Decoction with Additions & Subtractions)

INGREDIENTS: Semen Plantaginis (*Che Qian Zi*), Herba Lycopi Lucidi (*Ze Lan*), and Herba Leonuri Heterophylli (*Yi Mu Cao*), 30g each, Sclerotium Poriae Cocos (*Fu Ling*), 20g, Rhizoma Alismatis (*Ze Xie*), 15g, Radix Lateralis Praeparatus Aconiti Carmichaeli (*Fu Zi*), 9-15g, Rhizoma Atractylodis Macrocephalae (*Bai Zhu*), 9g, dry Rhizoma Zingiberis (*Gan Jiang*), Radix Albus Paeoniae Lactiflorae (*Bai Shao*), and Radix Glycyrrhizae (*Gan Cao*), 5g each, and Cortex Cinnamomi Cassiae (*Rou Gui*), 3g

ANALYSIS OF FORMULA: Vacuity cold is the cause of water rheum accumulation in this case. Therefore, one should warm and supplement yang and scatter cold with the three most powerful Chinese medicinals for those purposes: *Fu Zi, Gan Jiang,* and *Rou Gui. Fu Zi,* due to its travelling nature, goes to all 12 channels and drains cold everywhere in the body. *Gan Jiang* warms the center and transforms water rheum, especially if its origin is in the upper and middle burners, while *Rou Gui* helps promote the transformation of water rheum especially if its origin is in the middle and lower burners. *Fu Ling, Ze Xie,* and *Bai Zhu* seep and transform water rheum. These three medicinals are helped by *Che Qian Zi, Ze Lan,* and *Yi Mu Cao* by disinhibiting water. In addition, *Ze Lan* and *Yi Mu Cao* quicken the blood and transform stasis due to water rheum obstructing the chest.

ADDITIONS & SUBTRACTIONS: If there is marked qi vacuity, add 15 grams of Radix Astragali Membranacei (*Huang Qi*) and 12 grams of Radix Codonopsitis Pilosulae (*Dang Shen*). If there is concomitant blood vacuity, add nine grams each of Radix Angelicae Sinensis (*Dang Gui*) and cooked Radix Rehmanniae (*Shu Di*). If there is marked blood stasis, add 12 grams of Radix Salviae Miltiorrhizae (*Dan Shen*), nine grams of Flos Carthami Tinctorii (*Hong Hua*), and three grams of Radix Pseudoginseng (*San Qi*), powdered and taken with the strained decoction. For panting due to kidney failing to absorb the qi, add three grams of Gecko (*Ge Jie*), powdered and taken with the strained decoction, 12 grams of Fructus Psoraleae Corylifoliae (*Bu Gu Zhi*), and nine grams of Semen Juglandis Regiae (*Hu Tao Ren*). For scanty urination, add 12 grams of uncooked Cortex Rhizomatis Zingiberis (*Sheng Jiang Pi*) and 15 grams of Pericarpium Benincasae Hispidae (*Dong Gua Pi*). If there is incessant sweating, add nine grams of Fructus Corni Officinalis (*Shan Zhu Yu*), 20 grams of uncooked Concha Ostreae (*Mu Li*), and 15 grams of Semen Levis Tritici Aestivi (*Fu Xiao Mai*).

If there are water evils damaging the upper burner with panting, cough, dyspnea which prevents lying down, profuse, thin, white, foamy phlegm, heart palpitations, fearful throbbing, rapid breathing, restlessness, sweating, aversion to cold, dark purple lips and tongue with glossy tongue fur, and a rapid, racing pulse, replace *Zhen Wu Tang Jia Jian* with *Ting Li Da Zao Xie Fei Tang* (Lipidium & Red Dates Drain the Lungs Decoction) plus *Wu Ling San* (Five [Ingredients] Poria Powder) with additions and subtractions: Semen Lepidii Seu Descurainiae (*Ting Li Zi*) and Sclerotium Poriae Cocos (*Fu Ling*), 30g each, Sclerotium Polypori Umbellati (*Zhu Ling*) and Semen Plantaginis (*Che Qian Zi*), 20g each, Rhizoma Alismatis (*Ze Xie*) and Radix Salviae Miltiorrhizae (*Dan Shen*), 15g each, and Ramulus Cinnamomi Cassiae (*Gui Zhi*), Radix Lateralis Praeparatus Aconiti Carmichaeli (*Fu Zi*), and Flos Carthami Tinctorii (*Hong Hua*), and Radix Cyathulae (*Chuan Niu Xi*), 9g each. If there are no cold symptoms, subtract *Fu Zi.* If there is concomitant yang qi vacuity desertion, add 15 grams of Radix Panacis Ginseng (*Ren Shen*) and nine grams of dry Rhizoma Zingiberis (*Gan Jiang*). If there is phlegm heat, subtract *Fu Zi* and add nine grams of Radix Scutellariae Baicalensis (*Huang Qin*), 15 grams of Herba Houttuyniae Cordatae Cum Radice (*Yu Xing Cao*), and 12 grams of Pericarpium Trichosanthis Kirlowii (*Gua Lou Pi*). For marked blood stasis, add 12 grams of Radix Salviae Miltiorrhizae (*Dan Shen*) and three grams of Radix Pseudoginseng (*San Qi*), powdered and taken with the strained decoction.

ACUPUNCTURE & MOXIBUSTION: *Xin Shu* (Bl 15), *Ju Que* (CV 14), *Nei Guan* (Per 6), *Feng Long* (St 40), *Yin Ling Quan* (Sp 9), *Ming Men* (GV 4)

ANALYSIS OF FORMULA: *Xin Shu* is the back transport point of the heart, while *Ju Que* is the front alarm point of the heart. Supplementing these points plus moxibustion scatters cold and dispels phlegm, warms and supplements heart yang. *Nei Guan* is the network point on the pericardium channel. Draining it frees the network vessels of the heart and frees the flow of the chest qi, dispels phlegm and regulates cardiac rhythm, reinforces the left ventricle of the heart and treats CAD. Draining *Feng Long* transforms phlegm, while draining *Yin Ling Quan* disinhibits water. Supplementing *Ming Men* with moxibustion warms and supplements kidney yang to transform water rheum.

ADDITIONS & SUBTRACTIONS: If there is marked qi vacuity, add *Pi Shu* (Bl 20) and *Wei Shu* (Bl 21). If there is concomitant blood vacuity and/or blood stasis, add *San Yin Jiao* (Sp 6) and *Ge Shu* (Bl 17). For panting due to kidney failing to absorb the qi, add *Tai Xi* (Ki 3). For scanty urination, add *Guan Yuan* (CV 4). If there is incessant sweating, add *He Gu* (LI 4) and *Fu Liu* (Ki 7). If there are water evils damaging the upper burner, add *Dan Zhong* (CV 17), *Fei Shu* (Bl 13), and *Tai Yuan* (Lu 9).

9. HEART QI VACUITY PATTERN

MAIN SYMPTOMS: Heart palpitations, dull pain in the chest or an empty sensation in the heart region, easy fright, shortness of breath, fatigue, bodily weakness, worsening of the symptoms after activity, sweating, and a forceless, bound, or regularly interrupted pulse

TREATMENT PRINCIPLES: Boost the qi and settle the heart

Rx: *Yang Xin Tang Jia Jian* (Nourish the Heart Decoction with Additions & Subtractions)

INGREDIENTS: Radix Astragali Membranacei (*Huang Qi*), 15g, Radix Codonopsitis Pilosulae (*Dang Shen*), 12g, mix-fried Radix Glycyrrhizae (*Gan Cao*), Sclerotium Pararadicis Poriae Cocos (*Fu Shen*), Sclerotium Poriae Cocos (*Fu Ling*), Ramulus Cinnamomi Cassiae (*Gui Zhi*), and Fructus Schisandrae Chinensis (*Wu Wei Zi*), 9g each, and Radix Angelicae Sinensis (*Dang Gui*), Radix Ligustici Wallichii (*Chuan Xiong*), Radix Polygalae Tenuifoliae (*Yuan Zhi*), and Semen Zizyphi Spinosae (*Suan Zao Ren*), 5g each

ANALYSIS OF FORMULA: *Huang Qi, Dang Shen,* mix-fried *Gan Cao,* and *Wu Wei Zi* boost the qi of the heart. *Fu Shen, Fu Ling, Suan Zao Ren, Wu Wei Zi,* and *Yuan Zhi* supplement and settle the heart and stop palpitations. *Gui Zhi* warms and frees the flow of the vessels of the heart and prevents heart yang vacuity, while *Chuan Xiong* quickens the blood to prevent blood stasis. Finally, *Dang Gui* and *Suan Zao Ren* supplement and nourish heart blood.

ADDITIONS & SUBTRACTIONS: If there is a marked qi vacuity, add 12 grams of Rhizoma Atractylodis Macrocephalae (*Bai Zhu*) and replace *Dang Shen* with six grams of Radix Panacis Ginseng (*Ren Shen*). If there is blood vacuity, add nine grams of Semen Biotae Orientalis (*Bai Zi Ren*) and 15 grams of Caulis Milletiae Seu Spatholobi (*Ji Xue Teng*). If sweating is severe, add 18 grams of Semen Levis Tritici Aestivi (*Fu Xiao Mai*) and 15 grams each of uncooked Os Draconis (*Long Gu*) and uncooked Concha Ostreae (*Mu Li*). If there are abdominal distention and reduced food intake, add nine grams of Pericarpium Citri Reticulatae (*Chen Pi*) and six grams of Fructus Amomi (*Sha Ren*). For heart yang vacuity with aversion to cold, cold hands, more severe heart pain especially worsened with cold, and cold sweats, add nine grams of Radix Lateralis Praeparatus Aconiti Carmichaeli (*Fu Zi*) and 15 grams of Bulbus Allii (*Xie Bai*).

ACUPUNCTURE & MOXIBUSTION: *Xin Shu* (Bl 15), *Shen Men* (Ht 7), *Qi Hai* (CV 6), *Nei Guan* (Per 6)

ANALYSIS OF FORMULA: Supplementing *Xin Shu* and *Shen Men* with moxibustion supplements the heart qi. Supplementing *Qi Hai* with moxibustion strongly supplements the original or source qi. Draining *Nei Guan* frees the flow of the network vessels of the heart and quickens the blood to prevent blood stasis due to qi vacuity.

ADDITIONS & SUBTRACTIONS: If there is marked qi vacuity, add *Pi Shu* (Bl 20) and *Wei Shu* (Bl 21). If there is blood vacuity, add *Ge Shu* (Bl 17) and *Gan Shu* (Bl 18). If sweating is severe, add *He Gu* (LI 4) and *Fu Liu* (Ki 7). If there is abdominal distention and reduced food intake, add *Gong Sun* (Sp 4) and *Zhong Wan* (CV 12). For heart yang vacuity with aversion to cold, cold hands, more severe heart pain especially worsened with cold, and cold sweats, also moxa *Dan Zhong* (CV 17), *Guan Yuan* (CV 4), and *Zu San Li* (St 36) (heavy moxibustion).

10. HEART YIN VACUITY PATTERN

MAIN SYMPTOMS: Heart palpitations which are worse at night, fearful throbbing, heart and chest pain with sometimes a burning hot sensation, restlessness, insomnia, night sweats, heat in the heart of the palms of the hands and soles of the feet, a dry mouth, dizziness, a red tongue with scanty fur, and a thin or thin and rapid pulse

NOTE: This pattern is sometimes accompanied by easy anger, severe restlessness, a red facial complexion, aversion to heat, possible soreness of low back and weakness of lower limbs due to yin vacuity with yang hyperactivity. This is a very common condition in Western patients with CAD.

TREATMENT PRINCIPLES: Supplement and enrich heart yin

RX: *Tian Wang Bu Xin Dan Jia Jian* (Heavenly Emperor Supplement the Heart Elixir with Additions & Subtractions)

INGREDIENTS: Radix Salviae Miltiorrhizae (*Dan Shen*) and Radix Scrophulariae Ningpoensis (*Xuan Shen*), 20g each, Tuber Asparagi Cochinensis (*Tian Men Dong*), Sclerotium Poriae Cocos (*Fu Ling*), and Tuber Ophiopogonis Japonici (*Mai Men Dong*), 15g each, Radix Polygalae Tenuifoliae (*Yuan Zhi*), Radix Panacis Ginseng (*Ren Shen*), Radix Angelicae Sinensis (*Dang Gui*), Semen Zizyphi Spinosae (*Suan Zao Ren*), and Semen Biotae Orientalis (*Bai Zi Ren*), 12g each, and Fructus Schisandrae Chinensis (*Wu Wei Zi*), 9g

ANALYSIS OF FORMULA: *Mai Men Dong, Tian Men Dong,*

and *Wu Wei Zi* supplement the heart and enrich yin, while *Dang Gui, Dan Shen,* and *Suan Zao Ren* supplement the heart and nourish the blood. *Yuan Zhi, Bai Zi Ren, Wu Wei Zi,* and *Suan Zao Ren* supplement the heart, settle the heart, and quiet the spirit. *Fu Ling* and *Ren Shen* fortify the spleen and boost the qi to promote the transformation of essence blood. *Xuan Shen, Tian Men Dong,* and *Mai Men Dong* clear vacuity heat, while *Dan Shen* cools the blood.

ADDITIONS & SUBTRACTIONS: If there are severe heart palpitations, add 15 grams each of Magnetitum (*Ci Shi*), Os Draconis (*Long Gu*), and Concha Ostreae (*Mu Li*). For severe yin vacuity, add 12 grams each of Radix Rehmanniae (*Sheng Di*) and Radix Albus Paeoniae Lactiflorae (*Bai Shao*). For dizziness, tinnitus, and high blood pressure, add 18 grams of Concha Haliotidis (*Shi Jue Ming*), 12 grams of Ramulus Uncariae Cum Uncis (*Gou Teng*), and 24 grams of Flos Chrysanthemi Morifolii (*Ju Hua*). For low back pain and weakness of the lower limbs with high blood pressure, add 15 grams each of Ramulus Loranthi Seu Visci (*Sang Ji Sheng*) and Radix Achyranthis Bidentatae (*Niu Xi*) and 12 grams of Cortex Eucommiae Ulmoidis (*Du Zhong*). For easy anger, severe restlessness, a red facial complexion, and aversion to heat, add nine grams each of Spica Prunellae Vulgaris (*Xia Ku Cao*), Fructus Gardeniae Jasminoidis (*Zhi Zi*), and Cortex Radicis Moutan (*Dan Pi*). For night sweats and hot flashes in the face, add 12 grams each of Cortex Radicis Lycii Chinensis (*Di Gu Pi*), Cortex Radicis Moutan (*Dan Pi*), and Rhizoma Anemarrhenae Asphodeloidis (*Zhi Mu*). For dry mouth with profuse drinking and hyperglycemia, add 24 grams of Radix Trichosanthis Kirlowii (*Tian Hua Fen*) and 30 grams of Radix Dioscoreae Oppositae (*Shan Yao*). If there is concomitant phlegm heat, add 12 grams of Pericarpium Trichosanthis Kirlowii (*Gua Lou Pi*) and nine grams each of Rhizoma Pinelliae Ternatae (*Ban Xia*) and Radix Scutellariae Baicalensis (*Huang Qin*).

ACUPUNCTURE & MOXIBUSTION: *Xin Shu* (Bl 15), *Shen Men* (Ht 7), *Fu Liu* (Ki 7), *San Yin Jiao* (Sp 6), *Nei Guan* (Per 6)

ANALYSIS OF FORMULA: Supplementing *Xin Shu* and *Shen Men* supplements the heart, settles palpitations, and quiets the spirit. Supplementing *Fu Liu* and *San Yin Jiao* is added to more strongly enrich yin. Draining *Nei Guan* frees the flow of the network vessels of the heart and prevents blood stasis.

ADDITIONS & SUBTRACTIONS: If there are severe heart palpitations, add *Ju Que* (CV 14) and *Dan Zhong* (CV 17). For dizziness, tinnitus, and high blood pressure, add *Xing Jian* (Liv 2) and *Feng Chi* (GB 20). For low back pain and weakness of lower limbs, add *Tai Xi* (Ki 3) and *Shen Shu* (Bl 23). For easy anger, severe restlessness, a red facial complexion, and aversion to heat, add *Xing Jian* (Liv 2) and *Xia Xi* (GB 43). For night sweats and hot flashes in the face, add *Da Zhui* (GV 14) and *Yin Xi* (Ht 6). If there is concomitant phlegm heat, add *Feng Long* (St 40), *Nei Ting* (St 44), and *Zhong Wan* (CV 12).

REMARKS

1. The main disease mechanism of coronary heart disease is yang vacuity and yin congelation. However, simply resolving congelation only achieves a temporary effect. Therefore, it is necessary to warm and free the flow of yang at the same time. For this, Aconite is the medicinal of first choice. Because of the interrelationship of yin and yang, yang vacuity is often complicated by yin vacuity, and yin and yang vacuity are almost always complicated by liver depression.

2. Based on the saying, "Enduring disease enters the network vessels," and on the nature of the pain associated with CAD, blood stasis typically plays a role in all patterns of this disease. Therefore, Salvia is included in almost every formula described above. In addition, Sanguis Draconis (*Xue Jie*) and Radix Pseudoginseng (*San Qi*) usually achieve a prompt effect when treating angina pectoris. For this purpose, 1.5 grams of each powdered can be swallowed with any of the above decoctions.

3. As with hypertension below, the comprehensive Chinese medical treatment of CAD necessitates dietary and lifestyle regulation.

4. Chinese medicine may be used to increase the clinical effects of Western medicines for CAD as well as eliminate the side effects of Western drugs. In addition, it may also be used to help prevent or avoid surgery.

5. For loosening the chest and treating chest impediment, Pericarpium Trichosanthis Kirlowii (*Gua Lou Pi*) is more effective than Fructus Trichosanthis Kirlowii (*Gua Lou*).

6. No matter whether treating vacuity or repletion patterns, when treating CAD with acupuncture, one should prevent strong draining needle manipulation. On the other hand, even in vacuity patterns, one should also use a moderate draining method to free the flow of the network vessels of the heart, especially in this disease, vacuity engenders stasis. Therefore, the best method is the even supplementing-even draining method. Likewise, Chinese medicinal formulas for the treatment of this disease normally must supplement and drain, support and attack at the same time.

7. There are several point combinations which get especially good empirical results when treating patients suffering from CAD. The most famous combinations are: *Dan Zhong* (CV 17) and *Nei Guan* (Per 6); *Dan Zhong* (CV 17) and *Ge Shu* (Bl 17); *Nei Guan* (Per 6) and *Xin Shu* (Bl 15); *Jue Yin*

Shu (Bl 14) and *Nei Guan* (Per 6); *Gong Sun* (Sp 4) and *Nei Guan* (Per 6); *Xi Men* (Per 4) and *Nei Guan* (Per 6); and *Nei Guan* (Per 6) and *Dui Dan* (CV 27).

8. According to clinical experience, *Nei Guan* (Per 6) seems to be the single most important point for treating CAD with acupuncture. Other empirically effective points for treating cardiac diseases are *Ling Dao* (Ht 4), *Shen Men* (Ht 7), *Qu Ze* (Per 3), *Xi Men* (Per 4), *Zhi Yang* (GV 9), *Jue Yin Shu* (Bl 14), *Xin Shu* (Bl 15), *Ge Shu* (Bl 17), *Ju Que* (CV 14), *Dan Zhong* (CV 17), and T4 & 5 *Jia Ji* (M-BW-35).

9. *Jian Shen Tang* (Fortify the Body Decoction) is a modern Chinese formula which treats elderly patients with qi and blood, spleen-kidney yin and yang vacuity plus blood stasis. It is comprised of: Radix Codonopsitis Pilosulae (*Dang Shen*), Radix Astragali Membranacei (*Huang Qi*), and Radix Salviae Miltiorrhizae (*Dan Shen*), 15-30g each, Radix Polygoni Multiflori (*He Shou Wu*), Fructus Lycii Chinensis (*Gou Qi*), and Radix Ligustici Wallichii (*Chuan Xiong*), 15g each, Rhizoma Atractylodis Macrocephalae (*Bai Zhu*), Sclerotium Poriae Cocos (*Fu Ling*), Cortex Radicis Moutan (*Dan Pi*), and Herba Epimedii (*Yin Yang Huo*), 9g each, and Ramulus Cinnamomi Cassiae (*Gui Zhi*) and mix-fried Radix Glycyrrhizae (*Gan Cao*), 6g each. For predominant yin vacuity, subtract *Gui Zhi* and add 15 grams of uncooked Radix Rehmanniae (*Sheng Di*) and nine grams each of Tuber Ophiopogonis Japonici (*Mai Men Dong*) and Fructus Schisandrae Chinensis (*Wu Wei Zi*). For predominant yang vacuity, subtract *Dan Pi* and add nine grams of Radix Lateralis Praeparatus Aconiti Carmichaeli (*Fu Zi*) and Bulbus Allii (*Xie Bai*). For ascendant liver yang hyperactivity with essential hypertension, add 15 grams of Radix Albus Paeoniae Lactiflorae (*Bai Shao*), 12 grams of Ramulus Uncariae Cum Uncis (*Gou Teng*), and nine grams of Radix Cyathulae (*Chuan Niu Xi*) or 12 grams each of Cortex Eucommiae Ulmoidis (*Du Zhong*), Ramulus Loranthi Seu Visci (*Sang Ji Sheng*), and Radix Achyranthis Bidentatae (*Niu Xi*). For constipation, add 15 grams each of Fructus Trichosanthis Kirlowii (*Gua Lou*) and Herba Cistanchis Deserticolae (*Rou Cong Rong*) and nine grams of Radix Angelicae Sinensis (*Dang Gui*). For insomnia, add 15 grams of Semen Zizyphi Spinosae (*Suan Zao Ren*) and 30 grams of Caulis Polygoni Multiflori (*Ye Jiao Teng*). For severe heart palpitations or arrhythmia, add 30 grams of mix-fried Radix Glycyrrhizae (*Gan Cao*). For qi stagnation, add three grams each of Lignum Aquilariae Agallochae (*Chen Xiang*) and Lignum Santali Albi (*Tan Xiang*), powdered and taken with the strained decoction, and 15 grams of *Jing Ling Zi San* (Fructus Meliae Toosendan Powder). For liver depression, add 12 grams each of Radix Bupleuri (*Chai Hu*), Rhizoma Cyperi Rotundi (*Xiang Fu*), and Radix Albus Paeoniae Lactiflorae (*Bai Shao*). For severe heart pain, increase the dosage of *Dan Shen* up to 50 grams and add three grams of Radix Pseudoginseng (*San Qi*), powdered and taken with the strained decoction. For severe heart qi vacuity, increase the dosage of *Huang Qi* up to 50 grams. For damp phlegm, add 30 grams of Pericarpium Trichosanthis Kirlowii (*Gua Lou Pi*) and nine grams of Bulbus Allii (*Xie Bai*). For phlegm heat, add 30 grams each of Pericarpium Trichosanthis Kirlowii (*Gua Lou Pi*) and Radix Ilicis Pubescentis (*Mao Dong Qing*). For internal heat, add 30 grams of Radix Ilicis Pubescentis (*Mao Dong Qing*), 15 grams of Herba Siegesbeckiae (*Xi Xian Cao*), and nine grams of Radix Scutellariae Baicalensis (*Huang Qin*). For hyperlipoproteinemia, add 20 grams of Fructus Crataegi (*Shan Zha*) and 15 grams each of Ramulus Loranthi Seu Visci (*Sang Ji Sheng*) and Radix Polygoni Multiflori (*He Shou Wu*).

10. The best Chinese medicinals for treating CAD are Hirudo Seu Whitmania (*Shui Zhi*), Radix Ilicis Pubescentis (*Mao Dong Qing*), Radix Salviae Miltiorrhizae (*Dan Shen*), Radix Pseudoginseng (*San Qi*), Fructus Crataegi (*Shan Zha*), Fructus Trichosanthis Kirlowii (*Gua Lou*), Pollen Typhae (*Pu Huang*), Herba Epimedii (*Yin Yang Huo*), Radix Panacis Ginseng (*Ren Shen*), Radix Ligustici Wallichii (*Chuan Xiong*), and Flos Carthami Tinctorii (*Hong Hua*). In particular, *Shui Zhi* is typically found in most modern Chinese empirical formulas for CAD even though it is not found as an ingredient in textbook formulas such as those given above. Therefore, this ingredient should be a considered addition or replacement whenever CAD is accompanied by blood stasis.

11. Chinese blood-quickening medicinals may potentiate the effects of Western anticoagulants and blood-thinners. Therefore, practitioners should take care not to over treat blood stasis if Western drugs have already been prescribed for these purposes.

22

Crohn's Disease

Also called granulomatous ileitis and ileocolitis, Crohn's disease is a nonspecific chronic transmural inflammatory disease that mostly affects the distal ileum and colon but may affect any part of the gastrointestinal tract from the mouth to the anus. Although its etiology is unknown, it is suspected to be an autoimmune disease since no specific micro-organism has been clearly established as the cause. Dietary factors, including a low fiber diet, have also been investigated without conclusive outcomes. The diagnosis of Crohn's disease within Western medicine is only several decades old. Therefore, its increasing incidence in Western populations may, in part, be a reflection of more attention being paid to it. So, this diagnosis is most prevalent among those of Northen European and Anglo-Saxon descent and among Jews. In terms of sex, it is relatively equally distributed between men and women, and there is a familial tendency which overlaps with ulcerative colitis. The peak incidence of this disease in terms of age is in the 20s, and most cases occur before 40. Its signs and symptoms are chronic painful diarrhea, fever, anorexia, weight loss, and a right lower quadrant mass or fullness. The extraintestinal complications of Crohn's disease are roughly the same as ulcerative colitis.

The Western medical diagnosis of Crohn's disease is based on the patient's history, including family history, and their presenting signs and symptoms. Laboratory findings are nonspecific and may include anemia, leukocytosis, hypoalbuminemia, and increased levels of acute phase reactants. Definitive diagnosis is usually made by x-ray. There is no specific therapy for Crohn's disease within Western medicine. The same sorts of drugs are prescribed for diarrhea and cramping in Crohn's disease as for ulcerative colitis, such as anticholinergics, diphenoxylate, deordorized opium tincture, and codeine. Antibiotics are prescribed for bacterial complications, such as abscesses and infected fistulas, and corticosteriods may be used in acute stages of this disease. Immunosuppressive agents, such as cyclosporin E, are currently being investigated, and surgery is usually considered necessary when there is recurrent intestinal obstruction, intractable abscesses, or fistulas. In terms of prognosis, complete recovery may follow a single isolated attack of acute ileitis. However, chronic regional enteritis is characterized by lifelong exacerbations. Fatal complications from free perforation, sepsis, inanition, or carcinoma are rare.

Chinese disease categorization: This disease is categorized in Chinese medicine as *xie xie*, diarrhea, *tong xie*, painful diarrhea, *chi bai li*, red and white dysentery, *jiu li*, enduring dysentery, *chang pi*, intestinal afflux, *bian xue*, hemafecia, and *chang bi*, intestinal impediment. In addition, intestinal abscesses are categorized as *chang yong*, intestinal welling abscess, perianal abscesses are categorized as *gang yong*, anal welling abscesses, anal fistulas are called *gang lou*, and anal fissures are called *gang lie*.

Disease causes: The six environmental excesses, the seven affects, unregulated eating and drinking, and taxation fatigue

Disease mechanisms: Damp heat evils may invade the body from the outside or damp heat may be engendered internally due to over-eating hot, spicy, greasy, fried, fatty foods and drinking alcohol. If damp heat pours downward to the large intestine, it may affect the intestines' conveyance and conduction, thus resulting in diarrhea. If damp heat brews and damages the network vessels, there may be hemafecia. Damp heat may also be caused by liver depression transforming heat and spleen vacuity engendering dampness internally. If this dampness and heat combine, they may also form damp heat. The causes of liver depression are mainly unfulfilled desires and anger. However, liver depression may be aggravated by blood vacuity and/or yang vacuity. Spleen vacuity in Western patients is most commonly due to overeating sugars and sweets and uncooked, chilled foods, overthinking and especially worry and anxiety, too little exercise, too much fatigue, and prolonged or overuse of antibiotics. In addition, because of menstruation, gestation, and lactation, women are more prone to spleen vacuity than men, while both men's and women's spleens become vacuous and weak with age.

If spleen vacuity reaches kidney yang, spleen qi vacuity may evolve into a spleen-kidney dual vacuity. If blood and fluid loss damages yin, there may be a qi and yin dual vacuity. If damp heat, damp turbidity, or qi stagnation endure, they may become complicated by blood stasis. Likewise, either liver depression or spleen vacuity may also be complicated by food stagnation. Because of the typical right lower quadrant mass, blood stasis is even more commonly found as a complicating mechanism in Crohn's disease than colitis. Intestinal abscesses are usually a combination of damp heat stasis and stagnation. Anal abscesses, fistulas, and fissures are mostly associated with damp heat evils brewing heat toxins.

TREATMENT BASED ON PATTERN DISCRIMINATION:

For the treatment of the diarrhea, hemafecia, weight loss, and anorexia of Crohn's disease, please see the patterns and treatments under ulcerative colitis below. The patterns presented in this chapter specifically deal with intestinal abscess and perianal lesions.

1. DAMP HEAT STASIS & STAGNATION PATTERN (INTESTINAL ABSCESSES)

MAIN SYMPTOMS: Right-sided lower abdominal pain which is worse on pressure, a palpable lump in the lower right quadrant, possible distended skin in the affected area, a tendency to lie curled-up, aversion to cold, fever, nausea, vomiting, reduced appetite, possible inhibited defecation, a red tongue with yellow fur, and a bowstring, slippery, rapid pulse

TREATMENT PRINCIPLES: Clear heat and eliminate dampness, quicken the blood and transform stasis

RX: *Da Huang Mu Dan Pi Tang* (Rhubarb & Moutan Decoction) & *Hong Teng Jian* (Sargentodoxa Decoction) with additions and subtractions

INGREDIENTS: Rhizoma Corydalis Yanhusuo (*Yan Hu Suo*), Flos Lonicerae Japonicae (*Jin Yin Hua*), and Caulis Sargentodoxae (*Hong Teng*), 15g each, Semen Benincasae Hispidae (*Dong Gua Zi*) and Radix Et Rhizoma Rhei (*Da Huang*), 12g each, Semen Pruni Persicae (*Tao Ren*), Herba Patriniae Heterophyllae Cum Radice (*Bai Jiang Cao*), and Fructus Forsythiae Suspensae (*Lian Qiao*), 9g each, and Mirabilitum (*Mang Xiao*), Cortex Radicis Moutan (*Dan Pi*), Resina Olibani (*Ru Xiang*), and Resina Myrrhae (*Mo Yao*), 6g each

ANALYSIS OF FORMULA: *Jin Yin Hua, Hong Teng, Bai Jiang Cao*, and *Lian Qiao* clear heat and resolve toxins. In addition, *Bai Jiang Cao* and *Hong Teng* are empirically specific medicinals for treating intestinal abscess. *Da Huang* and *Mang Xiao* discharge fire, resolve toxins, and free the flow of the stools. In addition, *Da Huang* quickens the blood. *Yan Hu Suo, Hong Teng, Tao Ren, Bai Jiang Cao, Dan Pi, Ru Xiang,* and *Mo Yao* quicken the blood, transform stasis, and stop pain. *Tao Ren* and *Dong Gua Zi* expel pus.

ADDITIONS & SUBTRACTIONS: For heat damaging yin, add 12 grams each of uncooked Radix Rehmanniae (*Sheng Di*) and Herba Dendrobii (*Shi Hu*). For severe abdominal distention, add nine grams each of Cortex Magnoliae Officinalis (*Hou Po*) and Radix Auklandiae Lappae (*Mu Xiang*).

ACUPUNCTURE & MOXIBUSTION: *Lan Wei Xue* (M-LE-13), *Tian Shu* (St 25), *Nei Ting* (St 44), *San Yin Jiao* (Sp 6), *He Gu* (LI 4)

ANALYSIS OF FORMULA: *Lan Wei Xue* is a special empirical point for the treatment of intestinal abscess. It is drained. Draining *Tian Shu* and *Nei Ting* clears heat and rectifies the intestinal qi mechanism, thus stops pain. The combination of *San Yin Jiao* and *He Gu* quickens the blood and transforms stasis when needled with draining technique.

ADDITIONS & SUBTRACTIONS: For enduring intestinal abscess with intermittent attacks, subtract *Nei Ting* and add *Ge Shu* (Bl 17) and *Xue Hai* (Sp 10) to quicken the blood and transform stasis. For high fever, add *Qu Chi* (LI 11).

NOTE: Acupuncture may have to be performed more than once per day for acute intestinal abscess and the needles may need to be left in place for up to an hour each treatment. *Lan Wei* should only be needled if and where it is tender. Otherwise, use *Zu San Li* (St 36).

2. DAMP HEAT BREWING & BINDING PATTERN (ANAL FISSURES & FISTULAS)

MAIN SYMPTOMS: Anal pain, dripping of fresh red blood while defecating, a sagging, distended sensation in the anus, sticky stools, a small amount of pus in the fissures, dampness and possible itching around the anus, a red tongue with thick, slimy fur, and a bowstring, rapid pulse

TREATMENT PRINCIPLES: Clear heat and disinhibit dampness

RX: *Bei Xie Shen Shi Tang Jia Wei* (Dioscorea Hypoglauca Overcome Dampness Decoction with Added Flavors)

INGREDIENTS: Talcum (*Hua Shi*), 15g, Semen Coicis Lachryma-jobi (*Yi Yi Ren*), 12g, Rhizoma Dioscoreae Hypoglaucae (*Bei Xie*), Cortex Phellodendri (*Huang Bai*),

Sclerotium Rubrum Poriae Cocos (*Chi Fu Ling*), Rhizoma Alismatis (*Ze Xie*), and Rhizoma Atractylodis (*Cang Zhu*), 9g each, and Cortex Radicis Moutan (*Dan Pi*) and Rhizoma Coptidis Chinensis (*Huang Lian*), 6g each

ANALYSIS OF FORMULA: *Hua Shi, Chi Fu Ling, Ze Xie*, and *Yi Yi Ren* seep dampness and clear heat via urination. *Bei Xie* separates the clear from turbid, while *Cang Zhu* aromatically dries and transforms dampness. *Huang Bai* and *Huang Lian,* bitter and cold, clear heat and eliminate dampness, and *Dan Pi* quickens and clears heat from the blood. In addition, both *Yi Yi Ren* and *Cang Zhu* fortify the spleen, the root of damp engenderment.

ADDITIONS & SUBTRACTIONS: For severe anal bleeding, add nine grams each of Radix Sanguisorbae Officinalis (*Di Yu*) and Flos Immaturus Sophorae Japonicae (*Huai Hua*). For severe redness and swelling around the anus, add nine grams of Radix Rubrus Paeoniae Lactiflorae (*Chi Shao*), 15 grams of Flos Lonicerae Japonicae (*Jin Yin Hua*), and 12 grams of Herba Taraxaci Mongolici Cum Radice (*Pu Gong Ying*). For severe anal itching, add nine grams each of Fructus Kochiae Scopariae (*Di Fu Zi*) and Cortex Radicis Dictamni Dasycarpi (*Bai Xian Pi*). For tenesmus or a sagging sensation in the anus, add six grams each of Radix Auklandiae Lappae (*Mu Xiang*) and Semen Arecae Catechu (*Bing Lang*).

EXTERNAL TREATMENT: For marked anal itching, dampness, and swelling, powder equal amounts of the following Chinese medicinals: Cortex Phellodendri (*Huang Bai*), Rhizoma Coptidis Chinensis (*Huang Lian*), Folium Hibisci (*Fu Rong Ye*), Radix Et Rhizoma Rhei (*Da Huang*), and Folium Lycopi Lucidi (*Ze Lan Ye*). Mix together with petrolatum (50% powder, 50% petrolatum) and apply to the affected area. For predominant bleeding, finely powder Rhizoma Bletillae Striatae (*Bai Ji*). Mix with petrolatum (50:50) and apply to the affected area. Either can be used 2-3 times per day.

ACUPUNCTURE & MOXIBUSTION: *Chang Qiang* (GV 1), *Cheng Shan* (Bl 57), *Yin Ling Quan* (Sp 9), *San Yin Jiao* (Sp 6), *Da Chang Shu* (Bl 25)

ANALYSIS OF FORMULA: Draining *Chang Qiang* and *Cheng Shan* clears heat and stops pain in the anal area. Draining *Yin Ling Quan, San Yin Jiao,* and *Da Chang Shu* clears heat and disinhibits dampness, regulates and rectifies the intestinal qi mechanism.

ADDITIONS & SUBTRACTIONS: For fever and aversion to cold, add *He Gu* (LI 4). For poor appetite, add *Zhong Wan* (CV 12). For abdominal pain, add *Zu San Li* (St 36).

REMARKS

1. Based on the saying, "Different diseases, same treatment," the Chinese medical treatment of Crohn's disease and ulcerative colitis are basically the same. There are the same disease causes and mechanisms, the same patterns, and the same treatment principles. Therefore, the reader should also see the chapter on ulcerative colitis below for more patterns and their treatments. However, because Crohn's disease tends to attack a younger group of patients, there tends to be more repletion and less vacuity, more heat and less cold. There also tends to be more blood stasis.

2. Anal abscesses, fissures, and fistulas commonly require surgical treatment. However, the administration of internal Chinese medicinals treats the root of these conditions. Thus the conditions are less recalcitrant to surgical treatment and do not relapse as easily.

3. Intestinal abscesses in Crohn's disease may be mistaken for acute appendicitis or intestinal obstruction. However, their Chinese medical treatment is basically the same.

4. A clear bland diet and lifestyle modifications, including both more physical exercise and more mental-emotional relaxation, are necessary parts of an overall Chinese medical treatment plan for this condition.

23

CUSHING'S SYNDROME

Cushing's syndrome is a constellation of clinical abnormalities due to chronic exposure to excesses of cortisol or related corticosteriods. This chronic excessive exposure may be due to hypersecretion of ACTH by the pituitary, secretion of ACTH by a non-pituitary tumor, or administration of exogenous ACTH. Its clinical manifestations include fatigue, a rounded, moon-like face, fluid retention, truncal obesity with prominent supraclavicular and dorsal cervical fat pads, muscular weakness and wasting, thin, atrophic skin, poor wound healing, easy bruising, excessive sweating, and purple striae on the abdomen. Psychiatric disturbances, especially irritability, are common, while females usually have menstrual irregularities.

The Western medical diagnosis of this condition depends on several different laboratory tests: dexamethasone test, metyrapone test, ACTH stimulation test, and CRF test. In addition, CT scans may be used to determine the presence of pituitary or adrenal tumors. When Cushing's syndrome is due to prolonged administration of exogenous corticosteroids, there is an obvious history of their use. When Cushing's syndrome is due to hyperfunction of pituitary or adrenal glands, surgery is often used to excise or oblate tumors. When this condition is due to prolonged, excessive administration of exogenous corticosteroids, the patient should be weaned from this medicines. Unfortunately, however, these medicines may be necessary to control other disease processes in the body.

CHINESE DISEASE CATEGORIZATION: The main clinical manifestations of this condition are categorized as *neng shi shan ji*, ability to eat with rapid hungering, *shui zhong*, water swelling or edema, *fei pang*, obesity, *yi nu*, easy anger or irritability, *zi han*, spontaneous perspiration, *dao han*, thief sweating, *i.e.*, night sweats, and *shi mian*, loss of sleep, or *bu mian*, insomnia.

DISEASE CAUSES: Former heaven natural endowment insufficiency, internal damage by the seven affects, unregulated eating and drinking, over-taxation, aging, enduring disease, and iatrogenesis

DISEASE MECHANISMS: The clinical manifestations of this condition divide into two main categories. On the one hand there is spleen qi and kidney yang vacuity with dampness and phlegm, while, on the other, there is yin vacuity with effulgent fire. Spleen-kidney vacuity may be due to faulty diet, over-taxation, aging, enduring disease, and/or iatrogenesis. Kidney yin vacuity is commonly due to former heaven natural endowment insufficiency, aging, enduring disease, and/or iatrogenesis. Phlegm may be due to faulty diet. However, it may also be due to either long-term accumulation and congelation of water dampness in turn due to spleen-kidney vacuity or long-term heat stewing and steaming the fluids, thus also congealing phlegm.

When Cushing's syndrome is due to iatrogenesis, its mechanisms are essentially similar to overprescribing acrid, windy natured medicinals. Corticosteriods, such as prednisone, clear heat by out-thrusting it, while they stop pain by forcefully moving the qi. In this way, prednisone is something similar to Radix Bupleuri (*Chai Hu*). When acrid, windy, exterior-resolving medicinals are wrongly or overused, they A) outthrust and, therefore, damage yang qi and B) plunder and consume yin fluids. Thus their side effects are to cause qi and ultimately yang vacuity on the one hand, and yin vacuity with vacuity heat on the other, with phlegm congelation being associated with either or both of these two mechanisms.

TREATMENT BASED ON PATTERN DISCRIMINATION:

1. YIN VACUITY WITH ASCENDANT LIVER YANG HYPERACTIVITY PATTERN

MAIN SYMPTOMS: Obesity, a red, flushed face or malar flushing, dizziness or vertigo, headache, clouded spirit, tinnitus, oral dryness, rapid hungering, low back and knee soreness and limpness, scanty sleep, a red tongue with scanty fur, and a fine, bowstring, rapid pulse

TREATMENT PRINCIPLES: Enrich yin and subdue yang

RX: *Liu Wei Di Huang Wan Jia Wei* (Six Flavors Rehmannia Pills with Added Flavors)

INGREDIENTS: Ramulus Uncariae Cum Uncis (*Gou Teng*), 15g, Radix Achyranthis Bidentatae (*Niu Xi*) and cooked Radix Rehmanniae (*Shu Di*), 12g each, Radix Puerariae (*Ge Gen*), Radix Dioscoreae Oppositae (*Shan Yao*), Fructus Corni Officinalis (*Shan Zhu Yu*), and Sclerotium Poriae Cocos (*Fu Ling*), 9g each, and Cortex Radicis Moutan (*Dan Pi*) and Rhizoma Alismatis (*Ze Xie*), 6g each

ANALYSIS OF FORMULA: *Shu Di, Niu Xi, Shan Yao, Fu Ling,* and *Shan Zhu Yu* together nourish blood and enrich yin, supplement the liver and kidneys. *Ze Xie* downbears effulgent fire of the kidneys. *Dan Pi* clears the liver and cools the blood. *Ge Gen* clears heat, engenders fluids, and treats tinnitus. In addition, *Ge Gen* upbears clear yang. Paradoxically, the upbearing of clear yang helps to downbear ascendant liver yang hyperactivity at the same time as it out-thrusts the yang qi counterflowing upward along the du mai-tai yang. And *Gou Teng,* with the help of *Niu Xi,* subdues yang.

ADDITIONS & SUBTRACTIONS: For severe obesity, add 12 grams each of Radix Polygoni Multiflori (*He Shou Wu*) and Semen Cassiae Torae (*Jue Ming Zi*). For severe malar flushing, add nine grams each of Cortex Phellodendri (*Huang Bai*) and Rhizoma Anemarrhenae Asphodeloidis (*Zhi Mu*). For clouded spirit and/or tinnitus, add 9-12 grams of Rhizoma Acori Graminei (*Shi Chang Pu*). For thirst or oral dryness, add 12 grams each of Rhizoma Phragmitis Communis (*Lu Gen*) and Radix Trichosanthis Kirlowii (*Tian Hua Fen*). For rapid hungering, add 15 grams of Gypsum Fibrosum (*Shi Gao*) and nine grams of Rhizoma Anemarrhenae Asphodeloidis (*Zhi Mu*). For severe low back and knee soreness and limpness, add nine grams each of Ramulus Loranthi Seu Visci (*Sang Ji Sheng*) and Radix Polygoni Multiflori (*He Shou Wu*). For insomnia, add 15 grams each of Caulis Polygoni Multiflori (*Ye Jiao Teng*) and Semen Zizyphi Spinosae (*Suan Zao Ren*).

ACUPUNCTURE & MOXIBUSTION: *Fu Liu* (Ki 7), *San Yin Jiao* (Sp 6), *Tai Chong* (Liv 3), *Feng Chi* (GB 20)

ANALYSIS OF FORMULA: *Fu Liu* is the metal and, therefore, the mother point on the kidney channel. Supplementing it supplements the kidneys, enriches true yin, and engenders fluids. Supplementing *San Yin Jiao* (Sp 6) nourishes yin, blood, and essence and, therefore, helps *Fu Liu* to enrich true yin. Draining *Tai Chong* levels the liver and subdues yang. Draining *Feng Chi* subdues yang and opens the orifices.

ADDITIONS & SUBTRACTIONS: For a bitter taste in the mouth and easy anger, add *Yang Ling Quan* (GB 34). For headache or dizziness, add *Bai Hui* (GV 20). For clouded spirit, add *Si Shen Cong* (M-HN-1). For tinnitus, add *Ting Hui* (GB 2) and *Yi Feng* (TB 17). For rapid hungering, add *Zhong Wan* (CV 12) and *Nei Ting* (St 44). For severe low back and knee soreness and limpness, add *Shen Shu* (Bl 23) and *Zhi Shi* (Bl 52). For insomnia, add *Shen Men* (Ht 7). For night sweats, add *Yin Xi* (Ht 6).

2. YIN VACUITY-FIRE EFFULGENCE PATTERN

MAIN SYMPTOMS: An obese torso but emaciation of the limbs, a red, rounded, moon-like face, hot flashes in the face, vexatious heat in the five hearts, night sweats, dryness of mouth and throat, low back and knee soreness and limpness, restlessness, heart palpitations, insomnia, profuse dreams, thirst, scanty menstruation or amenorrhea, purple striae or macules on the lower abdomen and lower limbs, constipation, a red tongue, especially on the tip, with scanty fur, and a fine, deep, rapid pulse

TREATMENT PRINCIPLES: Supplement the kidneys and enrich yin, clear and drain ministerial fire

RX: *Zhi Bai Di Huang Wan Jia Jian* (Anemarrhena & Phellodendron Rehmannia Pills with Additions & Subtractions)

INGREDIENTS: Radix Salviae Miltiorrhizae (*Dan Shen*), uncooked Radix Rehmanniae (*Sheng Di*), and Rhizoma Polygonati (*Huang Jing*), 20g each, Fructus Lycii Chinensis (*Gou Qi Zi*), Caulis Polygoni Multiflori (*Ye Jiao Teng*), and Cortex Radicis Moutan (*Dan Pi*), 12g each, Rhizoma Anemarrhenae Asphodeloidis (*Zhi Mu*), Cortex Phellodendri (*Huang Bai*), and Radix Gentianae Scabrae (*Long Dan Cao*), 9g each, and Fructus Corni Officinalis (*Shan Zhu Yu*), 6g

ANALYSIS OF FORMULA: *Sheng Di, Gou Qi,* and *Shan Zhu Yu* supplement the kidneys and enrich yin. *Huang Jing* boosts the qi and fills the essence, supplements the spleen to support the kidneys. It is a well-known empirical medicinal for the treatment of Cushing's syndrome. *Huang Bai, Zhi Mu,* and *Long Dan Cao* clear and drain ministerial fire. *Long Dan Cao* is also a well-known empirical medicinal for Cushing's syndrome. *Dan Shen* quickens the blood and transforms stasis due to fire effulgence. *Ye Jiao Teng* nourishes heart and liver blood, calms the *hun* and quiets the spirit.

ADDITIONS & SUBTRACTIONS: For ascendant liver yang

hyperactivity with headache, head distention, easy anger, and irritability, add 12 grams of Ramulus Uncariae Cum Uncis (*Gou Teng*) and Flos Chrysanthemi Morifolii (*Ju Hua*). For insomnia, profuse dreams, impaired memory, and restlessness, add 15 grams each of Semen Zizyphi Spinosae (*Suan Zao Ren*) and Radix Polygalae Tenuifoliae (*Yuan Zhi*). For constipation, add nine grams of Semen Pruni (*Yu Li Ren*) or 6-9 grams of Radix Et Rhizoma Rhei (*Da Huang*). For concomitant spleen qi vacuity, add 15 grams of Radix Astragali Membranacei (*Huang Qi*) and nine grams of Radix Codonopsitis Pilosulae (*Dang Shen*). For restless legs, add 15 grams each of Radix Albus Paeoniae Lactiflorae (*Bai Shao*), Periostracum Cicadae (*Chan Tui*), and Bombyx Batryticatus (*Jiang Can*). For purple striae or macules on the lower abdomen and lower limbs or scanty menstruation and amenorrhea, add nine grams each of Flos Carthami Tinctorii (*Hong Hua*) and Semen Pruni Persicae (*Tao Ren*). For severe obesity, add 12 grams each of Radix Polygoni Multiflori (*He Shou Wu*) and Semen Cassiae Torae (*Jue Ming Zi*). For thirst or oral dryness, add 12 grams each of Rhizoma Phragmitis Communis (*Lu Gen*) and Radix Trichosanthis Kirlowii (*Tian Hua Fen*). For tinnitus, add 12 grams of Rhizoma Acori Graminei (*Shi Chang Pu*). For severe low back and knee soreness and limpness, add nine grams of Ramulus Loranthi Seu Visci (*Sang Ji Sheng*) and Radix Polygoni Multiflori (*He Shou Wu*).

ACUPUNCTURE & MOXIBUSTION: *Fu Liu* (Ki 7), *San Yin Jiao* (Sp 6), *Ran Gu* (Ki 2), *Bai Hui* (GV 20)

ANALYSIS OF FORMULA: *Fu Liu* is the metal point on the kidney channel. Supplementing it supplements the kidneys, enriches true yin, and engenders fluids. Supplementing *San Yin Jiao* nourishes yin, blood, and essence. Therefore, it helps *Fu Liu* enrich true yin. Draining *Ran Gu* clears and drains ministerial fire, while draining *Bai Hui* subdues yang, opens the orifices, and quiets the spirit.

ADDITIONS & SUBTRACTIONS: For liver yang hyperactivity with headache and distention, add *Feng Chi* (GB 20). For insomnia, profuse dreams, impaired memory, and restlessness, add *Shen Men* (Ht 7). For constipation, add *Zhi Gou* (TB 6). For concomitant spleen qi vacuity, add *Zu San Li* (St 36). For restless legs, add *He Gu* (LI 4) and *Tai Chong* (Liv 3). For purple striae or macules on the lower abdomen and lower limbs or scanty menstruation and amenorrhea, add *Xue Hai* (Sp 10). For tinnitus, add *Ting Hui* (GB 2) and *Yi Feng* (TB 17). For severe low back and knee soreness and limpness, add *Shen Shu* (Bl 23).

3. ASCENDANT LIVER YANG HYPERACTIVITY WITH PHLEGM FIRE PATTERN

MAIN SYMPTOMS: Obesity, a red, flushed face, head distention, dizziness and vertigo, throbbing headache, irritability, irascibility, chest oppression, heart vexation, profuse dreams, thirst, constipation, slimy, yellow tongue fur, and a slippery, bowstring, rapid pulse

TREATMENT PRINCIPLES: Level the liver and subdue yang, clear and transform phlegm heat

RX: *Er Ke Tang* (Two Shells Decoction)

INGREDIENTS: Concha Margaritiferae (*Zhen Zhu Mu*) and Concha Haliotidis (*Shi Jue Ming*), 20g each, Fructus Gardeniae Jasminoidis (*Zhi Zi*), Fructus Trichosanthis Kirlowii (*Tian Hua Fen*), Radix Scrophulariae Ningpoensis (*Xuan Shen*), Radix Puerariae (*Ge Gen*), and Herba Apocyni Veneti (*Lo Bu Ma Ye*), 9g each, bile-processed Rhizoma Arisaematis (*Dan Nan Xing*) and Radix Et Rhizoma Rhei (*Da Huang*), 6g each, and Rhizoma Coptidis Chinensis (*Huang Lian*), 3g

ANALYSIS OF FORMULA: *Zhen Zhu Mu*, *Shi Jue Ming*, and *Lo Bu Ma Ye* level the liver and subdue yang. *Zhi Zi* and *Huang Lian* clear the liver. *Tian Hua Fen* clears heat and engenders fluids. *Xuan Shen* clears specifically vacuity heat. *Dan Nan Xing* clears and transforms phlegm heat. *Da Huang* drains and discharges heat downward. *Ge Gen* out-thrusts the yang qi counterflowing upward along the du mai-tai yang.

ADDITIONS & SUBTRACTIONS: For severe obesity, add 12 grams each of Radix Polygoni Multiflori (*He Shou Wu*) and Semen Cassiae Torae (*Jue Ming Zi*). For head distention, dizziness, and vertigo, add 12 grams each of Rhizoma Gastrodiae Elatae (*Tian Ma*), Ramulus Uncariae Cum Uncis (*Gou Teng*), and Flos Chrysanthemi Morifolii (*Ju Hua*). For throbbing headache, add three grams each of Buthus Martensi (*Quan Xie*) and Scolopendra Subspinipes (*Wu Gong*), powdered and taken with the strained decoction. For irritability or irascibility, add six grams of Radix Gentianae Scabrae (*Long Dan Cao*). For thirst, add 12 grams each of Rhizoma Phragmitis Communis (*Lu Gen*) and Radix Trichosanthis Kirlowii (*Tian Hua Fen*).

ACUPUNCTURE & MOXIBUSTION: *Tai Chong* (Liv 3) through to *Yong Quan* (Ki 1), *Xia Xi* (GB 43), *Feng Chi* (GB 20), *Feng Long* (St 40)

ANALYSIS OF FORMULA: Needling *Tai Chong* through to *Yong Quan* with draining technique levels the liver and subdues yang. Draining *Xia Xi* clears the liver and gallbladder. Draining *Feng Chi* subdues yang and clears the head. Draining *Feng Long* transforms phlegm.

ADDITIONS & SUBTRACTIONS: For head distention, dizziness, and vertigo, add *Bai Hui* (GV 20). For throbbing headache, add *Tai Yang* (M-HN-9) and *Wai Guan* (TB 5). For irritability or irascibility, add *Gan Shu* (Bl 18) and *Hun Men* (Bl 47).

4. Yin vacuity with heat toxins pattern

Main symptoms: Suppurative pharyngitis, pneumonia, pleuritis, erysipelas, fever and chills, generalized body pain, oral dryness and thirst, reduced food intake, a red tongue with yellow fur, and a surging, rapid or slippery, rapid pulse

Note: This pattern is seen when using large doses of steroids which have compromised the immune system and there is secondary bacterial infection.

Treatment principles: Enrich yin and clear heat, quicken the blood and resolve toxins

Rx: *Wu Wei Xiao Du Yin Jia Jian* (Five Flavors Disperse Toxins Drink with Additions & Subtractions)

Ingredients: Herba Taraxaci Mongolici Cum Radice (*Pu Gong Ying*), Herba Violae Yedoensitis Cum Radice (*Zi Hua Di Ding*), and Radix Scrophulariae Ningpoensis (*Xuan Shen*), 15g each, uncooked Radix Rehmanniae (*Sheng Di*), 12g, Radix Achyranthis Bidentatae (*Niu Xi*), Cortex Radicis Moutan (*Dan Pi*), Flos Chrysanthemi Indici (*Ye Ju Hua*), and Rhizoma Anemarrhenae Aspheloidis (*Zhi Mu*), 9g each, and uncooked Radix Glycyrrhizae (*Gan Cao*), 3-6g

Analysis of formula: *Pu Gong Ying, Zi Hua Di Ding, Xuan Shen,* and *Ye Ju Hua* clear heat, resolve toxins, and dispel pus. In addition, *Xuan Shen* disinhibits the throat. *Zhi Mu* drains fire and nourishes yin. *Sheng Di* and *Niu Xi* enrich yin and supplement the kidneys. *Niu Xi* and *Dan Pi* quicken the blood and transform stasis. *Dan Pi* also clears heat from the blood. *Gan Cao* also clears heat, especially from the throat and lungs. It also harmonizes the other medicinals in this formula.

Additions & subtractions: For suppurative pharyngitis, add 12 grams each of Fructus Arctii Lappae (*Niu Bang Zi*), Fructus Forsythiae Suspensae (*Lian Qiao*), and Radix Istadis Seu Baphicacanthi (*Ban Lan Gen*). For pneumonia, add nine grams of Radix Scutellariae Baicalensis (*Huang Qin*) and 15 grams each of Herba Houttuyniae Cordatae Cum Radice (*Yu Xing Cao*) and Herba Patriniae Heterophyllae Cum Radice (*Bai Jiang Cao*). For pleuritis, add nine grams each of Semen Lepidii Seu Descurainiae (*Ting Li Zi*) and Flos Inulae (*Xuan Fu Hua*) and 20 grams each of Cortex Radicis Mori Albi (*Sang Bai Pi*) and Herba Houttuyniae Cordatae Cum Radice (*Yu Xing Cao*). For erysipelas, add nine grams each of Radix Scutellariae Baicalensis (*Huang Qin*), Fructus Forsythiae Suspensae (*Lian Qiao*), Radix Salviae Miltiorrhizae (*Dan Shen*), and Radix Istadis Seu Baphicacanthi (*Ban Lan Gen*).

Acupuncture & moxibustion: *He Gu* (LI 4), *Wai Guan* (TB 5), *San Yin Jiao* (Sp 6)

Analysis of formula: Draining *He Gu* and *Wai Guan* clears heat and resolves toxins, while supplementing *San Yin Jiao* enriches yin. However, in the case of this pattern, acupuncture is only an adjunctive treatment.

Additions & subtractions: For suppurative pharyngitis, add *Shao Shang* (Lu 11) and *Shang Yang* (LI 1). For pneumonia, add *Feng Men* (Bl 12), *Fei Shu* (Bl 13), and *Chi Ze* (Lu 5). For pleuritis, add *Dan Zhong* (CV 17), *Qi Men* (Liv 14), and *Qu Chi* (LI 11). For erysipelas, add *Qu Chi* (LI 11), *Xue Hai* (Sp 10), and *Wei Zhong* (Bl 40).

5. Spleen qi vacuity with phlegm dampness pattern

Main symptoms: Obesity, edema, fatigue, lack of strength, lassitude of the spirit, abdominal and ductal glomus and distention, torpid intake, cold hands and feet, loose stools, a pale facial complexion, a pale, fat tongue with slimy, white fur, and a fine, weak pulse

Treatment principles: Fortify the spleen and promote transportation, transform phlegm and eliminate dampness

Rx: *Zhi Shi Xiao Pi Wan Jia Jian* (Immature Aurantium Disperse Glomus Pills with Additions & Subtractions)

Ingredients: Fructus Crataegi (*Shan Zha*) and Radix Stephaniae Tetrandrae (*Han Fang Ji*), 30g each, Immaturus Citri Aurantii (*Zhi Shi*), Radix Codonopsitis Pilosulae (*Dang Shen*), and Semen Raphani Sativi (*Lai Fu Zi*), 15g each, Cortex Magnoliae Officinalis (*Hou Po*), Rhizoma Atractylodis Macrocephalae (*Bai Zhu*), Sclerotium Poriae Cocos (*Fu Ling*), Semen Sinapis Albae (*Bai Jie Zi*), and Rhizoma Alismatis (*Ze Xie*), 9g each, and mix-fried Radix Glycyrrhizae (*Gan Cao*), 6g

Analysis of formula: *Dang Shen, Bai Zhu, Fu Ling,* and mix-fried *Gan Cao* are the four ingredients of *Si Jun Zi Tang* (Four Gentlemen Decoction), a main formula for fortifying the spleen and supplementing the qi. *Shan Zha* and *Lai Fu Zi* disperse food and promote the transformative function of the spleen. *Han Fang Ji, Fu Ling,* and *Ze Xie* seep dampness. *Hou Po* moves the qi and transforms dampness. *Bai Jie Zi, Fu Ling,* and *Ze Xie* transform phlegm. *Zhi Shi* aids *Hou Po* in moving the qi to help disperse phlegm and dampness.

Additions & subtractions: If there is headache and dizziness, add nine grams of Flos Chrysanthemi Morifolii (*Ju Hua*) and 15 grams of Radix Ligustici Wallichii (*Chuan Xiong*). If there is constipation, add six grams of Mirabilitum (*Mang Xiao*) and up to 15 grams of Radix Et Rhizoma Rhei

(*Da Huang*). If spleen vacuity has reached the kidneys and there are more marked signs of vacuity cold, add nine grams of Radix Lateralis Praeparatus Aconiti Carmichaeli (*Fu Zi*) and six grams of dry Rhizoma Zingiberis (*Gan Jiang*).

For liver-spleen disharmony with phlegm dampness and obesity, edema, bright, shiny skin, pitting edema, chest oppression, abdominal fullness, heart palpitations, shortness of breath, dizziness, head distention, easy anger, mental depression, lack of happiness, frequent sighing, fatigue, hypersomnia or somnolence, scanty menstruation or amenorrhea, scanty urine, dry stools, a swollen tongue with slimy fur, and a deep, bowstring, slippery pulse, replace *Zhi Shi Xiao Pi Wan Jia Jian* with Radix Codonopsitis Pilosulae (*Dang Shen*), Sclerotium Poriae Cocos (*Fu Ling*), and Rhizoma Alismatis (*Ze Xie*), 15g each, and Radix Bupleuri (*Chai Hu*), Rhizoma Polygonati (*Huang Jing*), Fructus Immaturus Citri Aurantii (*Zhi Shi*), Cortex Magnoliae Officinalis (*Hou Po*), Rhizoma Atractylodis Macrocephalae (*Bai Zhu*), Rhizoma Pinelliae Ternatae (*Ban Xia*), Pericarpium Citri Reticulatae (*Chen Pi*), Fructus Crataegi (*Shan Zha*), and Radix Salviae Miltiorrhizae (*Dan Shen*), 9g each.

For liver-spleen disharmony with depressive heat and a red facial complexion, an obese torso but emaciation of the limbs, facial acne, headache, dizziness, easy anger, rib-side fullness or pain, tremor of hands, mental depression, frequent sighing, reduced appetite, loose stools, abdominal distention, fatigue, nausea, a possible bitter taste in the mouth, red tongue edges and tip, and a bowstring, fine pulse, replace *Zhi Shi Xiao Pi Wan Jia Jian* with *Dan Zhi Xiao Yao San Jia Jian* (Moutan & Gardenia Rambling Powder with Additions & Subtractions): Radix Bupleuri (*Chai Hu*), Radix Angelicae Sinensis (*Dang Gui*), Radix Albus Paeoniae Lactiflorae (*Bai Shao*), Sclerotium Poriae Cocos (*Fu Ling*), Rhizoma Polygonati (*Huang Jing*), Rhizoma Atractylodis Macrocephalae (*Bai Zhu*), mix-fried Radix Glycyrrhizae (*Gan Cao*), Cortex Radicis Moutan (*Dan Pi*), Fructus Gardeniae Jasminoidis (*Zhi Zi*), and Radix Ledebouriellae Divaricatae (*Fang Feng*), 9g each, Bombyx Batryticatus (*Jiang Can*) and Periostracum Cicadae (*Chan Tui*), 6g each, and dry Rhizoma Zingiberis (*Gan Jiang*) and Radix Gentianae Scabrae (*Long Dan Cao*), 3g each.

ACUPUNCTURE & MOXIBUSTION: *Zu San Li* (St 36), *Yin Ling Quan* (Sp 9), *Feng Long* (St 40), *Guan Yuan* (CV 4)

ANALYSIS OF FORMULA: Supplementing *Zu San Li* fortifies the spleen and boosts the qi. Draining *Yin Ling Quan* disinhibits dampness, while draining *Feng Long* transforms phlegm. Supplementing *Guan Yuan* with moxibustion warms and supplements the spleen and kidneys.

ADDITIONS & SUBTRACTIONS: If there is headache and dizziness, add *Bai Hui* (GV 20). If there is constipation, add *Zhi Gou* (TB 6). If spleen vacuity has reached the kidneys and there are more marked signs of vacuity cold, add *Shen Shu* (Bl 23). For liver-spleen disharmony with phlegm dampness, add *Nei Guan* (Per 6) and *Tai Chong* (Liv 3). For liver-spleen disharmony with depressive heat, add *Tai Chong* (Liv 3) and *He Gu* (LI 4). For severe edema, add *San Yin Jiao* (Sp 6) and *Shui Fen* (CV 9). For severe fatigue, lack of strength, and lassitude of the spirit, add *Tai Bai* (Sp 3). For venter and abdominal glomus and distention, add *Tian Shu* (St 25).

5. SPLEEN-KIDNEY YANG VACUITY PATTERN

MAIN SYMPTOMS: A somber white facial complexion, bodily edema, dizziness, aversion to cold and a liking for warmth, fatigue, weak limbs, heart palpitations, easy sweating, reduced appetite, scanty stools but profuse urine, impotence, reduced sexual desire, lusterless hair, soft bones, a pale tongue with thin fur, and a deep, soft pulse

TREATMENT PRINCIPLES: Fortify the spleen and boost the qi, supplement the kidneys and invigorate yang

RX: *Huang Qi Yi Yi Ren Fu Zi Tang* (Astragalus, Coix & Aconite Decoction)

INGREDIENTS: Semen Coicis Lachryma-jobi (*Yi Yi Ren*) and Radix Astragali Membranacei (*Huang Qi*), 20g each, Radix Codonopsitis Pilosulae (*Dang Shen*) and Sclerotium Poriae Cocos (*Fu Ling*), 15g each, Radix Lateralis Praeparatus Aconiti Carmichaeli (*Fu Zi*), Rhizoma Atractylodis Macrocephalae (*Bai Zhu*), Pericarpium Citri Reticulatae (*Chen Pi*), Rhizoma Pinelliae Ternatae (*Ban Xia*), and Pericarpium Arecae Catechu (*Da Fu Pi*), 9g each, dry Rhizoma Zingiberis (*Gan Jiang*) and mix-fried Radix Glycyrrhizae (*Gan Cao*), 6g each, and Fructus Zizyphi Jujubae (*Da Zao*), 6 pieces

ANALYSIS OF FORMULA: *Yi Yi Ren, Huang Qi, Fu Ling,* and *Da Fu Pi* seep dampness by disinhibiting urination. *Huang Qi, Dang Shen, Bai Zhu, Fu Ling, Da Zao,* and mix-fried *Gan Cao* all supplement the spleen and boost the qi. *Fu Zi* and *Gan Jiang* warm spleen and kidney yang, while *Ban Xia* and *Chen Pi* rectify the qi at the same time as dispelling dampness and turbidity.

ADDITIONS & SUBTRACTIONS: If there is impotence and reduced sexual desire, add nine grams each of Herba Epimedii (*Xian Ling Pi*) and Rhizoma Curculiginis Orchioidis (*Xian Mao*). If there is low back pain, add nine grams each of Cortex Eucommiae Ulmoidis (*Du Zhong*) and Radix Dipsaci (*Xu Duan*).

ACUPUNCTURE & MOXIBUSTION: *Fu Liu* (Ki 7), *San Yin Jiao* (Sp 6), *Zu San Li* (St 36), *Guan Yuan* (CV 4), *Ming Men* (GV 4)

ANALYSIS OF FORMULA: *Zu San Li* and *San Yin Jiao* supplement and boost the spleen qi. *Fu Liu* and *San Yin Jiao* supplement and invigorate kidney yang. The combination of *Guan Yuan* and *Ming Men* also supplements the kidneys and invigorates yang. Needle all these points with supplementing method and moxa *Guan Yuan* and *Ming Men*.

ADDITIONS & SUBTRACTIONS: If there is marked dampness, add *Yin Ling Quan* (Sp 9). For dizziness, add *Bai Hui* (GV 20). For tinnitus, add *Ting Hui* (GB 2). For heart palpitations and insomnia, add *Shen Men* (Ht 7). For persistent vaginal discharge, add *Dai Mai* (GB 26). For impotence and premature ejaculation, add *Zhi Shi* (Bl 52). For amenorrhea, add *Gui Lai* (St 29).

6. YIN & YANG DUAL VACUITY PATTERN

MAIN SYMPTOMS: Red face and eyes, malar flushing, a fat face and edematous body, especially in the lower limbs, spontaneous perspiration and night sweats, dizziness, tinnitus, heart palpitations, insomnia, weakness of the four limbs, low back and knee soreness and limpness, vexatious heat, cold feet, nocturia, persistent vaginal discharge, impotence, premature ejaculation, amenorrhea, a pale, fat, tender tongue with red tip or red tongue with scanty fur, and a fine, bowstring, possibly rapid pulse that may also be deep in either or both cubit positions

TREATMENT PRINCIPLES: Supplement the kidneys and nourish the liver, enrich yin and invigorate yang

RX: *Er Xian Tang Jia Jian* (Two Immortals Decoction with Additions & Subtractions)

INGREDIENTS: Radix Albus Paeoniae Lactiflorae (*Bai Shao*), 18g, uncooked Radix Rehmanniae (*Sheng Di*), 12g, and Rhizoma Anemarrhenae Aspheloidis (*Zhi Mu*), Cortex Phellodendri (*Huang Bai*), Rhizoma Curculiginis Orchioidis (*Xian Mao*), Herba Epimedii (*Xian Ling Pi*), and Radix Angelicae Sinensis (*Dang Gui*), 9g each

ANALYSIS OF FORMULA: *Sheng Di*, *Bai Shao*, and *Dang Gui* nourish liver blood and enrich kidney yin. *Zhi Mu* and *Huang Bai* drain fire and clear vacuity heat. *Xian Mao* and *Yin Yang Huo* warm and supplement kidney yang.

ADDITIONS & SUBTRACTIONS: If there is marked qi vacuity, add 15 grams of Radix Astragali Membranacei (*Huang Qi*) and nine grams of Radix Codonopsitis Pilosulae (*Dang Shen*). If there is marked dampness, add nine grams each of Rhizoma Atractylodis Macrocephalae (*Bai Zhu*), Sclerotium Poriae Cocos (*Fu Ling*), and Rhizoma Alismatis (*Ze Xie*).

ACUPUNCTURE & MOXIBUSTION: *Fu Liu* (Ki 7), *San Yin Jiao* (Sp 6), *Tai Xi* (Ki 3), *Guan Yuan* (CV 4), *Ming Men* (GV 4)

ANALYSIS OF FORMULA: *Fu Liu*, *San Yin Jiao*, *Tai Xi*, *Guan Yuan*, and *Ming Men* together supplement the kidneys and nourish the liver, enrich yin and invigorate yang. Needle all these points with supplementing method and moxa *Guan Yuan* and *Ming Men*.

ADDITIONS & SUBTRACTIONS: If there is marked qi vacuity, add *Zu San Li* (St 36). If there is marked dampness, add *Yin Ling Quan* (Sp 9). For spontaneous perspiration and night sweats, add *He Gu* (LI 4). For dizziness, add *Bai Hui* (GV 20). For tinnitus, add *Ting Hui* (GB 2). For heart palpitations and insomnia, add *Shen Men* (Ht 7). For persistent vaginal discharge, add *Dai Mai* (GB 26). For impotence and premature ejaculation, add *Zhi Shi* (Bl 52). For amenorrhea, add *Gui Lai* (St 29).

REMARKS

1. When attempting to get off corticosteroids, it is imperative that the patient be under the care of the prescribing physician and that the physician determine the schedule of withdrawal. Sudden discontinuance of corticosteroids may have dire consequences.

2. During steroid therapy, there is often rapid hungering and excessive appetite. When steroids are withdrawn, rapid hungering often swings to lack of appetite and torpid intake. In this case, lack of appetite is usually due to spleen vacuity but may be complicated by food stagnation and/or phlegm dampness.

3. Many patients prescribed steroids already suffer from qi and yin vacuity with damp heat, and steroids may aggravate any of these three disease mechanisms.

4. Cushing's syndrome may cause hypertension and hypercholesterolemia. Therefore, medicinals which are hypertensive, such as Radix Glycyrrhizae (*Gan Cao*), should either be used with care or avoided when treating this condition.

5. As with all other conditions in Chinese medicine, treatment should mainly be based on the patient's personal pattern discrimination. The above protocols are only meant as illustrative examples.

6. Some Chinese doctor's have recently suggested that iatrogenic Cushing's syndrome due to administration of corticosteroids should be seen as a type of kidney essence congestion and gathering resulting in both blood stasis and internal accumulation of water dampness. We believe that this suggested disease mechanism does not account for all the patterns presented in real-life by those with Cushing's syndrome and that it is based on an overly simplistic equation of steroids with kidney essence supplements. Such an equation fails to explain why steroids such as Prednisone are anti-inflammatory and pain-relieving.

24

Diabetes Mellitus

Diabetes mellitus (DM) is the name of a syndrome whose main characteristics are abnormal insulin secretion, elevated glucose levels, and a variety of complications, such as nephropathy, retinopathy, neuropathy, and accelerated atherosclerosis. Its etiology seems to be a variable interaction between hereditary, dietary, and environmental factors. Many Western scientists consider it an autoimmune disease. There are two main types of diabetes mellitus, Type I or insulin-dependent diabetes mellitus (IDDM) and Type II or noninsulin-dependent diabetes mellitus (NIDDM).

Type I patients are dependent upon exogenous insulin to prevent ketoacidosis and death. Seventy-five percent of Type I diabetics have antibodies to their own pancreatic cells, and viral infections may be responsible for initiating such an autoimmune response. Viruses which may induce this reaction include pertussis, hepatitis, rubella, coxsackie, Epstein-Barr viruses, cytomegalovirus, and herpes virus 6. Susceptibility to Type I diabetes may also be genetically predetermined. Ongoing immunologic research suggests that Type I diabetes occurs predominantly in persons with specific tissue types.[1]

Type II patients may or may not use exogenous insulin but do not need exogenous insulin for survival. Diet, obesity, allergies to certain foods, viral infections, and stress are all factors that can contribute to the onset of or aggravate Type II diabetes. An estimated 85% of Type II diabetics are overweight when diagnosed.[2] As Dr. Ernest Pfeiffer, Professor of Medicine at Ulm University in Germany says, "It's almost a law that any person 30% overweight for 30 years will become a [Type II] diabetic."[3]

There is also a third type of diabetes – gestational diabetes. This is where glucose intolerance develops or is discovered during pregnancy. Characterized by excessive hunger, thirst, and a need to urinate, it is a mild condition and often goes unnoticed. However, it is an important condition to treat because elevated blood sugar levels can damage the fetus. Gestational diabetes can usually be controlled with diet but may require insulin. This type of diabetes usually disappears or becomes subclinical following the end of pregnancy.

According to the U.S. Department of Health & Human Services, there are nearly 6,000,000 diabetics in the U.S. which was the seventh leading cause of death in 1991.

The earliest symptom of elevated blood glucose is polyuria. Continued hyperglycemia and glucosuria may lead to thirst, hunger, and weight loss. Glucosuria is also associated with an increased incidence of monilial vaginitis and itching. Accelerated fat catabolism in untreated insulin-dependent patients may produce ketoacidosis leading to anorexia, nausea, vomiting, air hunger, and, if left untreated, coma and death. The onset of this condition tends to be abrupt in children and insidious in older patients. In older patients, the age of onset is usually over 40. Diabetics are 3.5 times at higher risk to die of cardiovascular disease, 30% of diabetics develop peripheral vascular disease, and leg and foot amputations are five times more common in diabetics than in nondiabetic persons. A significant majority of these amputees have a history of smoking. Renal failure is seen in 50% of IDDM patients after 20-30 years of diabetes. Diabetic retinopathy is usually first detected five years or more after diagnosis of DM and is present in 50% of patients after 10 years. Impotence in the male is the most common symptom of neuropathy in DM, affecting 50-60% of male patients.

The Western medical diagnosis of diabetes mellitus is based on 1) unequivocal elevation of plasma glucose concentration along with the typical symptoms of polyuria, polydipsia, ketonuria, and rapid weight loss, 2) a fasting plasma glucose concentration equal to or above 140mg/dL, or 3) elevated plasma glucose concentration after an oral glucose challenge on more than one occasion. Unfortunately, the absence of a single precise marker for DM continues to be a problem within Western medicine.

The Western medical treatment of diabetes primarily relies on dietary avoidance of sugars and sweets, the regular scheduling of meals, weight loss (for NIDDM), and, when necessary, insulin replacement therapy. There are as many as seven different types of injectible insulin currently prescribed in the United States, each having their own time to onset of action, peak action, and duration of action. Complications of insulin treatment include insulin shock, *i.e.*, hypoglycemia, if too much insulin or too little food are taken, local reactions to insulin injections, such as heat, induration, erythema, and urticaria, and insulin resistance. Several oral sulfonylureates that lower blood glucose level may be used to treat selected patients. However, these are not adequate for treating IDDM patients. When hypertension complicates diabetes, diuretics and sympathetic inhibitors may accelerate or worsen impotence.

CHINESE DISEASE CATEGORIZATION: Diabetes mellitus is traditionally categorized as *xiao ke*, wasting thirst or wasting and thirsting. However, because polyphagia, polydipsia, and polyuria are three of the most common symptoms of this condition, it also falls under *duo shi*, profuse eating, *duo yin*, profuse drinking, and *duo niao*, profuse urination. Other conditions associated with this disease include *fei pang*, obesity, *yang wei*, impotence, *ma mu*, tingling and numbness, *chuang yang*, sores, and *qing mang*, clear-eyed blindness.

DISEASE CAUSES: Former heaven natural endowment insufficiency, aging, unregulated eating and drinking, and internal damage by the seven affects

DISEASE MECHANISMS: In juvenile-onset diabetes, the disease mechanism appears to be a natural endowment insufficiency, whereas, in adults, this disease typically begins with long-standing heat in the stomach coupled with spleen vacuity.[4] This heat may be due to over-eating hot, spicy, greasy, fatty, thick-flavored foods or alcohol or to depressive heat of the liver and stomach and gives rise to a large appetite and/or rapid hungering after meals. The spleen vacuity may be due to over-eating sugars and sweets and/or fatty, thick-flavored foods, too much thinking, too little exercise, and too much taxation fatigue. Spleen vacuity is responsible for obesity and fatigue initially and also for anorexia, emaciation, and muscular atrophy as this disease progresses. If heat endures, it eventually damages and consumes yin fluids in the stomach and lungs, giving rise to polydipsia. If lung-stomach yin vacuity reaches the kidneys and is complicated by yin vacuity due to aging, lung-stomach yin vacuity may evolve into kidney yin vacuity. If spleen qi vacuity evolves into kidney yang vacuity, there may be kidney yin and yang dual vacuity. Kidney yin and/or yang vacuity give rise to urinary problems as well as impotence. Because all adult diabetics also exhibit signs and symptoms of liver depression qi stagnation, long-term qi stagnation coupled with qi and blood vacuity, typically gives rise to blood stasis. In addition, spleen vacuity often also becomes complicated by damp heat which pours downward, resulting in sores, urinary disturbances, impotence, restless leg syndrome, and/or vaginitis.

TREATMENT BASED ON PATTERN DISCRIMINATION:

1. LUNG-STOMACH HEAT ACCUMULATION & FLUID DAMAGE PATTERN

MAIN SYMPTOMS: Vexatious thirst, polydipsia, a dry mouth and tongue, frequent urination which is excessive in amount, red tongue edges and tip, thin, yellow tongue fur, and a surging, rapid pulse

NOTE: This pattern is also referred to as upper wasting since its main symptom is excessive thirst. It typically corresponds to early stage diabetes.

TREATMENT PRINCIPLES: Clear heat from the lungs and stomach, engender fluids and stop thirst

RX: *Yang Yin Qing Fei Tang Jia Jian* (Nourish Yin & Clear the Lungs Decoction with Additions & Subtractions)

INGREDIENTS: Gypsum Fibrosum (*Shi Gao*), 18g, Radix Scrophulariae Ningpoensis (*Xuan Shen*), Radix Salviae Miltiorrhizae (*Dan Shen*), and uncooked Radix Rehmanniae (*Sheng Di*), 15g each, Tuber Ophiopogonis Japonicae (*Mai Dong*) and Tuber Asparagi Cochinensis (*Tian Dong*), 12g each, Herba Dendrobii (*Shi Hu*), Rhizoma Anemarrhenae Aspheloidis (*Zhi Mu*), Radix Trichosanthis Kirlowii (*Hua Fen*), Radix Albus Paeoniae Lactiflorae (*Bai Shao*), and Cortex Radicis Moutan (*Dan Pi*), 9g each, and Radix Glycyrrhizae (*Gan Cao*), 6g

ANALYSIS OF FORMULA: *Shi Gao* drains fire and clears heat from the lungs and stomach. *Mai Men Dong*, *Tian Men Dong*, and *Zhi Mu* clear heat, moisten the lungs, and engender fluids. *Sheng Di*, *Shi Hu*, and *Tian Hua Fen* clear heat, nourish yin, and engender fluids. *Xuan Shen* clears vacuity heat. *Bai Shao* nourishes the blood, remembering that blood and fluids share a common source. It also restrains the liver, remembering that the liver and lungs work hand in hand to control the flow of qi, and if one becomes vacuous and weak, the other tends to become exuberant and effulgent. *Dan Pi* quickens and clears heat from the blood. In this formula, it helps prevent flaring of ministerial fire due to mutual engenderment. *Gan Cao* harmonizes the other medicinals. *Mai Men Dong*,

Tian Men Dong, Zhi Mu, Sheng Di, Tian Hua Fen, and *Xuan Shen* have all also been shown to lower blood sugar.

Additions & subtractions: If there is liver depression qi stagnation, add nine grams each of Fructus Meliae Toosendan (*Chuan Lian Zi*) and Radix Auklandiae Lappae (*Mu Xiang*). If there is marked spleen vacuity with fatigue (as there most commonly is), add 20 grams of Radix Astragali Membranacei (*Huang Qi*) and Radix Dioscoreae Oppositae (*Shan Yao*) and nine grams of Radix Codonopsitis Pilosulae (*Dang Shen*). If there is polyphagia and rapid hungering after eating denoting even more effulgent stomach heat, increase the dosage of *Shi Gao* up to 30-50 grams and add 12 grams of Rhizoma Polygonati Odorati (*Yu Zhu*). For constipation, add 12-18 grams of Radix Et Rhizoma Polygoni Cuspidati (*Hu Zhang*). For heart palpitations, add 12 grams each of Semen Zizyphi Spinosae (*Suan Zao Ren*) and Semen Biotae Orientalis (*Bai Zi Ren*). For tongue sores and reddish urine showing that heat has also accumulated in the heart, add nine grams each of Fructus Gardeniae Jasminoidis (*Zhi Zi*) and Folium Bambusae (*Zhu Ye*).

Acupuncture & moxibustion: *Chi Ze* (Lu 5), *Fu Liu* (Ki 7), *Nei Ting* (St 44)

Analysis of formula: Based on the saying, "To treat upper wasting, moisten the lungs and clear the stomach," draining *Chi Ze* clears and moistens the lungs. Supplementing *Fu Liu* helps to more strongly nourish lung yin. In this case, *Fu Liu* is not being used to supplement the kidneys but to engender fluids. Clearing *Nei Ting* clears heat from the stomach.

Additions & subtractions: For severe dryness of the lungs, add *Fei Shu* (Bl 13) and *San Yin Jiao* (Sp 6). For severe heat, add *He Gu* (LI 4). For concomitant spleen qi vacuity, add *Zu San Li* (St 36). For constipation, add *Zhi Gou* (TB 6). For tongue sores and reddish urine, add *Tong Li* (Ht 5).

2. Intense & exuberant stomach heat pattern

Main symptoms: Polyphagia and rapid hungering after eating are the predominant symptoms of this pattern. These are then complicated by lesser degrees of thirst and polyuria, bodily emaciation, dry, bound stools, a red tongue with yellow fur, and a slippery, large, forceful pulse.

Note: This pattern is also called middle wasting.

Treatment principles: Clear the stomach and drain fire, moisten the intestines and free the flow of the stools

Rx: *Yan Shi Zhong Xiao Fang Jia Jian* (Master Yan's Middle Wasting Formula with Additions & Subtractions)

Ingredients: Uncooked Gypsum Fibrosum (*Shi Gao*) and Rhizoma Phragmitis Communis (*Lu Gen*), 30g each, Radix Scrophulariae Ningpoensis (*Xuan Shen*), 15g, Fructus Gardeniae Jasminoidis (*Shan Zhi*), Radix Et Rhizoma Rhei (*Da Huang*), Cortex Radicis Moutan (*Dan Pi*), Semen Pruni Persicae (*Tao Ren*), and Radix Scutellariae Baicalensis (*Huang Qin*), 9g each, and Rhizoma Coptidis Chinensis (*Huang Lian*), 3g

Analysis of formula: *Shi Gao* and *Lu Gen* clear the stomach and engender fluids. *Zhi Zi, Huang Qin*, and *Huang Lian* clear the stomach and drain fire. *Da Huang* clears heat and frees the flow of the stools. *Xuan Shen* clears vacuity heat, nourishes yin, and also frees the flow of the stools. *Dan Pi* and *Tao Ren* quicken the blood and transform stasis on the one hand, but *Tao Ren* also moistens the intestines to help *Da Huang* to free the flow of the stools.

Additions & subtractions: For severe constipation with dry stools, add 6-9 grams of Mirabilitum (*Mang Xiao*). For swollen, painful gums due to stomach fire, add nine grams each of Fructus Forsythiae Suspensae (*Lian Qiao*) and Radix Achyranthis Bidentatae (*Niu Xi*). For severe thirst and frequent urination, add 15 grams each of Radix Dioscoreae Oppositae (*Shan Yao*) and cooked Radix Rehmanniae (*Shu Di*) as well as nine grams each of Radix Glehniae Littoralis (*Sha Shen*) and Fructus Schisandrae Chinensis (*Wu Wei Zi*). For concomitant qi vacuity, add 20 grams each of Radix Dioscoreae Oppositae (*Shan Yao*) and Radix Astragali Membranacei (*Huang Qi*). Please also see the preceding pattern.

Acupuncture & moxibustion: *Zu San Li* (St 36), *Nei Ting* (St 44), *Fu Liu* (Ki 7)

Analysis of formula: Based on the saying, "To treat middle wasting, clear the stomach and enrich the kidneys," draining *Nei Ting* and *Zu San Li* clears the stomach and drains fire. Supplementing *Fu Liu* enriches kidney yin to protect the yin fluids of the stomach since the kidneys are the root of yin in the body.

Additions & subtractions: For severe constipation, add *Zhi Gou* (TB 6). For severe thirst, add *Fei Shu* (Bl 13) and *San Yin Jiao* (Sp 6). For severe heat, add *He Gu* (LI 4). For concomitant spleen qi vacuity, add *Pi Shu Li* (BL 20). For tongue sores and reddish urine, add *Tong Li* (Ht 5).

3. Qi & yin dual vacuity pattern

Main symptoms: Excessive thirst, frequent, copious, possibly turbid urination, frequent night-time urination, fatigue, lassitude of the spirit, shortness of breath, possible dry stools and constipation, a pale facial complexion with possible malar flushing, emaciation, possible heart palpitations, impaired memory, dizziness, vexatious heat in the five hearts, insomnia, profuse dreams, spontaneous perspiration and/or night sweats, a fat, swollen, red tongue with scanty fur and fluids, and a fine, weak pulse

TREATMENT PRINCIPLES: Boost the qi and engender fluids, moisten dryness and stop thirst

RX: *Yu Ye Tang* (Jade Humor Decoction)

INGREDIENTS: Radix Dioscoreae Oppositae (*Shan Yao*), 30g, Rhizoma Anemarrhenae Aspheloidis (*Zhi Mu*), 18g, Radix Astragali Membranacei (*Huang Qi*), 15g, Radix Trichosanthis Kirlowii (*Tian Hua Fen*), Fructus Schisandrae Chinensis (*Wu Wei Zi*), and Radix Puerariae (*Ge Gen*), 9g each, and Endothelium Corneum Gigeriae Galli (*Ji Nei Jin*), 6g

ANALYSIS OF FORMULA: *Huang Qi*, *Shan Yao*, and *Wu Wei Zi* boost the qi without damaging yin. *Zhi Mu*, *Wu Wei Zi*, *Tian Hua Fen*, and *Ge Gen* engender fluids, moisten dryness, and stop thirst. In addition, *Shan Yao* and *Wu Wei Zi* restrain urination, *Zhi Mu* clears vacuity heat, *Ge Gen* upbears the clear, and *Tian Hua Fen* clears heat. *Ji Nei Jin* helps the transformation of the spleen and also restrains urination.

ADDITIONS & SUBTRACTIONS: For more marked fatigue, add nine grams each of Radix Codonopsitis Pilosulae (*Dang Shen*) and Radix Pseudostellariae (*Tai Zi Shen*) as well as six grams of mix-fried Radix Glycyrrhizae (*Gan Cao*). For concomitant blood stasis, add 15 grams of Radix Salviae Miltiorrhizae (*Dan Shen*) and nine grams each of Semen Pruni Persicae (*Tao Ren*) and Cortex Radicis Moutan (*Dan Pi*). If there is liver depression qi stagnation, add nine grams each of Fructus Meliae Toosendan (*Chuan Lian Zi*) and Radix Auklandiae Lappae (*Mu Xiang*). For heart palpitations with a bound or regularly interrupted pulse, add 15 grams of Concha Ostreae (*Mu Li*), 12 grams of Semen Zizyphi Spinosae (*Suan Zao Ren*), and nine grams of Ramulus Cinnamomi Cassiae (*Gui Zhi*). For loose stools, add 15 grams of Semen Coicis Lachryma-jobi (*Yi Yi Ren*) and nine grams each of Sclerotium Poriae Cocos (*Fu Ling*) and Semen Plantaginis (*Che Qian Zi*). For constipation, add 12 grams each of Radix Scrophulariae Ningpoensis (*Xuan Shen*), uncooked Radix Rehmanniae (*Sheng Di*), and Tuber Ophiopogonis Japonici (*Mai Men Dong*). For predominant yin vacuity with fire effulgence, add 15 grams of Cortex Radicis Lycii Chinensis (*Di Gu Pi*) and nine grams of Cortex Phellodendri (*Huang Bai*).

ACUPUNCTURE & MOXIBUSTION: *Zu San Li* (St 36), *Fu Liu* (Ki 7), *San Yin Jiao* (Sp 6)

ANALYSIS OF FORMULA: Supplementing *Zu San Li* and *San Yin Jiao* fortifies the spleen and boosts the qi. Supplementing *Fu Liu* and *San Yin Jiao* supplement water and engender fluids. Together, these three points supplement the spleen, stomach, liver, and kidneys.

ADDITIONS & SUBTRACTIONS: If there are polyphagia and rapid hungering after eating, add *Nei Ting* (St 44). If there is severe thirst, add *Chi Ze* (Lu 5). For severe fatigue, add *Pi Shu* (Bl 20) and *Wei Shu* (Bl 21). If there is copious, frequent urination, especially at night, add *Shen Shu* (Bl 23). For heat palpitations or impaired memory, add *Shen Men* (Ht 7). For night sweats, add *Yin Xi* (Ht 6). For spontaneous perspiration, add *He Gu* (LI 4).

4. KIDNEY YIN VACUITY PATTERN

MAIN SYMPTOMS: Frequent urination which is excessive in amount, possible turbid urine like fat or grease, even more frequent urination at night, a dry mouth, a dark, blackish facial complexion, scorched, dry auricles, dizziness, tinnitus, low back and knee soreness and limpness, itching, impotence, premature ejaculation, a red tongue with scanty, yellow fur or scanty fluids, and a fine, bowstring pulse

NOTE: This pattern is also called lower wasting.

TREATMENT PRINCIPLES: Supplement the kidneys and enrich yin, nourish and quicken the blood

RX: *Mai Wei Di Huang Wan Jia Wei* (Ophiopogon & Schisandra Rehmannia Pills with Added Flavors)

INGREDIENTS: Cooked Radix Rehmanniae (*Shu Di*), 30g, Radix Dioscoreae Oppositae (*Shan Yao*) and Radix Salviae Miltiorrhizae (*Dan Shen*), 15g each, Tuber Ophiopogonis Japonicae (*Mai Dong*), 12g, and Fructus Schizandrae Chinensis (*Wu Wei Zi*), Cortex Radicis Moutan (*Dan Pi*), Sclerotium Poriae Cocos (*Fu Ling*), Fructus Corni Officinalis (*Shan Zhu Yu*), Rhizoma Alismatis (*Ze Xie*), and Flos Carthami Tinctorii (*Hong Hua*), 9g each

ANALYSIS OF FORMULA: *Shu Di*, *Shan Zhu Yu*, *Shan Yao*, *Ze Xie*, *Dan Pi*, and *Fu Ling* are the six ingredients of *Liu Wei Di Huang Wan* (Six Flavors Rehmannia Pills) which is a main formula for supplementing the kidneys and enriching yin. *Wu Wei Zi* supplements the kidneys and restrains urination, engenders fluids and stops thirst. *Mai Men Dong* nourishes yin and engenders fluids. *Dan Shen*, *Dan Pi*, and *Hong Hua* quicken the blood and transform stasis.

ADDITIONS & SUBTRACTIONS: For marked vacuity heat and fire effulgence, add nine grams each of Cortex Phellodendri (*Huang Bai*) and Rhizoma Anemarrhenae Aspheloidis (*Zhi Mu*). For pronounced qi vacuity, add 15 grams of Radix Astragali Membranacei (*Huang Qi*) and nine grams of Radix Codonopsitis Pilosulae (*Dang Shen*). For marked dizziness and tinnitus due to liver-kidney yin vacuity, add 12 grams each of Fructus Lycii Chinensis (*Gou Qi Zi*) and Fructus Ligustri Lucidi (*Nu Zhen Zi*). For severe thirst, add 20 grams of Radix Trichosanthis Kirlowii (*Tian Hua Fen*). For profuse urination, add 15 grams of Ootheca Mantidis (*Sang Piao Xiao*) and nine grams of Fructus Alpiniae Oxyphyllae (*Yi Zhi Ren*). For insomnia, add 15 grams each of Caulis Polygoni Multiflori (*Ye Jiao Teng*) and Fructus Ligustri Lucidi (*Nu Zhen Zi*).

If there is dual yin and yang vacuity, replace *Mai Wei Di Huang Wan* with *Shen Qi Wan Jia Wei* (Kidney Qi Pills with Added Flavors): Cooked Radix Rehmanniae (*Shu Di*), 25g, Radix Dioscoreae Oppositae (*Shan Yao*), 15g, Fructus Corni Officinalis (*Shan Zhu Yu*), Sclerotium Poriae Cocos (*Fu Ling*), Fructus Lycii Chinensis (*Gou Qi Zi*), Semen Cuscutae Chinensis (*Tu Si Zi*), and Radix Astragali Membranacei (*Huang Qi*), 12g each, Cortex Radicis Moutan (*Dan Pi*) and Rhizoma Alismatis (*Ze Xie*), 9g each, and Cortex Cinnamomi Cassiae (*Rou Gui*) and Radix Lateralis Praeparatus Aconiti Carmichaeli (*Fu Zi*), 6g each. For impotence, add 12 grams of Herba Epimedii (*Yin Yang Huo*). For frequent, copious urination, add 12 grams each of Fructus Alpiniae Oxyphyllae (*Yi Zhi Ren*) and Ootheca Mantidis (*Sang Piao Xiao*). For spermatorrhea or premature ejaculation, add 12 grams each of Semen Euryalis Ferocis (*Qian Shi*), Fructus Rubi Chingii (*Fu Pen Zi*), and Fructus Rosae Laevigatae (*Jin Ying Zi*). For edema, add 12 grams each of Rhizoma Atractylodis Macrocephalae (*Bai Zhu*) and Semen Plantaginis (*Che Qian Zi*). For diarrhea, add 12 grams of Rhizoma Atractylodis Macrocephalae (*Bai Zhu*) and Fructus Psoraleae Corylifoliae (*Bu Gu Zhi*) and six grams of Semen Myristicae Fragrantis (*Rou Dou Kou*). For low back pain, add nine grams each of Radix Dipsaci (*Xu Duan*) and Cortex Eucommiae Ulmoidis (*Du Zhong*). For concomitant blood stasis, add nine grams each of Radix Salviae Miltiorrhizae (*Dan Shen*) and Flos Carthami Tinctorii (*Hong Hua*).

ACUPUNCTURE & MOXIBUSTION: *Fu Liu* (Ki 7), *Tai Xi* (Ki 3), *Shen Shu* (Bl 23), *Tai Yuan* (Lu 9)

ANALYSIS OF FORMULA: Based on the saying, "To treat lower wasting, enrich the kidneys and supplement the lungs," supplementing *Fu Liu*, *Tai Xi*, and *Shen Shu* supplements the kidneys and enriches yin, while supplementing *Tai Yuan* supplements the lungs.

ADDITIONS & SUBTRACTIONS: If there is polyphagia and rapid hungering after eating, add *Nei Ting* (St 44). If there is severe thirst, add *Pi Shu* (Bl 20) and *Wei Shu* (Bl 21). If there is severe fatigue, add *Pi Shu* (Bl 20) and *Wei Shu* (Bl 21). If there is frequent, copious urination, especially at night, add *San Yin Jiao* (Sp 6). For heart palpitations or impaired memory, add *Shen Men* (Ht 7). For night sweats, add *Yin Xi* (Ht 6). For spontaneous perspiration, add *He Gu* (LI 4).

5. SPLEEN-STOMACH QI VACUITY PATTERN

MAIN SYMPTOMS: Excessive thirst, a normal or reduced appetite but, in all the cases, loose stools, devitalized essence spirit, abdominal distention, especially after meals, emaciation, weakness of the four limbs, fatigue, a pale tongue with dry, white fur, and a fine, forceless pulse.

NOTE: This pattern is sometimes a consequence of treatment with the kind of very cold, very bitter medicinals which are often used to treat heat patterns of wasting thirst. In Western clinics, it is rarely seen in this simple, discrete form. However, spleen qi vacuity commonly complicates other patterns of this disease. Here, the thirst is not due to heat but due to the spleen's failure to transport and transform fluids. Thus fluids are not upborne to the mouth but rather accumulate as dampness in the middle.

TREATMENT PRINCIPLES: Fortify the spleen and boost the qi, transform fluids and stop thirst

RX: *Qi Wei Bai Zhu San Jia Wei* (Seven Flavors Atractylodes Powder with Added Flavors)

INGREDIENTS: Radix Astragali Membranacei (*Huang Qi*) and Radix Dioscoreae Oppositae (*Shan Yao*), 20g each, Rhizoma Atractylodis Macrocephalae (*Bai Zhu*), Radix Puerariae (*Ge Gen*), and Sclerotium Poriae Cocos (*Fu Ling*), 12g each, Herba Agastachis Seu Pogostemi (*Huo Xiang*) and Radix Auklandiae Lappae (*Mu Xiang*), 9g each, and white Radix Panacis Ginseng (*Ren Shen*) and Radix Glycyrrhizae (*Gan Cao*), 6g each

ANALYSIS OF FORMULA: Within this formula, the four gentlemen (*i.e., Ren Shen, Fu Ling, Bai Zhu*, and *Gan Cao*) reinforced with *Huang Qi* and *Shan Yao* fortify the spleen and boost the qi. In addition, *Ren Shen, Fu Ling, Bai Zhu, Huang Qi, Shan Yao*, and *Ge Gen* are all empirically known to lower blood sugar. *Ge Gen* and *Huang Qi* upbear the clear, while *Huo Xiang* and *Mu Xiang* downbear the turbid. *Huo Xiang* arouses the spleen, and *Mu Xiang* moves the qi. All together, these medicinals harmonize the transportation and transformation of the spleen and the upbearing and downbearing of the center.

ADDITIONS & SUBTRACTIONS: If there is profuse urination, subtract *Fu Ling* and add nine grams each of Rhizoma Atractylodis (*Cang Zhu*), Galla Rhois Chinensis (*Wu Bei Zi*), and Fructus Alpiniae Oxyphyllae (*Yi Zhi Ren*). For concomitant kidney qi vacuity, add nine grams each of Herba Epimedii (*Yin Yang Huo*) and Semen Litchi Sinensis (*Li Zhi He*). For concomitant kidney yin vacuity, add 12 grams each of Fructus Lycii Chinensis (*Gou Qi Zi*) and Radix Polygoni Multiflori (*He Shou Wu*). For severe spleen qi vacuity, add 15 grams of Rhizoma Polygonati (*Huang Jing*) and 12 grams of Fructus Germinatus Hordei Vulgaris (*Mai Ya*).

ACUPUNCTURE & MOXIBUSTION: *Zu San Li* (St 36), *Tai Bai* (Sp 3), *San Yin Jiao* (Sp 6), *Qi Hai* (CV 6)

ANALYSIS OF FORMULA: Supplementing *Zu San Li*, *Tai Bai*, *San Yin Jiao*, and *Qi Hai* fortifies the spleen and boosts the qi, upbears the clear and downbears the turbid.

ADDITIONS & SUBTRACTIONS: If there is profuse urination add *Guan Yuan* (CV 4) with moxibustion. For concomitant kidney qi vacuity, add *Fu Liu* (Ki 7). For concomitant kidney yin vacuity, add *Tai Xi* (Ki 3). For severe spleen qi vacuity, add *Pi Shu* (Bl 20) and *Wei Shu* (Bl 21).

6. DAMP HEAT OBSTRUCTING THE CENTER PATTERN

MAIN SYMPTOMS: Thirst with a liking for profuse drinking, excessive eating with rapid hungering or only a feeling of hunger, ductal and abdominal glomus and oppression, possible nausea, yellow, slimy tongue fur, and a soggy or slippery, possibly rapid pulse

NOTE: This pattern is often a consequence of spleen vacuity which results in dampness which then transforms into heat.

TREATMENT PRINCIPLES: Clear heat and eliminate dampness

RX: *Huang Qin Hua Shi Tang Jia Jian* (Scutellaria & Talcum Decoction with Additions & Subtractions)

INGREDIENTS: Radix Scutellariae Baicalensis (*Huang Qin*), Talcum (*Hua Shi*), and Pericarpium Arecae Catechu (*Da Fu Pi*), 9g each, and Cortex Sclerotii Poriae Cocos (*Fu Ling Pi*), Rhizoma Alismatis (*Ze Xie*), Rhizoma Atractylodis (*Cang Zhu*), Cortex Phellodendri (*Huang Bai*), and Medulla Tetrapanacis Papyriferi (*Tong Cao*), 6g each

ANALYSIS OF FORMULA: *Huang Qin* and *Huang Bai* clear heat and dry dampness. *Cang Zhu* helps dry dampness. *Hua Shi*, *Zhu Ling*, and *Tong Cao* clear heat and disinhibit dampness. *Fu Ling* fortifies the spleen and seeps the dampness, and *Da Fu Pi* moves the qi and disinhibits dampness. *Huang Bai*, *Cang Zhu*, *Ze Xie*, and *Fu Ling* all are empirically known to lower blood sugar.

ADDITIONS & SUBTRACTIONS: For concomitant vacuity heat, add 12 grams each of Cortex Radicis Lycii Chinensis (*Di Gu Pi*) and Rhizoma Anemarrhenae Asphodeloidis (*Zhi Mu*). For damp heat damaging stomach yin, add 12 grams each of Tuber Ophiopogonis Japonici (*Mai Men Dong*) and Rhizoma Polygonati Odorati (*Yu Zhu*). For concomitant kidney yin vacuity, add 12 grams each of Fructus Lycii Chinensis (*Gou Qi Zi*) and Radix Polygoni Multiflori (*He Shou Wu*). For concomitant spleen vacuity, add 15 grams of Radix Dioscoreae Oppositae (*Shan Yao*), nine grams of Rhizoma Atractylodis Macrocephalae (*Bai Zhu*), and six grams of Radix Panacis Ginseng (*Ren Shen*). For thirst, add 12 grams each of Radix Puerariae (*Ge Gen*) and Radix Trichosanthis Kirlowii (*Tian Hua Fen*).

ACUPUNCTURE & MOXIBUSTION: *Zhong Wan* (CV 12), *Nei Ting* (St 44), *Yin Ling Quan* (Sp 9)

ANALYSIS OF FORMULA: Draining *Zhong Wan*, *Nei Ting*, and *Yin Ling Quan* clears heat and transforms dampness, especially in the middle burner. One can also use the formula *Qu Chi* (LI 11), *San Yin Jiao* (Sp 6), and *Yang Ling Quan* (GB 34). Please see remark #8 below.

ADDITIONS & SUBTRACTIONS: For concomitant vacuity heat, add *Fu Liu* (Ki 7) and *San Yin Jiao* (Sp 6). For damp heat damaging stomach yin, add *Wei Shu* (Bl 21) and *Fu Liu* (Ki 7). For concomitant kidney yin vacuity, add *Shen Shu* (Bl 23) and *Fu Liu* (Ki 7). For concomitant spleen vacuity, add *Zu San Li* (St 36). For thirst, add *Yu Ji* (Lu 10).

7. SPLEEN-KIDNEY YANG VACUITY PATTERN

MAIN SYMPTOMS: The three polys (polydipsia, polyphagia, and polyuria) are not very marked. Instead, there is aversion to cold, a possible chilly feeling in the abdomen, fatigued spirit, bodily weakness, shortness of breath, low back and knee soreness and limpness, tinnitus, deafness, seminal emission or impotence, spontaneous perspiration, frequent, clear, sometimes profuse urination or urinary incontinence, possible turbid urine, loose stools or fifth-watch diarrhea, a pale, swollen tongue with moist, white fur, and a deep, thin, forceless pulse, especially in the bar and cubit positions.

NOTE: This pattern is often seen in patients over 50 years old.

TREATMENT PRINCIPLES: Fortify the spleen and warm the kidneys, regulate yin and yang

RX: *Jian Pi Wen Shen Jiang Tang Fang* (Fortify the Spleen, Warm the Kidneys & Lower [Blood] Sugar Formula)

INGREDIENTS: Cooked Radix Rehmanniae (*Shu Di*), Fructus Lycii Chinensis (*Gou Qi*), and Radix Dioscoreae Oppositae (*Shan Yao*), 15g each, Radix Lateralis Praeparatus Aconiti Carmichaeli (*Fu Zi*), Fructus Corni Officinalis (*Shan Zhu Yu*), Fructus Psoraleae Corylifoliae (*Bu Gu Zhi*), Rhizoma Atractylodis (*Cang Zhu*), Rhizoma Atractylodis Macrocephalae (*Bai Zhu*), Semen Nelumbinis Nuciferae (*Lian Zi*), Endothelium Corneum Gigeriae Galli (*Ji Nei Jin*), and Galla Rhois Chinensis (*Wu Bei Zi*), 9g each, and dry Rhizoma Zingiberis (*Gan Jiang*), 5g

ANALYSIS OF FORMULA: *Shu Di*, *Gou Qi*, and *Shan Zhu Yu* enrich kidney yin to supplement kidney yang. *Fu Zi* and *Gan*

Jiang warm both the spleen and the kidneys. *Shan Yao, Cang Zhu, Bai Zhu, Ji Nei Jin,* and *Lian Zi* all fortify the spleen and boost the qi, while *Bu Gu Zhi, Shan Zhu Yu,* and *Lian Zi* supplement the kidneys and invigorate yang. In addition, *Lian Zi, Bu Gu Zhi,* and *Wu Bei Zi* stop diarrhea. Further, *Bai Zhu, Cang Zhu, Gou Qi, Shan Zhu Yu, Shan Yao,* and *Wu Bei Zi* are all empirically known to lower blood sugar.

ADDITIONS & SUBTRACTIONS: For a black facial complexion and cold limbs, add nine grams each of Ramulus Cinnamomi Cassiae (*Gui Zhi*), Radix Salviae Miltiorrhizae (*Dan Shen*), and Placenta Hominis (*Zi He Che*) and three grams of Cornu Cervi (*Lu Jiao*), powdered and taken with the strained decoction. For dribbling urination and nocturia, add 12 grams of Semen Ginkgonis Bilobae (*Bai Guo*). For cold lower back pain, add three grams of Cortex Cinnamomi Cassiae (*Rou Gui*) and 12 grams each of Ramulus Loranthi Seu Visci (*Sang Ji Sheng*), Radix Dipsaci (*Xu Duan*), and Herba Epimedii (*Yin Yang Huo*). For impotence, add 12 grams each of Radix Morindae Officinalis (*Ba Ji Tian*) and Herba Epimedii (*Yin Yang Huo*). For heart palpitations, add 12 grams each of Semen Zizyphi Spinosae (*Suan Zao Ren*), Sclerotium Pararadicis Poriae Cocos (*Fu Shen*), and Semen Biotae Orientalis (*Bai Zi Ren*) and six grams of Radix Polygalae Tenuifoliae (*Yuan Zhi*).

ACUPUNCTURE & MOXIBUSTION: *Guan Yuan* (CV 4), *Ming Men* (GV 4), *Fu Liu* (Ki 7), *San Yin Jiao* (Sp 6)

ANALYSIS OF FORMULA: Supplementing *Guan Yuan* and *Ming Men* with moxibustion warms and supplements spleen and kidney yang. Supplementing *Fu Liu* and *San Yin Jiao* boosts yin essence to engender yang from yin.

ADDITIONS & SUBTRACTIONS: For marked fatigue, add *Zu San Li* (St 36). For severe aversion to cold, moxa *Da Zhui* (GV 14) and *Zu San Li* (St 36). For seminal emission or impotence, add *Zhi Shi* (Bl 52). For spontaneous perspiration, add *He Gu* (LI 4). For loose stools or fifth-watch diarrhea, add *Yin Ling Quan* (Sp 9) and *Zu San Li* (St 36).

REMARKS

1. Blood stasis complicates most patterns of diabetes based on the saying, "Enduring diseases enter the network vessels." Therefore, blood-quickening medicinals have already been added as standard operating procedure to a number of the above formulas.

2. Most cases of diabetes exhibit symptoms of middle and lower wasting complicated by spleen vacuity. In other words, there is enduring heat in the middle burner with stomach and kidney yin vacuity at the same time as there is spleen qi vacuity. Then damp heat, liver depression, and/or blood stasis further complicate individual patient's patterns. Generally speaking, in adults, the early stage starts with dry heat which causes yin vacuity and even more replete heat. This then results in a dual qi and yin vacuity in the middle stage which then evolves into a yin and yang dual vacuity in the latter stage. This progression will vary depending on the patient's constitution and/or lifestyle.

3. Dietary therapy must be combined with acupuncture and/or Chinese medicinals for best results. This means A) totally eliminating refined sugar and sugar products, B) avoiding "junk" foods, C) eating snacks of protein between meals, D) eating complex carbohydrates, such as whole grains, legumes, fruits, and vegetables which release their sugars more slowly and evenly into the blood stream, E) reduce or eliminate alcohol, caffeine, and tobacco consumption, and F) lose weight through calorie reduction and increased exercise. In addition, food allergies to corn, wheat, and milk products may cause inflammatory responses which initiate or aggravate autoimmune reactions leading to diabetes.

A famous study conducted in Canada in 1991 clearly shows that the rate of diabetes is proportional to the quantity of milk consumed on average per individual. Thus, for example, in Japan where the milk consumption does not exceed the equivalent of 50 liters per person per year, the rate of new cases of diabetes per year is two per 100,000 youngsters 0-14 years old. In Denmark, with yearly milk consumption of 150 liters per person per year, the rate of new cases is 15 per year. In Finland, with a yearly consumption of 250 liters of milk per person per year, the rate is 30 new cases of diabetes per year. This study compared milk consumption to rates of new cases of diabetes in 12 Western countries, including the U.S., U.K., and New Zealand.[5]

4. Because acupuncture is not so efficient for treating yin vacuity and yin vacuity plays a part in most Western patients' diabetes, internally administered Chinese medicinals typically take precedence over acupuncture in the long-term treatment and maintenance of this disease.

5. In Chinese medicine there is a mnemonic saying about diabetes, "*san duo, yi shao.*" This translates as, "three polys and one lack." These refer to polydipsia, polyphagia, and polyuria combined with emaciation (*i.e.*, loss or lack of weight). Some doctors include weakness or lack of strength in this one lack. This saying describes both IDDM and NIDDM. However, it mostly describes only the late stage of NIDDM.

6. Chinese medicinals which have a proven ability to lower the blood sugar include: Bombyx Batryticatus (*Jiang Can*), Semen Litchi Sinensis (*Li Zhi He*), Stylus Zeae Maydis (*Yu Mi Xu*), Cortex Radicis Lycii Chinensis (*Di Gu Pi*), Rhizoma Atractylodis Macrocephalae (*Bai Zhu*), Rhizoma Atractylodis (*Cang Zhu*), Sclerotium Poriae Cocos (*Fu Ling*),

Radix Puerariae (*Ge Gen*), Fructus Lycii Chinensis (*Gou Qi Zi*), Radix Polygoni Multiflori (*He Shou Wu*), Radix Et Rhizoma Polygoni Cuspidati (*Hu Zhang*), Cortex Phellodendri (*Huang Bai*), Rhizoma Polygonati (*Huang Jing*), Radix Astragali Membranacei (*Huang Qi*), Tuber Ophiopogonis Japonici (*Mai Men Dong*), Fructus Germinatus Hordei Vulgaris (*Mai Ya*), Radix Panacis Ginseng (*Ren Shen*), Folium Mori Albi (*Sang Ye*), Fructus Corni Officinalis (*Shan Zhu Yu*), Radix Dioscoreae Oppositae (*Shan Yao*), uncooked Radix Rehmanniae (*Sheng Di*), Radix Trichosanthis Kirlowii (*Tian Hua Fen*), Galla Rhois Chinensis (*Wu Bei Zi*), Herba Agrimoniae Pilosae (*Xian He Cao*), Radix Scrophulariae Ningpoensis (*Xuan Shen*), Herba Epimedii (*Yin Yang Huo*), Rhizoma Polygonati Odorati (*Yu Zhu*), Rhizoma Alismatis (*Ze Xie*), and Rhizoma Anemarrhenae Asphodeloidis (*Zhi Mu*). These medicinals should be used according to the pattern discrimination.

7. The following formula is for spleen, liver, and kidney vacuity, qi and yin vacuity, replete heat (including damp heat), and dryness. This complex pattern is not infrequently seen in real-life clinical practice, especially in adults with enduring diabetes: *Xiao San Duo Tang* (Disperse the Three Profusions Decoction): Gypsum Fibrosum (*Shi Gao*), 30g, Rhizoma Polygonati (*Huang Jing*), Radix Albus Paeoniae Lactiflorae (*Bai Shao*), Radix Dioscoreae Oppositae (*Shan Yao*), and Radix Polygoni Multiflori (*He Shou Wu*) 15g each, Rhizoma Anemarrhenae Asphodeloidis (*Zhi Mu*), Rhizoma Coptidis Chinensis (*Huang Lian*), Gelatinum Corii Asini (*E Jiao*), Radix Trichosanthis Kirlowii (*Tian Hua Fen*), Tuber Ophiopogonis Japonici (*Mai Men Dong*), and Cortex Radicis Lycii Chinensis (*Di Gu Pi*), 9g each, and Radix Panacis Ginseng (*Ren Shen*), 5g. For upper wasting, add 9 grams each of Bulbus Lilii (*Bai He*) and Fructus Pruni Mume (*Wu Mei*). For middle wasting, increase the dosage of Gypsum Fibrosum (*Shi Gao*) up to 50g and add 15 grams of Rhizoma Anemarrhenae Asphodeloidis (*Zhi Mu*). For lower wasting, add 30 grams of Radix Dioscoreae Oppositae (*Shan Yao*), 15 grams of Fructus Lycii Chinensis (*Gou Qi*), and 9 grams each of Herba Ecliptae Prostratae (*Han Lian Cao*) and Fructus Corni Officinalis (*Shan Zhu Yu*).

8. In China, three points are considered particularly important in the treatment of diabetes mellitus: *Qu Chi* (LI 11), *San Yin Jiao* (Sp 6), and *Yang Ling Quan* (GB 34). One can add *Yu Ji* (Lu 10) and *Fu Liu* (Ki 7) to this basic formula when there is excessive thirst, *Zhong Wan* (CV 12) and *Nei Ting* (St 44) when there is excessive hunger, and *Guan Yuan* (CV 4) and *Tai Chong* (Liv 3) when there is excessive urination. Another approach is to add *Guan Yuan* (CV 4) for all types of diabetes and then *Yu Ji* (Lu 10) and *Fu Liu* (Ki 7) for upper wasting and thirsting, *Zhong Wan* (CV 12) and *Nei Ting* (St 44) for middle wasting and thirsting, and *Dai Mai* (GB 26) for lower wasting and thirsting.

9. Western MDs have known for years that insulin resistance (or inability to properly deal with dietary carbohydrates and sugars), abnormal blood lipids, obesity, and hypertension increase the risk of both heart disease and diabetes. Among progressive practitioners, this combination of conditions is known as syndrome X. Syndrome X is a diet-caused hormonal dyscrasia which mostly affects middle-aged adults, causing them to feel sluggish both physically and mentally, especially after meals. Insulin resistance and the syndrome X it results in is primarily due to eating a diet high in refined carbohydrates and simple sugars, saturated fat (as found in beef), omega-6 fatty acids (found in vegetable oils), and trans-fatty acids (found in margarine and foods with partially hydrogenated oils). In Chinese medicine, fatigue after meals is primarily a spleen vacuity symptom, while overeating fats and oils engenders both heat and dampness. Thus the core disease mechanisms of syndrome X are spleen vacuity with dampness and heat. In real life, if there is spleen vacuity, there is liver depression and vice versa. Therefore, in the overwhelming majority of syndrome X patients, there is also liver depression qi stagnation which aggravates and adds to the spleen vacuity, depressive heat, and damp evils. When these heat evils eventually damage the righteous yin of the stomach, lungs, and/or kidneys, syndrome X evolves into diabetes.

ENDNOTES

1 Pizzorno, J.E. & Murray, M.T., "Diabetes Mellitus," *Textbook of Natural Medicine*, John Bastyr College Publications, Seattle, WA, 1988

2 Forsham, P.H., "Treatment of Type I & Type II Diabetes," *Townsend Letter for Doctors*. #53, Dec., 1987, p. 390-393

3 Satter, D., "Diabetes Called Sure Fate for Obese People," *Los Angeles Times*, Sunday, Feb. 13, 1972, section C

4 As the incidence of juvenile obesity has gone up in developed countries, so has the incidence of juvenile-onset diabetes. More and more of these cases are now due to obvious faulty diet, *i.e.*, overeating sugars and sweets as well as fatty, greasy foods.

5 http://www.notmilk.comwww.notmilk.com/ailmenu.html and www.notmilk.com/deb/011099.html

25

DIVERTICULITIS

Diverticula are small pouches which bulge outward in the large intestine. When one has a number of these pouches, this is called diverticulosis. If these diverticula become inflammed, this is called diverticulitis. Fifty percent of Americans 60-80 years old have diverticulosis, and this number becomes 100% in those more than 80 years old. Ten to 25% of those with diverticulosis have diverticulitis. While the etiology of this condition is unknown, because it is most common in developed countries, there is speculation that it is related to a diet high in refined foods and low in fiber. Diverticulosis may be asymptomatic or there may be mild cramps, bloating, and constipation. Diverticulitis is characterized by abdominal pain and tenderness in the lower left abdomen. If the diverticula become infected, there may be fever, nausea, vomiting, chills, cramping, and constipation. This condition may lead to infections, perforations, tears, blockages, and bleeding.

The Western medical diagnosis of this condition is based on the patient's history and presenting complaints plus a digital rectal exam. The stools may be checked for blood, and lower GI x-rays may help confirm the diagnosis. Its Western medical treatment consists of a high fiber diet and mild pain medications. If there is infection, antibiotics may be prescribed. If attacks are severe or frequent, surgery may be used to remove a section of the colon.

CHINESE DISEASE CATEGORIZATION: Based on the symptoms of lower abdominal pain, distention, and constipation, this disease is categorized in Chinese medicine as *shao fu tong*, lesser abdominal pain, *xiao fu tong*, smaller abdominal pain, *xiao fu zhang tong*, smaller abdominal distention and pain, and *bian bi*, constipation.

DISEASE CAUSES: Habitual bodily vacuity weakness due to aging, unregulated diet

DISEASE MECHANISMS: Lower abdominal pain is the most prominent symptom of this condition, and the key statement of fact about pain in Chinese medicine is that, "If there is pain, there is no free flow." In this case, the pain tends to be fixed in location. This is one of the characteristics of blood stasis pain. Yan De-xin, one of the greatest living Chinese medical geriatric specialists believes that essentially all geriatric diseases are complicated by blood stasis. Such blood stasis is the result of a lifetime of damage due to external, internal, and neither external nor internal causes of disease. As Dr. Yan says, all diseases are diseases of the qi and blood. Further, it is said that, "Enduring disease enters the network vessels." This implies that chronic, enduring disease is associated with blood stasis in the network vessels.

It is also said in Chinese medicine, "In the elderly, blame the spleen." Most elderly patients exhibit signs and symptoms of qi and yin or yin and yang vacuity. When the spleen qi becomes vacuous and weak, it fails to upbear the clear. Instead, the unseparated clear and turbid fall downward to the lower burner. There, they block the free flow of qi and blood, giving rise to qi stagnation (abdominal distention) and blood stasis (fixed pain). Qi stagnation and blood stasis may give rise to depressive heat. If dampness becomes mixed with depressive heat, then there is damp heat stasis and stagnation. If damp heat brews and binds internally, it may give rise to heat toxins. In that case, abdominal cramps may be complicated by fever, chills, nausea, and vomiting. Sugars and sweets damage the spleen. However, so can refined carbohydrates. In the Yuan dynasty, Li Dong-yuan referred to these as "sodden wheat foods." A high fiber diet means the spleen-fortifying, stomach-boosting clear, bland diet of Chinese medicine.

If spleen vacuity reaches the kidneys, there may be kidney yang vacuity. In that case, vaçuity cold may further constrict and congeal the flow of qi, blood, and body fluids, thus resulting in both pain and constipation. On the other hand, yin vacuity may cause insufficient fluids in the large intestine. Thus, "the boat is not floated," and constipation occurs. In addition, both kidney yang vacuity and kidney yin vacuity cause or aggravate liver depression qi stagnation. If the liver fails to control coursing and discharge, the qi mechanism becomes inhibited, the spleen and stomach fail to upbear and downbear properly, and the large intestine's conduction and conveyance will be negatively affected.

TREATMENT BASED ON PATTERN DISCRIMINATION:

1. QI & YIN VACUITY WITH QI STAGNATION & BLOOD STASIS PATTERN

MAIN SYMPTOMS: Fatigue, lack of strength, lassitude of the spirit, shortness of breath, insomnia, heart palpitations, poor appetite, reduced food intake, a bland taste in the mouth or no flavor for food, slow digestion, constipation, dry skin, dry eyes, dry lips and mouth, a pale facial complexion with possible malar flushing, cold hands and feet and possible vexatious heat in the five hearts, tinnitus, dizziness, deafness, falling hair, decreased visual acuity, decreased memory power, loose or falling teeth, low back and knee soreness and limpness, lower abdominal distention and pain, a pale, tender tongue with possible red tip or a fat, red tongue with scanty or no fur and fluids, and a soggy, weak, or vacuous pulse depending upon whether qi or yin vacuity is most pronounced.

TREATMENT PRINCIPLES: Fortify the spleen and boost the qi, supplement the kidneys and nourish yin, free the flow of the stools and stop pain

RX: If spleen vacuity is more marked, *Bu Zhong Yi Qi Tang Jia Wei* (Supplement the Center & Boost the Qi Decoction with Added Flavors)

INGREDIENTS: Radix Astragali Membranacei (*Huang Qi*), 15g, cooked Radix Rehmanniae (*Shu Di*), Radix Polygoni Multiflori (*He Shou Wu*) and Tuber Ophiopogonis Japonicae (*Mai Dong*), 12g each, Radix Codonopsitis Pilosulae (*Dang Shen*), Rhizoma Atractylodis Macrocephalae (*Bai Zhu*), Radix Angelicae Sinensis (*Dang Gui*), Radix Achyranthis Bidentatae (*Niu Xi*), and Semen Pruni Persicae (*Tao Ren*), 9g each, Pericarpium Citri Reticulatae (*Chen Pi*) and mix-fried Radix Glycyrrhizae (*Gan Cao*), 6g each, Rhizoma Cimicifugae (*Sheng Ma*), 4.5g, and Radix Bupleuri (*Chai Hu*), 1-3g

ANALYSIS OF FORMULA: *Huang Qi, Dang Shen, Bai Zhu,* and mix-fried *Gan Cao* fortify the spleen and boost the qi. *Shu Di, He Shou Wu, Mai Men Dong,* and *Niu Xi* supplement the kidneys and nourish yin. *Sheng Ma* and *Chai Hu* upbear the clear. *Chen Pi* rectifies the qi, harmonizes the stomach, and stops pain. *Dang Gui* and *Tao Ren* together nourish the blood and transform stasis, moisten the intestines and free the flow of the stools.

ADDITIONS & SUBTRACTIONS: If there is more pronounced qi stagnation, add nine grams of Fructus Meliae Toosendan (*Chuan Lian Zi*) and six grams of Fructus Immaturus Citri Aurantii (*Zhi Shi*). If there is more marked blood stasis, add nine grams each of Radix Rubrus Paeoniae Lactiflorae (*Bai Shao*) and Cortex Radicis Moutan (*Dan Pi*). If there is concomitant depressive heat, add nine grams of Radix Scutellariae Baicalensis (*Huang Qin*). If there is concomitant vacuity heat, delete Bupleurum and add nine grams each of Rhizoma Anemarrhenae Asphleoidis (*Zhi Mu*) and Cortex Phellodendri (*Huang Bai*). If there is concomitant yang vacuity, add nine grams each of Herba Cistanchis Deserticolae (*Rou Cong Rong*) and Herba Cynomorii Songarici (*Suo Yang*). If there is more severe or enduring constipation, add nine grams each of Semen Cannabis Sativae (*Huo Ma Ren*) and Semen Pruni (*Yu Li*). If there is torpid intake and bad breath due to food stagnation, add nine grams each of Fructus Crataegi (*Shan Zha*) and Endothelium Corneum Gigeriae Galli (*Ji Nei Jin*).

If yin vacuity is more pronounced, *Liu Wei Di Huang Wan Jia Wei* (Six Flavors Rehmannia Pills with Added Flavors)

INGREDIENTS: Radix Astragali Membranacei (*Huang Qi*), 15g, cooked Radix Rehmanniae (*Shu Di*), 12g, Radix Dioscoreae Oppositae (*Shan Yao*), Fructus Corni Officinalis (*Shan Zhu Yu*), Sclerotium Poriae Cocos (*Fu Ling*), Fructus Schisandrae Chinensis (*Wu Wei Zi*), Radix Angelicae Sinensis (*Dang Gui*), and Semen Pruni Persicae (*Tao Ren*), 9g each, and Rhizoma Alismatis (*Ze Xie*) and Cortex Radicis Moutan (*Dan Pi*), 6g each

ANALYSIS OF FORMULA: *Huang Qi, Shan Yao,* and *Fu Ling* fortify the spleen and boost the qi. *Shu Di, Shan Zhu Yu,* and *Wu Wei Zi* supplement the kidneys and nourish yin. *Ze Xie* clears ministerial fire, while *Dan Pi* clears vacuity heat. *Dang Gui* and *Tao Ren* together nourish the blood and transform stasis, moisten the intestines and free the flow of the stools.

ADDITIONS & SUBTRACTIONS: If there is more severe qi vacuity, add 12 grams each of Radix Codonopsitis Pilosulae (*Dang Shen*) and Radix Pseudostellariae (*Tai Zi Shen*). If there is concomitant qi stagnation, add nine grams of Fructus Meliae Toosendan (*Chuan Lian Zi*) and six grams of Fructus Immaturus Citri Aurantii (*Zhi Shi*). If there is concomitant blood stasis, add 12 grams of Radix Cyathulae (*Chuan Niu Xi*) and nine grams of Radix Rubrus Paeoniae

Lactiflorae (*Chi Shao*). If there is vacuity heat, add nine grams each of Rhizoma Anemarrhenae Aspheloidis (*Zhi Mu*) and Cortex Phellodendri (*Huang Bai*). If there is concomitant yang vacuity, add nine grams each of Herba Cistanchis Deserticolae (*Rou Cong Rong*) and Herba Cynomorii Songarici (*Suo Yang*). If constipation is severe, add nine grams each of Semen Cannabis Sativae (*Huo Ma Ren*) and Semen Pruni (*Yu Li Ren*).

ACUPUNCTURE & MOXIBUSTION: *Zu San Li* (St 36), *Tian Shu* (St 25), *Qi Hai* (CV 6), *San Yin Jiao* (Sp 6), *Zhi Gou* (TB 6)

ANALYSIS OF FORMULA: *Zu San Li* is the master point of the abdomen, the uniting point of the stomach channel, and the earth point of the foot yang ming. Supplementing it fortifies the spleen and boosts the qi, harmonizes the stomach and intestines, supports the righteous or correct, and stops pain. *Tian Shu* is the alarm point of the large intestine. Draining it rectifies the qi in the intestines, frees the flow of the stools, and stops pain. Even supplementing-even draining *Qi Hai* supplements the kidneys and rectifies the qi in the lower abdomen. *San Yin Jiao* supplements the spleen, liver, and kidneys as well as supplements both the qi and the blood. *Zhi Gou* rectifies the qi in the three burners and frees the flow of the stools.

ADDITIONS & SUBTRACTIONS: For severe constipation, add *Zhao Hai* (Ki 6). For severe kidney yin vacuity, add *Fu Liu* (Ki 7). For concomitant yang vacuity, supplement and moxa *Qi Hai* (CV 6). For severe abdominal distention and flatulence, add *Nei Guan* (Per 6). For night sweats, add *Yin Xi* (Ht 6). For low back pain and abdominal distention, add *Gong Sun* (Sp 4). For undigested food in the stools or reduced food intake, add *Xuan Ji* (CV 21) and *Liang Men* (St 21). For severe qi vacuity, add *Tai Bai* (Sp 3).

2. QI VACUITY WITH DAMP HEAT STASIS & STAGNATION PATTERN

MAIN SYMPTOMS: Fatigue, lack of strength, lassitude of the spirit, shortness of breath, weak voice or disinclination to speak, fixed, burning pain on one side of the lower abdomen, dark-colored, bound stools, possible frequent but scanty, dark-colored urine, a dry mouth and throat, a fat or tender, pale or red tongue with slimy, yellow fur at its root, and a deep, bowstring, slippery, rapid pulse

TREATMENT PRINCIPLES: Fortify the spleen and boost the qi, clear heat and eliminate dampness, move the qi and quicken the blood

RX: *Bu Zhong Yi Qi Tang* (Supplement the Center & Boost the Qi Decoction) & *Yi Yi Fu Zi Bai Jiang San* (Coix, Aconite & Patrinia Powder) with additions and subtractions

INGREDIENTS: Semen Coicis Lachryma-jobi (*Yi Yi Ren*), 18g, Herba Patriniae Heterophyllae Cum Radice (*Bai Jiang Cao*), Caulis Sargentodoxae (*Hong Teng*), and Radix Astragali Membrancei (*Huang Qi*), 15g each, Radix Codonopsitis Pilosulae (*Dang Shen*), Rhizoma Atractylodis Macrocephalae (*Bai Zhu*), Radix Angelicae Sinensis (*Dang Gui*), Cortex Radicis Moutan (*Dan Pi*), Radix Rubrus Paeoniae Lactiflorae (*Chi Shao*), Radix Bupleuri (*Chai Hu*), and Fructus Immaturus Citri Aurantii (*Zhi Shi*), 9g each, Pericarpium Citri Reticulatae (*Chen Pi*) and mix-fried Radix Glycyrrhizae (*Gan Cao*), 6g each, and Rhizoma Cimicifugae (*Sheng Ma*), 4.5g

ANALYSIS OF FORMULA: *Huang Qi, Dang Shen, Bai Zhu,* and mix-fried *Gan Cao* fortify the spleen and boost the qi. *Yi Yi Ren, Chai Hu, Sheng Ma, Bai Jiang Cao,* and *Hong Teng* together clear heat and disinhibit dampness. Also, *Sheng Ma* and *Chai Hu* upbear the clear, *Yi Yi Ren* fortifies the spleen and expels pus, and *Bai Jiang Cao* and *Hong Teng* resolve toxins and quicken the blood. *Dang Gui, Dan Pi,* and *Chi Shao* quicken the blood and transform stasis, while *Chen Pi* and *Zhi Shi* move the qi.

ADDITIONS & SUBTRACTIONS: If there is concomitant yang vacuity, add six grams of Radix Lateralis Praeparatus Aconiti Carmichaeli (*Fu Zi*). If there is concomitant constipation, add nine grams of Semen Pruni Persicae (*Tao Ren*). For more severe pain, add 15 grams of Rhizoma Corydalis Yanhusuo (*Yan Hu Suo*) and Fructus Meliae Toosendan (*Chuan Lian Zi*). If enduring heat has damaged fluids, add 12 grams of Tuber Ophiopogonis Japonici (*Mai Men Dong*) and nine grams of Rhizoma Anemarrhenae Aspheloidis (*Zhi Mu*). For more severe heat, add nine grams each of Cortex Phellodendri (*Huang Bai*) and Radix Scutellariae Baicalensis (*Huang Qin*). If there is concomitant food stagnation, add nine grams each of Fructus Crataegi (*Shan Zha*) and Endothelium Corneum Gigeriae Galli (*Ji Nei Jin*).

ACUPUNCTURE & MOXIBUSTION: *Zu San Li* (St 36), *Tian Shu* (St 25), *Nei Guan* (Per 6), *Zhao Hai* (Ki 6), *Zhi Gou* (TB 6)

ANALYSIS OF FORMULA: *Zu San Li* is the master point of the abdomen, the uniting point of the stomach channel, and the earth point of the foot yang ming. Supplementing it fortifies the spleen, boosts the qi, and harmonizes the intestines. *Tian Shu* is the alarm point of the large intestine. Draining it rectifies the qi and clears the intestines, frees the flow of the stools and stops pain. Draining *Nei Guan* moves the qi, quickens the blood, and transforms stasis. *Zhao Hai* supplements the kidneys, nourishes the yin, and treats constipation. *Zhi Gou* rectifies the qi in the three burners, clears heat, and frees the flow of the stools.

ADDITIONS & SUBTRACTIONS: For severe kidney yin vacuity, add *San Yin Jiao* (Sp 6). For concomitant yang vacuity, add and moxa *Guan Yuan* (CV 4). For severe abdominal distention and flatulence, add *He Gu* (LI 4). For severe damp heat, add *Yin Ling Quan* (Sp 9) and *Nei Ting* (St 44). For night sweats, add *Yin Xi* (Ht 6). For low back pain and abdominal distention, add *Gong Sun* (Sp 4). For undigested food in the stools or reduced food intake, add *Xuan Ji* (CV 21) and *Liang Men* (St 21). For severe qi vacuity, add *Tai Bai* (Sp 3).

3. RIGHTEOUS QI VACUITY WEAKNESS WITH HEAT TOXINS BREWING & BINDING PATTERN

MAIN SYMPTOMS: Fatigue, lack of strength, lassitude of the spirit, shortness of breath, fever, possible nausea and vomiting, lower abdominal pain, constipation, a swollen, red or tender, red tongue with slimy, yellow tongue fur at the root, and a deep, bowstring, slippery, rapid pulse

TREATMENT PRINCIPLES: Support the righteous and expel (toxins from) the interior, cleat heat and stop pain

RX: *Tuo Li Xiao Du San Jia Wei* (Expel the Interior & Disperse Toxins Powder with Added Flavors)

INGREDIENTS: Radix Astragali Membranacei (*Huang Qi*), Fructus Forsythiae Suspensae (*Lian Qiao*), and Flos Lonicerae Japonicae (*Jin Yin Hua*), 15g each, Radix Codonopsitis Pilosulae (*Dang Shen*), Rhizoma Atractylodis Macrocephalae (*Bai Zhu*), Fructus Immaturus Citri Aurantii (*Zhi Shi*), Squama Manitis Pentadactylis (*Chuan Shan Jia*), Spina Gleditschiae Chinensis (*Zao Jiao Ci*), Semen Trichosanthis Kirlowii (*Gua Lou Ren*), Radix Angelicae Sinensis (*Dang Gui*), and Radix Ligustici Wallichii (*Chuan Xiong*), 9g each, Radix Angelicae Dahuricae (*Bai Zhi*) and mix-fried Radix Glycyrrhizae (*Gan Cao*), 6g each, and Rhizoma Cimicifugae (*Sheng Ma*), 3g

ANALYSIS OF FORMULA: *Huang Qi, Dang Shen, Bai Zhu,* and mix-fried *Gan Cao* fortify the spleen and boost the qi, while *Dang Gui* nourishes the blood. Together, they support the righteous. *Lian Qiao* and *Jin Yin Hua* clear heat and resolve toxins. *Zhi Shi* moves the qi, while *Chuan Shan Jia, Dang Gui,* and *Chuan Xiong* quicken the blood and transform stasis. *Bai Zhi, Zao Jiao Ci,* and *Gua Lou Ren* disperse swelling and expel pus from the interior. *Sheng Ma* both upbears the clear and clears the yang ming.

ADDITIONS & SUBTRACTIONS: For nausea and vomiting, delete *Sheng Ma* and add 12 grams of Rhizoma Phragmitis Communis (*Lu Gen*), nine grams of Caulis Bambusae In Taeniis (*Zhu Ru*), and two slices of uncooked Rhizoma Zingiberis (*Sheng Jiang*).

ACUPUNCTURE & MOXIBUSTION: Same as the preceding pattern, but replace *Zhao Hai* with *Nei Ting* (St 44).

ANALYSIS OF FORMULA: Please see the preceding pattern. *Nei Ting* clears heat from the yang ming.

ADDITIONS & SUBTRACTIONS: Please see the preceding pattern. If *Lan Wei Xue* (M-LE-13), *Shang Ju Xu* (St 37), or *Xia Ju Xu* (St 39) are tender, needle them.

REMARKS

1. The three constants in the Chinese pattern discrimination of diverticulitis are spleen vacuity, qi stagnation, and blood stasis. These are then complicated by yin vacuity, yang vacuity, and/or damp heat depending on age, body type, diet, etc. Damp heat may also sometimes evolve into heat toxins. In the very aged, it is not uncommon to find qi vacuity, yin and yang vacuity, and qi stagnation and blood stasis. In such complex cases, one should write the patterns in the order of their prominence, state the treatment principles necessary to rectify the disease mechanisms implied by the pattern in the same order as the statement of patterns, and then choose medicinals or acupoints to accomplish each of these principles.

2. While patients with diverticulitis need to eat a high fiber diet, they should not eat hard-to-digest foods. These include nuts and seeds. Since the overwhelming majority of diverticulitis sufferers exhibit significant spleen vacuity, they should also not eat uncooked and/or chilled foods. This latter point is quite important because many people trying to eat more fiber resort to eating a lot of uncooked salads. If there is damp heat brewing and binding, patients should also be advised to stay away from citrus fruits and juices.

26

Fibromyalgia Syndrome

Fibromyalgia, also called fibromyalgia syndrome or FMS, is a condition mostly affecting women between 20-50 years of age. It is characterized by chronic, widespread, severe muscular aching, pain, and stiffness accompanied by insomnia, fatigue, and depression. Unlike osteoarthritis, rheumatoid arthritis, and lupus erythmatosus, it is neither a rheumatic, inflammatory, progressive, or degenerative disorder. However, it is also not solely a psychosomatic or psychiatric disorder. In other words, it is not all in the patient's head. What it is, is a chronic, debilitating condition of unknown etiology or cause which is probably caused by a number of different factors involving a complex relationship between the psyche (the mind) and the soma (the body). In 1987, the American Medical Association (AMA) recognized FMS as a true illness and major cause of disability.[1]

Because this condition does not result in any physical damage to the body or its tissues, there is no one laboratory test or x-ray which can confirm this diagnosis. Because this condition is so commonly associated with chronic, enduring fatigue, it is often confused with chronic fatigue syndrome (CFS) or what is also known as chronic fatigue immune deficiency syndrome (CFIDS) in the U.S. However, unlike CFS, fibromyalgia sufferers usually experience much more significant muscle-joint aching and pain. It is estimated that as much as 75% of CFS-diagnosed patients actually fit the criteria for FMS.[2] Fibromyalgia can also be differentiated from other chronic muscle-joint pain by the presence of pain or tenderness upon pressure in at least 11 out of 18 specific points on the body.[3] In addition to the above characteristics, FMS sufferers are also typically hypersensitive to odors, bright lights, and loud noises. Headaches and jaw pain, also known as temporomandibular joint (TMJ) pain, are common.

The word syndrome in fibromyalgia syndrome means that this condition presents with a varying range of accompanying signs and symptoms besides just muscle and joint aching and pain. Although Western medicine cannot explain why these symptoms occur together as they do, Western doctors do recognize this constellation of symptoms as a clinical entity or disease. Some of these are listed below along with the rates of their occurrence.

Ninety to 100% of FMS sufferers have generalized body pain effecting all four quadrants of the body, fatigue, and muscular stiffness. These three symptoms are all typically worse in the morning. FMS patients often say their arms and legs feel "like tied to concrete blocks." The muscular pain associated with FMS is described as deep, burning, throbbing, shooting, and/or stabbing. And the fatigue may range from simple, random exhaustion to being unable to get out of bed.

Seventy to 90% of FMS sufferers will also have one or more of the following: post-exertional malaise, sleep disturbances, headaches, either migraine or tension, tenderness to pressure at certain, specific spots on the body, swollen feet, numbness and/or tingling, difficulty thinking and concentrating, also called "brain fog," dizziness, sensitivity to light, noise, and/or smells, hypersensitivity to stress, dysmenorrhea, or dry mouth. In terms of sleep disturbances, FMS sufferers are usually able to fall asleep but then are not able to sleep soundly or wake up too early in the morning. In terms of the swollen feet, the feet may actually be swollen or they may only feel swollen to the patient. The dizziness of FMS is often orthostatic hypotension, meaning dizziness when standing up. Dysmenorrhea may also be diagnosed as endometriosis.

Fifty to 70% of FMS sufferers will also have one or more of the following: irritable bowel syndrome (IBS), blurred vision, mood swings, heart palpitations, cold extremities, feverish feelings, or allergies. Irritable bowel syndrome refers to a constellation of symptoms including lower abdominal bloating, cramping, and pain, typically after eating, diarrhea and/or constipation, and mucus in the stools. It is sometimes also referred to as mucus colitis or allergic colitis. Based on our own clinical experience, we would add the words "night blindness" after blurred vision. Many women with this condition have decreased visual acuity at night which makes them reluctant or uncomfortable to drive at night even if, strictly speaking, they do not have the Western medical disease of nictolopia or night blindness.

Fifteen to 50% of FMS sufferers will also have one or more of the following: restless leg syndrome, muscle twitches, itchy skin, hearing disturbances, night sweats, breathing problems, proneness to infections, skin rashes, interstitial cystitis, TMJ pain, or multiple chemical sensitivities. Restless leg syndrome refers to a vague, hard to describe feeling of discomfort experienced in the legs, usually at night, characterized by the need to constantly move the legs in order to try and relieve this discomfort. Breathing problems include allergic rhinitis and allergic asthma. Interstitial cystitis is characterized by decreased urinary capacity and, therefore, frequent, painful urination and hematuria. Typically, this condition effects middle-aged women and may be either an allergic or autoimmune disease. Multiple chemical sensitivities are also referred to as environmental illness.

Less than 15% of FMS sufferers also display major depression. However, most FMS sufferers are mildly depressed. Other symptoms or conditions also reported in the FMS literature and which we have seen in a number of patients in our own practice are new or worsening PMS, fibrocystic breast disease (FBD), and mouth sores.

In order to qualify for a diagnosis of fibromyalgia, the above generalized muscle pain, stiffness, and fatigue have to have lasted for not less than three months. In addition, as stated above, at least 11 out of 18 specific tender points on the body should be painful to palpation. Because fibromyalgia involves a number of different symptoms, Western physicians try to treat this disorder by prescribing various medications and treatments for each of these different symptoms. In other words, because it has not yet identified the underlying cause of FMS, Western medicine has no single treatment for FMS *per se*. This means that antidepressants, such as Prozac, Elavil, Paxil, and Xanax, are commonly prescribed to treat the sleep and mood, while non-steroidal anti-inflammatories (NSAIDs), such as Ibuprofen, are prescribed for the pain. In addition, trigger points, *i.e.*, points that are hypersensitive to pressure, may be injected with lidocaine, a local anesthetic. Many FMS patients benefit from regular weekly massages, but few insurance companies will pay for this even when prescribed by an MD.

Unfortunately, not all patients tolerate antidepressants such as Prozac, Elavil, and Paxil without side effects. For instance, the side effects of Prozac include skin rashes, hives, and itching, headache, nervousness, insomnia, drowsiness and fatigue, tremors, dizziness, and impaired concentration.[4] In addition, many other patients simply do not want to take such Western psychotropic pharmaceuticals. NSAIDs can be very effective for acute pain relief, but they also have their own potential side effects, such as skin rashes, hives, and itching, headache, dizziness, blurred vision, ringing in the ears, depression, mouth sores, and gastrointestinal upset.[5] Ironically, some of these side effects include many of the symptoms of FMS. There are also some concerns about NSAIDs' effect on the kidneys when taken over a prolonged period of time.[6] Unfortunately, when used in the treatment of fibromyalgia, NSAIDs usually do have to be taken for such a prolonged time.

CHINESE DISEASE CATEGORIZATION: Fibromylagia is categorized as *ji bi*, muscle impediment in Chinese medicine. Most of the complaints associated with fibromylagia syndrome are disease categories in Chinese medicine in their own right. Therefore, when treating FMS, one should consider the patterns and treatments listed in this and other such books for these other Chinese disease categories. FMS's three main associated disease conditions besides fibromylagia *per se* are *xu lao*, vacuity taxation, *yu zheng*, depressive condition, and *shi mian*, insomnia.

DISEASE CAUSES: External contraction of the six environmental excesses, internal damage by the seven affects, unregulated eating and drinking, iatrogenesis, and aging

DISEASE MECHANISMS: In our experience, the core disease mechanisms at work in fibromylagia syndrome are a liver-spleen disharmony. Liver depression qi stagnation may be due to unfulfilled desires or anger damaging the liver. However, it may also be due to insufficient blood nourishing the liver or insufficient yang warming and steaming the liver. Spleen vacuity is due to either faulty diet, excessive taxation, excessive thinking and especially worry and anxiety, too little physical exercise, over-use of bitter, cold medicinals, including Western antibiotics, living in a damp, hot environment, and liver wood assailing spleen earth. If the liver becomes depressed, the qi and, therefore, blood and body fluids all will not flow smoothly and easily as they should. Liver qi symptoms include chest, breast, rib-side, and abdominal oppression, distention, fullness, and pain, emotional depression, irritability, headaches, PMS, and dysmenorrhea. Spleen qi vacuity symptoms include fatigue, lack of strength and/or warmth in the extremities, poor appetite, and loose stools. Damp accumulation symptoms include edema, abnormal vaginal discharge, damp skin lesions, and damp impediment. If dampness congeals into phlegm, there may be phlegm nodulation, phlegm in the lungs, or phlegm harassing and disquieting the heart spirit. Blood stasis may result in painful menstruation or any fixed location pain in the body.

Based on this core disease mechanism of liver-spleen disharmony, numerous other disease mechanisms may also be engendered. Since the defensive qi issues from the middle burner, spleen qi vacuity leads to defensive qi not securing with easy invasion of external evils. If spleen vacuity fails to transform and engender sufficient new blood, there will be heart and/or liver blood vacuity. If blood vacuity endures, it may give rise to yin vacuity, internal stirring of wind, worsening of liver depression, or blood stasis. If spleen vacuity endures, it may eventually reach the kidneys, damaging yang. In that case, there will be a spleen-kidney yang vacuity and vacuity cold which may constrict and congeal the blood, hence also causing blood stasis. In addition, if both the spleen and kidney yang are vacuous and weak, water metabolism must be even more negatively affected. If liver depression worsens or endures, qi depression may transform heat. This may give rise to liver fire flaming upward or ascendant liver yang hyperactivity. Heat in the liver may mutually engender heat in the stomach, spleen, heart, lungs, bladder, and/or blood. If heat endures it will damage and consume yin fluids. Further, when heat flares upward, it harasses the spirit and the clear orifices above. According to Li Dong-yuan, when heat flares upward from the lower and middle burners, it also consumes and damages the spleen qi. If dampness due to spleen vacuity and faulty diet unites with or engenders depressive heat, damp heat may pour downward, to the bladder, uterus, and lower limbs. It may also spill over into the space between the muscles and the skin. Damp heat pouring downward may damage liver and kidney yin at the same time as it stirs ministerial fire to flare upward. All of the signs and symptoms of FMS are due to some combination of these inter-related disease mechanisms.

TREATMENT BASED ON PATTERN DISCRIMINATION:

1. LIVER-SPLEEN DISHARMONY PATTERN

MAIN SYMPTOMS: Irritability, mental-emotional depression, constipation with thin, ribbon-like or small round stools or diarrhea alternating with constipation, burping and belching, chest, rib-side and abdominal distention or pain, premenstrual breast distention and pain, painful menstruation, fatigue, loss of strength in the extremities, reduced food intake, stomach and epigastric distention and fullness after eating, superficial edema, cold hands and feet, easy bruising, profuse menstruation or abnormal uterine bleeding, dizziness upon standing up, a pale facial complexion, a fat, pale yet dark tongue with thin, white fur, and a bowstring, fine pulse which is often soggy in the right bar position

NOTE: Although this pattern is the core of FMS, there usually must be at least one other disease mechanism before a patient exhibits FMS. By itself, this pattern does *not* correspond to FMS. However, we have presented it here to emphasize that this disease mechanism sits squarely in the center of all the other patterns which do describe various clinical aspects of FMS.

TREATMENT PRINCIPLES: Course the liver and rectify the qi, fortify the spleen and boost the qi

RX: *Xiao Yao San* (Rambling Powder)

INGREDIENTS: Radix Albus Paeoniae Lactiflorae (*Bai Shao*), 18g, Radix Bupleuri (*Chai Hu*), Rhizoma Atractylodis Macrocephalae (*Bai Zhu*), Sclerotium Poriae Cocos (*Fu Ling*), Radix Angelicae Sinensis (*Dang Gui*), 9g each, Herba Menthae Haplocalycis (*Bo He*) and mix-fried Radix Glycyrrhizae (*Gan Cao*), 6g each, and uncooked Rhizoma Zingiberis (*Sheng Jiang*), 2 slices

ANALYSIS OF FORMULA: *Bai Shao* and *Dang Gui* harmonize and emolliate the liver, while *Chai Hu* and *Bo He* course the liver and resolve depression. *Bai Zhu, Sheng Jiang, Fu Ling,* and mix-fried *Gan Cao* fortify the spleen, supplement the qi, and dry and transform dampness.

ADDITIONS & SUBTRACTIONS: If spleen vacuity is marked with fatigue and lack of strength or if the defensive qi is not securing, add 15 grams of Radix Astragali Membranacei (*Huang Qi*) and nine grams of Radix Codonopsitis Pilosulae (*Dang Shen*). If there is more pronounced dampness in the middle burner, add nine grams of Herba Agastachis Seu Pogostemi (*Huo Xiang*) and Fructus Amomi (*Sha Ren*). If dampness is spilling over into the extremities with puffy swelling, add nine grams each of Semen Plantaginis (*Che Qian Zi*) and Rhizoma Alismatis (*Ze Xie*). If there is phlegm dampness, add nine grams each of Rhizoma Pinelliae Ternatae (*Ban Xia*) and Pericarpium Citri Reticulatae (*Chen Pi*). If generalized blood vacuity is pronounced and there is malnourishment of the sinews, add 15 grams of Caulis Milletiae Seu Spatholobi (*Ji Xue Teng*) and 12 grams of cooked Radix Rehmanniae (*Shu Di*). If there is more serious liver blood vacuity, add nine grams of Fructus Lycii Chinensis (*Gou Qi Zi*) and 12 grams of Radix Polygoni Multiflori (*He Shou Wu*). If heart blood is vacuous and the spirit is disquieted, add 12 grams each of Semen Zizyphi Spinosae (*Suan Zao Ren*) and Semen Biotae Orientalis (*Bai Zi Ren*). If liver depression has transformed heat and that heat has entered the blood division, add nine grams each of Fructus Gardeniae Jasminoidis (*Zhi Zi*) and Cortex Radicis Moutan (*Dan Pi*). If there is heat specifically in the liver-gallbladder, lungs, stomach, and intestines, add nine grams of Radix Scutellariae Baicalensis (*Huang Qin*). If there is heat specifically in the liver-gallbladder, heart, stomach, and intestines, add 3-9 grams of Rhizoma Coptidis Chinensis (*Huang Lian*). If enduring heat has damaged stomach and/or lung fluids, add 12 grams of Tuber Ophiopogonis Japonici (*Mai Men Dong*). For more serious qi stagnation, add nine grams each of one or more of the following depending on the location, severity, and symptoms of qi stagnation: Rhizoma Cyperi Rotundi (*Xiang Fu*), Radix Auklandiae Lappae (*Mu Xiang*), Radix Linderae Strychnifoliae (*Wu Yao*), Fructus Citri Aurantii (*Zhi Ke*), Fructus Immaturus Citri Aurantii (*Zhi Shi*), Pericarpium Citri Reticulatae (*Chen Pi*), Pericarpium Citri Reticulatae Viride (*Qing Pi*), Semen Citri Reticulatae (*Ju He*), and Folium Citri Reticulatae (*Ju Ye*). If there is blood stasis, add nine grams each of Semen Pruni Persicae (*Tao Ren*) and Flos Carthami Tinctorii (*Hong Hua*). If there is painful diarrhea, add nine grams of Radix Ledebouriellae Divaricatae (*Fang Feng*) and six grams of Pericarpium Citri Reticulatae (*Chen Pi*).

ACUPUNCTURE & MOXIBUSTION: *Nei Guan* (Per 6), *Wai Guan* (TB 5), *Tai Chong* (Liv 3), *Zu San Li* (St 36), *Da Bao* (Sp 21)

ANALYSIS OF FORMULA: According to the ancients, the triple burner is the father of yang qi, while the pericardium is the mother of yin blood. Therefore, together, these two channels help smooth the flow of qi and blood in the whole body. *Wai Guan* is the network point of the triple burner channel and *Nei Guan* is the network point of the pericardium channel. Needling these two points harmonizes the qi and blood in the whole body. In addition, *Wai Guan* is the meeting point of the yang wei mai, while *Nei Guan* is the meeting point of the yin wei mai, two vessels which regulate the balance between yin and yang and the interior and exterior. *Tai Chong* is the source point of the liver channel. It courses the liver and rectifies the qi. *Zu San Li*, the uniting and earth point of the stomach channel, fortifies the spleen and boosts the qi. All these points should be drained, except *Zu San Li* which should be needled with the supplementing method. *Da Bao* is the great network point. According to the *Nei Jing (Inner Classic)*, it treats generalized body pain.

NOTE: In a few rare cases, acupuncture and massage can temporarily worsen the symptoms of fibromyalgia when pain is primarily due to malnourishment as opposed to stasis and stagnation.

ADDITIONS & SUBTRACTIONS: If spleen vacuity is marked with fatigue and lack of strength or if the defensive qi is not secure, add *Tai Bai* (Sp 3) and *He Gu* (LI 4). If there is more pronounced dampness in the middle burner, add *Yin Ling Quan* (Sp 9). If dampness is spilling over into the extremities with puffy swelling, also add *Yin Ling Quan* (Sp 9). If there is phlegm dampness, add *Feng Long* (St 40). If generalized blood vacuity is pronounced with malnourishment of the sinew vessels, add *San Yin Jiao* (Sp 6). If there is more serious liver blood vacuity, add *Ge Shu* (Bl 17) and *Gan Shu* (Bl 18). If heart blood is vacuous and the spirit is disquieted, add *Shen Men* (Ht 7) and *San Yin Jiao* (Sp 6). If liver depression has transformed heat and that heat has entered the blood division, add *Xue Hai* (Sp 10) and replace *Tai Chong* with *Xing Jian* (Liv 2). If there is heat specifically in the liver-gallbladder, lungs, stomach, and intestines, add *Yang Ling Quan* (GB 34) and *He Gu* (LI 4). If there is heat specifically in the liver-gallbladder, heart, stomach, and intestines, add *Yang Ling Quan* (GB 34), *Tong Li* (Ht 5), and *He Gu* (LI 4). If enduring heat has damaged stomach and/or lung fluids, add *Fu Liu* (Ki 7). If there is blood stasis, add *He Gu* (LI 4) and *San Yin Jiao* (Sp 6). If there is painful diarrhea, add *Tian Shu* (St 25). For pain or weakness in the lower limbs, add *Cheng Shan* (Bl 57). For pain in the upper limbs, add *Qu Chi* (LI 11).

For pain on palpation near *Feng Chi* (GB 20), needle *Feng Chi* (GB 20) or the *a shi* point. For pain on palpation near *Bai Lao* (M-HN-30), needle *Bai Lao* (M-HN-30) or the *a shi* point. For pain on palpation near *Tian Jing* (GB 21), needle *Tian Jing* (GB 21) or the *a shi* point. For pain on palpation near *Qu Yuan* (SI 13) or *Bing Feng* (SI 12), needle these points or the *a shi* point. For pain on palpation near *Yu Zhong* (Ki 26), needle *Yu Zhong* (Ki 26) or the *a shi* point. For pain on palpation near *Shou San Li* (LI 10), needle *Shou San Li* (LI 10) or the *a shi* point. For pain on palpation near *Bao Huang* (Bl 53), needle *Bao Huang* (Bl 53) or the *a shi* point. For pain on palpation on the greater trochanter posterior to the trochanteric prominence, needle the *a shi* point or eventually *Huan Tiao* (GB 30) or *Ju Liao* (GB 29). For pain on palpation near *Xue Hai* (Sp 10), needle *Xue Hai* (Sp 10) or the *a shi* point. However, usually *Da Bao* is sufficient to stop pain throughout the body.

2. DAMP HEAT PATTERN

MAIN SYMPTOMS: Loose stools or diarrhea, possibly dark, green-colored stools or light yellow, mustard-colored stools, a burning or acid feeling around the anus with or after defecation, foul-smelling stools, hot, possibly red, possibly swollen, painful limbs, red, hot, swollen, wet, or weeping skin lesions, hot, frequent, burning, and/or painful urination, red, hot swollen, wet or weeping external genitalia, thick white, curdy or creamy, yellow vaginal discharge, yellow-green nasal mucus, slimy, yellow tongue fur, and a slippery, rapid pulse

NOTE: Damp heat complicates most if not all cases of FMS. However, it is usually not the main pattern but rather complicates other patterns such as liver-spleen disharmony, qi and yin vacuity, and yin and yang vacuity. Damp heat manifests somewhat differently depending in which part of the body it is lodged. Areas of the body commonly effected by damp heat include the reproductive tract and external genitalia, the urinary tract, the digestive tract, the lower limbs, and the skin. Patients with damp heat typically exhibit that damp heat in two or more of these areas but rarely in all of them at the same time. It is common for damp heat to migrate from system to system within the body, sometimes manifesting as urinary tract damp heat, other times as gastrointestinal damp heat, and yet other times as dermatological damp heat. When damp heat causes impediment pain, this is also often called wind damp heat impediment. Because the heat of damp heat tends to waft upwards, damp heat below can also give rise to signs and symptoms of dry heat above, such as heat in the heart or dry mouth and throat and chapped lips.

TREATMENT PRINCIPLES: Clear heat and eliminate dampness

RX: For damp heat in the stomach and intestines, *Ban Xia Xie Xin Tang* (Pinelliae Drain the Heart Decoction)

INGREDIENTS: Rhizoma Pinelliae Ternatae (*Ban Xia*), 12g, Radix Codonopsitis Pilosulae (*Dang Shen*) and Radix Scutellariae Baicalensis (*Huang Qin*), 9g each, dry Rhizoma Zingiberis (*Gan Jiang*) and mix-fried Radix Glycyrrhizae (*Gan Cao*), 6g each Rhizoma Coptidis Chinensis (*Huang Lian*), 3g, and Fructus Zizyphi Jujubae (*Da Zao*), 3 pieces

ANALYSIS OF FORMULA: *Huang Qin* and *Huang Lian* clear heat, eliminate dampness, and resolve toxins. *Ban Xia* dries dampness and harmonizes the stomach and intestines. *Dang Shen, Gan Jiang, Da Zao,* and mix-fried *Gan Cao* fortify the spleen and prevent further damp accumulation which tends to transform into heat.

ADDITIONS & SUBTRACTIONS: For marked fatigue, add 18 grams of Radix Astragali Membranacei (*Huang Qi*). For diarrhea, add 18 grams of Radix Puerariae (*Ge Gen*).

ACUPUNCTURE & MOXIBUSTION: *Zhong Wan* (CV 12), *Tian Shu* (St 25), *Yin Ling Quan* (Sp 9), *Nei Ting* (St 44), *Da Bao* (Sp 21)

ANALYSIS OF FORMULA: Draining *Zhong Wan, Tian Shu, Shang Ju Xu,* and *Nei Ting* clears the stomach and intestines, clears and disinhibits dampness and heat. Draining *Da Bao* treats generalized body pain.

ADDITIONS & SUBTRACTIONS: Please see pattern #1 above.

For damp heat impediment, *Si Miao San Jia Wei* (Four Wonders Powder with Added Flavors)

INGREDIENTS: Uncooked Semen Coicis Lachryma-jobi (*Yi Yi Ren*), 21g, Radix Achyranthis Bidentatae (*Niu Xi*), 15g, and Rhizoma Atractylodis (*Can Zhu*), Cortex Phellodendri (*Huang Bai*), and Fructus Chaenomelis Lagenariae (*Mu Gua*), 9g each

ANALYSIS OF FORMULA: *Yi Yi Ren, Cang Zhu, Huang Bai,* and *Mu Gua* together clear heat and disinhibit dampness. *Yi Yi Ren* and *Mu Gua* eliminate dampness and free the flow of impediment, while *Cang Zhu* dispels wind dampness. *Niu Xi* supplements liver and kidneys and reinforces sinews and bones. In addition, it guides the other medicinals to move downward to the lower half of the body.

ADDITIONS & SUBTRACTIONS: For predominant dampness, add nine grams each of Scerotium Poriae Cocos (*Fu Ling*) and Rhizoma Alismatis (*Ze Xie*).

ACUPUNCTURE & MOXIBUSTION: *Yin Ling Quan* (Sp 9), *Qu Chi* (LI 11), *a shi* points, *Da Bao* (Sp 21)

ANALYSIS OF FORMULA: Draining *Yin Ling Quan* and *Qu Chi* clears and disinhibits dampness and heat, dispels wind dampness and frees the flow of impediment. Draining *a shi* points selected according to the location of pain frees the flow of the network vessels and disinhibits impediment. *Da Bao* treats generalized body pain.

ADDITIONS & SUBTRACTIONS: Please see pattern #1 above.

For damp heat in the bladder, *Ba Zheng San* (Eight Correcting [Ingredients] Powder) plus *Xiao Chai Hu Tang* (Minor Bupleurum Decoction) with additions & subtractions

INGREDIENTS: Talcum (*Hua Shi*), 18g, Sclerotium Poriae Cocos (*Fu Ling*) and Semen Plantaginis (*Che Qian Zi*) 12g each, Herba Dianthi (*Qu Mai*), Fructus Gardeniae Jasminoidis (*Zhi Zi*), Herba Polygoni Avicularis (*Bian Xu*), Radix Bupleuri (*Chai Hu*), Radix Scutellariae Baicalensis (*Huang Qin*), ginger stir-fried Rhizoma Pinelliae Ternatae (*Ban Xia*), and Radix Codonopsitis Pilosulae (*Dang Shen*), 9g each, and mix-fried Radix Glycyrrhizae (*Gan Cao*), 6g

ANALYSIS OF FORMULA: *Hua Shi, Che Qian Zi, Qu Mai,* and *Bian Xu* clear heat and eliminate dampness in the bladder and free the flow of urination. *Zhi Shi* and *Huang Qin* clear heat and dry dampness. *Fu Ling* seeps dampness and fortifies the spleen, while *Dang Shen* and mix-fried *Gan Cao* fortify the spleen and supplement the qi. *Ban Xia* transforms dampness and, therefore, helps fortify the spleen. *Chai Hu* courses the liver and rectifies the qi. It also clears depressive heat via out-thrusting.

ACUPUNCTURE & MOXIBUSTION: *Yin Ling Quan* (Sp 9), *Zhong Ji* (CV 3), *Xing Jian* (Liv 2), *Zu San Li* (St 36), *Da Bao* (Sp 21)

ANALYSIS OF FORMULA: Draining *Yin Ling Quan* and *Zhong Ji* clears and disinhibits dampness and heat in the bladder. Draining *Xing Jian* clears and eliminates damp heat from the liver channel, especially in the lower burner.

Supplementing *Zu San Li* fortifies the spleen to prevent further damp accumulation which tends to transform into heat. *Da Bao* treats generalized body pain.

ADDITIONS & SUBTRACTIONS: Please see pattern #1 above.

For damp heat in the uterus with abnormal vaginal discharge, *Er Huang San Bai Wan Jia Jian* (Two Yellows & Three Whites Pills with Additions & Subtractions)

INGREDIENTS: Rhizoma Atractylodis Macrocephalae (*Bai Zhu*), Radix Albus Paeoniae Lactiflorae (*Bai Shao*), Hallyositum Rubrum (*Chi Shi Zhi*), Radix Astragali Membranacei (*Huang Qi*), and Radix Angelicae Sinensis (*Dang Gui*), 9g each, Cortex Phellodendri (*Huang Bai*), Rhizoma Atractylodis (*Cang Zhu*), Radix Bupleuri (*Chai Hu*), and Cortex Toonae Sinensis (*Chun Gen Pi*), 6g each, and Rhizoma Coptidis Chinensis (*Huang Lian*) and Rhizoma Cimicifugae (*Sheng Ma*), 3g each

ANALYSIS OF FORMULA: *Huang Bai, Huang Lian, Sheng Ma, Cang Zhu,* and *Bai Zhu* together clear and dry damp heat. *Bai Shao* and *Chai Hu* course and harmonize the liver to prevent liver depression from transforming into heat. *Dang Gui* nourishes and quickens the blood. *Bai Zhu* and *Huang Qi* fortify the spleen and thus also prevent further damp accumulation from transforming into heat. *Chun Gen Pi* and *Chi Shi Zhi* astringe, secure, and stop abnormal vaginal discharge.

ACUPUNCTURE & MOXIBUSTION: *Qu Gu* (CV 2), *Yin Ling Quan* (Sp 9), *Dai Mai* (GB 26), *Xing Jian* (Liv 2), *Zu San Li* (St 36), *Da Bao* (Sp 21)

ANALYSIS OF FORMULA: Draining *Qu Gu* and *Yin Ling Quan* clears and disinhibits damp heat from the uterus. *Dai Mai* is an empirical point for the treatment of abnormal vaginal discharge. Draining *Xing Jian* clears and eliminates damp heat from the liver channel, especially in the lower burner. Supplementing *Zu San Li* fortifies the spleen to prevent further damp accumulation from transforming into heat. Draining *Da Bao* treats generalized body pain.

ADDITIONS & SUBTRACTIONS: Please see pattern #1 above.

For damp heat in the external genitalia with itching, *Yi Huang Tang Jia Jian* (Change the Yellow Decoction with Additions & Subtractions)

INGREDIENTS: Cortex Phellodendri (*Huang Bai*), Radix Sophorae Flavescentis (*Ku Shen*), Semen Plantaginis (*Che Qian Zi*), Radix Dioscoreae Oppositae (*Shan Yao*), Semen Euryalis Ferocis (*Qian Shi*), Semen Coicis Lachryma-jobi (*Yi Yi Ren*), Sclerotium Poriae Cocos (*Fu Ling*), Cortex Radicis Dictamni Dasycarpi (*Bai Xian Pi*), Radix Bupleuri (*Chai Hu*), Flos Lonicerae Japonicae (*Jin Yin Hua*), and Radix Codonopsitis Pilosulae (*Dang Shen*), 9g each, and mix-fried Radix Glycyrrhizae (*Gan Cao*), 3g

ANALYSIS OF FORMULA: *Huang Bai, Ku Shen, Che Qian Zi, Yi Yi Ren, Bai Xian Pi,* and *Jin Yin Hua* together clear and disinhibit dampness and heat in the lower burner, resolve toxins, dispel wind, and stop itching. *Shan Yao, Dang Shen, Qian Shi,* and mix-fried *Gan Cao* fortify the spleen to prevent damp accumulation from pouring downward. *Chai Hu* courses the liver and rectifies the qi as well as leads the other medicinals toward the liver channel in the external genital area.

ACUPUNCTURE & MOXIBUSTION: *Qu Gu* (CV 2), *Yin Ling Quan* (Sp 9), *Li Gou* (Liv 5), *Zu San Li* (St 36), *Da Bao* (Sp 21)

ANALYSIS OF FORMULA: Draining *Qu Gu* and *Yin Ling Quan* clears and disinhibits damp heat in the lower burner. *Li Gou* clears and disinhibits damp heat in the liver channel. It is also an empirical point for treating external genital itching. Supplementing *Zu San Li* fortifies the spleen to prevent further damp accumulation from transforming into heat. Draining *Da Bao* treats generalized body pain.

ADDITIONS & SUBTRACTIONS: Please see pattern #1 above.

For damp heat in the yang ming causing acne, *Yin Chen Hao Tang* (Artemisia Decoction) plus *Ban Xia Xie Xin Tang* (Pinelliae Drain the Heart Decoction) plus *Xiao Chai Hu Tang* (Minor Bupleurum Decoction) with additions & subtractions

INGREDIENTS: Herba Artemisiae Capillaris (*Yin Chen Hao*) and Flos Lonicerae Japonicae (*Jin Yin Hua*), 18g each, Flos Chrysanthemi Indici (*Ye Ju Hua*), Fructus Gardeniae Jasminoidis (*Zhi Zi*), Radix Scutellariae Baicalensis (*Huang Qin*), and Radix Rubrus Paeoniae Lactiflorae (*Chi Shao*), 9g each, Rhizoma Pinelliae Ternatae (*Ban Xia*), Radix Bupleuri (*Chai Hu*), Radix Codonopsitis Pilosulae (*Dang Shen*), and mix-fried Radix Glycyrrhizae (*Gan Cao*), 6g each, and Rhizoma Coptidis Chinensis (*Huang Lian*), 3g

ANALYSIS OF FORMULA: *Yin Chen Hao, Jin Yin Hua, Ye Ju Hua, Zhi Zi, Huang Qin,* and *Huang Lian* together clear heat in the stomach and intestines, dry dampness and resolve toxins. *Ban Xia* dries dampness and harmonizes the stomach and intestines. *Chi Shao* cools the blood and clears the liver. *Chai Hu* courses the liver and rectifies the qi. *Dang Shen* and mix-fried *Gan Cao* fortify the spleen to prevent further damp accumulation from transforming into heat.

ACUPUNCTURE & MOXIBUSTION: *Ling Tai* (GV 10), *Wei Zhong* (Bl 40), *Yin Ling Quan* (Sp 9), *He Gu* (LI 4), *Nei Ting* (St 44), *Da Bao* (Sp 21)

ANALYSIS OF FORMULA: Draining *Ling Tai* and *Wei Zhong* cools the blood and clears heat, especially in the skin. Draining *Yin Ling Quan*, *He Gu*, and *Nei Ting* clears and eliminates damp heat in the stomach and intestines. In addition, *He Gu* is the master point of the face where acne mainly occurs. Draining *Da Bao* treats generalized body pain.

ADDITIONS & SUBTRACTIONS: Please see pattern #1 above.

3. QI & YIN VACUITY WITH LIVER DEPRESSION & FIRE EFFULGENCE PATTERN

MAIN SYMPTOMS: Fatigue, lack of strength, scanty qi, disinclination to speak, low back pain and knee soreness, night-time urination, frequent but scanty, darkish urination, loose stools, dizziness, tinnitus, matitudinal insomnia, night sweats, tidal heat, a pale face but malar flushing, cold hands and feet alternating with vexatious heat in the five hearts, a fat, pale tongue with red tip and scanty, possibly dry and/or yellowish fur, and a fine, rapid, or floating, surging, rapid pulse

TREATMENT PRINCIPLES: Fortify the spleen and boost the qi, supplement the kidneys and enrich yin, clear heat and drain fire

RX: *Tian Wang Bu Xin Dan Jia Jian* (Heavenly Emperor Supplement the Heart Elixir with Additions & Subtractions)

INGREDIENTS: Uncooked Radix Rehmanniae (*Sheng Di*) and Radix Astragali Membranacei (*Huang Qi*), 15g each, Radix Codonopsitis Pilosulae (*Dang Shen*), Radix Scrophulariae Ningpoensis (*Xuan Shen*), Tuber Ophiopogonis Japonici (*Mai Dong*), and Tuber Asparagi Cochinensis (*Tian Men Dong*), 12g each, Fructus Schisandrae Chinensis (*Wu Wei Zi*), Radix Salviae Miltiorrhizae (*Dan Shen*), Radix Angelicae Sinensis (*Dang Gui*), Sclerotium Poriae Cocos (*Fu Ling*), Radix Dioscoreae Oppositae (*Shan Yao*), Radix Polygalae Tenuifoliae (*Yuan Zhi*), Radix Albus Paeoniae Lactiflorae (*Bai Shao*), Semen Zizyphi Spinosae (*Suan Zao Ren*), and Fructus Meliae Toosendan (*Chuan Lian Zi*), 9g each, Radix Platycodi Grandiflori (*Jie Geng*) and mix-fried Radix Glycyrrhizae (*Gan Cao*), 6g each, and Rhizoma Coptidis Chinensis (*Huang Lian*), 3g

ANALYSIS OF FORMULA: *Huang Qi, Dang Shen, Fu Ling, Shan Yao,* and mix-fried *Gan Cao* fortify the spleen and boost the qi. *Chuan Lian Zi* and *Bai Shao* course and harmonize the liver and resolve depression. *Sheng Di, Mai Men Dong,* and *Tian Men Dong* enrich yin, while *Dang Gui, Bai Shao,* and *Suan Zao Ren* nourish the blood, remembering that blood and essence share a common source. *Xuan Shen* clears heat and cools the blood, nourishes yin and eliminates vexation. *Wu Wei Zi, Mai Men Dong, Tian Men Dong, Dan Shen, Fu Ling, Yuan Zhi,* and *Suan Zao Ren* together nourish the heart and liver and quiet the ethereal soul and spirit. *Huang Lian* clears the heart and drains fire, thus indirectly quieting the spirit, and *Jie Geng* guides the other medicinals to the area of the chest and heart.

ADDITIONS & SUBTRACTIONS: For low back and knee soreness and pain, add nine grams each of Radix Achyranthis Bidentatae (*Niu Xi*), Cortex Eucommiae Ulmoidis (*Du Zhong*), and Ramulus Loranthi Seu Visci (*Sang Ji Sheng*). For night-time urination, add 12 grams each of Fructus Alpiniae Oxyphyllae (*Yi Zhi Ren*) and Fructus Rosae Laevigatae (*Jin Ying Zi*). For frequent but scanty, darkish urination, add nine grams each of Sclerotium Polypori Umbellati (*Zhu Ling*) and Rhizoma Alismatis (*Ze Xie*). For loose stools, add 12 grams of Rhizoma Atractylodis Macrocephalae (*Bai Zhu*). For dizziness, add 12 grams each of Radix Achyranthis Bidentatae (*Niu Xi*) and Fructus Lycii Chinensis (*Gou Qi Zi*). For night sweats, add 12 grams each of Semen Biotae Orientalis (*Bai Zi Ren*) and Semen Levis Tritici Aestivi (*Fu Xiao Mai*). If spleen vacuity is marked, increase the dosage of *Huang Qi* up to 25 grams and add 12 grams of Rhizoma Atractylodis Macrocephalae (*Bai Zhu*). If there is more serious kidney yin vacuity, add 12 grams of cooked Radix Rehmanniae (*Shu Di*). If there is more serious liver blood vacuity, add nine grams of Fructus Lycii Chinensis (*Gou Qi Zi*) and 12 grams of Radix Polygoni Multiflori (*He Shou Wu*). If heart blood is vacuous and the spirit is disquieted, add 12 grams each of Arillus Euphoriae Longanae (*Long Yan Rou*) and Semen Biotae Orientalis (*Bai Zi Ren*). If liver depression has transformed heat, add nine grams each of Fructus Gardeniae Jasminoidis (*Zhi Zi*) and Cortex Radicis Moutan (*Dan Pi*). If there is blood stasis, add nine grams each of Semen Pruni Persicae (*Tao Ren*) and Flos Carthami Tinctorii (*Hong Hua*). If there is painful diarrhea, add nine grams of Radix Ledebouriellae Divaricatae (*Fang Feng*) and six grams of Pericarpium Citri Reticulatae (*Chen Pi*).

ACUPUNCTURE & MOXIBUSTION: *San Yin Jiao* (Sp 6), *Fu Liu* (Ki 7), *Zu San Li* (St 36), *Tai Chong* (Liv 3), *Da Bao* (Sp 21)

ANALYSIS OF FORMULA: Supplementing *San Yin Jiao* and *Fu Liu* enriches yin and nourishes the blood, supplements the liver and boosts the kidneys. Supplementing *Zu San Li* and *San Yin Jiao* fortifies the spleen, boosts the qi, and disinhibits dampness. Draining *Tai Chong* courses the liver and resolves the depression. Draining *Da Bao* treats generalized body pain.

ADDITIONS & SUBTRACTIONS: For insomnia, add *Bai Hui* (GV 20) and *Shen Men* (Ht 7). If heart blood is vacuous and the spirit is disquieted, add *Shen Men* (Ht 7). For low back and knee pain and soreness, add *Gong Sun* (Sp 4) and *Shen Shu* (Bl 23). For night-time urination, add *Zhi Shi* (Bl 52). For frequent but scanty, darkish urination, add *Zhong Ji* (CV 3) and *Yin Ling Quan* (Sp 9). For loose stools, add *Yin*

Ling Quan (Sp 9). For dizziness, add *Feng Chi* (GB 20) and *Bai Hui* (GV 20). For night sweats, add *Yin Xi* (Ht 6). If spleen vacuity is marked, add *Tai Bai* (Sp 3). If there is more serious liver blood vacuity, add *Ge Shu* (Bl 17) and *Gan Shu* (Bl 18). If there is more serious kidney yin vacuity, add *Shen Shu* (Bl 23).

4. Spleen-kidney yang vacuity with liver depression pattern

Main symptoms: Fatigue, lack of strength, scanty qi, disinclination to speak, possible spontaneous perspiration, possible daybreak diarrhea but definitely a tendency to loose stools, low back and knee soreness and limpness, decreased sexual desire, frequent urination, nocturia, cold hands and feet, especially the feet, chest, abdominal, breast, rib-side oppression, distention, fullness, and pain, menstrual irregularities and especially a shortened luteal phase, possible dysmenorrhea, irritability, emotional depression, a pale but dark, fat, swollen tongue with thin, white or somewhat slimy fur, and a bowstring, fine, possibly deep, forceless pulse at least in the cubit positions

Note: This pattern is a typical complication of FMS in perimenopausal women. It most commonly shows up after 40 years of age.

Treatment principles: Fortify the spleen and boost the qi, supplement the kidneys and invigorate yang, course the liver and rectify the qi

Rx: *Bu Zhong Yi Qi Tang* (Supplement the Center & Boost the Qi Decoction) & *You Gui Yin* (Restore the Right [Kidney] Drink) with additions and subtractions

Ingredients: Radix Astragali Membranacei (*Huang Qi*), 15g, Semen Cuscutae Chinensis (*Tu Si Zi*) and Radix Dioscoreae Oppositae (*Shan Yao*), 12g each, cooked Radix Rehmanniae (*Shu Di*), Cortex Eucommiae Ulmoidis (*Du Zhong*), Fructus Lycii Chinensis (*Gou Qi Zi*), Fructus Corni Officinalis (*Shan Zhu Yu*), Rhizoma Atractylodis Macrocephalae (*Bai Zhu*), and Radix Bupleuri (*Chai Hu*), 9g each, and Radix Angelicae Sinensis (*Dang Gui*), Pericarpium Citri Reticulatae (*Chen Pi*) and mix-fried Radix Glycyrrhizae (*Gan Cao*), 6g each

Analysis of formula: *Huang Qi, Tu Si Zi, Shan Yao, Bai Zhu*, and mix-fried *Gan Cao* fortify the spleen and boost the qi. *Shu Di, Shan Yao, Tu Si Zi, Du Zhong, Gou Qi Zi*, and *Shan Zhu Yu* supplement the kidneys, enrich yin, and invigorate yang. *Chai Hu* courses the liver and, with *Chen Pi*, rectifies the qi. *Dang Gui* nourishes and quickens the blood, nourishes the sinews and harmonizes the liver.

Additions & subtractions: If there is blood vacuity failing to nourish the sinew vessels, add 15 grams each of Radix Salviae Miltiorrhizae (*Dan Shen*) and Caulis Milletiae Seu Spatholobi (*Ji Xue Teng*). For severe fatigue, add 12 grams of Radix Codonopsitis Pilosulae (*Dang Shen*) and increase the dosage of *Huang Qi* up to 30 grams. For daybreak diarrhea, add nine grams of Fructus Schisandrae Chinensis (*Wu Wei Zi*), six grams of Semen Myristicae Fragrantis (*Rou Dou Kou*), and three grams of Fructus Evodiae Rutecarpae (*Wu Zhu Yu*). For decreased sexual desire, add nine grams each of Herba Epimedii (*Yin Yang Huo*) and Rhizoma Curculiginis Orchioidis (*Xian Mao*). For frequent urination and nocturia, add 12 grams each of Fructus Alpiniae Oxyphyllae (*Yi Zhi Ren*) and Fructus Rosae Laevigatae (*Jin Ying Zi*). For chest, abdominal, breast, and rib-side oppression, distention, fullness, and pain due to liver depression, add nine grams each of Rhizoma Cyperi Rotundi (*Xiang Fu*), Radix Auklandiae Lappae (*Mu Xiang*), and Tuber Curcumae (*Yu Jin*). For menstrual irregularities, dysmenorrhea, and PMS, add nine grams each of Rhizoma Cyperi Rotundi (*Xiang Fu*) and Radix Ligustici Wallichii (*Chuan Xiong*).

Acupuncture & moxibustion: *San Yin Jiao* (Sp 6), *Zu San Li* (St 36), *Guan Yuan* (CV 4), *Tai Chong* (Liv 3), *Da Bao* (Sp 21)

Analysis of formula: Supplementing *San Yin Jiao* supplements the spleen, liver, and kidneys and regulates and rectifies the chong and ren. Supplementing *Zu San Li* fortifies the spleen and boosts the qi, supplements the latter heaven to support the former heaven, and, with moxibustion, warms yang. Supplementing *Guan Yuan* with moxibustion warms and supplements both spleen and kidney yang and regulates and rectifies the chong and ren. Draining *Tai Chong* courses the liver and resolves depression. Draining *Da Bao* treats generalized body pain.

Additions & subtractions: For severe fatigue, add *Tai Bai* (Sp 3). For daybreak diarrhea, add *Ming Men* (GV 4). For decreased sexual desire, add *Ming Men* (GV 4) and *Zhi Shi* (Bl 52). For chest, abdominal, breast, and rib-side oppression, distention, fullness, and pain due to liver depression, add *Nei Guan* (Per 6) and *Wai Guan* (TB 5). For menstrual irregularities, dysmenorrhea, and PMS, add *Jian Shi* (Per 5) and *Gui Lai* (St 29). For spontaneous perspiration, add *He Gu* (LI 4) and *Fu Liu* (Ki 7). For low back and knee soreness and limpness, add *Gong Sun* (Sp 4) and *Fu Liu* (Ki 7). For cold hands, add *He Gu* (LI 4). For cold lower limbs and feet, add *Cheng Shan* (Bl 57). For concomitant blood vacuity, add *Ge Shu* (Bl 17) and *Gan Shu* (Bl 18). If there is more serious kidney yang vacuity, add *Shen Shu* (Bl 23) with moxibustion.

5. Spleen qi and yin & yang vacuity with vacuity heat and liver depression pattern

Main symptoms: Fatigue, lack of strength, scanty qi, disinclination to speak, possible spontaneous perspiration and/or night sweats, loose stools or constipation, low back and knee soreness and limpness, decreased sexual desire, frequent urination, nocturia, cold hands and feet alternating with vexatious heat in the five centers, tidal heat, a pale face but malar flushing, chest, abdominal, breast, rib-side oppression, distention, fullness, and pain, menstrual irregularities and especially a shortened luteal phase, possible dysmenorrhea, irritability, emotional depression, a tender, swollen, red tongue with teeth-marks on its edges and scanty, possibly yellow fur, and a bowstring, fine, rapid pulse which is possibly deep and forceless at least in the right cubit position

TREATMENT PRINCIPLES: Fortify the spleen and boost the qi, supplement the kidneys and invigorate yang, enrich yin and clear heat, course the liver and rectify the qi

RX: *Bu Zhong Yi Qi Tang* (Supplement the Center & Boost the Qi Decoction) & *Er Xian Tang* (Two Immortals Decoction) with additions and subtractions

INGREDIENTS: Radix Astragali Membranacei (*Huang Qi*), 15g, Radix Codonopsitis Pilosulae (*Dang Shen*), Cortex Phellodendri (*Huang Bai*), Rhizoma Anemarrhenae Aspheloidis (*Zhi Mu*), Herba Epimedii (*Xian Ling Pi*), Rhizoma Curculiginis Orchioidis (*Xian Mao*), Radix Angelicae Sinensis (*Dang Gui*), Rhizoma Atractylodis Macrocephalae (*Bai Zhu*), and Fructus Meliae Toosendan (*Chuan Lian Zi*), 9g each, Pericarpium Citri Reticulatae (*Chen Pi*) and mix-fried Radix Glycyrrhizae (*Gan Cao*), 6g each, and Radix Bupleuri (*Chai Hu*), 1.5-3g

ANALYSIS OF FORMULA: *Huang Qi, Dang Shen, Bai Zhu,* and mix-fried *Gan Cao* fortify the spleen and boost the qi. *Zhi Mu* nourishes kidney yin and, with *Huang Bai,* clears vacuity heat. *Yin Yang Huo* and *Xian Mao* warm and supplement kidney yang. *Dang Gui* nourishes the blood and harmonizes the liver. *Chai Hu* and *Chuan Lian Zi* course the liver and, with *Chen Pi,* rectify the qi. In addition, *Chuan Lian Zi* clears heat and eliminates dampness.

ADDITIONS & SUBTRACTIONS: Add 21 grams of Fructus Levis Tritici Aestivi (*Fu Xiao Mai*) and 12 grams of Concha Ostreae (*Mu Li*) if there are night sweats and hot flashes. Add 12 grams each of Semen Zizyphi Spinosae (*Suan Zao Ren*) and Cortex Albizziae Julibrissinis (*He Huan Pi*) if there is insomnia. Add 15 grams each of Caulis Milletiae Seu Spatholobi (*Ji Xue Teng*), Radix Achyranthis Bidentatae (*Niu Xi*), and Cortex Radicis Acanthopanacis Gracilistylis (*Wu Jia Pi*) for malnourished sinews and body pain. Add 15 grams each of Radix Scrophulariae Ningpoensis (*Xuan Shen*) and Spica Prunellae Vulgaris (*Xia Ku Cao*), 12 grams each of Concha Ostreae (*Mu Li*), Semen Citri Reticulatae (*Ju He*), and Fructus Akebiae Trifoliatae (*Ba Yue Zha*), and nine grams each of Rhizoma Pinelliae Ternatae (*Ban Xia*), Herba Saragassii (*Hai Zao*), Bulbus Fritillariae Thunbergii (*Zhe Bei Mu*), and Sqauma Manitis Pentadactylis (*Chuan Shan Jia*) for fibrocystic breasts. For constipation, add six grams of Fructus Immaturus Citri Aurantii (*Zhi Shi*) and/or three grams of Radix Et Rhizoma Rhei (*Da Huang*). For daybreak diarrhea, add nine grams of Fructus Schisandrae Chinensis (*Wu Wei Zi*), six grams of Semen Myristicae Fragrantis (*Rou Dou Kou*), and three grams of Fructus Evodiae Rutecarpae (*Wu Zhu Yu*). For decreased sexual desire, add nine grams of Herba Cistanchis Deserticolae (*Rou Cong Rong*). For frequent urination and nocturia, add 12 grams each of Fructus Alpiniae Oxyphyllae (*Yi Zhi Ren*) and Fructus Rosae Laevigatae (*Jin Ying Zi*). For chest, abdominal, breast, and rib-side oppression, distention, fullness, and pain due to liver depression, add nine grams each of Rhizoma Cyperi Rotundi (*Xiang Fu*), Radix Auklandiae Lappae (*Mu Xiang*), and Tuber Curcumae (*Yu Jin*). For menstrual irregularities, dysmenorrhea, and PMS, add nine grams each of Rhizoma Cyperi Rotundi (*Xiang Fu*) and Radix Ligustici Wallichii (*Chuan Xiong*). For more marked kidney yin vacuity, add nine grams each of Radix Polygoni Multiflori (*He Shou Wu*), Fructus Ligustri Lucidi (*Nu Zhen Zi*), and Herba Ecliptae Prostratae (*Han Lian Cao*).

ACUPUNCTURE & MOXIBUSTION: *San Yin Jiao* (Sp 6), *Zu San Li* (St 36), *Guan Yuan* (CV 4), *Tai Chong* (Liv 3), *Fu Liu* (Ki 7), *Da Bao* (Sp 21)

ANALYSIS OF FORMULA: For the functions of *San Yin Jiao, Zu San Li, Guan Yuan,* and *Tai Chong,* please see the preceding pattern. Supplementing *Fu Liu* supplements the kidneys, enriches yin, and downbears vacuity heat. Draining *Da Bao* treats generalized body pain.

ADDITIONS & SUBTRACTIONS: Please see the preceding pattern. For vexatious heat in the five hearts or centers, tidal heat, and malar flushing, add *Yin Xi* (Ht 6) and *Da Zhui* (GV 14). For irritability and emotional depression, add *Nei Guan* (Per 6).

6. BLOOD STASIS PATTERN

MAIN SYMPTOMS: Fixed, sharp, stabbing and/or severe pain which is commonly worse in the evening and at night, engorged visible blood vessels, from large varicosities to spider nevi and cherry hemagiomas, engorged and distended sublingual veins, painful menstruation, blood clots in the menstruate, blood clots in any visible bleeding, a dark, sooty facial complexion, liver or age spots, a dark, possibly purplish tongue or static spots or black and blue marks on the tongue, and a bowstring, choppy, deep, slow, and/or irregular pulse

NOTE: This pattern only complicates other of the above patterns based on the saying, "New diseases are in the channels, and old diseases are in the network vessels."

TREATMENT PRINCIPLES: Quicken the blood and transform stasis, free the flow of the network vessels and stop pain

RX: *Shen Tong Zhu Yu Tang* (Body Pain Dispel Stasis Decoction)

INGREDIENTS: Semen Pruni Persicae (*Tao Ren*), Flos Carthami Tinctorii (*Hong Hua*), Radix Angelicae Sinensis (*Dang Gui*), and Radix Cyathulae (*Chuan Niu Xi*), 9g each, Radix Ligustici Wallichii (*Chuan Xiong*), Radix Et Rhizoma Notopterygii (*Qiang Huo*), Radix Gentianae Macrophyllae (*Qin Jiao*), Feces Trogopterori Seu Pteromi (*Wu Ling Zhi*), Lumbricus (*Di Long*), Resina Myrrhae (*Mo Yao*), and Rhizoma Cyperi Rotundi (*Xiang Fu*), 6g each, and Radix Glycyrrhizae (*Gan Cao*), 3g

ANALYSIS OF FORMULA: *Tao Ren, Hong Hua, Dang Gui, Chuan Xiong, Wu Ling Zhi*, and *Mo Yao* all quicken the blood, transform stasis, and stop pain. In addition, *Dang Gui* nourishes the blood. *Qiang Huo* and *Qin Jiao* dispel wind dampness, free the flow of the network vessels, and stop pain. In addition, *Qiang Huo* works in the upper part of the body, while *Qin Jiao* moves to the four limbs and spine. *Di Long* frees the flow of the network vessels and stops pain. *Xiang Fu* moves the qi to move the blood, and *Gan Cao* harmonizes the other medicinals in this formula.

ADDITIONS & SUBTRACTIONS: If there is low back pain, add nine grams each of Cortex Eucommiae Ulmoidis (*Du Zhong*) and Radix Morindae Officinalis (*Ba Ji Tian*). If there is concomitant qi vacuity with marked fatigue and lack of strength, add 15 grams of Radix Astragali Membranacei (*Huang Qi*) and nine grams of Radix Codonopsitis Pilosulae (*Dang Shen*). If there is accompanying dampness and heat, add nine grams each of Rhizoma Atractylodis (*Cang Zhu*) and Cortex Phellodendri (*Huang Bai*). If there is simultaneous blood vacuity, add 15 grams each of Radix Polygoni Multiflori (*He Shou Wu*) and Caulis Milletiae Seu Spatholobi (*Ji Xue Teng*).

ACUPUNCTURE & MOXIBUSTION: *He Gu* (LI 4), *San Yin Jiao* (Sp 6), *Jian Shi* (Per 5), *Wai Guan* (TB 5), *Da Bao* (Sp 21)

ANALYSIS OF FORMULA: Draining *He Gu* and *San Yin Jiao* quickens the blood in the whole body. Draining *Jian Shi* and *Wai Guan* moves the qi and quickens the blood in the whole body. *He Gu* works in the upper part of the body, *San Yin Jiao* works in the lower part of the body, *Jian Shi* works in the interior, and *Wai Guan* works in the exterior. In addition, *Jian Shi* moves the qi and quickens the blood in the anterior and posterior parts of the body. When treated with draining method, these points stop generalized body pain. Draining *Da Bao* also treats generalized body pain.

ADDITIONS & SUBTRACTIONS: Please see pattern #1 above.

7. PHLEGM NODULATION PATTERN

MAIN SYMPTOMS: Swollen lymphnodes, fibrocystic lumps in the breast, other hard, round, subcutaneous lumps and bumps

NOTE: Like static blood above, this pattern only complicates other patterns of FMS.

TREATMENT PRINCIPLES: Transform phlegm and scatter nodulation

RX: *Xiao Luo Wan* (Disperse Scrofula Pills) & *Er Chen Tang* (Two Aged [Ingredients]Decoction) with added flavors

INGREDIENTS: Radix Scrophulariae Ningpoensis (*Xuan Shen*), Spica Prunellae Vulgaris (*Xia Ku Cao*), and Bulbus Fritillariae Ningpoensis (*Zhe Bei Mu*), 15g each, Concha Ostreae (*Mu Li*), Herba Saragassii (*Hai Zao*), and Thallus Algae (*Kun Bu*), 12g each, Rhizoma Pinelliae Ternatae (*Ban Xia*), Sclerotium Poriae Cocos (*Fu Ling*), Pericarpium Citri Reticulatae (*Chen Pi*), 9g each, and mix-fried Radix Glycyrrhizae (*Gan Cao*), 3g

ANALYSIS OF FORMULA: *Ban Xia, Chen Pi, Fu Ling*, and mix-fried *Gan Cao* make up *Er Chen Tang* (Two Aged [Ingredients] Decoction) which is the main Chinese medicinal formula for transforming phlegm. With *Zhe Bei Mu, Hai Zao*, and *Kun Bu*, they transform phlegm and scatter nodulation. *Xuan Shen, Xia Ku Cao*, and *Mu Li* further soften the hard and scatter nodulation.

ADDITIONS & SUBTRACTIONS: For liver depression qi stagnation, add 9 grams each of Radix Bupleuri (*Chai Hu*), Radix Albus Paeoniae Lactiflorae (*Bai Shao*), and Pericarpium Citri Reticulatae Viride (*Qing Pi*). For phlegm heat with thirst, add 9 grams of Radix Trichosanthis Kirlowii (*Tian Hua Fen*).

ACUPUNCTURE & MOXIBUSTION: *Zu San Li* (St 36), *Feng Long* (St 40), *Da Bao* (Sp 21)

ANALYSIS OF FORMULA: Supplementing *Zu San Li* and draining *Feng Long* fortifies the spleen, disinhibits dampness, and transforms phlegm. Draining *Da Bao* treats generalized body pain.

ADDITIONS & SUBTRACTIONS: For liver depression qi stagnation, add *Tai Chong* (Liv 3) and *Jian Shi* (Per 5). For phlegm heat with thirst, add *Nei Ting* (St 44). For swollen lymphnodes, add *Que Pen* (St 12) and *Nao Hui* (TB 13). For fibrocystic lumps in the breast, add *Ru Gen* (St 18) and *Jian Shi* (Per 5). For subcutaneous lumps and bumps, place one needle in each corner and one needle right in the center of the lump.

REMARKS

1. As stated above, the core disease mechanism of FMS is a liver-spleen disharmony. This typically evolves into qi and yin vacuity and liver depression due to either body type or age, remembering that, "Yin is half consumed by 40 years of age." Likewise, it typically evolves into spleen-kidney yang vacuity with liver depression also due to age, this pattern being very common in Western perimenopausal women. Because yin and yang are mutually rooted, yin and yang vacuity with liver depression is also commonly seen.

2. When treating FMS, primary attention should be given to insomnia. Much of the body pain tends to disappear on its own if the patient's sleep can be improved. Insomnia may be due to yin and blood vacuity failing to nourish and quiet the spirit or the upward flaring of heat harassing the spirit. Most often it is due to a combination of both these mechanisms.

If the patient reports that she wakes in the middle of the night in a fright, startles easily, has heart palpitations, experiences phlegm in the back of her throat, and has a bowstring, slippery pulse this is gallbladder qi timidity or heart-gallbladder qi vacuity. Gallbladder qi timidity is shorthand for spleen vacuity engendering phlegm, liver depression qi stagnation, and phlegm harassing the heart. Heart-gallbladder qi vacuity is shorthand for worse qi vacuity now causing heart qi vacuity, heart blood vacuity, liver depression, and phlegm. Either of these two patterns may be complicated by depressive heat harassing the heart spirit. *Wen Dan Tang* (Warm the Gallbladder Decoction) is the usual guiding formula for gallbladder qi timidity, while *Shi Wei Wen Dan Tang* (Ten Flavors Warm the Gallbladder Decoction) is the formula for heart-gallbladder qi vacuity. If there is depressive heat, then Rhizoma Coptidis Chinensis (*Huang Lian*) may be added to either formula in order to clear heat from the heart.

3. When blood stasis or phlegm complicate any of the above patterns, medicinals should be added to those protocols which quicken the blood and transform stasis or transform phlegm. If there is phlegm nodulation, the treatment principles of softening the hard and scattering nodulation are also used.

4. Although many FMS patients benefit from regular weekly massage, others may experience a worsening of the muscular pain and stiffness 1-2 days after massage, even light massage. In that case, *a shi* points should be treated with non-scarring direct thread moxa.

5. The 18 points (all of which are bilateral) which are tender to palpation established by the American College of Rheumatology (ACR) are:

Occiput: At the suboccipital muscle insertion near *Feng Chi* (GB 20)

Lower cervical: At the lateral edges of the intervertebral spaces at C5-C7

Trapezius: At the midpoint of the upper border of the trapezius

Supraspinatus: At the origins above the scapular spine near the medial border

Second rib: At the second costochondral junctions just lateral to the junctions on the upper surfaces

Lateral epicondyle: 2cm distal to the epicondyles

Gluteal: In the upper and outer quadrants of the buttocks in the anterior fold of the muscle

Greater trochanter: Posterior to the trochanteric prominence

Knee: At the medial edge of the fat pad proximal to the joint line

ENDNOTES

[1] Starlanyl, Devin J., "FMS: Fibromyalgia Syndrome," www.sover.net/~devstar/fmsdef.htm, p. 1

[2] It was the Copenhagen Declaration published in 1990 that established the diagnostic criteria of pressure pain at a minimum of 11 of 18 specific points on the body.

[3] Long, James W., *The Essential Guide to Prescription Drugs*, Harper & Row, NY, 1990, p. 483

[4] *Ibid.*, p. 538

[5] Ronco, P. & Flahault, A., "Drug-induced End Stage Renal Disease," *New England Journal of Medicine*, Vol. 331, #25, 1994, p. 1711-1712

27

Gout

Formerly known as "the disease of kings," gout is caused by deposits of uric acid crystals in the joints of the hands, wrists, elbows, knees, ankles, and feet, and particularly the big toe. Symptoms include sudden, severe, pain and tenderness along with possible redness, warmth, and swelling in the affected joints. In 50% of cases, the first attack is characterized by intense pain in the first joint of the big toe. If the attack progresses, fever and chills will appear. Initial gout attacks usually strike at night and are preceded by a specific event, such as excessive consumption of alcohol, trauma, certain drugs, or surgery. Subsequent attacks are common, with most patients experiencing another attack within one year. However, seven percent of gout sufferers never have a second attack. Hyperuricemia leading to uric acid crystal formation is typically caused by either the body's overproduction of uric acid or the kidney's inability to eliminate uric acid fast enough. Uric acid may also collect under the skin as tophi or in the urinary tract as kidney stones. Attacks of gout are commonly precipitated by drinking alcohol, particularly beer and wine, or overeating rich, fatty foods, such as liver, anchovies, and gravy. In addition, this disease is strongly associated with obesity, hypertension, hyperlipidemia, and diabetes mellitus. This condition affects approximately three out of every 1,000 adults and is primarily a disease of adult men, 95% of gout sufferers being males over the age of 30.[1]

The Western medical diagnosis of gout begins with a physical examination and the patient's medical history in an effort to differentiate this type of arthritis from any other. However, definitive diagnosis depends on finding uric acid crystals in the joint fluid during an acute attack. Serum uric acid levels may also be tested and are often elevated. Unfortunately, uric acid levels in the blood alone are often misleading and may be transiently normal or even low. Additionally, uric acid levels are often elevated in individuals without gout. Although there is no cure for gout, colchicine has been the standard Western medical treatment for the pain of gout since the 1800s. While this drug is very effective, its common side effects when orally administered include nausea, vomiting, and diarrhea. These side effects are uncommon when this drug is administered intravenously. Because of the unpleasant side effects of colchicine, NSAIDs have become the treatment of choice for most acute attacks of gout. For patients with elevated serum uric acid, multiple attacks of gout, and tophi or urolithiasis, uric acid normalizing medicines such as probenecid and allopurinol may be prescribed. In addition, reducing obesity and eating a proper diet are essential for managing this disease.

Chinese disease categorization: Gout is a type of *bi zheng* or impediment condition which is specifically called *tong feng*, painful wind, in Chinese medicine. It may also be referred to as *guan jie wai tong feng*, joint external painful wind, or *tong feng xing guan jie yan*, gouty arthritis, in the more modern Chinese medical literature. Other common Chinese disease names for gout are *guan jie liu feng*, joint running wind, and *bai hu guan jie liu feng*, white tiger joint running wind.

Disease causes: Former heaven natural endowment (*i.e.*, sex), unregulated eating and drinking, enduring disease, and possible external contraction of evils

Disease mechanisms: As a species of impediment, gout is caused by either wind damp cold evils or wind damp heat evils. Damp heat evils are mainly internally engendered and are usually the result of or are associated with spleen damage due to unregulated eating and drinking. In particular, alcohol and greasy, fatty, thick-flavored foods tend to produce internal damp heat. Cold and dampness may be either internally engendered or externally contracted. For instance, living in a cold, damp environment may lead to wind damp cold impediment. However, the dampness of wind damp cold impediment may also be due to improper diet, and cold may be vacuity cold due to over-use of bitter, cold, heat-clearing medicinals, enduring disease, or age. Obviously, external evils may also take advantage of righteous vacuity to assail and enter the body. Hence there may be a combination of replete and vacuity evils. Because enduring impediment inhibits the free flow of qi and blood, this condition may be, and often is, complicated by blood stasis.

TREATMENT BASED ON PATTERN DISCRIMINATION:

1. WIND DAMP COLD IMPEDIMENT & BLOOD STASIS PATTERN

MAIN SYMPTOMS: Attacks of severe, acute joint pain which is fixed in location and which is worse on exposure to cold and better with warmth, possible deformation and hardening of the joint with restricted movement. In addition, although there may be swelling, there is no visible redness or heat, and there may be deformation and hardening of the joint with restricted movement. Other signs and symptoms include slimy, white tongue fur, and a slippery, deep, and bowstring or soggy, moderate (*i.e.*, slightly slow), and bowstring pulse.

TREATMENT PRINCIPLES: Dispel wind and eliminate dampness, warm the channels and free the flow of impediment

RX: *Ji Xue Fu Zi Nian Tong Tang* (Milletia & Aconite Assuage Pain Decoction)

INGREDIENTS: Caulis Milletiae Seu Spatholobi (*Ji Xue Teng*) and Caulis Lonicerae Japonicae (*Ren Dong Teng*), 50g each, Rhizoma Atractylodis (*Cang Zhu*), Herba Seu Flos Schizonepetae Tenuifoliae (*Jing Jie Sui*), Radix Ledebouriellae Divaricatae (*Fang Feng*), Radix Angelicae Pubescentis (*Du Huo*), Radix Et Rhizoma Notopterygii (*Qiang Huo*), Ramulus Cinnamomi Cassiae (*Gui Zhi*), Radix Gentianae Macrophyllae (*Qin Jiao*), Radix Clematidis Chinensis (*Wei Ling Xian*), Radix Achyranthis Bidentatae (*Niu Xi*), Radix Angelicae Sinensis (*Dang Gui*), Radix Ligustici Wallichii (*Chuan Xiong*), and Radix Rubrus Paeoniae Lactiflorae (*Chi Shao*), 15g each and, Resina Olibani (*Ru Xiang*), Resina Myrrhae (*Mo Yao*), Radix Lateralis Praeparatus Aconiti Carmichaeli (*Fu Zi*), and Radix Aconiti Carmichaeli (*Chuan Wu*), 6g each

ANALYSIS OF FORMULA: Within this formula, *Ji Xue Teng, Ren Dong Teng, Cang Zhu, Jing Jie Sui, Fang Feng, Du Huo, Qiang Huo, Qin Jiao, Wei Ling Xian*, and *Chuan Wu* all treat wind damp impediment pain. *Ji Xue Teng* also nourishes and quickens the blood, while *Cang Zhu* also dries dampness and fortifies the spleen. *Niu Xi, Dang Gui, Chuan Xiong, Chi Shao, Ru Xiang*, and *Mo Yao* all also nourish and/or quicken the blood. Further, *Niu Xi* leads the other medicinals downward to the lower extremities, and *Gui Zhi* and prepared *Chuan Wu* warm the channels and scatter cold.

ADDITIONS & SUBTRACTIONS: If there is marked qi vacuity, add 15 grams of Radix Astragali Membranacei (*Huang Qi*) and nine grams each of Radix Codonopsitis Pilosulae (*Dang Shen*) and Sclerotium Poriae Cocos (*Fu Ling*) and replace Rhizoma Atractylodis with Rhizoma Atractylodis Macrocephalae (*Bai Zhu*). If there is concomitant phlegm obstruction, add nine grams each of Semen Sinapis Albae (*Bai Jie Zi*) and Rhizoma Arisaematis (*Tian Nan Xing*). If wind is predominant and the pain is moving with itching and possible desquamation in the affected area, subtract *Chi Shao, Ru Xiang*, and *Mo Yao* and add 12 grams each of Radix Seu Rhizoma Cynanchi (*Xu Chang Qing*) and Fructus Xanthii Sibirici (*Cang Er Zi*). If cold is predominant with severe, fixed joint pain and restricted movement, subtract *Ren Dong Teng* and *Chi Shao* and add three grams of Herba Asari Cum Radice (*Xi Xin*) and nine grams of Caulis Piperis Futokadsurae (*Hai Feng Teng*). If dampness is predominant and the joint is swollen, painful, and heavy with numbness, and worsening of symptoms with rainy weather or damp environment, subtract *Jing Jie* and *Chi Shao* and add nine grams each of Radix Stephaniae Tetrandrae (*Han Fang Ji*), Rhizoma Dioscoreae Hypoglaucae (*Bei Xie*), and Rhizoma Smilacis Glabrae (*Tu Fu Ling*).

If there is a qi, blood, and yang vacuity with wind damp cold impediment and blood stasis, replace *Ji Xue Fu Zi Nian Tong Tang* with *Qing Hai Feng Teng Tang* (Sinomenium & Piper Hanceum Decoction): Caulis Milletiae Seu Spatholobi (*Ji Xue Teng*), 15g, Radix Achyranthis Bidentatae (*Niu Xi*), Cortex Eucommiae Ulmoidis (*Du Zhong*), Radix Dipsaci (*Xu Duan*), Fructus Ailanthi Altissimi (*Feng Yan Cao*), Rhizoma Sinomenii Acuti (*Qing Feng Teng*), Rhizoma Piperis Hancei (*Hai Feng Teng*), Radix Angelicae Sinensis (*Dang Gui*), cooked Radix Rehmanniae (*Shu Di*), Radix Astragali Membranacei (*Huang Qi*), Radix Albus Paeoniae Lactiflorae (*Bai Shao*), and Ramulus Cinnamomi Cassiae (*Gui Zhi*), 9g each.

If there is qi, blood, and yin vacuity with wind damp impediment, replace *Ji Xue Fu Zi Nian Tong Tang* with *Du Huo Ji Sheng Tang Jia Wei* (Angelica Pubescens & Loranthus Decoction with Added Flavors): cooked Radix Rehmanniae (*Shu Di*) and Ramulus Loranthi Seu Visci (*Sang Ji Sheng*), 15g each, Radix Achyranthis Bidentatae (*Niu Xi*) and Sclerotium Poriae Cocos (*Fu Ling*), 12g each, Radix Codonopsitis Pilosulae (*Dang Shen*), Radix Albus Paeoniae Lactiflorae (*Bai Shao*), Cortex Eucommiae Ulmoidis (*Du Zhong*), Radix Angelicae Sinensis (*Dang Gui*), Radix Angelicae Pubescentis (*Du Huo*) and Radix Gentianae Macrophyllae (*Qin Jiao*), 9g each, and Resina Olibani (*Ru Xiang*) and Resina Myrrhae (*Mo Yao*), 6g each.

ACUPUNCTURE & MOXIBUSTION: *He Gu* (LI 4), *San Yin Jiao* (Sp 6), distant channel and local points depending on the location of pain. Acupuncture can be helpful for relief of pain in the treatment of gout, but internally administered Chinese medicinals are better for the elimination of uric acid crystals.

ANALYSIS OF FORMULA: Draining *He Gu* and *San Yin Jiao* quickens the blood and frees the flow of the network vessels of the entire body. Draining distant channel and local points frees the flow of the network vessels and stops pain.

ADDITIONS & SUBTRACTIONS: For elbow impediment, add *Qu Chi* (LI 11), *Xiao Hai* (SI 8), *Zhou Liao* (LI 12), and *Shou San Li* (LI 10). For wrist impediment, add *Wai Guan* (TB 5), *Yang Chi* (TB 4), and *Wan Gu* (SI 4). For upper extremity phalangeal and metacarpal impediment, add *Bai Xie* (M-UE-22), *He Gu* (LI 4), and *Hou Xi* (SI 3). For knee impediment, add *Du Bi* (St 35), *Xi Yan* (M-LE-16a), *Qu Quan* (Liv 8), and *Wei Zhong* (Bl 40). For ankle impediment, choose between *Jie Xi* (St 41), *Shang Qiu* (Sp 5), *Qiu Xu* (GB 40), *Kun Lun* (Bl 60), *Tai Xi* (Ki 3), *Shen Mai* (Bl 62), and *Zhao Hai* (Ki 6). For metatarsal and lower extremity phalangeal impediment, add *Jie Xi* (St 41), *Gong Sun* (Sp 4), *Tai Chong* (Liv 3), *Zu Lin Qi* (GB 41), and *Ba Feng* (M-LE-8).

2. WIND DAMP HEAT IMPEDIMENT & BLOOD STASIS PATTERN

MAIN SYMPTOMS: Severe, acute joint aching and pain which is fixed in location and is accompanied by redness, swelling, and heat, possible fever, thirst, constipation, reddish yellow urine, a red tongue with yellow slimy fur, and a slippery, rapid, bowstring or soggy, rapid, bowstring pulse

TREATMENT PRINCIPLES: Clear heat and eliminate dampness, free the flow of the network vessels and stop pain

RX: *Ren Dong Pu Gong Er Miao San* (Caulis Lonicerae & Taraxacum Two Wonders Powder)

INGREDIENTS: Caulis Lonicerae Japonicae (*Ren Dong Teng*), Herba Taraxaci Mongolici Cum Radice (*Pu Gong Ying*), and Semen Coicis Lachryma-jobi (*Yi Yi Ren*), 30g each, Radix Angelicae Sinensis (*Dang Gui*) and Excrementum Bombycis Mori (*Can Sha*), 15g each, and *Liu Yi San* (Six to One Powder, *i.e.*, Talcum, *Hua Shi* and Radix Glycyrrhizae, *Gan Cao*), Semen Plantaginis (*Che Qian Zi*), Rhizoma Atractylodis (*Cang Zhu*), Cortex Phellodendri (*Huang Bai*), Caulis Trachelospermi (*Luo Shi Teng*), and Resina Myrrhae (*Mo Yao*), 9g each

ANALYSIS OF FORMULA: *Ren Dong Teng, Pu Gong Ying,* and *Huang Bai* clear heat and resolve toxins. *Ren Dong Teng* and *Luo Shi Teng* clear heat, free the flow of the network vessels, and stop pain. *Yi Yi Ren, Hua Shi, Che Qian Zi, Can Sha,* and *Cang Zhu* eliminate dampness and, combined with *Huang Bai,* clear and disinhibit dampness and heat. In addition, *Cang Zhu* and *Can Sha* specifically treat damp impediment. *Dang Gui* and *Mo Yao* quicken the blood, transform stasis, and stop pain, and *Gan Cao* harmonizes the other medicinals in this formula.

ADDITIONS & SUBTRACTIONS: For pain in the upper limbs, add nine grams each of Rhizoma Curcumae Longae (*Jiang Huang*) and Ramulus Mori Albi (*Sang Zhi*). For pain in the lower limbs, add nine grams of Radix Cyathulae (*Chuan Niu Xi*) and Fructus Chaenomelis Lagenariae (*Mu Gua*). For severe pain, add 15 grams of Rhizoma Corydalis Yanhusuo (*Yan Hu Suo*), six grams of Resina Olibani (*Ru Xiang*), and three grams of Buthus Martensis (*Quan Xie*), powdered and taken with the strained decoction. For fever, add 30 grams of Gypsum Fibrosum (*Shi Gao*) and nine grams each of Flos Lonicerae Japonicae (*Jin Yin Hua*) and Fructus Forsythiae Suspensae (*Lian Qiao*). For severe joint swelling, add nine grams each of Bulbus Shancigu (*Shan Ci Gu*), Radix Stephaniae Tetrandrae (*Han Fang Ji*), and Rhizoma Dioscoreae Hypoglaucae (*Bei Xie*). For constipation, add nine grams of Radix Et Rhizoma Rhei (*Da Huang*). For heat damaging yin with low-grade fever, night sweats, and dryness of the mouth, add 15 grams each of Herba Artemisiae Apiacae (*Qing Hao*), Radix Gentianae Macrophyllae (*Qin Jiao*), and Rhizoma Anemarrhenae Asphodeloidis (*Zhi Mu*). For restricted mobility, add 12 grams each of Herba Siegesbeckiae (*Xi Xian Cao*), Cortex Erythiniae (*Hai Tong Pi*), and Caulis Sargentodoxae (*Hong Teng*).

ACUPUNCTURE & MOXIBUSTION: *Da Zhui* (GV 14), *Qu Chi* (LI 11), *He Gu* (LI 4), distant channel and local points depending on the location of pain. Acupuncture can be helpful for pain in the treatment of gout, but internally administered Chinese medicinals are better for the elimination of uric acid crystals.

ANALYSIS OF FORMULA: Bleeding *Da Zhui* clears heat and dispels wind. Draining *Qu Chi* and *He Gu* clears heat because the yang ming channel has lots of qi and lots of blood. Draining the distant channel and local points moves the channel qi and frees the flow of the network vessels in the affected area to stop pain.

ADDITIONS & SUBTRACTIONS: Please see pattern #1 above.

3. QI STAGNATION & BLOOD STASIS PATTERN

MAIN SYMPTOMS: Severe, acute, fixed, lancinating pain as if being cut by a knife, a possibly dark or purple tongue or possible static macules or spots, and a bowstring and/or choppy pulse

NOTE: This pattern describes the acute, paroxysmal stage of gout. In addition, it does not typically present in this simple, discrete way but complicates other patterns.

TREATMENT PRINCIPLES: Quicken the blood and transform stasis, free the flow of the network vessels and stop pain

RX: *Wu Ling Di Long Tang* (Trogopterorus & Lumbricus Decoction)

INGREDIENTS: Lumbricus (*Di Long*), 12g, Feces Trogopterori Seu Pteromi (*Wu Ling Zhi*), Radix Achyranthis Bidentatae (*Niu Xi*), Radix Et Rhizoma Notopterygii (*Qiang Huo*), Semen Pruni Persicae (*Tao Ren*), Radix Angelicae Sinensis (*Dang Gui*), and Rhizoma Cyperi Rotundi (*Xiang Fu*), 9g each, and Resina Olibani (*Ru Xiang*) and uncooked Radix Glycyrrhizae (*Gan Cao*), 6g each

ANALYSIS OF FORMULA: Within this formula, *Tao Ren, Dang Gui, Wu Ling Zhi*, and *Niu Xi* all quicken the blood and transform stasis. In addition, *Dang Gui* nourishes the blood to prevent damage to the blood by the other attacking medicinals, while *Niu Xi* leads the other medicinals downward. *Qiang Huo* and *Xiang Fu* rectify the qi. *Qiang Huo* also treats wind damp impediment pain. *Ru Xiang* and *Di Long* free the flow of the network vessels and stop pain. *Gan Cao* harmonizes the rest of the medicinals in this formula.

ADDITIONS & SUBTRACTIONS: For pain in the upper limbs, add nine grams each of Rhizoma Curcumae Longae (*Jiang Huang*) and Ramulus Cinnamomi Cassiae (*Gui Zhi*). For pain in the lower limbs, add nine grams of Radix Angelicae Pubescentis (*Du Huo*) and Fructus Chaenomelis Lagenariae (*Mu Gua*). For severe pain, add 15 grams of Rhizoma Corydalis Yanhusuo (*Yan Hu Suo*) and three grams each of Buthus Martensis (*Quan Xie*) and Scolopendra Subspinipes (*Wu Gong*), powdered and taken with the strained decoction. For severe joint swelling, add nine grams each of Bulbus Shancigu (*Shan Ci Gu*), Radix Stephaniae Tetrandrae (*Han Fang Ji*), and Rhizoma Dioscoreae Hypoglaucae (*Bei Xie*). For restricted mobility, add 30 grams each of Caulis Milletiae Seu Spatholobi (*Ji Xue Teng*) and nine grams of Lumbricus (*Di Long*).

ACUPUNCTURE & MOXIBUSTION: *He Gu* (LI 4), *San Yin Jiao* (Sp 6), distant channel and local points depending on the site of pain. Acupuncture can be helpful for the relief of pain, but internally administered Chinese medicinals are better for the elimination of uric acid crystals.

ANALYSIS OF FORMULA: Please see pattern #1 above.

ADDITIONS & SUBTRACTIONS: Please see pattern #1 above.

4. TURBID DAMPNESS POURING DOWNWARD & BLOOD STASIS PATTERN

MAIN SYMPTOMS: Severe, acute joint aching and pain which is fixed in location and marked by pronounced swelling and distention of the affected joints

TREATMENT PRINCIPLES: Eliminate dampness and discharge turbidity, quicken the blood and transform stasis

RX: *Er Ze Tang* (Two Ponds Decoction)

INGREDIENTS: Rhizoma Smilacis Glabrae (*Tu Fu Ling*), Semen Coicis Lachryma-jobi (*Yi Yi Ren*), and Radix Clematidis Chinensis (*Wei Ling Xian*), 30g each, Rhizoma Dioscoreae Hypoglaucae (*Bei Xie*), 20g, Semen Plantaginis (*Che Qian Zi*), 12g, Rhizoma Alismatis (*Ze Xie*), Herba Lycopi Lucidi (*Ze Lan*), Semen Pruni Persicae (*Tao Ren*), and Radix Angelicae Sinensis (*Dang Gui*), 9g each

ANALYSIS OF FORMULA: Within this formula, *Tu Fu Ling* eliminates dampness and turbidity and treats joint pain due to predominant dampness. *Wei Ling Xian* likewise treats wind damp joint pain, *Bei Xie* promotes the division of the clear from the turbid and dispels wind dampness. It also relaxes the sinews and frees the flow of the network vessels in cases of wind damp impediment. *Yi Yi Ren, Ze Xie*, and *Che Qian Zi* all seep dampness, while *Ze Lan, Tao Ren*, and *Dang Gui* quicken the blood and transform stasis. Thus when all these medicinals are combined together, they dispel wind dampness and discharge turbid dampness as well as quicken the blood and transform stasis.

ADDITIONS & SUBTRACTIONS: If dampness pouring down is due to spleen vacuity which is relatively marked, replace *Er Ze Tang* with *Shen Ling Bai Zhu San Jia Jian* (Ginseng, Poria & Atractylodes Powder with Additions & Subtractions): Radix Astragali Membranacei (*Huang Qi*), Sclerotium Poriae Cocos (*Fu Ling*), Semen Coicis Lachryma-jobi (*Yi Yi Ren*), and Radix Stephaniae Tetrandrae (*Fan Ji*), 15g each, Rhizoma Dioscoreae Hypoglaucae (*Bei Xie*) and Talcum (*Hua Shi*), 12g each, Radix Codonopsitis Pilosulae (*Dang Shen*), Fructus Chaenomelis Lagenariae (*Mu Gua*), Radix Dioscoreae Oppositae (*Shan Yao*), Rhizoma Atractylodis Macrocephalae (*Bai Zhu*), Radix Angelicae Sinensis (*Dang Gui*), Radix Gentianae Macrophyllae (*Qin Jiao*), Herba Agastachis Seu Pogostemi (*Huo Xiang*), and Herba Eupatorii Fortunei (*Pei Lan*), 9g each, and Fructus Cardamomi (*Bai Dou Kou*), 6g.

ACUPUNCTURE & MOXIBUSTION: *Yin Ling Quan* (Sp 9), *Zu San Li* (St 36), distant channel and local points depending on the location of pain. Acupuncture can be helpful for the relief of pain, but internally administered Chinese medicinals are better for the elimination of uric acid crystals.

ANALYSIS OF FORMULA: Supplementing *Zu San Li* supplements the spleen, and the spleen governs the movement and transformation of water fluids in the body. Draining *Yin Ling Quan* seeps dampness. Draining the distant channel and local points moves the channel qi and frees the flow of the network vessels in the affected area to stop pain.

ADDITIONS & SUBTRACTIONS: Please see pattern #1 above.

5. PHLEGM & STASIS OBSTRUCTING NETWORK VESSELS PATTERN

MAIN SYMPTOMS: Enduring joint pain which sometimes is mild and sometimes is stronger but does not heal, recurrent attacks, swelling of the joint, restriction of movement, possible dark purple skin in the affected area, stiffness, hardening, and deformation of the joint, tophi under the skin (mainly on the face, ears, and joints) which are painless, a dark or purple tongue or possible static macules or spots, and a deep, fine, choppy, and/or bowstring pulse

TREATMENT PRINCIPLES: Transform phlegm and dispel stasis, free the flow of the network vessels and stop pain

RX: *Tao Hong Yin* (Persica & Carthamus Drink) plus *Er Chen Tang* (Two Aged [Ingredients] Decoction) with additions and subtractions

INGREDIENTS: Radix Clematidis Chinensis (*Wei Ling Xian*), 15g, Semen Pruni Persicae (*Tao Ren*), Flos Carthami Tinctorii (*Hong Hua*), Radix Ligustici Wallichii (*Chuan Xiong*), Radix Rubrus Paeoniae Lactiflorae (*Chi Shao*), Radix Angelicae Sinensis (*Dang Gui*), Pericarpium Citri Reticulatae (*Chen Pi*), Rhizoma Pinelliae Ternatae (*Ban Xia*), Semen Sinapis Albae (*Bai Jie Zi*), Bombyx Batryticatus (*Jiang Can*), and Lumbricus (*Di Long*), 9g each, and mix-fried Radix Glycyrrhizae (*Gan Cao*), 5g

ANALYSIS OF FORMULA: *Hong Hua, Tao Ren, Dang Gui, Chi Shao,* and *Chuan Xiong* all quicken the blood, transform stasis, and stop pain. *Wei Ling Xian* and *Di Long* free the flow of the network vessels and stop pain. *Ban Xia, Bai Jie Zi, Chen Pi,* and *Jiang Can* together transform phlegm and soften hardness.

ADDITIONS & SUBTRACTIONS: For severe or recalcitrant pain, add five grams each of Resina Olibani (*Ru Xiang*) and Resina Myrrhae (*Mo Yao*) and three grams each of Buthus Martensis (*Quan Xie*) and Scolopendra Subspinipes (*Wu Gong*), powdered and taken with the strained decoction. For pain in the upper limbs, add nine grams each of Rhizoma Curcumae Longae (*Jiang Huang*) and Ramulus Cinnamomi Cassiae (*Gui Zhi*). For pain in the lower limbs, add nine grams of Radix Angelicae Pubescentis (*Du Huo*) and Fructus Chaenomelis Lagenariae (*Mu Gua*). For severe joint swelling, add nine grams each of Bulbus Shancigu (*Shan Ci Gu*) and Rhizoma Dioscoreae Hypoglaucae (*Bei Xie*). For restricted mobility, add 30 grams of Caulis Milletiae Seu Spatholobi (*Ji Xue Teng*) and nine grams of Caulis Trachelospermi Jasminoidis (*Luo Shi Teng*).

If this pattern manifests mainly as tophi and hyperuricemia without swelling, pain, or joint deformation, replace *Tao Hong Yin* plus *Er Chen Tang* with *Xiao Tan Tang* (Disperse Phlegm Decoction) with additions and subtractions: Semen Sinapis Albae (*Bai Jie Zi*), Bulbus Fritillariae Thunbergii (*Zhe Bei Mu*), Sclerotium Poriae Cocos (*Fu Ling*), Radix Scrophulariae Ningpoensis (*Xuan Shen*), Bubus Shancigu (*Shan Ci Gu*), Radix Angelicae Sinensis (*Dang Gui*), and Radix Salviae Miltiorrhizae (*Dan Shen*), 12g each, Thallus Algae (*Kun Bu*), Herba Sargassii (*Hai Zao*), Rhizoma Pinelliae Ternatae (*Ban Xia*), and Radix Codonopsitis Pilosulae (*Dang Shen*), 9g each, and Rhizoma Arsiaematis (*Tian Nan Xing*), 6g. If the patient also tends to have stones in their urinary tract, add 15 grams each of Spora Lygodii Japonici (*Hai Jin Sha*) and Folium Pyrrosiae (*Shi Wei*).

ACUPUNCTURE & MOXIBUSTION: *Feng Long* (St 40), *Zu San Li* (St 36), *Zhong Wan* (CV 12), distant channel and local points depending on the location of pain.

ANALYSIS OF FORMULA: Draining *Feng Long* transforms phlegm and eliminates dampness. Supplementing *Zu San Li* and *Zhong Wan* fortifies the spleen and boosts the qi based on the saying, "the spleen is the root of phlegm engenderment." Draining the distant channel and local points moves the channel qi and frees the flow of the network vessels to stop pain.

ADDITIONS & SUBTRACTIONS: Please see pattern #1 above.

6. LIVER-KIDNEY YIN VACUITY PATTERN

MAIN SYMPTOMS: Enduring joint pain, low back and knee soreness and limpness, worsening of symptoms after taxation, lack of joint flexibility, night sweats, a dry mouth and throat, tinnitus, a red tongue with scanty fur, and a thin, rapid pulse

TREATMENT PRINCIPLES: Supplement and enrich the liver and kidneys, strengthen and reinforce the sinews and bones

RX: *Liu Wei Di Huang Wan Jia Wei* (Six Flavors Rehmannia Pills with Added Flavors)

INGREDIENTS: Radix Clematidis Chinensis (*Wei Ling Xian*) and Rhizoma Alismatis (*Ze Xie*), 15g each, cooked Radix Rehmanniae (*Shu Di*), Fructus Corni Officinalis (*Shan Zhu Yu*), Radix Dioscoreae Oppositae (*Shan Yao*), Sclerotium

Poriae Cocos (*Fu Ling*), Cortex Radicis Moutan (*Dan Pi*), Radix Achyranthis Bidentatae (*Niu Xi*), Fructus Psoraleae Corylifoliae (*Bu Gu Zhi*), and Cortex Eucommiae Ulmoidis (*Du Zhong*), 9g each

ANALYSIS OF FORMULA: *Shu Di, Shan Zhu Yu,* and *Niu Xi* supplement liver and kidney yin and essence. *Ze Xie* drains vacuity heat from the kidneys, and *Dan Pi* drains vacuity heat from the liver. *Shan Yao* and *Fu Ling* fortify the spleen which transforms the latter heaven essence to help nourish liver-kidney yin and blood. *Bu Gu Zhi, Du Zhong,* and *Niu Xi* supplement the liver and kidneys, strengthen and reinforce the sinews and bones. *Wei Ling Xian* frees the flow of the network vessels and stops pain.

ADDITIONS & SUBTRACTIONS: For joint swelling and distention, add nine grams of Rhizoma Atractylodis (*Cang Zhu*) and 15 grams of Semen Coicis Lachryma-jobi (*Yi Yi Ren*). For pain in the upper limbs, add nine grams each of Rhizoma Curcumae Longae (*Jiang Huang*) and Ramulus Cinnamomi Cassiae (*Gui Zhi*). For pain in the lower limbs, add nine grams each of Radix Angelicae Pubescentis (*Du Huo*) and Fructus Chaenomelis Lagenariae (*Mu Gua*). For restricted mobility, add 30 grams of Caulis Milletiae Seu Spatholobi (*Ji Xue Teng*) and nine grams of Caulis Trachelospermi Jasminoidis (*Luo Shi Teng*). For heat due to yin vacuity, add 15 grams each of uncooked Radix Rehmanniae (*Sheng Di*) and Cortex Phellodendri (*Huang Bai*). For dysuria, add 15 grams of Semen Plantaginis (*Che Qian Zi*). For severe or recalcitrant pain, add five grams each of Resina Olibani (*Ru Xiang*) and Resina Myrrhae (*Mo Yao*) and three grams each of Buthus Martensis (*Quan Xie*) and Scolopendra Subspinipes (*Wu Gong*), powdered and taken with the strained decoction. If the patient also tends to have stones in the urinary tract, add 15 grams each of Spora Lygodii Japonici (*Hai Jin Sha*) and Folium Pyrrosiae (*Shi Wei*).

ACUPUNCTURE & MOXIBUSTION: *Tai Xi* (Ki 3), *Fu Liu* (Ki 7), distant channel and local points depending on the location of pain. Acupuncture can be helpful for the relief of pain, but internally administered Chinese medicinals are better for the elimination of uric acid crystals.

ANALYSIS OF FORMULA: Supplementing *Tai Xi* and *Fu Liu* supplements the kidneys and enriches yin. Draining the distant channel and local points moves the channel qi and frees the flow of the network vessels to stop pain.

ADDITIONS & SUBTRACTIONS: Please see pattern #1 above.

REMARKS

1. The above patterns primarily describe the pattern discrimination of the symptoms experienced during an attack of gout. These patterns and treatments must be modified based on the patient's personal habitual bodily pattern. In other words, if there is obesity, phlegm and dampness must be taken into account, including the underlying causes of that phlegm and dampness. If there is liver-kidney yin vacuity, then one must nourish the liver and enrich the kidneys on top of treating the impediment. Likewise, there may be liver depression qi stagnation and/or yang vacuity, or there may be other, more complicated patterns due to other associated disease mechanisms. Therefore, the above treatment protocols are mainly for use during acute exacerbations or must be modified to more precisely fit all the concomitant patterns the patient presents.

2. Because this condition is an enduring one associated with paroxysms of severe, fixed pain, the treatment principles of freeing the flow of the network vessels and stopping pain should generally be considered. These principles suggest the use of medicinals which enter the network vessels and there quicken the blood and transform or dispel stasis. Therefore, the tree saps Resina Olibani (*Ru Xiang*) and Resina Myrrhae (*Mo Yao*) and insect medicinals, such as Lumbricus (*Di Long*), Buthus Martensis (*Quan Xie*), and Scolopendra Subspinipes (*Wu Gong*), are often added to formulas. In addition, because gout so commonly affects the large toe, medicinals which guide other medicinals downward to the lower extremities, such as Radix Achyranthis Bidentatae (*Niu Xi*) and Fructus Chaenomelis Lagenariae (*Mu Gua*) are often found in or added to prescriptions for gout.

3. Because Semen Strychnotis (*Ma Qian Zi*) is so powerful for disinhibiting the channels and stopping pain, it is often found in Chinese formulas for gout at dosages from 5-20g per day in decoction. However, this medicinal is very toxic and should be used with great care, especially in those with bodily weakness. Overdoses in humans have been reported from as little as 50mg of this medicinal. The symptoms of toxicity due to overdose with this medicinal include a crawling sensation in the cervical area, difficulty swallowing, and irritability. This may progress to convulsions and spasms of great force.

4. Because uric acid crystals may also play a part in the formation of urinary calculi, during the remission stage of gout, one should also consider adding the treatment principles of disinhibiting urination, freeing the flow of strangury, and dispersing stones. Frequently used medicinals for these purposes include Herba Desmodii Styrachifolii (*Jin Qiao Cao*), Spora Lygodii Japonici (*Hai Jin Sha*), Endothelium Corneum Gigeriae Galli (*Ji Nei Jin*), Talcum (*Hua Shi*), Herba Polygoni Avicularis (*Bian Xu*), Semen Plantaginis (*Che Qian Zi*), Caulis Akebiae (*Mu Tong*), and Radix Et Rhizoma Rhei (*Da Huang*). For further information on the treatment of urinary calculi see the chapter on urolithiasis. Regular consumption of green tea may also benefit gout

patients during periods of remission due to increasing uric acid output.

5. In most cases of gout, spleen movement has lost its harmony and the spleen has lost its power to move and transform water and foods. Fatty meats, rich-flavored food, and alcohol especially cannot be moved and transformed sufficiently. Therefore, it is extremely important to regulate diet during remissions, and diet is typically directly related to both treatment results and recurrences. This means that gout patients should avoid excessive fat and decrease their intake of such foods as animal liver, sardines, seafood in general, and beans. Fermented foods and drinks should be avoided altogether, and tobacco-smoking should also be stopped. Instead, one should eat plenty of vegetables and fruits so as to help expel turbidity and toxins.

6. In China, Semen Plantaginis (*Che Qian Zi*), Lumbricus (*Di Long*), Radix Stephaniae Tetrandrae (*Han Fang Ji*), and Bubus Shancigu (*Shan Ci Gu*) have the reputation as being especially good medicinals for treating gout.

7. Some Chinese doctors consider the purine metabolism dyscrasia which is often at the root of gout to be due to a natural endowment insufficiency. Therefore, there is almost always a vacuity at its root, and this root vacuity should be treated with appropriate supplementing medicinals during periods of remission.[2]

8. If the joints are swollen, red, and hot to the touch, one may also bleed around the affected joints to drain heat, disperse swelling, and help stop pain.

ENDNOTES

[1] Pizzorno, J.E. & Murray, M.T., *Encyclopedia of Natural Medicine*, Prima Publishing, Rocklin, CA, 1991

[2] Becker, Simon, personal communication, e-mail message, Jan. 17, 2001

28

Hashimoto's Thyroiditis

Hashimoto's disease is a form of autoimmune thyroiditis leading to hypothyroidism. It is also called lymphadenoid goiter, chronic lymphocytic thyroiditis, struma lymphomatosa, and Hashimoto's thyroiditis. It is a slowly developing, persistent inflammation of the thyroid resulting in decreased function of the gland. Although this condition may occur at any age, it is most common among middle-aged women. Its incidence is 1 out of 10,000. Risk factors, besides being a woman, include having a family history of thyroid disease. This condition is frequently associated with other autoimmune endocrine disorders, such as diabetes mellitus, Addison's disease, Grave's disease, hypoparathyroidism, hypopituitarism, and vitiligo Its symptoms include intolerance to cold, weight gain, fatigue, constipation, and an enlarged neck or the presence of goiter. Other symptoms which may be associated with this condition include joint stiffness and facial edema.

The Western medical diagnosis of this condition is primarily based on laboratory tests for determining thyroid function, such as T4, T3 resin uptake, serum TSH, and T3. Thyroid antibodies are frequently present, such as antithyroid microsomal antibody and antithyroglobulin antibody. This disease may also alter the results of the following tests: radioactive iodine uptake, blood differential, and antimitochondral antibody. Because its onset is slow and its symptoms may be caused by a number of other conditions, this disease is often not detected. If the thyroid is not or is only slightly enlarged and there is no sign of thyroid deficiency, Western treatment may only consist of regular monitoring and observation which obviously does nothing to alleviate the patient's symptoms. Thyroid hormone replacement therapy with levothyrosine may be given if there is a large goiter or if the hormone is deficient. If thyroiditis is severe, corticosteriods may be prescribed short-term to allay the inflammation.

Chinese disease categorization: Goiter in Chinese medicine is categorized as *ying liu*, *ying*, and *ying qi*. Fatigue is *pi juan* or *xu lao*, vacuity taxation, obesity is *fei pang*, constipation is *bian bi*, joint stiffness is *bi zheng*, impediment condition, and facial edema is *mian fu*.

Disease causes: Former heaven natural endowment insufficiency, unregulated eating and drinking, unregulated stirring and stillness, *i.e.*, activity and rest, internal damage by the seven affects, and aging

Disease mechanisms: In women, the blood rules. Because blood is either lost or consumed via menstruation, gestation, and/or lactation and the spleen is the source of blood engenderment and transformation, women are more prone to spleen vacuity than men. By the mid-30s, the spleen is becoming vacuous and weak in most Western women. This tendency is compounded by over-eating sugars and sweets, sodden wheat foods, *i.e.*, pastas and breads, and chilled, uncooked foods and drinks, too much thinking, worry, and anxiety, too much fatigue, and too little exercise. It may also be compounded by over-use of antibiotics. In addition, unfulfilled desires and/or anger may lead to liver depression, and a depressed liver may invade the spleen further weakening it. Because the spleen is the latter heaven source of qi engenderment and transformation, qi vacuity may lead to fatigue. Because yang is nothing other than a lot of qi, spleen qi vacuity may lead to yang vacuity, with yang vacuity resulting in fear of cold. Since the spleen governs the movement and transformation of water fluids in the body, spleen vacuity may lead to facial edema. If dampness collects and accumulates, it may congeal into phlegm, causing phlegm nodulation and goiter in the neck and obesity in general. Yang vacuity may lead to a defensive qi vacuity with easy entrance of wind, cold, and/or damp evils. If these evils lodge in the channels and network vessels obstructing the free flow of the qi and blood in the vicinity of the joints, joint pain and stiffness may occur.

Because of the inter-relationships between the qi and the blood, qi stagnation, dampness, and phlegm, may also easily give rise to blood stasis over time. Lack of yang qi to warm and move the intestinal qi mechanism plus lack of blood to moisten the intestines, may result in constipation.

TREATMENT BASED ON PATTERN DISCRIMINATION:

1. SPLEEN QI VACUITY WEAKNESS PATTERN

MAIN SYMPTOMS: Fatigue, cold hands and feet, obesity, puffy edema, a pale facial complexion, a tendency to loose stools, a fat, pale tongue with teeth-marks on its edges and thin, white fur, and a weak or soggy pulse

TREATMENT PRINCIPLES: Supplement the center and boost the qi

RX: *Bu Zhong Yi Qi Tang* (Supplement the Center & Boost the Qi Decoction)

INGREDIENTS: Radix Astragali Membranacei (*Huang Qi*), 18g, Radix Codonopsitis Pilosulae (*Dang Shen*) and Rhizoma Atractylodis Macrocephalae (*Bai Zhu*), 12g each, Radix Angelicae Sinensis (*Dang Gui*), mix-fried Radix Glycyrrhizae (*Gan Cao*), and Pericarpium Citri Reticulatae (*Chen Pi*), 6g each, Rhizoma Cimicifugae (*Sheng Ma*), 4.5g, and Radix Bupleuri (*Chai Hu*), 3g

ANALYSIS OF FORMULA: *Huang Qi, Dang Shen, Bai Zhu,* and mix-fried *Gan Cao* supplement the center and boost the qi. *Dang Gui* harmonizes the blood, while *Chen Pi* rectifies the qi. *Chai Hu* and *Sheng Ma* upbear the clear.

ADDITIONS & SUBTRACTIONS: If there is simultaneous liver depression, increase Radix Bupleuri (*Chai Hu*) to nine grams. If there is concomitant blood vacuity, increase Radix Angelicae Sinensis (*Dang Gui*) to nine grams. If there is both liver depression and blood vacuity, add nine grams of Radix Albus Paeoniae Lactiflorae (*Bai Shao*). If there is facial edema, add 12 grams of Sclerotium Poriae Cocos (*Fu Ling*). If there is constipation due to yang qi and blood vacuity, add *Ji Chuan Jian* (Flow the River Decoction): Radix Angelicae Sinensis (*Dang Gui*), 15g, Herba Cistanchis Deserticolae (*Rou Cong Rong*) and Radix Achyranthis Bidentatae (*Niu Xi*), 9g each, and Rhizoma Alismatis (*Ze Xie*) and Fructus Citri Aurantii (*Zhi Ke*), 6g each. If there is phlegm nodulation, add 15 grams each of Spica Prunellae Vulgaris (*Xiao Ku Cao*), Radix Scrophulariae Ningpoensis (*Xuan Shen*), Semen Citri Reticulatae (*Ju He*), and Concha Ostreae (*Mu Li*), 12 grams of Bulbus Fritillariae Thunbergii (*Zhe Bei Mu*), and nine grams each of Rhizoma Pinelliae Ternatae (*Ban Xia*), Herba Sargassii (*Hai Zao*), and Thallus Algae (*Kun Bu*). If there is simultaneous blood stasis, add 15 grams of Radix Salviae Miltiorrhizae (*Dan Shen*). If there is wind damp cold impediment, add 15 grams each of Cortex Radicis Acanthopanacis Gracilistylis (*Wu Jia Pi*) and Caulis Milletiae Seu Spatholobi (*Ji Xue Teng*). If there is depressive heat, add 9-12 grams of Radix Scutellariae Baicalensis (*Huang Qin*). If there are cold hands and feet, add 9 grams of Ramulus Cinnamomi Cassiae (*Gui Zhi*).

ACUPUNCTURE & MOXIBUSTION: *Zu San Li* (St 36), *Tai Bai* (Sp 3), *San Yin Jiao* (Sp 6)

ANALYSIS OF FORMULA: With moxibustion and supplementing method, *Zu San Li, Tai Bai,* and *San Yin Jiao* fortify the spleen and boost the qi.

ADDITIONS & SUBTRACTIONS: If there is simultaneous liver depression, add *Tai Chong* (Liv 3) needled toward *Yong Quan* (Ki 1). If there is concomitant blood vacuity, add *Ge Shu* (Bl 17) and *Pi Shu* (Bl 20). If there is facial edema, add *Yin Ling Quan* (Sp 9) and *Shui Gou* (GV 26). If there is constipation, add *Tian Shu* (St 25). If there is phlegm nodulation (*i.e.*, goiter), add *Que Pen* (St 12) and *Ren Ying* (St 9) or *Tian Chuang* (SI 16). If there is wind damp cold impediment, add *Qu Chi* (LI 11), *Yin Ling Quan* (Sp 9), and *a shi* points selected according to the location of pain. If there is depressive heat, add *Nei Ting* (St 44) or *Yang Ling Quan* (GB 34). If there are cold hands and feet, add *Wai Guan* (TB 5) and *Cheng Shan* (Bl 57).

2. SPLEEN-KIDNEY YANG VACUITY PATTERN

MAIN SYMPTOMS: All the above plus dizziness and tinnitus, decreased sexual desire, possible impotence or sterility in men and menstrual irregularities and/or infertility in women, low back and knee soreness and weakness, nighttime polyuria, more pronounced fear of cold, and colder feet than hands

TREATMENT PRINCIPLES: Fortify the spleen and boost the qi, supplement the kidneys and invigorate yang

RX: *Jia Wei Shen Qi Wan* (Added Flavors Kidney Qi Pills)

INGREDIENTS: Radix Astragali Membranacei (*Huang Qi*), 15g, cooked Radix Rehmanniae (*Shu Di*), 12g, Radix Codonopsitis Pilosulae (*Dang Shen*), Radix Dioscoreae Oppositae (*Shan Yao*), Fructus Corni Officinalis (*Shan Zhu Yu*), Sclerotium Poriae Cocos (*Fu Ling*), Radix Lateralis Praeparatus Aconiti Carmichaeli (*Fu Zi*), and Cortex

Cinnamomi Cassiae (*Rou Gui*), 9g each, and Cortex Radicis Moutan (*Dan Pi*) and Rhizoma Alismatis (*Ze Xie*), 6g each

ANALYSIS OF FORMULA: *Huang Qi, Dang Shen, Shan Yao,* and *Fu Ling* fortify the spleen and boost the qi. *Shu Di, Shan Zhu Yu, Dan Pi, Ze Xie, Fu Zi,* and *Rou Gui* together supplement kidney yin and yang. In addition, *Fu Ling* and *Ze Xie* disinhibit dampness.

ADDITIONS & SUBTRACTIONS: For marked kidney yang vacuity, add nine grams each of Herba Epimedii (*Yin Yang Huo*) and Rhizoma Curculiginis Orchioidis (*Xian Mao*). For constipation, add nine grams each of Herba Cynomorii Songarici (*Suo Yang*) and Herba Cistanchis Deserticolae (*Rou Cong Rong*). For loose stools, add nine grams each of Fructus Psoraleae Corylifoliae (*Bu Gu Zhi*) and Semen Cuscutae Chinensis (*Tu Si Zi*). For edema, increase the dosage of *Ze Xie* and *Fu Ling* up to 15 grams and add 12 grams each of Cortex Radicis Acanthopanacis Gracilistylis (*Wu Jia Pi*) and Rhizoma Atractylodis Macrocephalae (*Bai Zhu*). For marked low back and knee pain, add 12 grams each of Ramulus Loranthi Seu Visci (*Sang Ji Sheng*), Radix Achyranthis Bidentatae (*Niu Xi*), and Radix Dipsaci (*Xu Duan*). For spine and low back pain accompanied by a cold sensation, add 12 grams each of Rhizoma Cibotii Barometsis (*Gou Ji*), Radix Dipsaci (*Xu Duan*), and Cortex Eucommiae Ulmoidis (*Du Zhong*). For heart palpitations, replace *Rou Gui* with Ramulus Cinnamomi Cassiae (*Gui Zhi*) and add 12 grams each of Radix Salviae Miltiorrhizae (*Dan Shen*) and Radix Ligustici Wallichii (*Chuan Xiong*). For abdominal distention, add nine grams of Rhizoma Pinelliae Ternatae (*Ban Xia*) and six grams of Pericarpium Citri Reticulatae (*Chen Pi*). For poor appetite, add nine grams each of Massa Medica Fermentata (*Shen Qu*), Fructus Crataegi (*Shan Zha*), and Fructus Germinatus Hordei Vulgaris (*Mai Ya*) and six grams of Fructus Amomi (*Sha Ren*). If there is phlegm nodulation (*i.e.*, goiter), add 15 grams each of Spica Prunellae Vulgaris (*Xiao Ku Cao*), Radix Scrophulariae Ningpoensis (*Xuan Shen*), and Concha Ostreae (*Mu Li*), 12 grams of Bulbus Fritillariae Thunbergii (*Zhe Bei Mu*), and nine grams each of Herba Sargassii (*Hai Zao*), and Thallus Algae (*Kun Bu*). If there is simultaneous blood stasis, add 15 grams of Radix Salviae Miltiorrhizae (*Dan Shen*). If there is wind damp cold impediment, add 15 grams each of Cortex Radicis Acanthopanacis Gracilistylis (*Wu Jia Pi*) and Caulis Milletiae Seu Spatholobi (*Ji Xue Teng*). If there is depressive heat, add 9-12 grams of Radix Scutellariae Baicalensis (*Huang Qin*). If there is concomitant yin vacuity with easy fright, insomnia, night sweats, dizziness, hot flashes in the face, dry skin with possible desquamation, dry, lusterless hair, and constipation, add 12 grams each of Fructus Ligustri Lucidi (*Nu Zhen Zi*), Fructus Schisandrae Chinensis (*Wu Wei Zi*), and Herba Ecliptae Prostratae (*Han Lian Cao*) and increase the dosage of *Shu Di* up to 15-20g.

If there is a marked heart yang vacuity coupled with kidney yang vacuity, a combination often seen in hypothyroidism, accompanied by cardiac effusion, heart palpitations, an empty sensation in the heart, shortness of breath, possible chest oppression or pain, aversion to cold, cold limbs, a pale and puffy face, apathy and mental slowness, fatigue, dizziness, tinnitus, weak limbs, hypersomnia, a pale tongue with thin, white fur, and a deep, slow, weak, possibly bound or regularly interrupted pulse, replace *Jia Wei Shen Qi Wan* with *Zhi Gan Cao Tang Jia Jian* (Mix-fried Licorice Decoction with Additions & Subtractions): Radix Astragali Membranacei (*Huang Qi*), 30g, uncooked Radix Rehmanniae (*Sheng Di*), 20g, mix-fried Radix Glycyrrhizae (*Gan Cao*), 15g, and Radix Lateralis Praeparatus Aconiti Carmichaeli (*Fu Zi*), Radix Codonopsitis Pilosulae (*Dang Shen*), Radix Angelicae Sinensis (*Dang Gui*), Radix Ligustici Wallichii (*Chuan Xiong*), Ramulus Cinnamomi Cassiae (*Gui Zhi*), Radix Albus Paeoniae Lactiflorae (*Bai Shao*), Tuber Ophiopogonis Japonici (*Mai Men Dong*), and Fructus Schisandrae Chinensis (*Wu Wei Zi*), 9g each. If the pulse is weak, slow, and deep, add six grams of Herba Ephedrae (*Ma Huang*) and three grams of Herba Asari Cum Radice (*Xi Xin*). If the pulse is faint, bound, or regularly interrupted, add six grams of Fructus Immaturus Citri Aurantii (*Zhi Shi*) and replace *Dang Shen* with six grams of Radix Panacis Ginseng (*Ren Shen*). If there is chest oppression and pain, add 24 grams of Pericarpium Trichosanthis Kirlowii (*Gua Lou Pi*) and nine grams each of Bulbus Allii (*Xie Bai*), Rhizoma Corydalis Yanhusuo (*Yan Hu Suo*), and Radix Salviae Miltiorrhizae (*Dan Shen*).

ACUPUNCTURE & MOXIBUSTION: *Pi Shu* (Bl 20), *Shen Shu* (Bl 23), *Ming Men* (GV 4), *Guan Yuan* (CV 4)

ANALYSIS OF FORMULA: With moxibustion and supplementing method, *Pi Shu* and *Guan Yuan* supplement the latter heaven, while *Shen Shu* and *Ming Men* supplement the former heaven. Together, they fortify the spleen and boost the qi, supplement the kidneys and invigorate yang.

NOTE: This seemingly simple treatment achieves good result, but needs a long course (*e.g.*, 3-6 months). Moxibustion should use nonscarring direct thread moxa. Warming these points with a moxa roll is not adequate.

ADDITIONS & SUBTRACTIONS: If there is facial edema, add *Yin Ling Quan* (Sp 9) and *Shui Gou* (GV 26). If there is generalized edema, add *Yin Ling Quan* (Sp 9), *Shui Fen* (CV 9), and *San Yin Jiao* (Sp 6). If there is constipation, add *Tian Shu* (St 25). If there are loose stools, add *Zu San Li* (St 36). For spine and low back pain with a cold sensation, add *Da Zhui* (GV 14), *Ji Zhong* (GV 6), and *Chang Qiang* (GV 1). For heart palpitations, add *Nei Guan* (Per 6). For abdominal distention, add *Zhong Wan* (CV 12) and *Tian Shu* (St 25).

For poor appetite, add *Zu San Li* (St 36). If there is marked fatigue and weakness, add *Zu San Li* (St 36). If there is concomitant yin vacuity, add *Fu Liu* (Ki 7). If there is simultaneous liver depression, add *Tai Chong* (Liv 3) needled toward *Yong Quan* (Ki 1). If there is phlegm nodulation (*i.e.*, goiter), add *Que Pen* (St 12) and *Ren Ying* (St 9) or *Tian Chuang* (SI 16). If there is wind damp cold impediment, add *Qu Chi* (LI 11), *Yin Ling Quan* (Sp 9) and *a shi* points selected according to the location of pain. If there is depressive heat, add *Nei Ting* (St 44) or *Yang Ling Quan* (GB 34). If there are marked cold hands and feet, add *Wai Guan* (TB 5) and *Cheng Shan* (Bl 57).

3. LIVER DEPRESSION PHLEGM NODULATION PATTERN

MAIN SYMPTOMS: Swollen lumps in the front of the throat which are soft in consistency and not painful, a swollen feeling in the front of the throat or a plum pit sensation in the back of the throat, a tendency towards anger, chest oppression and a tendency to sighing, possible chest or rib-side pain, slimy, white tongue fur, and a bowstring pulse

NOTE: Although this pattern is almost always included in Chinese textbook discussions of hypothyroidism, it is never really seen in its pure form. Rather, liver depression and phlegm nodulation complicate other patterns contained herein.

TREATMENT PRINCIPLES: Rectify the qi and soothe depression, transform phlegm and scatter nodulation

Rx: *Si Hai Shu Yu Wan Jia Jian* (Four Seas Soothe Depression Pills with Additions & Subtractions)

INGREDIENTS: Herba Sargassii (*Hai Zao*), 15g, Pericarpium Citri Reticulatae (*Chen Pi*), Tuber Curcumae (*Yu Jin*), and Concha Cyclinae Meretricis (*Hai Ge Ke*), 12g each, Rhizoma Pinelliae Ternatae (*Ban Xia*), Radix Bupleuri (*Chai Hu*), Thallus Algae (*Kun Bu*), and Os Sepiae Seu Sepiellae (*Hai Piao Xiao*), 9g each, and Radix Auklandiae Lappae (*Mu Xiang*), 6g

ANALYSIS OF FORMULA: *Ban Xia, Chen Pi, Hai Zao, Kun Bu,* and *Hai Ge Ke* all transform phlegm. In addition, *Ban Xia, Hai Zao, Kun Bu, Hai Piao Xiao,* and *Hai Ge Ke* soften the hard and scatter nodulation. The last three medicinals are empirically known to treat goiter due to hypothyroidism. *Chen Pi, Yu Jin, Mu Xiang,* and *Chai Hu* rectify the qi and resolve depression.

ADDITIONS & SUBTRACTIONS: If there is neck discomfort, add 12 grams each of Radix Platycodi Grandiflori (*Jie Geng*) and Rhizoma Belamcandae (*She Gan*) and nine grams of Semen Pharbiditis (*Qian Niu Zi*). If there is depressive heat, add 15 grams each of Spica Prunellae Vulgaris (*Xiao Ku Cao*) and Radix Scrophulariae Ningpoensis (*Xuan Shen*). For concomitant spleen qi vacuity, add 30-60 grams of Radix Astragali Membranacei (*Huang Qi*) and 12 grams of Rhizoma Atractylodis Macrocephalae (*Bai Zhu*) and Sclerotium Poriae Cocos (*Fu Ling*). For concomitant kidney yang vacuity, add 12 grams each of cooked Radix Rehmanniae (*Shu Di*) and Herba Epimedii (*Yin Yang Huo*) and nine grams of Ramulus Cinnamomi Cassiae (*Gui Zhi*).

ACUPUNCTURE & MOXIBUSTION: *Tai Chong* (Liv 3), *Feng Long* (St 40), *Que Pen* (St 12), *Nao Hui* (TB 13), *Tian Chuang* (SI 16)

ANALYSIS OF FORMULA: Draining *Tai Chong* rectifies the qi and resolves depression. Draining *Feng Long* transforms phlegm. Draining *Que Pen* and *Tian Chuang* softens the hard and scatters nodulation. Draining *Nao Hui* courses and frees the flow of the three burners and disperses goiter qi.

ADDITIONS & SUBTRACTIONS: If there is neck discomfort, add *Lie Que* (Lu 7) and *Zhao Hai* (Ki 6). If there is depressive heat, add *Yang Ling Quan* (GB 34) and replace *Tai Chong* with *Xing Jian* (Liv 2). For concomitant spleen qi vacuity, add *Zu San Li* (St 36). For concomitant kidney yang vacuity, add *Tai Xi* (Ki 3).

4. PHLEGM CONGELATION & BLOOD STASIS PATTERN

MAIN SYMPTOMS: Hard goiter like stone which is immovable or sometimes moves slightly when one swallows, heavy disease nature, larger sized lumps, irregular surface to the lumps, possible accompanying aching and pain, hoarse voice, thin, white tongue fur, and a bowstring, possibly choppy pulse

NOTE: As with pattern #3 above, this pattern really only complicates other patterns and is not typically seen by itself in patients with hypothyroidism.

TREATMENT PRINCIPLES: Quicken the blood and transform stasis, soften the hard and scatter nodulation

RX: *Hai Zao Yu Hu Tang Jia Jian* (Sargassium Jade Flask Decoction with Additions & Subtractions)

INGREDIENTS: Radix Angelicae Sinensis (*Dang Gui*), 30g, Radix Salviae Miltiorrhizae (*Dan Shen*) and Sclerotium Poriae Cocos (*Fu Ling*), 20g each, Radix Ligustici Wallichii (*Chuan Xiong*), 18g, Herba Sargassii (*Hai Zao*), Semen Raphani Sativi (*Lai Fu Zi*), and Bulbus Fritillariae Thunbergii (*Zhe Bei Mu*), 15g each, Pericarpium Citri Reticulatae Viride (*Qing Pi*) and Tuber Curcumae (*Yu Jin*), 12g each, and Thallus Algae (*Kun Bu*), Rhizoma Sparganii

(*San Leng*), and Rhizoma Curcumae Zedoariae (*E Zhu*), 9g each

ANALYSIS OF FORMULA: *Zhe Bei Mu, Fu Ling, Hai Zao, Lai Fu Zi,* and *Kun Bu* all transform phlegm. In addition, *Zhe Bei Mu, Hai Zao,* and *Kun Bu* soften the hard and scatter nodulation. *Qing Pi* and *Yu Jin* rectify the qi and resolve depression. *Dang Gui, Dan Shen, Chuan Xiong, Yu Jin, San Leng,* and *E Zhu* quicken the blood and transform stasis. In addition, *San Leng* and *E Zhu* disperse concretions.

ADDITIONS & SUBTRACTIONS: If enduring depression has transformed heat, add 18 grams of Radix Scrophulariae Ningpoensis (*Xuan Shen*), 15 grams each of Spica Prunellae Vulgaris (*Xia Ku Cao*) and Rhizoma Anemarrhenae Aspheloidis (*Zhi Mu*), and 12 grams of Cortex Radicis Moutan (*Dan Pi*).

ACUPUNCTURE & MOXIBUSTION: *He Gu* (LI 4), *San Yin Jiao* (Sp 6), *Tian Ding* (LI 17), *Tian Rong* (SI 17), *Tian Tu* (CV 22)

ANALYSIS OF FORMULA: Draining *He Gu* and *San Yin Jiao* moves the qi, quickens the blood, and transforms stasis. Draining *Tian Ding, Tian Rong,* and *Tian Tu* softens the hard, scatters nodulation, and treats goiter.

ADDITIONS & SUBTRACTIONS: Please see the preceding patterns.

REMARKS

1. The most common presentation in Western middle-aged females with this condition is a combination of liver depression and spleen vacuity. If qi vacuity has reached yang, there is spleen-kidney yang vacuity. If qi stagnation has damaged the blood, there is blood stasis. If there are palpable lumps in the throat or a sensation of phlegm in the back of the throat, there is phlegm.

2. Although most of the signs and symptoms of this condition pertain to a yang qi vacuity, since there is liver depression, there is also often depressive heat.

3. Women with spleen-kidney yang vacuity and liver depression tend to be infertile due to a luteal phase deficiency and/or endometriosis. If there is phlegm nodulation, there may be polycystic ovaries as well as fibrocystic breast disease.

4. This condition usually responds well to Chinese medical treatment.

5. Because the spleen typically plays a central role in the disease mechanisms of this condition, attention to proper diet is usually quite important. This means eating warm, easy-to-digest foods. However, because many real-life cases are complicated by damp, depressive, or vacuity heat, it is usually also important to eat a clear bland diet.

6. Taking one's basal body temperature every morning for at least three days in a row is an easy way of determining the likelihood of hypothyroidism. If the BBT is consistently below 97.5° F, this suggests a thyroid problem. Typically, the lower the BBT, the greater the degree of hypothyroidism. Menstruating women should not take their BBT during the first several days of menstruation nor at midcycle during ovulation.

7. The patterns presented above cover all forms of hypothyroidism, whether due to autoimmune thyroiditis or not.

29

HEMORRHOIDS

Hemorrhoids, also called piles, are varicosities of the veins of the hemorrhoidal plexus in the region of the anus which are often complicated by inflammation, thrombosis, and bleeding. External hemorrhoids are located below the dentate line and are covered by squamous epithelium, while internal hemorrhoids are located above the dentate line and are lined by rectal mucosa. Hemorrhoids typically occur in the right anterior, right posterior, and left lateral zones and universally affect both adults and children. Although hemorrhoids may be asymptomatic, they often cause bleeding, protrusion, and pain. Hemorrhoids may regress spontaneously or be reduced manually. Only thrombosed or ulcerated hemorrhoids are painful. Ulcerated, edematous, or strangulated hemorrhoids can cause severe pain. Anal itching is usually not a symptom of hemorrhoids.

The Western medical diagnosis of thrombosed and ulcerated, edematous, strangulated hemorrhoids is through visual inspection of the rectum. Anoscopy may be used to evaluate painless hemorrhoids. The Western medical treatment of piles consists of administration of stool softeners and/or bulking agents, such as psyllium, in order to correct straining due to constipation. Pain due to thrombosed hemorrhoids is treated by warm sitz baths, anesthetic ointments, or witch hazel compresses. Bleeding hemorrhoids are treated, at least temporarily, by injection of 5% phenol in vegetable oil. Larger internal hemorrhoids or those that fail to respond to injection sclerotherapy are treated by rubber band ligation. One hemorrhoid is ligated once every two weeks with 3-6 treatments often being required. Laser destruction and various types of electrodestruction are currently under investigation. Hemorrhoidectomies are performed infrequently for bleeding hemorrhoids and those associated with incapacitating pain which fails to respond to more conservative therapy.

CHINESE DISEASE CATEGORIZATION: Hemorrhoids are referred to as *zhi chuang*, pile sores.

DISEASE CAUSES: Unregulated eating and drinking, unregulated stirring and stillness (*i.e.*, too much sitting or standing), internal damage by the seven affects, overwork taxation, enduring disease, aging, and pregnancy

DISEASE MECHANISMS: Dry heat may arise from excessive consumption of alcohol and spicy, hot foods. If internally engendered dry heat damages the fluids, the intestines may be deprived of moisture and the stools will become dry, leading to constipation. When these hard stools remain in the intestines for some time, they hinder and obstruct the free flow of qi and blood, causing blood vessel static binding and thus hemorrhoids.

If dampness either invades externally or is engendered internally, it usually lodges in the lower part of the body because of its heavy, stagnating nature. Because the anus is located in a place where there is poor ventilation, damp evils can easily take advantage of this to invade. If either external or internal dampness brews in the anus, over time, it will engender heat. If damp heat becomes congested in the anus, the network vessels there will be obstructed and the flow of qi and blood will become static and stagnant. This then gives rise to blood vessel static binding in the anus and thus hemorrhoids.

Qi stagnation and blood stasis usually develop from enduring sitting or standing, pregnancy, or liver depression due to emotional upset. If qi stagnation and blood stasis cause blood vessel stasis and binding in the region of the anus, hemorrhoids may occur.

Central qi falling downward, *i.e.*, spleen qi vacuity, often develops from enduring bleeding from hemorrhoids, enduring diarrhea, aging, or overwork taxation. Qi is responsible for keeping the viscera and bowels in their normal place, lifting and restraining them. Therefore, if, for any reason, the qi becomes vacuous and falls downward, the anus will not be kept in its normal place. Instead, it may sag downward. Such downward sagging hinders and obstructs the free flow of qi and blood through the local channels and network vessels. Hence, blood vessel static binding may give rise to hemorrhoids.

TREATMENT BASED ON PATTERN DISCRIMINATION:

1. DRY HEAT PATTERN

MAIN SYMPTOMS: Piles which possibly protrude beyond the anus, difficult defecation of dry stools, possible explosive discharge of fresh red blood from the anus, constipation, dry stools, abdominal distention or fullness, a dry mouth, oral thirst, dark-colored urination, a red tongue with scanty fluids and dry, yellow fur, and a rapid pulse

TREATMENT PRINCIPLES: Clear heat and moisten dryness, cool the blood and stop bleeding

RX: *Liang Xue Di Huang Tang Jia Jian* (Cool Blood Rehmannia Decoction with Additions & Subtractions)

INGREDIENTS: Uncooked Radix Rehmanniae (*Sheng Di*), 12g, Radix Angelicae Sinensis (*Dang Gui*), Radix Scutellariae Baicalensis (*Huang Qin*), Fructus Immaturus Sophorae Japonicae (*Huai Hua Mi*), Radix Sanguisorbae Officinalis (*Di Yu*), Herba Seu Flos Schizonepetae Tenuifoliae (*Jing Jie Sui*), Radix Rubrus Paeoniae Lactiflorae (*Chi Shao*), and Radix Trichosanthis Kirlowii (*Tian Hua Fen*), 9g each, and Fructus Citri Aurantii (*Zhi Ke*), Rhizoma Cimicifugae (*Sheng Ma*), uncooked Radix Et Rhizoma Rhei (*Da Huang*), and Rhizoma Coptidis Chinensis (*Huang Lian*), 6g each

ANALYSIS OF FORMULA: *Sheng Di, Tian Hua Fen,* and *Dang Gui* nourish yin and engender fluids, moisten dryness and stop bleeding. *Huang Qin* and *Huang Lian* clear the heat which has or is damaging fluids. *Huai Hua Mi, Di Yu, Jing Jie Sui,* and *Chi Shao* together cool blood and stop bleeding. *Da Huang* clears heat and frees the flow of the stools. *Zhi Ke* and *Sheng Ma* regulate the upbearing and downbearing movement of the qi and stop pain.

ADDITIONS & SUBTRACTIONS: For severe hemorrhoids, add nine grams of Fructus Aristolichiae (*Ma Dou Ling*) and six grams of Radix Ledebouriellae Divaricatae (*Fang Feng*). For severe bleeding, add nine grams each of Herba Seu Radix Cirsii Japonici (*Da Ji*) and Rhizoma Imperatae Cylindricae (*Bai Mao Gen*). For severe pain, add nine grams of Semen Arecae Catechu (*Bing Lang*) and 12 grams of Rhizoma Corydalis Yanhusuo (*Yan Hu Suo*).

For severe constipation with dry stools, temporarily replace *Liang Xue Di Huang Tang* with *Zeng Ye Cheng Qi Tang* (Increase Fluids & Order the Qi Decoction): uncooked Radix Rehmanniae (*Sheng Di*), 15g, Radix Scrophulariae Ningpoensis (*Xuan Shen*) and Tuber Ophiopogonis Japonici (*Mai Men Dong*), 12g each, Radix Et Rhizoma Rhei (*Da Huang*), 6-9g, and Mirabilitum (*Mang Xiao*), 3-6g.

EXTERNAL TREATMENT: Apply the ready-made Chinese ointment, *She Xiang Zhi Chuang Gao* (Musk Treat Hemorrhoids Ointment) or some similar external ointment.

ACUPUNCTURE & MOXIBUSTION: *Chang Qiang* (GV 1), *Cheng Shan* (Bl 57), *Er Bai* (M-UE-29), *Zhao Hai* (Ki 6), *Zhi Gou* (TB 6)

ANALYSIS OF FORMULA: *Chang Qiang, Cheng Shan,* and *Er Bai* is probably the strongest combination of acupuncture points for the treatment of hemorrhoids. When drained, these points rectify the qi and quicken the blood in the anal area, disperse swelling, and stop both pain and bleeding. In addition, supplementing *Zhao Hai* moistens dryness, while draining *Zhi Gou* clears heat. Together, these points treat constipation due to intestinal dryness.

ADDITIONS & SUBTRACTIONS: *Chang Qiang* (GV 1) can also be alternated with *Yao Shu* (GV 2) with moxibustion plus *Ba Liao* (Bl 31-32-33-34) with either electroacupuncture or five stars needle. For severe dryness, add *San Yin Jiao* (Sp 6). For severe heat, add *Nei Ting* (St 44) and *Qu Chi* (LI 11).

2. DAMP HEAT PATTERN

MAIN SYMPTOMS: Swollen, severely painful hemorrhoids, possible protrusion which looks dull red in color and ulcerated, anal discharge of turbid-colored blood, difficult defecation, a hot, burning, sagging, distended feeling in the anus, especially during defecation, itchy anus, tenesmus, abdominal distention, torpid intake, heavy body, fatigue, slimy, yellow tongue fur, and a slippery, rapid pulse

TREATMENT PRINCIPLES: Clear heat and disinhibit dampness, dispel stasis and scatter nodulation

RX: *Zhi Tong Ru Shen Tang Jia Wei* (Divinely Inspired Pain Stopping Decoction with Added Flavors)

INGREDIENTS: Radix Sanguisorbae Officinalis (*Di Yu*), Fructus Immaturus Sophorae Japonicae (*Huai Huai Mi*), Rhizoma Atractylodis (*Cang Zhu*), Cortex Phellodendri (*Huang Bai*), Radix Angelicae Sinensis (*Dang Gui*), and Semen Arecae Catechu (*Bing Lang*), 9g each, and Radix Ledebouriellae Divaricatae (*Fang Feng*), Rhizoma Alismatis (*Ze Xie*), Radix Et Rhizoma Rhei (*Da Huang*), Radix

Gentianae Macrophyllae (*Qin Jiao*), and Semen Pruni Persicae (*Tao Ren*), 6g each

ANALYSIS OF FORMULA: *Qin Jiao, Cang Zhu, Huang Bai,* and *Ze Xie* clear and eliminate damp heat in the lower burner. *Huai Hua Mi* and *Di Yu* cool the blood and, combined with *Fang Feng,* stop bleeding due to hemorrhoids. In addition, *Huai Hua Mi,* with *Da Huang, Tao Ren,* and *Dang Gui,* moistens the intestines and frees the flow of the stools. Further, *Tao Ren* and *Dang Gui* quicken the blood and stop pain. *Bing Lang* moves the qi to stop pain in the anus.

ADDITIONS & SUBTRACTIONS: For a severe hot, burning, sagging, and distended feeling in the anus and an ulcerated anus, add six grams each of Rhizoma Coptidis Chinensis (*Huang Lian*) and Radix Scutellariae Baicalensis (*Huang Qin*). For uneasy defecation, add nine grams of Fructus Immaturus Citri Aurantii (*Zhi Shi*). For severe hemorrhoids, add six grams of Herba Seu Flos Schizonepetae Tenuifoliae (*Jing Jie Sui*). For severe bleeding, add nine grams each of Herba Seu Radix Cirsii Japonici (*Da Ji*) and Rhizoma Imperatae Cylindricae (*Bai Mao Gen*). For severe pain, add nine grams of Semen Arecae Catechu (*Bing Lang*) and 12 grams of Rhizoma Corydalis Yanhusuo (*Yan Hu Suo*). If there is no constipation, dry stools, or uneasy defecation, subtract *Da Huang.*

EXTERNAL TREATMENT: Apply the ready-made Chinese ointment *She Xiang Zhi Chuang Gao* (Musk Treat Hemorrhoids Ointment), or, for a painful, burning, ulcerated anus, wash the affected part with a cool decoction made from nine grams each of Rhizoma Coptidis Chinensis (*Huang Lian*), Rhizoma Picrorrhizae (*Hu Huang Lian*), and Radix Sophorae Flavescentis (*Ku Shen*). Do this three times per day.

ACUPUNCTURE & MOXIBUSTION: *Chang Qiang* (GV 1), *Cheng Shan* (Bl 57), *Er Bai* (M-UE-29), *Yin Ling Quan* (Sp 9), *Shang Ju Xu* (St 37)

ANALYSIS OF FORMULA: As mentioned above, draining *Chang Qiang, Cheng Shan,* and *Er Bai* rectifies the qi and quickens the blood in the anal area, disperses swelling and stops both pain and bleeding. Draining *Yin Ling Quan* clears heat and disinhibits dampness in the lower burner. Draining *Shang Ju Xu* clears heat from the yang ming and, with *Yin Ling Quan,* eliminates damp heat in the large intestine.

ADDITIONS & SUBTRACTIONS: For severe heat, add *Nei Ting* (St 44) and *Qu Chi* (LI 11).

3. QI STAGNATION & BLOOD STASIS PATTERN

MAIN SYMPTOMS: Protruding hemorrhoids when defecating, discharge of blood, sagging, distended, and painful anus, difficult defecation, dark, swollen, mixed hemorrhoids which are comparatively large with severe pain, abdominal distention and fullness, a dark, purple tongue, and a bowstring pulse

TREATMENT PRINCIPLES: Rectify the qi and quicken the blood, disperse swelling and transform stasis

RX: *Tao He Cheng Qi Tang Jia Wei* (Persica Order the Qi Decoction with Added Flavors)

INGREDIENTS: Semen Pruni Persicae (*Tao Ren*), Radix Et Rhizoma Rhei (*Da Huang*), and Fructus Immaturus Sophorae Japonicae (*Huai Hua Mi*), 9g each, Fructus Citri Aurantii (*Zhi Ke*) and Ramulus Cinnamomi Cassiae (*Gui Zhi*), 6g each, and Mirabilitum (*Mang Xiao*) and mix-fried Radix Glycyrrhizae (*Gan Cao*), 3g each

ANALYSIS OF FORMULA: *Tao Ren* and *Da Huang* quicken the blood, transform and stop stasis. *Zhi Ke* moves the qi and stops pain. *Gui Zhi* frees the flow of yang to move qi and quicken the blood. *Huai Hua Mi* cools the blood and stops bleeding due to hemorrhoids. *Tao Ren, Da Huang,* and *Mang Xiao* moisten dryness and free the flow of the stools. *Gan Cao* harmonizes the other medicinals in this formula.

ADDITIONS & SUBTRACTIONS: If there is no constipation, subtract *Mang Xiao.* For stabbing pain in the anus, add nine grams each of Feces Trogopterori Seu Pteromi (*Wu Ling Zhi*) and Pollen Typhae (*Pu Huang*). For severe hemorrhoid bleeding, add three grams of Radix Pseudoginseng (*San Qi*) and nine grams each of Pollen Typhae (*Pu Huang*) and Radix Sanguisorbae Officinalis (*Di Yu*). For anal distention and pain, tenesmus, or abdominal fullness, add nine grams each of Radix Auklandiae Lappae (*Mu Xiang*) and Semen Arecae Catechu (*Bing Lang*). For severe protruding hemorrhoids, add 30 grams of Radix Astragali Membranacei (*Huang Qi*) and nine grams of Rhizoma Cimicifugae (*Sheng Ma*).

EXTERNAL TREATMENT: Apply the ready-made Chinese ointment *She Xiang Zhi Chuang Gao* (Musk Treat Hemorrhoids Ointment) or some such similar external remedy.

ACUPUNCTURE & MOXIBUSTION: *Chang Qiang* (GV 1), *Cheng Shan* (Bl 57), *Er Bai* (M-UE-29), *San Yin Jiao* (Sp 6), *Zhi Gou* (TB 6)

ANALYSIS OF FORMULA: Draining *Chang Qiang, Cheng Shan,* and *Er Bai* rectifies the qi and quickens the blood in the anal area, disperses swelling and stops both pain and bleeding. Draining *San Yin Jiao* cools and quickens the blood, transforms stasis and stops bleeding. Draining *Zhi Gou* moves the qi in the three burners and treats constipation.

ADDITIONS & SUBTRACTIONS: For severe pain, add *He Gu* (LI 4). For heat, add *Nei Ting* (St 44) and *Qu Chi* (LI 11).

4. CENTRAL QI FALLING DOWNWARD PATTERN

MAIN SYMPTOMS: Protruding hemorrhoids when defecating or when walking, coughing, sneezing, or standing for a long time, non-returning piles unless helped by the hands or lying flat, discharge of a large or small amount of pale-colored blood, forceless defecation, possible enduring diarrhea or frequent defecation, fatigue, lassitude of the spirit, a lusterless facial complexion, a pale tongue, and a fine, weak pulse

TREATMENT PRINCIPLES: Fortify the spleen and boost the qi, upbear yang and lift the fallen

RX: *Bu Zhong Yi Qi Tang Jia Jian* (Supplement the Center & Boost the Qi Decoction with Additions & Subtractions)

INGREDIENTS: Radix Astragali Membranacei (*Huang Qi*), 18g, Radix Codonopsitis Pilosulae (*Dang Shen*), 12g, Rhizoma Atractylodis Macrocephalae (*Bai Zhu*), Rhizoma Cimicifugae (*Sheng Ma*), Fructus Immaturus Sophorae Japonicae (*Huai Hua Mi*), and Radix Sanguisorbae Officinalis (*Di Yu*), 9g each, Pericarpium Citri Reticulatae (*Chen Pi*), Sclerotium Poriae Cocos (*Fu Ling*), and mix-fried Radix Glycyrrhizae (*Gan Cao*), 6g each, and Radix Bupleuri (*Chai Hu*), 3g

ANALYSIS OF FORMULA: *Huang Qi, Dang Shen, Bai Zhu, Fu Ling,* and mix-fried *Gan Cao* supplement the center and boost the qi. *Fu Ling, Bai Zhu,* and *Chen Pi* seep, dry, and move dampness to promote spleen transformation. *Huang Qi, Sheng Ma,* and *Chai Hu* upbear yang and lift the fallen. *Huai Hua Mi* and *Di Yu* cool the blood and stop bleeding due to hemorrhoids.

ADDITIONS & SUBTRACTIONS: For predominant distention and pain in the anus, subtract *Chen Pi* and add six grams each of Semen Arecae Catechu (*Bing Lang*), Fructus Citri Aurantii (*Zhi Ke*), and Radix Auklandiae Lappae (*Mu Xiang*).

For profuse bleeding without protrusion, pain, or distention, replace *Bu Zhong Yi Qi Tang* with *Gui Pi Tang Jia Jian* (Return the Spleen Decoction with Additions & Subtractions): Radix Astragali Membranacei (*Huang Qi*), 15g, Radix Codonopsitis Pilosulae (*Dang Shen*), Rhizoma Atractylodis Macrocephalae (*Bai Zhu*), Radix Angelicae Sinensis (*Dang Gui*), Arillus Euphoriae Longanae (*Long Yan Rou*), Gelatinum Corii Asini (*E Jiao*), and Fructus Immaturus Sophorae Japonicae (*Huai Hua Mi*), 9g each, blast-fried Rhizoma Zingiberis (*Pao Jiang*), 6g, and mix-fried Radix Glycyrrhizae (*Gan Cao*), 3g.

For hemorrhoids combined with enduring diarrhea, replace *Bu Zhong Yi Qi Tang* with *Huang Tu Tang* (Yellow Earth Decoction): Terra Flava Usta (*Fu Long Gan*), 24g, Radix Astragali Membranacei (*Huang Qi*), 18g, Rhizoma Atractylodis Macrocephalae (*Bai Zhu*), Radix Lateralis Praeparatus Aconiti Carmichaeli (*Fu Zi*), Rhizoma Cimicifugae (*Sheng Ma*), Fructus Sophorae Japonicae (*Huai Jiao*), and Radix Sanguisorbae Officinalis (*Di Yu*), 9g each, and blast-fried Rhizoma Zingiberis (*Pao Jiang*), 6g.

For qi and blood dual vacuity, replace *Bu Zhong Yi Qi Tang* with *Ti Gang Tang* (Lift the Anus Decoction): Radix Astragali Membranacei (*Huang Qi*), 18g, Rhizoma Cimicifugae (*Sheng Ma*), 15g, Radix Codonopsitis Pilosulae (*Dang Shen*), 12g, Rhizoma Atractylodis Macrocephalae (*Bai Zhu*), Radix Angelicae Sinensis (*Dang Gui*), Radix Albus Paeoniae Lactiflorae (*Bai Shao*), Fructus Immaturus Sophorae Japonicae (*Huai Hua Mi*), and Radix Sanguisorbae Officinalis (*Di Yu*), 9g each, and Radix Ligustici Wallichii (*Chuan Xiong*), 3g. For profuse white vaginal discharge, add 9 grams each of Semen Nelumbinis Nuciferae (*Lian Zi*) and Semen Euryalis Ferocis (*Qian Shi*). For concomitant spleen yang vacuity, add 6 grams of dry Rhizoma Zingiberis (*Gan Jiang*) and 3 grams of blasted Radix Lateralis Praeparatus Aconiti Carmichaeli (*Fu Zi*).

EXTERNAL TREATMENT: Apply a cool decoction of six grams of Galla Rhois Chinensis (*Wu Bei Zi*) and nine grams each of Fructus Rosae Laevigatae (*Jin Ying Zi*), Fructus Terminaliae Chebulae (*He Zi*), and Alumen (*Ming Fan*) three times per day as a compress.

ACUPUNCTURE & MOXIBUSTION: *Chang Qiang* (GV 1), *Cheng Shan* (Bl 57), *Er Bai* (M-UE-29), *Zu San Li* (St 36), *Bai Hui* (GV 20), *Qi Hai* (CV 6).

ANALYSIS OF FORMULA: Draining *Chang Qiang, Cheng Shan,* and *Er Bai* rectifies the qi and quickens the blood in the anal area, disperses swelling and stops both pain and bleeding. With heavy moxibustion, *Zu San Li, Bai Hui,* and *Qi Hai* fortify the spleen and boost the qi, upbear yang and lift the fallen.

ADDITIONS & SUBTRACTIONS: For severe bleeding, add *San Yin Jiao* (Sp 6). For heart palpitations, add *Xin Shu* (Bl 15). For dizziness, add *Xin Shu* (Bl 15) and *Pi Shu* (Bl 20). For poor appetite, add *Xuan Ji* (CV 21). For uterine leaking and spotting, add *San Yin Jiao* (Sp 6).

REMARKS

1. Central qi falling downward is characterized by worse hemorrhoidal pain and discomfort when fatigued or after standing for a long time. This is easy to question. It is also possible for hemorrhoids to be due to a combination of liver

depression, spleen vacuity, and damp heat. In that case, choose a guiding formula depending on which of these three elements is predominant. If liver depression is relatively pronounced, consider between either *Xiao Yao San* (Rambling Powder), *Dan Zhi Xiao Yao San* (Moutan & Gardenia Rambling Powder), or *Xiao Chai Hu Tang* (Minor Bupleurum Decoction) or modify *Bu Zhong Yi Qi Tang* (Supplement the Center & Boost the Qi Decoction) by increasing the dosage of Radix Bupleuri (*Chai Hu*) and Radix Angelicae Sinensis (*Dang Gui*). Most patterns of hemorrhoids are complicated by at least an element of blood stasis.

2. Acupuncture and moxibustion are effective for the symptomatic relief of hemorrhoidal swelling and pain. However, for severe cases, one should use a combined therapy of Chinese medicinals and acupuncture or consider banding or surgery. There are a number of special techniques for the treatment of hemorrhoids within acupuncture. These include 1) bleeding every *a shi* point on the back, 2) bleeding every dark red spot which does not lose color under pressure on the back, 3) bleeding every papule located on the frenulum of the upper lip, 4) bleeding every dark spot on the coccygeal area, and 5) bleeding *Yin Jiao* (GV 28). Other techniques include bleeding the hemorrhoid directly or doing direct moxibustion on top of the hemorrhoid. Although these are painful and embarrassing procedures, they are extremely effective.

3. The best points for bleeding hemorrhoids are *Er Bai* (M-UE-29), *Kong Zui* (Lu 6), and *Xi Men* (Per 4). The best points for hemorrhoidal pain are *Cheng Shan* (Bl 57), *Ci Liao* (Bl 32), *Yao Qi* (M-BW-29), and *Hui Yang* (Bl 35). However, the single best point to needle for hemorrhoids is *Chang Qiang* (GV 1).

4. Sometimes, in the case of hemorrhoids, the pattern discrimination may be confused due to an absence of specific symptoms. In this case, one can use the following simple Chinese medicinal protocol. If there is only bleeding, but no distention, pain, constipation, or other generalized symptoms, prescribe *Huai Hua San* (Sophora Flower Powder): Flos Immaturus Sophorae Japonicae (*Huai Hua Mi*) and Cacumen Biotae Orientalis (*Ce Bai Ye*), 12g each, and Herba Seu Flos Schizonepetae Tenuifoliae (*Jing Jie Sui*) and Fructus Citri Aurantii (*Zhi Ke*), 6g each. If there is bleeding, distention, and constipation but no pain, or other general symptoms, prescribe *Huai Jiao Wan* (Sophora Fruit Pills): Fructus Immaturus Sophorae Japonicae (*Huai Hua Mi*) and Radix Sanguisorbae Officinalis (*Di Yu*), 12g each, Radix Ledebouriellae Divaricatae (*Fang Feng*) and Radix Angelicae Sinensis (*Dang Gui*), 9g each, and Cortex Phellodendri (*Huang Bai*) and Fructus Citri Aurantii (*Zhi Ke*), 6g each. If there is bleeding, pain, and distention but no other generalized symptoms, prescribe *Di Yu San* (Sanguisorba Powder): Radix Sanguisorbae Officinalis (*Di Yu*), 12g, Fructus Immaturus Sophorae Japonicae (*Huai Hua Mi*) and Fructus Aristolichiae (*Ma Dou Ling*), 9g each, and Fructus Citri Aurantii (*Zhi Ke*), Semen Arecae Catechu (*Bing Lang*), and Radix Auklandiae Lappae (*Mu Xiang*), 6g each. In the last case, for constipation, add 3-9 grams of uncooked Radix Et Rhizoma Rhei (*Da Huang*). In all of the above cases, one can use *She Xiang Zhi Chuang Gao* (Musk Treat Hemorrhoids Ointment) externally.

5. Other first aid or folk remedy external treatments include making compresses from grated potatoes and white flour or grated taro root and white flour.

30

HERPES GENITALIA

Herpes genitalia refers to infection of the genital or anorectal skin or mucous membranes by either of two closely related herpes simplex viruses, HSV-1 or HSV-2, with HSV-2 accounting for 90% of genital herpes. This is the most common ulcerative sexually transmitted disease in developed countries. It is estimated that 25% of American adults have genital herpes. However, most do not know this because their symptoms are too mild to notice.[1] Genital herpes with or without symptoms currently affects approximately one in four females and one in five males in the total U.S. population of adults and adolescents. Within the past two decades, the number of genital herpes infections has increased 30% among Americans, with the most dramatic increase seen in young adults ages 20-29 and in Caucasian adolescents.[2] In fact, most persons infected with HSV-2 have no symptoms. When HSV-2 infection is symptomatic, primary lesions develop 4-7 days after contact. These typically appear as a small cluster of variably painful vesicles which then erode and form superficial, circular ulcers with red borders. These small ulcers may also coalesce into a single, larger lesion. After several days, these ulcers crust over and generally heal in 10 days, although they may also heal without crusting. Lesions may occur on the prepuce, glans penis, and penile shaft in males and on the labia, clitoris, perineum, vagina, and cervix in females. They may also occur perianally and in the rectum in homosexual men or in women who engage in rectal intercourse. These lesions may be accompanied by fever, malaise, painful urination, especially in females, headache, joint pain, cold sores around the mouth, and regional lymph node swelling and pain. Some people report pain and discomfort in the genital area after the lesions have healed. This pain is postherpetic neuralgia.

Approximately 40% of those infected with this virus who do show symptoms never have a second attack. However, because the virus chronically infects the sacral sensory nerve ganglia from which it reactivates and reinfects the skin, recurrences are common in the majority of those infected. Unfortunately, those antibodies which are produced early in the course of herpes infection do not prevent recurrence of the active phase of this disease since they do not affect intracellular viral replication and direct cell to cell viral transfer. Many with recurrent outbreaks have 4-5 recurrences per year. These recurrences are generally most common after sexual intercourse or masturbation causing trauma to the genital skin, after sunbathing, and during times of physical and emotional stress. Recurrent outbreaks may also be precipitated by faulty diet, such as ingestion of fatty meats, chocolate, and alcohol. During the initial outbreak, these lesions and their accompanying symptoms are typically more painful, widespread, and prolonged than in subsequent recurrent outbreaks. In females, recurrent outbreaks are often coordinated with the menstrual cycle with recurrences most commonly occurring before, during, or immediately after menstruation. In recurrent episodes, the outbreak of skin lesions is usually but not always preceded by itching, tingling, and/or burning and localized erythema. There may also be prodromal neurological pain radiating or beginning from the sacrum and/or perineum and traveling to the hips, genitalia, or down the legs. This pain may be severely uncomfortable and annoying. However, recurrent episodes are usually not accompanied by fever and severe malaise. Recurrences vary greatly in their severity and frequency and may continue for many years. Herpes simplex virus infection is a lifelong illness. In patients with depressed cell-mediated immunity due to HIV infection or other causes, prolonged or progressive lesions may last for weeks or longer.

Newborns may be infected during delivery with symptoms appearing 9-11 days after birth. These may include skin blisters, red eyes, and abnormal eye discharge. If the virus spreads through the baby's bloodstream to the brain, there may be lethargy, irritability, and seizures. If the virus spreads to the baby's lungs, there may be difficulty breathing requiring breathing assistance. However, the treatment of these symptoms are not discussed below. Because of fear of infection during vaginal delivery, pregnant women with genital herpes may be delivered by Caesarean section. Because the decision for Caesarean section is based on many factors, pregnant women with HSV infection should discuss the subject with their obstetrician as early as possible in pregnancy. If a pregnant woman in her third trimester feels a herpes outbreak coming on, she should call her doctor immediately.

Other complications of genital herpes include aseptic meningitis, transverse myelitis, autonomic nervous system dysfunction, or severe sacral neuralgia. During primary infection, hematogenous dissemination of the virus to the extragenital skin, joints, liver, or lungs occurs primarily in immunosuppressed or pregnant patients. Extragenital lesions in the buttocks, groin, or thigh may occur in recurrent disease by neuronal spread. Direct inoculation occasionally accounts for infections of the fingers and/or eyes.

A presumptive Western medical diagnosis of genital herpes is based on visual inspection of the affected area looking for characteristic lesions and finding characteristic multinucleated giant cells in Wright's-Giemsa-stained smears of cells taken from these lesions. This is referred to as the Tzanck test. Diagnosis is confirmed by culture, direct immunoflourescent assay, or serology. The appearance of genital herpes can vary from patient to patient. Further, HSV infection can mimic the appearance of other STDs and other STDs can mimic herpes. Therefore, the definitive Western medical diagnosis of this condition must rely on laboratory tests.

The Western medical treatment of genital herpes consists of antiviral therapy with acyclovir. This is used either remedially during acute outbreaks or prophylactically in order to try to suppress recurrences. The side effects of acyclovir include nausea, vomiting, and diarrhea (8% in long-term use), nervousness and depression (3%), and joint and muscle pain (3%). Other unusual, unexpected adverse reactions include skin rash, acne, and hair loss. It is also possible to develop strains of herpes virus which are resistant to this drug. Other antivirals used for less frequent but more severe recurrences include famcyclovir and valacyclovir. Postherpetic neuralgia is commonly treated with nonsteroidal anti-inflammatory drugs (NSAIDs). As of this writing, there is no Western medical cure for this disease.

CHINESE DISEASE CATEGORIZATION: Sores and ulcers on the genitals are referred to generically as *yin chuang*, genital sores. Sores which come and go like a fox darting its head in and out of its burrow are called *hu huo*, fox-like bewilderment, and this is the name given to herpes infections in general, including herpes infections of the oral cavity, eyes, and external genitalia. This name first occurs in Zhang Zhong-jing's *Jin Gui Yao Lue (Essentials of the Golden Cabinet)* where it says that lesions in the mouth region are called bewilderment, while lesions in the genital region are called fox-like. In the *Yi Zong Jin Jian (Golden Mirror of Ancestral Medicine)*, fox-like bewilderment of the anogenital region is also referred to as *xia gan*, lower *gan*.

DISEASE CAUSES: External invasion by damp heat evil toxins (in the primary infection stage) and deep-lying warm evils activated by righteous qi vacuity and/or internally engendered damp heat evils (in recurrent outbreaks)

DISEASE MECHANISMS: Due to external contraction of damp heat evil toxins, there is localized redness, swelling, pain, and ulceration when these damp heat toxins brew and putrify the skin and flesh. Because of exuberant heat toxins, there are also emission of heat (*i.e.*, fever) and malaise. Because of either the inherent strength or nature of these evil toxins or righteous qi vacuity, these warm evils may be retained and lie deeply in the blood aspect. If, for any reason, such as faulty diet, fatigue, or disease, the spleen becomes vacuous and weak, righteous qi may become vacuous and weak, thus allowing these hidden warm evils to become active again. It is also possible for these evil toxins to be activated by internally engendered damp heat due to faulty diet, such as overeating sugars and sweets, chocolate, fatty meats, hot, spicy foods, deep-fried foods, and/or alcohol. If damp heat evils linger and endure, they may eventually damage and consume yin fluids, this may give rise to yin vacuity fire flaring which stews and burns fluids and humors, also internally engendering damp heat.

In terms of recurrent herpes outbreaks in females associated with the menstrual cycle, dampness in the lower burner increases and accumulates premenstrually. This is because blood and fluids flow together, and when blood is sent downward to the uterus, fluids arrive there first. Postmenstrually, many women are left blood and yin vacuous and insufficient. This can thus give rise to damp heat lesions due to yin vacuity fire flaring. In addition, at midcycle, yin has reached its extreme and is transformed into yang. Therefore, heat in the body increases in general. If there is either accumulated dampness or qi depression, this may be transformed into damp heat.

TREATMENT BASED ON PATTERN DISCRIMINATION:

1. WIND HEAT PATTERN

MAIN SYMPTOMS: Fever, slight aversion to wind cold accompanied by generalized bodily discomfort, outbreak of water blisters on the two yin orifices and possibly on the mouth and nose area, slight pain or an itchy sensation, oral thirst, possible sore throat, a red tongue tip with thin, white or thin, yellow fur, and a floating, rapid pulse

NOTE: This pattern represents the initial outbreak before genital sores have ulcerated and when there is fear, malaise, and other flu-like symptoms.

RX: *Jing Fang Bai Du San Jia Jian* (Schizonepeta & Ledebouriella Vanquish Toxins Powder with Additions & Subtractions)

INGREDIENTS: Radix Gentianae Scabrae (*Long Dan Cao*), 20g, Radix Sophorae Flavescentis (*Ku Shen*), Herba Schizonepetae Tenuifoliae (*Jing Jie*), Radix Ledebouriellae Divaricatae (*Fang Feng*), Radix Bupleuri (*Chai Hu*), Radix Ligustici Wallichii (*Chuan Xiong*), and Periosticum Cicadae (*Chan Yi*), 15g each, Radix Et Rhizoma Notopterygii (*Qiang Huo*), Radix Angelicae Pubescentis (*Du Huo*), Fructus Citri Aurantii (*Zhi Ke*), Sclerotium Poriae Cocos (*Fu Ling*), Radix Peucedani (*Qian Hu*), and Radix Platycodi Grandiflori (*Jie Geng*), 9g each, and Radix Glycyrrhizae (*Gan Cao*), 6g

ANALYSIS OF FORMULA: *Long Dan Cao* and *Ku Shen* clear heat and eliminate dampness from the liver channel and skin respectively. *Jing Jie, Fang Feng, Chai Hu, Chan Yi, Qiang Huo,* and *Du Huo* all resolve the exterior and dispel wind. *Fu Ling* seeps dampness, while *Qian Hu* and *Jie Geng* clear heat and transform phlegm. *Chai Hu* and *Jie Geng* also upbear the clear so that the turbid may be more efficiently downborne. *Zhi Ke* moves and rectifies the qi, and *Chuan Xiong* moves and rectifies the blood. *Gan Cao* clears heat and resolves toxins at the same time as it harmonizes the other medicinals in this formula.

ADDITIONS & SUBTRACTIONS: If there is exterior repletion with interior vacuity, replace *Jing Fang Bai Du San Jia Jian* with *Ren Shen Bai Du San Jia Jian* (Ginseng Vanquish Toxins Powder with Additions & Subtractions): Radix Gentianae Scabrae (*Long Dan Cao*), 20g, Radix Sophorae Flavescentis (*Ku Shen*), Radix Bupleuri (*Chai Hu*), Radix Ligustici Wallichii (*Chuan Xiong*), and Periosticum Cicadae (*Chan Yi*), 15g each, Radix Et Rhizoma Notopterygii (*Qiang Huo*), Radix Angelicae Pubescentis (*Du Huo*), Radix Codonopsitis Pilosulae (*Dang Shen*), Fructus Citri Aurantii (*Zhi Ke*), Sclerotium Poriae Cocos (*Fu Ling*), Radix Peucedani (*Qian Hu*), and Radix Platycodi Grandiflori (*Jie Geng*), 9g each, and Radix Glycyrrhizae (*Gan Cao*), 6g

ACUPUNCTURE & MOXIBUSTION: *He Gu* (LI 4), *Qu Chi* (LI 11), *Da Zhui* (GV 14), *San Yin Jiao* (Sp 6), *Xing Jian* (Liv 2)

ANALYSIS OF FORMULA: Draining *He Gu, Qu Chi,* and *Da Zhui* resolves the exterior, scatters wind, and clears heat. Draining *San Yin Jiao* and *Xing Jian* clears heat and eliminates dampness from the liver channel in the genital region.

ADDITIONS & SUBTRACTIONS: If there is concomitant qi vacuity, add *Zu San Li.*

2. DAMP HEAT OBSTRUCTING THE NETWORK VESSELS PATTERN

MAIN SYMPTOMS: Water blisters and/or uclers with red margins on the genitals, perineum, or anorectal area, pain and/or burning in the affected area, possible fever, malaise, possible lumbosacral pain, reddish yellow urine, possible burning or painful urination, dry mouth and thirst, a red tongue with slimy, yellow fur, and a slippery, rapid or bowstring, rapid pulse

NOTE: This pattern describes the outbreak of red, hot, painful, water-filled vesicles and ulcers.

TREATMENT PRINCIPLES: Clear heat and eliminate dampness, resolve toxins and stop pain

RX: *Long Dan Xie Gan Tang Jia Jian* (Gentiana Scabra Drain the Liver Decoction with Additions & Subtractions)

INGREDIENTS: Uncooked Radix Rehmanniae (*Sheng Di*) and Radix Scutellariae Baicalensis (*Huang Qin*), 12g each, Fructus Gardeniae Jasminoidis (*Zhi Zi*), Rhizoma Alismatis (*Ze Xie*), Semen Plantaginis (*Che Qian Zi*), Extremitas Radicis Angelicae Sinensis (*Dang Gui Wei*), Radix Sophorae Flavescentis (*Ku Shen*), Cortex Radicis Dictamni Dasycarpi (*Bai Xian Pi*), and Radix Bupleuri (*Chai Hu*), 9g each, and Radix Glycyrrhizae (*Gan Cao*), 3g

ANALYSIS OF FORMULA: *Sheng Di* clears heat and cools the blood. It also prevents the other, bitter, cold medicinals from damaging yin fluids. *Huang Qin, Zhi Zi, Ku Shen,* and *Bai Xian Pi* clear heat and eliminate dampness, clear heat and resolve toxins, especially from the lower burner and skin. *Ze Xie* and *Che Qian Zi* seep dampness, thus helping clear and eliminate damp heat via urination. They also free the flow of strangury if there is painful, difficult urination. *Dang Gui Wei* quickens the blood and transforms stasis, thus helping to stop pain. *Chai Hu* courses and clears the liver, remembering that the liver channel courses and flows through the external genitalia. *Gan Cao* harmonizes the other medicinals in this formula.

ADDITIONS & SUBTRACTIONS: If there is fever, add 15 grams each of Flos Lonicerae Japonicae (*Jin Yin Hua*) and Fructus Forsythiae Suspensae (*Lian Qiao*). If there is lymphadenopathy, add 15 grams of Spica Prunellae Vulgaris (*Xia Ku Cao*) and 12 grams each of Concha Ostreae (*Mu Li*), Radix Scrophulariae Ningpeoensis (*Xuan Shen*), and Herba Saragassii (*Hai Zao*). If there is lumbosacral pain, add nine grams each of Radix Achyranthis Bidentatae (*Niu Xi*) and Cortex Eucommiae Ulmoidis (*Du Zhong*). If a diagnosis of herpes infection has been made, add 15 grams each of Radix Isatidis Seu Baphicacanthi (*Ban Lan Gen*) and Radix Lithospermi Seu Arnebiae (*Zi Cao*).

If there is damp heat brewing and binding with marked blood heat and blood stasis as evidenced by severe burning heat and redness as well as severe pain, replace *Long Dan Xie Gan Tang Jia Jian* with the following unnamed formula: Semen Phaseoli Calcarati (*Chi Xiao Dou*) and uncooked Semen Coicis Lachyrma-jobi (*Yi Yi Ren*), 25g each, Radix Sophorae Flavescentis (*Ku Shen*), Radix Scrophulariae Ningpoensis (*Xuan Shen*), Radix Rubrus Paeoniae Lactiflorae (*Chi Shao*), Radix Stephaniae Tetrandrae (*Fang Ji*), and Radix Lithopsermi Seu Arnebiae (*Zi Cao*), 12g each, Radix Angelicae Sinensis (*Dang Gui*), Cortex Phellodendri (*Huang Bai*), Cortex Radicis Moutan (*Dan Pi*), Semen Pruni Persicae (*Tao Ren*), and Rhizoma Atractylodis (*Cang Zhu*), 9g each, and Flos Carthami Tinctorii (*Hong Hua*), 6g.

If painful urination is marked, replace *Long Dan Xie Gan Tang Jia Jian* with *Ba Zheng San* (Eight Correcting [Ingredients] Powder): Talcum (*Hua Shi*), 20g, Fructus Gardeniae Jasminoidis (*Zhi Zi*), Herba Polygoni Avicularis (*Bian Xu*), Caulis Akebiae Mutong (*Mu Tong*), Herba Dianthi (*Qu Mai*), Semen Plantaginis (*Che Qian Zi*), and Radix Glycyrrhizae (*Gan Cao*), 9g each, Radix Et Rhizoma Rhei (*Da Huang*), 6-9g, and Medulla Junci Effusi (*Deng Xin Cao*), 3-6g.

If there is spleen vacuity engendering dampness and heat, replace *Long Da Xie Gan Tang Jia Jian* with *Gan Cao Xie Xin Tang* (Licorice Drain the Heart Decoction) and *Er Miao San* (Two Wonders Powder) with added flavors: Radix Scutellariae Baicalensis (*Huang Qin*) and uncooked Radix Glycyrrhizae (*Gan Cao*), 12g each, Rhizoma Pinelliae Ternatae (*Ban Xia*), Radix Codonopsitis Pilosulae (*Dang Shen*), Rhizoma Atractylodis (*Cang Zhu*), Radix Sophorae Flavescentis (*Ku Shen*), Cortex Radicis Dictamni Dasycarpi (*Bai Xian Pi*), and Cortex Phellodendri (*Huang Bai*), 9g each, dry Rhizoma Zingiberis (*Gan Jiang*), 6g, and Rhizoma Coptidis Chinensis (*Huang Lian*), 3-6g. If a diagnosis of herpes infection has been established, add 15 grams of Radix Isatidis Seu Baphicacanthi (*Ban Lan Gen*). If there is concomitant fatigue, add 15-30 grams of Radix Astragali Membranacei (*Huang Qi*). If there is concomitant liver depression, add 9 grams of Radix Bupleuri (*Chai Hu*).

If there is spleen vacuity engendering dampness and liver depression engendering heat, replace *Long Dan Xie Gan Tang Jia Jian* with *Xiao Chai Hu Tang Jia Wei* (Minor Bupleurum Decoction with Added Flavors): Radix Isatidis Seu Baphicacanthi (*Ban Lan Gen*) and Rhizoma Smilacis Glabrae (*Tu Fu Ling*), 15g each, Radix Scutellariae Baicalensis (*Huang Qin*) and Radix Glycyrrhizae (*Gan Cao*), 12g each, Radix Bupleuri (*Chai Hu*), Radix Codonopsitis Pilosulae (*Dang Shen*), Radix Sophorae Flavescentis (*Ku Shen*), Cortex Radicis Dictamni Dasycarpi (*Bai Xian Pi*), and Rhizoma Pinelliae Ternatae (*Ban Xia*), 9g each, Fructus Zizyphi Jujubae (*Da Zao*), 3 pieces, and uncooked Rhizoma Zingiberis (*Sheng Jiang*), 2 slices.

ACUPUNCTURE & MOXIBUSTION: *San Yin Jiao* (Sp 6), *Yin Ling Quan* (Sp 9), *Xue Hai* (Sp 10), *Xing Jian* (Liv 2)

ANALYSIS OF FORMULA: Draining *San Yin Jiao* and *Xue Hai* clears and quickens the blood and helps stop pain. Draining *San Yin Jiao* and *Yin Ling Quan* strongly clears heat and eliminates dampness from the lower burner. Draining *Xing Jian* clears heat from the liver channel.

ADDITIONS & SUBTRACTIONS: For sacral pain, add *Ba Liao* (Bl 31-34) and *Huan Tiao* (GB 30). For fever, add *Qu Chi* (LI 11) and *Wai Guan* (TB 5). If there is concomitant spleen vacuity, add *Zu San Li* (St 36) with supplementing method and use even supplementing-even draining on *San Yin Jiao*. If there is concomitant yin vacuity, add *Fu Liu* (Ki 7) with supplementing method and also use even supplementing-even draining on *San Yin Jiao*. One can also indirectly moxa the lesions themselves.

3. YIN VACUITY-FIRE FLARING ABOVE ENGENDERING DAMPNESS & HEAT BELOW PATTERN

MAIN SYMPTOMS: Postmenstrually, during enduring disease, or in the elderly, there are signs and symptoms of yin vacuity-fire flaring above with damp heat pouring downward, such as dizziness, tinnitus, malar flushing, night sweats, heart palpitations, vexation and agitation, insomnia, profuse dreams, a dry mouth and throat, low back pain and soreness, scanty, yellow urination, red, burning, painful, or itchy lesions on or around the genitalia which may or may not transform into vesicles and then ulcers, a red tongue with scanty, yellow or no fur, and a fine, rapid pulse

TREATMENT PRINCIPLES: Enrich yin and clear heat above, clear heat and eliminate dampness below

RX: *Zhi Bai Di Huang Wan Jia Wei* (Anemarrhena & Phellodendron Rehmannia Pills with Added Flavors)

INGREDIENTS: Uncooked Radix Rehmanniae (*Sheng Di*), 15g, Rhizoma Anemarrhenae Aspheloidis (*Zhi Mu*), 12g, Radix Dioscoreae Oppositae (*Shan Yao*), Fructus Corni Officinalis (*Shan Zhu Yu*), Sclerotium Poriae Cocos (*Fu Ling*), Rhizoma Alismatis (*Ze Xie*), Cortex Radicis Moutan (*Dan Pi*), Cortex Radicis Dictamni Dasycarpi (*Bai Xian Pi*), Radix Sophorae Flavescentis (*Ku Shen*), and Cortex Phellodendri (*Huang Bai*), 9g each

ANALYSIS OF FORMULA: *Sheng Di* clears heat and cools the blood at the same time as it enriches yin and engenders fluids. *Shan Yao* supplements the spleen and kidneys, while *Shan Zhu Yu* supplements the kidney qi. *Fu Ling* supplements the spleen qi, and former and latter heavens bolster and support each other. At the same time, *Fu Ling* assists *Ze Xie* in seeping dampness and disinhibiting urination. *Dan Pi* also clears and cools the blood. In addition, it quickens the blood and helps stop pain. *Bai Xian Pi, Ku Shen,* and *Huang Bai* clear heat and eliminate dampness, especially from the skin and/or the lower burner.

ADDITIONS & SUBTRACTIONS: If there is concomitant liver depression, add 9-12 grams of Fructus Meliae Toosendan (*Chuan Lian Zi*). If there is oral dryness, add nine grams each of Tuber Ophiopogonis Japonicae (*Mai Men Dong*) and Radix Trichosanthis Kirlowii (*Tian Hua Fen*). If pain is severe, add nine grams each of Resina Olibani (*Ru Xiang*) and Resina Myrrhae (*Mo Yao*). If there is difficult, choppy, astringent urination, delete *Shan Zhu Yu* and add nine grams of Semen Plantaginis (*Che Qian Zi*).

If there is marked yin and blood vacuity after menstruation, replace *Zhi Bai Di Huang Wan Jia Wei* with *Yi Guan Jian Jia Wei* (One Link Decoction with Added Flavors): uncooked Radix Rehmanniae (*Sheng Di*), 15g, Tuber Ophiopogonis Japonici (*Mai Men Dong*) and Radix Glehniae Littoralis (*Sha Shen*), 12 grams each, Radix Angelicae Sinensis (*Dang Gui*), Fructus Lycii Chinensis (*Gou Qi Zi*), Radix Sophorae Flavescentis (*Ku Shen*), Cortex Dictamni Dasycarpi (*Bai Xian Pi*), and Cortex Phellodendri (*Huang Bai*), 9g each, and Fructus Meliae Toosendan (*Chuan Lian Zi*), 6-9g. If there is lower abdominal pain, add 18 grams of Radix Albus Paeoniae Lactiflorae (*Bai Shao*) and 12 grams of Radix Glycyrrhizae (*Gan Cao*). If there is a bitter taste in the mouth, add three grams of Rhizoma Coptidis Chinensis (*Huang Lian*). If there is constipation, add nine grams of Semen Trichosanthis Kirlowii (*Gua Lou Ren*). If there are night sweats, add nine grams of Cortex Radicis Lycii Chinensis (*Di Gu Pi*). If there are swollen lymphnodes, add 12 grams of Radix Scrophulariae Ningpoensis (*Xuan Shen*) and nine grams of Bulbus Fritillariae Thunbergii (*Zhe Bei Mu*).

If there is qi and yin dual vacuity, replace *Zhi Bai Di Huang Wan Jia Jian* with *Ren Shen Gu Ben Wan Jia Jian* (Ginseng Secure the Root Pills with Additions & Subtractions): Radix Glehniae Littoralis (*Sha Shen*) and uncooked Radix Rehmanniae (*Sheng Di*), 15g each, Tuber Ophiopogonis Japonici (*Mai Men Dong*), Tuber Asparagi Cochinensis (*Tian Men Dong*), uncooked Semen Coicis Lachyrma-jobi (*Yi Yi Ren*), and Radix Dioscoreae Oppositae (*Shan Yao*), 12g each, Radix Astragali Membranacei (*Huang Qi*), Radix Glycyrrhizae (*Gan Cao*), stir-fried Radix Gentianae Scabrae (*Long Dan Cao*), Rhizoma Imperatae Cyclindricae (*Bai Mao Gen*), Herba Plantaginis (*Che Qian Zi*), and stir-fried Radix Albus Paeoniae Lactiflorae (*Bai Shao*), 9g each, and Rhizoma Cimicifugae (*Sheng Ma*) and Radix Isatidis Seu Baphicacanthi (*Ban Lan Gen*), 6g each. For recalcitrant lesions, add nine grams each of Radix Ampelopsis Japonicae (*Bai Lian*), Radix Cynanchi Atrati (*Bai Wei*), Radix Quinquefolii (*Xi Yang Shen*), and Testa Phaseoli Munginis (*Lu Dou Yi*). For severe itching and pain, add nine grams each of Radix Lithospermi Seu Arnebiae (*Zi Cao*) and Ramulus Uncariae Cum Uncis (*Gou Teng*) and 12 grams of Concha Haliotidis (*Shi Jue Ming*).

ACUPUNCTURE & MOXIBUSTION: *San Yin Jiao* (Sp 6), *Fu Liu* (Ki 7), *Yin Ling Quan* (Sp 9), *Xue Hai* (Sp 10)

ANALYSIS OF FORMULA: Supplementing *Fu Liu* and even supplementing-even draining *San Yin Jiao* supplements the kidneys and enriches yin. Draining *Yin Ling Quan* clears heat and eliminates dampness, while draining *Xue Hai* clears heat and cools the blood.

ADDITIONS & SUBTRACTIONS: For night sweats, add *Yin Xi* (Ht 6). For insomnia and profuse dreams, add *Shen Men* (Ht 7), *Bai Hui* (GV 20), and *Feng Chi* (GB 20). For oral thirst, add *Nei Ting* (St 44). For sacral pain, add *Ba Liao* (Bl 31-34) and *Huan Tiao* (GB 30). If there is concomitant qi vacuity, add *Zu San Li* (St 36). If there is marked blood vacuity, add *Ge Shu* (Bl 17) and *Gan Shu* (Bl 18).

REMARKS

1. The purpose of Chinese medical treatment is to A) prevent incipient outbreaks and B) help speed resolution and mitigate symptoms when outbreaks have occurred.

2. To help heal ulcerated sores, first wash in *Ku Shen Tang* (Sophora Decoction, *i.e.*, 30-45 grams of Radix Sophorae Flavescentis, *Ku Shen*, and water) and then apply Realgar (*Xiong Huang*) mixed with rubbing alcohol directly to the open ulcer. Do not get this paste on surrounding unulcerated tissue. Apply 2-3 times per day. Do not use if there are no ulcerated lesions. It is also possible to apply *Si Huang Powder* (Four Yellows Powder) to the affected area once the blisters have broken. This is made from a mixture of powdered equal portions of Rhizoma Coptidis Chinensis (*Huang Lian*), Radix Scutellariae Baicalensis (*Huang Qin*), Cortex Phellodendri (*Huang Bai*), and Radix Et Rhizoma Rhei (*Da Huang*).

3. At the first sign of recurrent episodes, take 15 grams or more of Radix Astragali Membranacei (*Huang Qi*) and 3-6 grams of powdered garlic and vitamin C per day and apply Tea Tree Oil to the area where sores typically recur. In addition, one should immediately change to a clear, bland diet and get plenty of rest. Since pain is a symptom of lack of free flow and herpetic neuralgia typically responds to blood-quickening medicinals, one can also take *Ge Xia Zhu Yu Tang* (Below the Diaphragm Dispel Stasis Decoction), *Shen Tong Zhu Yu Tang* (Body Pain Dispel Stasis Decoction), or other such blood-quickening, stasis-dispelling formulas in ready-made pill form to help abort incipient outbreaks characterized by herpetic neuralgia. From a Western pharmacodynamic point of view, blood-quickening Chinese medicinals

disperse inflammation and can regulate the immune system. With this or similar measures, it is possible to abort herpes outbreaks which are preceded by prodromal symptomology.

4. Most recurrent episodes of herpes genitalia tend to involve prominent spleen vacuity. Therefore, although most Chinese textbooks recommend *Long Dan Xie Gan Tang* as the guiding formula for acute occurrences of genital sores, this formula, at least unmodified, is often too attacking and draining, especially for Western patients. Rather than speeding healing, because this formula may damage and drain the righteous qi, its inappropriate, prolonged, or excessive use may actually prolong attacks. *Gan Cao Xie Xin Tang (Licorice Drain the Heart Decoction), Ban Xia Xie Xin Tang* (Pinellia Drain the Heart Decoction), or *Xiao Chai Hu Tang* (Minor Bupleurum Decoction) which drain and supplement at the same time are better choices as the guiding formula in many cases. These are then modified with additions and subtractions as necessary.

5. The overwhelming majority of genital herpes patients suffer from concomitant liver depression. Therefore, most patients require some liver-coursing, qi-rectifying medicinals in their formula. If there is no yin vacuity, this may be Radix Bupleuri (*Chai Hu*). If there is yin vacuity, this may be Fructus Meliae Toosendan (*Chuan Lian Zi*).

6. For marked pain, one can add nine grams each of Resina Olibani (*Ru Xiang*) and Resina Myrrhae (*Mo Yao*) and/or 15-18 grams of Rhizoma Corydalis Yanhusuo (*Yan Hu Suo*).

7. Although it may sound counterintuitive, another Chinese treatment for herpes genitalia is to indirectly moxa the sores with a moxa pole. This is done by straddling a lit moxa pole. Practitioners should remember that moxa can treat both hot and cold conditions, is indicated for all damp conditions, including damp heat, and does kill worms and resolve toxins.

8. The herpes virus is extremely contagious. Therefore one should take care not to touch any suspected herpes lesion even if such a lesion does not appear on the genitals. For instance, it is possible to have "genital" herpes outbreaks on the hips and buttocks. To help prevent the spread of genital herpes, persons who have the illness should abstain from sexual activity when they have symptoms of a herpes recurrence. They should also tell all sex partners about their herpes infection and use condoms during sexual activity. Unfortunately, the herpes virus can be transmitted via shedding even in the absence of visible lesions. Nevertheless, it is possible to not transmit this infection to long-term sexual partners if proper care and caution are taken.

9. Herpes infection has been suspected as a cofactor in certain urogenital cancers, such as cervical cancer. However, no absolute causal connection has been confirmed. Patients with genital herpes often have one or more other STDs, such as human papilloma virus (HPV) infection. In addition, HSV-2 infection may make it easier to catch HIV infection if one is exposed. Conversely, HSV-2 infection also makes it easier to transmit HIV infection to others in high-risk situations by those so infected.

ENDNOTES

1 "Herpes Statistics,"
www.herpes-coldsores-treatment pictures.com/hsv/herpes_statistics.htm

2 "GenitalHerpes,"
www.discoveryhealth.com/DH/ihtIH/WSDSC000/20726/10137.html

31

HERPES ZOSTER

Herpes zoster refers to infection by the varicella-zoster virus primarily involving the dorsal root ganglia and characterized by vesicular eruption and neuralgic pain in the dermatome of the affected root ganglia. Also called shingles, zona, and acute posterior ganglionitis, this condition tends to occur in immunosuppressed patients, such as the elderly, those with cancer, and those with HIV. Its signs and symptoms include prodromal pain along the site of the future eruption which typically precedes the appearance of lesions by 2-3 days. Characteristic groups of vesicles on an erythmatous base then appear following the cutaneous distribution of one or more adjacent dermatomes. The involved zone is usually hypersensitive and the pain may be severe. Eruptions occur most often in the thoracic and lumbar regions and are unilateral. Lesions continue to form for 3-5 days. Fewer than 4% of patients with herpes zoster experience recurrence, and most patients recover spontaneously. However, postherpetic neuralgia persisting for months or years is common in the elderly. This pain may be either sharp and intermittent or constant and debilitating.

The Western medical diagnosis of herpes zoster primarily depends on the visual recognition of the characteristic skin vesicles after they have erupted. The herpes zoster virus can be differentiated from herpes simplex virus serologically and by culture. Western medical treatment consists of wet compresses and analgesics for symptomatic pain relief. Acyclovir, valacyclovir, and famciclovir are all prescribed orally for the treatment of herpes zoster in immunosuppressed patients with the intention of speeding healing and decreasing postherpetic neuralgia.

CHINESE DISEASE CATEGORIZATION: Herpes zoster is referred to as *she chuan chuang*, snake string sores, *huo dai chuang*, fire belt sores, *zhi zhu chuang*, spider sores, *she ke chuang*, snake burrow sores, and *chan yao huo dan*, lumbus-binding fire cinnabar.

DISEASE CAUSES: External contraction of evil toxins, internal damage by the seven affects, unregulated eating and drinking, taxation fatigue, enduring disease, and aging

DISEASE MECHANISMS: Due to righteous qi vacuity, evil toxins may invade the body from outside or mental-emotional stress and frustration may damage the liver and gallbladder internally causing the engenderment of depressive heat. In addition, spleen dampness due to vacuity and over-eating sweet, fatty, spicy, hot, thick-flavored foods may smolder internally. If evil toxins, depressive fire, and/or damp heat struggle and bind, they may steam the skin, causing the engenderment of vesicles, and obstruct the channels and network vessels, causing pain. If evil qi or dampness and heat collect and endure, thus obstructing the qi and blood, qi stagnation and blood stasis must inevitably also be engendered.

TREATMENT BASED ON PATTERN DISCRIMINATION:

1. LIVER-GALLBLADDER DEPRESSIVE FIRE PATTERN

MAIN SYMPTOMS: Taut, red-colored skin vesicles which are like spots and dots of millet gathered into patches, burning heat, lancinating, pricking pain, a bitter taste in the mouth, dry throat, thirst with a predilection for chilled drinks, easy anger, vexation and agitation, dry stools or constipation, a red tongue with yellow fur, and a bowstring, rapid pulse

TREATMENT PRINCIPLES: Clear the liver and drain fire, quicken the blood and transform toxins

RX: *Long Dan Xie Gan Tang Jia Jian* (Gentiana Drain the Liver Decoction with Additions & Subtractions)

INGREDIENTS: Folium Daqingye (*Da Qing Ye*) and

uncooked Radix Rehmanniae (*Sheng Di*), 15g each, Radix Gentianae Scabrae (*Long Dan Cao*), Radix Scutellariae Baicalensis (*Huang Qin*), Cortex Radicis Moutan (*Dan Pi*), Radix Rubrus Paeoniae Lactiflorae (*Chi Shao*), Radix Lithopsermi Seu Arnebiae (*Zi Cao*), Flos Chrysanthemi Morifolii (*Ju Hua*), Flos Lonicerae Japonicae (*Yin Hua*), and Semen Pruni Persicae (*Tao Ren*), 9g each, and Rhizoma Coptidis Chinensis (*Huang Lian*), 3g

Analysis of formula: *Long Dan Cao, Huang Qin, Dan Pi, Chi Shao, Ju Hua,* and *Huang Lian* all clear the liver and drain fire. *Da Qing Ye, Huang Qin, Zi Cao, Jin Yin Hua,* and *Huang Lian* clear heat and resolve toxins. *Sheng Di, Dan Pi, Chi Shao,* and *Zi Cao* cool the blood, and *Tao Ren, Chi Shao,* and *Dan Pi* quicken the blood and stop pain.

Additions & subtractions: If there is concomitant constipation, add 6-9 grams of Radix Et Rhizoma Rhei (*Da Huang*). If there is a dry throat, add 15 grams of Radix Scrophulariae Ningpoensis (*Xuan Shen*). If the eruptions occur on the face, add 12 grams of Concha Haliotidis (*Shi Jue Ming*) and nine grams of Flos Chrysanthemi Morifolii (*Ju Hua*) or nine grams each of *Ju Hua* and Fructus Arctii Lappae (*Niu Bang Zi*). If dampness is exuberant, add nine grams each of Rhizoma Atractylodis (*Cang Zhu*) and Rhizoma Alismatis (*Ze Xie*). If the lesions are on the lower extremities, add nine grams each of Radix Achyranthis Bidentatae (*Niu Xi*) and Cortex Phellodendri (*Huang Bai*). If the lesions are on the chest or lower abdomen, add 12 grams of Radix Sophorae Flavescentis (*Ku Shen*). If there is aching and pain, add 12 grams of Rhizoma Corydalis Yanhusuo (*Yan Hu Suo*) and nine grams each of Resina Myrrhae (*Mo Yao*) and Resina Olibani (*Ru Xiang*). If there is itching, add nine grams of Bombyx Batryticatus (*Jiang Can*). If there is marked spleen vacuity with fatigue, add 15 grams of Radix Astragali Membranacei (*Huang Qi*) and nine grams of Radix Codonopsitis Pilosulae (*Dang Shen*).

Acupuncture & moxibustion: *Wai Guan* (TB 5), *Zu Lin Qi* (GB 41), *Ling Tai* (GV 10), *Xing Jian* (Liv 2)

Analysis of formula: *Wai Guan* and *Zu Lin Qi* are the paired meeting points of two of the eight extraordinary vessels which treat general disorders in the eyes, ears, face, cheeks, neck, or shoulders. Here, when needled with draining method, they are an empirical combination to clear the liver-gallbladder and drain fire, quicken the blood and resolve toxins to treat herpes zoster. Draining *Ling Tai* cools the blood and resolves toxins, especially in the skin division or aspect. *Xing Jian* clears and drains the liver.

Additions & subtractions: For herpes zoster located in the area of the eyes, add *Si Zhu Kong* (TB 23), *Zan Zhu* (Bl 2), and, eventually, *Tai Yang* (M-HN-9). For herpes zoster located on the face, add *He Gu* (LI 4). For herpes zoster located on the cheek area, add *Di Cang* (St 4) and *Jia Che* (St 6). For herpes zoster located in the temporal area, add *Tai Yang* (M-HN-9). For herpes zoster located on the upper part of the body, add *Qu Chi* (LI 11). For herpes zoster located on the lower part of the body, add *Yang Ling Quan* (GB 34). For blood heat, also bleed *Wei Zhong* (Bl 40) and then add *San Yin Jiao* (Sp 6) and *Ge Shu* (Bl 17). If severe pain and a burning sensation, bleed *Yin Bai* (Sp 1) and *Da Dun* (Liv 1). Then needle the head and tail of the eruption, *i.e.*, 2cm beyond the two ends of the lesion. Needle in direction of the line of eruptions. For a bitter taste in the mouth, irritability, and easy anger, add *Yang Ling Quan* (GB 34). For restlessness and insomnia due to pain, add *Shen Men* (Ht 7), *Bai Hui* (GV 20), and *Shen Ting* (GV 24). If there is itching, add *Xue Hai* (Sp 10) and *Qu Chi* (LI 11). For severe internal heat, add *Nei Ting* (St 44). For damp sores, add *Yin Ling Quan* (Sp 9).

2. Spleen dampness internally smoldering pattern

Main symptoms: Large, yellowish white skin vesicles filled with turbid fluid which easily break and seep, severe aching and pain after vesicular rupture, torpid intake, abdominal distention, loose stools, a fat, enlarged tongue with slimy, white or yellow fur, and a soggy or slippery, rapid pulse

Note: This pattern is also called spleen channel damp heat.

Treatment principles: Clear and disinhibit dampness and heat, quicken the blood and transform toxins

Rx: *Si Miao San Jia Wei* (Four Wonders Powder with Added Flavors)

Ingredients: Radix Isatidis Seu Baphicacanthi (*Ban Lan Gen*), uncooked Semen Coicis Lachryma-jobi (*Yi Yi Ren*), Rhizoma Smilacis Glabrae (*Tu Fu Ling*), and Herba Leonuri Heterophylli (*Yi Mu Cao*), 30g each, and Rhizoma Atractylodis (*Cang Zhu*), Rhizoma Atractylodis Macrocephalae (*Bai Zhu*), Cortex Phellodendri (*Huang Bai*), Radix Achyranthis Bidentatae (*Niu Xi*), *Liu Yi San* (Six to One Powder, *i.e.*, Talcum, *Hua Shi*, and Radix Glycyrrhizae, *Gan Cao*), Rhizoma Dioscoreae Hypoglaucae (*Bei Xie*), Cortex Radicis Moutan (*Dan Pi*), and Radix Lithospermi Seu Arnebiae (*Zi Cao*), 9g each

Analysis of formula: *Yi Yi Ren, Tu Fu Ling, Cang Zhu, Bai Zhu, Huang Bai, Bei Xie,* and *Liu Yi San* together clear and disinhibit dampness and heat. *Zi Cao, Dan Pi, Niu Xi,* and *Yi Mu Cao* together cool and quicken the blood. *Tu Fu Ling, Zi Cao, Ban Lan Gen,* and *Huang Bai* clear heat and resolve toxins.

ADDITIONS & SUBTRACTIONS: If there is marked spleen vacuity with fatigue, add 15 grams of Radix Astragali Membranacei (*Huang Qi*) and nine grams of Radix Codonopsitis Pilosulae (*Dang Shen*). For poor appetite, add nine grams each of Massa Medica Fermentata (*Shen Qu*) and Fructus Germinatus Hordei Vulgaris (*Mai Ya*). For abdominal distention and diarrhea, add nine grams each of Pericarpium Arecae Catechu (*Da Fu Pi*), Fructus Citri Aurantii (*Zhi Ke*), and Radix Auklandiae Lappae (*Mu Xiang*). For marked accumulation of dampness, add nine grams each of Herba Agastachis Seu Pogostemi (*Huo Xiang*), Pericarpium Arecae Catechu (*Da Fu Pi*), and Semen Plantaginis (*Che Qian Zi*). For marked heat, add 15 grams of Flos Lonicerae Japonicae (*Jin Yin Hua*) and nine grams of Fructus Gardeniae Jasminoidis (*Zhi Zi*).

ACUPUNCTURE & MOXIBUSTION: *Zu San Li* (St 36), *Yin Ling Quan* (Sp 9), *San Yin Jiao* (Sp 6), *He Gu* (LI 4), *Qu Chi* (LI 11)

ANALYSIS OF FORMULA: Draining *Zu San Li* and *Yin Ling Quan* disinhibits dampness, while draining *He Gu* and *Qu Chi* clears heat from the spleen and stomach. Draining *San Yin Jiao* cools and quickens the blood.

ADDITIONS & SUBTRACTIONS: Please see pattern #1 above.

3. QI STAGNATION & BLOOD STASIS PATTERN

MAIN SYMPTOMS: The base of the skin vesicles are dark and purple. The fluid contains bloody water. Aching and pain is severe and difficult to bear. The tongue is purple and dark or has static macules or spots. The pulse is bowstring and/or choppy.

NOTE: When this pattern describes postherpetic neuralgia, there may not be any remaining skin lesions or there may only be dark, purplish scars but no vesicles. In this case, the severe, fixed, lancinating pain may be the main or even the sole symptoms of blood stasis.

TREATMENT PRINCIPLES: Quicken the blood and transform toxins, move the qi and stop pain

RX: *She Chuan Fang* (Snake String Formula)

INGREDIENTS: Rhizoma Smilacis Glabrae (*Tu Fu Ling*), Semen Coicis Lachryma-jobi (*Yi Yi Ren*), and Herba Portulacae Oleraceae (*Ma Chi Xian*), 30g each, uncooked Radix Rehmanniae (*Sheng Di*) and Radix Salviae Miltiorrhizae (*Dan Shen*), 15g each, Lumbricus (*Di Long*), Radix Rubrus Paeoniae Lactiflorae (*Chi Shao*), Cortex Radicis Moutan (*Dan Pi*), and uncooked Pollen Typhae (*Pu Huang*), 9g each, and Hirudo (*Shui Zhi*), 3g

ANALYSIS OF FORMULA: *Dan Shen, Chi Shao, Dan Pi, Pu Huang,* and *Shui Zhi* quicken the blood, transform stasis, and stop pain. In addition, *Sheng Di, Dan Shen, Chi Shao,* and *Dan Pi* cool the blood. *Tu Fu Ling, Yi Yi Ren,* and *Ma Chi Xian* clear and disinhibit any lingering damp heat. *Tu Fu Ling* and *Ma Chi Xian* also clear heat and resolve toxins. *Di Long* clears heat, frees the flow of the network vessels, and stops pain.

ADDITIONS & SUBTRACTIONS: If there are no signs of remaining dampness and heat, delete *Tu Fu Ling, Yi Yi Ren,* and *Ma Chi Xian* and add 15 grams of Rhizoma Corydalis Yanhusuo (*Yan Hu Suo*) and nine grams each of Fructus Meliae Toosendan (*Chuan Lian Zi*), Radix Bupleuri (*Chai Hu*), and Tuber Curcumae (*Yu Jin*). If postherpetic neuralgia is severe, add 30 grams each of Concha Margaritiferae (*Zhen Zhu Mu*), Concha Ostreae (*Mu Li*), Dens Draconis (*Long Chi*), and Magnetitum (*Ci Shi*). If there is concomitant qi and blood vacuity, add 15 grams of Radix Astragali Membranacei (*Huang Qi*) and nine grams each of Radix Codonopsitis Pilosulae (*Dang Shen*) and Radix Angelicae Sinensis (*Dang Gui*).

ACUPUNCTURE & MOXIBUSTION: *San Yin Jiao* (Sp 6), *He Gu* (LI 4), *Zhi Gou* (TB 6), *Jian Shi* (Per 5), and one of the local treatments described under remark #5 below.

ANALYSIS OF FORMULA: *San Yin Jiao* and *He Gu* are a traditional combination to move the qi, quicken the blood, and stop pain. *Zhi Gou* and *Jian Shi* are also a traditional combination to move the qi and quicken the blood in the whole body in order to stop pain. Both sets of points are needled with draining method. Locally, use one of the methods described in remark #5 to quicken the blood, transform stasis, and stop pain.

ADDITIONS & SUBTRACTIONS: Please see pattern #1 above.

REMARKS

1. Most cases of herpes zoster in Western patients include spleen vacuity with damp heat and liver depression if not liver-gallbladder fire. In addition, most cases of herpes zoster also involve blood stasis. In elderly or seriously ill patients, there may also be qi and blood or yin and/or yang vacuity as well. If there is concomitant yin vacuity, add the Chinese ready-made medicines *Liu Wei Di Huang Wan* (Six Flavors Rehmannia Pills) or *Zhi Bai Di Huang Wan* (Anemarrhena & Phellodendron Rehmannia Pills). If there is yin and yang vacuity, add *Er Xian Wan* (Two Immortals Pills).

Da Yan Tang (Great Corydalis Decoction) is a modern Chinese formula for the acute stage of herpes zoster with a multipattern presentation. This formula clears and courses the liver, clears heat and resolves toxins, moves the qi and quickens the blood, disinhibits dampness and boosts the qi.

It is composed of: Rhizoma Corydalis Yanhusuo (*Yan Hu Suo*), Radix Istadis Seu Baphicacanthi (*Ban Lan Gen*), and Radix Astragali Membranacei (*Huang Qi*), 15g each, Folium Daqingye (*Da Qing Ye*), Flos Lonicerae Japonicae (*Jin Yin Hua*), Radix Codonopsitis Pilosulae (*Dang Shen*), Radix Lithospermi Seu Arnebiae (*Zi Cao*), and Radix Salviae Miltiorrhizae (*Dan Shen*), 12g each, Radix Scutellariae Baicalensis (*Huang Qin*), Radix Angelicae Dahuricae (*Bai Zhi*), and Cortex Radicis Dictamni Dasycarpi (*Bai Xian Pi*), 9g each, and Radix Stephaniae Tetrandrae (*Han Fang Ji*), Radix Bupleuri (*Chai Hu*), and Radix Glycyrrhizae (*Gan Cao*), 6g each.

2. According to some Chinese doctors' point of view, if the affected area is in the upper part of the body, *i.e.*, the head, face, or neck, herpes zoster is due to the heart and liver. If the affected area is in the middle part of the body, *i.e.*, the back, chest, abdomen, or rib-side, it is due to the spleen and liver. If the affected area is in the lower part of the body, *i.e.*, on the lower abdomen or lower limbs, it is due to the kidneys and liver.

3. If there is toxic, depressive, and/or damp heat, eating spicy, hot, greasy, fatty, or thick-flavored foods is prohibited as is drinking alcohol. If there is spleen vacuity, eating sugar and sweets as well as sodden wheat foods (*i.e.*, pasta and breads) is prohibited.

4. Before the lesions have ruptured, apply externally *Lu Hui Bing Zhu Wai Fu Ji* (Aloe, Borneol & Pearl External Application Prescription): one fresh Aloe leaf (*Lu Hui*) a few inches long, 0.3-1g of Borneolum (*Bing Pian*), and a pinch of powdered Margarita (*Zhen Zhu*). Mash these ingredients together and apply as a paste. Or use *Yu Lu Gao* (Jade Dew Ointment). This is made from Folium Seu Flos Hibisici Mutabilis (*Fu Rong Ye* or *Fu Rong Hua*) in an ointment base. *Fu Rong Ye* does have specific antiherpetic properties when applied externally.

After the lesions have ruptured, apply a small amount of *Er Wei Bai Du San* (Two Flavors Vanquish Toxins Powder), *i.e.*, equal parts Realgar (*Xiong Huang*) and Alumen (*Bai Fan*) mixed with water, directly to the open sores 1-2 times per day. Do not apply to the surrounding tissue and do not use this external application if there are no wet, open, glistening or weeping lesions.

For erosive lesions after rupture, decoct 30 grams each of Radix Sanguisorbae (*Di Yu*) and Herba Portulacae Oleraceae (*Ma Chi Xian*) and apply as a wet compress. After erosive surfaces have dried and scabs have formed, apply *Jin Huang Gao* (Golden Yellow Paste): Radix Trichosanthis Kirlowii (*Tian Hua Fen*), 200g, Radix Et Rhizoma Rhei (*Da Huang*), Cortex Phellodendri (*Huang Bai*), Rhizoma Curcumae Longae (*Jiang Huang*), and Radix Angelicae Dahuricae (*Bai Zhi*), 100g each, and Rhizoma Atractylodis (*Cang Zhu*), Cortex Magnoliae Officinalis (*Hou Po*), and Radix Glycyrrhizae (*Gan Cao*), 40g each. Grind all these ingredients into powder and mix with water and/or honey to form a paste.

After scabs have sloughed, apply *Xiao Feng Gao* (Disperse Wind Paste): Scolopendra Subspinipes (*Wu Gong*), 9 strips, Borneol (*Bing Pian*), 20g, petrolatum, 1000g. Fry the *Wu Gong* in the petrolatum till scorched, remove the dregs, and mix in the *Bing Pian* to form a paste.

5. Most cases of herpes zoster are self-limiting. However, Chinese medicinals and/or acupuncture can help relieve the symptoms and lessen the incidence and severity of postherpetic neuralgia.The following methods are several options for treating postherpetic neuralgia:

A. Warm the affected area with a moxa roll.
B. Encircle the painful line with 6-8 needles, including points 2cm beyond the head and tail of this line.
C. Use electroacupuncture on points 2cm beyond the head and tail of the line where the lesions had occurred.
D. Cotton moxibustion: Use as thin and light a layer of cotton wool as possible. However, this layer should be without holes. Light the cotton wool with a match or lighter. The patient may feel a slight burning sensation but this should not be a scald burn. Do this one time per day, with four treatments maximum equaling one course.

6. Radix Istadis Seu Baphicacanthi (*Ban Lan Gen*), Folium Daqingye (*Da Qing Ye*), Pulvis Indigonis (*Qing Dai*), three medicinals from the same plant, are often prescribed because they have an antiviral action and are known to be empirically effective for treating herpes zoster. Other medicinals often seen in modern Chinese medicinal formulas for herpes zoster are: Radix Lithospermi Seu Arnebiae (*Zi Cao*), Fructus Forsythiae Suspensae (*Lian Qiao*), Radix Et Rhizoma Polygoni Cuspidati (*Hu Zhang*), Herba Portulacae Oleraceae (*Ma Chi Xian*), Flos Lonicerae Japonicae (*Jin Yin Hua*), Radix Scutellariae Baicalensis (*Huang Qin*), and Rhizoma Corydalis Yanhusuo (*Yan Hu Suo*) for pain.

7. For herpes zoster after emotional stress such as anger, frustration, or humiliation causing depressive heat which then brews toxins, one can also use the following formula: *Jie Du Zhi Tong Tang* (Resolve Toxins & Stop Pain Decoction): Radix Istadis Seu Baphicacanthi (*Ban Lan Gen*) and Rhizoma Corydalis Yanhusuo (*Yan Hu Suo*), 25g each, Fructus Forsythiae Suspensae (*Lian Qiao*) and Bombyx Batryticatus (*Jiang Can*), 20g each, Radix Bupleuri (*Chai Hu*), Rhizoma Cyperi Rotundi (*Xiang Fu*), Fructus Meliae Toosendan (*Chuan Lian Zi*), Herba Menthae Haplocalysis (*Bo He*), Pericarpium Citri Reticulatae (*Chen Pi*), and mix-fried Radix Glycyrrhizae (*Zhi Gan Cao*), 15g each, and Radix Scutellariae Baicalensis (*Huang Qin*), 9g.

32

Hyperlipoproteinemia

Hyperlipoproteinema is the Western medical disease diagnosis of what most people refer more simply to as high cholesterol. This refers to abnormally elevated levels of lipids and their associated proteins in the blood. This may be due to genetic predisposition, endocrinopathy, specific organ failure, or external causes, such as excessive dietary intake of sugar and cholesterol. Because the incidence of coronary heart disease rises in a linear fashion with the level of serum cholesterol, this condition is seen as a precursor to coronary heart disease via atherosclerosis. The most common form of this condition found in adult American middle-aged males is type IV hyperlipoproteinemia, also known as endogenous hypertriglyceridemia or hyperprebetalipoproteinemia. This condition often runs in families and is characterized by variable elevations of serum triglycerides. It is also often frequently associated with mildly abnormal glucose tolerance curves showing a disturbance in carbohydrate metabolism and obesity. The serum is turbid and triglyceride levels are disproportionately elevated. Cholesterol may be only slightly increased secondary to stress, alcoholism, and dietary indiscretion.

The Western medical diagnosis of this condition is based on analysis of blood lipids and proteins. The optimum serum cholesterol for a middle-aged American man is probably 200mg/dL or less. The Western medical treatment of type IV hyperlipoproteinemia involves weight loss, dietary restriction of carbohydrates and alcohol, and internal administration of either niacin or gemfibrozil if blood lipids are not controllable by diet alone.

Chinese disease categorization: Because this condition as defined by Western medicine may be asymptomatic, it does not always correspond to a traditional Chinese disease category. Obesity is referred to as *fei pang*, fatty fatness. When this condition is associated with heart disease resulting in chest pain or pressure, it is referred to as *xiong bi*, chest impediment. When it is associated with hypertension, it is referred to as *tou tong*, headache, and/or *xuan yin*, dizziness.

Disease causes: Former heaven natural endowment with habitual bodily exuberance or insufficiency, undisciplined eating and drinking, internal damage by the seven affects, and aging

Disease mechanisms: Due to former heaven natural endowment, people may be either habitually bodily exuberant or vacuous and insufficient. As the *Ling Shu (Spiritual Axis)* states: "[Due to] the unfavorable and favorable [aspects of] the five body [types], it is said that people's bone joints may be large or small, their flesh may be firm or fragile, their skin may be thick or thin, their blood may be clear or turbid, or their qi may be slippery or choppy . . ." Therefore, some people have a predisposition to yang exuberance and phlegm dampness, while others are predisposed to yin vacuity. In addition, each person's viscera and bowels have an innate tendency towards vacuity or repletion. On top of such habitual bodily predispositions, over-eating fatty, sweet, thick-flavored foods may damage the spleen and stomach, which then lose their control over movement and transformation. This results in internal engenderment of phlegm dampness. Phlegm and dampness are yin depressions which may hinder and obstruct the free flow of qi, blood, and body fluids as well as confound and block the orifices of the heart and the upper clear orifices. If phlegm and dampness block the free flow of qi, blood, or body fluids, there may be distention and pain, swelling and edema, and/or malnourishment of the tissues and organs. In addition, it may also give rise to transformative heat which may cause yang to become hyperactive and may damage and consume yin. Other factors which may damage the spleen and lead to the engenderment of phlegm and dampness are too little exercise and too much thinking and worry.

On the other hand, unfulfilled desires or anger may damage the liver and cause it to lose its control over coursing and discharge. This may cause qi stagnation which may lead to blood stasis. It may cause transformative heat with its attendant yang hyperactivity and/or yin vacuity. And it may cause or aggravate damp accumulation and phlegm obstruction, since it is the qi which is responsible for moving and transforming both of these. In addition, liver repletion usually results in spleen vacuity since wood typically counterflows horizontally to invade the spleen when it becomes depressed. Unfortunately, the sweet flavor relaxes the liver. Therefore, people who are under emotional stress try to alleviate their liver depression by eating sweets. Sweet is the flavor which enters the spleen. In small amounts, it supplements the spleen, but in large amounts, it damages the spleen. Therefore, a liver-spleen disharmony is often the underlying imbalance predisposing one to this condition.

In addition, aging plays a role in the disease mechanisms of this disorder. Yin is half consumed by 40 and yang qi tends to become debilitated not very long after. Yin vacuity may fail to nourish and moisten the liver. Thus it tends to become even more depressed. Yang vacuity may fail to warm and steam the liver, thus also leading to liver depression. Spleen-kidney yang vacuity may also fail to warm and steam (*i.e.*, evaporate) body fluids. Hence yang vacuity commonly accelerates or aggravates a tendency towards phlegm damp accumulation. This is why many people become obese with age.

TREATMENT BASED ON PATTERN DISCRIMINATION:

1. LIVER DEPRESSION-SPLEEN VACUITY PATTERN

MAIN SYMPTOMS: Episodic bilateral rib-side pain which is not fixed in location, headache, dizziness, lassitude of the spirit, scanty food intake, emotional lability, a tendency to great sighing, loose stools, menstrual irregularities in females, breast distention and pain, a fat tongue with thin, white, slimy tongue fur, and a fine, bowstring pulse

TREATMENT PRINCIPLES: Course the liver and resolve depression, fortify the spleen and nourish the blood, lower fat

RX: *Xiao Yao San Jia Wei* (Rambling Powder with Added Flavors)

INGREDIENTS: Radix Bupleuri (*Chai Hu*), Radix Angelicae Sinensis (*Dang Gui*), Radix Albus Paeoniae Lactiflorae (*Bai Shao*), Sclerotium Poriae Cocos (*Fu Ling*), Rhizoma Atractylodis Macrocephalae (*Bai Zhu*), Fructus Trichosanthis Kirlowii (*Gua Lou*), and Fructus Crataegi (*Shan Zha*), 9g each, mix-fried Radix Glycyrrhizae (*Gan Cao*) and Herba Menthae Haplocalycis (*Bo He*), 6g each, and uncooked Rhizoma Zingiberis (*Sheng Jiang*), 2 slices

ANALYSIS OF FORMULA: *Chai Hu* and *Bo He* work on the yang aspect of the liver. They course the liver and resolve depression. *Bai Shao* and *Dang Gui* work on the yin aspect of the liver. They nourish liver blood. The liver can only perform its functions of coursing and discharging if it obtains sufficient blood to nourish it. This is because blood is the mother of qi. Together, these four medicinals harmonize the yin and yang aspects of the liver and resolve depression. *Bai Zhu, Fu Ling, Sheng Jiang,* and mix-fried *Gan Cao* fortify the spleen and boost the qi. According to the *Nei Jing (Inner Classic)*, when the liver is diseased, first treat the spleen. Although the liver controls the spleen, a strong spleen helps to keep the liver in check by preventing horizontal counterflow and wood assailing earth. In addition, because the spleen is the latter heaven root of qi and blood engenderment and transformation, supplementing the spleen helps to engender blood which can then nourish and emolliate the liver. *Gua Lou* disperses phlegm and loosens the chest, thus phlegm accumulation in the heart vessels of the chest. *Shan Zha* quickens the blood and lowers fat. It is empirically known to lower serum cholesterol.

ADDITIONS & SUBTRACTIONS: If there is damp accumulation, add nine grams each of Rhizoma Alismatis (*Ze Xie*) and Rhizoma Atractylodis (*Cang Zhu*). If there is severe liver depression, add 12 grams of Tuber Curcumae (*Yu Jin*). If liver depression transforms into fire, add nine grams each of Cortex Radicis Moutan (*Dan Pi*) and Fructus Gardeniae Jasminoidis (*Zhi Zi*). If there is a severe qi vacuity, add nine grams each of Rhizoma Polygonati (*Huang Jing*) and Ganoderma Lucidum (*Ling Zhi*), and six grams of Radix Panacis Ginseng (*Ren Shen*). For severe blood vacuity, add 15 grams of Radix Polygoni Multiflori (*He Shou Wu*). For blood stasis due to liver depression, add nine grams of Radix Salviae Miltiorrhizae (*Dan Shen*), and three grams of Radix Pseudoginseng (*San Qi*), powdered and taken with the strained decoction.

ACUPUNCTURE & MOXIBUSTION: *Zu San Li* (St 36), *Nei Guan* (Per 6), *Feng Long* (St 40), *Tai Chong* (Liv 3)

ANALYSIS OF FORMULA: Draining *Tai Chong* and *Nei Guan* courses the liver and resolves depression. Supplementing *Zu San Li* fortifies the spleen and boosts the qi, thus promoting the engenderment and transformation of blood. Draining *Feng Long* harmonizes the stomach and disinhibits dampness.

ADDITIONS & SUBTRACTIONS: If there is damp accumulation, add *Yin Ling Quan* (Sp 9). If there is severe liver depression, add *Gan Shu* (Bl 18) and *Zhang Men* (Liv 13). If liver depression transforms into fire, add *Xing Jian* (Liv 2). If there is a severe qi vacuity, add *Tai Bai* (Sp 3) and *Pi Shu* (Bl 20). For severe blood vacuity, add *Xin Shu* (Bl 15), *Ge Shu* (Bl 17), and *Gan Shu* (Bl 18). For blood stasis due to liver depression, add *San Yin Jiao* (Sp 6).

2. DAMPNESS & HEAT BREWING INTERNALLY

MAIN SYMPTOMS: Dizziness, headache, heavy-headedness, vexatious heat, chest oppression, stomach duct fullness, nausea, bodily fatigue, encumbered limbs, a bitter taste in the mouth and a dry throat, bodily obesity, possible constipation, yellow urine, a reddish tongue with slimy, yellow fur, and a slippery, rapid pulse

TREATMENT PRINCIPLES: Clear and disinhibit dampness and heat, lower fat

RX: *Jue Ming Xie Gan Jiang Zhi Tang* (Cassia Tora Drain the Liver & Lower Fat Decoction)

INGREDIENTS: Semen Cassiae Torae (*Jue Ming Zi*), 30g, Fructus Crataegi (*Shan Zha*), 18g, Rhizoma Alismatis (*Ze Xie*), Rhizoma Sclerotium Poriae Cocos (*Fu Ling*), and Herba Artemisiae Capillaris (*Yin Chen Hao*), 15g each, Semen Plantaginis (*Che Qian Zi*), 12g, Radix Bupleuri (*Chai Hu*), 9g, and wine-fried Radix Et Rhizoma Rhei (*Da Huang*), 3g

ANALYSIS OF FORMULA: *Ze Xie, Fu Ling, Yin Chen Hao, Che Qian Zi,* and *Da Huang* clear heat and disinhibit dampness. In addition, *Ze Xie, Da Huang,* and *Yin Chen Hao* lower fat. *Jue Ming Zi* and *Chai Hu* clear the liver. *Jue Ming Zi* also disinhibits dampness and lowers fat. *Shan Zha* quickens the blood and lowers fat.

ADDITIONS & SUBTRACTIONS: If there is severe damp heat accumulation, add nine grams each of Radix Et Rhizoma Polygoni Cuspidati (*Hu Zhang*) and Tuber Curcumae (*Yu Jin*). If there is yin damage due to damp heat, add nine grams of Rhizoma Polygonati Odorati (*Yu Zhu*). If there is concomitant liver depression, add 12 grams of Tuber Curcumae (*Yu Jin*). If there is concomitant qi vacuity, add 12 grams of Fructificatio Ganodermae Lucidi (*Ling Zhi*) and 6 grams of Radix Panacis Ginseng (*Ren Shen*). If there is concomitant blood vacuity, add 15 grams of Radix Polygoni Multiflori (*He Shou Wu*).

An alternative treatment is *Xiao Shi Tang* (Disperse Fat Decoction): Semen Cassiae Torae (*Jue Ming Zi*), Sclerotium Poriae Cocos (*Fu Ling*), Caulis Lonicerae Japonicae (*Ren Dong Teng*), and Semen Coicis Lachryma-jobi (*Yi Yi Ren*), 15g each, Folium Nelumbinis Nuciferae (*He Ye*) and Flos Chrysanthemi Morifolii (*Ju Hua*), 12g each, and Stylus Zeae Maydis (*Yu Mi Xu*), 9g.

ACUPUNCTURE & MOXIBUSTION: *Zu San Li* (St 36), *Nei Guan* (Per 6), *Yin Ling Quan* (Sp 9), *Nei Ting* (St 44)

ANALYSIS OF FORMULA: With draining method and in combination with *Nei Ting,* the spring point of the stomach channel, *Zu San Li* clears the yang ming and disinhibits damp heat. In addition, draining *Zu San Li* is empirically known to lower fat. Draining *Yin Ling Quan* rectifies the triple burner, *i.e.,* the water pathways of the whole body, and disinhibits damp heat, especially when combined with *Nei Ting,* a key point for internal heat. Draining *Nei Guan* moves the qi and lowers fat.

ADDITIONS & SUBTRACTIONS: For dizziness and headache, add *Feng Chi* (GB 20). If there is severe damp heat accumulation, add *Zhi Gou* (TB 6) and *Yang Ling Quan* (GB 34). If there is yin damage due to damp heat, add *Fu Liu* (Ki 7). For yin vacuity and effulgent fire, add *Ran Gu* (Ki 2). If there is nausea, poor appetite, or stomach venter fullness, add *Gong Sun* (Sp 4). If there is phlegm heat, add *Feng Long* (St 40) and *Zhong Wan* (CV 12). If there is concomitant liver depression, add *Tai Chong* (Liv 3). If there is concomitant qi vacuity, add *Tai Bai* (Sp 3) and *San Yin Jiao* (Sp 6) and supplement *Zu San Li.* If there is concomitant blood vacuity, add *Xin Shu* (Bl 15), *Ge Shu* (Bl 17), and *Gan Shu* (Bl 18).

3. PHLEGM & DAMPNESS INTERNALLY OBSTRUCTING PATTERN

MAIN SYMPTOMS: Obesity, an addiction to fatty, sweet foods, head dizziness, distention, and heaviness, chest and ductal glomus and oppression, nausea and a desire to vomit, a sticky feeling in the mouth and no thirst, fatigue and/or heaviness of the four limbs, numbness, abdominal distention, torpid intake, glossy, slimy tongue fur, and a bowstring, slippery pulse

TREATMENT PRINCIPLES: Fortify the spleen and transform phlegm, dispel dampness and lower fat

RX: *Er Chen Tang Jia Jian* (Two Aged [Ingredients] Decoction with Additions & Subtractions)

INGREDIENTS: Sclerotium Poriae Cocos (*Fu Ling*), Semen Coicis Lachryma-jobi (*Yi Yi Ren*), Fructus Trichosanthis Kirlowii (*Gua Lou*), and Rhizoma Alismatis (*Ze Xie*), 15g each, and Pericarpium Rhizoma Pinelliae Ternatae (*Ban Xia*), Citri Reticulatae (*Chen Pi*), Rhizoma Atractylodis (*Cang Zhu*), Rhizoma Atractylodis Macrocephalae (*Bai Zhu*), Semen Pruni Armeniacae (*Xing Ren*), Herba Saragassii (*Hai Zao*), and Cortex Magnoliae Officinalis (*Hou Po*), 9g each

ANALYSIS OF FORMULA: *Ban Xia, Chen Pi, Fu Ling, Hai Zao,* and *Ze Xie* together transform phlegm. *Xing Ren* and *Gua Lou* disperse phlegm, especially phlegm in the chest. In addition, *Gua Lou* treats chest impediment and prevents heart disease. *Chen Pi* and *Hou Po* move the qi to move the dampness and disperse the phlegm. *Fu Ling, Yi Yi Ren,* and *Ze Xie* disinhibit dampness, while *Bai Zhu, Cang Zhu,* and *Hou Po* dry dampness. Because the spleen is averse to dampness, all these medicinals fortify the spleen indirectly, while *Bai Zhu* supplements the spleen directly. *Ze Xie* and *Hai Zao* are empirically known to lower blood fat.

ADDITIONS & SUBTRACTIONS: If there is severe dizziness, add 12 grams each of Rhizoma Gastrodiae Elatae (*Tian Ma*) and Bombyx Batryticatus (*Jiang Can*). If there is concomitant liver depression, add 12 grams of Tuber Curcumae (*Yu Jin*). If there is severe qi vacuity, add 12 grams of Fructificatio Ganodermae Lucidi (*Ling Zhi*) and six grams of Radix Panacis Ginseng (*Ren Shen*). If there is concomitant blood vacuity, add nine grams each of Radix Polygoni Multiflori (*He Shou Wu*) and Radix Angelicae Sinensis (*Dang Gui*). For concomitant heart blood stasis or chest impediment with chest pain and heart palpitations, add 12 grams of Radix Salviae Miltiorrhizae (*Dan Shen*), nine grams of Bulbus Allii (*Xie Bai*), and three grams of Radix Pseudoginseng (*San Qi*), powdered and taken with the strained decoction.

ACUPUNCTURE & MOXIBUSTION: *Zu San Li* (St 36), *Nei Guan* (Per 6), *Feng Long* (St 40), *Yin Ling Quan* (Sp 9)

ANALYSIS OF FORMULA: Draining *Yin Ling Quan* rectifies the triple burner, *i.e.*, the water pathways of the entire body, and disinhibits dampness. It is a main point for the treatment of dampness. Draining *Feng Long* harmonizes the stomach and transforms phlegm. It is a main point for treating phlegm. Together, they are a main combination for treating phlegm dampness. Supplementing *Zu San Li* fortifies the spleen and boosts the qi, transforms dampness and prevents phlegm accumulation. The first two points treat the branch repletion, *i.e.*, the phlegm, the latter point treats the root vacuity, *i.e.*, the spleen. Draining *Nei Guan* moves the qi to disperse the phlegm. In addition, it treats chest impediment and prevents heart disease.

ADDITIONS & SUBTRACTIONS: If there is concomitant liver depression, add *Tai Chong* (Liv 3) and *Zhang Men* (Liv 13). If there is severe qi vacuity, add *Tai Bai* (Sp 3) and *Pi Shu* (Bl 20). If there is blood vacuity, add *Xin Shu* (Bl 15), *Ge Shu* (Bl 17), and *Gan Shu* (Bl 18). If there is blood stasis, add *San Yin Jiao* (Sp 6). If there is dizziness and headache, add *Feng Chi* (GB 20). If there is nausea, poor appetite, or stomach venter fullness, add *Gong Sun* (Sp 4) and, if necessary, *Zhong Wan* (CV 12).

4. PHLEGM HEAT BOWEL REPLETION PATTERN

MAIN SYMPTOMS: A strong, replete body or even obesity, constipation, chest oppression, abdominal distention, increased intake and rapid hungering, possible thirst, head dizziness, distention, and/or pounding pain, emotional rashness and impetuosity, a bitter taste in the mouth, heart vexation, a red face and eyes, anxiety and restlessness, a red tongue with slimy, yellow fur, and a bowstring, slippery, forceful, rapid pulse

NOTE: The name of this pattern is an abbreviation for phlegm accumulation and stomach heat bowel accumulation.

TREATMENT PRINCIPLES: Clear heat and transform phlegm, free the flow of the bowels and disperse accumulation

RX: *Da Cheng Qi Tang Jia Jian* (Major Order the Qi Decoction with Additions & Subtractions)

INGREDIENTS: Radix Scutellariae Baicalensis (*Huang Qin*), 15g, Cortex Magnoliae Officinalis (*Hou Po*), Fructus Immaturus Citri Aurantii (*Zhi Shi*), Rhizoma Picrorrhizae (*Hu Huang Lian*), Rhizoma Acori Graminei (*Shi Chang Pu*), Rhizoma Anemarrhenae Aspheloidis (*Zhi Mu*), and Fructus Crataegi (*Shan Zha*), 9g each, and Radix Et Rhizoma Rhei (*Da Huang*) and Radix Glycyrrhizae (*Gan Cao*), 6g each

ANALYSIS OF FORMULA: *Huang Qin* and *Hu Huang Lian* clear heat and eliminate dampness, while *Zhi Mu* drains fire and enriches yin, thus alleviating dryness and thirst. *Hou Po* moves the qi, transforms dampness, and disperses stagnation. *Zhi Shi* strongly rectifies the qi, especially of the lower burner intestines. Together, these two medicinals strongly rectify the intestinal qi and disperse distention and fullness. *Da Huang* both descends and precipitates yang ming accumulation and heat. *Shan Zha* disperses food and lowers fat, while *Shi Chang Pu* transforms phlegm. This latter ingredient also promotes the division of clear and turbid, and fat is often described as phlegm turbidity in Chinese medicine. *Gan Cao* harmonizes the other medicinals in this formula.

ADDITIONS & SUBTRACTIONS: If there is damp heat accumulation, add nine grams each of Radix Et Rhizoma Polygoni Cuspidati (*Hu Zhang*) and Tuber Curcumae (*Yu Jin*). If there is yin damage due to replete heat, add nine grams each of Rhizoma Polygonati Odorati (*Yu Zhu*) and Radix Polygoni Multiflori (*He Shou Wu*). If there is concomitant liver depression, add 12 grams of Tuber Curcumae (*Yu Jin*). If there is concomitant qi vacuity, add 12 grams of Fructificatio Ganodermae Lucidi (*Ling Zhi*) and six grams of Radix Panacis Ginseng (*Ren Shen*). If there is concomitant blood vacuity, add nine grams each of Radix Polygoni Multiflori (*He Shou Wu*) and Radix Angelicae Sinensis (*Dang Gui*).

ACUPUNCTURE & MOXIBUSTION: *Fei Shu* (Bl 13), *Chi Ze* (Lu 5), *Feng Long* (St 40), *Da Chang Shu* (Bl 25), *He Gu* (LI 4), *Qu Chi* (LI 11)

ANALYSIS OF FORMULA: *Fei Shu* is the back transport point of the lungs. The tai yin lungs share an interior/exterior relationship with the yang ming large intestine. In addition, the lungs govern the qi of the whole body and especially downbearing and depuration. To promote depurating and downbearing, this point should be drained. *Chi Ze* is the child-water or draining point of the lungs. Therefore, draining it can drain heat from the lungs and upper burner wafting upward from the middle and lower burners. Because the lungs are the upper source of water, clearing and rectifying the lung qi can also disinhibit the water passageways, thus helping eliminate dampness and turbidity. Draining *Feng Long* harmonizes the stomach and is a main point for transforming phlegm. *Da Chang Shu* is the back transport point of the large intestine. Draining it drains large intestine accumulation. When *He Gu* and *Qu Chi* are both drained, they strongly drain replete heat from both the upper and lower burners. Because they are transport points on the hand yang ming, they also strongly rectify the large intestine qi.

ADDITIONS & SUBTRACTIONS: To more forcefully descend and precipitate heat binding and accumulating in the yang ming, add *Nei Ting* (St 44) and *Tian Shu* (St 25). To more strongly downbear turbidity and transform phlegm, add *Zhong Wan* (CV 12). For phlegm heat harassing the heart, add *Lao Gong* (Per 8).

5. SPLEEN-KIDNEY YANG VACUITY PATTERN

MAIN SYMPTOMS: A typically older patient with low back pain, lack of strength, fear of cold, chilled limbs, abdominal fullness, torpid intake, loose stools, shortness of breath, disinclination to speak, tinnitus, blurred vision, a fat, pale tongue with thin, white fur, and a deep, fine pulse

TREATMENT PRINCIPLES: Warm yang and transform turbidity, fortify the spleen and supplement the kidneys

RX: *You Gui Wan Jia Jian* (Restore the Right [Kidney] Pills with Additions & Subtractions)

INGREDIENTS: Fructus Lycii Chinensis (*Gou Qi Zi*) and Sclerotium Poriae Cocos (*Fu Ling*), 20g each, cooked Radix Rehmanniae (*Shu Di*), processed Radix Polygoni Multiflori (*He Shou Wu*), Cortex Eucommiae Ulmoidis (*Du Zhong*), and Radix Dioscoreae Oppositae (*Shan Yao*), 15g each, Radix Morindae Officinalis (*Ba Ji Tian*), Fructus Psoraleae Corylifoliae (*Bu Gu Zhi*), Radix Codonopsitis Pilosulae (*Dang Shen*), and Rhizoma Atractylodis Macrocephalae (*Bai Zhu*), 9g each, and Radix Lateralis Praeparatus Aconiti Carmichaeli (*Fu Zi*), 6g

ANALYSIS OF FORMULA: *Gou Qi*, *Shu Di*, and *He Shou Wu* enrich the kidneys and supplement yin to bolster yang. This is because, "Yin and yang are mutually rooted," and "Yang is generated from yin." *Fu Ling*, *Shan Yao*, *Dang Shen*, and *Bai Zhu* fortify the spleen and boost the qi. They supplement the latter heaven to support the former heaven. *Du Zhong*, *Ba Ji Tian*, *Bu Gu Zhi*, and *Fu Zi* warm and supplement kidney yang. *He Shou Wu* and *Du Zhong* are empirically known to lower fat.

ADDITIONS & SUBTRACTIONS: If there is edema, damp accumulation, or phlegm, add nine grams of Rhizoma Alismatis (*Ze Xie*). If there is severe spleen qi vacuity, add nine grams of Rhizoma Polygonati (*Huang Jing*) and six grams of mix-fried Radix Glycyrrhizae (*Gan Cao*) and replace *Dang Shen* with five grams of Radix Panacis Ginseng (*Ren Shen*). If there is concomitant liver depression, add 12 grams of Tuber Curcumae (*Yu Jin*). If there is concomitant blood vacuity, add nine grams of Radix Angelicae Sinensis (*Dang Gui*). For concomitant blood stasis, add 12 grams of Radix Salviae Miltiorrhizae (*Dan Shen*) and three grams of Radix Pseudoginseng (*San Qi*), powdered and taken with the strained decoction.

ACUPUNCTURE & MOXIBUSTION: *Zu San Li* (St 36), *Nei Guan* (Per 6), *Ming Men* (GV 4), *Guan Yuan* (CV 4)

ANALYSIS OF FORMULA: When treated with moxibustion and supplementing method, *Zu San Li* fortifies the spleen and boosts the qi, transforms dampness and prevents phlegm accumulation. In addition, it supplements the latter heaven to support the former heaven and it lowers fat. Draining *Nei Guan* moves the qi, lowers fat, and prevents heart disease. *Zu San Li* and *Nei Guan* together, are an empirically effective combination for treating hyperlipoproteinemia. When treated with moxibustion and supplementing method, *Guan Yuan* and *Ming Men* warm and supplement the kidneys from the yin and yang aspects respectively.

ADDITIONS & SUBTRACTIONS: If there is phlegm, add *Feng Long* (St 40) and *Yin Ling Quan* (Sp 9). If there is concomitant liver depression, add *Tai Chong* (Liv 3) and *Zhang Men* (Liv 13). If there is severe spleen qi vacuity, add *Tai Bai* (Sp 3) and *Pi Shu* (Bl 20). If there is severe kidney vacuity, add *Shen Shu* (Bl 23) and *Fu Liu* (Ki 7). If there is blood vacuity, add *Xin Shu* (Bl 15), *Ge Shu* (Bl 17), and *Gan Shu* (Bl 18). If there is blood stasis, add *San Yin Jiao* (Sp 6). If there is dizziness and headache, add *Feng Chi* (GB 20). If there is nausea, poor appetite, or stomach venter fullness, add *Gong Sun* (Sp 4) and, if necessary, *Zhong Wan* (CV 12).

6. LIVER-KIDNEY YIN VACUITY PATTERN

MAIN SYMPTOMS: Low back and knee soreness and limpness, vexatious heat in the five hearts, advanced years bodily weakness, dizziness, tinnitus, night sweats, a dry mouth and throat, a red tongue with scanty fur, and a fine, rapid pulse

TREATMENT PRINCIPLES: Enrich and nourish the liver and kidneys

RX: *Qi Ju Di Huang Wan Jia Jian* (Lycium & Chrysanthemum Rehmannia Pills with Additions & Subtractions)

INGREDIENTS: Processed Radix Polygoni Multiflori (*He Shou Wu*), uncooked Radix Rehmanniae (*Sheng Di*), Fructus Lycii Chinensis (*Gou Qi Zi*), Ramulus Loranthi Seu Visci (*Sang Ji Sheng*), and Rhizoma Alismatis (*Ze Xie*), 15g each, and Fructus Ligustri Lucidi (*Nu Zhen Zi*), Flos Chrysanthemi Morifolii (*Ju Hua*), Radix Salviae Miltiorrhizae (*Dan Shen*), and Folium Mori Albi (*Sang Ye*), 9g each

ANALYSIS OF FORMULA: *He Shou Wu, Sheng Di, Gou Qi, Sang Ji Sheng,* and *Nu Zhen Zi* all nourish yin and supplement the liver and kidneys. *Ze Xie* drains kidney fire, *i.e.,* vacuity heat from yin vacuity. *Ju Hua* and *Sang Ye* clear and drain the liver and treat ascendant liver yang hyperactivity due to liver-kidney yin vacuity. *Dan Shen* quickens the blood and prevents heart disease. *He Shou Wu, Sang Ji Sheng, Nu Zhen Zi, Ze Xie,* and *Dan Shen* are all empirically known to lower the fat and treat hyperlipoproteinemia.

ADDITIONS & SUBTRACTIONS: If there is ascendant liver yang hyperactivity with marked headache or head distention, add 30 grams of Semen Cassiae Torae (*Jue Ming Zi*) and 18 grams each of Ramulus Uncariae Cum Uncis (*Gou Teng*) and Radix Puerariae (*Ge Gen*). If there is simultaneous qi and blood vacuity, add 15 grams of Radix Astragali Membranacei (*Huang Qi*) and 12 grams of Radix Angelicae Sinensis (*Dang Gui*). If there is either numbness or aching and pain in the limbs and body, add 12 grams of Rhizoma Gastrodiae Elatae (*Tian Ma*) and 30 grams each of Ramulus Mori Albi (*Sang Zhi*) and Caulis Milletiae Seu Spatholobi (*Ji Xue Teng*). If there is concomitant spleen vacuity, add five grams of Radix Panacis Ginseng (*Ren Shen*) and nine grams of Rhizoma Polygonati (*Huang Jing*). For concomitant kidney yang vacuity, add nine grams each of Cortex Eucommiae Ulmoidis (*Du Zhong*) and Herba Epimedii (*Yin Yang Huo*).

ACUPUNCTURE & MOXIBUSTION: *Zu San Li* (St 36), *Nei Guan* (Per 6), *Shen Shu* (Bl 23), *Fu Liu* (Ki 7)

ANALYSIS OF FORMULA: Supplementing *Zu San Li* fortifies the latter heaven to support the former heaven. In addition, it lowers fat. Draining *Nei Guan* moves the qi, lowers fat, and prevents heart disease. When combined together, *Zu San Li* and *Nei Guan* are empirically known to treat hyperlipoproteinemia. Supplementing *Shen Shu* and *Fu Liu* enrichs yin and supplements the kidneys.

ADDITIONS & SUBTRACTIONS: If there is ascendant liver yang hyperactivity, add *Tai Chong* (Liv 3) and *Feng Chi* (GB 20). If there is concomitant spleen qi vacuity, add *Tai Bai* (Sp 3). If there is severe liver-kidney yin vacuity, add *Gan Shu* (Bl 18) and *San Yin Jiao* (Sp 6). If there is concomitant blood vacuity, add *Xin Shu* (Bl 15), *Ge Shu* (Bl 17), and *Gan Shu* (Bl 18). If there is blood stasis, add *San Yin Jiao* (Sp 6).

7. STATIC BLOOD OBSTRUCTING & STAGNATING PATTERN

MAIN SYMPTOMS: Precordial pain, chest pain radiating to the upper back which is sometimes worse with taxation, dizziness, eye pain, a dark, purplish tongue or possible static macules or spots, and a bowstring, choppy pulse

TREATMENT PRINCIPLES: Quicken the blood and transform stasis, discharge turbidity and lower fat

RX: *Fu Yuan Huo Xue Tang Jia Jian* (Restore the Source & Quicken the Blood Decoction with Additions & Subtractions)

INGREDIENTS: Radix Salviae Miltiorrhizae (*Dan Shen*), 30g, Radix Angelicae Sinensis (*Dang Gui*), 15g, Fructus Trichosanthis Kirlowii (*Gua Lou*), Radix Bupleuri (*Chai Hu*), Tuber Curcumae (*Yu Jin*), Pollen Typhae (*Pu Huang*), Feces Trogopterori Seu Pteromi (*Wu Ling Zhi*), and Radix Ligustici Wallichii (*Chuan Xiong*), 9g each, and Radix Et Rhizoma Rhei (*Da Huang*), 6g

ANALYSIS OF FORMULA: *Dan Shen, Dang Gui, Pu Huang, Wu Ling Zhi, Yu Jin,* and *Chuan Xiong* all quicken the blood and transform stasis so as to treat heart pain and chest impediment. *Gua Lou* moves the qi and loosens the chest. It likewise treats chest impediment. *Chai Hu* and *Yu Jin* move the qi to quicken the blood. *Da Huang* discharges turbidity and lowers fat. In addition, *Dan Shen, Dang Gui, Yu Jin, Pu Huang,* and *Da Huang* are all empirically known to lower fat and treat hyperlipoproteinemia.

ADDITIONS & SUBTRACTIONS: If there is chest impediment with heart pain and palpitations, add 12 grams each of Fructus Crataegi (*Shan Zha*) and Bulbus Allii (*Xie Bai*) and three grams of Radix Pseudoginseng (*San Qi*), powdered and taken with the strained decoction. If there is dizziness and headache, add 12 grams of Rhizoma Gastrodiae Elatae (*Tian Ma*). If there is concomitant spleen qi vacuity, add nine grams of Rhizoma Polygonati (*Huang Jing*) and six grams of mix-fried Radix Glycyrrhizae (*Gan Cao*) and replace *Dang Shen* with five grams of Radix Panacis Ginseng (*Ren Shen*). If there is concomitant blood vacuity, add nine grams of Radix Polygoni Multiflori (*He Shou Wu*).

If there is heart blood stasis due to heart qi vacuity, replace *Fu Yuan Huo Xue Tang Jia Jian* with *Shu Xin Huo Xue Tang* (Soothe the Heart & Quicken the Blood Decoction): Radix Astragali Membranacei (*Huang Qi*), Radix Codonopsitis Pilosulae (*Dang Shen*), Radix Angelicae Sinensis (*Dang Gui*), and Pollen Typhae (*Pu Huang*), 9g each, and Flos Carthami Tinctorii (*Hong Hua*), 5g.

ACUPUNCTURE & MOXIBUSTION: *Zu San Li* (St 36), *Nei Guan* (Per 6), *San Yin Jiao* (Sp 6), *He Gu* (LI 4)

ANALYSIS OF FORMULA: Draining *Zu San Li* and *He Gu* moves the qi to quicken the blood and transform stasis. In addition, it discharges turbidity and lowers fat. Draining *Nei Guan* moves the qi and quickens the blood, transforms stasis, treats chest impediment, and prevents heart disease. *San Yin Jiao* quickens the blood of the whole body and transforms stasis. *Zu San Li* and *Nei Guan* are empirically known to treat hyperlipoproteinemia.

ADDITIONS & SUBTRACTIONS: If there is severe heart pain, add *Ju Que* (CV 14) and *Xin Shu* (Bl 15). If there is severe blood stasis, add *Xin Shu* (Bl 15) and *Ge Shu* (Bl 17). If there is ascendant liver yang hyperactivity, add *Tai Chong* (Liv 3) and *Feng Chi* (GB 20). If there is concomitant spleen qi vacuity, add *Tai Bai* (Sp 3). If there is concomitant blood vacuity, add *Xin Shu* (Bl 15), *Ge Shu* (Bl 17), and *Gan Shu* (Bl 18). If there is concomitant phlegm accumulation in the chest, add *Feng Long* (St 40).

8. PHLEGM & STASIS MUTUALLY BINDING PATTERN

MAIN SYMPTOMS: Chest oppression and pain, lassitude of the spirit, torpid intake, abdominal fullness, nausea, a dark, purplish tongue or possible static macules or spots and slimy, white fur, and a deep, bowstring, slippery pulse

TREATMENT PRINCIPLES: Transform phlegm and discharge turbidity, quicken the blood and transform stasis

RX: *Gua Lou Xie Bai Ban Xia Tang* (Trichosanthes, Allium & Pinellia Decoction) & *Shi Xiao San* (Loose a Smile Powder) with additions and subtractions

INGREDIENTS: Radix Salviae Miltiorrhizae (*Dan Shen*), 30g, Sclerotium Poriae Cocos (*Fu Ling*) and Rhizoma Alismatis (*Ze Xie*), 15g each, and Fructus Trichosanthis Kirlowii (*Gua Lou*), Bulbus Allii (*Xie Bai*), Pollen Typhae (*Pu Huang*), Feces Trogopterori Sei Pteromi (*Wu Ling Zhi*), Tuber Curcumae (*Yu Jin*), Pericarpium Citri Reticulatae (*Chen Pi*), and Folium Nelumbinis Nuciferae (*He Ye*), 9g each

ANALYSIS OF FORMULA: *Dan Shen, Pu Huang, Wu Ling Zhi,* and *Yu Jin* quicken the blood and transform stasis. *Fu Ling, Ze Xie, Chen Pi,* and *Gua Lou* transform phlegm and discharge turbidity. *He Ye* also discharges turbidity. *Gua Lou* and *Xie Bai* loosen the chest and treat impediment. *Dan Shen, Pu Huang, Yu Jin* and *Ze Xie* treat hyperlipoproteinemia.

ADDITIONS & SUBTRACTIONS: If there is chest impediment with heart pain and palpitations, add 12 grams each of Fructus Crataegi (*Shan Zha*) and three grams of Radix Pseudoginseng (*San Qi*), powdered and taken with the strained decoction. If there is dizziness and headache, add 12 grams of Rhizoma Gastrodiae Elatae (*Tian Ma*). If there is concomitant spleen qi vacuity, add nine grams of Rhizoma Polygonati (*Huang Jing*) and six grams of mix-fried Radix Glycyrrhizae (*Gan Cao*) and replace *Dang Shen* with five grams of Radix Panacis Ginseng (*Ren Shen*). If there is concomitant blood vacuity, add nine grams of Radix Polygoni Multiflori (*He Shou Wu*).

ACUPUNCTURE & MOXIBUSTION: *Zu San Li* (St 36), *Nei Guan* (Per 6), *San Yin Jiao* (Sp 6), *He Gu* (LI 4), *Feng Long* (St 40)

ANALYSIS OF FORMULA: Supplementing *Zu San Li* fortifies the spleen in order to promote the transformation of phlegm based on the saying, "The spleen is the root of phlegm engenderment." Draining *He Gu* moves the qi to quicken the blood and transform stasis. In addition, it discharges turbidity and lowers fat. Draining *Nei Guan* moves the qi and quickens the blood, transforms stasis, treats chest impediment, and prevents heart disease. *San Yin Jiao* quickens the blood of the whole body and transforms stasis. *Zu San Li* and *Nei Guan* are empirically known to treat hyperlipoproteinemia. In addition, draining *Feng Long* transforms phlegm and also treats hyperlipoproteinemia.

ADDITIONS & SUBTRACTIONS: If there is concomitant liver depression, add *Tai Chong* (Liv 3) and *Zhang Men* (Liv 13). If there is dizziness and headache, add *Feng Chi* (GB 20). If there is nausea, poor appetite, or stomach venter fullness, add *Gong Sun* (Sp 4) and, if necessary, *Zhong Wan* (CV 12). If there is severe heart pain, add *Ju Que* (CV 14) and *Xin Shu* (Bl 15). If there is severe blood stasis, add *Xin Shu* (Bl 15) and *Ge Shu* (Bl 17). If there is concomitant spleen qi vacuity, add *Tai Bai* (Sp 3) and *Pi Shu* (Bl 20). If there is concomitant blood vacuity, add *Xin Shu* (Bl 15), *Ge Shu* (Bl 17) and *Gan Shu* (Bl 18).

REMARKS

1. In most cases of hyperlipoproteinemia, there are disease mechanisms involving both the liver and spleen. Liver mechanisms may include depression, depressive heat, flaring fire, liver blood and yin vacuity, yang hyperactivity, and even wind. Spleen mechanisms include spleen vacuity as well as dampness and phlegm based on the saying, "The spleen is the root of phlegm engenderment." Because of qi stagnation, phlegm, and/or dampness, there is a tendency to blood stasis. Because of age, there is a tendency to yin and yang vacuities. Therefore, most patients display a combination of the above patterns as opposed to the discrete symptoms of only a single pattern.

2. While reducing dietary cholesterol is emphasized by most Western MDs and the popular press, it is our experience that eating sugar and refined carbohydrates is at least as large a part of this condition as is over-eating fats and oils. Cholesterol is manufactured in the body as a precursor to various hormones, and it is the hormones that control the endocrine system, with the pancreas being part of the endocrine system. Cholesterol may remain abnormally high as long as the patient continues to eat sugar and sweets even after they have eliminated all or almost all dietary fats and oils. Likewise, the body may produce cholesterol in response to stress. Therefore, when treating patients with this condition, it is not just enough to avoid foods high in dietary cholesterol. One should also eliminate sweets and refined carbohydrates as well as control stress. The latter may be done by changing one's lifestyle within the limits possible but also by doing a combination of daily deep relaxation and exercise.

3. Three acupuncture points have especially demonstrated incontestable effectiveness for hyperlipoproteinemia: *Zu San Li* (St 36), *Feng Long* (St 40), and *Nei Guan* (Per 6).

4. Several new, modern formulas have demonstrated good results for lowering fat and treating hyperlipoproteinemia in multitpattern presentations. For instance:

Yin Chen Jiang Zhi Tang (Artemisia Capillaris Downbear Fat Decoction): Herba Artemisiae Capillaris (*Yin Chen Hao*), 30g, Fructus Crataegi (*Shan Zha*) and Fructus Germinatus Hordei Vulgaris (*Mai Ya*), 15g each. This formula is for liver damp heat and spleen vacuity pattern hyperlipoproteinemia.

Fu Fang Jiang Zhi Tang (Compound Downbear Fat Decoction): Radix Polygoni Multiflori (*He Shou Wu*) and Rhizoma Polygonati (*Huang Jing*), 20g each, Ramulus Loranthi Seu Visci (*Sang Ji Sheng*) 18g. This formula is for liver-kidney-spleen vacuity or qi and blood vacuity.

Other interesting empirical formulas for multipattern presentations are:

Bao Xin Jiang Zhi Tang (Protect Heart & Downbear Fat Decoction): Radix Salviae Miltiorrhizae (*Dan Shen*), 20g, Radix Polygoni Multiflori (*He Shou Wu*), Radix Puerariae (*Ge Gen*), Ramulus Loranthi Seu Visci (*Sang Ji Sheng*), and Rhizoma Polygonati (*Huang Jing*), 10g each, and Radix Glycyrrhizae (*Gan Cao*), 6g. This formula is for chest impediment with liver-kidney yin vacuity, spleen vacuity, and heart blood stasis.

Jiang Zhi Dan (Downbear Fat Elixir): Ramulus Loranthi Seu Visci (*Sang Ji Sheng*), Herba Epimedii (*Yin Yang Huo*), Rhizoma Alismatis (*Ze Xie*), Rhizoma Polygonati Odorati (*Yu Zhu*), Semen Leonuri Heterophylli (*Chong Wei Zi*), and Fructus Crataegi (*Shan Zha*), 15g each. This formula is especially for hyperlipoproteinemia with hypertension due to dual kidney yin and yang vacuity with blood stasis.

5. The following are those Chinese medicinals which have all demonstrated pronounced empirical abilities to lower fat and treat hyperlipoproteinemia: Bulbus Allii Sativi (*Da Suan*), Cordyceps Chinensis (*Dong Chong Xia Cao*), Cortex Eucommiae Ulmoidis (*Du Zhong*), Flos Lonicerae Japonicae (*Jin Yin Hua*), Fructus Crataegi (*Shan Zha*), Fructus Ligustri Lucidi (*Nu Zhen Zi*), Fructificatio Ganodermae Lucidi (*Ling Zhi*), Herba Sargassii (*Hai Zao*), Pollen Typhae (*Pu Huang*), Radix Angelicae Sinensis (*Dang Gui*), Radix Et Rhizoma Polygoni Cuspidati (*Hu Zhang*), Radix Et Rhizoma Rhei (*Da Huang*), Radix Glycyrrhizae (*Gan Cao*), Radix Panacis Ginseng (*Ren Shen*), Radix Polygoni Multiflori (*He Shou Wu*), Radix Pseudoginseng (*San Qi*), Radix Puerariae (*Ge Gen*), Radix Salviae Miltiorrhizae (*Dan Shen*), Ramulus Loranthi Seu Visci (*Sang Ji Sheng*), Rhizoma Alismatis (*Ze Xie*), Rhizoma Dioscoreae Hypoglaucae (*Bei Xie*), Rhizoma Gastrodiae Elatae (*Tian Ma*), Rhizoma Polygonati (*Huang Jing*), Rhizoma Polygonati Odorati (*Yu Zhu*), Semen Cassiae Torae (*Jue Ming Zi*), and Tuber Curcumae (*Yu Jin*).

6. In Chinese medicine, certain foods are reputed to help regulate serum cholesterol. These include garlic, shiitake mushroom, soybeans, various types of seaweed, black Chinese tree fungus, and water chestnuts.

33

HYPERTENSION

Hypertension refers to elevated systolic and/or diastolic blood pressure. When this is due to unknown etiology, it is called essential hypertension and accounts for 85-90% of all diagnosed hypertension. The other type of hypertension is secondary hypertension when damage to the kidneys or endocrine dysfunction cause the blood pressure to rise. It is estimated that there are more than 35 million hypertensives in the United States, and high blood pressure occurs twice as often in African Americans than in white Americans. There is no consistent difference in the prevalence of diastolic hypertension between men and women. However, diastolic pressure does increase with age, at least until 55-60 years, and systolic pressure increases with age until at least 80. More than 50% of both white and African Americans suffer from some form of hypertension over age 65. Until complications develop, primary hypertension is asymptomatic. When signs and symptoms do arise, they include dizziness, facial flushing, headache, fatigue, epistaxis, and nervousness. However, none of these are pathognomonic for hypertension and all are due to some complication involving one or more target organs.

Although the causes of essential hypertension are unknown according to Western medicine, there are a number of factors which are associated with or lead to this condition. The main cause seems to be a diet high in animal fat and sodium chloride, especially if sodium chloride is high in relation to potassium and magnesium. Recent studies in remote areas of China, New Guinea, Panama, Brazil, and Africa where low fat, low sodium diets are the norm show virtually no evidence of hypertension, even with advanced age. However, when individuals in these groups moved to more industrialized areas and changed their diet to include more animal fat and salt, the incidence of hypertension increased proportionately to increases in body mass and fat.[1] Lifestyle choices also seem to play a role in the development of hypertension, including smoking tobacco and drinking alcohol and coffee. Even moderate alcohol consumption can produce hypertension in certain individuals, and chronic alcohol intake is one of the strongest predictors of high blood pressure. Smoking is a contributing factor to hypertension due to the fact that smokers are more prone to increased sugar, alcohol, and caffeine consumption. In addition, environmental factors, such as lead contamination from drinking water as well as residues from cadmium, have been shown to promote hypertension. People whose hypertension has been left untreated have been shown to have blood cadmium levels 3-4 times higher than those with normal blood pressure.[2]

The Western medical diagnosis of hypertension is based on measuring systolic and diastolic blood pressure using a blood pressure cuff. Since blood pressure may fluctuate, at least two blood pressure readings should be taken on separate days, and care should be taken to insure the proper sized cuff for the size of the arm. For instance, using too small a cuff on a larger than normal arm will tend to read hypertensive. The upper limit of normal blood pressure in adults is 140/90mm/Hg.

If patients have mild hypertension and no heart problems, diet and lifestyle changes may suffice if carried out with determination. Such diet and lifestyle modifications include weight loss, restricted intake of sodium, exercise, and relaxation. For more severe hypertension or for mild cases that do not respond to changes in diet and lifestyle within one year, drug treatment is usually considered necessary. Antihypertensive medications typically fall into one of five categories: diuretics, ACE inhibitors, beta-blockers, vasodilators, and calcium channel blockers. Diuretics cause the body to excrete water and salt. There are three main types of antihypertensive diuretics: thiazides, loop diuretics, and potassium-sparing agents. There are many different thiazides used for the treatment of hypertension, such as hydrochlorothiazide and chlorthalidone. Thiazides often serve as the basis for the treatment of hypertension, taken either alone or in combination with other types of drugs. Loop diuretics block sodium transport in parts of the kidneys. They act faster than thiazides and have a stronger diuretic effect. Loop diuretics include bumetanide, furosemide, and ethacrynic acid. Both thiazides and loop diuretics may deplete the body's supply of potassium and thus lead to heart arrhythmias. Potassium-sparing diuretics include amiloride, spironolactone, and triamterene. ACE inhibitors block angiotensin-converting enzyme (ACE), an enzyme that indirectly causes blood vessels to constrict. ACE inhibitors include captoril, enalapil, and lisinopril. Beta-blockers block the effects of adrenalin, thus easing the heart's pumping action and widening the blood vessels. They are very effective and are currently recommended along with or instead of diuretics for initial treatment. However, they are not as effective as ACE inhibitors in people with or at risk for kidney disease, such as diabetics. There are a number of beta-blockers now available, including propranol, acebutolo, atenolol, betaxolol, and cartedolol. Vasodilators expand the blood vessels and are often used with a diuretic or beta-blocker. Representative vasodilators include hydralazine, prazosin, clonidine, and minoxidil. Calcium channel blockers help decrease the contractions of the heart and widen blood vessels. They have an immediate effect on reducing blood pressure, but they have been linked to some severe problems. These drugs include diltiazem, amlodipine, verapami, nisoldipine, etc.

Nearly 15% of persons with hypertension are not currently on medication, and untreated hypertensives are at great risk for developing disabling or fatal heart disease, cerebral hemorrhage or infarction, or renal failure. Hypertension is the most important risk factor predisposing a person to stroke. However, of those hypertensives on antihypertensive medication, only 27% of American adults with high blood pressure have it under control. The rest are on medication which is not controlling their blood pressure. Unfortunately, all Western antihypertensive medicines have side effects. Some of these side effects are distressing, such as loss of sex drive, urinary incontinence, cold extremities, heart arrhythmias, fatigue, constipation, and allergic symptoms, and, therefore, achieving patient compliance is difficult, especially since treatment is life-long. In addition, some physicians are concerned about the long-term effects of antihypertensive medicines such as calcium channel blockers and loop diuretics on mental processes. These types of antihypertensive medications may result in depression and memory loss. On the plus side, one major study found that people taking blood pressure medication did not experience any greater decline in general quality of life or daily functioning over five years than did people who were not on blood pressure medication.[3]

CHINESE DISEASE CATEGORIZATION: Like hyperlipoproteinemia above, hypertension may be asymptomatic as far as Chinese medicine is concerned. When it is asymptomatic, it does not correspond to any traditional Chinese disease category. When hypertension is complicated and, therefore, there are signs and symptoms, it is mainly categorized as *tou tong*, headache, *tou zhang*, head distention, *xuan yun*, dizziness, *xin ji*, heart palpitations, *bu mian*, insomnia, and *ma mu*, numbness and tingling.

DISEASE CAUSES & MECHANISMS: Due to former heaven natural endowment, people may be either habitually bodily exuberant or vacuous and insufficient. As the *Ling Shu (Spiritual Axis)* states: "[Due to] the unfavorable and favorable [aspects of] the five body [types], it is said that people's bone joints may be large or small, their flesh may be firm or fragile, their skin may be thick or thin, their blood may be clear or turbid, or their qi may be slippery or choppy . . ." Therefore, some people have a predisposition to yang exuberance and phlegm dampness, while others are predisposed to yin vacuity. In addition, each person's viscera and bowels have an innate tendency towards vacuity or repletion. On top of such habitual bodily predispositions, overeating fatty, sweet, thick-flavored foods may damage the spleen and stomach, which then lose their control over movement and transformation. This results in internal engenderment of phlegm dampness. Phlegm and dampness are yin depressions which may hinder and obstruct the free flow of qi, blood, and body fluids as well as confound and block the orifices of the heart and the upper clear orifices. If phlegm and dampness block the free flow of qi, blood, or body fluids, there may be distention and pain, swelling and edema, and/or malnourishment of the tissues and organs. In addition, it may also give rise to transformative heat which may cause yang to become hyperactive and may damage and consume yin. Other factors which may damage the spleen and lead to the engenderment of phlegm and dampness are too little exercise and too much thinking and worry.

On the other hand, unfulfilled desires or anger may damage the liver and cause it to lose its control over coursing and discharge. This may cause qi stagnation which may lead to blood stasis. It may cause transformative heat with its attendant yang hyperactivity and/or yin vacuity. And it may cause or aggravate damp accumulation and phlegm obstruction, since it is the qi which is responsible for moving and transforming both of these. In addition, liver repletion usually results in spleen vacuity since wood typically counterflows horizontally to invade the spleen when it becomes depressed. Unfortunately, the sweet flavor relaxes the liver. Therefore, people who are under emotional stress try to alleviate their liver depression by eating sweets. Sweet is the flavor which enters the spleen. In small amounts, it supplements the spleen, but in large amounts, it damages the spleen. Therefore, a liver-spleen disharmony is often the underlying imbalance predisposing one to this condition.

In addition, aging plays a role in the disease mechanisms of this disorder. Yin is half consumed by 40 and yang qi tends to become debilitated not very long after. Yin vacuity may fail to nourish and moisten the liver. Thus it tends to become even more depressed. Yang vacuity may fail to warm and steam the liver, thus also leading to liver depression. Spleen-kidney yang vacuity may also fail to warm and steam (*i.e.*, evaporate) body fluids. Hence yang vacuity commonly accelerates or aggravates a tendency towards phlegm damp accumulation. This is why many people become obese with age.

TREATMENT BASED ON PATTERN DISCRIMINATION:

1. ASCENDANT LIVER YANG HYPERACTIVITY PATTERN

MAIN SYMPTOMS: Dizziness, head distention and pain, vertigo, a red facial complexion, tinnitus, ringing in the brain, vexation and agitation, easy anger, scanty sleep, a bitter taste in the mouth, a red tongue tip and/or edges with yellow fur, and a bowstring pulse

TREATMENT PRINCIPLES: Level the liver, subdue yang, and lower pressure

RX: *Tian Ma Gou Teng Yin Jia Jian* (Gastrodia & Uncaria Drink with Additions & Subtractions)

INGREDIENTS: Concha Haliotidis (*Shi Jue Ming*), Concha Ostreae (*Mu Li*), Os Draconis (*Long Gu*), Spica Prunellae Vulgaris (*Xia Ku Cao*), Ramulus Loranthi Seu Visci (*Sang Ji Sheng*), and Ramulus Uncariae Cum Uncis (*Gou Teng*), 15g each, Cortex Eucommiae Ulmoidis (*Du Zhong*), Rhizoma Gastrodiae Elatae (*Tian Ma*), and Radix Achyranthis Bidentatae (*Niu Xi*), 12g each, and Flos Chrysanthemi Morifolii (*Ju Hua*) and Radix Scutellariae Baicalensis (*Huang Qin*), 9g each

ANALYSIS OF FORMULA: *Sang Ji Sheng, Du Zhong,* and *Niu Xi* nourish kidney yin to check liver yang. *Shi Jue Ming, Long Gu,* and *Mu Li* level the liver and subdue yang. *Xia Ku Cao, Gou Teng, Ju Hua,* and *Huang Qin* drain the liver and clear heat. *Tian Ma* and *Gou Teng* settle the liver and extinguish wind. *Huang Qin, Xia Ku Cao, Shi Jue Ming, Du Zhong, Niu Xi, Sang Ji Sheng, Ju Hua,* and *Gou Teng* all have a direct hypotensive action according to Western pharmacodynamics.

ADDITIONS & SUBTRACTIONS: If there is constipation, add six grams of Radix Et Rhizoma Rhei (*Da Huang*). If dizziness is severe, add 15 grams of Concha Margaritiferae (*Zhen Zhu Mu*). For dry mouth and throat, add 15 grams of uncooked Radix Rehmanniae (*Sheng Di*) and nine grams of Radix Scrophulariae Ningpoensis (*Xuan Shen*). If there is numbness of the extremities, add nine grams each of Lumbricus (*Di Long*) and Herba Siegesbeckiae (*Xi Xian Cao*).

For more pronounced symptoms of heat and wind with red face and eyes, trembling hands, and numbness of the tongue, lips, and/or limbs, replace *Tian Ma Gou Teng Yin* with *Long Dan Xie Gan Tang Jia Jian* (Gentiana Drain the Liver Decoction with Additions & Subtractions): Concha Ostreae (*Mu Li*) and Concha Margaritiferae (*Zhen Zhu Mu*), 30g each, uncooked Radix Rehmanniae (*Sheng Di*) and Ramulus Uncariae Cum Uncis (*Gou Teng*), 15g each, Folium Et Ramulus Clerodendri (*Chou Wu Tong*), 12g, Radix Gentianae Scabrae (*Long Dan Cao*), Fructus Gardeniae Jasminoidis (*Zhi Zi*), Radix Scutellariae Baicalensis (*Huang Qin*), Flos Chrysanthemi Morifolii (*Ju Hua*), Fructus Tribuli Terrestris (*Bai Ji Li*), Herba Siegesbeckiae (*Xi Xian Cao*), and Lumbricus (*Di Long*), 9g each, and Rhizoma Gastrodiae Elatae (*Tian Ma*), 6g. If there is severe headache, add 12 grams of Radix Ligustici Wallichii (*Chuan Xiong*). If there is nausea or vomiting, add nine grams each of Caulis Bambusae In Taeniis (*Zhu Ru*) and Rhizoma Pinelliae Ternatae (*Ban Xia*).

ACUPUNCTURE & MOXIBUSTION: *Yang Fu* (GB 38), *Tai Chong* (Liv 3), *Tai Xi* (Ki 3), *Feng Chi* (GB 20), *Zu San Li* (St 36), *Qu Chi* (LI 11)

ANALYSIS OF FORMULA: Draining *Yang Fu* and *Tai Chong* level the liver and subdue yang, while supplementing *Tai Xi* nourishes kidney yin to check liver yang. Using even supplementing-even draining technique at *Feng Chi* levels the liver and extinguishes wind. Draining *Zu San Li* and *Qu Chi* are a commonly used empirical pair for lowering blood pressure since they drain yang evils from the entire body.

ADDITIONS & SUBTRACTIONS: *Qiu Xu* (GB 40) and *Xia Xi* (GB 43) can be alternated with *Yang Fu.* For severe hypertension, subtract *Feng Chi* and add *Da Zhui* (GV 14). For liver fire, add *Xing Jian* (Liv 2). For nausea or vomiting, add *Nei Guan* (Per 6). For heart palpitations, also add *Nei Guan* (Per 6). For hypertension appearing especially at night, add *Zhao Hai* (Ki 6). For headache in the corner of the head, add *Tou Wei* (St 8). For headache in the temple, needle and then bleed *Tai Yang* (M-HN-9). For headache in the occiput or tension in the neck, add *Shu Gu* (Bl 65). For dizziness, add *Bai Hui* (GV 20). For tension in the trapezius, add *Tian Jing* (GB 21). For severe liver-kidney yin vacuity, add *San Yin Jiao* (Sp 6). An alternative treatment is to drain *Xuan Zhong* (GB 39) and supplement *San Yin Jiao* (Sp 6), then needle *Feng Chi* (GB 20) with even supplementing-even draining technique if there is headache or dizziness.

2. PHLEGM FIRE HARASSING ABOVE PATTERN

MAIN SYMPTOMS: Dizziness, head distention, chest and ductal glomus and oppression, nausea and vomiting, profuse phlegm, a bitter taste in the mouth, torpid intake, profuse dreams, heart palpitations, a pale tongue with red tip and/or sides and slimy, yellow fur, and a bowstring, slippery, rapid pulse

TREATMENT PRINCIPLES: Clear heat and transform phlegm, clear the liver and lower pressure

RX: *Huang Lian Wen Dan Tang Jia Jian* (Coptis Warm the Gallbladder Decoction with Additions & Subtractions)

INGREDIENTS: Spica Prunellae Vulgaris (*Xia Ku Cao*), 15g, Semen Cassiae Torae (*Jue Ming Zi*) and Herba Siegesbeckiae (*Xi Xian Cao*), 12g each, Radix Scutellariae Baicalensis (*Huang Qin*), Rhizoma Pinelliae Ternatae (*Ban Xia*), Rhizoma Acori Graminei (*Shi Chang Pu*), and Sclerotium Poriae Cocos (*Fu Ling*), 9g each, and bile-processed Rhizoma Arisaematis (*Dan Nan Xing*), Pericarpium Citri Reticulatae (*Chen Pi*), and Caulis Bambusae In Taeniis (*Zhu Ru*), 6g each

ANALYSIS OF FORMULA: *Xia Ku Cao, Huang Qin,* and *Jue Ming Zi* clear the liver and lower pressure. When used together, *Ban Xia, Chen Pi, Fu Ling, Huang Qin, Dan Nan Xing,* and *Zhu Ru* clear heat and transform phlegm. In addition, *Dan Nan Xing* extinguishes wind. *Xi Xian Cao* clears heat and lowers pressure. *Shi Chang Pu* harmonizes the center and transforms phlegm, opens the orifices and arouses the spirit.

ADDITIONS & SUBTRACTIONS: If there is concomitant liver fire, add nine grams each of Fructus Gardeniae Jasminoidis (*Zhi Zi*) and Ramulus Uncariae Cum Uncis (*Gou Teng*). If there is phlegm fire, add three grams of Rhizoma Coptidis Chinensis (*Huang Lian*). If there is constipation, add six grams of Radix Et Rhizoma Rhei (*Da Huang*). If dizziness is severe, add 15 grams of Concha Margaritiferae (*Zhen Zhu Mu*). If there is numbness of the upper extremities, add nine grams each of Lumbricus (*Di Long*) and Ramulus Mori Albi (*Sang Zhi*). If there is numbness of the lower extremities, add nine grams each of Lumbricus (*Di Long*) and Radix Cyathulae (*Chuan Niu Xi*). For rigidity of the neck, add 15 grams of Radix Puerariae (*Ge Gen*). For chest pain, add 20 grams of Fructus Trichosanthis Kirlowii (*Gua Lou*) and nine grams of Tuber Curcumae (*Yu Jin*).

ACUPUNCTURE & MOXIBUSTION: *Tai Chong* (Liv 3), *Feng Chi* (GB 20), *Zu San Li* (St 36), *Qu Chi* (LI 11), *Feng Long* (St 40), *Nei Ting* (St 44)

ANALYSIS OF FORMULA: Draining *Tai Chong* levels and clears the liver. Even supplementing-even draining *Feng Chi* levels the liver, extinguishes wind, and clears the head. Draining *Zu San Li* and *Qu Chi* drain yang evils from the entire body. Draining *Feng Long* transforms phlegm, while draining *Nei Ting* drains interior heat. Together, these last two treat phlegm heat.

ADDITIONS & SUBTRACTIONS: For severe hypertension, subtract *Feng Chi* and add *Da Zhui* (GV 14). For liver fire, replace *Tai Chong* with *Xing Jian* (Liv 2). For nausea or vomiting, add *Nei Guan* (Per 6). For heart palpitations, also add *Nei Guan* (Per 6). For hypertension appearing especially at night, add *Zhao Hai* (Ki 6). For headache in the corner of the head, add *Tou Wei* (St 8). For headache in the temple, needle, then bleed *Tai Yang* (M-HN-9). For headache in the occiput or tension in the neck, add *Shu Gu* (Bl 65). For dizziness, add *Bai Hui* (GV 20). For tension in the trapezius, add *Tian Jing* (GB 21).

3. LIVER-KIDNEY YIN VACUITY PATTERN

MAIN SYMPTOMS: Dizziness, tinnitus, blurred vision, insomnia, devitalized essence spirit, decreased memory, heart palpitations, bilateral eye dryness and roughness, numbness in the extremities, a dry mouth, low back and knee soreness and limpness, seminal emission in males and menstrual irregularities in females, bilateral afternoon malar flushing, a red, tender tongue with scanty or no fur, and a fine, rapid pulse

TREATMENT PRINCIPLES: Enrich the kidneys, supplement the liver, and lower pressure

RX: If there are mainly kidney yin vacuity symptoms, *Qi Ju Di Huang Wan Jia Wei* (Lycium & Chrysanthemum Pills with Added Flavors)

INGREDIENTS: Plastrum Testudinis (*Gui Ban*) and Concha Ostreae (*Mu Li*), 30g each, cooked Radix Rehmanniae (*Shu Di*), 24g, Radix Dioscoreae Oppositae (*Shan Yao*) and Fructus Corni Officinalis (*Shan Zhu Yu*), 12g each, and Rhizoma Alismatis (*Ze Xie*), Cortex Radicis Moutan (*Dan Pi*), Sclerotium Poriae Cocos (*Fu Ling*), Fructus Lycii Chinensis (*Gou Qi Zi*), and Flos Chrysanthemi Morifolii (*Ju Hua*), 9g each

ANALYSIS OF FORMULA: *Shu Di, Shan Yao, Shan Zhu Yu, Ze Xie, Dan Pi,* and *Fu Ling* are the six flavors of *Liu Wei Di Huang Wan* (Six Flavors Rehmannia Pills) which together supplement kidney yin and drain heat evils. When the yin is exuberant, it is able to check yang and prevent ascension of vacuity heat. *Gui Ban* and *Gou Qi Zi* help the six flavors to nourish liver-kidney yin. *Ju Hua, Gui Ban,* and *Mu Li* subdue yang.

ADDITIONS & SUBTRACTIONS: If dizziness is severe with numbness of the limbs, add 12 grams each of Ramulus Uncariae Cum Uncis (*Gou Teng*) and Lumbricus (*Di Long*) and nine grams of Rhizoma Gastrodiae Elatae (*Tian Ma*). If there are dry, bound stools, add 15 grams each of black Semen Sesami Indici (*Hei Zhi Ma*) and Semen Biotae Orientalis (*Bai Zi Ren*). If there is concomitant liver depression, add 12 grams of Fructus Meliae Toosendan (*Chuan Lian Zi*). If there is concomitant blood stasis, add 12 grams each of Radix Salviae Miltiorrhizae (*Dan Shen*) and Radix Angelicae Sinensis (*Dang Gui*).

If there are mainly liver yin vacuity symptoms, *Shou Wu Yan Shou Dan Jia Jian* (Polygonum Multiflorum Extend Longevity Elixir with Additions & Subtractions)

INGREDIENTS: Magnetitum (*Ci Shi*), 30g, Radix Polygoni Multiflori (*He Shou Wu*), Gelatinum Plastri Testudinis (*Gui Ban Jiao*), Ramulus Loranthi Seu Visci (*Sang Ji Sheng*), and Radix Achyranthis Bidentatae (*Niu Xi*), 15g each, stir-fried Semen Zizyphi Spinosae (*Suan Zao Ren*), uncooked Radix Rehmanniae (*Sheng Di*), and Fructus Lycii Chinensis (*Gou Qi Zi*), 12g each, and Cortex Eucommiae Ulmoidis (*Du Zhong*) and Flos Chrysanthemi Morifolii (*Ju Hua*), 9g each

ANALYSIS OF FORMULA: *He Shou Wu, Gui Ban, Sang Ji Sheng, Niu Xi, Suan Zao Ren, Sheng Di,* and *Gou Qi Zi* nourish both liver yin and blood. In addition, *Gui Ban* subdues yang, while *Sang Ji Sheng* and *Niu Xi* lower the blood pressure. *Ci Shi* nourishes yin and subdues yang. *Du Zhong* supplements kidney yin and yang equally and also lowers pressure. *Ju Hua* levels the liver, subdues yang, and lowers pressure.

ADDITIONS & SUBTRACTIONS: If there is chest oppression and heart pain, add 15 grams each of Radix Salviae Miltiorrhizae (*Dan Shen*) and Fructus Trichosanthis Kirlowii (*Gua Lou*).

If there are heart-kidney yin vacuity symptoms, *Tian Wang Bu Xin Dan Jia Jian* (Heavenly Emperor Supplement the Heart Elixir with Additions & Subtractions)

INGREDIENTS: Concha Ostreae (*Mu Li*) and Os Draconis (*Long Gu*), 30g each, uncooked Radix Rehmanniae (*Sheng Di*), 15g, Radix Scrophulariae Ningpoensis (*Xuan Shen*), Tuber Ophiopogonis Japonici (*Mai Dong*), Tuber Asparagi Cochinensis (*Tian Men Dong*), Semen Zizyphi Spinosae (*Suan Zao Ren*), and Semen Biotae Orientalis (*Bai Zi Ren*), 12g each, Radix Salviae Miltiorrhizae (*Dan Shen*), Radix Angelicae Sinensis (*Dang Gui*), Sclerotium Poriae Cocos (*Fu Ling*), and Radix Polygalae Tenuifoliae (*Yuan Zhi*), 9g each, Radix Platycodi Grandiflori (*Jie Geng*) and Radix Panacis Ginseng (*Ren Shen*), 6g each, and Rhizoma Coptidis Chinensis (*Huang Lian*), 3g

ANALYSIS OF FORMULA: *Sheng Di, Mai Men Dong,* and *Tian Men Dong* nourish heart yin. *Sheng Di* and *Tian Men Dong* nourish kidney yin. *Dang Gui* nourishes the heart blood. *Xuan Shen* clears vacuity heat due to heart yin insufficiency and lowers pressure. *Suan Zao Ren, Yuan Zhi, Bai Zi Ren, Fu Ling* and *Ren Shen* all nourish the heart and calm the spirit. *Long Gu* and *Mu Li* subdue yang and quiet the spirit. *Huang Lian* clears heart fire to help calm the spirit and lower pressure. Within this formula, *Jie Geng* is a messenger which leads the other medicinals to the upper burner where the root of the disease is located.

ADDITIONS & SUBTRACTIONS: Same as above.

If vacuity fire is flaming upward, *Zhi Bai Di Huang Wan Jia Jian* (Anemarrhena & Phellodendron Rehmannia Pills with Additions & Subtractions)

INGREDIENTS: Concha Haliotidis (*Shi Jue Ming*), 30g, Concha Ostreae (*Mu Li*), 18g, uncooked Radix Rehmanniae (*Sheng Di*), 15g, Radix Polygoni Multiflori (*He Shou Wu*), Ramulus Loranthi Seu Visci (*Sang Ji Sheng*), Fructus Ligustri Lucidi (*Nu Zhen Zi*), and Plastrum Testudinis (*Gui Ban*), 12g each, and cooked Radix Rehmanniae (*Shu Di*), Fructus Corni Officinalis (*Shan Zhu Yu*), Cortex Radicis Moutan (*Dan Pi*), Rhizoma Anemarrhenae Aspheloidis (*Zhi Mu*), Cortex Phellodendri (*Huang Bai*), and Radix Albus Paeoniae Lactiflorae (*Bai Shao*), 9g each

ANALYSIS OF FORMULA: *He Shou Wu, Sang Ji Sheng, Nu Zhen Zi, Gui Ban, Shan Zhu Yu,* and *Shu Di* all enrich yin and supplement the kidneys. *Shi Jue Ming* and *Mu Li* subdue yang. *Sheng Di, Gui Ban, Dan Pi, Zhi Mu,* and *Huang Bai* clear vacuity heat and downbear fire. *Bai Shao* levels the liver, constrains yin, and stops sweating. *Sang Ji Sheng, Shi Jue Ming,* and *Dan Pi* lower the pressure.

ADDITIONS & SUBTRACTIONS: Same as above.

ACUPUNCTURE & MOXIBUSTION: *Tai Xi* (Ki 3), *San Yin Jiao* (Sp 6), *Xuan Zhong* (GB 39), *Zu San Li* (St 36), *Qu Chi* (LI 11)

ANALYSIS OF FORMULA: Supplementing *Tai Xi* and *San Yin Jiao* nourishes and enriches liver-kidney blood and yin. Draining *Xuan Zhong* downbears fire. When combined with *San Yin Jiao,* these two points are a special empirical combination for lowering blood pressure. Draining *Zu San Li* and *Qu Chi* are another famous empirical combination for lowering blood pressure by draining yang evils from the entire body.

ADDITIONS & SUBTRACTIONS: For predominant kidney yin vacuity, add *Shen Shu* (Bl 23). For predominant liver blood vacuity, add *Gan Shu* (Bl 18). For heart yin vacuity, add *Shen Men* (Ht 7). For vacuity fire flaming upward, add *Ran Gu* (Ki 2). For concomitant ascendant liver yang hyperactivity, add *Feng Chi* (GB 20). For severe hypertension, add *Da Zhui* (GV 14). For nausea or vomiting, add *Nei Guan* (Per 6). For heart palpitations, add *Nei Guan* (Per 6). For hypertension appearing especially at night, add *Zhao Hai* (Ki 6). For headache in the corner of the head, add *Tou Wei* (St 8). For headache in the temple, needle, then bleed *Tai Yang*

(M-HN-9). For headache in the occiput or tension in the neck, add *Shu Gu* (Bl 65). For dizziness, add *Bai Hui* (GV 20). For tension in the trapezius, add *Tian Jing* (GB 21).

4. CHONG & REN DISREGULATION PATTERN

MAIN SYMPTOMS: Women's perimenopausal hypertension accompanied by dizziness, headache, heart vexation, easy anger, hot flashes, night sweats, a dry mouth and throat, scanty sleep, generalized bodily discomfort, low back and knee soreness and weakness, a pale red tongue with scanty fur, and a bowstring fine pulse

NOTE: This pattern is made up of liver-kidney yin and yang vacuity with fire effulgence or yang hyperactivity.

TREATMENT PRINCIPLES: Regulate and rectify the chong and ren

RX: *Er Xian Tang Jia Wei* (Two Immortals Decoction with Added Flavors)

INGREDIENTS: Cortex Eucommiae Ulmoidis (*Du Zhong*) and Radix Achyranthis Bidentatae (*Niu Xi*), 12g each, and Rhizoma Curculiginis Orchioidis (*Xian Mao*), Herba Epimedii (*Xian Ling Pi*), Radix Morindae Officinalis (*Ba Ji Tian*), Radix Angelicae Sinensis (*Dang Gui*), Cortex Phellodendri (*Huang Bai*), and Rhizoma Anemarrhenae Aspheloidis (*Zhi Mu*), 9g each

ANALYSIS OF FORMULA: *Niu Xi* nourishes liver-kidney yin. *Dang Gui* nourishes liver blood and rectifies and regulates the chong and ren. *Xian Ling Pi*, *Xian Mao*, and *Ba Ji Tian* warm and supplement kidney yang. *Huang Bai* and *Zhi Mu* clear vacuity heat and downbear fire. Although *Du Zhong* and *Xian Ling Pi* are warm in nature and supplement yang, they lower the blood pressure.

ADDITIONS & SUBTRACTIONS: If there is simultaneous qi vacuity, add 15 grams of Radix Astragali Membranacei (*Huang Qi*) and nine grams of Radix Codonopsitis Pilosulae (*Dang Shen*). If there are night sweats and hot flashes, add 21 grams of Fructus Levis Tritici Aestivi (*Fu Xiao Mai*) and 12 grams of Concha Ostreae (*Mu Li*). If there is spleen vacuity with loose stools, add nine grams each of Sclerotium Poriae Cocos (*Fu Ling*) and Radix Dioscoreae Oppositae (*Shan Yao*). If there is concomitant blood stasis, add nine grams each of Semen Pruni Persicae (*Tao Ren*) and Flos Carthami Tinctorii (*Hong Hua*). If there is liver depression qi stagnation, add nine grams of Fructus Meliae Toosendan (*Chuan Lian Zi*).

ACUPUNCTURE & MOXIBUSTION: *Qi Hai* (CV 6), *Guan Yuan* (CV 4), *San Yin Jiao* (Sp 6), *Xing Jian* (Liv 2), *Nei Guan* (Per 6)

ANALYSIS OF FORMULA: Supplementing *San Yin Jiao* nourishes and enriches liver-kidney blood and yin as well as rectifies and regulates the chong and ren. Supplementing *Qi Hai* and *Guan Yuan* warms and supplements kidney yang. They also rectify and regulate the chong and ren. Draining *Xing Jian* levels the liver and subdues yang, while draining *Nei Guan* courses the liver, resolves depression, and protects the heart.

ADDITIONS & SUBTRACTIONS: If there is no chest pain or heart palpitations, subtract *Nei Guan* and add *Da Zhui* (GV 14). For vacuity fire flaming upward instead of ascendant liver yang hyperactivity, replace *Xing Jian* with *Ran Gu* (Ki 2). For severe yin vacuity, add *Tai Xi* (Ki 3). For hot flashes or severe hypertension, add *Da Zhui* (GV 14). For night sweats, add *Yin Xi* (Ht 6). For hypertension appearing especially at night, add *Zhao Hai* (Ki 6). For headache in the corner of the head, add *Tou Wei* (St 8). For headache in the temple, needle, then bleed *Tai Yang* (M-HN-9). For headache in the occiput or tension in the neck, add *Shu Gu* (Bl 65). For dizziness, add *Bai Hui* (GV 20). For tension in the trapezius, add *Tian Jing* (GB 21).

5. STATIC BLOOD OBSTRUCTING THE NETWORK VESSELS PATTERN

MAIN SYMPTOMS: Enduring, non-healing dizziness and headache, fixed, unmovable pain, visible varicosities, spider nevi, cherry hemangiomas, a dark, sooty facial complexion, numerous age spots, a dark, purplish tongue or possible static macules or spots, and a bowstring, choppy pulse

NOTE: As in so many other conditions, blood stasis most often complicates other patterns.

TREATMENT PRINCIPLES: Quicken the blood and transform stasis

RX: *Xue Fu Zhu Yu Tang Jia Jian* (Blood Mansion Dispel Stasis Decoction with Additions & Subtractions)

INGREDIENTS: Carapax Amydae Chinensis (*Bie Jia*), Plastrum Testudinis (*Gui Ban*), and Radix Salviae Miltiorrhizae (*Dan Shen*), 15g each, Semen Pruni Persicae (*Tao Ren*), uncooked Radix Rehmanniae (*Sheng Di*), and Radix Cyathulae (*Chuan Niu Xi*), 12g each, Flos Carthami Tinctorii (*Hong Hua*), Radix Angelicae Sinensis (*Dang Gui*), Radix Ligustici Wallichii (*Chuan Xiong*), Radix Rubrus Paeoniae Lactiflorae (*Chi Shao*), Tuber Curcumae (*Yu Jin*), and Fructus Citri Aurantii (*Zhi Ke*), 9g each, and Radix Platycodi Grandiflori (*Jie Geng*), 6g

ANALYSIS OF FORMULA: *Tao Ren*, *Dan Shen*, *Chuan Niu Xi*, *Hong Hua*, *Dang Gui*, *Chuan Xiong*, and *Chi Shao* quicken the blood and transform stasis. *Bei Jia* and *Gui Ban* also dispel stasis at the same time as they subdue yang. *Sheng Di* nourishes yin. *Chuan Niu Xi* downbears the blood. *Yu Jin* and *Zhi Ke* move the qi to quicken the blood. *Hong Hua* and *Dan Shen* specifically lower blood pressure. *Jie Geng* leads the other medicinals in the formula to the upper burner to promote the dispersion of heart blood stasis.

ADDITIONS & SUBTRACTIONS: For chest pain, add *Shi Xiao San* (Loose a Smile Powder), *i.e.*, Feces Trogopterori Seu Pteromi (*Wu Ling Zhi*) and Pollen Typhae (*Pu Huang*), nine grams each. For cyanotic lips and nails and frequent racing heart, add three grams of Radix Pseudoginseng (*San Qi*), powdered and taken with the strained decoction. For qi vacuity, add 15 grams of Radix Astragali Membranacei (*Huang Qi*) and nine grams of Radix Codonopsitis Pilosulae (*Dang Shen*).

ACUPUNCTURE & MOXIBUSTION: *San Yin Jiao* (Sp 6), *Ge Shu* (Bl 17), *Nei Guan* (Per 6), *Zu San Li* (St 36), *Qu Chi* (LI 11)

ANALYSIS OF FORMULA: Draining *San Yin Jiao* and *Ge Shu* quickens the blood and transforms stasis. They are also empirical points for lowering blood pressure. Draining *Zu San Li* and *Qu Chi* are a famous empirical pair for lowering pressure by draining yang evils from the entire body. Draining *Nei Guan* moves the qi and quickens the blood, protects the heart and lowers pressure.

ADDITIONS & SUBTRACTIONS: For concomitant kidney yin vacuity, add *Shen Shu* (Bl 23). For concomitant liver blood vacuity, add *Gan Shu* (Bl 18). For concomitant heart yin vacuity, add *Shen Men* (Ht 7). For concomitant vacuity fire flaming upward, add *Ran Gu* (Ki 2). For concomitant ascendant liver yang hyperactivity, add *Feng Chi* (GB 20). For concomitant liver fire, add *Xing Jian* (Liv 2). For severe hypertension add *Da Zhui* (GV 14). For hypertension appearing especially at night, add *Zhao Hai* (Ki 6). For headache in the corner of the head, add *Tou Wei* (St 8). For headache in the temple, needle, then bleed *Tai Yang* (M-HN-9). For headache in the occiput or tension in the neck, add *Shu Gu* (Bl 65). For dizziness, add *Bai Hui* (GV 20). For tension in the trapezius, add *Tian Jing* (GB 21).

6. PHLEGM TURBIDITY OBSTRUCTING THE CENTER PATTERN

MAIN SYMPTOMS: Head and eye clouding and covering, dizziness heavy-headedness, chest and ductal glomus and oppression, possible nausea, reduced appetite, mostly an obese body, fatigue, somnolence, profuse phlegm and drool, thick, white, slimy tongue fur, and a bowstring, slippery pulse

NOTE: This pattern also tends to complicate other patterns of hypertension.

TREATMENT PRINCIPLES: Dispel dampness, transform phlegm, and lower pressure

RX: *Ban Xia Bai Zhu Tian Ma Tang Jia Jian* (Pinelliae, Atractylodes & Gastrodia Decoction with Additions & Subtractions)

INGREDIENTS: Rhizoma Atractylodis Macrocephalae (*Bai Zhu*) and Semen Coicis Lachryma-jobi (*Yi Yi Ren*), 15g each, Rhizoma Pinelliae Ternatae (*Ban Xia*), Sclerotium Poriae Cocos (*Fu Ling*), and Rhizoma Gastrodiae Elatae (*Tian Ma*), 9g each, Exocarpium Citri Erythrocarpae (*Ju Hong*), 6g, Radix Glycyrrhizae (*Gan Cao*), 3g, uncooked Rhizoma Zingiberis (*Sheng Jiang*), 3 slices, and Fructus Zizyphi Jujubae (*Da Zao*), 3 pieces

ANALYSIS OF FORMULA: *Ban Xia*, *Ju Hong*, and *Fu Ling* transform phlegm and downbear counterflow. With *Tian Ma*, they transform wind phlegm, while *Tian Ma* treats dizziness. *Bai Zhu*, *Yi Yi Ren*, *Fu Ling*, *Zhi Gan Cao*, *Sheng Jiang*, and *Da Zao* fortify the spleen to prevent further phlegm production. In addition, *Sheng Jiang* is a "holy medicinal for vomiting." With *Ban Xia*, it harmonizes the stomach and downbears counterflow.

ADDITIONS & SUBTRACTIONS: For more prominent wind, delete the *Sheng Jiang* and *Da Zao* and add 15 grams of Ramulus Uncariae Cum Uncis (*Gou Teng*) and nine grams each of Rhizoma Acori Graminei (*Shi Chang Pu*) and Bombyx Batryticatus (*Jiang Can*). For concomitant blood stasis, add 15 grams of Radix Salviae Miltiorrhizae (*Dan Shen*) and nine grams of Radix Ligustici Wallichii (*Chuan Xiong*).

ACUPUNCTURE & MOXIBUSTION: *Zu San Li* (St 36), *Qu Chi* (LI 11), *Nei Guan* (Per 6), *Feng Long* (St 40), *Yin Ling Quan* (Sp 9)

ANALYSIS OF FORMULA: *Zu San Li* and *Qu Chi* are a famous empirical combination for lowering pressure by draining yang evils. In this case, using even supplementing-even draining technique on *Zu San Li* also fortifies the spleen to prevent further phlegm accumulation. Draining *Nei Guan* moves the qi to help the transformation of phlegm. It also protects the heart, lowers the blood pressure, and lowers high cholesterol. *Feng Long* is the main or ruling point for transforming phlegm, while *Yin Ling Quan* is a key point for disinhibiting dampness. Together, when drained, they are a main combination for treating phlegm dampness no matter what the disease.

ADDITIONS & SUBTRACTIONS: Please see pattern #5 above.

7. QI & YIN DUAL VACUITY PATTERN

MAIN SYMPTOMS: Dizziness which is provoked or aggravated by exertion, tinnitus, bilateral dry, rough eyes, a dry throat, tidal heat, fatigue, lack of strength, sweating and/or shortness of breath on slight exertion, a fat, pale tongue with teeth-marks on its edges and scanty or no fur, and a fine, forceless, possibly rapid pulse

TREATMENT PRINCIPLES: Supplement both the qi and yin

RX: *Shen Zhe Zhen Qi Tang* (Ginseng & Hematite Settle the Qi Decoction) & *Er Zhi Wan* (Two Ultimates Pills) with additions and subtractions

INGREDIENTS: Os Draconis (*Long Gu*), Concha Ostreae (*Mu Li*), Haemititum (*Dai Zhe Shi*), Radix Astragali Membranacei (*Huang Qi*), and Fructus Ligustri Lucidi (*Nu Zhen Zi*), 15g each, Radix Albus Paeoniae Lactiflorae (*Bai Shao*), Herba Ecliptae Prostratae (*Han Lian Cao*), Radix Dioscoreae Oppositae (*Shan Yao*), and Fructus Corni Officinalis (*Shan Zhu Yu*), 12g each, and Fructus Perillae Frutescentis (*Zi Su Zi*) and Radix Codonopsitis Pilosulae (*Dang Shen*), 9g each

ANALYSIS OF FORMULA: *Huang Qi*, *Dang Shen*, and *Shan Yao* fortify the spleen and boost the qi. *Nu Zhen Zi*, *Han Lian Cao*, and *Shan Zhu Yu* supplement yin to check yang. *Long Gu*, *Mu Li*, and *Dai Zhe Shi* subdue yang. *Bai Shao* nourishes the blood, levels the liver, and constrains yin. *Zi Su Zi* descends the qi, supplements vacuity taxation, and disinhibits both urination and defecation, thus leading yang downward. This treatment also disperses phlegm and moistens the heart and lungs.

ADDITIONS & SUBTRACTIONS: If complicated by blood stasis, add 15 grams each of Carapax Amydae Chinensis (*Bie Jia*) and Radix Salviae Miltiorrhizae (*Dan Shen*). If there is simultaneous liver depression, add nine grams of Fructus Meliae Toosendan (*Chuan Lian Zi*). If there is simultaneous damp heat, add nine grams of Radix Sophorae Flavescentis (*Ku Shen*) and Cortex Phellodendri (*Huang Bai*).

ACUPUNCTURE & MOXIBUSTION: *Fu Liu* (Ki 7), *San Yin Jiao* (Sp 6), *Zu San Li* (St 36), *Bai Hui* (GV 20)

ANALYSIS OF FORMULA: Supplementing *Fu Liu* and *San Yin Jiao* nourishes yin to check yang. Supplementing *Zu San Li* fortifies the spleen, boosts the qi, and upbears the clear. Supplementing *Bai Hui* with moxibustion upbears the yang and leads the qi and blood to the head to nourish the sea of marrow. Also it stops dizziness.

ADDITIONS & SUBTRACTIONS: For night sweats, add *Yin Xi* (Ht 6). For marked kidney yin vacuity, add *Shen Shu* (Bl 23). For marked liver blood vacuity, add *Gan Shu* (Bl 18). For marked heart yin vacuity, add *Shen Men* (Ht 7). For concomitant vacuity fire flaming upward, add *Ran Gu* (Ki 2). For concomitant ascendant liver yang hyperactivity, add *Tai Chong* (Liv 3). For severe dizziness, add *Feng Chi* (GB 20). For severe hypertension, add *Da Zhui* (GV 14). For hypertension appearing especially at night, add *Zhao Hai* (Ki 6). For headache in the corner of the head, add *Tou Wei* (St 8). For headache in the temple, needle and then bleed *Tai Yang* (M-HN-9). For headache in the occiput or tension in the neck, add *Shu Gu* (Bl 65).

8. YIN & YANG DUAL VACUITY PATTERN

MAIN SYMPTOMS: Dizziness, tinnitus, deafness, vexatious heat in the five hearts, possible fear of cold, puffy swelling of the lower limbs, especially around the ankles, impotence, decreased sexual desire, seminal emission, frequent nighttime urination, a pale, tender tongue with possible red tip and/or swollen, red papillae on the tongue root, and a deep, slow, and forceless, floating, surging, or fine, rapid pulse depending on the predominance of yin and yang vacuities

NOTE: The difference between this pattern and disregulation of the chong and ren above is that there are less signs of effulgent fire above and more marked vacuity cold below. This pattern is usually only seen in the elderly.

TREATMENT PRINCIPLES: Foster yin, invigorate yang, and lower pressure

RX: *Shen Qi Wan* (Kidney Qi Pills) & *Er Xian Tang* (Two Immortals Decoction) with additions and subtractions

INGREDIENTS: Plastrum Testudinis (*Gui Ban*), 18g, Ramulus Loranthi Seu Visci (*Sang Ji Sheng*), 15g, Cortex Eucommiae Ulmoidis (*Du Zhong*), 12g, Herba Epimedii (*Xian Ling Pi*), Fructus Corni Officinalis (*Shan Zhu Yu*), cooked Radix Rehmanniae (*Shu Di*), and Cortex Cinnamomi Cassiae (*Rou Gui*), 9g each, and Radix Lateralis Praeparatus Aconiti Carmichaeli (*Fu Zi*), 6g

ANALYSIS OF FORMULA: *Shu Di*, *Shan Zhu Yu*, *Gui Ban*, and *Sang Ji Sheng* nourish kidney yin to check yang. In addition, *Gui Ban* subdues yang and downbears effulgent fire above, while *Sang Ji Sheng* lowers blood pressure. *Rou Gui*, *Du Zhong*, *Xian Ling Pi*, *Shan Zhu Yu*, and *Fu Zi* warm and supplement kidney yang. In addition, *Du Zhong* and *Xian Ling Pi* lower blood pressure. Note that *Rou Gui* and *Fu Zi*, despite their hot natures, do not necessarily raise blood pressure. On the contrary, when used in the right patterns, these two medicinals actually lower the blood pressure.

ACUPUNCTURE & MOXIBUSTION: *Tai Xi* (Ki 3), *San Yin Jiao* (Sp 6), *Shi Men* (CV 5), *Zu San Li* (St 36)

ANALYSIS OF FORMULA: Together, supplementing *Tai Xi* and *San Yin Jiao* nourishes yin and downbears yin vacuity effulgent heat. Supplementing *Zu San Li* fortifies the latter heaven to support the former heaven and also lowers blood pressure. *Shi Men* is an empirical point for lowering blood pressure. When moxaed or warm-needled, it warms the kidneys and boosts the essence.

ADDITIONS & SUBTRACTIONS: Please see pattern #7 above.

REMARKS

1. Acupuncture is usually very effective for bringing down a high systolic pressure within 15-20 minutes of insertion of the needles. It is less effective for reducing an elevated diastolic pressure. Further, it is more effective for draining repletion patterns of hypertension than for supplementing vacuity patterns. A simple but often very effective acupuncture formula for immediately lowering the blood pressure is *Zu San Li* (St 36), *Qu Chi* (LI 11) and *Nei Guan* (Per 6). If there is ascendant liver yang hyperactivity, add *Tai Chong* (Liv 3). If there is yin vacuity, add *San Yin Jiao* (Sp 6). Ear acupuncture with intradermal needles left in place between regularly scheduled body acupuncture sessions may improve the therapeutic effect of acupuncture. It is also possible to use "ion pellets" or radish seeds taped over the selected ear points which the patient stimulates several times per day with finger pressure.

2. Diet, exercise, weight loss, and deep relaxation are all extremely important for the comprehensive treatment of this condition. Some patients also find biofeedback very helpful. Weight loss reduces blood pressure in those with and without hypertension and should be a goal for all hypertensives who are obese or moderately overweight. Because exercise reduces both stress and blood pressure, it is highly recommended as a regular part of a person's lifestyle.

3. Some patients have labile hypertension, and their blood pressure goes up every time they walk into a doctor's office or have their blood pressure taken. This is called "white coat hypertension." If this is suspected, have the patient run in place for 10 minutes and then take their pressure. Then have the patient do a deep relaxation technique for another 10 minutes and take their pressure again. If their blood pressure comes down significantly after either of these short exercises, a diagnosis of labile hypertension should be considered.

4. When taking the blood pressure, it is important to use the right size cuff for the patient's build. If one uses too small a cuff for a patient with a large diameter upper arm, one will get a higher reading than is true. Therefore, one should have several sizes of blood pressure cuffs on hand if one intends to measure patients' blood pressure.

5. Radix Glycyrrhizae (*Gan Cao*) can raise the blood pressure. Therefore, it should be used with care or avoided in patients with hypertension. Radix Panacis Ginseng (*Ren Shen*) can also raise the blood pressure if taken by patients with habitual bodily exuberance and repletion and especially by those with ascendant liver yang hyperactivity and phlegm fire uncomplicated by qi vacuity. In contradistinction, the most common substitute for *Ren Shen*, *i.e.*, Radix Codonopsitis Pilosulae (*Dang Shen*), lowers the blood pressure. Other medicinals which raise the blood pressure include Herba Ephedrae (*Ma Huang*), Cornu Parvum Cervi (*Lu Rong*), Fructus Immaturus Citri Aurantii (*Zhi Shi*), Pericarpium Citri Reticulatae Viride (*Qing Pi*), Radix Angelicae Dahuricae (*Bai Zhi*), Folium Artemisiae Argyii (*Ai Ye*), Fructus Psoraleae Corylifoliae (*Bu Gu Zhi*), Herba Asari Cum Radice (*Xi Xin*), Herba Portulacae Oleraceae (*Ma Chi Xian*), and Folium Menthae Haplocalysis (*Bo He Ye*).

6. Erroneous taiji and qigong practice can actually raise the blood pressure even though these systems of exercise and relaxation are often prescribed to lower the pressure. (Erroneous taiji and qigong can also cause neurological and psychiatric conditions.) Therefore, patients using these systems should be under the direct supervision of a qualified teacher. If blood pressure becomes high while practicing either taiji or qigong, patients should stop their practice until a qualified teacher can assess and modify their practice.

7. According to Chinese dietary therapy, the following common foods and herbs can all help reduce blood pressure: hawthorn fruit, chrysanthemum flower, celery, onion, garlic, carrot, shepherd's purse, apple, pear, and tangerine. Hawthorn fruit is useful for the treatment of essential hypertension accompanied by hyperlipidemia and coronary heart disease. Chrysanthemum flower, celery, and shepherd's purse are used for essential hypertension presenting either liver fire flaming upward or yin vacuity-yang hyperactivity patterns. Onion and garlic can both prevent and lower hypertension.

8. Chinese medicine does not achieve perfectly satisfactory results in lowering the blood pressure and keeping it low. Therefore, the combination of Chinese and Western medicines is often the treatment of choice. In this case, Chinese medicinals may be used to treat those aspects of the patient's condition not covered by the Western medication or can be used to treat the side effects of Western antihypertensive medications. In either cases, one should simply do a pattern discrimination of the patient's signs and symptoms *while on their Western drugs* and proceed accordingly. If the combination of Western and Chinese therapies achieves good reduction in blood pressure, it may be possible for the patient to use a lower dose of their Western medication or even rely solely on Chinese medicinals. However, while this may be both the patient and practitioner's goal, it may not always be possible.

ENDNOTES

[1] He, J. *et al.*, "Effect of Migration on Blood Pressure: The Yi People Study," *Epidemiology*, #2, March, 1991, p. 88-97

[2] Glauser, S.C., Bello, C.T. & Gauser, E.M., "Blood-Cadmium Levels in Normotensive & Untreated Hypertensive Humans," *Lancet*, #1, April, 1976, p. 717-718

[3] "What Are the Drug Treatments for High Blood Pressure?" WebMDHealth, http://my.webmd.com/content/dmk/dmk_article_5462194

34

HYPERTHYROIDISM

Hyperthyroidism is a clinical condition encompassing several specific diseases. Also called thyrotoxicosis, it is characterized by hypermetabolism and elevated serum levels of free thyroid hormones. Some of the diseases which may cause increased synthesis and secretion of thyroid hormones are Grave's disease, an autoimmune disease, anterior pituitary tumors stimulating TSH secretion, molar pregnancy, choriocarcinoma, and various types of thyroiditis. However, the signs and symptoms of hyperthyroidism are the same for almost all types. Common signs and symptoms are goiter, tachycardia, warm, fine, moist skin, tremors, palpitations, nervousness, increased activity, increased sweating, hypersensitivity to heat, increased appetite, weight loss, insomnia, fatigue, weakness, and increased frequency of bowel movements. Eye signs associated with hyperthyroidism include staring, lid lag, lid retraction, and mild degrees of conjunctival injection. Thyroid storm refers to the abrupt onset of more florid symptoms of hyperthyroidism, such as fever, marked weakness and muscle wasting, extreme restlessness and emotional lability, confusion, psychosis, and even coma.

The Western medical diagnosis of hyperthyroidism is based on the patient's history, physical examination, and routine thyroid function tests. Once hyperthyroidism has been established, a thyroid radioactive iodine uptake test may be performed to determine the cause of the hyperthyroidism. In Grave's disease, blood analysis may reveal antibodies against the thyroid TSH receptors. Depending upon its etiology, the Western medical treatment of hyperthyroidism may consist of administration of iodine. Propylthiouracil and methimazole are both antithyroid drugs which decrease the organification of iodine and impair the coupling reaction. Beta-blockers, such as propranolol, may help control the symptoms of hyperthyroidism due to adrenergic stimulation. In the United States, radioactive sodium iodine is the most common treatment of hyperthyroidism. It is the treatment of choice for Grave's disease and toxic nodular goiter. It works by ablating all or part of the thyroid. Consequently, 25% of patients prescribed this drug go on to become hypothyroid within one year of its use, with the incidence of hypothyroidism continuing to increase yearly thereafter. Surgical treatment, *i.e.*, ablation, is indicated for younger patients with Grave's disease whose disease has recurred after courses of antithyroid drug and who refuse radioactive sodium iodine.

CHINESE DISEASE CATEGORIZATION: Hyperthyroidism mainly comes under the category of *ying qi* or *qi ying*, goiter, in Chinese medicine. In terms of its main clinical manifestations, it may also be categorized as *xiao ke*, wasting and thirsting, *shi yi*, eating again, as in rapid hungering after eating, *jing ji*, fright palpitations, *zheng chong*, fearful throbbing, etc.

DISEASE CAUSES: Internal damage by the seven affects, unregulated eating and drinking, aging, enduring disease

DISEASE MECHANISMS: The mechanisms of this disease are closely related to the liver. Mostly it is due to internal damage by the seven affects. If liver depression is not outthrust, the qi mechanism may become depressed and stagnant. Then dampness and phlegm may congeal and bind. It is also possible for enduring depression to transform into fire. If phlegm is drafted up to the heart by depressive heat, the orifices of the heart may be confounded by phlegm and the heart spirit may be harassed by fire. If depressive heat or fire endure, they may burn and damage yin fluids, thus resulting in yin vacuity with fire effulgence. Since "strong fire eats qi," this may further result in qi and yin both becoming damaged. If liver fire assails the stomach, the stomach may become hot. If a replete liver assails the spleen, the spleen becomes vacuous and weak. Therefore, though the liver is typically at the center of the disease mechanisms associated with the production of all the clinical manifestations of this disease, it also involves the heart, stomach, spleen, and kidneys.

In particular, goiter tends to be due to a combination of liver depression and phlegm. Heart palpitations, agitation, and restlessness are mostly due to phlegm and heat harassing the heart spirit. Excessive appetite and rapid hungering are due to stomach heat. Weakness and fatigue are due to spleen vacuity. Tremors and shaking are due to liver heat stirring wind and to liver-kidney yin vacuity not nourishing the sinew vessels. Staring eyes (actually bulging eyes) are due to liver fire, phlegm, and qi counterflowing upward and congealing and gathering in the eyes. And loose stools are due to liver wood assailing the spleen.

TREATMENT BASED ON PATTERN DISCRIMINATION:

1. QI STAGNATION & PHLEGM CONGELATION PATTERN

MAIN SYMPTOMS: Goiter swelling in the front of the neck which is soft and not painful, possible nodulations on the thyroid gland, possible exophthalmia or a sensation of distention in the eyes, emotional depression, frequent suspicion, irritability, easy anger, a tendency to taciturnity, chest oppression, rib-side pain, a tendency to great sighing, a pale red tongue with thin, slimy fur, and a bowstring, slippery pulse

TREATMENT PRINCIPLES: Course the liver and rectify the qi, transform phlegm and scatter nodulation

RX: *Xiao Chai Hu Tang* (Minor Bupleurum Decoction) & *Xiao Yao San* (Rambling Powder) with additions and subtractions

INGREDIENTS: Spica Prunellae Vulgaris (*Xia Ku Cao*), 15g, Concha Ostreae (*Mu Li*), Bulbus Fritillariae Thunbergii (*Zhe Bei Mu*), and Sclerotium Poriae Cocos (*Fu Ling*), 12g each, Radix Bupleuri (*Chai Hu*), Radix Codonopsitis Pilosulae (*Dang Shen*), Rhizoma Atractylodis Macrocephalae (*Bai Zhu*), Radix Angelicae Sinensis (*Dang Gui*), Radix Albus Paeoniae Lactiflorae (*Bai Shao*), Thallus Algae (*Kun Bu*), and Rhizoma Pinelliae Ternatae (*Ban Xia*), 9g each, Pericarpium Citri Reticulatae (*Chen Pi*) and mix-fried Radix Glycyrrhizae (*Gan Cao*), 6g each Fructus Zizyphi Jujubae (*Da Zao*), 3 pieces, and uncooked Rhizoma Zingiberis (*Sheng Jiang*), 3 slices

ANALYSIS OF FORMULA: *Chai Hu*, *Bai Shao*, and *Xia Ku Cao* course and harmonize the liver, thus resolving depression. *Zhe Bei Mu*, *Kun Bu*, *Fu Ling*, *Ban Xia*, and *Chen Pi* transform phlegm, while *Dang Shen*, *Bai Zhu*, *Fu Ling*, mix-fried *Gan Cao*, and *Sheng Jiang* fortify the spleen and dry dampness to prevent further phlegm engenderment. In addition, *Xia Ku Cao*, *Mu Li*, *Zhe Bei Mu*, and *Kun Bu* soften the hard, scatter nodulation, and treat goiter.

ADDITIONS & SUBTRACTIONS: If there is not just depression but depressive heat, add 15 grams of Radix Scrophulariae Ningpoensis (*Xuan Shen*) and 12 grams of Radix Scutellariae Baicalensis (*Huang Qin*). If enduring heat has damaged stomach fluids, add 12 grams of Tuber Ophiopogonis Japonici (*Mai Dong*) and Radix Trichosanthis Kirlowii (*Tian Hua Fen*). If there is vexation and agitation and heart palpitations, add 12 grams of Os Draconis (*Long Gu*) and 3-6 grams of Rhizoma Coptidis Chinensis (*Huang Lian*). For insomnia, add 12 grams each of Cortex Albizziae Julibrissinis (*He Huan Pi*), Caulis Polygoni Multiflori (*Ye Jiao Teng*), and Semen Zizyphi Spinosae (*Suan Zao Ren*). For fatigue, add 20 grams of Radix Astragali Membranacei (*Huang Qi*). For increased appetite, add 15 grams of Gypsum Fibrosum (*Shi Gao*) and nine grams of Rhizoma Anemarrhenae Asphodeloidis (*Zhi Mu*). For aversion to heat with sweating, add nine grams each of Fructus Gardeniae Jasminoidis (*Zhi Zi*) and Radix Salviae Miltiorrhizae (*Dan Shen*). For loose stools, increase the dosage of *Dang Shen*, *Bai Zhu*, *Fu Ling*, and *Chen Pi*. For tremors of the hand or fingers, add 15 grams each of Bombyx Batryticatus (*Jiang Can*) and Periostracum Cicadae (*Chan Tui*). For severe goiter, add nine grams each of Rhizoma Dioscoreae Bulberiferae (*Huang Yao Zi*), Rhizoma Sparganii (*San Leng*), and Rhizoma Curcumae Zedoariae (*E Zhu*). For concomitant blood vacuity, add nine grams each of Radix Angelicae Sinensis (*Dang Gui*) and Radix Salviae Miltiorrhizae (*Dan Shen*). For leukopenia, add 15 grams each of Radix Astragali Membranacei (*Huang Qi*) and Caulis Milletiae Seu Spatholobi (*Ji Xue Teng*) and nine grams of Gelatinum Cornu Cervi (*Lu Jiao Jiao*). For a sensation of throat obstruction, add 12 grams of Rhizoma Belamcandae Chinensis (*She Gan*). For severe liver depression qi stagnation, add six grams of Pericarpium Citri Reticulatae Viride (*Qing Pi*).

ACUPUNCTURE & MOXIBUSTION: *Tai Chong* (Liv 3), *Feng Long* (St 40), *Nao Hui* (TB 13), *Tian Chuang* (SI 16), *Tian Ding* (LI 17), *Tian Rong* (SI 17), *Tian Tu* (CV 22)

ANALYSIS OF FORMULA: *Tai Chong* rectifies the qi and resolves depression. *Feng Long* transforms phlegm. *Tian Chuang*, *Tian Ding*, *Tian Rong*, and *Tian Tu* soften the hard and scatter nodulation. *Nao Hui* courses and frees the flow of the three burners and disperses goiter qi. Needle all these points with draining method.

ADDITIONS & SUBTRACTIONS: For severe liver depression, add *Yang Ling Quan* (GB 34). If there is depressive heat, add *Yang Ling Quan* (GB 34) and replace *Tai Chong* with *Xing Jian* (Liv 2). For concomitant spleen qi vacuity with fatigue and loose stools, add *Zu San Li* (St 36). For exophthalmia or a sensation of distention in the eyes, add *Jing Ming* (Bl 1), *Feng Chi* (GB 20), and *Tai Yang* (M-HN-9). For marked irritability, easy anger, and emotional depression, add *Jian Shi* (Per 5) and *Shen Ting* (GV 24). For insomnia and heart palpitations, add *Nei Guan* (Per 6) and *Shen Men* (Ht 7). For increased appetite, add *Zhong Wan* (CV 12) and *Nei Ting* (St 44). For aversion to heat with sweating, also add *He Gu* (LI 4) and *Nei Ting* (St 44). For tremors of the hands or fingers, add *He Gu* (LI 4).

2. LIVER FIRE HYPERACTIVITY & EXUBERANCE PATTERN

MAIN SYMPTOMS: Marked goiter which is soft and not painful, possible nodulations, possible exophthalmia, emotional tension, irritability, impetuosity, a red face and eyes, headache, dizziness, head distention, tinnitus, tongue and hand shaking and trembling, heart palpitations, insomnia, dread of heat, profuse sweating, rapid hungering with increased food intake, oral thirst with profuse drinking, a bitter taste in the mouth, a red tongue with yellow fur, and a bowstring, rapid pulse

NOTE: In this case, although the pattern name does not say so, there is still phlegm nodulation.

TREATMENT PRINCIPLES: Clear the liver and drain fire, transform phlegm and scatter nodulation

RX: *Long Dan Xie Gan Tang Jia Jian* (Gentiana Scabra Drain the Liver Decoction with Additions & Subtractions)

INGREDIENTS: Spica Prunellae Vulgaris (*Xia Ku Cao*) and Radix Scrophulariae Ningpoensis, 15g each, uncooked Radix Rehmanniae (*Sheng Di*), Concha Ostreae (*Mu Li*), Os Draconis (*Long Gu*), Rhizoma Pinelliae Ternatae (*Ban Xia*), Sclerotium Poriae Cocos (*Fu Ling*), and Bulbus Fritillariae Thunbergii (*Zhe Bei Mu*), 12g each, Radix Bupleuri (*Chai Hu*), Radix Scutellariae Baicalensis (*Huang Qin*), Fructus Gardeniae Jasminoidis (*Zhi Zi*), Extremitas Radicis Angelicae Sinensis (*Dang Gui Wei*), Herba Sargassii (*Hai Zao*), and Thallus Algae (*Kun Bu*), 9g each, Pericarpium Citri Reticulatae (*Chen Pi*), 6g, and uncooked Radix Glycyrrhizae (*Gan Cao*), 3g

ANALYSIS OF FORMULA: *Xia Ku Cao*, *Huang Qin*, and *Zhi Zi* clear the liver and drain fire. *Ban Xia*, *Fu Ling*, *Zhe Bei Mu*, *Hai Zao*, and *Kun Bu* transform phlegm. *Mu Li* and *Long Gu* level the liver and subdue yang. *Chai Hu* courses the liver and resolves depression. *Dang Gui Wei* quickens the blood and transforms stasis. *Chen Pi* rectifies the qi. *Sheng Di* nourishes and protects liver yin. *Xia Ku Cao*, *Xuan Shen*, *Mu Li*, *Ban Xia*, *Zhe Bei Mu*, *Hai Zao*, and *Kun Bu* soften the hard, scatter nodulation, and treat goiter, and *Gan Cao* harmonizes the other medicinals in this formula.

ADDITIONS & SUBTRACTIONS: If the stomach is strong and hot and the spleen is vacuous and weak, replace *Long Dan Xie Gan Tang* with *Bai Hu Jia Ren Shen Tang* (White Tiger Plus Ginseng Decoction) plus *Xiang Sha Liu Jun Zi Tang* (Auklandia & Amomum Six Gentlemen Decoction) with additions and subtractions: Gypsum Fibrosum (*Shi Gao*), 30g, Rhizoma Anemarrhenae Aspheloidis (*Zhi Mu*) and Rhizoma Pinelliae Ternatae (*Ban Xia*), 12g each, Radix Codonopsitis Pilosulae (*Dang Shen*), Rhizoma Atractylodis Macrocephalae (*Bai Zhu*), and Sclerotium Poriae Cocos (*Fu Ling*), 9g each, Pericarpium Citri Reticulatae (*Chen Pi*), Radix Auklandiae Lappae (*Mu Xiang*), and mix-fried Radix Glycyrrhizae (*Gan Cao*), 6g each. If there is concomitant phlegm nodulation, add 15 grams each of Spica Prunellae Vulgaris (*Xia Ku Cao*) and Radix Scrohulariae Ningpoensis (*Xuan Shen*), 12 grams of Bulbus Fritillariae Thunbergii (*Zhe Bei Mu*), and nine grams each of Concha Ostreae (*Mu Li*), Thallus Algae (*Kun Bu*), and Herba Sargassii (*Hai Zao*). For severe goiter, add nine grams each of Rhizoma Dioscoreae Bulberiferae (*Huang Yao Zi*), Rhizoma Sparganii (*San Leng*), and Rhizoma Curcumae Zedoariae (*E Zhu*). For hand shaking and trembling, add 15 grams of Concha Haliotidis (*Shi Jue Ming*), and nine grams each of Ramulus Uncariae Cum Uncis (*Gou Teng*) and Radix Albus Paeoniae Lactiflorae (*Bai Shao*). For insomnia, emotional tension, irritability, and impetuosity add 12 grams each of Cortex Albizziae Julibrissinis (*He Huan Pi*), Caulis Polygoni Multiflori (*Ye Jiao Teng*), and Semen Zizyphi Spinosae (*Suan Zao Ren*). For fatigue add 20 grams of Radix Astragali Membranacei (*Huang Qi*). For increased appetite due to stomach heat, add 15 grams of uncooked Radix Rehmanniae (*Sheng Di*) and nine grams of Rhizoma Anemarrhenae Asphodeloidis (*Zhi Mu*). For constipation, add 6-9 grams of Radix Et Rhizoma Rhei (*Da Huang*). For loose stools due to spleen vacuity, add 12 grams of Radix Codonopsitis Pilosulae (*Dang Shen*) and Rhizoma Atractylodis Macrocephalae (*Bai Zhu*). For a sensation of throat obstruction, add 12 grams of Rhizoma Belamcandae Chinensis (*She Gan*). For oral thirst with profuse drinking, add 12 grams each of Tuber Ophiopogonis Japonici (*Mai Men Dong*) and Radix Trichosanthis Kirlowii (*Tian Hua Fen*). For profuse sweating, add 15 grams each of Semen Levis Tritici Aestivi (*Fu Xiao Mai*) and Fructus Schisandrae Chinensis (*Wu Wei Zi*). For a sensation of pain and distention in the eyes, add 15 grams each of Radix Angelicae Dahuricae (*Bai Zhi*) and Fructus Lycii Chinensis (*Gou Qi Zi*) and nine grams each of Rhizoma Acori Graminei (*Shi Chang Pu*) and Fructus Tribuli Terrestris (*Bai Ji Li*).

ACUPUNCTURE & MOXIBUSTION: *Xing Jian* (Liv 2), *Yang Ling Quan* (GB 34), *Nao Hui* (TB 13), *Tian Chuang* (SI 16), *Tian Ding* (LI 17), *Tian Rong* (SI 17), *Tian Tu* (CV 22)

ANALYSIS OF FORMULA: *Xing Jian* and *Yang Ling Quan* clear the liver and drain fire, rectify the qi and resolve depression. *Tian Chuang*, *Tian Ding*, *Tian Rong*, and *Tian Tu* transform phlegm, soften the hard, and scatter nodulation. *Nao Hui* courses and frees the flow of the three burners and disperses the goiter. Needle all these points with draining method.

ADDITIONS & SUBTRACTIONS: For exophthalmia or a sensation of distention in the eyes, add *Jing Ming* (Bl 1), *Feng Chi* (GB 20), and *Tai Yang* (M-HN-9). For marked irritability, easy anger, and emotional depression, add *Jian Shi* (Per 5) and *Shen Ting* (GV 24). For insomnia and heart palpitations, add *Nei Guan* (Per 6) and *Shen Men* (Ht 7). For loose stools and fatigue, add *Zu San Li* (St 36). For constipation, add *Zhi Gou* (TB 6). For increased appetite, add *Zhong Wan* (CV 12) and *Nei Ting* (St 44). For aversion to heat with sweating, add *He Gu* (LI 4) and *Nei Ting* (St 44). For tremors of the hands or fingers, add *He Gu* (LI 4). For a sensation of throat obstruction, add *Liang Quan* (CV 23) and *Tong Li* (Ht 5). For profuse sweating, add *Fu Liu* (Ki 7) and *He Gu* (LI 4).

3. YIN VACUITY, YANG HYPERACTIVITY PATTERN

MAIN SYMPTOMS: Large or small goiter, possible nodulations, possible exopthalmia or a tense feeling in the region of the eyes, vexatious heat in the five hearts, insomnia or scanty sleep, profuse dreams, dizziness, blurred vision, heart palpitations, restlessness, easy sweating, dread of heat, hot flashes, a red facial complexion, shaking hands, tinnitus, rough eyes, low back and knee soreness and limpness, increased food intake but emaciation, lack of strength, dryness of the mouth and throat, a red tongue with scanty fur, and a bowstring, fine, rapid pulse

NOTE: As with the pattern above, there is no mention of phlegm nodulation in the pattern name. However, if there is palpable enlargement or nodulation of the thyroid, there is phlegm nodulation. In addition, there is also still liver depression.

TREATMENT PRINCIPLES: Enrich yin and subdue yang, transform phlegm and scatter nodulation

RX: *Tian Wan Bu Xin Dan* (Heavenly Emperor Supplement the Heart Elixir) & *Yi Guan Jian* (One Link Decoction) with additions and subtractions

INGREDIENTS: Uncooked Radix Rehmanniae (*Sheng Di*), Radix Scrophulariae Ningpoensis (*Xuan Shen*), and Rhizoma Dioscoreae Bulbiferae (*Huang Yao Zi*), 15g each, Tuber Ophiopogonis Japonici (*Mai Dong*), Tuber Asparagi Cochinensis (*Tian Men Dong*), Fructus Lycii Chinensis (*Gou Qi Zi*), Semen Zizyphi Spinosae (*Suan Zao Ren*), Os Draconis (*Long Gu*), Concha Ostreae (*Mu Li*), and Sclerotium Poriae Cocos (*Fu Ling*), 12g each, Fructus Meliae Toosendan (*Chuan Lian Zi*), Radix Polygalae Tenuifoliae (*Yuan Zhi*), Fructus Schisandrae Chinensis (*Wu Wei Zi*), Semen Biotae Orientalis (*Bai Zi Ren*), Rhizoma Pinelliae Ternatae (*Ban Xia*), Herba Sargassii (*Hai Zao*), and Thallus Algae (*Kun Bu*), 9g each, Pericarpium Citri Reticulatae (*Chen Pi*), 6g, and Rhizoma Coptidis Chinensis (*Huang Lian*), 3g

ANALYSIS OF FORMULA: *Sheng Di, Mai Men Dong, Tian Men Dong, Gou Qi Zi, Suan Zao Ren, Yuan Zhi, Wu Wei Zi,* and *Bai Zi Ren* supplement the yin and blood of the heart and liver. *Long Gu* and *Mu Li* level the liver, subdue yang, and quiet the spirit. *Xuan Shen, Huang Yao Zi, Mu Li, Hai Zao,* and *Kun Bu* soften the hard, scatter nodulation, and treat goiter, while *Ban Xia, Chen Pi,* and *Fu Ling* transform phlegm. *Chuan Lian Zi* courses the liver and resolves depression, and *Huang Lian* clears the stomach, heart, and liver.

ADDITIONS & SUBTRACTIONS: If yin vacuity is severe, add 12 grams each of Plastrum Testudinis (*Gui Ban*), Radix Polygoni Multiflori (*He Shou Wu*), and Fructus Ligustri Lucidi (*Nu Zhen Zi*). If effulgent fire is severe, add nine grams of Cortex Phellodendri (*Huang Bai*). If liver yang rises up suddenly giving engendering internal wind, add 15 grams of Ramulus Uncariae Cum Uncis (*Gou Teng*) and nine grams of Bombyx Batryticatus (*Jiang Can*). If there is concomitant qi vacuity, add nine grams of Radix Codonopsitis Pilosulae (*Dang Shen*). For concomitant liver depression transforming into heat or for severe goiter, add 12 grams of Spica Prunellae Vulgaris (*Xia Ku Cao*). For marked liver-kidney yin vacuity, add 15 grams each of Radix Achyranthis Bidentatae (*Niu Xi*) and Ramulus Loranthi Seu Visci (*Sang Ji Sheng*). For marked ascendant liver yang hyperactivity, add 15 grams of Concha Margaritiferae (*Zhen Zhu Mu*) and nine grams of Ramulus Uncariae Cum Uncis (*Gou Teng*). For dizziness, add 15 grams each of Rhizoma Gastrodiae Elatae (*Tian Ma*) and Radix Polygoni Multiflori (*He Shou Wu*). For protrusion of the eyes, add 12 grams each of Semen Cassiae Torae (*Jue Ming Zi*) and Semen Celosiae Argentae (*Qing Xiang Zi*). For thirst, add nine grams each of Fructus Pruni Mume (*Wu Mei*) and Herba Dendrobii (*Shi Hu*). For leukopenia, add 12 grams each of Radix Et Rhizoma Polygoni Cuspidati (*Hu Zhang*) and Plastrum Testudinis (*Gui Ban*). For rapid hungering and thirst, add 15 grams of Gypsum Fibrosum (*Shi Gao*) and nine grams of Rhizoma Anemarrhenae Asphodeloidis (*Zhi Mu*). For constipation, add 6-9 grams of Radix Et Rhizoma Rhei (*Da Huang*). For loose or frequent stools, add 15 grams of Rhizoma Atractylodis Macrocephalae (*Bai Zhu*).

ACUPUNCTURE & MOXIBUSTION: *Tai Chong* (Liv 3), *Shen Men* (Ht 7), *Fu Liu* (Ki 7), *Nao Hui* (TB 13), *Tian Chuang* (SI 16), *Tian Ding* (LI 17), *Tian Rong* (SI 17), *Ren Ying* (St 9)

ANALYSIS OF FORMULA: *Tai Chong* levels the liver and subdues yang. *Shen Men* nourishes the heart and quiets the spirit. *Fu Liu* nourishes true yin to check ascendant yang. *Tian Chuang, Tian Ding, Tian Rong,* and *Ren Ying* transform phlegm, soften the hard, and scatter nodulation. *Nao Hui* courses and frees the flow of the three burners and disperses goiter. Needle all these points with draining method except *Shen Men* and *Fu Liu* which should be supplemented.

ADDITIONS & SUBTRACTIONS: For dizziness, add *Feng Chi* (GB 20). For rough eyes and blurred vision, add *Guang Ming* (GB 37). For hot flashes in the face, add *Yin Xi* (Ht 6) and *Da Zhui* (GV 14). For tinnitus, add *Ting Hui* (GB 2). For low back and knee soreness and limpness, add *Shen Shu* (Bl 23). For exopthalmia or a sensation of distention in the eyes, add *Jing Ming* (Bl 1), *Feng Chi* (GB 20), and *Tai Yang* (M-HN-9). For marked heart palpitations, add *Nei Guan* (Per 6). For lack of strength and frequent or loose stools due to spleen vacuity, add *Zu San Li* (St 36). For constipation, add *Zhi Gou* (TB 6). For increased appetite, add *Zhong Wan* (CV 12) and *Nei Ting* (St 44). For aversion to heat with sweating, add *He Gu* (LI 4) and *Nei Ting* (St 44). For tremors of the hands or fingers, add *He Gu* (LI 4). For a sensation of throat obstruction, add *Liang Quan* (CV 23) and *Tong Li* (Ht 5). For profuse sweating, add *He Gu* (LI 4).

4. QI & YIN DUAL VACUITY PATTERN

MAIN SYMPTOMS: Essence spirit lassitude and fatigue, shortness of breath, dizziness, tinnitus, heart palpitations, emaciation, lack of strength, dry, rough eyes with a possible distended feeling, a pale, lusterless facial complexion with possible malar flushing, restlessness, insomnia, impaired memory, a dry mouth and parched throat, a tasteless feeling in the mouth, low back and knee soreness and weakness, low-grade fever or heat in the hands, feet, and heart, possible sweating, possible tremors of the hands and tongue, scanty intake, abdominal distention after eating, loose stools, a red tongue with thin or peeled, shedding fur, and a vacuous, rapid pulse

TREATMENT PRINCIPLES: Boost the qi and nourish yin

RX: *Jia Kang Zhong Fang* (Heavy Hyperthyroid Formula)

INGREDIENTS: Radix Astragali Membranacei (*Huang Qi*), 30-45g, Spica Prunellae Vulgaris (*Xia Ku Cao*), 30g, Radix Polygoni Multiflori (*He Shou Wu*), 20g, uncooked Radix Rehmanniae (*Sheng Di*), 15g, and Radix Albus Paeoniae Lactiflorae (*Bai Shao*) and Rhizoma Cyperi Rotundi (*Xiang Fu*), 12g each

ANALYSIS OF FORMULA: *Huang Qi* fortifies the spleen and boosts the qi. *He Shou Wu, Sheng Di,* and *Bai Shao* nourish the blood and enrich yin, supplement and boost the liver and kidneys. *Xia Ku Cao* clears the liver, softens the hard, and scatters nodulation, and *Xiang Fu* courses the liver and resolves depression.

ADDITIONS & SUBTRACTIONS: For spleen vacuity loose stools, delete uncooked *Sheng Di* and add 12 grams of Radix Dioscoreae Oppositae (*Shan Yao*), nine grams of Rhizoma Atractylodis Macrocephalae (*Bai Zhu*), and 6 grams of Massa Medica Fermentata (*Shen Qu*). If there are bulging, swollen, distended eyes, add 15 grams of Fructus Lycii Chinensis (*Gou Qi Zi*) and nine grams each of Semen Sinapis Albae (*Bai Jie Zi*), Rhizoma Alismatis (*Ze Xie*), Semen Raphani Sativi (*Lai Fu Zi*), Cortex Radicis Lycii Chinensis (*Di Gu Pi*), and Fructus Tribuli Terrestris (*Bai Ji Li*). If there is heart fire effulgence, add 6-9 grams of Rhizoma Coptidis Chinensis (*Huang Lian*). If there is liver fire effulgence, add six grams of Radix Gentianae Scabrae (*Long Dan Cao*). For severe heart palpitations, fatigue, and shortness of breath, add *Sheng Mai San* (Engender the Pulse Powder), *i.e.,* Radix Panacis Ginseng (*Ren Shen*), 6g, Tuber Ophiopogonis Japonici (*Mai Men Dong*), 9g, and Fructus Schisandrae Chinensis (*Wu Wei Zi*), 6g, plus 12 grams of Semen Zizyphi Spinosae (*Suan Zao Ren*). For severe sweating, add 30 grams of Semen Levis Tritici Aestivi (*Fu Xiao Mai*) and 12 grams of Radix Ephedrae (*Ma Huang Gen*). For severe goiter, add nine grams each of Rhizoma Dioscoreae Bulberiferae (*Huang Yao Zi*) and Radix Scrophulariae Ningpoensis (*Xuan Shen*) and 30 grams of Concha Ostreae (*Mu Li*). For dizziness, add 15 grams each of Fructus Lycii Chinensis (*Gou Qi Zi*) and Flos Chrysanthemi Morifolii (*Ju Hua*). For yin vacuity with internal stirring of wind, add 15 grams each of Plastrum Testudinis (*Gui Ban*), Carapax Amydae Sinensis (*Bie Jia*), and Concha Margaritiferae (*Zhen Zhu Mu*).

ACUPUNCTURE & MOXIBUSTION: *Xin Shu* (Bl 15), *Gan Shu* (Bl 18), *Pi Shu* (Bl 20), *Shen Shu* (Bl 23), *Nao Hui* (TB 13), *Tian Chuang* (SI 16), *Tian Ding* (LI 17), *Tian Rong* (SI 17)

ANALYSIS OF FORMULA: Supplementing, *Xin Shu, Gan Shu,* and *Shen Shu* nourishes the yin of the heart, liver, and kidneys, while *Pi Shu* fortifies the spleen and boosts the qi. Draining *Tian Chuang, Tian Ding,* and *Tian Rong* soften the hard and scatter nodulation, while draining *Nao Hui* courses and frees the flow of the three burners and disperses goiter.

ADDITIONS & SUBTRACTIONS: For marked heart yin vacuity, add *Shen Men* (Ht 7). For marked liver-kidney yin vacuity, add *Fu Liu* (Ki 7). For marked spleen qi vacuity, add *Zu San Li* (St 36). For essence spirit lassitude and fatigue with poor memory, add *Si Shen Cong* (M-HN-1). For dizziness, add *Feng Chi* (GB 20). For rough eyes and/or blurred vision, add *Guang Ming* (GB 37). For hot flashes in the face, add *Yin Xi* (Ht 6) and *Da Zhui* (GV 14). For tinnitus, add *Ting Hui* (GB 2). For low back and knee soreness and limpness, add *Zhi Shi* (Bl 52). For exopthalmia or a sensation of distention in the eyes, add *Jing Ming* (Bl 1), *Feng Chi* (GB 20), and *Tai Yang* (M-HN-9). For marked heart palpitations, add *Nei Guan* (Per 6). For increased appetite, add *Zhong Wan* (CV 12) and *Nei Ting* (St 44). For tremors of the hands or fingers, add *He Gu* (LI 4) and *Tai Chong* (Liv 3). For a sensation of throat obstruction, add *Liang Quan* (CV 23) and *Tong Li* (Ht 5). For profuse sweating, add *He Gu* (LI 4) and *Fu Liu* (Ki 7).

REMARKS

1. The disease mechanisms of this condition are a combination of vacuity and repletion. The root vacuities in this condition are mainly yin vacuity, qi vacuity, and, if severe, yang vacuity. The branch repletions are qi stagnation, phlegm congelation, and blood stasis.

2. During the initial stage of this disease, liver depression and phlegm nodulation is the most common pattern. Therefore, one should mainly out-thrust depressed wood. During the middle stage, the emphasis is usually on clearing the liver and draining heat. At this stage, the disease is mostly in the liver, heart, and stomach. During the latter stage, the emphasis is mostly on supplementing qi and yin vacuities. At this stage, the disease is primarily in the liver, heart, spleen, and kidneys.

3. Medicinals which scatter phlegm nodulation in the region of the throat include Spica Prunellae Vulgaris (*Xia Ku Cao*), Radix Scrophulariae Ningpoensis (*Xuan Shen*), and Rhizoma Dioscoreae Bulbiferae (*Huang Yao Zi*). Prunella tends to be used more for repletion patterns, while Dioscoreae Bulberifera is used more for vacuity patterns and especially qi vacuity. Scrophulariae can be used for either repletion or vacuity. Medicinals which transform phlegm and scatter nodulation include Rhizoma Pinelliae Ternatae (*Ban Xia*), Semen Sinapis Albae (*Bai Jie Zi*), and Bulbus Fritillariae Thunbergii (*Zhe Bei Mu*). And medicinals which soften the hard and scatter nodulation include Os Draconis (*Long Gu*), Concha Ostreae (*Mu Li*), Concha Meretricis (*Hai Ge Ke*), Pumice (*Hai Fu Shi*), Thallus Algae (*Kun Bu*), Herba Sargassii (*Hai Zao*), and Herba Laminariae (*Hai Dai*).

4. When Radix Astragali Membranacei (*Huang Qi*) is used in heavy doses (25-50g), it can lower T3 & T4, and effectively treats hyperthyroidism. Rhizoma Dioscoreae Bulberiferae (*Huang Yao Zi*) is another important medicinal for hyperthyroidism. However, it is hepatotoxic. Therefore, its dose should not exceed 10 grams and should only be used for a limited period of time.

5. Because hyperthyroidism is basically a yin-yang imbalance with yang surplus causing heat and stirring and yin vacuity resulting in lack of stillness and quiet, it is important to also modify the diet and lifestyle in cases of hyperthyroidism. In terms of lifestyle, stress and taxation should both be minimized. In terms of diet, one should avoid acrid, hot, drying, and stimulating foods, such as hot spices, alcohol, coffee and strong tea, etc. On the other hand, if there are spleen vacuity and phlegm, one should avoid uncooked, chilled foods as well as oils and fats, including those in dairy products such as milk and cheese.

6. The following modern formulas all treat complex multi-pattern presentations:

Ping Ying Fu Fang (Level Goiter Compound Formula) treats a yin blood vacuity with qi and blood stagnation and phlegm nodulation. It consists of: Concha Ostreae (*Mu Li*), 20g, Spica Prunellae Vulgaris (*Xia Ku Cao*), 15g, Concha Arcae (*Wa Leng Zi*), Radix Scrophulariae Ningpoensis (*Xuan Shen*), Radix Albus Paeoniae Lactiflorae (*Bai Shao*), Cortex Radicis Moutan (*Dan Pi*), uncooked Radix Rehmanniae (*Sheng Di*), Radix Angelicae Sinensis (*Dang Gui*), and Sclerotium Poriae Cocos (*Fu Ling*), 12g each, and Fructus Corni Officinalis (*Shan Zhu Yu*), Bulbus Fritillariae Thunbergii (*Zhe Bei Mu*), Pericarpium Citri Reticulatae Viride (*Qing Pi*), Pericarpium Citri Reticulatae (*Chen Pi*), Rhizoma Sparganii (*San Leng*), and Rhizoma Curcumae Zedoariae (*E Zhu*), 9g each.

Jia Kang Ping (Hyperthyroidism Balancer) treats qi and yin vacuity with phlegm nodulation. It consists of: Radix Pseustellariae Heterophyllae (*Tai Zi Shen*) and Concha Ostreae (*Mu Li*), 30g each, uncooked Radix Rehmanniae (*Sheng Di*) and Concha Cyclinae Sinensis (*Hai Ge Ke*), 15g each, Herba Dendrobii (*Shi Hu*), Bulbus Fritillariae Thunbergii (*Zhe Bei Mu*), and Spica Prunellae Vulgaris (*Xia Ku Cao*), 12g each, and Tuber Ophiopogonis Japonici (*Mai Men Dong*) and Radix Scrophulariae Ningpoensis (*Xuan Shen*), 9g each.

Jia Kang Jian Tang (Hyperthyroidism Decoction) treats qi and yin vacuity with liver depression transforming heat and phlegm nodulation. It consists of: Radix Albus Paeoniae Lactiflorae (*Bai Shao*), Fructus Pruni Mume (*Wu Mei*), Fructus Chaenomelis Lagenariae (*Mu Gua*), Radix Glehniae Littoralis (*Sha Shen*), Tuber Ophiopogonis Japonici (*Mai Men Dong*), Herba Dendrobii (*Shi Hu*), Semen Dolichoris Lablab (*Bai Bian Dou*), and Semen Nelumbinis Nuciferae (*Lian Zi*), 12g each, Thallus Algae (*Kun Bu*) and Herba Sargassii (*Hai Zao*), 9g each, and Radix Bupleuri (*Chai Hu*), Folium Mori Albi (*Sang Ye*), and Fructus Gardeniae Jasminoidis (*Zhi Zi*), 6g each.

35

HYPOGLYCEMIA

Hypoglycemia refers to an abnormally low blood glucose level or to abnormal fluctuations of blood sugar levels secondary to an oversecretion of insulin by the pancreas. Mostly this is due to a reaction in response to a meal or specific nutrients. In that case, this is called reactive hypoglycemia and is the most common type of this condition. The characteristics of reactive hypoglycemia are the development of faintness, weakness, tremulousness, heart palpitations, sweating, hunger, and nervousness 2-4 hours after a meal. In addition, there may be headache, confusion, visual disturbances, motor weakness, ataxia, and marked personality changes. The symptoms of recurrent episodes of hypoglycemia in the same patient tend to be repetitive. However, their severity may vary. Most cases of reactive hypoglycemia are due to overeating sugars, sweets, and carbohydrates. In terms of specific nutrients which inhibit glucose output, these include fructose, galactose, and leucine. Reactive hypoglycemia occurs during the early stages of adrenal stress and blood sugar imbalance problems. It can exist by itself and may be the early stages of pancreatic and diabetic problems.

Other factors that may be involved in reactive hypoglycemia are food allergies, low thyroid, nutrient deficiencies, especially of those that increase insulin sensitivity, such as vitamin B_6, chromium, zinc, and essential fatty acids, excessive exercise, stress, missing a meal or irregular eating habits, excessive alcohol, drug, or tobacco consumption, poor protein digestion, insufficient dietary protein, poor digestion due to other factors, low digestive enzymes, and an excessively refined and processed diet. For instance, cigarette smoking greatly aggravates blood sugar lability, while skipping breakfast, drinking too many caffeinated beverages in the morning, or eating a low fiber, high sugar breakfast may create periods of low blood sugar in the mid to late afternoon with symptoms such as fatigue, poor concentration, and irritability – what are popularly called the "sugar blues."

Hypoglycemia may also be drug-induced. Drugs which may cause hypoglycemia include exogenous insulin; insulin plus certain other drugs, such as beta-adrenergic receptor blockers; sufonylureas; sufonylureas plus other drugs, such as phenylbutazone; phenformin; pentamidine; disopyramide; quinine; salicylates; haloperidol; chlorpromazine; aminobenzoic acid; and alcohol. Insulin, alcohol, and sulfonylureas account for more than 50% of all hospitalized cases of hypoglycemia. Other, nondrug causes of hypoglycemia include: fasting, islet cell adenoma or carcinoma, severe liver or kidney disease, endotoxic shock, and hypopituitarism. If hypoglycemia is severe, CNS disturbances may progress to loss of consciousness, convulsion, coma, and death.

The Western medical diagnosis of hypoglycemia depends on documentation of plasma glucose levels equal to or below 50mg/dL associated with the above signs and symptoms which are relieved by ingestion of sugar or other food. The Western treatment of acute or severe episodes of hypoglycemia with epinephrine-like or CNS symptoms consists of oral ingestion of glucose or sucrose. The treatment of hypoglycemia following meals is more complex. This consists of a diet high in proteins and low in carbohydrates. For functional, *i.e.*, essential or idiopathic, hypoglycemia, stress reduction techniques may occasionally be successful. Diabetic patients taking insulin should always carry sugar lumps or candy for first aid relief of hypoglycemic symptoms.

CHINESE DISEASE CATEGORIZATION: Reactive hypoglycemia after meals is mainly categorized as *tou xuan tong*, dizziness and headache, *xuan diao*, dizziness and shaking, *pi juan*, fatigue, *xin ji*, heart palpitations, *han chu*, sweating, *neng shi shan ji*, rapid hungering despite ability to eat, *you lu bu jue*, anxiety and indecision, and *yi nu*, easy anger or irritability.

DISEASE CAUSES: Unregulated eating and drinking, internal damage by the seven affects, iatrogenesis

DISEASE MECHANISMS: The sweet flavor is moderating, *i.e.*, relaxing. Therefore, it is often craved by people under stress as a first aid method of coursing the liver and rectifying the qi. The sweet flavor also enters the spleen where it boosts the qi. Hence people who, due to whatever reason, suffer from spleen vacuity also typically crave sweets and carbohydrates whose flavor is sweet. In other words, if liver wood depresses spleen earth, one desires the sweet flavor to harmonize the liver and spleen. However, the sweet flavor also engenders dampness which may further damage the spleen, remembering that the spleen is averse to dampness. The main symptom of liver depression is irritability or easy anger. The main symptom of spleen vacuity is fatigue and bodily weakness. Further, if the spleen fails to upbear the clear qi and/or fails to engender and transform the blood, the heart may also become vacuous and insufficient. This then results in heart palpitations, impaired memory, lack of mental clarity, confusion, anxiety, etc. Therefore, the disease mechanisms at the core of most hypoglycemics' condition is a liver-spleen disharmony with a heart qi and/or blood vacuity. Then, depending on age, bodily constitution, disease course and severity, etc., there may be yin and/or yang vacuity, dampness and phlegm, damp heat, cold dampness, blood stasis, hidden or retained evils, defensive qi insecurity, etc., etc.

TREATMENT BASED ON PATTERN DISCRIMINATION:

1. LIVER-SPLEEN DISHARMONY PATTERN

MAIN SYMPTOMS: Weakness and discomfort with nervousness and irritability 2-4 hours after a meal, possible headache, reduced appetite, fatigue, rib-side, chest, breast, and diaphragmatic distention and pain, a tendency to depression or changes of mood, possible spontaneous perspiration, loose stools, and abdominal fullness, especially after meals, which are worse with stress or emotional upset, orthostatic hypotension, menstrual irregularities in women, a pale tongue with thin, white fur, and a fine, bowstring pulse

TREATMENT PRINCIPLES: Course the liver and rectify the qi, fortify the spleen and boost the qi

RX: *Xiao Yao San Jia Jian* (Rambling Powder with Additions & Subtractions)

INGREDIENTS: Radix Angelicae Sinensis (*Dang Gui*), Radix Albus Paeoniae Lactiflorae (*Bai Shao*), Radix Codonopsitis Pilosulae (*Dang Shen*), and Rhizoma Cyperi Rotundi (*Xiang Fu*), 9g each, and Rhizoma Atractylodis Macrocephalae (*Bai Zhu*), Sclerotium Poriae Cocos (*Fu Ling*), Radix Bupleuri (*Chai Hu*), Radix Auklandiae Lappae (*Mu Xiang*), and mix-fried Radix Glycyrrhizae (*Gan Cao*), 6g each.

ANALYSIS OF FORMULA: *Chai Hu* and *Xiang Fu* work on the yang aspect of the liver. They course the liver and resolve depression. *Bai Shao* and *Dang Gui* work on the yin aspect of the liver. They nourish liver blood to prevent further liver depression and qi stagnation. Together, these four medicinals harmonize both the yin and yang apsects of the liver and resolve depression. *Dang Shen, Bai Zhu, Fu Ling,* and *Gan Cao* fortify the spleen and boost the qi. They support the transformation function of the spleen. *Mu Xiang* harmonizes the stomach and rectifies the qi.

NOTE: In the beginning, this treatment can increase the appetite but reduce faintness. In this case, the patient must not increase the number of meals, avoid sugar and sweets, and leave at least four hours between each meal.

ADDITIONS & SUBTRACTIONS: For nausea, add nine grams of Rhizoma Pinelliae Ternatae (*Ban Xia*) and Pericarpium Citri Reticulatae (*Chen Pi*). For frequent hunger and thirst, add 15 grams of Gypsum Fibrosum (*Shi Gao*) and nine grams of Rhizoma Anemarrhenae Asphodeloidis (*Zhi Mu*). For severe fatigue, weakness after meals, or spontaneous perspiration, add 15 grams of Radix Astragali Membranacei (*Huang Qi*).

If liver depression transforms into heat with frequent anger, permanent irritability, a bitter taste in the mouth, red sides of the tongue, and thin, yellow fur, replace *Xiao Yao San Jia Jian* with *Xiao Chai Hu Tang Jia Jian* (Minor Bupleurum Decoction with Additions & Subtractions): Rhizoma Atractylodis Macrocephalae (*Bai Zhu*), 12g, Rhizoma Pinelliae Ternatae (*Ban Xia*), Pericarpium Citri Reticulatae (*Chen Pi*), Sclerotium Poriae Cocos (*Fu Ling*), Radix Codonopsitis Pilosulae (*Dang Shen*), Radix Scutellariae Baicalensis (*Huang Qin*), and Fructus Gardeniae Jasminoidis (*Zhi Zi*), 9g each, and mix-fried Radix Glycyrrhizae (*Gan Cao*), 6g.

ACUPUNCTURE & MOXIBUSTION: *Zu San Li* (St 36), *Tai Bai* (Sp 3), *Nei Guan* (Per 6), *Tai Chong* (Liv 3)

ANALYSIS OF FORMULA: Supplementing *Zu San Li* and *Tai Bai* supplements the spleen and boosts the qi. Draining *Nei Guan* and *Tai Chong* rectifies the qi and courses the liver.

ADDITIONS & SUBTRACTIONS: For nausea, add *Gong Sun* (Sp 4). For frequent hunger and thirst, add *Nei Ting* (St 44). For severe fatigue and weakness after meals, add *Pi Shu* (Bl 20) and *Wei Shu* (Bl 21). If liver depression transforms into heat, replace *Tai Chong* with *Xing Jian* (Liv 2). For dizziness, add *Bai Hui* (GV 20). For tremors, add *He Gu* (LI 4). For spontaneous perspiration, add *Fu Liu* (Ki 7) and *He Gu* (LI 4).

2. QI VACUITY & PHLEGM ACCUMULATION PATTERN

MAIN SYMPTOMS: Mental confusion, faintness, weakness, dizziness, heavy-headedness, especially 2-4 hours after a meal, poor appetite, the sound of phlegm in the throat, possible vomiting of clear fluids or drool, lassitude of the spirit, somnolence, tremor of the limbs, slimy, white tongue fur, and a slippery, bowstring pulse

TREATMENT PRINCIPLES: Fortify the spleen and boost the qi, dry dampness and transform phlegm

RX: *Di Tan Tang Jia Jian* (Flush Phlegm Decoction with Additions & Subtractions)

INGREDIENTS: Rhizoma Acori Graminei (*Shi Chang Pu*), 15g, Radix Codonopsitis Pilosulae (*Dang Shen*), 12g, Rhizoma Pinelliae Ternatae (*Ban Xia*), Rhizoma Arsiaematis (*Tian Nan Xing*), Sclerotium Poriae Cocos (*Fu Ling*), Fructus Immaturus Citri Aurantii (*Zhi Shi*), Rhizoma Atractylodis (*Cang Zhu*), 9g each, and mix-fried Radix Glycyrrhizae (*Gan Cao*), 3g

ANALYSIS OF FORMULA: *Ban Xia, Tian Nan Xing, Shi Chang Pu,* and *Fu Ling* together transform phlegm. In addition, *Fu Ling* seeps dampness and supplements the heart, *Shi Chang Pu* dries dampness and opens the orifices. *Chen Pi* and *Zhi Shi* move the qi based on the saying, "To treat phlegm, first treat the qi", *i.e.*, move the qi to disperse the phlegm and prevent further damp accumulation. *Cang Zhu* strongly dries the dampness which is the precursor of phlegm dampness. *Dang Shen, Fu Ling,* and mix-fried *Gan Cao* fortify the spleen, boost the qi, and prevent the engenderment of new phlegm.

ADDITIONS & SUBTRACTIONS: For severe heavy-headedness and dizziness, add nine grams each of Rhizoma Atractylodis Macrocephalae (*Bai Zhu*) and Rhizoma Gastrodiae Elatae (*Tian Ma*). For vomiting of clear fluids or drool, add nine grams each of uncooked Rhizoma Zingiberis (*Sheng Jiang*) and Cortex Magnoliae Officinalis (*Hou Po*). For severe fatigue and weakness, add 15 grams of Radix Astragali Membranacei (*Huang Qi*) and five grams of Rhizoma Cimicifugae (*Sheng Ma*). For tremors of the limbs, add 12 grams each of Periostracum Cicadae (*Chan Tui*) and Rhizoma Gastrodiae Elatae (*Tian Ma*).

ACUPUNCTURE & MOXIBUSTION: *Zu San Li* (St 36), *Yin Ling Quan* (Sp 9), *Feng Long* (St 40), *Bai Hui* (GV 20)

ANALYSIS OF FORMULA: Supplementing *Zu San Li* boosts the qi, while draining *Yin Ling Quan* disinhibits dampness. Draining *Feng Long* transforms phlegm, and even supplementation-even draining at *Bai Hui* upbears the clear and opens the orifices.

ADDITIONS & SUBTRACTIONS: For severe heavy-headedness and dizziness, add *Feng Chi* (GB 20). For vomiting of clear fluids or drool, add *Zhong Wan* (CV 12). For severe fatigue and weakness, add *Pi Shu* (Bl 20) and *Wei Shu* (Bl 21). For tremors of the limbs, add *He Gu* (LI 4) and *Tai Chong* (Liv 3). For somnolence, add *San Jian* (LI 3). For poor appetite, add *Xuan Ji* (CV 21) and *Liang Men* (St 21).

3. STOMACH REPLETION-SPLEEN WEAKNESS PATTERN

MAIN SYMPTOMS: Rapid hungering after eating, sweating, hunger, and nervousness 2-4 hours after a meal, emaciation, thirst, clamoring stomach, abdominal fullness after eating, restlessness coupled with fatigue, loose stools or constipation, lassitude of the spirit, an enlarged tongue with lateral cracks and yellow fur especially in the middle, and a fine, bowstring, possibly rapid pulse

TREATMENT PRINCIPLES: Regulate and rectify the spleen and stomach, clear the stomach and fortify the spleen

RX: *Ban Xia Xie Xin Tang Jia Jian* (Pinellia Drain the Heart Decoction with Additions & Subtractions)

INGREDIENTS: Radix Codonopsitis Pilosulae (*Dang Shen*), 12g, Rhizoma Pinelliae Ternatae (*Ban Xia*), Radix Scutellariae Baicalensis (*Huang Qin*), and Rhizoma Atractylodis Macrocephalae (*Bai Zhu*), 9g each, Fructus Gardeniae Jasminoidis (*Zhi Zi*), Rhizoma Coptidis Chinensis (*Huang Lian*), Sclerotium Poriae Cocos (*Fu Ling*), and mix-fried Radix Glycyrrhizae (*Gan Cao*), 6g each, and dry Rhizoma Zingiberis (*Gan Jiang*), 3g

ANALYSIS OF FORMULA: *Dang Shen, Bai Zhu, Fu Ling,* and mix-fried *Gan Cao* fortify the spleen and boost the qi, while *Gan Jiang* warms the spleen. *Huang Qin, Huang Lian,* and *Zhi Zi* clear the stomach and dry dampness. In addition, *Huang Lian* clears the heart and *Zhi Zi* eliminates vexation. *Ban Xia* regulates and rectifies the spleen and stomach.

ADDITIONS & SUBTRACTIONS: For frequent hunger, add 20 grams of Gypsum Fibrosum (*Shi Gao*) and nine grams of Rhizoma Anemarrhenae Asphodeloidis (*Zhi Mu*). For thirst, add nine grams each of Rhizoma Phragmitis Communis (*Lu Gen*) and Radix Trichosanthis Kirlowii (*Tian Hua Fen*). For spontaneous perspiration or severe fatigue, add 15 grams of Radix Astragali Membranacei (*Huang Qi*).

ACUPUNCTURE & MOXIBUSTION: *Zu San Li* (St 36), *San Yin Jiao* (Sp 6), *Zhong Wan* (CV 12), *Nei Ting* (St 44)

ANALYSIS OF FORMULA: Supplementing *Zu San Li* and *San Yin Jiao* fortifies the spleen and boosts the qi. Draining

Zhong Wan and *Nei Ting* clears the stomach and harmonizes the center.

ADDITIONS & SUBTRACTIONS: For spontaneous perspiration, add *Fu Liu* (Ki 7) and *He Gu* (LI 4). For loose stools, add *Yin Ling Quan* (Sp 9). For constipation, add *Zhi Gou* (TB 6). For abdominal fullness after eating, add *Nei Guan* (Per 6) and *Gong Sun* (Sp 4). For severe fatigue, add *Tai Bai* (Sp 3).

4. QI & BLOOD DUAL VACUITY PATTERN

MAIN SYMPTOMS: Heart palpitations, faintness, sweating and nervousness 2-4 hours after a meal, a pale white or sallow yellow facial complexion, restlessness, dizziness, shortness of breath, weakness, fatigue, spontaneous perspiration, poor appetite, pale lips and nails, impaired memory, a pale tongue with white fur, and a fine, weak pulse

TREATMENT PRINCIPLES: Supplement and nourish the qi and blood, nourish the heart and quiet the spirit

RX: *Ba Zhen Tang Jia Wei* (Eight Pearls Decoction with Added Flavors)

INGREDIENTS: Radix Codonopsitis Pilosulae (*Dang Shen*), Arillus Euphoriae Longanae (*Long Yan Rou*), and cooked Radix Rehmanniae (*Shu Di*), 30g each, Rhizoma Atractylodis Macrocephalae (*Bai Zhu*), Sclerotium Poriae Cocos (*Fu Ling*), Radix Ligustici Wallichii (*Chuan Xiong*), Radix Albus Paeoniae Lactiflorae (*Bai Shao*), Radix Angelicae Sinensis (*Dang Gui*), and Fructus Corni Officinalis (*Shan Zhu Yu*), 9g each, and mix-fried Radix Glycyrrhizae (*Gan Cao*), 4,5g

ANALYSIS OF FORMULA: *Dang Shen, Bai Zhu, Fu Ling*, and mix-fried *Gan Cao* supplement the qi and reinforce transportation, replenish the source of engenderment and transformation of the qi and blood. *Shu Di, Bai Shao, Dang Gui*, and *Chuan Xiong* nourish the blood and harmonize the constructive. *Long Yan Rou* fortifies the spleen, nourishes the heart, and quiets the spirit. *Shan Zhu Yu* supplements the liver and kidneys and restrains the heart qi.

ADDITIONS & SUBTRACTIONS: For cold limbs and long, clear urination, add 0.5-1 gram of Cornu Parvum Cervi (*Lu Rong*). For severe heart palpitations or impaired memory, add 12 grams each of Semen Biotae Orientalis (*Bai Zi Ren*) and Semen Zizyphi Spinosae (*Suan Zao Ren*). For severe qi vacuity, add 15 grams of Radix Astragali Membranacei (*Huang Qi*). For spontaneous perspiration, add 15 grams of Fructus Schisandrae Chinensis (*Wu Wei Zi*) and nine grams of Fructus Pruni Mume (*Wu Mei*). For insomnia and restlessness, add 15 grams of Caulis Polygoni Multiflori (*Ye Jiao Teng*) and replace *Fu Ling* with Sclerotium Pararadicis Poriae Cocos (*Fu Shen*). For concomitant food stagnation, add nine grams each of Fructus Crataegi (*Shan Zha*), Massa Medica Fermentata (*Shen Qu*), and Fructus Germinatus Hordei Vulgaris (*Mai Ya*).

ACUPUNCTURE & MOXIBUSTION: *Zu San Li* (St 36), *San Yin Jiao* (Sp 6), *Shen Men* (Ht 7)

ANALYSIS OF FORMULA: Supplementing *Zu San Li* fortifies the spleen and boosts the qi. Supplementing *San Yin Jiao* supplements the qi and nourishes the blood, while supplementing *Shen Men* nourishes the heart and quiets the spirit.

ADDITIONS & SUBTRACTIONS: For severe blood vacuity, add *Ge Shu* (Bl 17). For severe qi vacuity, add *Tai Bai* (Sp 3). For cold limbs and long, clear urination, add *Guan Yuan* (CV 4) with moxibustion. For severe heart palpitations, add *Nei Guan* (Per 6). For spontaneous perspiration, add *He Gu* (LI 4) and *Fu Liu* (Ki 7). For insomnia and restlessness, add *Bai Hui* (GV 20). For food stagnation, add *Liang Men* (St 21).

REMARKS

1. The above patterns are merely the most common core patterns in patients with hypoglycemia. These core patterns may then be complicated by any number of other, related patterns or disease mechanisms, such as blood stasis as a complication of either qi stagnation of blood vacuity, damp encumbrance as a complication of spleen vacuity, depressive heat as a complication of liver or any other depression, yin vacuity as a complication of blood vacuity, and yang vacuity as a complication of spleen vacuity. In that case, formulas and acupoints should be chosen accordingly.

2. Because reactive hypoglycemia is commonly associated with faulty diet, especially overeating sugars, sweets, and carbohydrates, dietary therapy is generally a must in the overall treatment of this condition. Typically, this means eating frequent, small meals comprised of protein as opposed to carbohydrates. Such protein-rich foods include lean meats, eggs, fish, and cheese if there is not concomitant dampness. In addition, carbohydrates should be complex carbohydrates which take longer to digest and, therefore, release sugars into the blood stream more slowly. Similarly, eating plenty of vegetables allows sugar to arrive more slowly in the blood and helps to avoid the brutal peaks and troughs of reactive hypoglycemia.

3. Because the eating of sweets is often a stress reaction, efforts should also be taken to reduce stress through exercise and relaxation as well as through lifestyle modifcation. It is typically when people are stressed that they crave or gravitate towards "comfort" foods.

4. Sugars and sweets are emotionally addicting if not physi-

cally so. Therefore, when "kicking" the sugar habit, patients typically report cravings for sugar and sweets for several days. However, these cravings also typically disappear after 3-4 days, until or unless the person indulges them again, and this can set off another spiralling round of sugar and sweet consumption. Hence, perserverance is a must in dealing with this or any other addiction and abstinence should usually be complete to avoid recidivism.

5. Chinese medicinals with empirically known hyperglycemic effects include Radix Codonopsitis Pilosulae (*Dang Shen*), Herba Dendrobii (*Shi Hu*), Radix Scutellariae Baicalensis (*Huang Qin*), Radix Gentianae Macrophyllae (*Qin Jiao*), Folium Bambusae (*Zhu Ye*), uncooked Rhizoma Zingiberis (*Sheng Jiang*), Flos Sophorae Japonicae (*Huai Hua*), and Radix Gentianae Scabrae (*Long Dan Cao*).

36

HYPOTENSION

Hypotension refers to lower than normal blood pressure. In modern Western medicine, low blood pressure, for instance 60/90, is not considered a problem. Rather, because high blood pressure is known to be such a killer, many Western health care providers tell patients with chronically low blood pressure that this is good. However, in Chinese medicine, low blood pressure is considered a disease and it is routinely treated. The two subtypes of hypotension which Western medicine does recognize and attempt to treat are idiopathic orthostatic hypotension and Shy-Drager syndrome. Idiopathic orthostatic hypotension is a syndrome of symptoms due to degeneration of postganglionic sympathetic neurons confined to the autonomic nervous system. Shy-Drager syndrome is due to multiple systems degeneration with more widespread neurologic damage, including autonomic dysfunction with cerebrellar atraxia, parkinsonism, corticospinal and corticobulbar tract dysfunction, and amyotrophy. Western medical treatment of these two conditions includes administration of steroids, salt supplementation, and ephedrine in an effort to constrict blood vessels and increase blood pressure. Unfortunately, metoclopramide, one of the drugs used by Western physicians, may exacerbate parkinsonian symptoms and long-term use may lead to tardive dyskinesia, dystonia, or akathisia.

CHINESE DISEASE CATEGORIZATION: Like hypertension, hypotension may be asymptomatic as far as Chinese medicine is concerned. When it is asymptomatic, it does not correspond to any traditional Chinese disease category. When hypotension is complicated and, therefore, there are signs and symptoms, it is mainly categorized as *xu lao*, vacuity taxation, *xuan yun*, dizziness, and *xin ji*, heart palpitations.

DISEASE CAUSES & MECHANISMS: The most common clinical symptoms of low blood pressure are orthostatic hypotension, fatigue, and cold hands and feet. These are mainly spleen qi vacuity symptoms and, therefore, we can say that the core disease mechanism of hypotension is nothing other than spleen qi vacuity. However, in clinical practice, spleen qi vacuity may be complicated by a number of other disease mechanisms. These include yin and/or yang vacuity, dampness, qi stagnation, and blood stasis.

TREATMENT BASED ON PATTERN DISCRIMINATION:

1. SPLEEN QI VACUITY PATTERN

MAIN SYMPTOMS: A pale, lusterless facial complexion, fatigue which is often worse after large meals, weak limbs, diminished qi, a weak voice and disinclination to speak due to speaking being fatiguing, aversion to cold, dizziness, loose stools, commonly a craving for sweets, a swollen tongue with teeth-marks on its edges, and a fine, forceless, sometimes slow or moderate (*i.e.*, slightly slow) pulse

TREATMENT PRINCIPLES: Fortify the spleen and boost the qi

RX: *Sheng Ya Tang* (Upbear the [Blood] Pressure Decoction)

INGREDIENTS: Radix Astragali Membranacei (*Huang Qi*) and Radix Codonopsitis Pilosulae (*Dang Shen*), 30g each, Fructus Schisandrae Chinensis (*Wu Wei Zi*), 20g, Tuber Ophiopogonis Japonici (*Mai Men Dong*), 9g, and Radix Bupleuri (*Chai Hu*), 3g

ANALYSIS OF FORMULA: *Sheng Ya Tang* is a modification of *Sheng Mai San* (Engender the Pulse Powder). *Ren Shen*, *Mai Men Dong*, and *Wu Wei Zi* strongly boost the qi and engender the pulse, while *Huang Qi* and *Chai Hu* boost the qi and upbear the clear.

ADDITIONS & SUBTRACTIONS: For heart yang vacuity

with heart palpitations, an empty feeling in the heart region, cold hands, and purple nails and lips, add 15 grams of Os Draconis (*Long Gu*) and nine grams each of mix-fried Radix Glycyrrhizae (*Gan Cao*) and Ramulus Cinnamomi Cassiae (*Gui Zhi*). For concomitant blood vacuity, add 15 grams each of Radix Angelicae Sinensis (*Dang Gui*) and cooked Radix Rehmanniae (*Shu Di*). For concomitant yin vacuity-fire effulgence, add nine grams each of uncooked Radix Rehmanniae (*Sheng Di*) and Radix Scrophulariae Ningpoensis (*Xuan Shen*) and three grams of Rhizoma Coptidis Chinensis (*Huang Lian*). For loose stools and fatigue which is often worse after large meals, add 12 grams each of Sclerotium Poriae Cocos (*Fu Ling*) and Rhizoma Atractylodis Macrocephalae (*Bai Zhu*). For concomitant liver depression, add 12 grams of Radix Albus Paeoniae Lactiflorae (*Bai Shao*) and increase the dosage of *Chai Hu* up to nine grams.

ACUPUNCTURE & MOXIBUSTION: *Zu San Li* (St 36), *San Yin Jiao* (Sp 6), *Bai Hui* (GV 20), *Qi Hai* (CV 6)

ANALYSIS OF FORMULA: Supplementing *Zu San Li* fortifies the spleen, boosts the qi, and raises the pressure. Supplementing *San Yin Jiao* fortifies the spleen, boosts the qi, and nourishes the blood. Supplementing *Bai Hui* and *Qi Hai* with moxibustion is a special combination for upbearing the clear and treating hypotension. Together, these points lift the yang qi to nourish the clear cavity, arouse the brain and open the orifices.

ADDITIONS & SUBTRACTIONS: For heart yang vacuity with heart palpitations, an empty feeling in the heart, cold hands, and purple nails and lips, add *Xin Shu* (Bl 15), *Ge Shu* (Bl 17), and *Nei Guan* (Per 6). For concomitant blood vacuity, add *Ge Shu* (Bl 17) and *Pi Shu* (Bl 20). For concomitant yin vacuity-fire effulgence, add *Zhao Hai* (Ki 6). For loose stools and fatigue which is often worse after large meals, add *Tai Bai* (Sp 3). For concomitant liver depression, add *Gan Shu* (Bl 18) and *Hun Men* (Bl 47).

2. QI & YIN DUAL VACUITY PATTERN

MAIN SYMPTOMS: Dizziness which appears or is worse on exertion, fatigue, lack of strength, sweating and/or shortness of breath on slight exertion, night sweats, a dry mouth and throat, especially in the afternoon and night, heart palpitations, constipation, a pale tongue with teeth-marks on its edges and a red tip plus scanty or no fur, and a fine, forceless, possibly rapid pulse

TREATMENT PRINCIPLES: Boost the qi and nourish yin

RX: *Jia Wei Sheng Mai San* (Added Flavors Engender the Pulse Powder).

INGREDIENTS: Radix Codonopsitis Pilosulae (*Dang Shen*), Tuber Ophiopogonis Japonici (*Mai Men Dong*), Fructus Schisandrae Chinensis (*Wu Wei Zi*), uncooked Radix Rehmanniae (*Sheng Di*), Fructus Corni Officinalis (*Shan Zhu Yu*), Fructus Lycii Chinensis (*Gou Qi Zi*), and mix-fried Radix Glycyrrhizae (*Gan Cao*), 12g each

ANALYSIS OF FORMULA: *Dang Shen*, *Wu Wei Zi*, and *Mai Men Dong* boost the qi and nourish yin. In addition, *Sheng Di* clears heat and cools the blood, nourishes the blood and engenders fluids. *Shan Zhu Yu* and *Gou Qi Zi* supplement and boost the liver and kidneys, enrich yin and fill the essence.

ADDITIONS & SUBTRACTIONS: For concomitant yang vacuity, add two grams of Cortex Cinnamomi Cassiae (*Rou Gui*). For predominant qi vacuity, add 20 grams of Radix Astragali Membranacei (*Huang Qi*) and 15 grams of Rhizoma Polygonati (*Huang Jing*). For spontaneous perspiration, add 20 grams each of Semen Levis Tritici Aestivi (*Fu Xiao Mai*) and Radix Astragali Membranacei (*Huang Qi*). For night sweats, add 12 grams each of Radix Albus Paeoniae Lactiflorae (*Bai Shao*) and Semen Zizyphi Spinosae (*Suan Zao Ren*). For dry mouth and throat, add nine grams each of Rhizoma Anemarrhenae Asphodeloidis (*Zhi Mu*) and Rhizoma Polygonati Odorati (*Yu Zhu*). For heart palpitations, add 12 grams each of Sclerotium Pararadicis Poriae Cocos (*Fu Shen*), Semen Zizyphi Spinosae (*Suan Zao Ren*), and Radix Salviae Miltiorrhizae (*Dan Shen*). For concomitant liver depression, add nine grams each of Radix Bupleuri (*Chai Hu*), Radix Albus Paeoniae Lactiflorae (*Bai Shao*), and Cortex Albizziae Julibrissinis (*He Huan Pi*).

If there is primarily liver-kidney yin vacuity, replace *Jia Wei Sheng Mai San* with *Liu Wei Di Huang Wan Jia Wei* (Six Flavors Rehmannia Pills with Added Flavors): Rhizoma Polygonati (*Huang Jing*), 30g, cooked Radix Rehmanniae (*Shu Di*), 20g, Radix Dioscoreae Oppositae (*Shan Yao*), Fructus Corni Officinalis (*Shan Zhu Yu*), Fructus Lycii Chinensis (*Gou Qi Zi*), Radix Scrophulariae Ningpoensis (*Xuan Shen*), Tuber Ophiopogonis Japonici (*Mai Men Dong*), and Radix Astragali Membranacei (*Huang Qi*), 15g each, Cortex Radicis Moutan (*Dan Pi*), Rhizoma Alismatis (*Ze Xie*), and Sclerotium Poriae Cocos (*Fu Ling*), 9g each. If there is severe dizziness, add 12 grams each of Rhizoma Gastrodiae Elatae (*Tian Ma*) and Ramulus Uncariae Cum Uncis (*Gou Teng*). For blurred vision, add 12 grams each of Fructus Ligustri Lucidi (*Nu Zhen Zi*) and Fructus Mori Albi (*Sang Shen Zi*). For impaired memory, heart palpitations, and insomnia, add 12 grams each of Semen Zizyphi Spinosae (*Suan Zao Ren*), Rhizoma Acori Graminei (*Shi Chang Pu*), and Radix Polygalae Tenuifoliae (*Yuan Zhi*). For concomitant liver depression, add nine grams each of Radix Bupleuri (*Chai Hu*), Radix Albus Paeoniae Lactiflorae (*Bai Shao*), and Cortex Albizziae Julibrissinis (*He Huan Pi*).

ACUPUNCTURE & MOXIBUSTION: *Fu Liu* (Ki 7), *San Yin Jiao* (Sp 6), *Zu San Li* (St 36), *Bai Hui* (GV 20)

ANALYSIS OF FORMULA: Supplementing *Fu Liu* and *San Yin Jiao* enriches yin and nourishes the blood. Supplementing *Zu San Li* fortifies the spleen, boosts the qi, and upbears the clear. With moxibustion and supplementing method, *Bai Hui* upbears the clear and leads the qi, blood, and essence to the head to nourish the sea of marrow.

ADDITIONS & SUBTRACTIONS: For concomitant yang vacuity, add *Qi Hai* (CV 6) with moxibustion. For spontaneous perspiration, add *He Gu* (LI 4). For night sweats, add *Yin Xi* (Ht 6). For dry mouth and throat, add *Zhao Hai* (Ki 6). For heart palpitations, add *Shen Men* (Ht 7) and *Nei Guan* (Per 6). For marked kidney yin vacuity, add *Shen Shu* (Bl 23). For marked liver blood vacuity, add *Gan Shu* (Bl 18). For marked heart yin vacuity, add *Shen Men* (Ht 7). For concomitant vacuity fire flaming upward, add *Ran Gu* (Ki 2). For dizziness, add *Feng Chi* (GB 20).

3. SPLEEN-KIDNEY YANG VACUITY PATTERN

MAIN SYMPTOMS: Dizziness, a pale, lusterless facial complexion, impaired memory, fatigue, aversion to cold, cold limbs, heart palpitations, shortness of breath, reduced food intake, loose stools, low back and knee soreness and limpness, decreased sexual desire, infertility and menstrual irregularities in women, a swollen tongue with teeth-marks on its edges and slimy, white fur, and a deep, moderate (*i.e.*, slightly slow) pulse

TREATMENT PRINCIPLES: Warm and supplement the spleen and kidneys as well as reinforce heart yang

RX: *Jin Gui Shen Qi Wan Jia Jian* (*Golden Cabinet* Kidney Qi Pills with Additions & Subtractions)

INGREDIENTS: Cooked Radix Rehmanniae (*Shu Di*), Radix Astragali Membranacei (*Huang Qi*), and Radix Dioscoreae Oppositae (*Shan Yao*), 20g each, Fructus Corni Officinalis (*Shan Zhu Yu*), Sclerotium Poriae Cocos (*Fu Ling*), Fructus Psoraleae Corylifoliae (*Bu Gu Zhi*), and Fructus Trichosanthis Kirlowii (*Gua Lou*), 12g each, Radix Lateralis Praeparatus Aconiti Carmichaeli (*Fu Zi*), Cortex Radicis Moutan (*Dan Pi*), Ramulus Cinnamomi Cassiae (*Gui Zhi*), and dry Rhizoma Zingiberis (*Gan Jiang*), 9g each, and mix-fried Radix Glycyrrhizae (*Gan Cao*), 6g

ANALYSIS OF FORMULA: *Shu Di* and *Shan Zhu Yu* enrich yin to supplement yang. *Shan Yao, Fu Ling, Gan Jiang, Huang Qi, Gui Zhi,* and mix-fried *Gan Cao* warm and supplement spleen yang and boost the qi. *Shan Zhu Yu, Fu Zi,* and *Gui Zhi* warm and supplement kidney yang. In addition, *Fu Zi* and *Gui Zhi* reinforce heart yang. *Gua Lou* and *Dan Pi* loosen the chest and quicken the blood of the heart.

ADDITIONS & SUBTRACTIONS: For impaired memory, add six grams of Radix Panacis Ginseng (*Ren Shen*). For severe fatigue, add 15 grams of Radix Codonopsitis Pilosulae (*Dang Shen*). For severe heart palpitations, add 15 grams each of Os Draconis (*Long Gu*) and Dens Draconis (*Long Chi*). For reduced food intake and loose stools, add 12 grams of Rhizoma Atractylodis Macrocephalae (*Bai Zhu*). For low back and knee soreness and limpness, add nine grams each of Radix Dipsaci (*Xu Duan*) and Cortex Eucommiae Ulmoidis (*Du Zhong*). For concomitant liver depression, add nine grams each of Radix Bupleuri (*Chai Hu*), Radix Albus Paeoniae Lactiflorae (*Bai Shao*), and Cortex Albizziae Julibrissinis (*He Huan Pi*).

ACUPUNCTURE & MOXIBUSTION: *Qi Hai* (CV 6), *Bai Hui* (GV 20), *Guan Yuan* (CV 4), *Zu San Li* (St 36)

ANALYSIS OF FORMULA: Supplementing *Bai Hui* and *Qi Hai* with moxibustion is a special combination for upbearing the clear and raising the pressure. They lift the yang qi to nourish the clear cavity, arouse the brain, and open the orifices. Supplementing *Guan Yuan* with moxibustion warms and supplements kidney yang, while supplementing *Zu San Li* with moxibustion warms and supplements spleen yang.

ADDITIONS & SUBTRACTIONS: Please see pattern #1 above. For impaired memory, add *Si Shen Cong* (M-HN-1). For severe fatigue, add *Tai Bai* (Sp 3). For severe heart palpitations, add *Nei Guan* (Per 6). For reduced food intake and loose stools, add *Liang Men* (St 21) and *Yin Ling Quan* (Sp 9). For low back and knee soreness and limpness, add *Fu Liu* (Ki 7). For concomitant liver depression, add *Jian Shi* (Per 5).

4. SPLEEN VACUITY MIXED WITH DAMPNESS PATTERN

MAIN SYMPTOMS: Dizziness, headache, chest oppression, nausea, ductal glomus, reduced food intake, slight swelling of the four limbs which is more severe in the lower limbs, short, scanty urination, loose stools, a pale, possible fat tongue, and a soggy, moderate (*i.e.*, slightly slow), forceless pulse

TREATMENT PRINCIPLES: Fortify the spleen and boost the qi, move the qi and transform dampness

RX: *Shen Zhu Yi Qi Shen Shi Tang* (Ginseng & Atractylodes Boost the Qi & Seep Dampness Decoction)

INGREDIENTS: Coicis Lachryma-jobi (*Yi Yi Ren*), 18g, Radix Codonopsitis Pilosulae (*Dang Shen*), 12g, Rhizoma

Atractylodis Macrocephalae (*Bai Zhu*), Cortex Radicis Acanthopanacis Gracilistylis (*Wu Jia Pi*), Sclerotium Poriae Cocos (*Fu Ling*), and Rhizoma Alismatis (*Ze Xie*), 9g each, Fructus Immaturus Citri Aurantii (*Zhi Shi*), 6g, and Fructus Cardamomi (*Bai Dou Kou*), 4.5g

ANALYSIS OF FORMULA: *Dang Shen, Bai Zhu,* and *Wu Jia Pi* fortify the spleen and boost the qi. *Fu Ling, Yi Yi Ren,* and *Ze Xie* disinhibit water and seep dampness, and *Bai Dou Kou* and *Zhi Shi* regulate and ease the flow of the qi mechanism.

ADDITIONS & SUBTRACTIONS: For concomitant liver depression, add nine grams each of Radix Bupleuri (*Chai Hu*) and Radix Albus Paeoniae Lactiflorae (*Bai Shao*). For more serious orthostatic hypotension and fatigue, add 15 grams of Radix Astragali Membranacei (*Huang Qi*). For persistent loose stools and orthostatic hypotension, add six grams of Rhizoma Cimicifugae (*Sheng Ma*) and three grams of Radix Bupleuri (*Chai Hu*). For concomitant blood vacuity, add six grams of ginger stir-fried Radix Angelicae Sinensis (*Dang Gui*) and nine grams of Radix Albus Paeoniae Lactiflorae (*Bai Shao*).

ACUPUNCTURE & MOXIBUSTION: *Bai Hui* (GV 20), *Zu San Li* (St 36), *Zhong Wan* (CV 12), *Feng Long* (St 40), *Shang Qiu* (Sp 5)

ANALYSIS OF FORMULA: Supplementing *Zu San Li* and *Bai Hui* with moxibustion upbears clear yang, arouses the brain, and raises the pressure. Draining *Zhong Wan, Feng Long,* and *Shang Qiu* drys and transforms dampness and turbidity.

ADDITIONS & SUBTRACTIONS: For more marked spleen qi vacuity, add *Pi Shu* (Bl 20) and *Wei Shu* (Bl 21). For concomitant blood vacuity, add *Ge Shu* (Bl 17), *Gan Shu* (Bl 18), and *Pi Shu* (Bl 20). For liver depression qi stagnation, add *Tai Chong* (Liv 3) and *Nei Gong* (Per 6). For heart palpitations, add *Nei Guan* (Per 6) and *Shen Men* (Ht 7).

5. QI VACUITY & BLOOD STASIS PATTERN

MAIN SYMPTOMS: Either low blood pressure or blood pressure which is sometimes low and sometimes high, relatively high blood lipids, dizziness, headache, chest oppression, piercing pain, heart fluster, shortness of breath, lassitude of the spirit, lack of strength, a dark tongue and/or possible static macules or spots, and a bowstring, moderate (*i.e.*, slightly slow), choppy pulse

NOTE: Although the name of this pattern does not say so, this pattern includes an element of phlegm turbidity due to the spleen qi's failure to divide clear from turbid.

TREATMENT PRINCIPLES: Transform phlegm and downbear turbidity, boost the qi and quicken the blood

RX: *Huang Jing Dang Shen Sheng Ya Tang* (Polygonatum & Codonopsis Upbear the [Blood] Pressure Decoction)

INGREDIENTS: Radix Puerariae (*Ge Gen*) and Radix Ligustici Wallichii (*Chuan Xiong*), 18g each, Rhizoma Polygonati (*Huang Jing*) and Radix Codonopsitis Pilosulae (*Dang Shen*), 12g each, lime-processed Rhizoma Pinelliae Ternatae (*Ban Xia*), Sclerotium Poriae Cocos (*Fu Ling*), Rhizoma Acori Graminei (*Shi Chang Pu*), Fructus Crataegi (*Shan Zha*), Radix Rubrus Paeoniae Lactiflorae (*Chi Shao*), and Semen Cassiae Torae (*Jue Ming Zi*), 9g each

ANALYSIS OF FORMULA: *Huang Jing* and *Dang Shen* nourish the heart and boost the qi. *Ban Xia, Fu Ling,* and *Shi Chang Pu* dispel phlegm and transform turbidity. *Chuan Xiong, Ge Gen, Shan Zha, Chi Shao,* and *Jue Ming Zi* move the qi and quicken the blood, expand the arteries and raise the pressure.

ADDITIONS & SUBTRACTIONS: For marked fatigue, add 18 grams of Radix Astragali Membranacei (*Huang Qi*). For concomitant liver depression qi stagnation, add 9 grams each of Radix Bupleuri (*Chai Hu*) and Radix Albus Paeoniae Lactiflorae (*Bai Shao*). For concomitant blood vacuity, add 18 grams of Caulis Milletiae Seu Spatholobi (*Ji Xue Teng*) and 9 grams of Radix Angelicae Sinensis (*Dang Gui*).

ACUPUNCTURE & MOXIBUSTION: *Bai Hu* (GV 20), *Zu San Li* (St 36), *San Yin Jiao* (Sp 6), *Ge Shu* (Bl 17)

ANALYSIS OF FORMULA: Supplementing *Zu San Li* and *Bai Hui* with moxibustion upbears clear yang, arouses the brain, and raises the pressure. Draining *San Yin Jiao* and *Ge Shu* quickens the blood and transforms stasis.

ADDITIONS & SUBTRACTIONS: For marked spleen vacuity, add *Tai Bai* (Sp 3) and *Pi Shu* (Bl 20). For heart fluster and chest oppression, add *Nei Guan* (Per 6) and *Shen Men* (Ht 7). For more marked phlegm turbidity, add *Feng Long* (St 40) and *Zhong Wan* (CV 12). For concomitant blood vacuity, use even supplementing-even draining method on *San Yin Jiao* and *Ge Shu* and add supplementing method at *Gan Shu* (Bl 18) and *Pi Shu* (Bl 20). For concomitant liver depression, add *Tai Chong* (Liv 3) and *Nei Guan* (Per 6).

REMARKS

1. Low blood pressure typically responds well to Chinese medical treatment, whether acupuncture-moxibustion or Chinese medicinal. When patients are treated for low blood pressure with Chinese medicine, they typically report more energy and warmer hands and feet.

2. Because low blood pressure always involves spleen qi vacuity and because spleen qi vacuity is typically complicated by

liver depression qi stagnation, *Bu Zhong Yi Qi Tang* (Supplement the Center & Boost the Qi Decoction) can be used as the guiding formula for most cases of low blood pressure when modified appropriately for each case. In this case, a larger dose of Radix Bupleuri (*Chai Hu*) can not only upbear the yang but also course the liver and rectify the qi, while a larger dose of Radix Angelicae Sinensis (*Dang Gui*) can emolliate and, therefore, harmonize the liver.

3. Chinese medicinals with a known empirical effect of raising blood pressure include: Herba Ephedrae (*Ma Huang*), Fructus Immaturus Citri Aurantii (*Zhi Shi*), Radix Angelicae Dahuricae (*Bai Zhi*), Folium Artemisiae Argyii (*Ai Ye*), Fructus Psoraleae Corylifoliae (*Bu Gu Zhi*), Fructificatio Ganodermae Lucidi (*Ling Zhi*), Herba Cephalanoploris Segeti (*Xiao Ji*), Herba Portulacae Oleraceae (*Ma Chi Xian*), Flos Carthami Tinctorii (*Hong Hua*), Herba Asari Cum Radice (*Xi Xin*), Radix Astragali Membranacei (*Huang Qi*), Cornu Cervi Parvum (*Lu Rong*), Radix Panacis Ginseng (*Ren Shen*), and Fructus Schisandrae Chinensis (*Wu Wei Zi*). Some of these medicinals also are known to lower blood pressure. In other words, depending on the patient's individual pattern discrimination, those medicinals which can either raise or lower blood pressure actually regulate the blood pressure.

37

IDIOPATHIC THROMBOCYTOPENIC PURPURA

Idiopathic or immunologic thrombocytopenic purpura (ITP) is an autoimmune hemorrhagic disorder involving the spleen and unassociated with other systemic disease. In children and adolescents, this condition is typically acute and self-limiting and is thought to be triggered by a viral antigen associated with the surface of the platelets. In adults, ITP is usually chronic and results from the development of an autoantibody against a structural platelet antigen. Like many other autoimmune diseases, the chronic, adult form of ITP seems to attack women more often than men.

The Western medical diagnosis of this disease is based upon the presence of petechiae, purpura, and mucosal bleeding which may either be minimal or profuse. In adults, the spleen is commonly enlarged, but the bone marrow is basically normal (there may be increased numbers of megakaryocytes). In the acute type, blood tests show a sharp reduction in platelet count and platelet life is markedly shorter than normal. In the adult form, platelet counts are often found to be in the 30-80 x 10^9/L range (normal is 130-400 x 10^9/L). In both cases, bleeding time is prolonged because of poor contraction of blood clots. In terms of the Western medical treatment of ITP, treatment of adults usually begins with oral corticosteroids. In responding patients, platelet counts rise to normal in 2-6 weeks, and steroid administration is tapered off. However, most patients fail to respond or relapse as soon as the dosage of the steroids is reduced. In that case, splenectomy achieves remission in 50-60% of patients whose ITP is refractory to corticosteroids. At this point in time, according to the authors of *The Merck Manual*, the long-term clinical course of chronic ITP is unknown. In patients with ITP and life-threatening bleeding, platelet transfusions are combined with intravenous immunoglobulin and/or high doses of methylprednisolone.

CHINESE DISEASE CATEGORIZATION: Thrombocytopenic purpura is categorized as *xue zheng*, bleeding condition, *ji xue*, spontaneous bleeding of the flesh, *fa ban*, macular eruption, *zi ban*, purple macules, *pu tao yi*, grape epidemic, and *xu lao*, vacuity taxation.

DISEASE CAUSES: External contraction of evils, internal damage by the seven affects, unregulated eating and drinking, taxation fatigue, enduring disease, and aging

DISEASE MECHANISMS: In Chinese medicine, this disease is mainly due to either heat toxins hiding internally in the constructive and blood or viscera and bowel qi, and blood debility and vacuity, and, in clinical practice, these two mechanisms are typically intermingled. Replete evils may result in righteous vacuity, or righteous vacuity may result in replete evils. In terms of replete disease evils, heat and stasis are the two main culprits. Heat damages yin and consumes the qi, while static blood impedes the engenderment of fresh blood. In terms of disease location, it is mainly in the liver, spleen, and kidneys. The various types of righteous vacuity that may be seen in this disease are spleen qi vacuity weakness, liver-kidney yin vacuity, and spleen-kidney yang vacuity. Bleeding is mostly due to either heat causing the blood to move frenetically outside its vessels or qi vacuity failing to contain the blood within its channels. However, subdermal bleeding takes the form of dark-colored petechiae and purple macules (hence the name "purpura"). Therefore, when there is subdermal bleeding, there is also blood stasis. Because the blood flows normally only when it is canalized within the channels and vessels, any time there is bleeding, and especially when there is chronic bleeding, there is the likelihood that the bleeding itself will cause blood stasis. To make matters worse, blood stasis is yet another cause of pathological bleeding. It forces the blood to move outside its proper pathways.

TREATMENT BASED ON PATTERN DISCRIMINATION:

1. HEAT TOXINS DEPRESSED WITHIN THE CONSTRUCTIVE PATTERN

MAIN SYMPTOMS: Relatively acute onset initially beginning with cold and heat, oral thirst, a dry throat, vexation, agitation, and restlessness, reddish urine, constipation, lots of deep-colored purpurae, dizziness, possible accompanying epistaxis, bleeding gums, hematuria, hemafecia, and hematemesis, in women, excessive menstruation like a flood, fresh red blood, a red crimson tongue with either slimy or dry, yellow or brownish yellow fur, and a bowstring, rapid or slippery rapid pulse. In children, purple lines in the wind and/or qi bars or gates.

NOTE: This pattern describes the initial outbreak of acute thrombocytopenic purpura.

TREATMENT PRINCIPLES: Clear heat and resolve toxins, cool the blood and stop bleeding

RX: *Xi Jiao Di Huang Tang Jia Jian* (Rhinoceros Horn & Rehmannia Decoction with Additions & Subtractions)

INGREDIENTS: Cornu Bubali (*Shui Niu Jiao*) and Herba Cephalanoploris Segeti (*Xiao Ji*), 30g each, uncooked Radix Rehmanniae (*Sheng Di*), 20g, Fructus Forsythiae Suspensae (*Lian Qiao*), 15g, Radix Lithospermi Seu Arnebiae (*Zi Cao*), 12g, and Radix Rubrus Paeoniae Lactiflorae (*Chi Shao*), Cortex Radicis Moutan (*Dan Pi*), and Radix Scrophulariae Ningpoensis (*Xuan Shen*), 9g each.

ANALYSIS OF FORMULA: *Shui Niu Jiao, Xiao Ji, Sheng Di, Zi Cao, Chi Shao, Dan Pi*, and *Xuan Shen* cool the blood, clear the constructive, and stop bleeding. *Lian Qiao* and *Xuan Shen* clear heat and resolve toxins. In addition, *Zi Cao* and *Shui Niu Jiao* disperse purple macules, while *Chi Shao* and *Dan Pi* quicken the blood and transform stasis.

ADDITIONS & SUBTRACTIONS: If bleeding is profuse, add 30 grams of Herba Agrimoniae Pilosae (*Xian He Cao*) and 15 grams of Radix Rubiae Cordifoliae (*Qian Cao Gen*). If there is oral thirst with a liking for chilled drinks, add 30 grams of Gypsum Fibrosum (*Shi Gao*) and nine grams of Rhizoma Anemarrhenae Aspheloidis (*Zhi Mu*). If there is vexation and agitation and constipation, add six grams of Radix Et Rhizoma Rhei (*Da Huang*). For epistaxis, add nine grams each of Radix Scutellariae Baicalensis (*Huang Qin*), Radix Cyathulae (*Chuan Niu Xi*), and Cacumen Biotae Orientalis (*Ce Bai Ye*). For bleeding gums, add 30 grams of Gypsum Fibrosum (*Shi Gao*) and six grams of Rhizoma Coptidis Chinensis (*Huang Lian*). For hemafecia, add nine grams each of Radix Sanguisorbae Officinalis (*Di Yu*) and Fructus Sophorae Japonicae (*Huai Jiao*). For hematuria, add 30 grams of Nodus Rhizomatis Nelumbinis Nuciferae (*Ou Jie*) and 15 grams of Herba Seu Radix Cirsii Japonici (*Da Ji*). For hematemesis, add 15 grams each of Rhizoma Imperatae Cylindricae (*Bai Mao Gen*) and Cacumen Biotae Orientalis (*Ce Bai Ye*) and five grams of Rhizoma Bletillae Striatae (*Bai Ji*), powdered and taken with the strained decoction. For excessive menstruation like a flood, add 12 grams of Pollen Typhae (*Pu Huang*) and nine grams of Gelatinum Corii Asini (*E Jiao*). For severe heat toxins with a red, painful, swollen throat, add 15 grams each of Radix Sophorae Subprostratae (*Shan Dou Gen*), Radix Istadis Seu Baphicacanthi (*Ban Lan Gen*), and Rhizoma Belamcandae Chinensis (*She Gan*). For heat entering in the pericardium with restlessness, insomnia, deranged speech, and confusion, add nine grams each of Fructus Gardeniae Jasminoidis (*Zhi Zi*) and Plumula Nelumbinis Nuciferae (*Lian Xin*) and six grams of Rhizoma Coptidis Chinensis (*Huang Lian*). For fever, add 30 grams of Flos Lonicerae Japonicae (*Jin Yin Hua*). For fatigue and weakness, add 12 grams each of Radix Astragali Membranacei (*Huang Qi*) and Radix Codonopsitis Pilosulae (*Dang Shen*).

ACUPUNCTURE & MOXIBUSTION: *Ge Shu* (Bl 17), *Xue Hai* (Sp 10), *San Yin Jiao* (Sp 6), *Yong Quan* (Ki 1)

ANALYSIS OF FORMULA: *Ge Shu* is the meeting point of the blood. Draining it cools the blood and clears the constructive, quickens the blood and stops bleeding mainly in the upper part of the body. *Xue Hai's* name is the sea of blood. Draining it cools the blood and clears the constructive, quickens the blood and stops bleeding mainly in the lower part of the body. Draining *San Yin Jiao* also cools the blood and clears the constructive, quickens the blood and stops bleeding. However, it stops bleeding anywhere in the body. *Yong Quan* clears heat and abates fever. It is also an empirical point for the treatment of ITP. Acupuncture for the acute stage of ITP should only be seen as an auxiliary therapy.

ADDITIONS & SUBTRACTIONS: For epistaxis, add *Kong Zui* (Lu 6). For bleeding gums, add *He Gu* (LI 4). For hemafecia, add *Shang Ju Xu* (St 37). For hematuria, add *Zhong Ji* (CV 3). For hematemesis, add *Xi Men* (Per 4). For excessive menstruation like a flood, add *Zhong Du* (Liv 6). For fever, add *He Gu* (LI 4) and *Wai Guan* (TB 5). If there is vexation and agitation and constipation, add *Zhi Gou* (TB 6). For severe heat toxins with a red, painful, swollen throat, add *Yu Ji* (Lu 10) and *Chi Ze* (Lu 5). For heat entering in the pericardium with restlessness, insomnia, deranged speech, and confusion, add *Lao Gong* (Per 8) and *Shen Men* (Ht 7). For fatigue and weakness, add *Zu San Li* (St 36) or *Pi Shu* (Bl 20). For splenomegaly, add *Zhang Men* (Liv 13).

2. YIN VACUITY, FIRE EFFULGENCE PATTERN

MAIN SYMPTOMS: Insidious onset or prolonged course, skin purpurae sometimes light, sometimes heavy, purple red or dark red in color, epistaxis, bleeding gums, hemafecia, hematuria, dark red blood, vexatious heat in the five hearts, tidal fever, low-grade fever, night sweats, hot flashes in the face, generalized lack of strength, oral thirst, a dry throat, dizziness, tinnitus, excessively profuse menstruation in women which dribbles and drips and does not stop and which is dark red, sticky, and thick in consistency, low back pain and weakness in the lower limbs, dry stools, a red tongue with scanty, no fur, or peeled fur, and a fine, rapid pulse

NOTE: This pattern is mostly seen in chronic thrombocytopenic purpura or as the sequela of the acute disease.

TREATMENT PRINCIPLES: Nourish yin and clear heat, cool the blood and stop bleeding

RX: *Da Bu Yin Wan Jia Jian* (Greatly Supplementing Yin Pills with Additions & Subtractions)

INGREDIENTS: Uncooked Radix Rehmanniae (*Sheng Di*) and cooked Radix Rehmanniae (*Shu Di*), 20g each, Plastrum Testudinis (*Gui Ban*) and Herba Ecliptae Prostratae (*Han Lian Cao*), 15g each, Rhizoma Anemarrhenae Aspheloidis (*Zhi Mu*) and Fructus Ligustri Lucidi (*Nu Zhen Zi*), 12g each, and Cortex Phellodendri (*Huang Bai*), Gelatinum Corii Asini (*E Jiao*), Cortex Radicis Moutan (*Dan Pi*), Cortex Radicis Lycii Chinensis (*Di Gu Pi*), and Cacumen Biotae Orientalis (*Ce Bai Ye*), 9g each

ANALYSIS OF FORMULA: *Sheng Di, Shu Di, Gui Ban, Han Lian Cao, Nu Zhen Zi,* and *E Jiao* all nourish yin blood, and essence. In addition, *E Jiao* and *Gui Ban* stop bleeding, while *Sheng Di, Han Lian Cao, Dan Pi,* and *Ce Bai Ye* cool the blood and stop bleeding. *Zhi Mu, Huang Bai, Di Gu Pi,* and *Dan Pi* clear vacuity heat.

ADDITIONS & SUBTRACTIONS: For severe purpura, add 15 grams of Radix Rubiae Cordifoliae (*Qian Cao Gen*) and 12 grams Radix Lithospermi Seu Arnebiae (*Zi Cao*). For epistaxis, add nine grams each of Radix Scutellariae Baicalensis (*Huang Qin*), and Radix Cyathulae (*Chuan Niu Xi*). For bleeding gums, add 30 grams of Gypsum Fibrosum (*Shi Gao*) and six grams of Rhizoma Coptidis Chinensis (*Huang Lian*). For hemafecia, add nine grams each of Radix Sanguisorbae Officinalis (*Di Yu*) and Fructus Sophorae Japonicae (*Huai Jiao*). For hematuria, add 30 grams of Nodus Rhizomatis Nelumbinis Nuciferae (*Ou Jie*) and 15 grams of Herba Seu Radix Cirsii Japonici (*Da Ji*). For hematemesis, add 15 grams of Rhizoma Imperatae Cylindricae (*Bai Mao Gen*) and five grams of Rhizoma Bletillae Striatae (*Bai Ji*), powdered and taken with the strained decoction. For excessive menstruation like a flood, add 12 grams of Pollen Typhae (*Pu Huang*). For low-grade fever or tidal fever, add nine grams each of Radix Stellariae Dichotomae (*Yin Chai Hu*), Radix Cynanchi Baiwai (*Bai Wai*), and Rhizoma Picrorrhizae (*Hu Huang Lian*). For heat damaging fluids with dryness of the mouth, eyes, skin, and stools, add nine grams each of Tuber Ophiopogonis Japonici (*Mai Men Dong*), Radix Trichosanthis Kirlowii (*Tian Hua Fen*), and Radix Scrophulariae Ningpoensis (*Xuan Shen*). For ascendant liver yang hyperactivity, add 30 grams of Concha Ostreae (*Mu Li*) and 18 grams of Radix Albus Paeoniae Lactiflorae (*Bai Shao*).

ACUPUNCTURE & MOXIBUSTION: *Ge Shu* (Bl 17), *Shen Shu* (Bl 23), *San Yin Jiao* (Sp 6), *Yong Quan* (Ki 1)

ANALYSIS OF FORMULA: Supplementing *Ge Shu* harmonizes the blood and stops bleeding. Supplementing *San Yin Jiao* supplements the liver and kidneys, nourishes yin and stops bleeding. Draining *Yong Quan* subdues yang and downbears counterflow. It is also an empirical point for the treatment of ITP.

ADDITIONS & SUBTRACTIONS: For severe purpura, add *Xue Hai* (Sp 10). For epistaxis, add *Kong Zui* (Lu 6). For bleeding gums, add *He Gu* (LI 4). For hemafecia, add *Shang Ju Xu* (St 37). For hematuria, add *Zhong Ji* (CV 3). For hematemesis, add *Xi Men* (Per 4). For excessive menstruation like a flood, add *Zhong Du* (Liv 6). For low-grade fever, add *Da Zhui* (GV 14). If there is vexation and agitation and constipation, add *Zhi Gou* (TB 6). For fatigue and weakness, add *Zu San Li* (St 36) or *Pi Shu* (Bl 20). For heat damaging fluids with dryness of the mouth, eyes, skin, and stools, add *Zhao Hai* (Ki 6). For ascendant liver yang hyperactivity, add *Tai Chong* (Liv 3) and *Feng Chi* (GB 20). For splenomegaly, add *Zhang Men* (Liv 13).

3. SPLEEN QI DEBILITY & VACUITY PATTERN

MAIN SYMPTOMS: Insidious onset, disease condition worsened by taxation and fatigue, purpurae which come and go and which are scattered in location and pale in color, epistaxis, bleeding gums, lassitude of the spirit, lack of strength, heart palpitations, shortness of breath, dizziness, a lusterless facial complexion, devitalized eating and drinking, long, profuse menstruation with pale-colored, watery blood in women, abdominal fullness, loose stools, a possible bland taste in the mouth, a pale tongue with teeth-marks on its edges, and a fine, weak pulse

NOTE: This pattern is seen in chronic ITP.

TREATMENT PRINCIPLES: Fortify the spleen and boost the qi, lead the blood back to flow within its channels

RX: *Gui Pi Tang Jia Jian* (Return the Spleen Decoction with Additions & Subtractions)

INGREDIENTS: Radix Astragali Membranacei (*Huang Qi*), 20g, Radix Codonopsitis Pilosulae (*Dang Shen*), 15g, Herba Ecliptae Prostratae (*Han Lian Cao*), 12g, Rhizoma Atractylodis Macrocephalae (*Bai Zhu*), Sclerotium Poriae Cocos (*Fu Ling*), Radix Angelicae Sinensis (*Dang Gui*), Radix Albus Paeoniae Lactiflorae (*Bai Shao*), Arillus Euphoriae Longanae (*Long Yan Rou*), Gelatinum Corii Asini (*E Jiao*), 9g each, mix-fried Radix Glycyrrhizae (*Gan Cao*), 6g, and Fructus Zizyphi Jujubae (*Da Zao*), 5 pieces

ANALYSIS OF FORMULA: *Huang Qi, Dang Shen, Bai Zhu, Fu Ling, Long Yan Rou, Da Zao*, and mix-fried *Gan Cao* fortify the spleen and boost the qi. *Dang Gui, Han Lian Cao, Bai Shao*, and *E Jiao* nourish and enrich yin blood and lead the blood back to flow within its channels, *i.e.,* stop bleeding.

ADDITIONS & SUBTRACTIONS: For persistent purpurae which are hard to disperse and splenomegaly, add three grams of powdered Radix Pseudoginseng (*San Qi*) swallowed with the decoction. If the disease course has been prolonged and there is fear of cold, chilled limbs, low back pain, and loose stools, add six grams of Radix Lateralis Praeparatus Aconiti Carmichaeli (*Fu Zi*). For purpurae without splenomegaly, add 30 grams of Herba Agrimoniae Pilosae (*Xian He Cao*) and nine grams of Radix Lithospermi Seu Arnebiae (*Zi Cao*). For epistaxis, add 15 grams of Herba Agrimoniae Pilosae (*Xian He Cao*) and nine grams of Folium Artemisiae Argyi (*Ai Ye*). For bleeding gums, add 15 grams of Herba Agrimoniae Pilosae (*Xian He Cao*). For hemafecia, add 15 grams of Terra Falva Ustae (*Fu Long Gan*). For hematuria, add nine grams each of Herba Seu Radix Cirsii Japonici (*Da Ji*) and Herba Cephalanoploris Segeti (*Xiao Ji*). For hematemesis, add nine grams of blast-fried Rhizoma Zingiberis (*Pao Jiang*) and five grams of Rhizoma Bletillae Striatae (*Bai Ji*), powdered and taken with the strained decoction. For excessive menstruation like a flood, add 12 grams each of Pollen Typhae (*Pu Huang*) and Folium Artemisiae Argyi (*Ai Ye*). For reduced appetite and loose stools, add nine grams each of Massa Medica Fermentata (*Shen Qu*), Fructus Germinatus Hordei Vulgaris (*Mai Ya*), and Fructus Crataegi (*Shan Zha*) and six grams of Fructus Amomi (*Sha Ren*).

ACUPUNCTURE & MOXIBUSTION: *Pi Shu* (Bl 20), *Ge Shu* (Bl 17), *San Yin Jiao* (Sp 6), *Zu San Li* (St 36)

ANALYSIS OF FORMULA: Supplementing *Ge Shu* harmonizes the blood and stops bleeding. Supplementing *San Yin Jiao* boosts the qi and nourishes the blood, supplements the spleen and stops bleeding. *Pi Shu* and *Zu San Li* are, respectively, the back transport point of the spleen and uniting point of the stomach channel. Supplementing them boosts the qi to contain the blood.

ADDITIONS & SUBTRACTIONS: For severe purpura, add *Xue Hai* (Sp 10). For epistaxis, add *Kong Zui* (Lu 6). For bleeding gums, add *He Gu* (LI 4). For hemafecia, add *Shang Ju Xu* (St 37). For hematuria, add *Zhong Ji* (CV 3). For hematemesis, add *Xi Men* (Per 4). For excessive menstruation like a flood, add *Zhong Du* (Liv 6). If the disease course has been prolonged and there is fear of cold, chilled limbs, low back pain, and loose stools, add *Shen Shu* (Bl 23) and *Ming Men* (GV 4). For reduced appetite and loose stools, add *Liang Men* (St 21). For splenomegaly, add *Zhang Men* (Liv 13).

4. STATIC BLOOD OBSTRUCTING THE NETWORK VESSELS PATTERN

MAIN SYMPTOMS: Enduring disease course, non-healing nature, static macules which are dark and purple in color and which disperse slowly, excessively profuse menstruation which is dark in color and contains blood clots, bilateral ribside swelling and lumps, aching and pain, a soot black facial complexion, possible low-grade fever, a dry mouth but no particular desire to drink, possible black stools, a dark, purple tongue or possible static macules or spots, and a fine, choppy pulse

NOTE: This pattern mostly complicates other patterns of chronic, enduring ITP.

TREATMENT PRINCIPLES: Quicken the blood and transform stasis, cool the blood and stop bleeding

RX: *Xue Fu Zhu Yu Tang Jia Jian* (Blood Mansion Dispel Stasis Decoction with Additions & Subtractions)

INGREDIENTS: Radix Salviae Miltiorrhizae (*Dan Shen*), 18g, Semen Pruni Persicae (*Tao Ren*) and uncooked Radix Rehmanniae (*Sheng Di*), 12g each, Flos Carthami Tinctorii (*Hong Hua*), Radix Angelicae Sinensis (*Dang Gui*), Radix Rubrus Paeoniae Lactiflorae (*Chi Shao*), Cortex Radicis Moutan (*Dan Pi*), Tuber Curcumae (*Yu Jin*), Radix Ligustici Wallichii (*Chuan Xiong*), and Radix Bupleuri (*Chai Hu*), 9g each, Fructus Citri Aurantii (*Zhi Ke*) and Lignum Dalbergiae Odoriferae (*Jiang Xiang*), 6g each, and Radix Glycyrrhizae (*Gan Cao*), 3g

ANALYSIS OF FORMULA: *Dan Shen, Tao Ren, Hong Hua, Dang Gui, Chi Shao, Dan Pi, Yu Jin, Chuan Xiong*, and *Jiang Xiang* all quicken the blood and transform stasis. *Sheng Di* nourishes the blood and stops bleeding. *Chai Hu* and *Zhi Ke* move the qi to quicken the blood, and *Gan Cao* harmonizes the other medicinals in this formula.

ADDITIONS & SUBTRACTIONS: If there is concomitant qi vacuity, add 15 grams each of Radix Astragali Membranacei (*Huang Qi*), Herba Agrimoniae Pilosae (*Xian He Cao*), and Herba Leonuri Heterophylli (*Yi Mu Cao*). For splenomegaly, add 15 grams of Carapax Amydae Sinensis (*Bie Jia*). For constipation, add 6-9 grams of Radix Et Rhizoma Rhei (*Da Huang*). For incessant bleeding, subtract *Hong Hua, Tao Ren,* and *Chuan Xiong* and add 15 grams each of Pollen Typhae (*Pu Huang*) and Herba Agrimoniae Pilosae (*Xian He Cao*).

ACUPUNCTURE & MOXIBUSTION: *Ge Shu* (Bl 17), *Xue Hai* (Sp 10), *San Yin Jiao* (Sp 6), *Yong Quan* (Ki 1)

ANALYSIS OF FORMULA: Draining *Ge Shu* quickens the blood, transforms stasis, and stops bleeding mainly in the upper part of the body. Draining *Xue Hai* quickens the blood, transforms stasis, and stops bleeding mainly in the lower part of the body. Draining *San Yin Jiao* quickens the blood, transforms stasis, and stops bleeding in the whole body. *Yong Quan* is an empirical point for the treatment of ITP.

ADDITIONS & SUBTRACTIONS: For epistaxis, add *Kong Zui* (Lu 6). For bleeding gums, add *He Gu* (LI 4). For hemafecia, add *Shang Ju Xu* (St 37). For hematuria, add *Zhong Ji* (CV 3). For hematemesis, add *Xi Men* (Per 4). For excessive menstruation like a flood, add *Zhong Du* (Liv 6). For splenomegaly, add *Zhang Men* (Liv 13). For constipation, add *Zhi Gou* (TB 6). For fatigue and weakness, add *Zu San Li* (St 36) or *Pi Shu* (Bl 20).

5. SPLEEN-KIDNEY YANG VACUITY PATTERN

MAIN SYMPTOMS: Not very pronounced bleeding signs, dizziness, lack of strength, heart palpitations, tinnitus, dread of chill, a somber white facial complexion, spontaneous perspiration, purple macules which come and go but tend to be brought on by over-taxation, low back and lower leg soreness and limpness, loose stools, torpid intake, a pale tongue with thin, glossy fur, and a deep, fine, forceless pulse

TREATMENT PRINCIPLES: Warm and supplement the spleen and kidneys, nourish the blood and stop bleeding

RX: *Gui Fu Ba Wei Tang* (Cinnamon & Aconite Eight Flavors Decoction) & *Huang Tu Tang* (Yellow Earth Decoction)

INGREDIENTS: Uncooked Radix Rehmanniae (*Sheng Di*), 20g, Terra Flava Usta (*Fu Long Gan*), 18g, Fructus Corni Officinalis (*Shan Zhu Yu*) and Rhizoma Atractylodis Macrocephalae (*Bai Zhu*), 15g each, Radix Dioscoreae Oppositae (*Shan Yao*), Sclerotium Poriae Cocos (*Fu Ling*), Gelatinum Corii Asini (*E Jiao*), Radix Scutellariae Baicalensis (*Huang Qin*), and Cortex Radicis Moutan (*Dan Pi*), 9g each, and Radix Lateralis Praeparatus Aconiti Carmichaeli (*Fu Zi*), Cortex Cinnamomi Cassiae (*Rou Gui*), Rhizoma Alismatis (*Ze Xie*), and mixed-friedRadix Glycyrrhizae (*Gan Cao*), 6g each

ANALYSIS OF FORMULA: *Shan Zhu Yu, Shan Yao, Fu Zi,* and *Rou Gui* together warm and supplement kidney yang. In addition, *Shan Zhu Yu* stops bleeding. *Bai Zhu, Shan Yao, Fu Ling,* and mix-fried *Gan Cao* fortify the spleen and boost the qi to contain the blood. *Fu Long Gan* warms the spleen and stops bleeding. *Ze Xie* seeps dampness, while *Dan Pi* quickens the blood. *Sheng Di* and *E Jiao* nourish the blood and stop bleeding. *Huang Qin* cools the blood and stops bleeding. Within this formula, *Huang Qin* prevents the acrid warm ingredients from excessively warming the blood and, thus, aggravating bleeding. Hence it functions as a harmonizing ingredient.

ADDITIONS & SUBTRACTIONS: For more severe qi vacuity, add 15 grams of Radix Astragali Membranacei (*Huang Qi*) and nine grams of Radix Codonopsitis Pilosulae (*Dang Shen*). For metrorrhagia, add nine grams each of Folium Artemisiae Argyi (*Ai Ye*), blast-fried Rhizoma Zingiberis (*Pao Jiang*), and Fructus Schisandrae Chinensis (*Wu Wei Zi*). For black stools, add three grams of Rhizoma Bletillae Striatae (*Bai Ji*), powdered and taken with the strained decoction. For diarrhea, add 12 grams each of Fructus Psoraleae Corylifoliae (*Bu Gu Zhi*) and Semen Cuscutae Chinensis (*Tu Si Zi*) and six grams of Semen Myristicae Fragrantis (*Rou Dou Kou*). For severe bleeding, add nine grams of Gelatinum Cornu Cervi (*Lu Jiao Jiao*). For marked kidney yang vacuity, add 0.3 grams of Cornu Parvum Cervi (*Lu Rong*), powdered and taken with the strained decoction.

ACUPUNCTURE & MOXIBUSTION: *Ge Shu* (Bl 17), *Pi Shu* (Bl 20), *Shen Shu* (Bl 23), *San Yin Jiao* (Sp 6)

ANALYSIS OF FORMULA: Supplementing *Ge Shu* harmonizes the blood and stops bleeding. Supplementing *San Yin Jiao* fortifies the spleen and boosts the qi, supplements the kidneys and nourishes the blood, and stops bleeding. *Pi Shu* and *Shen Shu* are, respectively, the back transport points of the spleen and kidneys. Supplementing them with moxibustion warms and supplements the yang of the spleen and kidneys.

ADDITIONS & SUBTRACTIONS: For more severe qi vacuity, add *Zu San Li* (St 36). For epistaxis, add *Kong Zui* (Lu 6). For bleeding gums, add *He Gu* (LI 4). For hemafecia, add *Shang Ju Xu* (St 37). For hematuria, add *Zhong Ji* (CV 3). For hematemesis, add *Xi Men* (Per 4). For excessive menstruation like a flood, add *Zhong Du* (Liv 6). For splenomegaly, add *Zhang Men* (Liv 13). For diarrhea, add *Yin Ling Quan* (Sp 9) and *Zu San Li* (St 36). For marked kidney yang vacuity, add *Ming Men* (GV 4).

6. LIVER FIRE EFFULGENCE & EXUBERANCE PATTERN

MAIN SYMPTOMS: Fresh red purpurae which are large and plaque-like, nose and/or gum-bleeding, red face and eyes, tension, agitation, easy anger, a dry mouth with a bitter taste, constipation, excessively profuse menstruation like a flood, a red tongue with yellow fur, and a bowstring, rapid pulse

NOTE: This pattern is seen in acute thrombocytopenic purpura or in chronic ITP whose nature has become heavier.

TREATMENT PRINCIPLES: Clear the liver and drain fire, cool the blood and stop bleeding

RX: *Wen Qing Yin Jia Jian* (Warming & Clearing Drink with Additions & Subtractions)

INGREDIENTS: Uncooked Radix Rehmanniae (*Sheng Di*), 30g, Radix Albus Paeoniae Lactiflorae (*Bai Shao*) and Rhizoma Imperatae Cylindricae (*Bai Mao Gen*), 18g each, Radix Angelicae Sinensis (*Dang Gui*), Radix Rubrus Paeoniae Lactiflorae (*Chi Shao*), Radix Ligustici Wallichii (*Chuan Xiong*), Fructus Gardeniae Jasminoidis (*Zhi Zi*), Radix Scutellariae Baicalensis (*Huang Qin*), and Cortex Phellodendri (*Huang Bai*), 9g each, Radix Auklandiae Lappae (*Mu Xiang*), Radix Gentianae Scabrae (*Long Dan Cao*), and Radix Et Rhizoma Rhei (*Da Huang*), 6g each, and Rhizoma Coptidis Chinensis (*Huang Lian*), 3g

ANALYSIS OF FORMULA: *Chi Shao, Zhi Zi, Huang Qin, Long Dan Cao,* and *Huang Lian* clear the liver and drain fire. In addition, *Huang Qin* and *Huang Lian* with *Huang Bai* clear fire from all three burners. *Sheng Di, Chi Shao, Bai Shao,* and *Bai Mao Gen* cool the blood and stop bleeding. *Dang Gui, Chi Shao,* and *Chuan Xiong* quicken the blood and transform stasis to avoid further bleeding. *Da Huang* discharges fire and quickens the blood, and *Mu Xiang* rectifies the qi.

ADDITIONS & SUBTRACTIONS: If there is concomitant qi vacuity, add 15 grams of Radix Astragali Membranacei (*Huang Qi*) and six grams of uncooked Radix Glycyrrhizae (*Gan Cao*).

ACUPUNCTURE & MOXIBUSTION: *Ge Shu* (Bl 17), *Gan Shu* (Bl 18), *San Yin Jiao* (Sp 6), *Xue Hai* (Sp 10), *Yong Quan* (Ki 1)

ANALYSIS OF FORMULA: Draining *Ge Shu* cools the blood and clears the constructive, quickens the blood and stops bleeding mainly in the upper part of the body. Draining *Xue Hai* cools the blood and clears the constructive, quickens the blood and stops bleeding mainly in the lower part of the body. Draining *San Yin Jiao* cools the blood and clears the constructive, quickens the blood and stops bleeding in the whole body. *Gan Shu* clears the liver and drains fire. *Yong Quan* downbears liver fire and subdues liver yang. It is also an empirical point for the treatment of ITP. Acupuncture for the acute stage of ITP should only be used as an auxiliary therapy.

ADDITIONS & SUBTRACTIONS: For epistaxis, add *Kong Zui* (Lu 6). For bleeding gums, add *He Gu* (LI 4). For hemafecia, add *Shang Ju Xu* (St 37). For hematuria, add *Zhong Ji* (CV 3). For hematemesis, add *Xi Men* (Per 4). For excessive menstruation like a flood, add *Zhong Du* (Liv 6). For splenomegaly, add *Zhang Men* (Liv 13). For severe liver fire, add *Xing Jian* (Liv 2).

REMARKS

1. In all cases of chronic ITP, one should expect that there is concomitant liver depression qi stagnation simply due to the patient being an adult and being chronically ill. In that case, there will be a bowstring pulse. Therefore, one or more qi-rectifying medicinals should usually be added to the above formulas which do not accomplish rectification of the qi or harmonization of the liver as part of their standard functions.

2. Thrombocytopenic purpura may also be present in HIV disease or secondary to collagen vascular disorders, such as SLE. Drug-related immune thrombocytopenias, such as to quinidine, have clinical findings identical to ITP except for the history of drug ingestion. It is also possible to develop thrombocytopenia as a reaction to heparin. Drug-related thrombocytopenias usually remit spontaneously after the offending drug is withdrawn, with platelet counts beginning to increase in 1-7 days. Although this chapter specifically deals with idiopathic thrombocytopenic purpura, all types of thrombocytopenic purpura are included in the above Chinese medical discussion based on the dictum: "Same disease, different treatments; different diseases, same treatment."

3. Thrombotic thrombocytopenic purpura (TTP) often complicates acute renal failure. This is then refered to as TTP and hemolytic-uremic syndrome (TTP-HUS). This is typically an acute, potentially fatal disorder. For more information on the Chinese medical pattern discrimination and treatment of uremia and kidney failure, see the chapter on chronic renal failure above.

4. In real-life practice, chronic ITP is mainly a mixture of qi and yin dual vacuity with fire effulgence and blood stasis. If there is qi and yin vacuity with blood stasis, there must also be liver depression qi stagnation.

5. Chinese medicinals with a marked empirical effect on ITP include: uncooked Radix Glycyrrhizae (*Gan Cao*), 15-30g per day, Fructus Forysthiae Suspensae (*Lian Qiao*), 18g per day, Cordyceps Sinensis (*Dong Chong Xiao Cao*), 3g of powder per day, and Radix Rumecis (*Yang Ti Gen*), 10-15g per day. Other medicinals with a demonstrated effect on ITP include: Radix Angelicae Sinensis (*Dang Gui*), Fructus Corni Officinalis (*Shan Zhu Yu*), Gelatinum Corii Asini (*E Jiao*), Fructus Gardeniae Jasminoidis (*Zhi Zi*), Gelatinum Cornu Cervi (*Lu Jiao Jiao*), Fructificatio Ganodermae Lucidi (*Ling Zhi*), and Herba Agrimoniae Pilosae (*Xian He Cao*). Although Radix Astragali Membranacei (*Huang Qi*) is not mentioned in the research literature as being a specific for ITP, it is present in almost all modern Chinese medicinal formulas, with a heavy dosage of 15-60g per day.

38

INTERSTITIAL CYSTITIS

Interstitial cystitis (IC), also called painful bladder syndrome and frequency-urgency-dysuria syndrome, is a complex, chronic disorder of unknown etiology characterized by inflammation and irritation of the bladder wall which can lead to scarring and stiffening of the bladder, decreased bladder capacity, pinpoint bleeding, and, in rare cases, ulceration of the bladder lining. Ninety percent of patients are women, and, although it may strike at any age, two-thirds of sufferers are between 20-40 years old. It is estimated that there may be a half million sufferers in the U.S. This disease may be an autoimmune condition as a reaction to a leaky bladder lining. Seventy percent of IC patients do have a leaky bladder.

Interstitial cystitis is divided into two types. The first is non-ulcerative IC. It primarily affects young and middle-aged women. Ulcerative IC affects middle-aged to older women. In general, the symptoms of IC are decreased bladder capacity, an urgent need to urinate, urinary frequency both day and night, pressure, pain, and tenderness around the bladder and perineum, painful intercourse, and worsening of pain around menstruation. There is no definitive Western medical test for interstitial cystitis, and its diagnosis depends mostly on ruling out other diseases, such as endometriosis, kidney stones, STD, chronic bacterial and nonbacterial prostatitis, urinary tract infections, and vaginal tract infections. Likewise, there is no specific Western medical treatment for IC. Like other autoimmune diseases, IC is spontaneously remittent. Western medications and treatments are mainly aimed at symptomatic relief. These include DMSO administered through catheter, antihistamines, and pain medications, such as amitryptline (Elavil). Transcutaneous electrical nerve stimulation (TENS) may also be used as well as surgery. Foods which may aggravate this condition include alcohol, tomatoes, spices, chocolate, caffeinated and citrus beverages, and high acid foods.

CHINESE DISEASE CATEGORIZATION: Frequent urination is called *xiao bian shuo* and *niao pin* in Chinese. Urinary urgency is *niao ji*. Painful intercourse is *nu xing xing jiao tong*, women's sexual intercourse pain, and lower abdominal pain is *xiao fu tong*.

DISEASE CAUSES: Former heaven natural endowment insufficiency, unregulated eating and drinking, unregulated stirring and stillness, *i.e.*, activity and rest, internal damage by the seven affects, iatrogenesis, and aging

DISEASE MECHANISMS: The disease mechanisms of interstitial cystitis are mainly spleen and kidney vacuity with damp heat pouring downward. Spleen vacuity may be due to sex, age, faulty diet, too much work, too little exercise, excessive thinking, worry, and anxiety, or iatrogenesis. Because the spleen and kidneys mutually bolster and support each other, spleen qi vacuity often evolves into spleen-kidney yang vacuity, especially in women in their late 30s and throughout their 40s. The spleen and kidneys are two of the three viscera who control water fluids in the body. If, due to vacuity weakness, the spleen and/or kidney qi fails to move and transform fluids, these may collect and transform into dampness. If dampness pours downward, it may further inhibit the bladder's qi mechanism. In addition, depressive dampness may engender depressive heat and hence give rise to damp heat. The heat of damp heat will tend to force the fluids in the bladder to move frenetically, while qi vacuity of the spleen and/or kidneys may fail to contain and restrain the fluids within the body. In addition, there will typically be the complication of liver depression qi stagnation which may give rise to pain in the lower abdomen.

TREATMENT BASED ON PATTERN DISCRIMINATION:

1. DAMP HEAT POURING DOWNWARD PATTERN

MAIN SYMPTOMS: Frequent, urgent, painful urination with

a burning hot feeling in the urethra, short, dark-colored, turbid urination, a sticky, dry mouth, thirst without desire to drink, lower abdominal distention and fullness, constipation, a red tongue with slimy, yellow fur, and a slippery, rapid pulse

NOTE: In real-life, most Western patients with IC do not exhibit this pattern. While damp heat may complicate some patients' patterns, it is usually damp heat due to a liver-spleen disharmony.

TREATMENT PRINCIPLES: Clear heat and disinhibit dampness

RX: *Ba Zheng San* (Eight Correcting [Ingredients] Powder)

INGREDIENTS: Talcum (*Hua Shi*), 18g, Semen Plantaginis (*Che Qian Zi*), 12g, Herba Dianthi (*Qu Mai*), cooked Radix Et Rhizoma Rhei (*Da Huang*), Fructus Gardeniae Jasminoidis (*Zhi Zi*), and Herba Polygoni Avicularis (*Bian Xu*), 9g each, and Radix Tenuis Glycyrrhizae (*Gan Cao Shao*) and Caulis Akebiae (*Mu Tong*), 6g each

ANALYSIS OF FORMULA: *Ba Zheng San* is a main Chinese medicinal formula for the treatment of cystitis due to damp heat pouring downward. *Hua Shi*, *Che Qian Zi*, *Qu Mai*, cooked *Da Huang*, *Bian Xu*, *Mu Tong*, *Zhi Zi*, and *Gan Cao Shao* together clear and disinhibit dampness in the bladder. Unlike other forms of *Da Huang*, cooked enters the bladder and treats damp heat. Likewise, *Gan Cao Shao* is the only form of *Gan Cao* which disinhibits dampness. Because this formula is very bitter, it should only be used for a short period of time until damp heat is cleared and eliminated.

ADDITIONS & SUBTRACTIONS: For nausea from taking this formula, subtract *Mu Tong* and *Da Huang* and add six grams each of uncooked Rhizoma Zingiberis (*Sheng Jiang*) and ginger-processed Rhizoma Pinelliae Ternatae (*Ban Xia*). For concomitant qi vacuity with fatigue, abdominal distention after meals, and loose stools, subtract *Mu Tong* and *Da Huang*, and add 15 grams each of Radix Astragali Membranacei (*Huang Qi*), Radix Codonopsitis Pilosulae (*Dang Shen*), and Sclerotium Poriae Cocos (*Fu Ling*). For concomitant liver depression, add nine grams each of Radix Bupleuri (*Chai Hu*), Radix Albus Paeoniae Lactiflorae (*Bai Shao*), and Fructus Meliae Toosendan (*Chuan Lian Zi*). For concomitant kidney vacuity, add nine grams of Semen Cuscutae Chinensis (*Tu Si Zi*) and one gram of Cortex Cinnamomi Cassiae (*Rou Gui*). For alternating fever and chills, a bitter taste in the mouth, dry throat, and nausea, add *Xiao Chai Hu Tang* (Minor Bupleurum Decoction): uncooked Radix Bupleuri (*Chai Hu*), uncooked Radix Scutellariae Baicalensis (*Huang Qin*), and ginger stir-fried Rhizoma Pinelliae Ternatae (*Ban Xia*), 9g each, Radix Codonopsitis Pilosulae (*Dang Shen*) and uncooked Rhizoma Zingiberis (*Sheng Jiang*), 6g each, and Fructus Zizyphi Jujubae (*Da Zao*), 4 pieces. For hematuria, add 15 grams each of Herba Cephalanoploris Segeti (*Xiao Ji*), Herba Seu Radix Cirsii Japonici (*Da Ji*), and Rhizoma Imperatae Cylindricae (*Bai Mao Gen*). For constipation, add nine grams of Fructus Immaturus Citri Aurantii (*Zhi Shi*) and replace cooked *Da Huang* with uncooked *Da Huang*. For damp heat damaging yin with thirst and a desire to drink, and a dry mouth and throat, subtract *Da Huang* and add nine grams each of Rhizoma Anemarrhenae Asphodeloidis (*Zhi Mu*), uncooked Radix Rehmanniae (*Sheng Di*), and Rhizoma Imperatae Cylindricae (*Bai Mao Gen*). If this formula is too bitter and heat-clearing as written above, one can subtract *Mu Tong* and *Da Huang*, increase the dosage of *Hua Shi* up to 25 grams, and add nine grams each of Sclerotium Poriae Cocos (*Fu Ling*) and Fructus Zizyphi Jujubae (*Da Zao*).

ACUPUNCTURE & MOXIBUSTION: *Zhong Ji* (CV 3), *Zhi Bian* (Bl 54), *San Yin Jiao* (Sp 6), *Qu Quan* (Liv 8)

ANALYSIS OF FORMULA: Draining *Zhong Ji* and *San Yin Jiao* is a basic combination for clearing and disinhibiting dampness and heat from the bladder. Draining *Zhi Bian* is a key empirical point for treating urinary tract infection and cystitis. Draining *Qu Quan* disinhibits dampness, frees the flow, and stops pain in the liver channel which penetrates the lower abdomen and encircles the urogenital organs.

ADDITIONS & SUBTRACTIONS: For fever, a bitter taste in the mouth, nausea, and vomiting, add *San Jiao Shu* (Bl 22) and *Ye Men* (TB 3). For constipation, add *Zhao Hai* (Ki 6) and *Zhi Gou* (TB 6). For fever, add *Qu Chi* (LI 11). For colicky pain in the abdomen and low back, add *Xiao Chang Shu* (Bl 27). For severely painful and/or burning urination, add *Shui Quan* (Ki 5). For concomitant qi vacuity, add *Tai Bai* (Sp 3) and *Zu San Li* (St 36). For concomitant liver depression, add *Xing Jian* (Liv 2) and *Jian Shi* (Per 5). For concomitant kidney vacuity, add *Tai Xi* (Ki 3). For hematuria, add *Xue Hai* (Sp 10). For nausea, add *Shang Wan* (CV 13) or *Nei Guan* (Per 6).

2. LIVER DEPRESSION & DAMP ACCUMULATION PATTERN

MAIN SYMPTOMS: Frequent urination, an unfinished feeling after voiding, rib-side discomfort, lower abdominal distention and fullness, irritability, possible premenstrual or menstrual breast distention and pain, menstrual lower abdominal distention and pain, a normal or possibly dark, somewhat swollen tongue with slimy, white fur, and a bowstring pulse

TREATMENT PRINCIPLES: Course the liver and rectify qi, eliminate dampness and disinhibit urination

RX: *Chai Hu Shu Gan San Jia Wei* (Bupleurum Course the Liver Powder with Added Flavors)

INGREDIENTS: Talcum (*Hua Shi*), 18g, Semen Plantaginis (*Che Qian Zi*), 12g, Radix Bupleuri (*Chai Hu*), Radix Albus Paeoniae Lactiflorae (*Bai Shao*), Fructus Citri Aurantii (*Zhi Ke*), Rhizoma Cyperi Rotundi (*Xiang Fu*), Fructus Meliae Toosendan (*Chuan Lian Zi*), Rhizoma Alismatis (*Ze Xie*), and Tuber Curcumae (*Yu Jin*), 9g each, and Pericarpium Citri Reticulatae (*Chen Pi*), Radix Ligustici Wallichii (*Chuan Xiong*), and Radix Glycyrrhizae (*Gan Cao*), 6g each

ANALYSIS OF FORMULA: *Hua Shi, Che Qian Zi,* and *Ze Xie* clear heat, eliminate dampness, and disinhibit urination. *Chai Hu, Bai Shao, Zhi Ke, Xiang Fu, Chuan Lian Zi,* and *Yu Jin* course the liver and rectify the qi. In addition, *Bai Shao* combined with *Gan Cao* relieve spasm. *Xiang Fu* and *Chuan Lian Zi* are empirical medicinals for the treatment of cystitis. *Yu Jin* with *Chuan Xiong* quicken the blood and stop pain, *Chai Hu* upbears the clear, while the first group of medicinals downbear the turbid. *Gan Cao* harmonizes the other medicinals in this formula.

ADDITIONS & SUBTRACTIONS: For blood stasis signs and symptoms such as a dark purple tongue or static macules on the tip and edges of the tongue, add nine grams each of Radix Rubrus Paeoniae Lactiflorae (*Chi Shao*) and Radix Salviae Miltiorrhizae (*Dan Shen*) and six grams of Flos Carthami Tinctorii (*Hong Hua*). For acid regurgitation, dry throat, and a red tongue, add nine grams each of uncooked Fructus Gardeniae Jasminoidis (*Zhi Zi*) and Cortex Radicis Moutan (*Dan Pi*). For depressive heat in the liver and stomach, add 9-12 grams of Radix Scutellariae Baicalensis (*Huang Qin*). For painful menstruation, add nine grams each of Herba Leonuri Heterophylli (*Yi Mu Cao*) and Radix Angelicae Sinensis (*Dang Gui*). For chest oppression, add nine grams of Radix Platycodi Grandiflori (*Jie Geng*). For frequent belching, add three grams of Lignum Aquilariae Agallochae (*Chen Xiang*) and nine grams of Flos Inulae Racemosae (*Xuan Fu Hua*). For severe liver depression, add six grams of Pericarpium Citri Reticulatae Viride (*Qing Pi*) and nine grams of Fructus Citri Sacrodactylis (*Fo Shou*). For concomitant spleen qi vacuity, add nine grams each of Rhizoma Atractylodis Macrocephalae (*Bai Zhu*), Sclerotium Poriae Cocos (*Fu Ling*), and mix-fried Radix Codonopsitis Pilosulae (*Dang Shen*). For severe lower abdominal distention and pain, add nine grams of Rhizoma Corydalis Yanhusuo (*Yan Hu Suo*). If the condition gets worse with emotional disturbances, such as anger, frustration, and depression, add 12 grams each of Semen Zizyphi Spinosae (*Suan Zao Ren*), Cortex Albizziae Julibrissinis (*He Huan Pi*), and Caulis Polygoni Multiflori (*Ye Jiao Teng*).

ACUPUNCTURE & MOXIBUSTION: *Xing Jian* (Liv 2), *Zhong Feng* (Liv 4), *Qu Quan* (Liv 8), *Qu Gu* (CV 2), *Zhi Bian* (Bl 54)

ANALYSIS OF FORMULA: Draining *Xing Jian, Zhong Feng,* and *Qu Quan* courses the liver and frees the flow in the liver channel which penetrates the lower abdomen and circles the urogenital organs. *Xing Jian* and *Zhong Feng* are both well-known points for the treatment of strangury conditions, while *Qu Gu* and *Zhi Bian* are empirical points which clear and disinhibit dampness and heat and treat urinary tract infections and cystitis when needled with draining method.

ADDITIONS & SUBTRACTIONS: For concomitant blood stasis, add *Xue Hai* (Sp 10) and *San Yin Jiao* (Sp 6). For depressive heat in the liver and stomach, add *Nei Ting* (St 44). For painful menstruation, add *Gui Lai* (St 29). For chest oppression, add *Nei Guan* (Per 6). For frequent belching, add *Jiu Wei* (CV 15). For severe liver depression, add *Jian Shi* (Per 5). For concomitant spleen qi vacuity, add *Zu San Li* (St 36). For severely painful and/or burning urination, add *Shui Quan* (Ki 5). For lower abdominal distention and pain, add *Yin Bao* (Liv 9). For frequent sighing, add *Yang Ling Quan* (GB 34). For rib-side pain, add *Qi Men* (Liv 14). For a bitter taste in the mouth due to depressive heat, add *Xia Xi* (GB 43).

3. SPLEEN QI VACUITY PATTERN

MAIN SYMPTOMS: Frequent, long, clear urination, possible urinary incontinence or enuresis, pale lips, a pale facial complexion, fatigue, lassitude of the spirit, lack of strength, dizziness, shortage of qi, lack of warmth in the four limbs, possible facial edema, reduced food intake, loose stools, a pale, fat tongue with white fur, and a vacuous, weak pulse

TREATMENT PRINCIPLES: Fortify the spleen and boost the qi

RX: *Bu Zhong Yi Qi Tang Jia Wei* (Supplement the Center & Boost the Qi Decoction with Added Flavors)

INGREDIENTS: Radix Astragali Membranacei (*Huang Qi*), 15g, Radix Codonopsitis Pilosulae (*Dang Shen*), Rhizoma Atractylodis Macrocephalae (*Bai Zhu*), Fructus Schisandrae Chinensis (*Wu Wei Zi*), and Sclerotium Poriae Cocos (*Fu Ling*), 9g each, Radix Angelicae Sinensis (*Dang Gui*), Pericarpium Citri Reticulatae (*Chen Pi*), and mix-fried Radix Glycyrrhizae (*Gan Cao*), 6g each, Rhizoma Cimicifugae (*Sheng Ma*), 4.5g, and Radix Bupleuri (*Chai Hu*), 3g

ANALYSIS OF FORMULA: *Huang Qi, Dang Shen, Bai Zhu, Fu Ling,* and mix-fried *Gan Cao* fortify the spleen, boost the qi, and upbear the clear. In addition, *Huang Qi, Bai Zhu, Chen Pi,* and *Fu Ling* dry and/or seep dampness and downbear turbidity. *Chai Hu* and *Sheng Ma* help the first group of medicinals upbear yang qi. *Chen Pi* rectifies the qi, while *Dang Gui* harmonizes the blood. *Wu Wei Zi* supplements the qi and astringes urination.

ADDITIONS & SUBTRACTIONS: For severe frequent urination due to spleen disease reaching the kidneys, add nine grams each of Semen Euryalis Ferocis (*Qian Shi*), Fructus Rosae Laevigatae (*Jin Ying Zi*), and Semen Cuscutae Chinensis (*Tu Si Zi*). For susceptibility to common cold, add nine grams of Radix Ledebouriellae Divaricatae (*Fang Feng*). For phlegm dampness obstructing the lungs manifesting as cough with white phlegm, add nine grams each of Rhizoma Pinelliae Ternatae (*Ban Xia*) and Radix Platycodi Grandiflori (*Jie Geng*). For food stagnation with loss of appetite, abdominal distention, and loss of taste, add six grams each of Fructus Germinatus Hordei Vulgaris (*Mai Ya*), Semen Raphani Sativi (*Lai Fu Zi*), and stir-fried Fructus Crataegi (*Shan Zha*).

For heart-spleen dual vacuity, replace *Bu Zhong Yi Qi Tang* with modified *Gui Pi Tang* (Return the Spleen Decoction): Radix Astragali Membranacei (*Huang Qi*), 15g, uncooked Rhizoma Atractylodis Macrocephalae (*Bai Zhu*), 12g, stir-fried Radix Angelicae Sinensis (*Dang Gui*), Arillus Euphoriae Longanae (*Long Yan Rou*), Radix Codonopsitis Pilosulae (*Dang Shen*), and Fructus Alpiniae Oxyphyllae (*Yi Zhi Ren*), 9g each, Radix Auklandiae Lappae (*Mu Xiang*), Semen Zizyphi Spinosae (*Suan Zao Ren*), Radix Polygalae Tenuifoliae (*Yuan Zhi*), and Sclerotium Poriae Cocos (*Fu Ling*), 6g each, and mix-fried Radix Glycyrrhizae (*Gan Cao*), 3g.

For both qi and blood vacuity, replace *Bu Zhong Yi Qi Tang* with modified *Ba Zhen Tang* (Eight Pearls Decoction): cooked Radix Rehmanniae (*Shu Di*), 18g, Rhizoma Atractylodis Macrocephalae (*Bai Zhu*) and Radix Astragali Membranacei (*Huang Qi*), 15g each, Radix Albus Paeoniae Lactiflorae (*Bai Shao*), Radix Angelicae Sinensis (*Dang Gui*), and Radix Codonopsitis Pilosulae (*Dang Shen*), 9g each, and Sclerotium Poriae Cocos (*Fu Ling*), Ramulus Cinnamomi Cassiae (*Gui Zhi*), Radix Ligustici Wallichii (*Chuan Xiong*), and mix-fried Radix Glycyrrhizae (*Gan Cao*), 6g each.

ACUPUNCTURE & MOXIBUSTION: *Guan Yuan* (CV 4), *Qi Hai* (CV 6), *Bai Hui* (GV 20), *Zu San Li* (St 36), *San Yin Jiao* (Sp 6)

ANALYSIS OF FORMULA: Supplementing *Guan Yuan, Qi Hai,* and *Bai Hui* with moxibustion boosts the qi and upbears the clear, while supplementing *Zu San Li* and *San Yin Jiao* fortifies the spleen, boosts the qi, and upbears the clear.

ADDITIONS & SUBTRACTIONS: For severe frequent urination, add *Zhong Ji* (CV 3) with supplementing method. For susceptibility to common cold, add *He Gu* (LI 4) and *Da Zhui* (GV 14). For phlegm dampness obstructing the lungs manifesting as cough with profuse white phlegm, add *Feng Men* (Bl 12) and *Fei Shu* (Bl 13). For food stagnation, add *Liang Men* (St 21). For concomitant kidney qi vacuity, add *Tai Xi* (Ki 3). For heart-spleen dual vacuity, add *Shen Men* (Ht 7).

4. STRAITENED SPLEEN PATTERN

MAIN SYMPTOMS: Frequent, possibly dark-colored urination, a tendency to dry, hard stools, rapid hungering and large appetite, possible abdominal fullness, possible fatigue, a fat, enlarged tongue with yellow, possibly dry tongue fur, and a slippery, bowstring pulse which is often also floating in the right bar

NOTE: Straitened spleen refers to a replete stomach with a vacuous spleen. It is said that the kidneys are the sluicegate of the stomach. Therefore, there is a close reciprocal relationship between the stomach and kidneys. If the stomach is hot, it hyperfunctions. Since one of its functions are to downbear turbidity, a hyperfunctioning stomach disperses food too quickly on the one hand, while downbears fluids too quickly to the bladder on the other. This gives rise to rapid hungering and frequent urination accompanied by a tendency to constipation. This is a common pattern in Western clinical practice. In real-life, it is typically complicated by liver depression/depressive heat.

TREATMENT PRINCIPLES: Clear the stomach and moisten the intestines, fortify the spleen and supplement the qi, move the qi and free the flow of the stools

RX: *Xiao Chai Hu Tang* (Minor Bupleurum Decoction) & *Ma Zi Ren Wan* (Cannabis Seed Pills) with additions and subtractions

INGREDIENTS: Radix Scutellariae Baicalensis (*Huang Qin*), 12g, Radix Bupleuri (*Chai Hu*), Radix Codonopsitis Pilosulae (*Dang Shen*), Rhizoma Pinelliae Ternatae (*Ban Xia*), Semen Cannabis Sativae (*Huo Ma Ren*), Cortex Magnoliae Officinalis (*Hou Po*), and Radix Albus Paeoniae Lactiflorae (*Bai Shao*), 9g each, Fructus Immaturus Citri Aurantii (*Zhi Shi*), Semen Pruni Armeniacae (*Xing Ren*), and mix-fried Radix Glycyrrhizae (*Gan Cao*), 6g each, and Fructus Zizyphi Jujubae (*Da Zao*), 3 pieces

ANALYSIS OF FORMULA: *Huang Qin* clears the stomach and liver. *Chai Hu* and *Bai Shao* course the liver and resolve depression. *Dang Shen*, mix-fried *Gan Cao*, and *Da Zao* fortify the spleen and boost the qi. *Ban Xia* harmonizes the stomach. *Hou Po* and *Zhi Shi* move the qi of the large intestine, while *Huo Ma Ren* and *Xing Ren* moisten the intestines and free the flow of the stools.

ADDITIONS & SUBTRACTIONS: If constipation is severe, add six grams of Radix Et Rhizoma Rhei (*Da Huang*). If there are no dry stools, delete *Huo Ma Ren* and *Xing Ren*. If spleen vacuity with dampness is marked, add nine grams each of Rhizoma Atractylodis Macrocephalae (*Bai Zhu*) and Sclerotium Poriae Cocos (*Fu Ling*). If *Huo Ma Ren* is difficult to find, replace with Semen Pruni Persicae (*Tao Ren*).

ACUPUNCTURE & MOXIBUSTION: *Wei Shu* (Bl 21), *Zhao Hai* (Ki 6), *San Yin Jiao* (Sp 6), *Nei Ting* (St 44), *Zhi Gou* (TB 6)

ANALYSIS OF FORMULA: Supplementing *Wei Shu, Zhao Hai,* and *San Yin Jiao* together fortify the spleen, boost the qi, and moisten the intestines, while draining *Nei Ting* and *Zhi Gou* clears the stomach, moves the qi, and frees the flow of the stools.

ADDITIONS & SUBTRACTIONS: For concomitant dysuria, painful urination, and constipation, add *Zhi Bian* (Bl 54). For concomitant liver depression, add *Zhong Feng* (Liv 4) and *Qu Quan* (Liv 8). For abdominal pain, add *Da Heng* (Sp 15). For bad breath, add *Jie Xi* (St 41). For heart vexation, add *Shen Men* (Ht 7). If constipation is severe, add *Shang Ju Xu* (St 37). If there are no dry stools, subtract *Zhao Hai.* If spleen vacuity with dampness is marked, add *Yin Ling Quan* (Sp 9) and *Tai Bai* (Sp 3). For severely painful and/or burning urination, add *Shui Quan* (Ki 5). For lower abdominal distention and pain, add *Yin Bao* (Liv 9). For rib-side pain, add *Qi Men* (Liv 14). For a bitter taste in the mouth due to depressive heat, add *Xia Xi* (GB 43).

5. BLOOD STASIS OBSTRUCTING INTERNALLY PATTERN

MAIN SYMPTOMS: Frequent, painful urination with dark-colored, turbid urine and possible purple clots in the urine, dribbling urination, lower abdominal distention and pain which refuses pressure, a dark tongue with static macules or spots, and a bowstring and/or choppy pulse

NOTE: This pattern mainly complicates other patterns associated with frequent urination.

TREATMENT PRINCIPLES: Quicken the blood and transform stasis, free the flow of and disinhibit urination

RX: *Shao Fu Zhu Yu Tang Jia Wei* (Lower Abdomen Dispel Stasis Decoction with Added Flavors)

INGREDIENTS: Semen Plantaginis (*Che Qian Zi*), 12g, Radix Angelicae Sinensis (*Dang Gui*), Radix Ligustici Wallichii (*Chuan Xiong*), Radix Rubrus Paeoniae Lactiflorae (*Chi Shao*), Pollen Typhae (*Pu Huang*), Trogopterori Seu Pteromi (*Wu Ling Zhi*), Rhizoma Corydalis Yanhusuo (*Yan Hu Suo*), Resina Myrrhae (*Mo Yao*), Rhizoma Alismatis (*Ze Xie*), and Sclerotium Polypori Umbellati (*Zhu Ling*), 9g each, Fructus Foeniculi Vulgaris (*Xiao Hui Xiang*), 6g, andCortex Cinnamomi Cassiae (*Rou Gui*), 3g

ANALYSIS OF FORMULA: *Chuan Xiong, Dang Gui, Chi Shao, Pu Huang, Wu Ling Zhi, Yan Hu Suo,* and *Mo Yao* quicken the blood, transform stasis, and stop pain. In addition, *Pu Huang, Che Qian Zi, Ze Xie,* and *Zhu Ling* free the flow of and disinhibit urination. *Xiao Hui Xiang* moves the qi in the lower abdomen and helps *Rou Gui* to stimulate the qi transformation of the bladder.

ADDITIONS & SUBTRACTIONS: For hematuria, subtract *Rou Gui* and add three grams of Radix Pseudoginseng (*San Qi*) and one gram of Succinum (*Hu Po*), powdered and taken with the strained decoction. For painful urination, add nine grams each of Herba Lophatheri Graqcilis (*Dan Zhu Ye*) and Radix Tenuis Glycyrrhizae (*Gan Cao Shao*) and 15 grams of Talcum (*Hua Shi*). For absence of cold and the presence of heat, subtract *Xiao Hui Xiang* and *Rou Gui* and add nine grams each of Cortex Radicis Moutan (*Dan Pi*) and Radix Salviae Miltiorrhizae (*Dan Shen*). For severe pain, add 12 grams each of Radix Albus Paeoniae Lactiflorae (*Bai Shao*) and Herba Lysimachiae Seu Desmodii (*Jin Qian Cao*) and nine grams of Radix Glycyrrhizae (*Gan Cao*).

ACUPUNCTURE & MOXIBUSTION: *Zhong Ji* (CV 3), *Zhi Bian* (Bl 54), *San Yin Jiao* (Sp 6), *Shui Quan* (Ki 5)

ANALYSIS OF FORMULA: Draining *Zhong Ji, Zhi Bian, San Yin Jiao,* and *Shui Quan* quickens the blood, and transforms stasis, disinhibits urination and stops pain.

ADDITIONS & SUBTRACTIONS: For concomitant urethral distention and pain, add *Zhong Fu* (Liv 4). For lower abdominal or umbilical region distention and pain, add *Qi Hai* (CV 6). For stone strangury, add *Wei Yang* (Bl 39) and *Ran Gu* (Ki 2).

6. KIDNEY YIN VACUITY PATTERN

MAIN SYMPTOMS: Frequent, short, dark-colored urination, tinnitus, dizziness, a dry throat and mouth, red cheeks and lips, vacuity vexation and insomnia, low back and knee soreness and limpness, steaming bones and taxation fever, vexatious heat in the five hearts, night sweats, dry stools, a red tongue with scanty fur, and a fine, rapid pulse

TREATMENT PRINCIPLES: Enrich yin and downbear fire

RX: *Zhi Bai Di Huang Wan Jia Wei* (Anemarrhena & Phellodendron Rehmannia Pills with Added Flavors)

INGREDIENTS: Cooked Radix Rehmanniae (*Shu Di*), 12g, and Fructus Corni Officinalis (*Shan Zhu Yu*), Radix Dioscoreae Oppositae (*Shan Yao*), Sclerotium Poriae Cocos (*Fu Ling*), Cortex Radicis Moutan (*Dan Pi*), Rhizoma Alismatis (*Ze Xie*), Rhizoma Anemarrhenae Asphodeloidis (*Zhi Mu*), Cortex Phellodendri (*Huang Bai*), and Radix Achyranthis Bidentatae (*Niu Xi*), 9g each

ANALYSIS OF FORMULA: *Shu Di, Shan Zhu Yu, Shan Yao,*

and *Niu Xi* together supplement the kidneys and enrich yin. In addition, *Shan Zhu Yu* and *Shan Yao* secure the kidneys and reduce urination. *Huang Bai* and *Zhi Mu* clear vacuity heat and downbear ministerial fire. *Dan Pi* cools the blood and transforms stasis. *Fu Ling* and *Ze Xie* seep dampness. In addition, *Ze Xie* helps *Zhi Mu* and *Huang Bai* to downbear ministerial fire, and *Fu Ling* helps *Shan Yao* to fortify the spleen so as to avoid 1) damp accumulation and 2) further upward stirring of ministerial fire which would eat the qi of the middle burner.

ADDITIONS & SUBTRACTIONS: For tidal heat and steaming bones, add nine grams each of Cortex Radicis Lycii Chinensis (*Di Gu Pi*), Herba Artemisiae Apiaciae (*Qing Hao*), and Radix Stellariae Dichotomae (*Yin Chai Hu*). For night sweats, add 12 grams each of Fructus Schisandrae Chinensis (*Wu Wei Zi*) and Semen Zizyphi Spinosae (*Suan Zao Ren*). For thirst and a dry mouth and throat at night, add 12 grams each of Radix Scrophulariae Ningpoensis (*Xuan Shen*) and Tuber Ophiopogonis Japonici (*Mai Men Dong*). For severe kidney yin vacuity, add *Er Zhi Wan* (Two Ultimate Pills), *i.e.*, 15 grams each of Fructus Ligustri Lucidi (*Nu Zhen Zi*) and Herba Ecliptae Prostratae (*Han Lian Cao*). For vexatious heat in the chest, add nine grams of Fructus Gardeniae Jasminoidis (*Zhi Zi*). For insomnia, add 12 grams of Semen Zizyphi Spinosae (*Suan Zao Ren*). For concomitant spleen qi vacuity, add 15 grams of Radix Astragali Membranacei (*Huang Qi*) and nine grams each of Radix Codonopsitis Pilosulae (*Dang Shen*) and Rhizoma Atractylodis Macrocephalae (*Bai Zhu*). If there is concomitant liver depression, add nine grams of Fructus Meliae Toosendan (*Chuan Lian Zi*). For concomitant kidney yang vacuity with cold limbs, aversion to cold, and decreased sexual desire, add three grams each of bland Radix Lateralis Praeparatus Aconiti Carmichaeli (*Fu Zi*) and Cortex Cinnamomi Cassiae (*Rou Gui*) and nine grams of Radix Morindae Officinalis (*Ba Ji Tian*).

For damaged yin from enduring damp heat remaining in the yin division, replace *Liu Wei Di Huang Wan* with modified *E Jiao San* (Donkey Skin Glue Powder): uncooked Radix Rehmanniae (*Sheng Di*) and Talcum (*Hua Shi*), 15g each, Semen Plantaginis (*Che Qian Zi*) and Herba Cephalanoploris Segeti (*Xiao Ji*), 12g each, and Sclerotium Polypori Umbellati (*Zhu Ling*), Rhizoma Alismatis (*Ze Xie*), Sclerotium Rubrum Poriae Cocos (*Chi Fu Ling*), Gelatinum Corii Asini (*E Jiao*), and Herba Ecliptae Prostratae (*Han Lian Cao*), 9g each.

ACUPUNCTURE & MOXIBUSTION: *Fu Liu* (Ki 7), *Zhao Hai* (Ki 6), *Ran Gu* (Ki 2), *San Yin Jiao* (Sp 6), *Guan Yuan* (CV 4)

ANALYSIS OF FORMULA: Supplementing *Fu Liu*, *Zhao Hai*, *Ran Gu*, *San Yin Jiao*, and *Guan Yuan* boosts the origin and enriches yin, downbears ministerial fire and disinhibits urination.

ADDITIONS & SUBTRACTIONS: For heart palpitations and insomnia, add *Xin Shu* (Bl 15). For just insomnia, add *Shen Men* (Ht 7). For vexatious heat of the five hearts and night sweats, add *Yin Xi* (Ht 6). For seminal emission, add *Zhi Shi* (Bl 52). For scanty menstruation or blocked menstruation, *i.e.*, amenorrhea, add *Xue Hai* (Sp 10) and *Gui Lai* (St 29). For severe kidney yin vacuity with effulgent fire, add *Yin Gu* (Ki 10), *Zhao Hai* (Ki 6), and *Jiao Xing* (Ki 8) to enrich yin, downbear fire, and free the flow of urination. For hematuria, add *Xue Hai* (Sp 10).

7. KIDNEY YANG VACUITY PATTERN

MAIN SYMPTOMS: Frequent, long, clear urination, possible urinary incontinence or enuresis, a bright white facial complexion, dizziness, tinnitus, shortage of qi, lack of strength in the low back and knees, lack of warmth in the limbs, a pale, fat tongue with thin, white fur, and a deep, fine, weak pulse

TREATMENT PRINCIPLES: Supplement the kidneys and invigorate yang

RX: *You Gui Wan Jia Wei* (Restore the Right [Kidney] Pills with Added Flavors)

INGREDIENTS: Cooked Radix Rehmanniae (*Shu Di*) and Semen Cuscutae Chinensis (*Tu Si Zi*), 12g each, Radix Dioscoreae Oppositae (*Shan Yao*), Fructus Corni Officinalis (*Shan Zhu Yu*), Fructus Lycii Chinensis (*Gou Qi Zi*), Cortex Eucommiae Ulmoidis (*Du Zhong*), Fructus Alpiniae Oxyphyllae (*Yi Zhi Ren*), and Ootheca Mantidis (*Sang Piao Xiao*), 9g each, Radix Angelicae Sinensis (*Dang Gui*) and Gelatinum Cornu Cervi (*Lu Jiao Jiao*), 6g each, and Radix Lateralis Praeparatus Aconiti Carmichaeli (*Fu Zi*) and Cortex Cinnamomi Cassiae (*Rou Gui*), 3g each

ANALYSIS OF FORMULA: *Shu Di* and *Gou Qi* nourish yin to engender yang. *Tu Si Zi*, *Shan Yao*, *Shan Zhu Yu*, *Du Zhong*, *Yi Zhi Ren*, *Sang Piao Xiao*, *Lu Jiao Jiao*, *Rou Gui*, and *Fu Zi* all supplement either the kidney qi or yang. In addition, *Tu Si Zi*, *Shan Yao*, *Shan Zhu Yu*, *Yi Zhi Ren*, and *Sang Piao Xiao* secure the kidneys and reduce urination.

ADDITIONS & SUBTRACTIONS: For severe frequent, long, clear urination, enuresis, urinary incontinence, or nocturia, add nine grams each of Fructus Rosae Laevigatae (*Jin Ying Zi*) and Fructus Rubi Chingii (*Fu Pen Zi*). For heart palpitations and a bound or regularly intermittent pulse, add nine grams each of mix-fried Radix Glycyrrhizae (*Gan Cao*) and Radix Salviae Miltiorrhizae (*Dan Shen*). For hasty panting and spontaneous perspiration, add six grams of Radix Panacis Ginseng (*Ren Shen*) and nine grams of Fructus Schisandrae Chinensis (*Wu Wei Zi*). For seminal emission, vaginal discharge, or diarrhea, add nine grams of Fructus Psoraleae Corylifoliae (*Bu Gu Zhi*). For lower limb edema, subtract *Yi Zhi Ren, Tu Si Zi,* and *Sang Piao Xiao* and add 12 grams each of Cortex Radicis Acanthopanacis Gracistylis (*Wu Jia Pi*) and Rhizoma Alismatis (*Ze Xie*) and nine grams of Sclerotium Poriae Cocos (*Fu Ling*). For decreased sexual desire or impotence, add nine grams each of Rhizoma Curculiginis Orchioidis (*Xian Mao*) and Herba Epimedii (*Xian Ling Pi*). For liver depression qi stagnation, increase *Chai Hu* to nine grams. For spleen vacuity, add 15 grams of Radix Astragali Membranacei (*Huang Qi*) and nine grams each of Radix Codonopsitis Pilosulae (*Dang Shen*) and Rhizoma Atractylodis Macrocephalae (*Bai Zhu*).

ACUPUNCTURE & MOXIBUSTION: *Tai Xi* (Ki 3), *Guan Yuan* (CV 4), *Shen Shu* (Bl 23), *Zhi Shi* (Bl 52)

ANALYSIS OF FORMULA: Supplementing *Tai Xi, Guan Yuan, Shen Shu,* and *Zhi Shi* with moxibustion warms and supplements the lower origin, secures and astinges the kidney qi.

ADDITIONS & SUBTRACTIONS: For panting counterflow, add *Ran Gu* (Ki 2). For dribbling urination, add *Pang Guang Shu* (Bl 28). For frequent night-time urination, add *Zhao Hai* (Ki 6). For clear, thin vaginal discharge, add *Dai Mai* (GB 26).

REMARKS

1. Practitioners should take care not to allow the word "cystitis" in interstitial cystitis to seduce them into immediately thinking of damp heat strangury. Most patients with interstitial cystitis do not exhibit the signs and symptoms of an acute damp heat pattern, such as burning hot urinary pain, even though this is the first pattern listed under this disease category.

2. A liver-spleen disharmony is the central disease mechanism of this condition in most Western patients. This may then be complicated by either damp heat or stomach heat. If spleen vacuity has reached the kidneys, there may be spleen-kidney yang vacuity. If qi stagnation has damaged the blood, there may be blood stasis. If enduring heat has damaged yin, there may be yin vacuity. In perimenopausal women, there is often spleen qi and kidney yin vacuity or yin and yang vacuity.

3. Whether qi vacuity or replete heat is the main disease mechanism associated with frequent urination depends largely on constitution and age. Those who have a habitual yang exuberant body and are younger are more likely to have stomach or damp heat. Those who are habitually less yang exuberant and are older tend to have more qi and yang vacuity. Because many Westerners have a hot, dry stomach and vacuous, damp spleen, it is important to assess these two organs separately, not assuming that every case of spleen vacuity is a spleen-stomach vacuity weakness.

4. Do not use securing and astringing medicinals if there is replete heat frequent urination.

5. Chinese reports confirm the effectiveness of *Zhi Bian* (Bl 54) for the treatment of acute and chronic cystitis. However, according to modern Chinese style acupuncture, one should needle this point deeply to induce a strong qi sensation in the lower abdomen or genitals.

6. Caulis Akebiae (*Mu Tong*) should not be used for a long time, even in small amounts, due to concerns over nephrotoxicity from aristolochic acid. This is because Caulis Aristolochiae Manchurensis is commonly substituted for Caulis Akebiae Trifoliatae Seu Quinatae. When one can be sure they are prescribing Caulis Akebiae, then this is not a concern. However, one can rarely be so sure.

39

Irritable Bowel Syndrome

Irritable bowel syndrome (IBS), a.k.a. spastic colon or mucus colitis, is a motility disorder involving the small intestine and large bowel associated with variable degrees of abdominal pain, constipation, or diarrhea, largely as a reaction to stress in susceptible individuals. The abdominal pain tends to be triggered by eating and may be relieved after a bowel movement. It may be accompanied by other gastrointestinal complaints, such as bloating, flatulence, nausea, passage of mucus, a feeling of incomplete emptying, or pain in the anus and rectum. Irritable bowel syndrome also has a range of symptoms that are not digestive in nature. Among these are headache, fatigue, lassitude, depression, anxiety, and poor concentration. Luckily, any given person with IBS will not experience all these symptoms. Most people tend to experience a few of them, usually pretty much the same ones, periodically.

Irritable bowel syndrome is one of the purely *functional* gastrointestinal disorders. Although this disorder has always existed, it was not recognized by Western medicine until about 50 years ago and has only become a common diagnosis in the last 20 years. By definition in Western medical theory, a functional disorder is one where there is *no* known structural (meaning anatomical), biochemical, or infectious cause. When such a disorder presents as a group of symptoms which tend to occur together, it is called a "syndrome." The symptoms of IBS are similar to those of other common diseases, some of which can be quite serious. Conditions that may be confused with IBS include lactose intolerance, bacterial or parasitic infection, and colon or ovarian cancers, to name just a few. For this reason, depending on the severity of a person's symptoms, their age, and their general health, testing may be required to rule out other possible conditions before a diagnosis of IBS is reached.

It is estimated that 10-20% of all American adults experience symptoms of IBS. Even though only half of these visit a doctor, patients with IBS account for one-half of all GI referrals or initial visits for GI complaints. Irritable bowel syndrome affects three times as many women as men, and, after the common cold, is the next most common cause of missed school and work.[1] The symptoms of IBS are caused by abnormal motility (or movement) and increased pain sensitivity of the gut. Motor function may be lower than normal, causing diarrhea. Increased frequency and strength of contractions in the colon cause constipation. Pain is caused both by increased contractions or spasms and by heightened sensitivity of the nerves in the intestinal tract. People with IBS may experience pain even from normal contractions and normal amounts of intestinal gas.

Both initial and subsequent episodes of IBS can be triggered by emotional factors, foods, some medicines, and hormones. Many people with IBS have a history of either parasitic infections or early trauma, including physical or sexual abuse.

No one knows why some people develop heightened sensitivity of the GI tract, at least in terms of Western medicine, but researchers are working on the theory that there are direct links between the GI tract and the central nervous system. Such a brain-gut connection would explain why emotional upsets affect the intestines and why intestinal symptoms affect mood. In addition, in an effort to more completely understand irritability of the bowel, researchers are developing more sophisticated and sensitive techniques to measure physiological activity in the gastrointestinal tract.

Western MDs usually treat IBS using a combination of diet and lifestyle changes coupled with a prescription for one or more Western pharmaceuticals which are used as needed to treat the symptoms of constipation, diarrhea, pain, and mental-emotional discomfort. For constipation, a fiber supplement, such as bran or psyllium seeds, is recommended to increase the diameter of the colon and reduce the pressure inside. This takes 1-2 months to work. Therefore, other medication may be prescribed on a temporary basis to relieve spastic pain. An anticholinergic agent, alone or in combination with a mild tranquilizer or sedative, may be used for this purpose. Diarrhea is treated with medications that slow peristalsis and reduce intestinal spasm. Tranquilizers and antidepressants are used to deal with nervousness, anxiety, and depression.Unfortunately, many people experience side effects from any or all of these types of Western medication.

Propantheline, the anticholinergic agent suggested by the authors of *The Merck Manual* for treating spastic pain accompanying constipation, may actually cause constipation as well as difficulty in urination, skin rash or hives, headache, eye pain, sensitivity to light, blurred vision, nausea, vomiting, dry mouth, loss of taste, flushing, fever, drowsiness, weakness, and sleeplessness.[2] Loperamide (Immodium) and diphenoxylate (Lomotil) may be used to treat diarrhea. The most common side effect of Immodium is constipation. Occasionally, it may cause nausea, abdominal pain, dizziness, or dry mouth.[3] Likewise, Lomotil commonly causes gastrointestinal symptoms such as nausea, vomiting, and abdominal distention and may cause other side effects, such as drowsiness, dizziness, numbness of the extremities, blurred vision, weakness, and mental depression. Symptoms of overdosage with this medication, which may not show up for 24-30 hours after it is taken, include tachycardia, dry nose, throat and mouth, flushing, and fever.[4] Amitriptyline, more commonly known as Elavil, is the cyclic antidepressant *The Merck Manual* recommends it for IBS, in low doses for its anticholinergic effects and often in higher doses for depression. The *AARP Prescription Drug Handbook* lists over 60 possible side effects for Elavil. Of particular relevance to those with IBS is that Elavil can cause either constipation or diarrhea.[5] Thus, many people cannot take or do not want to take these types of Western pharmaceuticals.

Happily, many Western clinicians recognize that diet and lifestyle play a part in the cause, treatment, and prevention of IBS. In terms of diet, Western MDs typically make recommendations based on symptoms. When abdominal distention and flatulence are a problem, typically MDs advise reducing or eliminating beans, cabbage, and other foods high in fermentable carbohydrates, such as fruit juices and dried fruits. A low fat diet with increased protein is recommended for those who have abdominal pain after eating. Bland bulking agents, such as the bran and psyllium previously mentioned, are suggested for those with constipation, and those with lactose intolerance are obviously advised to avoid dairy products.

In terms of lifestyle, many Western clinicians today are aware of the mind-body connection that plays such a large role in IBS. Therefore, they may recommend some form of stress reduction, counseling, or possibly psychotherapy. Regular exercise is often recommended to reduce stress and to normalize bowel function in those who are constipated. Later on, we will also talk about these from the Chinese point of view.

CHINESE DISEASE CATEGORIZATION: This disease is mostly categorized as *xie tong*, painful diarrhea. If there is abdominal distention, this is categorized as *fu zhang*, while constipation is *bian bi*. The symptoms of headache, fatigue, depression, and anxiety are all also disease categories in their own right in Chinese medicine.

DISEASE CAUSES: Internal damage by the seven affects, unregulated eating and drinking, unregulated stillness (*i.e.*, rest) and stirring (*i.e.*, activity), iatrogenesis, and habitual bodily vacuity due to former heaven natural endowment, enduring disease, and/or aging

DISEASE MECHANISMS: The modern Chinese medical literature is unanimous in saying that the root cause of IBS is always a disharmony between the liver and spleen. Due to emotional stress and frustration, the liver may become depressed and the qi become stagnant. Qi stagnation then results in abdominal distention and pain. Due to worry, lack of exercise, overfatigue, improper diet, or over or prolonged use of antibiotics, the spleen may become vacuous and weak. Spleen qi vacuity results in fatigue, lack of strength, and downward diarrhea. In addition, these two disease mechanisms mutually engender each other. When the liver becomes depressed, it commonly counterflows horizontally to assail the spleen, thus causing or worsening spleen vacuity weakness. Conversely, if the spleen is vacuous and weak, this may cause or worsen liver depression. This is because spleen qi vacuity may lead to blood vacuity, and the liver can only function when it receives an adequate supply of blood to nourish it. Hence liver depression and spleen vacuity typically go hand in hand in clinical practice. In addition, because of their monthly loss of blood, women's spleens must work harder at producing blood than men's spleens must. This also predisposes women in particular to spleen vacuity and explains why three times as many women as men suffer from IBS.

If the liver becomes depressed and the qi becomes stagnant, this stagnation may eventually transform into depressive heat. Over time, this pathological heat will damage and consume the blood, body fluids, and ultimately kidney yin. Spleen vacuity may also lead to blood and, therefore, yin vacuity because the spleen is the root of blood engenderment and the blood and essence share a common source. Since yin is supposed to control yang, if kidney yin becomes vacuous and weak, liver yang may become hyperactive. Since fire burns upward and the heart and lungs are located above the liver, this pathological heat may also accumulate in the heart and/or lungs, disturbing either or both heart and lung function.

Because the spleen is also in charge of moving and transforming liquids, if the spleen becomes weak, water dampness may accumulate. Dampness which is yin, being thick, heavy and turbid, tends to percolate downward and may further block the free flow of qi which is yang, thus aggravating liver depression. Dampness may also give rise to depressive heat which then may cause the dampness to become damp heat. It is also possible for liver depression/transformative heat to stew the juices and give rise to damp heat.

In addition, if qi becomes stagnant and the spleen becomes weak, food stagnation is easily engendered. Food stagnation means food which sits in the stomach undigested. Such food stagnation may also transform into depressive heat.

If qi stagnation fails to move the blood, the blood will stop and become static. Thus, if liver depression is bad enough or lasts long enough, it may give rise to blood stasis. Blood stasis is mainly associated with pain, such as abdominal pain, headache, or other relatively severe aches and pains which are fixed in location and tend to be sharp or piercing in nature.

If spleen vacuity endures, it may eventually reach the kidneys, thus resulting in spleen qi and kidney yang vacuity. This commonly occurs in perimenopausal women and then again later in life in both men and women. Because kidney yang warms and steams the liver, kidney yang vacuity tends to aggravate liver depression. Because kidney yang also warms and steams (*i.e.*, evaporates) body fluids, kidney yang vacuity also aggravates any accumulation of evil dampness. Further, because yang vacuity causes vacuity cold and cold's nature is to contract and constrict, kidney yang vacuity tends to cause or aggravate blood stasis.

TREATMENT BASED ON PATTERN DISCRIMINATION:

LIVER-SPLEEN DISHARMONY PATTERN

MAIN SYMPTOMS: Abdominal distention and painful diarrhea which are worse with stress or emotional upset, chest, breast, and rib-side distention and pain, irritability, fatigue, lack of strength, cold hands and feet, orthostatic hypotension, easy bruising, menstrual irregularities in women, a pale but dark, possibly swollen tongue with thin, white fur, and a fine, bowstring pulse

TREATMENT PRINCIPLES: Course the liver and rectify the qi, fortify the spleen and boost the qi

RX: *Tong Xie Yao Fang* (Essential Formula for Painful Diarrhea)

INGREDIENTS: Rhizoma Atractylodis Macrocephalae (*Bai Zhu*), Radix Albus Paeoniae Lactiflorae (*Bai Shao*), and Radix Ledebouriellae Divaricatae (*Fang Feng*), 9g each, and Pericarpium Citri Reticulatae (*Chen Pi*), 6g

ANALYSIS OF FORMULA : *Bai Zhu*, bitter, sweet, and warm, fortifies the spleen, dries dampness, and treats earth vacuity. It is the sovereign medicinal in this formula. *Bai Shao*, sour and cool, nourishes the blood, emolliates the liver, and treats wood repletion. It is the minister. Together, these two medicinals harmonize the liver and spleen, supplementing the spleen and draining the liver. *Chen Pi*, acrid, bitter, and warm, rectifies the qi, dries dampness, and helps *Bai Shao* to harmonize the liver and *Bai Zhu* to fortify the spleen. It is the assistant. *Fang Feng* rectifies the qi of the liver and intestines, overcomes the dampness, and stops pain. Together, these medicinals regulate liver and spleen, harmonize intestines and stomach, and stop painful diarrhea.

ADDITIONS & SUBTRACTIONS: If spleen vacuity is more pronounced, add 15 grams of Radix Astragali Membranacei (*Huang Qi*), nine grams each of Radix Codonopsitis Pilosulae (*Dang Shen*) and Sclerotium Poriae Cocos (*Fu Ling*), and six grams of mix-fried Radix Glycyrrhizae (*Gan Cao*). If the central qi has fallen due to chronic, enduring diarrhea, also add six grams of Fructus Immaturus Citri Aurantii (*Zhi Shi*), 4.5 grams of Rhizoma Cimicifugae (*Sheng Ma*), and three grams of Radix Bupleuri (*Chai Hu*). If there are cold hands and feet, add nine grams of Ramulus Cinnamomi Cassiae (*Gui Zhi*) and/or six grams of dry Rhizoma Zingiberis (*Gan Jiang*). If there is marked dampness, add nine grams each of Rhizoma Atractylodis (*Cang Zhu*), Semen Plantaginis (*Che Qian Ze*), and Rhizoma Alismatis (*Ze Xie*) and three slices of uncooked Rhizoma Zingiberis (*Sheng Jiang*). If qi stagnation is more pronounced, add nine grams each of Radix Bupleuri (*Chai Hu*), Rhizoma Cyperi Rotundi (*Xiang Fu*), and Radix Auklandiae Lappae (*Mu Xiang*). If there is depressive or damp heat, add nine grams of Radix Scutellariae Baicalensis (*Huang Qin*) and three grams of Rhizoma Coptidis Chinensis (*Huang Lian*). If there is concomitant food stagnation, add nine grams of Massa Medica Fermentata (*Shen Qu*) and 15 grams of Fructus Germinatus Hordei Vulgaris (*Mai Ya*) for cereal foods accumulation, or nine grams each of Fructus Crataegi (*Shan Zha*) and Endothelium Corneum Gigeriae Galli (*Ji Nei Jin*) for fatty, meaty food accumulation. If enduring heat has damaged stomach fluids with oral thirst, add 12 grams of Tuber Ophiopogonis Japonici (*Mai Men Dong*) and nine grams of Radix Puerariae (*Ge Gen*). If there is concomitant blood vacuity, add nine grams of Radix Angelicae Sinensis (*Dang Gui*). If enduring spleen vacuity has reached the kidneys and damaged the kidney qi, add nine grams of Fructus Pruni Mume (*Wu Mei*), Fructus Terminaliae Chebulae (*He Zi*), and Fructus Myristicae Fragrantis (*Rou Dou Kou*). If enduring spleen vacuity has reached the kidneys and damaged kidney yang, add nine grams each of Radix Dioscoreae Oppositae (*Shan Yao*), Semen Cuscutae Chinensis (*Tu Si Zi*), and Fructus Psoraleae Corylifoliae (*Bu Gu Zhi*). If enduring depression has engendered stasis, add 15 grams of Rhizoma Corydalis Yanhusuo (*Yan Hu Suo*) and nine grams of Radix Rubrus Paeoniae Lactiflorae (*Chi Shao*). If damp heat has bound with qi stagnation and blood stasis, add 21 grams of Semen Coicis Lachryma-jobi (*Yi Yi Ren*), 15 grams each of Herba Patriniae Heterophyllae Cum Radicis (*Bai Jiang Cao*) and Caulis Sargentodoxae (*Hong Teng*), and nine grams each of Fructus Meliae Toosendan (*Chuan Lian Zi*) and Cortex Radicis Moutan (*Dan Pi*). If there is frequent anger, depression, insomnia, or emotional tension, add 15 grams each of Caulis Polygoni Multiflori (*Ye Jiao Teng*) and Cortex Albizziae Julibrissinis (*He Huan Pi*). If there are night sweats, pale lips and nails, anger, and emotional tension, add 15 grams each of Semen Zizyphi Spinosae (*Suan Zao Ren*) and Sclerotium Pararadicis Poriae Cocos (*Fu Shen*) and six grams of Radix Angelicae Sinensis (*Dang Gui*). For anxiety as well as poor memory and concentration, add 12 grams each of Sclerotium Pararadicis Poriae Cocos (*Fu Shen*), Semen Biotae Orientalis (*Bai Zi Ren*), and Semen Zizyphi Spinosae (*Suan Zao Ren*). For mental confusion, add nine grams each of Tuber Curcumae (*Yu Jin*) and Rhizoma Acori Graminei (*Shi Chang Pu*) and six grams of Radix Polygalae Tenuifoliae (*Yuan Zhi*).

ACUPUNCTURE & MOXIBUSTION: *Nei Guan* (Per 6), *Zu San Li* (St 36), *Tian Shu* (St 25), *Shui Fen* (CV 9), *Qi Hai* (CV 6), *Tai Chong* (Liv 3), *Si Shen Cong* (M-HN-1)

ANALYSIS OF FORMULA: Supplementing *Zu San Li*, the master point of the abdomen, supplements earth and boosts the qi. Draining *Tai Chong*, the source point of the liver channel, courses the liver and resolves depression. *Nei Guan* helps *Tai Chong* to course the liver and rectify the qi, stop abdominal pain and quiet the heart spirit. With even supplementing-even draining method, *Tian Shu*, *Shui Fen*, and *Qi Hai* locally harmonize the intestines, rectify the qi, and stop pain. *Si Shen Cong* quiets the spirit. This is an example of a point above being used to treat a disease below. Its use is based on the relationship between the emotional condition and the intestinal symptoms.

ADDITIONS & SUBTRACTIONS: For diarrhea, add *Yin Ling Quan* (Sp 9). For constipation, add *Zhi Gou* (TB 6). For cold symptoms, add moxibustion on *Zu San Li*, *Tian Shu*, *Shui Fen*, and *Qi Hai*. For heat symptoms, replace *Zu San Li* with *Shang Ju Xu* (St 37), add *Nei Ting* (St 44), and delete *Qi Hai*. For damp heat symptoms, add *Yin Ling Quan* (Sp 9) and *Nei Ting* (St 44) and subtract *Qi Hai*. For severe spleen qi vacuity, add *Tai Bai* (Sp 3). For food stagnation, add *Xuan Ji* (CV 21) and *Liang Men* (St 21). For kidney qi or yang vacuity, add *Ming Men* (GV 4) with moxibustion. For kidney yin vacuity, add *Fu Liu* (Ki 7). For liver depression transforming heat, subtract *Tai Chong* and *Nei Guan* and add *Xing Jian* (Liv 2) and *Yang Ling Quan* (GB 34). For severe emotional tension and a tendency to mental depression, add *Shen Ting* (GV 24) and *Shen Men* (Ht 7).

REMARKS

1. The modern Chinese medical literature is virtually unanimous in stating that a liver-spleen disharmony is the core disease mechanism of this disease. Further, every published Chinese medicinal formula we are aware of for this condition is based on *Tong Xie Yao Fang*. However, the possible modifications of that formula are legion. Therefore, the above additions and subtractions are only meant as suggestions. While all Western patients with IBS manifest a liver-spleen disharmony, many manifest simultaneous damp heat. Therefore, supplementing and draining, hot and cold medicinals must be used at the same time. In that case, one often winds up with a prescription which is a combination of *Tong Xie Yao Fang*, *Xiao Chai Hu Tang* (Minor Bupleurum Decoction), and *Ban Xia Xie Xin Tang* (Pinellia Drain the Heart Decoction) with additions and subtractions.

2. Comprehensive Chinese medical treatment of this condition typically requires a combination of Chinese medicinal therapy, Chinese dietary therapy, and lifestyle modifications, including more exercise and more relaxation. A clear, bland diet is usually an important aspect of the overall Chinese treatment plan, especially if damp heat evils are marked.

ENDNOTES

[1] http://www.broadwing.medunc.edu/medicine/fgidc UNC Functional Gastrointestinal Disorders Center, Douglas A. Drossman, MD, and William E. Whitehead, MD, co-directors.

[2] *AARP Pharmacy Service Prescription Drug Handbook*, Second Edition, Nancy J. Olins, MA, senior editor, HarperCollins Publishers, Inc., New York, NY, 1992, pp. 382-385

[3] Clayton, Bruce D., *Mosby's Handbook of Pharmacology*, Fourth edition, The C.V. Mosby Company, St. Louis, MO, 1987, p. 721

[4] *Ibid.*, p. 711

[5] *AARP Prescription Drug Handbook*, *op. cit.*, pp. 622-623

40

LATERAL EPICONDYLITIS

Lateral epicondylitis, also called tenosynovitis and, more colloquially, tennis elbow, consists of inflammation of the tendons attached to the lateral side of the elbow at the epicondyle of the humerus. Patients with tennis elbow experience pain in the lateral aspect of the elbow which may radiate into the forearm and occasionally into the hand. The pain occurs with grasping activities and may be accompanied by a sense of weakness. An achy discomfort may also be present at rest or at night after activity. This inflammation may be caused by sudden violent injury or by repetitive strain or micro-trauma. Tennis elbow occurs equally in men and women and is most commonly seen between the ages of 35-50. Tennis elbow is not only found in tennis players but in baseball players, swimmers, carpenters, plumbers, meat cutters, musicians, or anyone who repeats an arm motion over and over.

The Western medical diagnosis of lateral epicondylitis mainly consists of physical examination of the affected area eliciting abnormal tenderness to palpation over the lateral epicondyle. X-rays may show calcium deposits on the lateral epicondyle but are not typically required to make this diagnosis. Bone spurs only occur in 20% of tennis elbow patients. The Western medical treatment of tennis elbow mainly consists of rest, anti-inflammatory medication, and the application of ice. This is supplemented by stretching and strengthening exercises, straps, wrist braces, and cortisone shots. Surgery is indicated in approximately 5% of cases when all the above measures have failed over a course of several months and pain continues to prevent activity. In general, tennis elbow surgery achieves excellent relief of pain in 85-95% of patients.[1] However, patients typically require 3-6 weeks recuperation before returning to work and several months before returning to sports or heavy use of the arm.

CHINESE DISEASE CATEGORIZATION: Tennis elbow is called *zhou lao*, elbow taxation, *zhou tong*, elbow pain, and *shang jin*, damaged sinews, in Chinese medicine.

DISEASE CAUSES: Taxation detriment with possible contraction of wind cold evils

DISEASE MECHANISMS: Overwork taxation causes detriment and damage to the sinews and vessels of the elbow. On the one hand, there is insufficient blood to nourish the sinews, while, on the other hand, there is blood stasis obstructing the free flow of the vessels. This may then be complicated by external contraction of wind cold evils due to defensive qi vacuity.

TREATMENT BASED ON PATTERN DISCRIMINATION:

QI & BLOOD VACUITY WITH WIND COLD IMPEDIMENT PATTERN

MAIN SYMPTOMS: Recurrent or enduring pain which is worse on exertion, worse on exposure to cold, and better on obtaint of heat

TREATMENT PRINCIPLES: Boost the qi and nourish the blood, warm the channels and free the flow of impediment

RX: *Huang Qi Gui Zhi Wu Wu Tang* (Astragalus & Cinnamon Twig Five Materials Decoction)

INGREDIENTS: Uncooked Rhizoma Zingiberis (*Sheng Jiang*) and Radix Astragali Membranacei (*Huang Qi*), 12g each, Radix Albus Paeoniae Lactiflorae (*Bai Shao*) and Ramulus Cinnamomi Cassiae (*Gui Zhi*), 9g each, and Fructus Zizyphi Jujubae (*Da Zao*), 12 pieces

ANALYSIS OF FORMULA: Within this formula, *Huang Qi* boosts the qi, while *Bai Shao* nourishes the blood. *Sheng*

Jiang and *Gui Zhi* scatter cold and free the flow of the channels. *Da Zao* aids both *Huang Qi* and *Bai Shao* in supplementing the qi and blood. Since *Gui Zhi* and *Sheng Jiang* move the qi, they may be used whether or not this condition is complicated by wind cold. In addition, *Bai Shao* relaxes cramping.

ADDITIONS & SUBTRACTIONS: For concomitant blood vacuity and/or blood stasis, add 15 grams of Caulis Milletiae Seu Spatholobi (*Ji Xue Teng*) and nine grams of Radix Angelicae Sinensis (*Dang Gui*). For marked wind cold dampness, add nine grams each of Cortex Radicis Acanthpanacis Gracistylis (*Wu Jia Pi*), Radix Clematidis Chinensis (*Wei Ling Xian*), and Radix Et Rhizoma Notopterygii (*Qiang Huo*). For bone weakness and sinew fatigue, add nine grams each of Cortex Eucommiae Ulmoidis (*Du Zhong*) and Radix Dipsaci (*Xu Duan*).

For severe blood stasis due to acute trauma or repetitive strain or micro-trauma, replace *Huang Qi Gui Zhi Wu Wu Tang* with *Huo Ying Zhi Tong Tang Jia Jian* (Quicken the Constructive & Stop Pain Decoction with Additions & Subtractions): Radix Dipsaci (*Xu Duan*) and Rhizoma Corydalis Yanhusuo (*Yan Hu Suo*), 12g each, Extremitas Radicis Angelicae Sinensis (*Dang Gui Wei*), Radix Rubrus Paeoniae Lactiflorae (*Chi Shao*), Radix Ligustici Wallichii (*Chuan Xiong*), Lignum Sappan (*Su Mu*), Pericarpium Citri Reticulatae (*Chen Pi*), Semen Pruni Persicae (*Tao Ren*), and Radix Linderae Strychnifoliae (*Wu Yao*), 9g each, Resina Myrrhae (*Mo Yao*), Resina Olibani (*Ru Xiang*), and Radix Glycyrrhizae (*Gan Cao*), 6g each.

If there is mainly blood vacuity failing to nourish the sinews, replace *Huang Qi Gui Zhi Wu Wu Tang* with *Dang Gui Jian Zhong Tang* (Dang Gui Fortify the Center Decoction): Maltose (*Yi Tang*) and Radix Albus Paeoniae Lactiflorae (*Bai Shao*), 18g each, Ramulus Cinnamomi Cassiae (*Gui Zhi*), Radix Angelicae Sinensis (*Dang Gui*), and uncooked Rhizoma Zingiberis (*Sheng Jiang*), 9g each, mix-fried Radix Glycyrrhizae (*Gan Cao*), 6g, and Fructus Zizyphi Jujubae (*Da Zao*), 12 pieces.

If there is blood vacuity with marked cold impediment, replace *Huang Qi Gui Zhi Wu Wu Tang* with *Dang Gui Si Ni Tang* (Dang Gui Four Counterflows Decoction): Radix Angelicae Sinensis (*Dang Gui*), Radix Albus Paeoniae Lactiflorae (*Bai Shao*), and Ramulus Cinnamomi Cassiae (*Gui Zhi*), 9g each, Herba Asari Cum Radice (*Xi Xin*), Caulis Akebiae (*Mu Tong*), and mix-fried Radix Glycyrrhizae (*Gan Cao*), 6g each, and Fructus Zizyphi Jujubae (*Da Zao*), 25 pieces.

If qi and blood vacuity are pronounced, replace *Huang Qi Gui Zhi Wu Wu Tang* with *Shi Quan Da Bu Tang Jia Wei* (Ten [Ingredients] Completely & Greatly Supplementing Decoction with Added Flavors): cooked Radix Rehmanniae (*Shu Di*), Caulis Milletiae Seu Spatholobi (*Ji Xue Teng*), and Radix Astragali Membranacei (*Huang Qi*), 12g each, Radix Albus Paeoniae Lactiflorae (*Bai Shao*), Radix Angelicae Sinensis (*Dang Gui*), Radix Codonopsitis Pilosulae (*Dang Shen*), Rhizoma Atractylodis Macrocephalae (*Bai Zhu*), and Sclerotium Poriae Cocos (*Fu Ling*), 9g each, and Radix Ligustici Wallichii (*Chuan Xiong*), mix-fried Radix Glycyrrhizae (*Gan Cao*), and Ramulus Cinnamomi Cassiae (*Gui Zhi*), 6g each.

ACUPUNCTURE & MOXIBUSTION: *Zhou Liao* (LI 12), *Shou San Li* (LI 10), *Shou Wu Li* (LI 13), *He Gu* (LI 4), local *a shi* points

ANALYSIS OF FORMULA: Draining *Zhou Liao, Shou San Li, Shou Wu Li*, and any *a shi* points frees the flow of the channels and network vessels in the local area. *He Gu* is the source point on the hand yang ming, and the pain of tennis elbow is usually located on this channel. Draining this important distal point on this channel helps free the flow of the qi and blood within the hand yang ming. Use warm needle technique on all local points if there is prominent cold.

ADDITIONS & SUBTRACTIONS: If qi and blood vacuity are marked, add *Zu San Li* (St 36) and *Ge Shu* (Bl 17) with supplementing technique. If there is concomitant liver-kidney vacuity, add *Tai Xi* (Ki 3), *San Yin Jiao* (Sp 6), *Ge Shu* (Bl 17), and *Gan Shu* (Bl 18) with supplementing technique. If there are signs and symptoms of systemic blood stasis, add *Xue Hai* (Sp 10). If there is phlegm obstructing the channels, add *Feng Long* (St 40) and *Zu San Li* (St 36).

REMARKS

1. In real life, most patients with tennis elbow also have liver depression qi stagnation either simply due to being an adult or due to the frustration of not being able to work or play. Therefore, one will typically have to add appropriate qi-rectifying medicinals to the above formulas or use a liver-spleen harmonizing formula, such as *Xiao Yao San* (Rambling Powder) and then modify that for blood vacuity, blood stasis, and/or wind cold impediment. In addition, if the patient clearly has a pattern based on their habitual bodily constitution, then one should choose a formula for that constitution and modify it for tennis elbow, keeping in mind the main mechanisms of this disease. In other words, if a person had a liver blood-kidney yin vacuity bodily constitution, then one might start with *Liu Wei Di Huang Wan* (Six Flavors Rehmannia Pills). If one has a phlegm damp bodily constitution, then one might modify *Er Chen Tang* (Two Aged [Ingredients] Decoction), etc.

2. In order to get a satisfactory result with tennis elbow, the patient needs to refrain from all activities, be they work or play, that aggravate this condition. Until or unless the patient

is willing to allow the inflammation of their lateral epicondyle to heal, no amount of acupuncture or Chinese medicinals are going to get a satisfactory effect. If the cause of this inflammation is work related, the patient should be advised to modify their equipment or their work habits. This may mean using a lighter hammer or tennis racket or seeking professional advice from an ergonomic specialist or kinesiologist. For instance, Alexander Technique™ therapists and Aston Patterners™ can help identify and correct faulty work postures.

3. While ice is indicated within Chinese medicine for recent traumatic injuries and acute inflammations with redness, swelling, and palpable heat, it is usually contraindicated for tennis elbow. Even though Western medicine defines lateral epicondylitis as a species of inflammation, it does not usually present heat signs and symptoms according to Chinese pattern discrimination. In fact, given the common age range of patients with tennis elbow and its Chinese name, elbow taxation, this condition is usually a vacuity condition complicated by cold and/or blood stasis, all of which may be worsened by the application of cold.

Instead of ice, patients may also be given warming and moving, impediment-assuaging Chinese medical liniments, plasters, or compresses for home use between regularly scheduled office visits, or they may be taught how to do indirect pole moxa at home. Such self-administered treatments are especially important in the U.S. where most patients cannot afford to receive more than one professionally administered acupuncture treatment per week.

4. Rest and moxibustion seem to be the best treatments for enduring tennis elbow. While direct nonscarring thread moxibustion is our preferred technique, indirect moxibustion with a roll, on a medicinal cake, or on a slice of ginger are also very effective. In addition, it is very important not to forget to treat the *a shi* point of pain. This can be treated with either acupuncture, moxibustion, seven star needle, or tuina. For instance, one can use chicken claw needling at the point of pain. This refers to inserting a needle perpendicularly and shallowly at the *a shi* point, then needling obliquely on both sides of the point following the channel pathway. In both the premodern and contemporary Chinese literature, the most frequently used points for tenosynovitis are: *Qu Chi* (LI 11), *Shou San Li* (LI 10), *He Gu* (LI 4), *Chi Ze* (Lu 5), the *a shi* point, *Zhou Liao* (LI 12), *Shou Wu Li* (LI 13), and *Zhou Jian* (M-UE-46). If pain is recalcitrant to acupuncture and moxibustion, one may then use electroacupuncture or magnetotherapy with not less than a 2000 gauss magnet on the site pain.

5. For pain of the epitrochlea or "internal tennis elbow," one can use the same overall therapeutic strategy, but with different acupoints: *Xiao Hai* (SI 8) and *Shao Hai* (Ht 3) as local points, and *Yang Lao* (SI 6) and *Hou Xi* (SI 3) as distant points.

ENDNOTES

[1] McFarland, Ed & Curl, Lee Ann, "Patient Guide to Tennis Elbow," Johns Hopkins Sports Medicine, www.med.jhu.edu/ortho/sports/tenelbow.htm p. 4

41

LUMBAR DISK HERNIATION

Lumbar disk herniation refers to degenerative changes, with or without trauma, resulting in protrusion or rupture of the nucleus of the intervertebral disks in the lumbar region. Thus the nucleus moves either posterolaterally or posteriorly into the extradural space. If the herniated nucleus compresses or irritates the nerve root, there may be either sudden, severe, or insidious pain, paresthesias or numbness, and eventual muscular weakness and atrophy. Pain is aggravated by movement or anything else, such as coughing, laughing, or defecating, which puts increased pressure on the vertebral disk.

This condition is diagnosed in Western medicine by x-rays which show narrowing of the space between the lumbar vertebrae. CT scan may also show disk protrusion, and myelography best defines the size and location of the herniation. Western medical treatment consists of an initial two weeks of strict bed rest with analgesics and mild tranquilizers. If the condition persists or worsen, decompressive laminectomy may be performed.

CHINESE DISEASE CATEGORIZATION: This condition is mainly categorized as *yao tong*, lumbar pain. However, it is also sometimes referred to as *yao tui tong*, low back and leg pain, and *yao tong lian xi*, lumbar pain linking with the knee.

DISEASE CAUSES: Traumatic injury, invasion by external wind, cold, damp, or heat evils, and/or habitual bodily vacuity due to aging, taxation fatigue, excessive sexual activity, or enduring disease

DISEASE MECHANISMS: Invasion by wind, cold, and/or damp evils may obstruct the channels and network vessels traversing the low back. Likewise, obstruction may occur due to either externally invading or internally engendered damp heat evils. If these evils inhibit the flow of qi and blood, there will be pain. If there is habitual bodily vacuity due to either aging, enduring disease, overwork, or excessive sexual activity, the sinews and vessels of the low back may fail to receive sufficient nourishment. In that case, the sinews will become dry and contract, resulting in stiffness, while the vessels will become inhibited, resulting in pain. If there is kidney yang vacuity, vacuity cold may further lead to pain due to cold's constricting and contracting nature. Because the low back is the mansion of the kidneys, kidney vacuity, whether yin, yang, or both, is the main vacuity leading to lumbar pain. If the flow of qi and blood are inhibited for some time, this may give rise to blood stasis no matter whether the inhibition was due to the presence of replete evils or righteous vacuity. Blood stasis may also be the result of traumatic injury severing the channels and vessels in the region of the low back.

TREATMENT BASED ON PATTERN DISCRIMINATION:

1. COLD DAMP IMPEDIMENT PATTERN

MAIN SYMPTOMS: Chilly pain in the lower and upper back, a heavy sensation in the low back or feeling as if one were sitting in cold water or carrying a heavy weight, chilled limbs and lack of strength, definite points tender to palpation, increased pain on exposure to cold, decreased pain on obtaint of warmth, long, clear urination, a pale tongue with thin, white or slimy fur, and a deep, tight pulse

TREATMENT PRINCIPLES: Warm the channels and scatter cold, dispel dampness and stop pain

RX: *Wu Tou Ma Xin Gui Jiang Tang Jia Wei* (Aconite, Ephedra, Asarum, Cinnamon & Ginger Decoction with Added Flavors)

INGREDIENTS: Processed Radix Aconiti Carmichaeli (*Chuan Wu*), Radix Lateralis Praeparatus Aconiti

Carmichaeli (*Fu Zi*), Ramulus Cinnamomi Cassiae (*Gui Zhi*), Radix Angelicae Pubescentis (*Du Huo*), Radix Puerariae (*Ge Gen*), and dry Rhizoma Zingiberis (*Gan Jiang*), 9g each, Herba Ephedrae (*Ma Huang*) and Radix Glycyrrhizae (*Gan Cao*), 6g each, and Herba Asari Cum Radice (*Xi Xin*), 3g

Analysis of formula: *Ma Huang, Gui Zhi, Ge Gen, Xi Xin,* and *Du Huo* dispel wind and scatter cold. In addition, *Gui Zhi* and *Du Huo* warm the channels and treat impediment pain. *Du Huo* dispels evils especially in the lower part of the body, while *Ge Gen* resolves the muscles, especially in the bladder channels in the upper back. *Du Huo* and *Ge Gen* are probably the best Chinese medicinals to dispel wind and stop pain in the back, with *Ge Gen* better for the upper back and *Du Huo* better for the lower back. *Chuan Wu, Fu Zi, Gan Jiang, Xi Xin,* and *Gui Zhi* scatter cold, dispel dampness, and stop pain. *Fu Zi* and *Xi Xin* are very powerful for stopping pain. *Gan Cao* harmonizes all the other medicinals of this formula and controls the toxicity of *Fu Zi*.

Additions & subtractions: If there is concomitant kidney vacuity, add nine grams each of Ramulus Loranthi Seu Visci (*Sang Ji Sheng*) and Radix Dipsaci (*Xu Duan*). If there is a severe heavy sensation in the low back, add nine grams of Rhizoma Atractylodis (*Cang Zhu*). For concomitant spleen vacuity, add 12 grams each of Rhizoma Atractylodis Macrocephalae (*Bai Zhu*) and Sclerotium Poriae Cocos (*Fu Ling*). For concomitant blood stasis, add nine grams of Radix Rubrus Paeoniae Lactiflorae (*Chi Shao*) and six grams each of Resina Olibani (*Ru Xiang*) and Resina Myrrhae (*Mo Yao*). For concomitant wind cold with migrant pain or pain radiating to the leg or rib-side, add nine grams each of Radix Et Rhizoma Notopterygii (*Qiang Huo*) and Radix Ledebouriellae Divaricatae (*Fang Feng*).

Acupuncture & moxibustion: The following method may be used if modern investigations (*i.e.*, x-rays, CT scan, or myelography) show precisely the location of the herniation:

A. If the nucleus has moved posteriorly into the extradural space, needle bilateraly the *Jia Ji* (M-BW-35) corresponding to the affected vertebra plus the *Jia Ji* above and below the affected vertebra. In other words, for herniation of the nucleus between L2 and L3, needle the *Jia Ji* of L1, 2, and 3. Use even supplementing-even draining method and moxibustion.

B. If the nucleus has moved posterolaterally and is putting pressure on the rachidian nerve, needle the *Jia Ji* (M-BW-35) on the opposite side of the vertebra with the herniation plus the *Jia Ji* above and below the affected vertebra, always in the opposite side of the herniation. In other words, for herniation of the nucleus between L2 and L3, needle the *Jia Ji* of L1, 2, and 3 but only on the opposite side of the herniation. Use even supplementing-even draining method and moxibustion.

Then add to the *Jia Ji* other local points according to the location of pain, such as: *Ming Men* (GV 4), *Yao Yang Guan* (GV 3), *Xuan Shu* (GV 5), *San Jiao Shu* (Bl 22), *Shen Shu* (Bl 23), *Qi Hai Shu* (Bl 24), *Da Chang Shu* (Bl 25), *Guan Yuan Shu* (Bl 26), or *a shi* point(s). Use moxibustion and draining method.

Analysis of formula: All these points warm the channels, scatter cold, and dispel dampness, free the flow of the network vessels and stop pain.

Additions & subtractions: For lateral pain on the bladder channel, add *Wei Zhong* (Bl 40) or *Kun Lun* (Bl 60). For central pain on the governing vessel, add *Chang Qiang* (GV 1), *Shui Gou* (GV 26), or *Hou Xi* (SI 3). For both lateral and central pain, add *Shen Mai* (Bl 62) plus *Hou Xi* (SI 3). For buttock pain, add *Zhi Bian* (Bl 54) or *Huan Tiao* (GB 30). For cold pain in the low back, buttocks, and lower limbs, moxa *Zhi Bian* (Bl 54), *Cheng Fu* (Bl 36), and *Cheng Shan* (Bl 57). For pain radiating to the lateral side of the thigh, add *Feng Shi* (GB 31). For pain radiating to the posterior side of the thigh, add *Yin Men* (Bl 37). For pain radiating to the lateral side of the lower leg, add *Yang Ling Quan* (GB 34) or *Xuan Zhong* (GB 39). For pain radiating to the calf, add *Cheng Shan* (Bl 57). For severe cold pain and cold limbs, moxa *Ming Men* (GV 4). For lack of strength in the low back and knees, add *Fu Liu* (Ki 7). For digestive troubles, add *Gong Sun* (Sp 4). For lumbar and hip pain, add *Bai Huan Shu* (Bl 30) and *Ju Liao* (GB 29). For lumbosacral and coccygeal pain, add *Yin Bao* (Liv 9) and *Ci Liao* (Bl 32) or other *Ba Liao* points.

2. Wind damp impediment pattern

Main symptoms: Lower and upper back pain which is not fixed in location but migrates around. The pain in the low back is often accompanied by heaviness and can radiate to the lower extremities. This is accompanied by numbness of the skin, changes in the condition associated with changes in the weather, slight aversion to wind and cold, bodily heaviness, a pale tongue with thin, white or thin, yellow fur, and a floating, fine, bowstring pulse.

Note: In this pattern, wind cold evils are associated with qi and blood vacuity which have allowed these evils to invade.

Treatment principles: Dispel wind and eliminate dampness, diffuse impediment and free the flow of the network vessels

Rx: *Du Huo Ji Sheng Tang* (Angelica Pubescens & Loranthus Decoction)

INGREDIENTS: Ramulus Loranthi Seu Visci (*Sang Ji Sheng*), 18g, cooked Radix Rehmanniae (*Shu Di*), 15g, Radix Angelicae Sinensis (*Dang Gui*), Radix Codonopsitis Pilosulae (*Dang Shen*), Sclerotium Poriae Cocos (*Fu Ling*), Gentianae Macrophyllae (*Qin Jiao*), and Cortex Eucommiae Ulmoidis (*Du Zhong*), 12g each, Radix Angelicae Pubescentis (*Du Huo*), Radix Ledebouriellae Divaricatae (*Fang Feng*), Radix Ligustici Wallichii (*Chuan Xiong*), Radix Albus Paeoniae Lactiflorae (*Bai Shao*), and Radix Achyranthis Bidentatae (*Niu Xi*), 9g each, and Herba Asari Cum Radice (*Xi Xin*), Cortex Cinnamomi Cassiae (*Rou Gui*), and Radix Glycyrrhizae (*Gan Cao*), 3g each

ANALYSIS OF FORMULA: *Sang Ji Sheng, Du Huo, Qin Jiao, Fang Feng, Xi Xin,* and *Chuan Xiong* dispel wind and eliminate dampness, diffuse impediment and free the flow of the network vessels. *Sang Ji Sheng, Shu Di,* and *Niu Xi* supplement the liver and kidneys, boost the marrow, and reinforce the bones. *Shu Di, Dang Gui,* and *Bai Shao* nourish liver blood so as to strengthen the sinews. *Du Zhong* gently supplements both kidney yin and yang, strengthens the sinews and reinforces the bones. *Rou Gui* warms the channels, frees the flow of the network vessels, and diffuses impediment. *Dang Shen, Fu Ling,* and mix-fried *Gan Cao* boost the latter heaven to engender acquired essence and replenish the former heaven. In addition, *Du Huo* especially treats the lower part of the body, while *Niu Xi* leads the action of the other medicinals to the lower part of the body. *Xi Xin* stops pain very effectively. *Bai Shao* relaxes cramping. *Du Zhong* is the master Chinese medicinal for the treatment of low back pain. When combined with other Chinese medicinals appropriate to the pattern, it can be used for any kind of low back pain.

ADDITIONS & SUBTRACTIONS: If there is a severe heavy sensation, add nine grams each of Rhizoma Atractylodis (*Cang Zhu*) and Radix Clematidis Chinensis (*Wei Ling Xian*). If there is restriction of mobility, add nine grams each of Caulis Trachelospermi Jasminoidis (*Luo Shi Teng*) and Caulis Piperis Futokadsurae (*Hai Feng Teng*). For severe kidney vacuity, add nine grams each of Rhizoma Cibotii Barometsis (*Gou Ji*) and Radix Dipsaci (*Xu Duan*). For concomitant spleen vacuity, add 12 grams of Rhizoma Atractylodis Macrocephalae (*Bai Zhu*). For concomitant blood stasis, add nine grams of Radix Rubrus Paeoniae Lactiflorae (*Chi Shao*) and six grams each of Resina Olibani (*Ru Xiang*) and Resina Myrrhae (*Mo Yao*).

ACUPUNCTURE & MOXIBUSTION: Please see pattern #1 above.

3. DAMP HEAT IMPEDIMENT PATTERN

MAIN SYMPTOMS: Low back pain often accompanied by a hot sensation, low back soreness and heaviness, inability to bend forward and backward, possible vexatious heat, spontaneous perspiration, thirst, short voidings of dark-colored urine, painful urination, loose stools, slimy, yellow tongue fur, and a soggy, rapid or slippery, rapid pulse

TREATMENT PRINCIPLES: Clear heat and disinhibit dampness, diffuse impediment and stop pain

RX: *Jia Wei Si Miao Wan* (Added Flavors Four Wonders Pills)

INGREDIENTS: Semen Coicis Lachryma-jobi (*Yi Yi Ren*), 30g, Rhizoma Atractylodis (*Cang Zhu*) and Radix Achyranthis Bidentatae (*Niu Xi*), 12g each, and Cortex Phellodendri (*Huang Bai*) and Radix Gentianae Macrophyllae (*Qin Jiao*), 9g each

ANALYSIS OF FORMULA: *Cang Zhu* strongly dries dampness. It is probably the most drying medicinal in the Chinese materia medica. *Huang Bai* also dries dampness. However, more importantly, it clears heat, especially in the lower burner. Together, these two medicinals effectively dry and clear dampness and heat in the lower burner. In this formula, *Niu Xi* is mainly the messenger which leads the other medicinals to work in the lower part of the body. *Yi Yi Ren* helps the preceding medicinals to disinhibit dampness. It also treats wind damp impediment pain. In addition, *Cang Zhu* with *Qin Jiao* diffuses impediment and stops pain. *Qin Jiao* is well known for its empirical effect on conditions affecting the spinal column.

ADDITIONS & SUBTRACTIONS: If there is severe distention and heaviness in the low back, add nine grams each of Radix Stephaniae Tetrandrae (*Han Fang Ji*) and Fructus Chaenomelis Lagenariae (*Mu Gua*). If there is predominant heat with thirst and red urine, add nine grams each of Fructus Forsythiae Suspensae (*Lian Qiao*) and Fructus Gardeniae Jasminoidis (*Zhi Zi*) and three grams of Caulis Akebiae (*Mu Tong*). If there is yin vacuity with dry throat and mouth which are worse at night, low back weakness, and vexatious heat in the five hearts, add 12 grams of uncooked Radix Rehmanniae (*Sheng Di*) and nine grams each of Fructus Ligustri Lucidi (*Nu Zhen Zi*) and Herba Ecliptae Prostratae (*Han Lian Cao*). If there is restricted mobility, add nine grams each of Caulis Trachelospermi Jasminoidis (*Luo Shi Teng*) and Caulis Piperis Futokadsurae (*Hai Feng Teng*). If there is severe kidney vacuity, add nine grams each of Rhizoma Cibotii Barometsis (*Gou Ji*) and Radix Dipsaci (*Xu Duan*). For concomitant spleen vacuity, add 12 grams each of Rhizoma Atractylodis Macrocephalae (*Bai Zhu*) and Sclerotium Poriae Cocos (*Fu Ling*). For concomitant blood stasis, add nine grams of Radix Rubrus Paeoniae Lactiflorae (*Chi Shao*) and six grams each of Resina Olibani (*Ru Xiang*) and Resina Myrrhae (*Mo Yao*).

ACUPUNCTURE & MOXIBUSTION: Please see pattern #1 above but do not use moxibustion and add *Yin Ling Quan*

(Sp 9) and *Nei Ting* (St 44) alternated with *Xing Jian* (Liv 2) and *Yang Ling Quan* (GB 34).

ANALYSIS OF FORMULA: *Yin Ling Quan* is a key point for disinhibiting dampness, while *Nei Ting* is a key point for clearing internal heat. Together, they treat damp heat in the whole body. *Xing Jian* is the fire point on the liver channel, while *Yang Ling Quan* is the uniting point on the gallbladder channel. Together, they treat damp heat, especially in the wood phase.

ADDITIONS & SUBTRACTIONS: Please see pattern #1 above .

4. KIDNEY YIN VACUITY PATTERN

MAIN SYMPTOMS: Dull lower back pain which is also often so limp and lacking strength that it hinders walking and/or standing, pained worsened by fatigue and improved by lying down, rest, pressure, and massage, vexatious heat in the five centers, possible afternoon tidal heat, night sweats, a dry mouth, a red tongue with scanty fluids, and a fine, rapid pulse

TREATMENT PRINCIPLES: Supplement the kidneys and enrich yin, clear heat and harmonize the network vessels

RX: *Zuo Gui Wan Jia Jian* (Restore the Left [Kidney] Pills with Additions & Subtractions)

INGREDIENTS: Cooked Radix Rehmanniae (*Shu Di*) and Cortex Eucommiae Ulmoidis (*Du Zhong*), 12g each, Radix Dioscoreae Oppositae (*Shan Yao*), Fructus Corni Officinalis (*Shan Zhu Yu*), Fructus Lycii Chinensis (*Gou Qi Zi*), Radix Achyranthis Bidentatae (*Niu Xi*), Semen Cuscutae Chinensis (*Tu Si Zi*), and Ramulus Loranthi Seu Visci (*Sang Ji Sheng*), 9g each, Gelatinum Cornu Cervi (*Lu Jiao Jiao*) and Gelatinum Plastri Testudinis (*Gui Ban Jiao*), 6g each

ANALYSIS OF FORMULA: *Shu Di*, *Shan Yao*, and *Shan Zhu Yu* are the three supplementing medicinals of *Liu Wei Di Huang Wan* (Six Flavors Rehmannia Pills) which supplement and enrich kidney yin. *Gou Qi Zi*, *Niu Xi*, *Sang Ji Sheng*, and *Gui Ban Jiao* help the preceding medicinals to strongly boost the essence and supplement yin so as to reinforce the bones. *Lu Jiao Jiao*, *Du Zhong*, and *Tu Si Zi* supplement the kidneys and invigorate yang, reinforce the bones and strengthen the low back. *Lu Jiao Jiao*, *Gui Ban Jiao*, *Tu Si Zi*, *Shu Di*, and *Gou Qi Zi* boost the essence to nourish the marrow which thus engenders the bones. *Du Zhong* is the master Chinese medicinal for all types of low back pain. With *Sang Ji Sheng*, it treats herniation. *Niu Xi* leads the other medicinals to the lower part of the body.

ADDITIONS & SUBTRACTIONS: If there is dizziness, tinnitus, heart palpitations, and insomnia, add 12 grams of Concha Haliotidis (*Shi Jue Ming*) and 15 grams each of uncooked Os Draconis (*Long Gu*) and uncooked Concha Ostreae (*Mu Li*). If there is vacuity heat with dry throat and mouth, vexatious heat, and night sweats, add nine grams each of Cortex Phellodendri (*Huang Bai*) and Rhizoma Anemarrhenae Asphodeloidis (*Zhi Mu*). If there is restriction of mobility, add nine grams each of Fasciculus Vascularis Luffae Cylindricae (*Si Gua Luo*) and Caulis Trachelospermi Jasminoidis (*Luo Shi Teng*). If there is concomitant qi stagnation and blood stasis, add six grams each of Resina Olibani (*Ru Xiang*) and Resina Myrrhae (*Mo Yao*). If there is concomitant wind cold dampness, add 12 grams each of Radix Gentianae Macrophyllae (*Qin Jiao*) and Radix Et Rhizoma Notopterygii (*Qiang Huo*). For concomitant spleen vacuity, add 12 grams each of Rhizoma Atractylodis Macrocephalae (*Bai Zhu*) and Sclerotium Poriae Cocos (*Fu Ling*).

ACUPUNCTURE & MOXIBUSTION: Please see pattern #1 above and add *Fu Liu* (Ki 7) and *San Yin Jiao* (Sp 6).

ANALYSIS OF FORMULA: When *Fu Liu*, and *San Yin Jiao* are combined, they supplement the kidneys, enrich yin, and clear heat.

ADDITIONS & SUBTRACTIONS: Same as for pattern #1 above. For effulgent fire of the heart and kidneys manifest by reduced sleep, seminal emission, and short voidings of dark-colored urine, add *Yong Quan* (Ki 1) and *Xin Shu* (Bl 15) to downbear heart fire. For tinnitus, add *Ting Hui* (GB 2). For sore throat, add *Zhao Hai* (Ki 6).

5. KIDNEY YANG VACUITY PATTERN

MAIN SYMPTOMS: Dull, lingering low back pain that is worsened by overwork and improved by lying down, rest, pressure, warmth, and massage, low back soreness and limpness, weakness of the lower limbs which sometimes prevents walking or standing, lack of warmth in the hands and feet, fear of cold especially below the waist, possible shortness of breath, a bright white facial complexion, long, clear urine, a pale tongue with white fur, and a deep, fine, forceless pulse

TREATMENT PRINCIPLES: Supplement the kidneys and invigorate yang, warm the channels and scatter cold

RX: *You Gui Wan Jia Jian* (Restore the Right [Kidney] Pills with Additions & Subtractions)

INGREDIENTS: Cooked Radix Rehmanniae (*Shu Di*), 12g, Cortex Eucommiae Ulmoidis (*Du Zhong*), Semen Cuscutae Chinensis (*Tu Si Zi*), Radix Dipsaci (*Xu Duan*), Gelatinum Cornu Cervi (*Lu Jiao Jiao*), Radix Dioscoreae Oppositae (*Shan Yao*), Fructus Lycii Chinensis (*Gou Qi Zi*), Rhizoma Cibotii Barometsis (*Gou Ji*), and Fructus Corni Officinalis (*Shan Zhu Yu*), 9g each, Radix Angelicae Sinensis (*Dang

Gui), 6g, and Radix Lateralis Praeparatus Aconiti Carmichaeli (*Fu Zi*), 3g

Analysis of formula: *Shu Di*, *Shan Yao*, and *Shan Zhu Yu* are the three supplementing medicinals of *Liu Wei Di Huang Wan* (Six Flavors Rehmannia Pills) which supplement the kidneys and enrich yin. With *Gou Qi Zi*, they nourish yin to supplement yang based on the sayings, "Yin and yang are mutually rooted" and, "Yang is engendered from yin." *Lu Jiao Jiao*, *Du Zhong*, *Tu Si Zi*, *Xu Duan*, *Gou Ji*, and *Fu Zi* all warm and supplement kidney yang and all reinforce the low back. In addition, *Xu Duan* quickens the blood and knits the bones. *Du Zhong* is the master Chinese medicinal for low back pain. *Gou Ji* works especially on the spinal column, and *Lu Jiao Jiao* boosts the essence and reinforces the bones. *Fu Zi* warms the 14 channels and stops pain. *Dang Gui* quickens the blood to transform stasis and stop pain. It also nourishes liver blood to nourish the sinews.

Additions & subtractions: If there is central qi fall with a falling sensation in the low back and a continuous sensation of hollow pain, subtract *Gou Qi Zi* and *Dang Gui* and add 12 grams of Radix Astragali Membranacei (*Huang Qi*) and nine grams each of Radix Codonopsitis Pilosulae (*Dang Shen*) and Rhizoma Atractylodis Macrocephalae (*Bai Zhu*), and three grams each of Radix Bupleuri (*Chai Hu*) and Rhizoma Cimicifugae (*Sheng Ma*). If there is qi stagnation and blood stasis, add six grams each of Resina Olibani (*Ru Xiang*) and Resina Myrrhae (*Mo Yao*) and increase *Dang Gui* to nine grams. If there is concomitant wind cold dampness, add nine grams each of Radix Gentianae Macrophyllae (*Qin Jiao*), Radix Angelicae Pubescentis (*Du Huo*), and Radix Et Rhizoma Notopterygii (*Qiang Huo*). For concomitant spleen vacuity, add 12 grams each of Rhizoma Atractylodis Macrocephalae (*Bai Zhu*) and Sclerotium Poriae Cocos (*Fu Ling*).

Acupuncture & moxibustion: Please see pattern #1 above and add *Ming Men* (GV 4) and *Fu Liu* (Ki 7).

Analysis of formula: *Ming Men* and *Fu Liu* warm the kidneys and scatter cold when needled with supplementing method and moxa is burned on the heads of the needles.

Additions & subtractions: Please see pattern #1 above. For tinnitus, moxa *Er Men* (TB 21) indirectly. For dizziness, moxa *Bai Hui* (GV 20). For seminal emission, moxa *Zhi Shi* (Bl 52). For yang exhaustion, add *Tai Xi* (Ki 3) and *San Yin Jiao* (Sp 6) to supplement yang by nourishing yin.

6. Qi stagnation & blood stasis pattern

Main symptoms: Sharp, lancinating low back and leg pain which is fixed in location and which is better during the day but worse at night. Pressure sometimes makes the spinal pain unbearable. Possible pain radiating to the lower leg accompanied by numbness, a possible history of traumatic injury, difficulty turning, vexation and agitation, dry stools, a purple, dark tongue or possible static macules or spots, and a deep, bowstring, choppy pulse

Treatment principles: Move the qi and quicken the blood, dispel stasis and quicken the network vessels to stop pain

Rx: *Shen Tong Zhu Yu Tang Jia Jian* (Body Pain Dispel Stasis Decoction with Additions & Subtractions)

Ingredients: Radix Dipsaci (*Xu Duan*), 12g, Rhizoma Drynariae (*Gu Sui Bu*), Radix Ligustici Wallichii (*Chuan Xiong*), Semen Pruni Persicae (*Tao Ren*), Flos Carthami Tinctorii (*Hong Hua*), Radix Et Rhizoma Notopterygii (*Qiang Huo*), Resina Olibani (*Ru Xiang*), Radix Angelicae Sinensis (*Dang Gui*), Radix Cyathulae (*Chuan Niu Xi*), Lumbricus (*Di Long*), and Radix Gentianae Macrophyllae (*Qin Jiao*), 9g each, Rhizoma Cyperi Rotundi (*Xiang Fu*), 6g, and Radix Glycyrrhizae (*Gan Cao*), 3g

Analysis of formula: *Tao Ren*, *Hong Hua*, *Ru Xiang*, *Dang Gui*, *Chuan Xiong*, and *Chuan Niu Xi* quicken the blood, dispel stasis, and stop pain. *Xu Duan* and *Gu Sui Bu* also quicken the blood but supplement the kidneys and reinforce the bones as well. *Xiang Fu* moves the qi to quicken the blood. *Qiang Huo*, *Chuan Xiong*, and *Qin Jiao* diffuse impediment and stop pain. *Ru Xiang* and *Di Long* quicken the network vessels to stop pain, while *Gan Cao* harmonizes the other medicinals in this formula.

Additions & subtractions: If there is qi stagnation and blood stasis due to wind damp, add nine grams each of Radix Angelicae Pubescentis (*Du Huo*), Radix Clematidis Chinensis (*Wei Ling Xian*), and Radix Ledebouriellae Divaricatae (*Fang Feng*). If there has been traumatic injury to the low back, add three grams of Radix Pseudoginseng (*San Qi*), 12 grams of Radix Rubiae Cordifoliae (*Qian Cao*), and nine grams of Lignum Sappan (*Su Mu*) or *Yun Nan Bai Yao* (Yunnan White Medicine, a Chinese ready-made medicine).

If there is low back pain with menstrual irregularity, replace *Shen Tong Zhu Yu Tang* with modified *Tao Hong Si Wu Tang* (Persica & Carthamus Four Materials Decoction): Radix Dipsaci (*Xu Duan*), Radix Angelicae Sinensis (*Dang Gui*), and Radix Ligustici Wallichii (*Chuan Xiong*), 12g each, Semen Pruni Persicae (*Tao Ren*), Flos Carthami Tinctorii (*Hong Hua*), cooked Radix Rehmanniae (*Shu Di*), Radix Albus Paeoniae Lactiflorae (*Bai Shao*), and Rhizoma Cyperi Rotundi (*Xiang Fu*), 9g each, and Radix Bupleuri (*Chai Hu*), 6g. For concomitant kidney vacuity, add 15 grams of Cortex Radicis Acanthopanacis Gracilistylis (*Wu Jia Pi*) and nine grams each of Ramulus Loranthi Seu Visci (*Sang Ji Sheng*) and Rhizoma Cibotii Barometsis (*Gou Ji*). For concomitant spleen vacuity, add 12 grams each of Rhizoma Atractylodis Macrocephalae (*Bai Zhu*) and Sclerotium Poriae Cocos (*Fu Ling*). For stubborn pain with numbness in the lower limbs, add six grams each of Eupolyphaga Seu Opisthoplatia (*Tu Bie Chong*) and Zaocys Dhumnades (*Wu Shao She*) and three grams of Scolopendra Subspinipes (*Wu Gong*).

Acupuncture & moxibustion: *A shi* points, *Shui Gou* (GV 26), *Wei Zhong* (Bl 40)

Note: Needle the *a shi* points moderately for 20 minutes. Then withdraw the needles. After withdrawal, needle *Shui Gou* and *Wei Zhong* with draining method and ask the patient to do some movement, such as turning, bending, and stretching until the pain is relieved. If three successive treatments fail to achieve an effect, add *San Yin Jiao* (Sp 6) and *He Gu* (LI 4) while subtracting *Shui Gou* and *Wei Zhong.*

Analysis of formula: The *a shi* points quicken the network vessels, while *Shui Gou* and *Wei Zhong* free the flow in the governing vessel and foot tai yang bladder channel respectively.

Additions & subtractions: Please see pattern #1 above. For concomitant menstrual irregularity, add *Xue Hai* (Sp 10) and *Di Ji* (Sp 8). For a fine pulse, add *San Yin Jiao* (Sp 6) and *Zu San Li* (St 36) to nourish the blood. For pain in the rib-side region, add *Dai Mai* (GB 26).

Remarks

1. If there is chronic low back pain, there will be concomitant liver depression qi stagnation. In that case, add appropriate qi-rectifying medicinals to any of the above formulas.

2. In Western patients and especially women, spleen vacuity may complicate any of the above patterns. Since the defensive qi issues from the middle burner, spleen vacuity may be responsible for easy invasion of external evils. Since the spleen controls the movement and transformation of water fluids in the body, spleen vacuity may be responsible for the dampness in either wind dampness, cold dampness, or damp heat. And kidney yang vacuity in Western patients with low back pain is most commonly due to spleen vacuity reaching the kidneys. Therefore, the overwhelming majority of cases of kidney yang vacuity are complicated by spleen qi vacuity. In addition, one should also not overlook the extremely common combined pattern of spleen qi and kidney yin vacuity.

3. Damp heat may result in either spleen vacuity, liver-kidney yin vacuity, or kidney yang vacuity. It also tends to bind with blood stasis and qi stagnation. Because it is often associated with a vacuity pattern, its manifestations may not be as extreme as the signs and symptoms listed above under wind damp heat impediment.

4. Blood stasis should be suspected in all cases of enduring low back pain no matter what the main disease mechanism or pattern. It should also be suspected in all cases of low back pain in the elderly.

5. Adjunctive treatment with Chinese medicinal tincture and plasters is often beneficial in both chronic and acute conditions.

6. During acute attacks of lumbar pain precipitated by strain or traumatic injury, one should lie in bed on a firm mattress or surface for one or more days. Be careful not to massage the affected area too vigorously so as to avoid causing further muscle spasm. During acute attacks due to muscular strain or injury, cold packs may also be beneficial for the first 24-48 hours.[1] Heat is generally contraindicated unless there are clear-cut symptoms of cold. Western sedatives and muscle-relaxants may be combined with Chinese medicinals and acupuncture for quicker relief as can gentle, passive and active reduction of any spinal subluxations.

7. For low back pain associated with digestive troubles, the key point is *Gong Sun* (Sp 4) which is very effective in that case. It can be combined with *Guan Yuan* (CV 4) to make its effect even stronger.

8. Other points which give good result in clinic for lumbar pain are: *Jing Ming* (Bl 1), *Zan Zhu* (Bl 2), *Zhi Yin* (Bl 67), *Yao Tong* (N-UE-19), *Yao Yan* (M-BW-24), *Yin Tang* (M-HN-3), *Yang Lao* (SI 6), *Tian Zhu* (Bl 10), *Cheng Shan* (Bl 57), *Da Bao* (Sp 21), *Zhi Gou* (TB 6), *Fei Yang* (Bl 58), and *Zhong Zhu* (TB 3).

9. Several Chinese medicinals work very well for the spinal column, especially for herniation. The best are: Rhizoma Cibotii Barometsis (*Gou Ji*), especially for yang vacuity; Ramulus Loranthi Seu Visci (*Sang Ji Sheng*), especially for yin vacuity; Cortex Eucommiae Ulmoidis (*Du Zhong*) for both yin or yang vacuity; and Radix Gentianae Macrophyllae (*Qin Jiao*), especially for wind damp or vacuity heat. Because low back pain is most often combined with kidney vacuity and because Cortex Eucommiae Ulmoidis (*Du Zhong*) is the major medicinal in Chinese medicine for low back pain, this medicinal can be added to any formula for low back pain. As the ancients said: "[For] low back pain, one must [use] *Du Zhong.*" In fact, *Du Zhong* can be used for both vacuity and repletion, hot and cold.

10. For wind damp cold taking advantage of kidney vacuity and complicated by qi stagnation and blood stasis, use *Zhuang Yao Qu Feng Zhen Tong Tang* (Invigorate the Low Back, Dispel Wind & Settle Pain Decoction): Radix Clematidis Chinensis (*Wei Ling Xian*), 15g, Cortex Eucommiae Ulmoidis (*Du Zhong*), Rhizoma Cibotii Barometsis (*Gou Ji*), cooked Radix Rehmanniae (*Shu Di*),

Radix Et Rhizoma Notopterygii (*Qiang Huo*), Radix Angelicae Pubescentis (*Du Huo*), Radix Gentianae Macrophyllae (*Qin Jiao*), Radix Ligustici Wallichii (*Chuan Xiong*), and Zaocys Dhumnades (*Wu Shao She*), 9g each, and Buthus Martensis (*Quan Xie*), Scolopendra Subspinipes (*Wu Gong*), processed Radix Aconiti Carmichaeli (*Chuan Wu*), and processed Radix Aconiti Kusnezofii (*Cao Wu Tou*), 5g each. For difficult turning or restricted stretching and bending, add Radix Achyranthis Bidentatae (*Niu Xi*), Fructus Chaenomelis Lagenariae (*Mu Gua*), Herba Lycopodii (*Shen Jin Cao*), and Caulis Trachelospermi Jasminoidis (*Luo Shi Teng*). For a history of traumatic injury or fixed pain, add Radix Angelicae Sinensis (*Dang Gui*), Flos Carthami Tinctorii (*Hong Hua*), Semen Pruni Persicae (*Tao Ren*), and Radix Rubrus Paeoniae Lactiflorae (*Chi Shao*). For numbness and heaviness of the limbs which suggest cold and dampness, add Rhizoma Atractylodis (*Cang Zhu*), Rhizoma Atractylodis Macrocephalae (*Bai Zhu*), and Sclerotium Poriae Cocos (*Fu Ling*). For muscle wilting and weakness in the lower limbs, add Radix Astragali Membranacei (*Huang Qi*) and Radix Codonopsitis Pilosulae (*Dang Shen*).

11. Lumbar disk herniation may be associated with bone spurs in the low back area. The key Chinese medicinals for the treatment of vertebral disk herniation are, interestingly, also the key Chinese medicinals used for the treatment of bone spurs. Therefore, even in this case, one does not need to do anything other than prescribe treatment based on the patient's personal pattern discrimination.

ENDNOTES

[1] According to Simon Becker in a personal communication dated Jan. 17, 2001, his teacher, Dr. Li, recommended ice for the first 12 hours, then no external therapy for 12-24 hours, and heat thereafter. Becker says that he has seen this protocol strictly adhered to in China and has personally found it to be very effective even though it contradicts contemporary Western medical practice.

42

LYME DISEASE

Lyme disease is a tick-transmitted, spirochetal, inflammatory disorder causing a characteristic rash that may be followed weeks or months later by neurologic, cardiac, or joint abnormalities. The disease was first recognized in 1975 because of a close clustering of cases in Lyme, Conneticut. It has since been reported in 49 states, but more than 90% of cases occur from Massachusetts to Maryland, and in Wisconsin and Minnesota, and in California and Oregon. Lyme disease also occurs in Europe, across the former Soviet Union, and in China and Japan. Onset is typically in the summer and fall, and most patients are children and young adults living and playing in heavily wooded areas.

There are five groups of symptoms in Lyme disease. The hallmark and best clinical indicator of this disease is erythema migrans which develops in at least 75% of patients. This begins as a red macule or papule between the third and 32nd day after being bit by the tick. The erythematous area expands, often with central clearing, up to a diameter of 50cm. Soon thereafter, 50% of untreated patients develop multiple, smaller lesions without indurated centers. The second group of symptoms are flu-like. These include malaise, fatigue, chills, fever, headache, stiff neck, and muscle-joint pain. These symptoms are characteristically intermittent and changing, and malaise and fatigue may linger for weeks. The third group of symptoms are neurological abnormalities, such as lymphocytic meningitis, meningoencephalitis, and cranial neuritis. These only affect 15% of patients. The fourth group of symptoms are myocardial abnormalities, such as A-V block. These only affect 8% of patients. And the fifth group of symptoms all have to do with arthritis. Sixty percent of Lyme's disease sufferers develop intermittent swelling and pain of the large joints, especially the knees, within weeks to months of onset. Affected joints are painful, swollen, hot, but rarely red. Baker's cysts may form and rupture. About 10% of patients develop chronic knee involvement.

The Western medical diagnosis of Lyme's disease in patient's with typical erythema migrans in an endemic area usually does not require laboratory confirmation, However, this disease must be distinguished from a host of others, including Reiter's syndrome, RA, Bell's palsy, and chronic fatigue. Cryoprecipitates and circulating immune complexes often occur early, and the ESR may be elevated. Hematocrit and WBCs are usually normal. Rheumatoid and antinuclear antibodies are rarely present. X-ray findings are usually limited to soft tissue swelling. The Western medical treatment of Lyme disease rests mainly on the administration of various antibiotics depending on the presence or absence of the above five classes of abnormalities. Unfortunately, the time to complete resolution of this disease may extend well beyond the period of antibiotic treatment which may last anywhere from 21-30 days depending on the regime. Aspirin and other NSAIDs are administered for symptomatic relief. Complete heart block may require a temporary pacemaker. Aspiration of synovial fluids and crutches may be used for tense knee joints. Patients with arthritis of the knee that persists despite antibiotic therapy may respond to arthroscopic synovectomy. A vaccine for prophylaxis against *Borrelia burgdorferi* is currently under investigation.

CHINESE DISEASE CATEGORIZATION: The erythema migrans of Lyme's disease is categorized as *huo dan*, fire cinnabar, or *dan du*, cinnabar toxins. The flu-like symptoms fall under the category of *gan mao*, *i.e.*, flu, but, literally, contraction and encroachment. The joint pain of Lyme's disease is categorized as *bi zheng*, impediment condition. Facial neuritis comes under the category of *mian tong*, face pain, and *mian tan*, facial paralysis.

DISEASE CAUSES: External contraction of wind, damp, heat evils

DISEASE MECHANISMS: Wind, damp, heat evils enter

the exterior causing disharmony between the defensive and constructive. This results in headache, fever, aversion to chills, malaise, and muscle-joint pain and soreness. When heat evils enter the blood division, they cause erythema. When heat evils flow to and lodge in the channels and vessels of the joints, they cause pain, heat, swelling, and occasionally redness. Because damp heat easily damages the spleen, there is marked fatigue. If the condition persists, there will be liver depression due to frustration and inactivity. If impediment endures, it will eventually give rise to blood stasis. In addition to damaging the spleen, enduring heat evils may also consume yin fluids, in which case there is typically a qi and yin vacuity with lingering heat evils.

TREATMENT BASED ON PATTERN DISCRIMINATION:

1. WIND DAMP HEAT & EVIL TOXINS PATTERN

MAIN SYMPTOMS: Erythematous skin rash, fever, chills, aversion to wind, muscle-joint pain and soreness, oral dryness with a liking for chilled drinks, a red tongue with slimy, yellow fur, and a possibly floating, bowstring, slippery, rapid pulse

NOTE: This pattern corresponds to the initial stage of rash and flu-like symptoms.

TREATMENT PRINCIPLES: Clear heat and resolve toxins, cool and quicken the blood

RX: *Wu Wei Xiao Du Yin* (Five Flavors Disperse Toxins Drink) & *Wu Shen Tang* (Five Spirits Decoction)

INGREDIENTS: Herba Taraxaci Mongolici Cum Radice (*Pu Gong Ying*), Flos Lonicerae Japonicae (*Jin Yin Hua*), and Herba Violae Yedoensitis Cum Radice (*Zi Hua Di Ding*), 30g each, Sclerotium Poriae Cocos (*Fu Ling*) and Semen Plantaginis (*Che Qian Zi*), 24g each, Flos Chrysanthemi Indici (*Ye Ju Hua*), 15g, Radix Achyranthis Bidentatae (*Niu Xi*), 12g, and Tuber Semiaquilegiae (*Tian Kui Zi*), 9g

ANALYSIS OF FORMULA: *Jin Yin Hua* dispels wind, clears heat, and resolves toxins. *Pu Gong Ying, Zi Hua Di Ding*, and *Tian Kui Zi* clear heat and resolve toxins, especially in the skin division or aspect. *Fu Ling, Che Qian Zi,* and *Tian Kui Zi* clear and disinhibit dampness and heat, and *Niu Xi* quickens and descends the blood, thus leading yang to follow the blood downward.

ADDITIONS & SUBTRACTIONS: If there is marked fatigue, add 15-18 grams of Radix Astragali Membranacei (*Huang Qi*), nine grams of Radix Angelicae Sinensis (*Dang Gui*), and six grams of mix-fried Radix Glycyrrhizae (*Gan Cao*). If red rash is pronounced, add 15 grams of Radix Lithospermi Seu Arnebiae (*Zi Cao*) and nine grams each of Cortex Radicis Moutan (*Dan Pi*) and Radix Rubrus Paeoniae Lactiflorae (*Chi Shao*). For marked muscle-joint soreness and pain, add 18 grams of Radix Puerariae (*Ge Gen*).

ACUPUNCTURE & MOXIBUSTION: *Qu Chi* (LI 11), *Xue Hai* (Sp 10), *Feng Shi* (GB 31), *Wei Zhong* (Bl 40)

ANALYSIS OF FORMULA: Draining *Qu Chi* and *Xue Hai* is a special combination for dispelling wind, clearing heat, and disinhibiting dampness, especially in the skin aspect. Draining *Feng Shi* helps these first two points dispel wind and treat skin disease, especially in the lower limbs where this disease often begins. Draining *Wei Zhong* cools and quickens the blood.

ADDITIONS & SUBTRACTIONS: If there is marked fatigue, add *Zu San Li* (St 36). If a red rash is pronounced, add *Ling Tai* (GV 10). For marked muscle-joint soreness and pain, add *Yin Ling Quan* (Sp 9) and *a shi* points.

2. HEAT TOXINS WITH RIGHTEOUS QI VACUITY PATTERN

MAIN SYMPTOMS: Swelling, heat, and pain in the joints with possible redness, oral dryness and thirst, marked fatigue, a tender, swollen, light red tongue with yellow, slimy fur, and a surging, rapid pulse

TREATMENT PRINCIPLES: Clear heat and resolve toxins, support the righteous and out-thrust the interior

RX: *Tuo Li San Jia Jian* (Out-thrust the Interior Powder with Additions & Subtractions)

INGREDIENTS: Uncooked Radix Rehmanniae (*Shu Di*), 30g, Radix Astragali Membranacei (*Huang Qi*), 18g, Flos Lonicerae Japonicae (*Jin Yin Hua*), 15g, Tuber Ophiopogonis Japonici (*Mai Dong*), 12g each, Radix Et Rhizoma Notopterygii (*Qiang Huo*), Radix Ledebouriellae Divaricatae (*Fang Feng*), Radix Stephaniae Tetrandrae (*Fang Ji*), Radix Angelicae Sinensis (*Dang Gui*), Radix Scutellariae Baicalensis (*Huang Qin*), Radix Codonopsitis Pilosulae (*Dang Shen*), Sclerotium Polypori Umbellati (*Zhu Ling*), Fructus Chaenomelis Lagenariae (*Mu Gua*), Radix Achyranthis Bidentatae (*Niu Xi*), Cortex Phellodendri (*Huang Bai*), and Fructus Gardeniae Jasminoidis (*Zhi Zi*), 9g each, Pericarpium Citri Reticulatae (*Chen Pi*) and mix-fried Radix Glycyrrhizae (*Gan Cao*), 6g each, and Rhizoma Coptidis Chinensis (*Huang Lian*), 3g

ANALYSIS OF FORMULA: Uncooked *Sheng Di* clears heat and cools the blood. *Huang Qin, Huang Lian,* and *Zhi Zi* clear heat and eliminate dampness. *Jin Yin Hua* clears heat and resolves toxins. *Huang Qi, Dang Shen,* and mix-fried

Gan Cao fortify the spleen and supplement the qi. *Dang Gui* nourishes and quickens the blood. *Niu Xi* also quickens the blood, but it clears damp heat from the lower burner and guides the other medicinals to the lower body as well. *Zhu Ling* seeps dampness. So does *Fang Ji*. However, *Fang Ji, Fang Feng,* and *Qiang Huo* also treat wind dampness and alleviate impediment. *Mu Gua* frees the flow of the channels and vessels, especially in the lower extremities. *Mai Men Dong* clears heat from the heart and engenders fluids. The heat of damp heat always wafts upward where it may accumulate in the lungs and heart, consuming and damaging yin fluids there. In addition, the inclusion of *Mai Men Dong* prevents the windy, acrid, drying medicinals in this formula from also damaging yin. It is a grace note to this formula. And *Chen Pi* transforms dampness but also rectifies the qi, disinhibiting the qi mechanism.

ADDITIONS & SUBTRACTIONS: For Baker's or popliteal cysts, add nine grams each of Radix Angelicae Dahuricae (*Bai Zhi*), Spina Gleditschiae Chinensis (*Zao Jiao Ci*), and Squama Manitis Pentadactylis (*Chuan Shan Jiao*) to outthrust pus. If there is constipation, add six grams of uncooked Radix Et Rhizoma Rhei (*Da Huang*). For concomitant blood stasis, add three grams each of Resina Olibani (*Ru Xiang*) and Resina Myrrhae (*Mo Yao*) or nine grams of Lignum Sappan (*Su Mu*). If there is concomitant liver depression qi stagnation, add nine grams of Radix Auklandiae Lappae (*Mu Xiang*).

ACUPUNCTURE & MOXIBUSTION: *Qu Chi* (LI 11), *Yin Ling Quan* (Sp 9), *Zu San Li* (St 36), *a shi* points

ANALYSIS OF FORMULA: Draining *Qu Chi* and *Yin Ling Quan* dispels wind and clears heat, disinhibits dampness and frees the flow of impediment. Draining any *a shi* points frees the flow of the network vessels, disperses swelling, and stops pain. Supplementing *Zu San Li* boosts the qi and supports the righteous.

ADDITIONS & SUBTRACTIONS: For jaw impediment, add *Xia Guan* (St 7), *Yin Feng* (TB 17), and *He Gu* (LI 4). For cervical impediment, add *Feng Chi* (GB 20), *Wan Gu* (GB 12), and *Tian Zhu* (Bl 10). For thoracic vertebral impediment, add *Jia Ji* (M-BW-35) at the level of involvement. For sacrococcygeal impediment, add *Da Chang Shu* (Bl 25), *Ming Men* (GV 4), *Ba Liao* (Bl 31-34), and *Wei Zhong* (Bl 40). For shoulder impediment, add *Jian Yu* (LI 15), *Tian Zong* (SI 11), and *Ji Quan* (Ht 1). For elbow impediment, add *Qu Chi* (LI 11), *Xiao Hai* (SI 8), *Zhou Liao* (LI 12), and *Shou San Li* (LI 10). For wrist impediment, add *Wai Guan* (TB 5), *Yang Chi* (TB 4), and *Wan Gu* (SI 4). For upper extremity phalangeal and metacarpal impediment, add *Bai Xie* (M-UE-22), *He Gu* (LI 4), and *Hou Xi* (SI 3). For sacroiliac impediment, add *Guan Yuan Shu* (Bl 26), *Xiao Chang Shu* (Bl 27), *Bai Huan Shu* (Bl 30), *Huan Tiao* (GB 30), *Zhi Bian* (Bl 54), and *Ju Liao* (GB 29). For hip impediment, add *Huan Tiao* (GB 30) and *Yang Ling Quan* (GB 34). For knee impediment, add *Du Bi* (St 35), *Xi Yan* (M-LE-16a), *Qu Quan* (Liv 8), and *Wei Zhong* (Bl 40). For ankle impediment, choose between *Jie Xi* (St 41), *Shang Qiu* (Sp 5), *Qiu Xu* (GB 40), *Kun Lun* (Bl 60), *Tai Xi* (Ki 3), *Shen Mai* (Bl 62), and *Zhao Hai* (Ki 6). For metatarsal and lower extremity phalangeal impediment, add *Jie Xi* (St 41), *Gong Sun* (Sp 4), *Tai Chong* (Liv 3), *Zu Lin Qi* (GB 41), and *Ba Feng* (M-LE-8).

3. QI & YIN VACUITY WITH LINGERING DAMP HEAT EVILS PATTERN

MAIN SYMPTOMS: Fatigue, lassitude of the spirit, lack of strength, dizziness, tinnitus, low back and knee soreness and limpness, swelling, heat, and pain, dry mouth and throat, afternoon tidal heat, malar flushing, vexatious heat in the five hearts, a swollen, enlarged, red tongue with scanty fur and/or fluids, and a bowstring, fine, rapid pulse

NOTE: The difference between this pattern and the preceding one is the reversal of the proportions between evil heat and righteous vacuity. Further, in this pattern, there is not just qi and blood vacuity but qi and yin vacuity.

TREATMENT PRINCIPLES: Supplement the qi and enrich yin, clear heat and eliminate dampness

RX: *Dang Gui Nian Tong Tang* (Dang Gui Assuage Pain Decoction) & *San Miao San* (Three Wonders Powder) with additions and subtractions

INGREDIENTS: Cooked Radix Rehmanniae (*Shu Di*) and Radix Astragali Membranacei (*Huang Qi*), 18g each, Radix Puerariae (*Ge Gen*), 15g, Radix Codonopsitis Pilosulae (*Dang Shen*), Radix Angelicae Sinensis (*Dang Gui*), Rhizoma Anemarrhenae Aspheloidis (*Zhi Mu*), Cortex Phellodendri (*Huang Bai*), Radix Sophorae Flavescentis (*Ku Shen*), Herba Artemisiae Capillaris (*Yin Chen Hao*), Radix Et Rhizoma Notopterygii (*Qiang Huo*), Radix Ledebouriellae Divaricatae (*Fang Feng*), Rhizoma Atractylodis Macrocephalae (*Bai Zhu*), Rhizoma Atractylodis (*Cang Zhu*), Fructus Chaenomelis Lagenariae (*Mu Gua*), and Sclerotium Poriae Cocos (*Fu Ling*), 9g each, Rhizoma Alismatis (*Ze Xie*) and mix-fried Radix Glycyrrhizae (*Gan Cao*), 6g each, and Rhizoma Cimicifugae (*Sheng Ma*), 3g

ANALYSIS OF FORMULA: *Huang Qi, Dang Shen, Bai Zhu, Cang Zhu, Fu Ling,* and mix-fried *Gan Cao* all fortify the spleen and boost the qi. In addition, *Bai Zhu* and *Cang Zhu* strongly dry dampness, while *Fu Ling* and *Ze Xie* seep dampness. *Huang Bai, Ku Shen,* and *Yin Chen Hao* all clear heat and eliminate dampness. *Yin Chen Hao* also courses the liver and rectifies the qi without damaging fluids the way Radix Bupleuri (*Chai Hu*) often does. *Ge Gen, Fang Feng,* and

Qiang Huo all course wind and eliminate dampness in the treatment of wind damp impediment problems. In addition, *Ge Gen* upbears yang, thus benefiting the spleen, and engenders fluids, hence protecting yin from damage by the windy, acrid, drying medicinals in this formula. *Shu Di* and *Zhi Mu* enrich yin. *Zhi Mu* also drains fire. *Dang Gui* nourishes the blood, thus also supporting yin fluids, at the same time as it quickens the blood. *Mu Gua* soothes the sinews and frees the flow of the channels, especially in the lower extremities. *Sheng Ma* both raises clear yang and clears heat and resolves toxins, especially those deep-lying in the blood division.

ADDITIONS & SUBTRACTIONS: For concomitant blood stasis, add nine grams each of Cortex Radicis Moutan (*Dan Pi*) and Radix Rubrus Paeoniae Lactiflorae (*Chi Shao*). For afternoon tidal fever and vexatious heat, add 15 grams each of Cortex Radicis Lycii Chinensis (*Di Gu Pi*) and Cortex Radicis Moutan (*Dan Pi*).

ACUPUNCTURE & MOXIBUSTION: *Ge Shu* (Bl 17), *Gan Shu* (Bl 18), *Pi Shu* (Bl 20), *Wei Shu* (Bl 21), *Shen Shu* (Bl 23)

ANALYSIS OF FORMULA: Supplementing *Ge Shu*, *Gan Shu*, *Pi Shu*, *Wei Shu*, and *Shen Shu* together boosts the qi and nourishes the blood, enriches yin and supplements the spleen, liver, and kidneys.

ADDITIONS & SUBTRACTIONS: Please see pattern #2 above.

REMARKS

1. Because the latter stages of Lyme disease often resemble rheumatoid arthritis, SLE, chronic fatigue syndrome, and/or fibromyalgia, readers should refer to those sections for more ideas about alternative treatments based on the Chinese saying, "Different diseases, same treatment." For the treatment of heat or damp heat impediment, one may also see the heat impediment section under osteoarthritis.

2. Because the standard Western treatment of Lyme disease is a relatively strong and relatively prolonged course of antibiotics and antibiotics run the risk of damaging the spleen, Chinese medicinals may either be used to prevent or remedy such damage. It is our clinical experience that combined Western-Chinese medicine for Lyme disease achieves a quicker and better effect than Western medicine alone. In addition, the symptoms of Lyme's disease often continue long after antibiotic therapy has been discontinued. During this stage, Western medicine can typically only offer symptomatic relief with NSAIDs, whereas Chinese medicine has been successfully addressing such conditions as fatigue and impediment for hundreds of years.

3. As in all cases of spleen vacuity and damp heat, a clear, bland diet is of paramount importance.

4. Rocky Mountain spotted fever (RMSF) is an acute febrile disease which is also transmitted by ticks. Although initially recognized in the Rocky Mountain area of the United States, it occurs in practically all U.S. states (except Maine, Hawaii, and Alaska) and is now especially prevalent in the Atlantic states. Infection occurs mainly from May to September, although in southern states it may occur all year round. The incidence of this disease is high in children below 15 years of age and in others who frequent tick infested areas for work or recreation. After an incubation period of 2-12 days, onset of symptoms is abrupt, with severe headache, fever and chills, prostration, muscular pain, and cough. Fever may remain high for 15-20 days in severe cases, although morning remissions may occur. Between the first and sixth days of fever, most patients develop a rash on their wrists, ankles, palms, and soles which rapidly expands to the neck, face, axilla, buttocks, and trunk. After approximately four days, these lesions become petechial and may coalesce to form large hemorrhagic areas that later ulcerate. Complications may include encephalitis, hypotension, hepatomegaly, pneumonia, tissue necrosis, and circulatory failure.

The modern Western medical treatment of RMSF is the administration of antibiotics as soon as clinical signs and symptoms appear, such as fever, headache, malaise, or rash. Such antibiotic treatment has reduced mortality due to RMSF from 20 to seven percent. In terms of Chinese medicine, one can treat RMSF based on pattern discrimination similar to Lyme disease. Initially there is most commonly a wind damp heat with exuberant toxins pattern followed by heat toxins and qi vacuity. If fever endures and does not abate, heat may consume yin fluids, thus giving rise to qi and yin vacuity with possible lingering heat or damp heat evils. Integrated Chinese-Western treatment for RMSF makes use of the speed and aggressiveness of antibiotics and the righteous-supporting, whole person qualities of Chinese medicine.

5. Other increasingly common exotic diseases which share many similar clincial features with both Lyme disease and RMSF are Rift Valley fever (fever, malaise, headaches, and myalgia), West Nile fever (fever, malaise, headaches, myalgia, lymphadenopathy, and rash), and Hanta virus (fever, malaise, headaches, myalgia, and hemorrhage). These likewise should be treated with a combination of Chinese and Western medicines with the Chinese medical treatment predicated primarily on pattern discrimination.

43

Macular Degeneration

Also called senile or age-related macular degeneration, this condition is a leading cause of visual loss in the elderly. It is found equally in both men and women. However, it is much more common in whites than in those of African descent. According to Western medicine, there is no predisposing systemic risk factor for the development of this condition, but it may be hereditary. In this condition, the central area of the retina deteriorates, resulting in the loss of sharp vision. It is the leading cause of severe visual loss in North America and Europe for those 55 years of age and older, and it is the third leading cause of impaired vision in those over 65.[1]

There are two forms of this condition. In atrophic macular degeneration, a.k.a. the dry form, there is pigmentary disturbance in the macular region but no elevated macular scar and no hemorrhage or exudation in the region of the macula. In exudative macular degeneration, the so-called wet form, there is formation of a subretinal network of choroidal neovascularization often associated with intraretinal hemorrhage, subretinal fluid, pigment epithelial detachment, and hyperpigmentation. Eventually, this complex contracts, leaving a distinct elevated scar at the posterior pole of the retina. This second form of macular degeneration is much less common than the first form. Both forms are typically bilateral.

The signs and symptoms of macular degeneration are slow or sudden, painless loss of central visual acuity. Occasionally, the first symptom is visual distortion in one eye. Funduscopy reveals pigmentary or hemorrhagic disturbance in the macular region of the involved eye. Fluorescein angiography may demonstrate a neovascular membrane beneath the retina.

There is no corrective Western medical treatment for this condition unless fluorescein angiography demonstrates a neovascular network outside the fovea. In that case, this may be treated with laser photocoagulation. Patients with age-related macular degeneration, although often legally blind, have good peripheral vision and useful color vision and do not typically lose all sight.

Chinese disease categorization: Macular degeneration is a type of *qing mang* or clear-eye blindness. This refers to loss of visual acuity without any obvious externally visible changes in the eyes.

Disease causes: Former heaven natural endowment insufficiency, enduring disease, and aging

Disease mechanisms: The Chinese medical disease mechanisms of this disease are either nonconstruction and malnourishment of the eyesight due to insufficiency, or blockage and obstruction of the clear orifices of the eyes by qi and blood stasis and stagnation. Vision is a result of the essence qi of the five viscera constructing and nourishing the eyesight. The main visceral vacuities involved are those of the spleen, liver, and kidneys.

Treatment based on pattern discrimination:

1. Liver-kidney yin debility pattern

Main symptoms: Decreased visual acuity, possible rough, dry eyes, tinnitus, dizziness, low back and knee soreness and weakness, a dry throat, red cheeks, vexatious heat in the five hearts, profuse dreams, insomnia, night sweats, a pale tongue with a red tip or a red tongue with scanty fur and moisture, and a fine, rapid pulse

Treatment principles: Enrich and nourish the liver and kidneys and brighten the eyes

Rx: *Ming Mu Di Huang Wan Jia Jian* (Brighten the Eyes Rehmannia Pills with Additions & Subtractions)

INGREDIENTS: Cooked Radix Rehmanniae (*Shu Di*), uncooked Radix Rehmanniae (*Sheng Di*), and Radix Salviae Miltiorrhizae (*Dan Shen*), 18g each, Fructus Corni Officinalis (*Shan Zhu Yu*), Fructus Lycii Chinensis (*Gou Qi Zi*), and Flos Chrysanthemi Morifolii (*Ju Hua*), 12g each, and Radix Dioscoreae Oppositae (*Shan Yao*), Rhizoma Alismatis (*Ze Xie*), Sclerotium Pararadicis Poriae Cocos (*Fu Shen*), Radix Bupleuri (*Chai Hu*), Radix Angelicae Sinensis (*Dang Gui*), and Fructus Schisandrae Chinensis (*Wu Wei Zi*), 9g each

ANALYSIS & FORMULA: *Sheng Di, Shu Di, Gou Qi Zi, Dang Gui*, and *Wu Wei Zi* nourish the blood and enrich the yin of the liver and kidneys. *Gou Qi Zi* also brightens the eyes. *Dang Gui* both nourishes and quickens the blood, while *Dan Shen* both quickens and nourishes the blood. Since this condition is age-related and since blood stasis is such a common factor in geriatric diseases, the addition of at least some blood-quickening medicinals is indicated. *Shan Zhu Yu* supplements the kidneys and the spleen, while *Shan Yao* supplements both the spleen and kidneys. The use of these two medicinals is based on the relationship between former and latter heavens. *Fu Shen* supplements the heart and spleen at the same time as it quiets the spirit. *Chai Hu* courses the liver and resolves depression at the same time as it guides the effects of the other medicinals to the eyes. This is based on the saying, "The liver opens into the orifices of the eyes," and the fact that *Chai Hu* is a main medicinal for the liver. *Ze Xie* seeps dampness, as does to a lesser extent *Fu Shen*. Seeping dampness helps lead ministerial fire back down to its lower source. *Ju Hua* clears the liver and brightens the eyes.

ADDITIONS & SUBTRACTIONS: If there are profuse dreams and insomnia, add 12 grams each of Semen Biotae Orientalis (*Bai Zi Ren*) and Semen Zizyphi Spinosae (*Suan Zao Ren*). If there is low back and knee soreness and weakness, add 12 grams of Ramulus Loranthi Seu Visci (*Sang Ji Sheng*) and nine grams of Cortex Eucommiae Ulmoidis (*Du Zhong*). If there are night sweats and heart palpitations, add 30 grams of Fructus Levis Tritici Aestivi (*Fu Xiao Mai*) and 12 grams of Concha Ostreae (*Mu Li*).

ACUPUNCTURE & MOXIBUSTION: *Fu Liu* (Ki 7), *San Yin Jiao* (Sp 6), *Jing Ming* (Bl 1), *Qiu Hou* (M-HN-8), *Cheng Qi* (St 1)

ANALYSIS OF FORMULA: Supplementing *Fu Liu* supplements the kidneys and enriches water. Supplementing *San Yin Jiao* nourishes and supplements liver blood and kidney yin. Supplementing *Jing Ming, Qiu Hou*, and/or *Cheng Qi* brightens the eyes.

ADDITIONS & SUBTRACTIONS: If there are night sweats, add *He Gu* (LI 4). If there is dizziness and tinnitus, add *Feng Chi* (GB 20). If there is insomnia and profuse dreams, add *Shen Men* (Ht 7) and *Feng Chi* (GB 20). If there is low back pain, add *Shen Shu* (Bl 23). If there is concomitant liver depression, add *He Gu* (LI 4) and *Tai Chong* (Liv 3).

2. SPLEEN-KIDNEY YANG VACUITY PATTERN

MAIN SYMPTOMS: Decreased visual acuity, a cold body and chilled limbs, aversion to cold, shortness of breath on slight exertion, faint or weak voice, fatigue, bodily weakness, frequent urination at night, decreased intake, loose stools, possible cockcrow diarrhea, low back and knee soreness and weakness, tinnitus, dizziness, a pale, typically enlarged tongue with white fur, and a deep, fine, forceless pulse

TREATMENT PRINCIPLES: Warm and supplement the spleen and kidneys and brighten the eyes

RX: *Gui Fu Ba Wei Wan* (Aconite & Cinnamon Eight Flavors Pills) & *Li Zhong Tang* (Rectify the Center Decoction) with additions and subtractions

INGREDIENTS: Fructus Corni Officinalis (*Shan Zhu Yu*) and Flos Immaturus Buddleiae Officinalis (*Mi Meng Hua*), 15g each, cooked Radix Rehmanniae (*Shu Di*), 12g, Radix Dioscoreae Oppositae (*Shan Yao*), Rhizoma Atractylodis Macrocephalae (*Bai Zhu*), Sclerotium Poriae Cocos (*Fu Ling*), Rhizoma Alismatis (*Ze Xie*), Cortex Cinnamomi Cassiae (*Rou Gui*), and Cortex Radicis Moutan (*Dan Pi*), 9g each, Radix Panacis Ginseng (*Ren Shen*), Radix Lateralis Praeparatus Aconiti Carmichaeli (*Fu Zi*), and mix-fried Radix Glycyrrhizae (*Gan Cao*), 6g each

ANALYSIS OF FORMULA: *Mi Meng Hua* benefits and brightens the eyes no matter whether there is vacuity or repletion. *Ren Shen, Shan Yao, Bai Zhu, Fu Ling*, and mix-fried *Gan Cao* fortify the spleen and supplement the qi. *Shu Di, Shan Yao*, and *Shan Zhu Yu* supplement the kidneys. In addition, *Shan Zhu Yu* secures and astringes the essence, urine, and stools. *Fu Zi* and *Rou Gui* strongly warm and invigorate spleen and kidney yang. *Fu Ling* and *Ze Xie* seep dampness and prevent ministerial fire from stirring upward, and *Dan Pi* quickens the blood and transforms stasis.

ADDITIONS & SUBTRACTIONS: If there is liver depression qi stagnation, add nine grams each of Radix Bupleuri (*Chai Hu*) and Radix Albus Paeoniae Lactiflorae (*Bai Shao*). If there is downward falling of the spleen qi, add 4.5 grams of Rhizoma Cimicifugae (*Sheng Ma*) and three grams of Radix Bupleuri (*Chai Hu*). If there is concomitant blood stasis, add nine grams of Radix Salviae Miltiorrrhizae (*Dan Shen*). If there is concomitant phlegm misting the clear orifices, add nine grams of Rhizoma Acori Graminei (*Shi Chang Pu*). If there is more marked fatigue and bodily weakness, add up to 30 grams of Radix Astragali Membranacei (*Huang Qi*). If there is low back pain and weakness, add nine grams each of Radix Dipsaci (*Xu Duan*) and Cortex Eucommiae Ulmoidis (*Du Zhong*). If there is decreased sexual desire and impotence, add nine grams each of Rhizoma Curculiginis Orchioidis (*Xian Mao*) and Herba Epimedii (*Xiang Ling Pi*).

ACUPUNCTURE & MOXIBUSTION: *Zu San Li* (St 36), *San Yin Jiao* (Sp 6), *Pi Shu* (Bl 20), *Wei Shu* (Bl 21), *Shen Shu* (Bl 23), *Jing Ming* (Bl 1), *Qiu Hou* (M-HN-8), *Cheng Qi* (St 1)

ANALYSIS OF FORMULA: Supplementing *Zu San Li, San Yin Jiao, Pi Shu,* and *Wei Shu* fortifies the spleen and boosts the qi. Supplementing *San Yin Jiao* and *Shen Shu* supplements the kidneys and invigorates yang. Supplementing *Jing Ming, Qiu Hou,* and/or *Cheng Qi* brightens the eyes. Also use moxibustion at *Pi Shu, Wei Shu,* and *Shen Shu.*

ADDITIONS & SUBTRACTIONS: For more marked spleen qi vacuity, add *Tai Bai* (Sp 3). For concomitant liver depression, add *Tai Chong* (Liv 3) and *He Gu* (LI 4). For concomitant blood stasis, use even supplementing-even draining technique at *San Yin Jiao* and drain *He Gu.* If blood stasis is even more marked, also drain *Ge Shu* (Bl 17). For more marked kidney yang vacuity, add moxibustion at *Guan Yuan* (CV 4) and *Ming Men* (GV 4).

3. QI & BLOOD DUAL VACUITY WITH QI STAGNATION & BLOOD STASIS PATTERN

MAIN SYMPTOMS: Decreased visual acuity, dizziness, fatigue, bodily weakness, shortness of breath, a pale white, sallow yellow, or dark, sooty facial complexion, irritability, emotional depression, taciturnity and disinclination to stir or speak, dry, scaly skin, brittle nails, dry, falling hair, itching, age spots, cherry hemangiomas, spider nevi, or other varicosities, possible constipation, loose stools, or alternating constipation and loose stools, a pale, enlarged but darkish tongue with possible static macules and/or spots, and a fine, forceless but yet bowstring pulse

TREATMENT PRINCIPLES: Boost the qi and upbear yang, course and harmonize the liver, nourish and quicken the blood, and brighten the eyes

RX: *Yi Qi Sheng Yang Bu Xue Fang* (Boost the Qi, Upbear Yang & Supplement the Blood Formula)

INGREDIENTS: Radix Albus Paeoniae Lactiflorae (*Bai Shao*) and Radix Salviae Miltiorrhizae (*Dan Shen*), 15g each, Radix Codonopsitis Pilosulae (*Dang Shen*), Radix Astragali Membranacei (*Huang Qi*), Radix Angelicae Sinensis (*Dang Gui*), cooked Radix Rehmanniae (*Shu Di*), Radix Rubrus Paeoniae Lactiflorae (*Chi Shao*), Tuber Curcumae (*Yu Jin*), and Cortex Radicis Moutan (*Dan Pi*), 12g each, Rhizoma Atractylodis Macrocephalae (*Bai Zhu*), Pericarpium Citri Reticulatae (*Chen Pi*), Fructus Lycii Chinensis (*Gou Qi Zi*), and Semen Pruni Persicae (*Tao Ren*), 9g each, Radix Bupleuri (*Chai Hu*) and Rhizoma Acori Graminei (*Shi Chang Pu*), 6g each, and Rhizoma Cimcifugae (*Sheng Ma*), 3g

ANALYSIS OF FORMULA: This formula is a modification of *Bu Zhong Yi Qi Tang* (Supplement the Center & Boost the Qi Decoction). *Dang Shen, Huang Qi,* and *Bai Zhu* fortify the spleen and supplement the qi. *Bai Shao, Dan Shen, Dang Gui, Gou Qi Zi,* and *Shu Di* supplement the liver and nourish the blood. In addition, *Gou Qi Zi* brightens the eyes. *Dan Shen, Dang Gui, Yu Jin, Dan Pi, Chi Shao,* and *Tao Ren* quicken the blood and transform stasis. *Chai Hu, Chen Pi,* and *Sheng Ma* regulate and rectify the qi mechanism, upbearing the clear and downbearing the turbid. *Shi Chang Pu* transforms phlegm and opens the orifices.

ADDITIONS & SUBTRACTIONS: For concomitant dampness and phlegm, add nine grams each of Sclerotium Poriae Cocos (*Fu Ling*) and Rhizoma Pinelliae Ternatae (*Ban Xia*).

ACUPUNCTURE & MOXIBUSTION: *Zu San Li* (St 36), *San Yin Jiao* (Sp 6), *Tai Chong* (Liv 3), *He Gu* (LI 4), *Ge Shu* (Bl 17), *Gan Shu* (Bl 18), *Jing Ming* (Bl 1), *Qiu Hou* (M-HN-8), *Cheng Qi* (St 1)

ANALYSIS OF FORMULA: Supplementing *Zu San Li* supplements the spleen and boosts the qi. Even supplementing-even draining *San Yin Jiao* helps *Zu San Li* supplement the qi at the same time as it quickens the blood and transforms stasis. Draining *Tai Chong* and *He Gu* moves the qi and quickens the blood of the whole body, especially when combined with *San Yin Jiao.* Even supplementing-even draining *Ge Shu* and *Gan Shu* both nourishes and quickens the blood as well as helps *Tai Chong* course the liver and rectify the qi. Even supplementing-even draining *Jing Ming, Qiu Hou,* and/or *Cheng Qi* opens the orifices and brightens the eyes.

ADDITIONS & SUBTRACTIONS: For phlegm confounding the clear orifices, add *Feng Long* (St 40). For chest pain or oppression, add *Nei Guan* (Per 6) and *Dan Zhong* (CV 17). For more marked liver depression, add *Guang Ming* (GB 37) and *Feng Chi* (GB 20). For more marked spleen qi vacuity, add *Tai Bai* (Sp 3).

4. QI, BLOOD, YIN & YANG VACUITY PATTERN

MAIN SYMPTOMS: Decreased visual acuity which is worse at night and when fatigued, a pale, possibly sallow yellow facial complexion, fatigue, lack of strength, shortness of breath on slight exertion, dry skin, brittle nails, low back and knee soreness and weakness, tinnitus, dizziness, impaired memory, decreased auditory acuity, decreased sexual desire, cold hands and feet, upper back chill, aversion to cold, nocturia, possible seminal emission, constipation, spider nevi, cherry hemangiomas, or other varicosities, age spots on the skin, a pale, enlarged or enlarged, red, dry tongue with scanty fur, and a fine, deep, weak pulse

NOTE: If qi and blood, yin and yang are all truly vacuous and insufficient, there will have to be complications associated with liver depression and blood stasis at the least even if the name of this pattern does not say so.

TREATMENT PRINCIPLES: Enrich the kidneys and invigorate yang, nourish the blood and boost the qi, quicken the blood and free the flow of the network vessels

RX: *Wang Yi Jian* (Retinal Changes Decoction)

INGREDIENTS: Caulis Milletiae Seu Spatholobi (*Ji Xue Teng*), 30g, Radix Codonopsitis Pilosulae (*Dang Shen*), 20g, cooked Radix Rehmanniae (*Shu Di*), Semen Cuscutae Chinensis (*Tu Si Zi*), Fructus Liquidambaris Taiwaniae (*Lu Lu Tong*), and Flos Immaturus Buddleiae Officinalis (*Mi Meng Hua*), 15g each, Fructus Ligustri Lucidi (*Nu Zhen Zi*), Fructus Lycii Chinensis (*Gou Qi Zi*), Radix Lateralis Praeparatus Aconiti Carmichaeli (*Fu Zi*), Radix Morindae Officinalis (*Ba Ji Tian*), and Semen Leonuri Heterophylli (*Chong Wei Zi*), 12g each, Radix Angelicae Sinensis (*Dang Gui*), Radix Albus Paeoniae Lactiflorae (*Bai Shao*), Semen Pruni Persicae (*Tao Ren*), and Flos Carthami Tinctorii (*Hong Hua*), 9g each, Rhizoma Cimicifugae (*Sheng Ma*), 6g, and Radix Glycyrrhizae (*Gan Cao*), 3g

ANALYSIS OF FORMULA: *Ji Xue Teng, Shu Di, Dang Gui, Bai Shao, Nu Zhen Zi,* and *Gou Qi Zi* all supplement the liver and nourish the blood. *Shu Di, Gou Qi Zi,* and *Tu Si Zi* supplement the kidneys and help foster essence. In addition, *Tu Si Zi, Nu Zhen Zi,* and *Gou Qi Zi* brighten the eyes. *Tu Si Zi* also secures and astringes essence and urine. *Ba Ji Tian* supplements the kidneys and invigorates yang, while *Fu Zi* warms and invigorates yang. *Ji Xue Teng, Dang Gui, Hong Hua, Chong Wei Zi, Lu Lu Tong,* and *Tao Ren* quicken the blood and transform stasis. *Tao Ren* also moistens the intestines and frees the flow of the stools. *Dang Shen* fortifies the spleen and supplements the qi. *Sheng Ma* upbears the clear, thus aiding in the rectification of the qi mechanism and the supplementation of the qi. *Mi Meng Hua* generally benefits and brightens the eyes, being used for either replete or vacuity patterns of eye problems. *Gan Cao* harmonizes all the other medicinals in this formula.

ADDITIONS & SUBTRACTIONS: If there is liver depression qi stagnation, add nine grams of Radix Bupleuri (*Chai Hu*). If there is yin vacuity-fire effulgence, add nine grams each of Cortex Phellodendri (*Huang Bai*) and Rhizoma Anemarrhenae Aspheloidis (*Zhi Mu*). If there is more marked fatigue and bodily weakness, add up to 30 grams of Radix Astragali Membranacei (*Huang Qi*). If there is low back pain, add 12 grams each of Cortex Eucommiae Ulmoidis (*Du Zhong*) and Ramulus Loranthi Seu Visci (*Sang Ji Sheng*). If there is phlegm misting the clear orifices, add nine grams of Rhizoma Acori Graminei (*Shi Chang Pu*). For decreased sexual desire, add nine grams each of Rhizoma Curculiginis Orchioidis (*Xian Mao*) and Herba Epimedii (*Yin Yang Huo*).

ACUPUNCTURE & MOXIBUSTION: *Zu San Li* (St 36), *Fu Liu* (Ki 7), *San Yin Jiao* (Sp 6), *Ge Shu* (Bl 17), *Gan Shu* (Bl 18), *Pi Shu* (Bl 20), *Shen Shu* (Bl 23), *Jing Ming* (Bl 1), *Qiu Hou* (M-HN-8), *Cheng Qi* (St 1)

ANALYSIS OF FORMULA: Supplementing *Zu San Li, San Yin Jiao,* and *Pi Shu* fortifies the spleen and boosts the qi. Supplementing *Ge Shu* and *Gan Shu* supplements the liver and nourishes the blood. Supplementing *Fu Liu,* the metal-mother point of the kidneys, supplements the kidneys and enriches yin. Supplementing *Shen Shu* with moxibustion supplements the kidneys and invigorates yang. Supplementing *Jing Ming, Qiu Hou,* and/or *Cheng Qi* brightens the eyes.

ADDITIONS & SUBTRACTIONS: If there is marked blood stasis, needle *Ge Shu* and *San Yin Jiao* with even supplementing-even draining technique. If there is marked qi vacuity, add *Tai Bai* (Sp 3). If there is marked yang vacuity, also moxa *Guan Yuan* (CV 4) and *Ming Men* (GV 4).

REMARKS

1. Vision degeneration problems are often difficult to treat satisfactorily with either fine needle acupuncture or internally administered Chinese medicinals. One explanation for this is that there is blood stasis in the grandchild network vessels which nourish the eyes, and fine needles are not so good for freeing the flow of the network vessels, especially in this region. Therefore, daily local self-massage, including tapotement around the orbits of the eyes, is recommended as local adjunctive therapy. Likewise, cupping, *gua sha,* and bleeding therapy may also be helpful adjunctively as these are more successful for freeing the flow of the network vessels and dispelling stasis.

2. Some Chinese textbooks also give the pure patterns of spleen qi vacuity, liver depression qi stagnation, and qi stagnation and blood stasis for this disorder. However, since this condition is a geriatric disease, such pure patterns are not clinically realistic. According to Yan De-xin, we can expect blood stasis to play a part in all diseases of the elderly. Likewise, if there is qi, blood, yin, and/or yang vacuity with

a chronic, enduring disease, then there will be liver depression qi stagnation. In addition, because A) blood and body fluids flow together and B) aging is closely associated with spleen and kidney decline and debility and the spleen and kidneys are two of the three viscera which control water fluids, phlegm turbidity often complicates any and all of the above patterns.

ENDNOTES

[1] Pizzorno, J.E. & Murray, M.T., *A Textbook of Natural Medicine*, John Bastyr College Publications, Seattle, WA, 1989

44

MENIERE'S DISEASE

Meniere's disease is characterized by recurrent dizziness and vertigo, tinnitus, and sensory hearing loss. Its etiology is unknown, and it mostly occurs in the middle-aged. Attacks of vertigo appear suddenly and last from a few to 24 hours before gradually subsiding. These attacks are typically associated with nausea and vomiting. In addition, there may often be a feeling of recurrent fullness or pressure in the affected ear. Eighty to 90% of cases are one-sided, and tinnitus may be either constant or intermittent, possibly worsening before, during, or after attacks. The Western medical treatment of Meniere's disease is mostly based on providing symptomatic relief with anticholinergic agents, antihistamines, or barbituates. Diazepam (*i.e.*, Valium) is also used to relieve the distress of severe vertigo. Several different surgeries may be used in patients with disabling severe, recurrent vertigo.

CHINESE DISEASE CATEGORIZATION: Meniere's disease is mainly categorized as *xuan yun*, dizziness, *xuan mao*, veiling dizziness, *tou xuan*, head dizziness, and *tou feng xuan*, head wind dizziness. Nausea is categorized as *e xin*, nausea, literally "malign heart," and *ou e*, nausea and vomiting.

DISEASE CAUSES: External contraction of the six environmental excesses, internal damage by the seven affects, unregulated eating and drinking, taxation fatigue, and loss of blood

DISEASE MECHANISMS: In patients who have a habitual bodily yang exuberance, emotional stress, frustration, or anger and/or over-eating spicy, acrid, hot, fatty foods or drinking alcohol may result in liver yang becoming effulgent. If extreme, this may engender wind and transform into fire. It is also possible for unfulfilled desires or anger to anger damage the liver, resulting in liver depression which may also transform into fire. Further, due to aging, enduring disease, taxation fatigue, drug use, or excessive sexual activity, yin vacuity may lead to yang hyperactivity with subsequent wind and fire. In all these cases, wind and fire may ascend and harass the clear orifices above, thus resulting in dizziness.

Enduring disease or taxation fatigue may consume and damage the qi and blood, excessive thinking or worry and anxiety may damage the spleen, or simple blood loss may all result in qi and blood dual vacuity. If the qi becomes vacuous, the clear yang will become devitalized. If the blood becomes vacuous, the brain will fail to receive sufficient nourishment. In either case, there may be dizziness.

Former heaven natural endowment insufficiency, aging, enduring disease, drug use, and excessive sexual activity may all result in kidney essence insufficiency. Essence engenders the marrow which gathers in the brain. If kidney essence insufficiency fails to fill the brain with marrow, dizziness may occur.

If, due to over-eating fatty, sweet foods or drinking alcohol, dampness is engendered internally, this dampness may transform into phlegm. It is also possible for excessive worry and anxiety to damage the spleen which may fail to do its duty of moving and transforming fluids in the body. If fluids collect, they may transform into evil dampness. If dampness endures, it may transform into phlegm. No matter how it is engendered, phlegm dampness or phlegm turbidity may obstruct the center, thus preventing clear yang from being upborne and turbid yin from being downborne. Rather, phlegm dampness may confound and block the clear orifices and hence cause dizziness. If phlegm turbidity becomes depressed and engenders heat or transforms into fire, phlegm and fire may ascend to assail the clear orifices. This can cause even more serious dizziness.

TREATMENT BASED ON PATTERN DISCRIMINATION:

1. LIVER YANG HARASSING ABOVE PATTERN

MAIN SYMPTOMS: Dizziness, tinnitus with a loud noise, possible diminished hearing, head distention and pain, easy anger, taxation fatigue worsening the condition, insomnia, profuse dreams, a bitter taste in the mouth, a flushed red facial complexion, a red tongue with yellow fur, and a bowstring, fine, rapid pulse

TREATMENT PRINCIPLES: Level the liver and subdue yang, enrich and nourish the liver and kidneys

RX: *Tian Ma Gou Teng Yin* (Gastrodia & Uncaria Drink)

INGREDIENTS: Rhizoma Gastrodiae Elatae (*Tian Ma*), Ramulus Uncariae Cum Uncis (*Gou Teng*), Radix Achyranthis Bidentatae (*Niu Xi*), and Herba Leonuri Heterophylli (*Yi Mu Cao*), 15g each, Concha Haliotidis (*Shi Jue Ming*), Cortex Eucommiae Ulmoidis (*Du Zhong*), and Ramulus Loranthi Seu Visci (*Sang Ji Sheng*), 12g each, and Radix Scutellariae Baicalensis (*Huang Qin*), Fructus Gardeniae Jasminoidis (*Zhi Zi*), Sclerotium Pararadicis Poriae Cocos (*Fu Shen*), and Caulis Polygoni Multiflori (*Ye Jiao Teng*), 9g each

ANALYSIS OF FORMULA: *Gou Teng, Tian Ma*, and *Shi Jue Ming* level the liver and subdue yang. *Sang Ji Sheng, Du Zhong*, and *Niu Xi* supplement liver and kidney yin to check liver yang. In addition, *Niu Xi* downbears the blood to lead fire back to its lower source. *Huang Qin* and *Zhi Zi* clear depressive liver heat due to emotional disturbance. *Yi Mu Cao* quickens the blood and disinhibits water, thus also leading fire back down to its lower source via urination. *Ye Jiao Teng* nourishes liver blood, and *Fu Shen* supplements the heart. Together, they quiet the ethereal soul and calm the spirit.

ADDITIONS & SUBTRACTIONS: If there is liver fire hyperactivity and exuberance with dizziness, severe headache, deafness, sudden tinnitus, red eyes, a bitter taste in the mouth, a red tongue with dry, yellow fur, and a rapid pulse, delete *Du Zhong* and *Sang Ji Sheng* and add nine grams each of Radix Gentianae Scabrae (*Long Dan Cao*), Cortex Radicis Moutan (*Dan Pi*), and Flos Chrysanthemi Morifolii (*Ju Hua*) and 15 grams of Spica Prunellae Vulgaris (*Xia Ku Cao*). If the stools are constipated, the urine is reddish yellow, and the pulse is bowstring and rapid, add *Dang Gui Long Hui Wan* (Dang Gui, Gentiana & Aloe Pills, a Chinese ready-made medicine) in order to free the flow of the bowels, discharge and drain. If dizziness is severe, there is repeated vomiting, and there is severe numbness of the hands and feet similar to Raynaud's phenomenon, add 12 grams each of Concha Margaritiferae (*Zhen Zhu Mu*), Os Draconis (*Long Gu*), Concha Ostreae (*Mu Li*), and Cornu Caprae (*Shan Yang Jiao*) to settle the liver and extinguish wind.

If there is liver fire attacking the stomach with the same symptoms as above but accompanied by severe nausea and vomiting, replace *Tian Ma Gou Teng Yin* with *Wen Dan Tang Jia Jian* (Warm the Gallbladder Decoction with Additions & Subtractions): Rhizoma Atractylodis (*Cang Zhu*), 12g, Rhizoma Pinelliae Ternatae (*Ban Xia*), Caulis Bambusae In Taeniis (*Zhu Ru*), Radix Scutellariae Baicalensis (*Huang Qin*), Fructus Immaturus Citri Aurantii (*Zhi Shi*), Fructus Gardeniae Jasminoidis (*Zhi Zi*), and Ramulus Uncariae Cum Uncis (*Gou Teng*), 9g each, Pericarpium Citri Reticulatae (*Chen Pi*), 6g, and Radix Gentianae Scabrae (*Long Dan Cao*) and Radix Glycyrrhizae (*Gan Cao*), 3g each.

If liver depression transforms into fire with the same symptoms as above but with less heat and more liver depression symptoms, replace *Tian Ma Gou Teng Yin* with *Dan Zhi Xiao Yao San Jia Wei* (Moutan & Gardenia Rambling Powder with Added Flavors): Rhizoma Gastrodiae Elatae (*Tian Ma*), Ramulus Uncariae Cum Uncis (*Gou Teng*), and Radix Albus Paeoniae Lactiflorae (*Bai Shao*), 15g each, Radix Bupleuri (*Chai Hu*), Radix Angelicae Sinensis (*Dang Gui*), Rhizoma Atractylodis Macrocephalae (*Bai Zhu*), Sclerotium Poriae Cocos (*Fu Ling*), Cortex Radicis Moutan (*Dan Pi*), Fructus Gardeniae Jasminoidis (*Zhi Zi*), and Fructus Tribuli Terrestris (*Bai Ji Li*), 9g each, mix-fried Radix Glycyrrhizae (*Gan Cao*) and Herba Menthae Haplocalycis (*Bo He*), 6g each, and uncooked Rhizoma Zingiberis (*Sheng Jiang*), 3 slices.

If liver-kidney yin vacuity is relatively severe with more severe dizziness accompanied by low back and knee soreness and limpness, seminal emission, a red tongue, and a bowstring, fine, rapid pulse, replace *Tian Ma Gou Teng Yin* with *Da Ding Feng Zhu* (Major Stabilize Wind Pearls) to foster yin and subdue yang: uncooked Radix Rehmanniae (*Sheng Di*), Radix Albus Paeoniae Lactiflorae (*Bai Shao*), and Tuber Ophiopogonis Japonici (*Mai Dong*), 18g each, mix-fried Radix Glycyrrhizae (*Gan Cao*), Plastrum Testudinis (*Gui Ban*), Carapax Amydae Sinensis (*Bie Jia*), and Concha Ostreae (*Mu Li*), 12g each, Gelatinum Corii Asini (*E Jiao*), 9g, Fructus Schisandrae Chinensis (*Wu Wei Zi*) and Semen Cannabis Sativae (*Huo Ma Ren*), 6g each, and chicken egg yolk (*Ji Zi Huang*), 2 pieces.

ACUPUNCTURE & MOXIBUSTION: *Tai Chong* (Liv 3), *Feng Chi* (GB 20), *San Yin Jiao* (Sp 6), *Tai Xi* (Ki 3)

ANALYSIS OF FORMULA: *Tai Chong* is the source point of the liver channel. Draining it levels the liver and subdues yang, extinguishes the wind and treats dizziness and headache. *Feng Chi* is the intersection point of the yang wei mai, yang qiao mai, gallbladder, and triple burner channels. Draining it levels the liver and subdues yang, clears the head and promotes the hearing. It also treats both dizziness and headache. *San Yin Jiao* is the intersection point of the three foot yin. Supplementing it supplements the spleen, liver and kidneys, boosts the qi, and nourishes and supplements yin blood. *Tai Xi* is the source point of the kidney's channel. Supplementing it enriches kidney yin and essence and also downbears vacuity heat. When combined with *San Yin Jiao*, it supplements liver yin to check liver yang.

ADDITIONS & SUBTRACTIONS: For tinnitus or deafness, add *Ting Gong* (SI 19), *Ting Hui* (GB 2), or *Er Men* (TB 21). For headache at the vertex, add *Bai Hui* (GV 20) and *Yong Quan* (Ki 1). For temporal headache and/or red eyes, add *Tai Yang* (M-HN-9). For severe dizziness and tinnitus, add *Shuai Gu* (GB 8), *Yi Feng* (TB 17), and *Chi Mai* (TB 18). For low back pain, add *Zhi Shi* (Bl 52). For nausea and vomiting, add *Nei Guan* (Per 6). For restlessness and emotional upset, add *Yin Tang* (M-HN-3) and *Nei Guan* (Per 6).

2. QI & BLOOD DUAL VACUITY PATTERN

MAIN SYMPTOMS: Dizziness and vertigo made worse by movement, taxation fatigue causing recurrent attacks, a marked somber white facial complexion during attacks, otherwise either a somber white or sallow yellow facial complexion, heart palpitations, insomnia, lassitude of the spirit and a desire to sleep, slight but continuous tinnitus, decreased hearing, disinclination to speak, devitalized eating and drinking, cold hands and feet, a fat, pale tongue with teeth-marks on its edges, and a fine, weak pulse

TREATMENT PRINCIPLES: Supplement and boost the qi and blood, fortify the spleen and harmonize the stomach

RX: *Gui Pi Tang* (Restore the Spleen Decoction)

INGREDIENTS: Radix Astragali Membranacei (*Huang Qi*), Radix Angelicae Sinensis (*Dang Gui*), and Rhizoma Atractylodis Macrocephalae (*Bai Zhu*), 15g each, Sclerotium Poriae Cocos (*Fu Ling*), 12g, Arillus Euphoriae Longanae (*Long Yan Rou*), Radix Codonopsitis Pilosulae (*Dang Shen*), Semen Zizyphi Spinosae (*Suan Zao Ren*), and Radix Polygalae Tenuifoliae (*Yuan Zhi*), 9g each, and Radix Auklandiae Lappae (*Mu Xiang*) and mix-fried Radix Glycyrrhizae (*Gan Cao*), 6g each

ANALYSIS OF FORMULA: *Huang Qi, Bai Zhu, Fu Ling, Dang Shen,* and mix-fried *Gan Cao* supplement the center and boost the qi. In addition, *Bai Zhu* and *Fu Ling* fortify the spleen and eliminate dampness. *Dang Gui, Long Yan Rou,* and *Suan Zao Ren* nourish the blood and quiet the spirit. *Yuan Zhi* also quiets the spirit. *Mu Xiang* moves the qi to promote qi transformation and prevents supplementation from causing stagnation. In addition, the combination of *Huang Qi* plus *Dang Gui* strongly supplements the blood.

ADDITIONS & SUBTRACTIONS: If there is qi vacuity with damp exuberance accompanied by diarrhea or loose stools, increase the dosage of *Fu Ling* and *Bai Zhu* and add 15 grams of Semen Coicis Lachryma-jobi (*Yi Yi Ren*) and nine grams each of Rhizoma Alismatis (*Ze Xie*) and Semen Dolichoris Lablab (*Bai Bian Dou*). For cold body and chilled limbs, add nine grams of Ramulus Cinnamomi Cassiae (*Gui Zhi*) and six grams of dry Rhizoma Zingiberis (*Gan Jiang*) to warm the spleen and boost the qi. If blood vacuity is severe, add 12 grams of cooked Radix Rehmanniae (*Shu Di*) and nine grams each of Gelatinum Corii Asini (*E Jiao*) and Placenta Hominis (*Zi He Che*).

For central qi insufficiency and devitalized clear yang with shortness of breath, lack of strength, torpid intake, lassitude of the spirit, loose stools falling down, and a forceless pulse, replace *Gui Pi Tang* with *Bu Zhong Yi Qi Tang* (Supplement the Center & Boost the Qi Decoction): Radix Astragali Membranacei (*Huang Qi*), 18g, Radix Codonopsitis Pilosulae (*Dang Shen*), 12g, Rhizoma Atractylodis (*Bai Zhu*), 9g, Radix Angelicae Sinensis (*Dang Gui*), mix-fried Radix Glycyrrhizae (*Gan Cao*), and Pericarpium Citri Reticulatae (*Chen Pi*), 6g each, Rhizoma Cimicifugae (*Sheng Ma*), 4.5g, and Radix Bupleuri (*Chai Hu*), 3g. For spleen-kidney yang vacuity, use *Bu Zhong Yi Qi Tang* plus *Zhen Wu Tang* (True Warrior Decoction), *i.e.*, add 15 grams of Sclerotium Poriae Cocos (*Fu Ling*), nine grams each of Radix Lateralis Praeparatus Aconiti Carmichaeli (*Fu Zi*) and Radix Albus Paeoniae Lactiflorae (*Bai Shao*), and three slices of uncooked Rhizoma Zingiberis (*Sheng Jiang*).

If there is qi and blood dual vacuity but without marked heart blood vacuity, replace *Gui Pi Tang* with *Ba Zhen Tang Jia Wei* (Eight Pearls Decoction with Added Flavors): Radix Astragali Membranacei (*Huang Qi*) and cooked Radix Rehmanniae (*Shu Di*), 15g each, Radix Codonopsitis Pilosulae (*Dang Shen*), Radix Albus Paeoniae Lactiflorae (*Bai Shao*), wine stir-fried Radix Angelicae Sinensis (*Dang Gui*), Rhizoma Atractylodis Macrocephalae (*Bai Zhu*), Sclerotium Poriae Cocos (*Fu Ling*), and Rhizoma Acori Graminei (*Shi Chang Pu*), 9g each, and Radix Ligustici Wallichii (*Chuan Xiong*) and mix-fried Radix Glycyrrhizae (*Gan Cao*), 6g each.

ACUPUNCTURE & MOXIBUSTION: *Ge Shu* (Bl 17), *Pi Shu* (Bl 20), *Wei Shu* (Bl 21), *Bai Hui* (GV 20)

ANALYSIS OF FORMULA: *Ge Shu* is the meeting point of the blood. It is the point where the blood of the heart above the diaphragm and of the liver below the diaphragm collect. *Pi Shu* and *Wei Shu* are the back transport points of the spleen and stomach respectively. Because the spleen and stomach are the root of qi and blood engenderment and transformation, these points boost the qi and supplement the blood. *Bai Hui* is at the very top of the body. Moxaing it brings qi and blood upward to nourish the clear cavity and thus stop dizziness and tinnitus. All these points should be needled with supplementing method and warmed with indirect moxibustion.

ADDITIONS & SUBTRACTIONS: For severe qi vacuity, add *Zu San Li* (St 36). For severe blood vacuity, add *San Yin Jiao* (Sp 6). For tinnitus or deafness, add *Ting Gong* (SI 19), *Ting Hui* (GB 2), or *Er Men* (TB 21). For temporal headache, add *Tai Yang* (M-HN-9). For severe dizziness and tinnitus, add

Shuai Gu (GB 8), *Yi Feng* (TB 17), and *Chi Mai* (TB 18). For nausea and vomiting, add *Nei Guan* (Per 6). For restlessness and emotional upset, add *Yin Tang* (M-HN-3) and *Nei Guan* (Per 6). For concomitant spleen-kidney yang vacuity, subtract *San Yin Jiao* and add *Ming Men* (GV 4) and *Shen Shu* (Bl 23) with moxibustion. For insomnia and heart palpitations, add *Shen Men* (Ht 7).

3. Kidney essence insufficiency pattern

Main symptoms: Dizziness, continuous tinnitus which increases during attacks, marked decrease in hearing during attacks, devitalized essence spirit, impaired memory, insomnia, profuse dreams, low back and knee soreness and limpness, and premature ejaculation. If yin vacuity is predominant, there is vexatious heat in the five hearts, a red tongue, and a fine, rapid pulse. If kidney yang vacuity is predominant, there is lack of warmth in the four limbs, aversion to cold, decreased sexual desire, a pale tongue, and a deep, fine, forceless pulse.

Treatment principles: Supplement the kidneys and fill the essence. If tending to yin vacuity, also enrich yin. If tending to yang vacuity, also invigorate yang.

Rx: If tending to yin vacuity, *Zuo Gui Wan* (Restore the Left [Kidney] Pills)

Ingredients: Cooked Radix Rehmanniae (*Shu Di*), Semen Cuscutae Chinensis (*Tu Si Zi*), Radix Achyranthis Bidentatae (*Niu Xi*), and Fructus Corni Officinalis (*Shan Zhu Yu*), 15g each, Radix Dioscoreae Oppositae (*Shan Yao*) and Fructus Lycii Chinensis (*Gou Qi Zi*), 12g each, and Gelatinum Cornu Cervi (*Lu Jiao Jiao*) and Gelatinum Pastri Testudinis (*Gui Ban Jiao*), 9g each

Analysis of formula: *Shu Di*, *Shan Yao*, and *Shan Zhu Yu* are the three supplementing medicinals of *Liu Wei Di Huang Wan* (Six Flavors Rehmannia Pills) which supplement and enrich kidney yin. *Gou Qi Zi*, *Niu Xi*, and *Gui Ban Jiao* help the preceding medicinals to strongly boost the essence and supplement yin. *Lu Jiao Jiao* and *Tu Si Zi* invigorate yang and boost the essence. *Lu Jiao Jiao*, *Gui Ban Jiao*, *Tu Si Zi*, *Shu Di*, and *Gou Qi Zi* all boost the essence to nourish the marrow which thus engenders the sea of marrow.

If tending to yang vacuity, *You Gui Wan* (Restore the Right [Kidney] Pills)

Ingredients: Fructus Lycii Chinensis (*Gou Qi Zi*), cooked Radix Rehmanniae (*Shu Di*), Fructus Corni Officinalis (*Shan Zhu Yu*), Radix Angelicae Sinensis (*Dang Gui*), Gelatinum Cornu Cervi (*Lu Jiao Jiao*), and Radix Dioscoreae Oppositae (*Shan Yao*), 15g each, Cortex Eucommiae Ulmoidis (*Du Zhong*) and Semen Cuscutae Chinensis (*Tu Si Zi*), 9g each, and Radix Lateralis Praeparatus Aconiti Carmichaeli (*Fu Zi*) and Cortex Cinnamomi Cassiae (*Rou Gui*), 6g each

Analysis of formula: *Shu Di*, *Shan Yao*, and *Shan Zhu Yu* are the three supplementing medicinals of *Liu Wei Di Huang Wan* (Six Flavors Rehmannia Pills) which supplement and enrich kidney yin. With *Dang Gui* and *Gou Qi Zi*, they nourish yin to supplement yang, based on the sayings, "Yin and yang are mutually rooted," and, "Yang is engendered from yin." *Lu Jiao Jiao*, *Du Zhong*, *Tu Si Zi*, *Rou Gui*, and *Fu Zi* all warm and supplement kidney yang. In addition, *Shu Di*, *Gou Qi Zi*, *Tu Si Zi*, and *Lu Jiao Jiao* boost the essence to engender the marrow, especially the sea of marrow.

Additions & subtractions: If cold symptoms are not marked, subtract *Rou Gui* and *Fu Zi* from *You Gui Wan* and add nine grams each of Radix Morindae Officinalis (*Ba Ji Tian*) and Herba Epimedii (*Yin Yang Huo*). If kidney vacuity is not able to grasp or absorb the qi and there is shortness of breath, coughing and panting, and sweating, add six grams of Radix Panacis Ginseng (*Ren Shen*), and nine grams each of Semen Juglandis Regiae (*Hu Tao Rou*) and Gecko (*Ge Jie*). If water is spilling over into the lower limbs causing swelling due to yang vacuity, add 15 grams of Ramulus Cinnamomi Cassiae (*Gui Zhi*) and nine grams each of Sclerotium Poriae Cocos (*Fu Ling*) and Rhizoma Alismatis (*Ze Xie*). If there are loose stools, abdominal distention, and scanty eating due to spleen vacuity, add nine grams each of Rhizoma Atractylodis Macrocephalae (*Bai Zhu*) and Sclerotium Poriae Cocos (*Fu Ling*). For severe dizziness add 18 grams of Radix Albus Paeoniae Lactiflorae (*Bai Shao*) and 15 grams of Fructus Tribuli Terrestris (*Bai Ji Li*). For enduring tinnitus, add 15 grams of Magnetitum (*Ci Shi*) and nine grams of Rhizoma Acori Graminei (*Shi Chang Pu*).

Acupuncture & moxibustion: If tending to yin vacuity: *Fu Liu* (Ki 7), *Shen Shu* (Bl 23), *Zhi Shi* (Bl 52), *Bai Hui* (GV 20). If tending to yang vacuity: *Tai Xi* (Ki 3), *Guan Yuan* (CV 4), *Qi Hai* (CV 6), *Bai Hui* (GV 20)

Analysis of formula: Supplementing *Fu Liu*, *Shen Shu*, and *Zhi Shi* supplements and enriches kidney yin, boost the essence and engenders the marrow. *Bai Hui* is located at the very top of the body. Moxaing it draws yin essence upward to nourish the clear cavity and thus stop dizziness and tinnitus. Supplementing with moxibustion *Tai Xi*, *Guan Yuan*, and *Qi Hai* warms and supplements kidney yang to engender the essence. Moxaing *Bai Hui* draws yang essence upward to nourish the clear cavity and stop dizziness and tinnitus.

Additions & subtractions: For tinnitus or deafness, add *Ting Gong* (SI 19), *Ting Hui* (GB 2), or *Er Men* (TB 21).

For temporal headache, add *Tai Yang* (M-HN-9). For severe dizziness and tinnitus, add *Shuai Gu* (GB 8), *Yi Feng* (TB 17), and *Chi Mai* (TB 18). For severe essence vacuity, add *Zu San Li* (St 36) and *San Yin Jiao* (Sp 6). For restlessness and emotional upset, add *Yin Tang* (M-HN-3) and *Nei Guan* (Per 6). For insomnia and heart palpitations, add *Shen Men* (Ht 7).

4. PHLEGM TURBIDITY OBSTRUCTING THE CENTER PATTERN

MAIN SYMPTOMS: Dizziness, vertigo, tinnitus with a low sound, decreased hearing, profuse phlegm, heavy-headedness, chest oppression, nausea, vomiting, devitalized eating and drinking, possible heart palpitations, slimy, white tongue fur, and a soggy, moderate (*i.e.*, slightly slow) pulse

TREATMENT PRINCIPLES: Transform phlegm and eliminate dampness, harmonize the stomach and stop vomiting

Rx: *Ban Xia Tian Ma Bai Zhu Tang Jia Jian* (Pinellia, Gastrodia & Atractylodes Decoction with Additions & Subtractions)

INGREDIENTS: Sclerotium Poriae Cocos (*Fu Ling*), Radix Ligustici Wallichii (*Chuan Xiong*), and Pericarpium Citri Reticulatae (*Chen Pi*), 15g each, Rhizoma Pinelliae Ternatae (*Ban Xia*), Rhizoma Atractylodis Macrocephalae (*Bai Zhu*), and Ramulus Uncariae Cum Uncis (*Gou Teng*), 12g each, Fructus Viticis (*Man Jing Zi*) and mix-fried Radix Glycyrrhizae (*Gan Cao*), 6g each, uncooked Rhizoma Zingiberis (*Sheng Jiang*), 5 slices, and Fructus Zizyphi Jujubae (*Da Zao*), 5 pieces

ANALYSIS OF FORMULA: *Ban Xia, Chen Pi, Fu Ling,* and mix-fried *Gan Cao* are the four ingredients of *Er Chen Tang* (Two Aged [Ingredients] Decoction), the main Chinese medicinal formula for the treatment of phlegm dampness. In addition, *Chen Pi* and *Ban Xia* harmonize the stomach and stop vomiting. *Bai Zhu,* mix-fried *Gan Cao, Sheng Jiang,* and *Da Zao* fortify the spleen to prevent further damp accumulation which might transform into phlegm. *Gou Teng* with *Ban Xia* treats wind phlegm which may confound and block the clear orifices and hence cause dizziness. *Gou Teng* has been proven to be more empirically effective than Rhizoma Gastrodiae Elatae (*Tian Ma*), a standard ingredient of *Ban Xia Tian Ma Bai Zhu Tang,* for the treatment of Meniere's disease. *Man Jing Zi* clears the head, and *Chuan Xiong* quickens the blood in order to help the dispersion of phlegm at the same time as it guides the other medicinals in this formula upward to the head.

ADDITIONS & SUBTRACTIONS: If there is stomach loss of harmony and downbearing with frequent vomiting, add 12 grams each of Haemititum (*Dai Zhe Shi*) and Caulis Bambusae In Taeniis (*Zhu Ru*). If there is damp obstruction and qi stagnation with venter oppression, no eating, and severe abdominal distention, add nine grams each of Fructus Cardamomi (*Bai Dou Kou*) and Fructus Amomi (*Sha Ren*). If dampness is encumbering spleen yang with heavy limbs and slimy tongue fur, add nine grams each of Herba Agastachis Seu Pogostemi (*Huo Xiang*) and Herba Eupatorii Fortunei (*Pei Lan*) and six grams of Rhizoma Acori Graminei (*Shi Chang Pu*). If phlegm dampness is blocking and obstructing the clear orifices with tinnitus and hardness of hearing, add nine grams each of Bulbus Allii Fistulosi (*Cong Bai*), Tuber Curcumae (*Yu Jin*), and Rhizoma Acori Graminei (*Shi Chang Pu*) to free the flow of yang and open the orifices. If phlegm is obstructing the qi mechanism and depression is transforming heat, one can add three grams of Rhizoma Coptidis Chinensis (*Huang Lian*) and nine grams of Caulis Bambusae In Taeniis (*Zhu Ru*) to transform phlegm and clear heat. If phlegm dampness has damaged spleen yang with abdominal distention, diarrhea, and slimy, white tongue fur, one can add six grams each of dry Rhizoma Zingiberis (*Gan Jiang*) and Fructus Cardamomi (*Bai Dou Kou*) to warm yang and stop diarrhea. If phlegm turbidity is confounding and covering heart yang with heart palpitations and fearful throbbing, one can add nine grams of Rhizoma Acori Graminei (*Shi Chang Pu*) to free the flow of yang, transform phlegm, and quiet the spirit. If there is profuse phlegm, add nine grams each of Rhizoma Alismatis (*Ze Xie*) and Rhizoma Arsiaematis (*Tian Nan Xing*) to even more strongly dry dampness. If there is severe dizziness, add nine grams each of Bombyx Batryticatus (*Jiang Can*), Rhizoma Gastrodiae Elatae (*Tian Ma*), and bile-processed Rhizoma Arisaematis (*Dan Nan Xing*) to transform phlegm and extinguish wind. If there is marked qi vacuity with fatigue and weakness of the limbs, add 15 grams of Radix Astragali Membranacei (*Huang Qi*) and nine grams of Radix Codonopsitis Pilosulae (*Dang Shen*) to fortify the spleen and supplement the qi.

ACUPUNCTURE & MOXIBUSTION: *Feng Long* (St 40), *Yin Ling Quan* (Sp 9), *Zu San Li* (St 36), *Bai Hui* (GV 20), *Nei Guan* (Per 6)

ANALYSIS OF FORMULA: *Feng Long* is the key point in Chinese acupuncture for the treatment of phlegm. *Yin Ling Quan* is the key point for treating dampness. *Zu San Li* is the key point for supplementing the spleen. Together, these are a key combination for treating phlegm dampness due to spleen vacuity. In addition, *Feng Long* downbears counterflow of the stomach. *Nei Guan* harmonizes the stomach and downbears counterflow, transforms phlegm and stops vomiting. Draining *Bai Hui* opens the orifices and clears the head, thus dispelling evils to stop dizziness and tinnitus. Drain *Feng Long, Yin Ling Quan, Nei Guan,* and *Bai Hui* and supplement *Zu San Li.*

ADDITIONS & SUBTRACTIONS: For severe nausea or vomiting, add *Shang Wan* (CV 13). For tinnitus or deafness, add *Ting Gong* (SI 19), *Ting Hui* (GB 2), or *Er Men* (TB 21). For temporal headache, add *Tai Yang* (M-HN-9). For severe dizziness and tinnitus, add *Shuai Gu* (GB 8), *Yi Feng* (TB 17), and *Chi Mai* (TB 18). For a heavy sensation, in the head, add *Feng Chi* (GB 20). For restlessness and emotional upset, add *Yin Tang* (M-HN-3) and *Nei Guan* (Per 6). For insomnia and heart palpitations, add *Shen Men* (Ht 7). For hypersomnia or somnolence, add *San Jian* (LI 3).

REMARKS

1. Any or all of these patterns may occur in combination with each other. In that case, determine which pattern and, therefore, disease mechanism is most pronounced and modify its treatment protocol with additions and subtractions taken from the other patterns. A good example of a treatment which addresses a mixture of disease mechanisms is *Zhi Yun Tang* (Stop Dizziness Decoction), a modern formula especially for the treatment of Meniere's disease: Rhizoma Alismatis (*Ze Xie*), 15-30g, uncooked Radix Rehmanniae (*Sheng Di*), 15g, Flos Chrysanthemi Morifolii (*Ju Hua*), 12g, Gypsum Fibrosum (*Shi Gao*), 12-30g, Sclerotium Poriae Cocos (*Fu Ling*), 12-25g, Rhizoma Atractylodis Macrocephalae (*Bai Zhu*), 12-20g, Ramulus Cinnamomi Cassiae (*Gui Zhi*), Radix Scutellariae Baicalensis (*Huang Qin*), Pericarpium Citri Reticulatae (*Chen Pi*), and Rhizoma Pinelliae Ternatae (*Ban Xia*), 9g each, Os Draconis (*Long Gu*) and Concha Ostreae (*Mu Li*), 25g each, and Radix Glycyrrhizae (*Gan Cao*), 6g. This formula treats liver depression and spleen vacuity transforming heat and dryness in the liver and stomach as well as phlegm dampness.

2. The following acupuncture formula can be used to good effect in most cases of Meniere's disease no matter what the pattern discrimination: *Bai Hui* (GV 20), *Tai Chong* (Liv 3), *San Yin Jiao* (Sp 6), *Feng Long* (St 40), *He Gu* (LI 4), *Nei Guan* (Per 6), and *Ting Gong* (SI 19).

3. Because wind is the main cause of dizziness and dizziness is such an important pathognomonic symptom of Meniere's disease, Ramulus Uncariae Cum Uncis (*Gou Teng*) can be used in all cases of this condition. Also, because tinnitus and/or decrease in hearing is very common in this disease, Rhizoma Acori Graminei (*Shi Chang Pu*) can be used on a regular basis. And finally, because nausea and vomiting are often present and because phlegm mixed with wind is the most common cause of dizziness, Rhizoma Pinelliae Ternatae (*Ban Xia*) should also be routinely used.

4. Recently, large doses of certain Chinese medicinals have been used to treat Meniere's disease with good success. These include: A) Herba Agrimoniae Pilosae (*Xian He Cao*), 60g or more per day used alone; B) Herba Dianthi (*Qu Mai*), as in *Qu Long Tang* (Dianthus & Earthworm Decoction): Herba Dianthi (*Qu Mai*), 20-50g, Lumbricus (*Di Long*) and Radix Puerariae (*Ge Gen*), 20g each, Rhizoma Acori Graminei (*Shi Chang Pu*), 15g, Rhizoma Cimicifugae (*Sheng Ma*), 6g, and Scolopendra Subspinipes (*Wu Gong*), 2 strips; and Rhizoma Alismatis (*Ze Xie*), 60-120g, combined with Rhizoma Pinelliae Ternatae (*Ban Xia*), 18-30g, and Rhizoma Atractylodis Macrocephalae (*Bai Zhu*) and Ramulus Uncariae Cum Uncis (*Gou Teng*), 9g each.

45

MIGRAINE HEADACHES

Migraines are a type of recurrent, paroxysmal, neurovascular headache with or without associated visual and gastrointestinal disturbances. Their etiology is unknown, but a genetic predisposition is strongly suspected since a family history is obtained in more than 50% of cases. One theory favored by many researchers is that migraines are due to vulnerability of the nervous system to sudden changes either internally within the body or in the external environment. This vulnerability may be due to inheriting a more sensitive nervous system than most people. According to Elaine Aron, 15-20% of people have such a highly sensitive nervous system.[1] Biochemically, this heightened sensitivity seems to be associated with serotonin (5-hydroxytryptamine or 5-HT) metabolism. It seems that serotonin levels in the blood fall at the onset of a migraine headache but are normal between attacks and that urinary excretion of serotonin metabolite 5-hydroxy indoleacetic acid also increases during an attack and return to normal afterward.[2]

Migraines may occur at any age but usually begin between the ages of 10-30 years. They also occur more often in women than in men. Attacks may or may not be preceded by a prodrome. Such prodromal symptoms include a short period of depression, irritability, restlessness, anorexia, scintillating scotomas, visual field defects such as tunnel vision, paresthesias, and, more rarely, hemiparesis. These symptoms may disappear shortly before the pain begins or may merge with it. Certain factors can provoke or trigger a migraine in some people. Among the foods which may trigger a migraine are alcohol, especially red wine, foods containing monosodium glutamate (MSG), foods that contain tyramine, such as aged cheeses, and preserved meats with nitrates and nitrites. Other factors include too much or too little sleep, fluctuations in female hormones, stress and anxiety, and environmental factors, such as weather or temperature changes, glaring or flourescent lights, computer screens, strong odors, and high altitude.

Pain is either hemilateral or generalized. When pain is one-sided, it may or may not always occur on the same side. Untreated attacks may last for hours or days. Nausea, vomiting, and photophobia are common. Some migraineurs experience a climax culminating in vomiting and diarrhea after which the pain subsides. Other migraine sufferers find their headaches disappear only after sleeping. Attacks may occur daily or only once in several months. In women, attacks may occur either before, during, or after menstruation or at ovulation. Some women's migraines begin at puberty and end at menopause, while other women's migraines begin at menopause. It is estimated that 25% of all people experience a migraine headache at some point in their life.

The Western medical diagnosis of migraines is largely based on the patient's personal and family history and the presenting signs and symptoms plus an absence of any intracranial pathological changes. The Western medical management of migraines can be divided into nonspecific therapy with analgesics and specific therapy with serotonin receptor agonists. It can also be divided into remedial treatment during an attack and preventive treatment between attacks. There are a number of nonspecific analgesics available for the treatment of the pain associated with migraine. These drugs can be broadly subdivided into low-range, mid-range, and high-range analgesics depending on their strength, side effects, and potential for habituation. Low-range analgesics include simple over-the-counter analgesics or prescription nonsteroidal anti-inflammatory drugs (NSAIDs) alone or in combinations that include caffeine. Examples of low-range analgesics include aspirin, acetaminophen, naproxen, ketorolac, and indomethacin. Although NSAIDs have been found to diminish both the severity and duration of migraine attacks, no NSAID has been found to be more effective than another. The most common side effects of NSAIDs are gastrointestinal, ranging from mild dyspepsia to gastric bleeding. Mid-range analgesics include the sedative butalbital combined with either aspirin or acetaminophen. These medicines must be used cautiously as rebound headaches can develop if the recommended dosage is exceded. High-range analgesics include aspirin or acetaminophen in combination with an opiod/narcotic analgesic or an opiod medication alone. Although the prescription of opiods for the treatment of migraine is controversial, surveys suggest that codeine, meperidine, and oxycodone are commonly prescribed for this purpose.[3]

Specific therapy is based on drugs which act at 5-HT receptor sites. These drugs activate a variety of 5-HT receptors which then blocks the release of neuropetides and prevents neurogenic inflammation. Dihydroergotamine (DHE) is the current ergotamine derivative of choice since it is considered safer than the previous migraine stand-by ergotamine. Although DHE has less peripheral vasoconstrictor activity than ergotamine, the contraindications to DHE are similar, including Prinzmetal's angina, ischemic heart disease, uncontrolled hyertension, peripheral arterial disease, and impaired liver or kidney function. Selective serotonin receptor agonists, such as sumatriptan, naratriptan, rizatriptan, and zolmitriptan have broadened the treatment options for specific therapy. However, these medications should also not be used in patients with ischemic heart disease or uncontrolled hypertension.

Prophylactic therapy is usually recommended for patients who experience more than 2-3 headaches per month with disability lasting three days or more. Some of the drugs or drug classes which have been used for preventive therapy include: beta-blockers, tricyclic antidepressants, anticonvulsants, NSAIDs, calcium channel blockers, methysergide (an ergot derivative), and monamine oxidase (MAO) inhibitors. However, prophylactic therapy is rarely effective in completely eliminating headaches and may only minimally affect the severity and duration of the headaches that do occur. In fact, preventive therapy is considered effective if it only reduces attacks by 50%. Because it may take four weeks before the initial response of prophylactic therapy to be observed and this effect continues to increase for three months, many patients discontinue preventive therapy after only 1-2 weeks.

CHINESE DISEASE CATAGORIZATIONS: One-sided migraines are called *pian tou tong*, one-sided headaches, and *tou feng*, head wind, or *pian tou feng*, side head wind. Generalized migraines are simply called *tou tong*. Nausea and vomiting are categorized as *ou tu*.

DISEASE CAUSES: Internal damage by the seven affects, unregulated eating and drinking, and the exuberance and debility of maturation and aging as well as the waxing and waning of yin and yang with the menstrual cycle

DISEASE MECHANISMS: The main disease mechanisms of migraine headaches all involve the liver. If the liver becomes depressed due to emotional stress, the qi will become stagnant. Because qi is yang and the liver is a yin viscus, either this yang qi will tend to follow the liver channel upward to the eyes and vertex or shift into the shao yang channel to rise to the sides of the head, congesting in and inhibiting the channels and vessels there. If liver depression counterflows horizontally, it may assail the stomach, resulting in nausea and vomiting. If liver depression transforms into heat, heat may flare upward to harass the clear portals above. If heat is extreme, it may transform into fire which may then engender wind which also tends to counterflow upward. Because the head is a bony box, counterflowing yang qi, heat or fire, and wind, arriving in the head, have little or no exit. Therefore, they stagnate and congest, inhibiting the free flow of qi and blood, thus causing pain.

Frequently, upward counterflow of the liver is associated with women's menstrual cycles. At mid-cycle, yin reaches its apogee and transforms into yang. Ministerial fire becomes exuberant, and this exuberance may facilitate or aggravate liver depression transforming heat. During the premenstruum, blood is sent down from the heart to the uterus. If there is a blood vacuity, A) the sinews' vessels in the upper body may not receive sufficient moistening and nourishment, and B) the liver may not receive its proper nourishment. If the liver fails to be nourished and emolliated, the liver cannot course and discharge properly, and yet again liver depression may result in upward counterflow or depressive heat may flare upward. Since the sea of blood discharges and is empty during and after the menses, blood vacuity or even yin vacuity may aggravate liver depression or liver yang ascendant hyperactivity during those times as well. As we have seen above, when the liver becomes depressed, it typically assails spleen and stomach earth. When it assails the spleen, the spleen becomes damaged and vacuous and fails to engender sufficient blood. The spleen may also be damaged by excessive thinking as well as worry and anxiety. Perimenopausally, liver blood and kidney yin are exhausted. So this is also a time when liver depression with upward counterflow, liver yang ascendant hyperactivity, and liver fire and wind are all more likely.

Besides failing to engender sufficient blood, it is also possible for spleen vacuity and/or faulty diet to result in internal engenderment of phlegm dampness. If this phlegm dampness obstructs the qi mechanism in the middle burner, the clear yang may not be upborne and the turbid yin may not be downborne. Instead, phlegm and dampness may ascend, confounding the clear orifices and blocking the channels and network vessels. Such upward movement by phlegm and dampness is all the more likely if liver qi or internally engendered fire or wind draft it upwards.

If the flow of qi and blood is inhibited for a long time or recurrently over a long period of time, blood stasis may further complicate any of the above scenarios, in which case static blood enters the network vessels causing localized, sharp, or severe pain.

TREATMENT BASED ON PATTERN DISCRIMINATION:

1. LIVER DEPRESSION-QI & BLOOD VACUITY PATTERN

MAIN SYMPTOMS: One-sided headache most often occurring in females perimenstrually, blurred vision, tunnel vision, photophobia, numbness and tingling of the fingers or face, chest, rib-side, and/or breast distention and fullness, a tendency to sighing, headaches caused or aggravated by emotional stimulation, emotional depression, fatigue, lack of strength, cold hands and feet, menstrual irregularities, possible lower abdominal distention and pain, alternating constipation and diarrhea or loose stools, a pale but dark tongue with white fur, and a bowstring, fine pulse

NOTE: This pattern describes a liver-spleen disharmony complicated by blood vacuity.

TREATMENT PRINCIPLES: Harmonize the liver and resolve depression, fortify the spleen and supplement the qi

RX: *Xiao Yao San Jia Wei* (Rambling Powder with Added Flavors)

INGREDIENTS: Radix Albus Paeoniae Lactiflorae (*Bai Shao*), 18g, Radix Ligustici Wallichii (*Chuan Xiong*) and Radix Angelicae Dahuricae (*Bai Zhi*), 15g each, Radix Bupleuri (*Chai Hu*), Radix Angelicae Sinensis (*Dang Gui*), Rhizoma Atractylodis Macrocephalae (*Bai Zhu*), and Sclerotium Poriae Cocos (*Fu Ling*), 9g each, mix-fried Radix Glycyrrhizae (*Gan Cao*) and Herba Menthae Haplocalycis (*Bo He*), 6g each, and uncooked Rhizoma Zingiberis (*Sheng Jiang*), 3 slices

NOTE: Because of its ascendant, upbearing nature, *Chai Hu* is usually forbidden in case of upward counterflow of liver qi, yang, or fire. However, it is an essential medicinal to resolve depression. Therefore, it is important when using this medicinal for the treatment of headache to use either stir-fried or vinegar stir-fried *Chai Hu* and to combine *Chai Hu* with *Bai Shao*. Using correctly processed *Chai Hu* and combining it with *Bai Shao* will prevent this medicinal's upbearing nature from causing unwanted side effects.

ANALYSIS OF FORMULA: *Chai Hu* and *Bo He* work on the yang aspect of the liver. They course the liver and resolve depression. *Bai Shao* and *Dang Gui* work on the yin aspect of the liver. They nourish liver blood to prevent further liver depression and qi stagnation. Together, these four medicinals harmonize the liver and resolve depression. *Bai Zhu, Fu Ling, Sheng Jiang,* and mix-fried *Gan Cao* fortify the spleen and boost the qi so as to keep the liver qi in its rightful place. If the spleen is strong, the liver cannot counterflow horizontally onto it. Since the spleen is the root of qi and blood engenderment and transformation, these medicinals also help engender the blood so that the liver can function correctly. *Chuan Xiong* and *Dang Gui* quicken the blood and stop pain. In addition, *Chuan Xiong, Bai Zhi,* and *Bo He* free the flow of the network vessels in the head and stop pain.

ADDITIONS & SUBTRACTIONS: If liver depression has transformed heat, add 15 grams each of Spica Prunellae Vulgaris (*Xia Ku Cao*) and Flos Chyrsanthemi Morifolii (*Ju Hua*) and nine grams each of Cortex Radicis Moutan (*Dan Pi*) and Fructus Gardeniae Jasminoidis (*Zhi Zi*). If there is concomitant blood stasis, add 15 grams of Radix Salviae Miltiorrhizae (*Dan Shen*) and nine grams each of Semen Pruni Persicae (*Tao Ren*) and Flos Carthami Tinctorii (*Hong Hua*). If enduring disease has entered the network vessels, add nine grams each of Buthus Martensis (*Quan Xie*) and Scolopendra Subspinipes (*Wu Gong*). If spleen qi vacuity is more pronounced with marked fatigue, add 15 grams of Radix Astragali Membranacei (*Huang Qi*) and nine grams of Radix Codonopsitis Pilosulae (*Dang Shen*). If blood vacuity is more pronounced, add 15 grams of Caulis Milletiae Seu Spatholobi (*Ji Xue Teng*) and 12 grams of Radix Polygoni Multiflori (*He Shou Wu*). If phlegm dampness is obstructing the network vessels, add nine grams each of Rhizoma Arisaematis (*Tian Nan Xing*) and Semen Sinapis Albae (*Bai Jie Zi*). During acute attacks, if there is marked pain at the vertex, nausea and vomiting, and counterflow chilling, nine grams each of Fructus Evodiae Rutecarpae (*Wu Zhu Yu*), Rhizoma Pinelliae Ternatae (*Ban Xia*), and Pericarpium Citri Reticulatae (*Chen Pi*) may be added. Between attacks, only add *Ban Xia* and *Chen Pi*. If perimenstrually there is concomitant low back soreness and pain, add 15 grams of Radix Achyranthis Bidentatae (*Niu Xi*) and nine grams of Cortex Eucommiae Ulmoidis (*Du Zhong*). If there is accompanying dizziness, add 15 grams of Ramulus Uncariae Cum Uncis (*Gou Teng*) and nine grams of Rhizoma Gastrodiae Elatae (*Tian Ma*).

ACUPUNCTURE & MOXIBUSTION: *Tai Chong* (Liv 3), *Nei Guan* (Per 6), local points according to the location of pain, distant points according to the channel affected. For local points according to the site of pain, select 1-3 points per treatment from among: *Jiao Sun* (TB 20), *Shuai Gu* (GB 8), *Yang Bai* (GB 14), *Tai Yang* (M-HN-9), *Bai Hui* (GV 20), *Feng Chi* (GB 20), *Yi Feng* (TB 17), *Yin Tang* (M-HN-3), and *a shi* points. Direct the tip of the needle to the site where the pain is most severe. For distant points according to the channel affected, select one hand and one foot point from among: *Wai Guan* (TB 5), *Zhong Zhu* (TB 3), *Ye Men* (TB 2), *Xuan Zhong* (GB 39), and *Yang Ling Quan* (GB 34) for the gallbladder channel. For the bladder channel, add *Hou Xi* (SI 3) and *Shu Gu* (Bl 65). For the liver channel causing pain at the vertex, add *Yong Quan* (Ki 1), and for pain on the stomach channel, add *He Gu* (LI 4).

ANALYSIS OF FORMULA: Draining *Tai Chong* and *Nei Guan* courses the liver and resolves depression. Draining *Nei Guan* also harmonizes the stomach and stops vomiting. All the other local and distant points are well-known empirical points for the treatment of migraine. The local points free the flow of the network vessels to stop pain, while the distant points move the channel qi of the affected channel to stop pain. Use draining method on all points.

ADDITIONS & SUBTACTIONS: During the headache itself, use only "side three needles" technique with draining method. This means to needle *Tai Yang* (M-HN-9) in the direction of *Quan Liao* (SI 18), *He Gu* (LI 4) perpendicularly, and *Tai Chong* (Liv 3) in the direction of *Yong Quan* (Ki 1). For photophobia or visual migraine, add *Si Zhu Kong* (TB 23) and *Yu Yao* (M-HN-6). For nausea, add *Shang Wan* (CV 13). For tension or pain in the solar plexus region, add *Jiu Wei* (CV 15). For tension in the trapezius, add *Tian Jing* (GB 21). For severe qi vacuity, add *Zu San Li* (St 36) with supplementing method.

2. ASCENDANT LIVER YANG HYPERACTIVITY PATTERN

MAIN SYMPTOMS: Headache, distention, and pain often located in the eye and/or the temporal region, dizziness, extremely severe, possibly bilateral temporal pain, headaches occurring mostly in older patients which tend to get worse at night or begin during sleep, scintillating scotomas, photophobia, heart vexation, easy anger, restless sleep at night, dizziness, tinnitus, a dry mouth with a bitter taste, a red tongue with thin, yellow fur, and a bowstring, forceful pulse

TREATMENT PRINCIPLES: Level the liver and subdue yang

RX: *Tian Ma Gou Teng Yin* (Gastrodia & Uncaria Drink)

INGREDIENTS: Ramulus Uncariae Cum Uncis (*Gou Teng*), 15g, Ramulus Loranthi Seu Visci (*Sang Ji Sheng*), 12g, Rhizoma Gastrodiae Elatae (*Tian Ma*), Cortex Eucommiae Ulmoidis (*Du Zhong*), Radix Cyathulae (*Chuan Niu Xi*), Radix Scutellariae Baicalensis (*Huang Qin*), Fructus Gardeniae Jasminoidis (*Zhi Zi*), Herba Leonuri Heterophylli (*Yi Mu Cao*), Caulis Polygoni Multiflori (*Ye Jiao Teng*), and Sclerotium Pararadicis Poriae Cocos (*Fu Shen*), 9g each, and Concha Haliotidis (*Shi Jue Ming*), 6g

ANALYSIS OF FORMULA: *Gou Teng*, *Tian Ma*, and *Shi Jue Ming* level the liver and subdue yang. *Sang Ji Sheng*, *Du Zhong*, and *Chuan Niu Xi* supplement liver and kidney yin to check liver yang. In addition, *Chuan Niu Xi* downbears the blood and thus leads yang back down to its lower source. *Huang Qin* and *Zhi Zi* clear depressive liver heat due to emotional disturbance. *Yi Mu Cao* quickens the blood and disinhibits the water, thus also leading yang back downward via urination. *Ye Jiao Teng* nourishes liver blood, and *Fu Shen* supplements the heart. Together, these two medicinals quiet the ethereal soul and calm the spirit.

ADDITIONS & SUBTRACTIONS: If there is concomitant blood stasis, add 15 grams of Radix Salviae Miltiorrhizae (*Dan Shen*) and nine grams each of Semen Pruni Persicae (*Tao Ren*) and Flos Carthami Tinctorii (*Hong Hua*). If enduring disease has entered the network vessels, add nine grams each of Buthus Martensis (*Quan Xie*) and Scolopendra Subspinipes (*Wu Gong*). If there is concomitant yin vacuity, add 12 grams each of cooked Radix Rehmanniae (*Shu Di*), Plastrum Testudinis (*Gui Ban*), and Carapax Amydae Sinensis (*Bie Jia*) and nine grams of Fructus Lycii Chinensis (*Gou Qi Zi*). If there is simultaneous qi vacuity, add nine grams each of Radix Astragali Membranacei (*Huang Qi*), Radix Codonopsitis Pilosulae (*Dang Shen*), and Radix Dioscoreae (*Shan Yao*). If there are hot flashes in the face, add 12 grams each of uncooked Radix Rehmanniae (*Sheng Di*) and Flos Chrysanthemi Morifolii (*Ju Hua*). For marked liver-kidney yin vacuity, add nine grams each of Rhizoma Anemarrhenae Asphodeloidis (*Zhi Mu*), cooked Radix Rehmanniae (*Shu Di*), and Fructus Lycii Chinensis (*Gou Qi Zi*).

If there is simultaneous heart vacuity and liver depression with fatigue, lassitude of the spirit, chest oppression, abdominal distention, and more pronounced insomnia, heart vexation, and irritability, replace *Tian Ma Gou Teng Yin* with *Wu Shi Tong Yu Fang* (Master Wu's Pain-healing Formula): Os Draconis (*Long Gu*), Concha Ostreae (*Mu Li*), Tuber Curcumae (*Yu Jin*), and Fructus Tritici Aestivi (*Huai Xiao Mai*), 30g each, Radix Albus Paeoniae Lactiflorae (*Bai Shao*), Radix Ligustici Wallichii (*Chuan Xiong*), Fructus Viticis (*Man Jing Zi*), Rhizoma Cimicifugae (*Sheng Ma*), and Cortex Albizziae Julibrissinis (*He Huan Pi*), 15g each, Flos Chrysanthemi Morifolii (*Ju Hua*), 12g, Rhizoma Gastrodiae Elatae (*Tian Ma*), Radix Polygalae Tenuifoliae (*Yuan Zhi*), Rhizoma Acori Graminei (*Shi Chang Pu*), Fructus Citri Aurantii (*Zhi Ke*), and mix-fried Radix Glycyrrhizae (*Gan Cao*), 9g each, and Fructus Zizyphi Jujubae (*Da Zao*), 5 pieces.

If there is pure liver fire flaming upward instead of ascendant liver yang hyperactivity, with severe distention and pain in the temporal area, pain which pounds as if it were a heart in the *Tai Yang* (M-HN-9) area, possible pain in the whole head, emotional tension during the attack and habitual easy anger, a red facial complexion, red eyes, photophobia, nausea and vomiting, dryness and a bitter taste in the mouth, a red tongue with yellow fur, and a rapid, bowstring pulse, replace *Tian Ma Gou Teng Yin* with *Yi Dan Ju Yin* (Repress the Gallbladder Chrysanthemum Drink): Spica Prunellae Vulgaris (*Xia Ku Cao*), Ramulus Uncariae Cum Uncis (*Gou Teng*), and Concha Margaritiferae (*Zhen Zhu Mu*), 30g each, Radix Scutellariae Baicalensis (*Huang Qin*), Flos Chrysanthemi Morifolii (*Ju Hua*), Rhizoma Gastrodiae Elatae (*Tian Ma*), Radix Angelicae Dahuricae (*Bai Zhi*), Radix Ligustici Wallichii (*Chuan Xiong*), Cortex Radicis Moutan (*Dan Pi*), and Fructus Gardeniae Jasminoidis (*Zhi Zi*), 12 grams each, and Lumbricus (*Di Long*) and Buthus Martensi (*Quan Xie*), 9 grams each. In this case, for nausea, add 12 grams each of Haemititum (*Dai Zhe Shi*) and Caulis Bambusae In Taeniis (*Zhu Ru*). For phlegm, add nine grams each of Rhizoma Pinelliae Ternatae (*Ban Xia*) and bile-processed Rhizoma Arisaematis (*Dan Nan Xing*). For enduring pain entering the network vessels, add 12 grams each of Semen Pruni Persicae (*Tao Ren*) and Radix Rubrus Paeoniae Lactiflorae (*Chi Shao*). For constipation, add 6-9 grams of Radix Et Rhizoma Rhei (*Da Huang*).

ACUPUNCTURE & MOXIBUSTION: *Xing Jian* (Liv 2), *Tai Xi* (Ki 3), local points according to the location of pain, distant points according to the affected channel. Local points are the same as for pattern #1 above. However, prick to bleed any hot or painful channel or *a shi* points. Distant points are the same as for pattern #1 above.

ANALYSIS OF FORMULA: *Xing Jian* is the fire point on the liver channel. Draining it clears and levels the liver and subdues yang. Supplementing *Tai Xi* nourishes yin to check yang. Once the frequency of attacks is decreased, one should pay less attention to the local treatment of pain and pay more attention to nourishing liver-kidney yin. In this case, medicinals are more effective than acupuncture.

ADDITIONS & SUBTRACTIONS: Please see pattern #1 above. During attacks, use only "side three needle" technique with draining method, *i.e.*, *Tai Yang* (M-HN-9) in the direction of *Quan Liao* (SI 18), *He Gu* (LI 4) perpendicularly, and *Tai Chong* (Liv 3) in the direction of *Yong Quan* (Ki 1).

3. COLD REVERSAL PATTERN

MAIN SYMPTOMS: Severely painful headache at the vertex, a chilly, icy sensation at the time of pain, aversion to wind, possible vomiting of clear liquids, counterflow chilling of the four limbs, glossy, white tongue fur, and a fine, bowstring pulse

NOTE: These signs and symptoms are due to an extremely severe attack of liver wood on spleen earth. This pattern describes the acute paroxysmal attack of migraine headache itself.

TREATMENT PRINCIPLES: Harmonize wood and earth, warm the spleen and scatter cold, downbear counterflow and stop pain

RX: *Wu Zhu Yu Tang* (Evodia Decoction)

INGREDIENTS: Uncooked Rhizoma Zingiberis (*Sheng Jiang*), 18g, Fructus Evodiae Rutecarpae (*Wu Zhu Yu*), 12g, Radix Panacis Ginseng (*Ren Shen*), 9g, and Fructus Zizyphi Jujubae (*Da Zao*), 5 pieces

NOTE: This formula is only to be used during acute attacks. It is not for preventive use.

ANALYSIS OF FORMULA: *Sheng Jiang* and *Wu Zhu Yu* warm the spleen and scatter cold, downbear counterflow and stop pain. In addition, *Wu Zhu Yu* harmonizes wood and earth and treats jue yin channel headache. *Ren Shen* and *Da Zao* supplement the spleen.

ADDITIONS & SUBTRACTIONS: If vomiting is severe, add nine grams each of Rhizoma Pinelliae Ternatae (*Ban Xia*), Pericarpium Citri Reticulatae (*Chen Pi*), and Fructus Amomi (*Sha Ren*). If headache is severe, add 15 grams each of Radix Et Rhizoma Ligustici Chinensis (*Gao Ben*), Radix Ligustici Wallichii (*Chuan Xiong*), and Radix Angelicae Dahuricae (*Bai Zhi*) and nine grams of Radix Angelicae Sinensis (*Dang Gui*).

ACUPUNCTURE & MOXIBUSTION: *Tai Yang* (M-HN-9) needled in the direction of *Quan Liao* (SI 18), *He Gu* (LI 4) needled perpendicularly, *Tai Chong* (Liv 3) needled in the direction of *Yong Quan* (Ki 1) plus *Bai Hui* (GV 20) and/or *Yong Quan* (Ki 1).

ANALYSIS OF FORMULA: *He Gu, Tai Chong,* and *Tai Yang* are all famous points for treating migraine headaches. Draining *He Gu* frees the flow of the network vessels of the whole head because it is the master point of the face and head. Draining *Tai Yang* subdues yang, quiets the spirit, and frees the flow of the network vessels in the temporal region of the head. Draining *Tai Chong* moves the channel qi of the liver. *Bai Hui* and *Yong Quan* both are empirical points for the treatment of headache at the vertex. *Bai Hui* should be drained and *Yong Quan* supplemented.

ADDITIONS & SUBTRACTIONS: For a severe cold sensation, moxa *Zu San Li* (St 36) or *Qi Hai* (CV 6) and also moxa *Bai Hui* (GV 20) and *Yong Quan* (Ki 1). For nausea, needle *Nei Guan* (Per 6) and moxa *Shang Wan* (CV 13).

4. PHLEGM REVERSAL PATTERN

MAIN SYMPTOMS: Headache, dizziness, and heavy-headedness, the feeling of a tight band wrapped around the head, nausea, possible vomiting of phlegm drool, chest oppression, fatigued limbs, numbness of the extremities, lack of appetite, a fat tongue with teeth-marks on its edges and thick, slimy tongue fur, and a bowstring, slippery pulse

NOTE: Although this pattern may be seen in clinical practice in this pure form, phlegm dampness more commonly complicates other patterns.

TREATMENT PRINCIPLES: Dispel phlegm and downbear counterflow

RX: *Ban Xia Bai Zhu Tian Ma Tang Jia Jian* (Pinellia, Atractylodes & Gastrodia Decoction with Additions & Subtractions)

INGREDIENTS: Radix Ligustici Wallichii (*Chuan Xiong*) and Radix Angelicae Dahuricae (*Bai Zhi*), 15g each, Rhizoma Pinelliae Ternatae (*Ban Xia*), 12g, Rhizoma Gastrodiae Elatae (*Tian Ma*), Rhizoma Typhonii Gigantei (*Bai Fu Zi*), Rhizoma Atractylodis Macrocephalae (*Bai Zhu*), and Sclerotium Poriae Cocos (*Fu Ling*), 9g each, mix-fried Radix Glycyrrhizae (*Gan Cao*), 3g, uncooked Rhizoma Zingiberis (*Sheng Jiang*), 3 slices, and Fructus Zizyphi Jujubae (*Da Zao*), 3 pieces

ANALYSIS OF FORMULA: *Ban Xia* and *Fu Ling* transform phlegm and downbear counterflow. With *Tian Ma*, they transform wind phlegm, while *Tian Ma* by itself treats headache and downbears counterflow. With *Bai Fu Zi*, these medicinals transform phlegm causing obstruction of the channels in the head. In addition, *Bai Fu Zi* treats headache. With *Chuan Xiong* and *Bai Zhi*, they transform phlegm confounding the clear orifices and blocking the channels and network vessels in the head. In addition, *Chuan Xiong* and *Bai Zhi* treat headache, the former in the temporal area, the latter on the forehead and corner of the head. *Bai Zhu*, *Fu Ling*, mix-fried *Gan Cao*, *Sheng Jiang*, and *Da Zao* fortify the spleen to prevent further engenderment of phlegm. And finally, *Sheng Jiang*, a "holy medicinal for vomiting" with *Ban Xia* harmonizes the stomach and downbears counterflow.

ADDITIONS & SUBTRACTIONS: If there is marked spleen vacuity fatigue and lack of strength or if the headache is brought on or aggravated by taxation fatigue, add 15 grams of Radix Astragali Membranacei (*Huang Qi*) and nine grams of Radix Codonopsitis Pilosulae (*Dang Shen*). To eliminate dampness more through drying and seeping, add nine grams each of Rhizoma Atractylodis (*Cang Zhu*) and Rhizoma Alismatis (*Ze Xie*). For enduring disease entering the network vessels, add nine grams each of Buthus Martensis (*Quan Xie*) and Scolopendra Subspinipes (*Wu Gong*). For phlegm depression transforming heat, add nine grams each of Radix Scutellariae Baicalensis (*Huang Qin*) and bile-processed Rhizoma Arisaematis (*Dan Nan Xing*). For vomiting of clear, thin phlegm, add nine grams each of Ramulus Cinnamomi Cassiae (*Gui Zhi*) and Pericarpium Citri Reticulatae (*Chen Pi*) and six grams of dry Rhizoma Zingiberis (*Gan Jiang*).

ACUPUNCTURE & MOXIBUSTION: *Feng Long* (St 40), *Yin Ling Quan* (Sp 9), *Zu San Li* (St 36), local points according to the location of pain, distant points according to the affected channel. Please see pattern #1 above.

ANALYSIS OF FORMULA: *Feng Long* is a key point for treating phlegm. It should be drained. *Yin Ling Quan* is a key point for treating dampness. It should also be drained. *Zu San Li* is the key point for supplementing the spleen. It should be supplemented. Together, they are a key combination for treating phlegm dampness due to spleen vacuity. In addition, *Feng Long* downbears counterflow of the stomach

ADDITIONS & SUBTRACTIONS: Please see pattern #1 above.

5. BLOOD STASIS OBSTRUCTING THE NETWORK VESSELS PATTERN

MAIN SYMPTOMS: Enduring headache that will not heal, immovable, fixed pain, piercing, lancinating pain, possible history of traumatic injury to the head, a purple, dark tongue or possible static macules or spots, and a fine, bowstring, choppy pulse

NOTE: As with phlegm reversal above, this pattern mostly complicates other patterns of migraine.

TREATMENT PRINCIPLES: Quicken the blood and transform stasis, free the flow of the network vessels and stop pain

RX: *Tong Qiao Huo Xue Tang Jia Wei* (Free the Flow of the Orifices & Quicken the Blood Decoction with Added Flavors)

INGREDIENTS: Radix Ligustici Wallichii (*Chuan Xiong*) and Rhizoma Corydalis Yanhusuo (*Yan Hu Suo*), 15g each, Radix Rubrus Paeoniae Lactiflorae (*Chi Shao*), Semen Pruni Persicae (*Tao Ren*), Flos Carthami Tinctorii (*Hong Hua*), and Tuber Curcumae (*Yu Jin*), 9g each, Rhizoma Acori Graminei (*Shi Chang Pu*), 6g, uncooked Rhizoma Zingiberis (*Sheng Jiang*), 2 slices, and Fructus Zizyphi Jujubae (*Da Zao*), 2 pieces

ANALYSIS OF FORMULA: *Chuan Xiong*, *Yan Hu Suo*, *Chi Shao*, *Tao Ren*, *Hong Hua*, and *Yu Jin* all quicken the blood and transform stasis, free the flow of the network vessels and stop pain. In addition, *Chuan Xiong* especially treats pain in the temporal region, and *Yan Hu Suo* is well-known for stopping pain. *Yu Jin* also opens the orifices. *Shi Chang Pu* opens the nine orifices, disinhibits the clear cavity, and helps stop pain in the head. *Sheng Jiang* and *Da Zao* harmonize the other medicinals in this formula and promote transformation.

ADDITIONS & SUBTRACTIONS: If enduring disease has entered the network vessels, add 15 grams of Fasciculus Vascularis Luffae Cylindricae (*Si Gua Luo*), nine grams each of Buthus Martensis (*Quan Xie*) and Scolopendra Subspinipes (*Wu Gong*), and three grams of Herba Asari Cum Radice (*Xi Xin*). If there is concomitant phlegm, add nine grams each of Semen Sinapis Albae (*Bai Jie Zi*) and Rhizoma Pinelliae Ternatae (*Ban Xia*). For concomitant liver depression, add nine grams each of Rhizoma Cyperi Rotundi (*Xiang Fu*), Fructus Meliae Toosendan (*Chuan Lian Zi*), and Radix Albus Paeoniae Lactiflorae (*Bai Shao*). For concomitant qi vacuity, add 15 grams of Radix Astragali Membranacei (*Huang Qi*) and nine grams of Radix Codonopsitis Pilosulae (*Dang Shen*).

ACUPUNCTURE & MOXIBUSTION: *He Gu* (LI 4), *San Yin Jiao* (Sp 6), local points according to the location of pain, distant points according to the affected channel same as pattern #1 above.

ANALYSIS OF FORMULA: Draining *He Gu* moves the qi above, while draining *San Yin Jiao* quickens the blood below. When the qi moves, the blood moves. In addition, *He Gu* is the ruling or master point of the face and head which stops pain in the head. *San Yin Jiao* can also regulate menstruation in women who experience migraines perimenstrually.

ADDITIONS & SUBTRACTIONS: Please see pattern #1 above.

REMARKS

1. Because blood stasis obstructing the network vessels commonly complicates most cases of enduring migraine, worm and insect medicinals, such as Buthus Martensis (*Quan Xie*), Scolopendra Subspinipes (*Wu Gong*), Lumbricus (*Di Long*), and Bombyx Batryticatus (*Jiang Can*) are very important in the treatment of this condition. Other medicinals which enter the network vessels and stop pain include Herba Asari Cum Radice (*Xi Xin*) and Fasiculus Vascularis Luffae Cylindricae (*Si Gua Luo*). Further, some Chinese doctors add up to 30 grams each of Radix Ligustici Wallichii (*Chuan Xiong*) and Radix Angelicae Dahuricae (*Bai Zhi*) for any kind of migraine, although 30 grams of *Chuan Xiong* may cause vomiting in some patients.

2. Most cases of migraine involve the liver, whether liver depression-spleen vacuity, liver depression-depressive heat, ascendant liver yang hyperactivity, liver wind stirring internally, or liver blood-kidney yin vacuity with fire effulgence. Phlegm dampness and static blood then complicate these main patterns. While external evils often play a part in other types of headaches, they are not so common in migraines. Some Chinese doctors posit the existence of retained or deep-lying wind evils lodged in the channels when they want to use exterior-resolving, wind-treating medicinals which enter the tai yang, such as Radix Et Rhizoma Notopterygii (*Qiang Huo*), Radix Ledebouriella Divaricatae (*Fang Feng*), Ramulus Cinnamomi Cassiae (*Gui Zhi*), and Radix Et Rhizoma Ligustici Chinensis (*Gao Ben*). However, their use may just as easily be rationalized in terms of moving the qi and stopping pain in the regions traversed by the tai yang.

3. As in modern Western medicine, the Chinese medical treatment of migraines should be divided into two phases: A) preventive treatment between attacks and B) treatment during the acute episodes themselves. *Wu Zhu Yu Tang* (Evodia Decoction) is typically only used during acute attacks. Patients who display cold reversal symptoms during their headaches may be given a packet or two of this formula to keep on hand for attacks. This formula may actually provoke vomiting in those who are severely nauseous. However, in that case, vomiting is commonly followed by diminishment of the headache.

Another formula for treating acute attacks is *Lu Tong Yin* (Skull Pain Drink): Concha Haliotidis (*Shi Jue Ming*), 50g, Ramulus Uncariae Cum Uncis (*Gou Teng*) and Radix Ligustici Wallichii (*Chuan Xiong*), 30g each, Radix Albus Paeoniae Lactiflorae (*Bai Shao*), 20g, and Herba Asari Cum Radice (*Xi Xin*), 15g. Because of the very high dosage of *Xi Xin,* this formula should be used for only 1-3 days for the acute crisis, and the patient should be very well observed to avoid toxicity from this medicinal. To be safe, one can also lower the dosage of *Xi Xin* down to three grams but add 15 grams of Radix Angelicae Dahuricae (*Bai Zhi*) and three grams each of Buthus Martensis (*Quan Xie*), and Scolopendra Subspinipes (*Wu Gong*).

In addition, acupuncture can also often relieve migraine head pain and nausea on a first aid basis.

4. Although some Western MDs question whether foods, such as chocolate, cheese, wine, and coffee, trigger migraines, in Chinese medicine, there are sound theoretical reasons why these foods might. Therefore, Chinese dietary therapy is usually an important part of any overall Chinese medical treatment plan for migraine headache.

5. Many times migraines occur on weekends or after periods of special stress are over. In this case, stagnant qi counterflows upward when the person relaxes and the liver attempts to start coursing and discharging.

6. Migraines may sometimes be aborted by anything which leads the qi to move downward. This includes treading in cold water, soaking the hands in cold water, eating, and even sex.

7. Daily deep relaxation and regular exercise are also important components in any over-all treatment plan for this condition. Biofeedback may also be beneficial for many patients.

8. *Gua sha* treatment of the nape of the neck and upper back can often help improve treatment outcomes for migraine, especially when blood stasis is playing a part. If *gua sha* results in revealing purple *sha*, it should be done one or two more times, 1-2 weeks apart.

9. Patients with frequent headaches often overuse simple over-the-counter analgesics, prescription opiod analgesics, and specific antimigraine agents, such as ergotamine. Such medication overuse by headache-prone patients can frequently evolve into a pattern of chronic daily headache with dependence on symptomatic medications. These types of headaches are referred to as drug-induced rebound headaches. Therefore, practitioners should carefully question their headache patients about their use of prescription pain-relievers, ergotamine, sumatriptan, and OTC medications. Analgesic rebound contributes to the chonicity of headache and reduces the effectiveness of other pharmacological and nonpharmacological therapies. The possibility of analgesic rebound headache should be considered if a patient reports analgesic use more than three times per week for headaches and especially if daily use is reported.

ENDNOTES

1 Aron, Elaine, "Overwhelmed by the World?" *Utne Reader*, Nov.-Dec. 2000, p. 90

2 Larkin, Marilynn, "The Role of Serotonin in Migraine," *JAMA Migraine Information Center*, www.ama-assn.org/special/migraine/newsline/briefing/serotoni.htm

3 "Managing Migraine Today (II): Pharmacologic and Nonpharmacologic Treatment," *JAMA Migraine Information Center*, www.ama-assn.org/special/migraine/treatmnt/managmig/migdrug.htm

46

MULTIPLE SCLEROSIS

Multiple sclerosis (MS), also called disseminated sclerosis, is a slowly progressive autoimmune disease characterized by disseminated patches of demyelination in the brain and spinal cord. This results in multiple and varied neurological symptoms. The onset of this disease is usually insidious, and its course is marked by alternating periods of remission and exacerbation. As with so many other autoimmune diseases, the etiology of this condition is unknown. In other words, biologists have yet to pin-point the initial triggering factor for the body's autoimmune attack against its own tissue. However, some, as yet unknown environmental factor seems to play a role in this disease since its incidence is five times higher in temperate than in tropical climates and its occurrence has been linked to the location where a patient spent their first 15 years. Slightly more women than men suffer from this disease, and its age of diagnosis is usually between 20-40 years. Some authorities believe that, by the time this condition has been diagnosed, it is well established, having actually begun in adolescence or even childhood.

The most frequently presenting symptoms of MS are 1) numbness in one or more extremities, in the trunk, or on the side of the face, 2) weakness or clumsiness of a hand or leg, 3) or visual disturbances, such as partial blindness, pain in one eye, double vision, dimness of vision, or scotomas. Other common early symptoms include fleeting ocular palsy, transient weakness of one or more extremities, slight stiffness or fatigability of a limb, minor gait disturbances, difficulties with bladder control, vertigo, and mild emotional disturbances. Excess heat may aggravate any or all of the symptoms. As demyelination progresses, any or all of these symptoms may get worse, with paralysis and muscular atrophy leading to the patient becoming wheelchair-bound or bedridden.

In terms of Western medical diagnosis, the cerebral spinal fluid in more than 55% of MS patients is abnormal, in which case, gamma globulin is more than 13% and lymphocyte and protein content is slightly increased. However, these findings are not, in and of themselves, pathognomonic. MRI may show many plaques. Lesions may also be visible using contrast-enhanced CT scans. Western medicine has no specific treatment for MS. Spontaneous remissions make the effectiveness difficult to evaluate. Prednisone is often given during acute attacks in an attempt to hasten recovery. However, long-term corticosteriod treatment is rarely justified. As for prognosis, the course of this disease is highly varied and unpredictable. At first, months and years may separate acute episodes. Unfortunately, as the disease progresses, these periods of remission typically grow shorter and eventually progressive and even permanent disability occur. The average duration of this disease probably exceeds 25 years, but it is occasionally fatal within one year.

Although the cause of MS is as yet undetermined, many researchers and practitioners think that it is a complex, multifactorial condition. People with MS typically have nutritional deficiencies. Studies show that essential fatty acids, the building blocks of the brain and nervous system, are commonly missing in MS patients.[1]

Foods which are low in essential fatty acids include meats, dairy products, processed foods, and coconut and palm oils. As it turns out, MS is most prevalent in countries where the diet is high in foods that are low in essential fatty acids. However, other studies have shown that, even with a balanced diet, people with MS tend to have difficulty absorbing essential nutrients, such as vitamin B_1, vitamin B_6, vitamin B_{12}, magnesium, zinc, folic acid, amino acids, manganese, selenium, and essential fatty acids. Intolerances to certain foods are common in MS sufferers, such as to milk and diary products, caffeine, tannin, yeast, sugar, fungi, wheat, gluten, corn, food additives, and fermented products, such as ketchup, vinegar, and wine. Environmental toxins have also been suggested as triggering antibody reactions that cross-react with myelin. Some of the environmental toxins so implicated are carbon monoxide, diesel fumes, fumes from domestic gas water heaters, solvents, aresol sprays, and out-gassing from chipboard and foam-filled furniture. Multiple sclerosis patients have also been found to have seven times higher levels of mercury in their cerebrospinal fluid as compared to neurologically healthy patients.[2] It has also been noted that, initial episodes of MS often follow either physical trauma or a period of emotional stress and that the initial symptoms sometimes occur at the site of a previous trauma. Further, medical researchers have long suspected a viral involvement in MS, with the Epstein-Barr virus being the leading suspect. This virus interferes with the body's ability to metabolize essential fatty acids, causing a partial breakdown in the body's immune system. And finally, although MS is not considered hereditary, it is familial, with first generation relatives of MS patients showing a 30-50 times greater risk of developing this disease than the general population.

DISEASE CATEGORIZATION: The main Chinese disease categorization of this disease is *wei zheng*, wilting condition. However, different of its symptoms are their own disease categories in Chinese medicine, *e.g. ma mu*, numbness and tingling, *fa li*, lack of strength, *zhi juan*, fatigued limbs, *ban shen bu sui*, hemiplegia, *shi yi wei er*, double vision, *mu hu*, blurred vision, *zhen chan*, tremors or spasticity, *xuan yun*, dizziness, and *niao shi jin*, urinary incontinence.

DISEASE CAUSES: External invasion or internal engenderment of damp heat evils, unregulated diet, over-taxation, and former heaven natural endowment insufficiency

DISEASE MECHANISMS: Damp heat evils due to either external invasion or internal engenderment may brew and steam internally, thus damaging the qi and consuming yin at the same time as possibly congealing dampness into phlegm. It is also possible for prolonged or extreme over-taxation to consume blood and yin. Hence, the sinew vessels fail to receive adequate moistening and nourishing. Lack of blood and yin may give rise to internally stirring of wind, with consequent spasms and contractures. Extreme or prolonged yin vacuity may reach yang, giving rise to kidney yang insufficiency. Kidney yang insufficiency may also be due to over-taxation, former heaven natural endowment insufficiency, or overuse of steroids.

TREATMENT BASED ON PATTERN DISCRIMINATION:

1. PHLEGM HEAT INTERNALLY BREWING PATTERN

MAIN SYMPTOMS: Atrophy, wilting, and weakness of the extremities either accompanying the onset of fever or as the sequelae of a fever, possible limb numbness and insensitivity tending toward paralysis, head distention, chest oppression, tinnitus, possible decreased visual acuity, nausea, vomiting, oral thirst but no desire to drink, profuse, yellow-colored, thick, sticky phlegm, a red tongue with yellow, or slimy, yellow fur, and a bowstring, slippery or slippery, rapid pulse

NOTE: This pattern is usually only seen as the main pattern of this disease in obese patients. Otherwise, phlegm tends to be only a complicating factor in a number of other patterns.

TREATMENT PRINCIPLES: Clear heat and transform phlegm, open the orifices and free the flow of the network vessels

RX: *Di Tan Tang Jia Jian* (Flush Phlegm Decoction with Additions & Subtractions)

INGREDIENTS: Bile-processed Rhizoma Arisaematis (*Dan Xing*), 6g, Pericarpium Citri Reticulatae (*Chen Pi*), 9g, Rhizoma Pinelliae Ternatae (*Ban Xia*), 8g, Sclerotium Poriae Cocos (*Fu Ling*), 15g, Fructus Immaturus Citri Aurantii (*Zhi Shi*), 6g, Lumbricus (*Di Long*), 9g, Fascicularis Vascularis Luffae Cylindricae (*Xi Gua Luo*), 12g, and Succus Bambusae (*Zhu Li*), 30ml

ANALYSIS OF FORMULA: *Dan Nan Xing, Ban Xia, Fu Ling, Zhi Shi, Chen Pi*, and *Zhu Li* together dry and/or seep dampness, move the qi to dispel phlegm, clear heat and transform phlegm. In addition, *Dan Nan Xing* and *Zhu Li* treat wind phlegm, especially that obstructing the network vessels. *Di Long* clears heat and, when combined with *Xi Gua Luo,* frees the flow of the network vessels.

ADDITIONS & SUBTRACTIONS: One can substitute Concretio Silicea Bambusae (*Tian Zhu Huang*) and Fructus Gleditschiae Chinensis (*Zao Jiao*) for *Zhu Li.* For marked yellow phlegm or other symptoms of heat, add nine grams of Radix Scutellariae Baicalensis (*Huang Qin*). For chest distention, add nine grams of Rhizoma Typhonii Gigantei (*Bai Fu Zi*). For chest oppression, add nine grams of Radix Platycodi Grandiflori (*Jie Geng*). For nausea or vomiting, add nine grams of Caulis Bambusae In Taeniis (*Zhu Ru*) and six grams of uncooked Rhizoma Zingiberis (*Sheng Jiang*). For concomitant qi vacuity, add nine grams each of Rhizoma Atractylodis Macrocephalae (*Bai Zhu*) and Radix Codonopsitis Pilosulae (*Dang Shen*) and 15 grams of Radix Astragali Membranacei (*Huang Qi*).

ACUPUNCTURE & MOXIBUSTION: 1. *Shen Ting* (GV 24), *Bai Hui* (GV 20), *Feng Fu* (GV 16), *Da Zhui* (GV 14), *Ling Tai* (GV 10), *Ji Zhong* (GV 6), *Ming Men* (GV 4), *Chang Qiang* (GV 1). 2. *Feng Long* (St 40), *Nei Ting* (St 44), *Yin Ling Quan* (Sp 9). 3. Please see the additions and subtractions below.

ANALYSIS OF FORMULA: With even supplementing-even draining method, the first group of points regulate the governing vessel and harmonize yin and yang, open the orifices and quiet the spirit, extinguish wind, support the righteous, and free the flow of the network vessels. *Bai Hui*, *Feng Fu*, *Da Zhui*, and *Chang Qiang* are indispensable for these purposes. The second group of points treat the root of the disease, linking with the pattern discrimination. Therefore, draining *Feng Long*, *Nei Ting*, and *Yin Ling Quan* transforms phlegm and clears heat. The third group of points treat the branches of the disease. In other words, they treat the symptoms of MS. These points should be chosen on the basis of the patient's symptoms from the additions and subtractions.

ADDITIONS & SUBTRACTIONS: For visual disturbances, add *Jing Ming* (Bl 1) or *Zan Zhu* (Bl 2) and *Tai Yang* (M-HN-9). For tremors in or contractions of the limbs, add *Tai Chong* (Liv 3) and *He Gu* (LI 4). For dizziness, add *Feng Chi* (GB 20). For fatigue, add *Zu San Li* (St 36) and *Qi Hai* (CV 6). If Western medical diagnosis can precisely identify plaques of demyelination in the spinal cord, add *Jia Ji* (M-BW-35) corresponding to the affected area. For atrophy, wilting, weakness, numbness, and/or insensitivity of the upper extremities, add *Jian Yu* (LI 15), *Bi Nao* (LI 14), *Qu Chi* (LI 11), *Shou San Li* (LI 10), *He Gu* (LI 4), and *Wai Guan* (TB 5). Select 2-3 points per treatment. For atrophy, wilting, weakness, numbness, and/or insensitivity of the lower extremities, add *Bi Guan* (St 31), *Fu Tu* (St 32), *Liang Qiu* (St 34), *Zu San Li* (St 36), *Shang Ju Xu* (St 37), and/or *Jie Xi* (St 41). Select 2-3 points per treatment. For weakness of the wrist, add *Yang Chi* (TB 4) and *Yang Xi* (LI 5). For weakness of the hand, add *He Gu* (LI 4) through to *Hou Xi* (SI 3) using the penetrating needle method. For weakness or numbness of the fingers, add *Ba Xie* (M-UE-22). For weakness of the knees, add *Wei Zhong* (Bl 40) and *Qu Quan* (Liv 8). For weakness of the feet or numbness of the toes, add *Ba Feng* (M-LE-8). For talipes equinus due to weakness of the sinew vessels of the foot yang ming, foot shao yang, and foot jue yin, use *Shang Ju Xu* (St 37), *Jie Xi* (St 41), *Qiu Xu* (GB 40), *Zhong Feng* (Liv 4), and/or *Yang Ling Quan* (GB 34). For talipes varus due to weakness of the sinew vessels of the foot tai yang and foot shao yang, add *Kun Lun* (Bl 60), *Shen Mai* (Bl 62), *Xuan Zhong* (GB 39), and *Qiu Xu* (GB 40). For talipes valgus due to weakness of the sinew vessels of the foot tai yin and foot shao yin, add *Gong Sun* (Sp 4), *San Yin Jiao* (Sp 6), *Tai Xi* (Ki 3), and *Zhao Hai* (Ki 6). For nausea or vomiting, add *Shang Wan* (CV 13) and *Nei Guan* (Per 6). For head distention, add *Tai Yang* (M-HN-9). For chest oppression, add *Nei Guan* (Per 6). For tinnitus, add *Ting Hui* (GB 2).

2. DAMP HEAT DAMAGING THE SINEWS PATTERN

MAIN SYMPTOMS: In the early stage, there is abnormal sensitivity, heaviness, and a cumbersome sensation or numbness in the limbs. This is then followed by wilting and weak limbs, drooping of the hands and feet, and loss of use of the limbs. Other symptoms may include chest and abdominal glomus and oppression, sticky, foul-smelling, dark-colored or bright yellow stools with burning around the anus, hot, astringent, painful urination with dark-colored urine, a red tongue with yellow, slimy fur, and a slippery, rapid pulse.

NOTE: This pattern rarely presents in this pure form in Western patients. However, damp heat is a common complication in many Western patients with MS. This dampness and heat are usually internally engendered and are almost always found in combination with spleen vacuity and liver depression. Therefore, treatment for damp heat is usually secondary or tertiary to other treatment principles.

TREATMENT PRINCIPLES: Clear heat and eliminate dampness

RX: *Jia Wei Er Miao San* (Added Flavors Two Wonders Powder)

INGREDIENTS: Plastrum Testudinis (*Gui Ban*), 12g, and Cortex Phellodendri (*Huang Bai*), Rhizoma Atractylodis (*Cang Zhu*), Radix Angelicae Sinensis (*Dang Gui*), Radix Stephaniae Tetrandrae (*Han Fang Ji*), Radix Achyranthis Bidentatae (*Niu Xi*), and Rhizoma Dioscoreae Hypoglaucae (*Bei Xie*), 9g each

ANALYSIS OF FORMULA: *Huang Bai*, *Cang Zhu*, *Han Fang Ji*, and *Bei Xie* together clear heat and eliminate dampness. *Dang Gui* and *Niu Xi* nourish liver blood and enrich kidney yin and also quicken the blood. In addition, *Niu Xi* leads the other medicinals downward to the lower limbs. *Gui Ban* supplements the kidneys and strengthens the sinews and bones.

ADDITIONS & SUBTRACTIONS: If there is severe damp heat, add six grams of Radix Scutellariae Baicalensis (*Huang Qin*) and nine grams each of Sclerotium Poriae Cocos (*Fu Ling*) and Rhizoma Alismatis (*Ze Xie*). If damp heat has damaged yin, add nine grams each of Radix Dioscoreae Oppositae (*Shan Yao*), Radix Glehniae Littoralis (*Sha Shen*), and Radix Trichosanthis Kirlowii (*Tian Hua Fen*). If there is liver-kidney vacuity, add 15 grams of cooked Radix Rehmanniae (*Shu Di*) and nine grams of Cortex Radicis Acanthopanacis Gracilistylis (*Wu Jia Pi*). And for abnormal vaginal discharge, add nine grams each of Sclerotium Poriae Cocos (*Fu Ling*) and Cortex Toonae Sinensis (*Chun Gen Pi*).

ACUPUNCTURE & MOXIBUSTION: 1. Same as in pattern #1 above. 2. *Zhong Wan* (CV 12), *Zhong Ji* (CV 3), *Yin Ling Quan* (Sp 9). 3. Same as in pattern #1 above.

ANALYSIS OF FORMULA: *Zhong Wan*, *Zhong Ji*, and *Yin Ling Quan* clear heat and eliminate dampness.

ADDITIONS & SUBTRACTIONS: Please see pattern #1 above.

3. Blood vacuity with wind hyperactivity Pattern

Main symptoms: Weak eyesight, if extreme, insomnia, lack of strength in the four limbs, movement and standing not steady, quivering of the limbs, dizziness, tinnitus, a lusterless facial complexion, pale nails, a pale tongue with white fur, and a bowstring, fine pulse

Note: While blood vacuity and wind hyperactivity may be the proximal disease mechanisms of most MS patients' visual weakness and muscular spasticity, blood vacuity and wind hyperactivity usually are only two of a number of interrelated patterns in most Western MS patients' over-all pattern discrimination. Blood vacuity is mostly due to spleen vacuity not engendering and transforming the blood sufficiently.

Treatment principles: Enrich yin and nourish the blood, subdue yang and extinguish wind

Rx: *Tian Ma Gou Teng Yin Jia Jian* (Gastrodia & Uncaria Drink with Additions & Subtractions)

Ingredients: Uncooked Concha Haliotidis (*Shi Jue Ming*), 24g, uncooked Radix Rehmanniae (*Sheng Di*), Ramulus Loranthi Seu Visci (*Sang Ji Sheng*), and Fructus Lycii Chinensis (*Gou Qi Zi*), 15g each, and Rhizoma Gastrodiae Elatae (*Tian Ma*), Ramulus Uncariae Cum Uncis (*Gou Teng*), Fructus Tribuli Terrestris (*Bai Ji Li*), Radix Albus Paeoniae Lactiflorae (*Bai Shao*), Radix Angelicae Sinensis (*Dang Gui*), Flos Chrysanthemi Morifolli (*Ju Hua*), mix-fried Plastrum Testudinis (*Gui Ban*), and Semen Biotae Orientalis (*Bai Zi Ren*), 9g each

Analysis of formula: *Sheng Di, Bai Shao, Dang Gui, Sang Ji Sheng, Gou Qi Zi, Gui Ban,* and *Bai Zi Ren* together nourish liver blood and enrich kidney yin. *Tian Ma, Gou Teng, Shi Jue Ming, Bai Ji Li,* and *Gui Ban* together subdue yang and extinguish wind. In addition, *Bai Zi Ren* quiets the spirit and treats insomnia, *Gou Qi Zi* and *Dang Gui* brighten the eyes, and *Gui Ban* and *Sang Ji Sheng* strengthen the sinews and bones.

Additions & subtractions: For severely weak eyesight, add nine grams each of Fructus Mori Albi (*Sang Shen*), Radix Polygoni Multiflori (*He Shou Wu*), and Fructus Ligustri Lucidi (*Nu Zhen Zi*). For severe insomnia, add 12 grams of Semen Zizyphi Spinosae (*Suan Zao Ren*) and 15 grams of Caulis Polygoni Multiflori (*Ye Jiao Teng*). For lack of strength in the four limbs with unsteady moving and standing, add 12 grams each of Cortex Radicis Acanthopanacis Gracilistylis (*Wu Jia Pi*), Cortex Eucommiae Ulmoidis (*Du Zhong*), and Radix Achyranthis Bidentatae (*Niu Xi*). For severe pale lips, nails, and facial complexion, add nine grams each of Radix Polygoni Multiflori (*He Shou Wu*), Fructus Mori Albi (*Sang Shen*), and Radix Achyranthis Bidentatae (*Niu Xi*). For concomitant spleen qi vacuity, add 15 grams of Radix Astragali Membranacei (*Huang Qi*), nine grams each of Radix Codonopsitis Pilosulae (*Dang Shen*) and Rhizoma Atractylodis Macrocephalae (*Bai Zhu*), and six grams of mix-fried Radix Glycyrrhizae (*Gan Cao*). For concomitant liver depression, add nine grams each of Radix Bupleuri (*Chai Hu*) and Fructus Meliae Toosendan (*Chuan Lian Zi*) and increase the dosage of *Bai Shao* up to 15 grams.

Acupuncture & moxibustion: 1. Please see pattern #1 above. 2. *Ge Shu* (Bl 17), *Gan Shu* (Bl 18), *Pi Shu* (Bl 20), *Shen Shu* (Bl 23). 3. Please see pattern #1 above.

Analysis of formula: *Ge Shu, Gan Shu, Pi Shu,* and *Shen Shu* enrich yin and nourish the blood.

Additions & subtractions: Please see pattern #1 above.

4. Liver blood-kidney yin vacuity pattern

Main symptoms: Dizziness, tinnitus, double vision, blurred vision, unsteady stepping, low back and knee soreness and weakness, emaciated body, vexatious heat in the five hearts, yellow urination, dry stools, a red tongue with scanty fur, and a fine, rapid pulse

Note: The difference between this pattern and the one above is that there are no signs of stirring wind, *i.e.*, tremor, in this pattern.

Treatment principles: Supplement the kidneys and nourish the liver, supplement the blood and enrich yin

Rx: *Zuo Gui Wan Jia Jian* (Restore the Left [Kidney] Pills with Additions & Subtractions)

Ingredients: Radix Dioscoreae Oppositae (*Shan Yao*), 20g, Radix Polygoni Multiflori (*He Shou Wu*), 12g, cooked Radix Rehmanniae (*Shu Di*), Fructus Lycii Chinensis (*Gou Qi Zi*), Fructus Corni Officinalis (*Shan Zhu Yu*), Gelatinum Cornu Cervi (*Lu Jiao Jiao*), Gelatinum Plastri Testudinis (*Gui Ban Jiao*), Radix Cyathulae (*Chuan Niu Xi*), Fructus Ligustri Lucidi (*Nu Zhen Zi*), and Fructus Schisandrae Chinensis (*Wu Wei Zi*), 9g each, and uncooked Radix Glycyrrhizae (*Gan Cao*), 5g

Analysis of formula: *Shu Di, Gou Qi Zi, Shan Zhu Yu, Nu Zhen Zi, Wu Wei Zi,* and *He Shou Wu* supplement the kidneys and nourish the liver, nourish the blood and enrich yin. *Lu Jiao Jiao* and *Gui Ban Jiao* enrich yin and invigorate yang, nourish the blood and boost the essence. *Shan Yao* fortifies the latter heaven to support the former heaven. *Chuan Niu Xi* quickens the blood and leads the other medicinals downward to the lower limbs. *Gan Cao* harmonizes the other medicinals in this formula.

ADDITIONS & SUBTRACTIONS: For dizziness, add 12 grams of Rhizoma Gastrodiae Elatae (*Tian Ma*) and replace *Chuan Niu Xi* with Radix Achyranthis Bidentatae (*Niu Xi*). For tinnitus, add 15 grams of Magnetitum (*Ci Shi*) and nine grams of Rhizoma Acori Graminei (*Shi Chang Pu*). For blurred vision, add nine grams each of Fructus Mori Albi (*Sang Shen*), Radix Polygoni Multiflori (*He Shou Wu*), and Fructus Ligustri Lucidi (*Nu Zhen Zi*). For unsteady stepping and lack of strength in the lower limbs, add 12 grams each of Cortex Radicis Acanthopanacis Gracilistylis (*Wu Jia Pi*) and Cortex Eucommiae Ulmoidis (*Du Zhong*) and replace *Chuan Niu Xi* with Radix Achyranthis Bidentatae (*Niu Xi*). For low back and knee soreness and weakness, add 12 grams each of Rhizoma Cibotii Barometsis (*Gou Ji*) and Cortex Eucommiae Ulmoidis (*Du Zhong*). For severe vacuity heat, add nine grams each of Rhizoma Alismatis (*Ze Xie*), Cortex Radicis Moutan (*Dan Pi*), Cortex Phellodendri (*Huang Bai*), and Rhizoma Anemarrhenae Asphodeloidis (*Zhi Mu*). For concomitant kidney yang vacuity, add nine grams each of Herba Epimedii (*Yin Yang Huo*), Rhizoma Curculiginis Orchioidis (*Xian Mao*), and Radix Morindae Officinalis (*Ba Ji Tian*). For concomitant spleen qi vacuity, add 15 grams of Radix Astragali Membranacei (*Huang Qi*) and nine grams each of Radix Codonopsitis Pilosulae (*Dang Shen*) and Rhizoma Atractylodis Macrocephalae (*Bai Zhu*). For concomitant liver depression, add nine grams each of Radix Bupleuri (*Chai Hu*), Fructus Meliae Toosendan (*Chuan Lian Zi*), and Radix Albus Paeoniae Lactiflorae (*Bai Shao*).

ACUPUNCTURE & MOXIBUSTION: 1. Please see pattern #1 above. 2. *Tai Xi* (Ki 3), *Fu Liu* (Ki 7), *Gan Shu* (Bl 18), *Shen Shu* (Bl 23). 3. Please see pattern #1 above.

ANALYSIS OF FORMULA: *Tai Xi, San Yin Jiao, Gan Shu,* and *Shen Shu* supplement the kidneys and nourish the liver, supplement the blood and enrich yin.

ADDITIONS & SUBTRACTIONS: Please see pattern #1 above.

5. QI & YIN DUAL VACUITY PATTERN

MAIN SYMPTOMS: Fatigue, lack of strength in the four limbs, possible torpid intake and scanty eating, possible abdominal distention, possible easy bruising, orthostatic hypotension, either scanty or profuse menstruation in females, loose stools or diarrhea, tinnitus, dizziness, low back and knee soreness and weakness, possible emaciation, night sweats, tidal malar flushing, a pale, swollen tongue with red tip or a swollen, red tongue, dry or scanty, yellow tongue fur, and a fine, bowstring, rapid pulse

NOTE: Yin blood insufficiency results in delayed, scanty, or blocked menstruation, *i.e.*, amenorrhea. However, spleen qi not containing or vacuity heat forcing the blood to move frenetically may result in profuse and early menstruation. Whether there is scanty or profuse menstruation depends on whether vacuity is complicated by heat.

TREATMENT PRINCIPLES: Fortify the spleen and boost the qi, supplement the kidneys and enrich yin

RX: *Si Jun Zi Tang* (Four Gentlemen Decoction), *Er Zhi Wan* (Two Ultimates Pills) & *San Miao San* (Three Wonders Powder) with additions and subtractions

INGREDIENTS: Radix Astragali Membranacei (*Huang Qi*) and Caulis Milletiae Seu Spatholobi, 15g, Carapax Amydae Sinensis (*Bei Jia*), Radix Codonopsitis Pilosulae (*Dang Shen*), Herba Ecliptae Prostratae (*Han Lian Cao*), Fructus Ligustri Lucidi (*Nu Zhen Zi*), and Radix Achyranthis Bidentatae (*Niu Xi*), 12g each, Rhizoma Atractylodis Macrocephalae (*Bai Zhu*), Sclerotium Poriae Cocos (*Fu Ling*), Rhizoma Anemarrhenae Aspheloidis (*Zhi Mu*), and Cortex Phellodendri (*Huang Bai*), 9g each, and mix-fried Radix Glycyrrhizae (*Gan Cao*), 3g

ANALYSIS OF FORMULA: *Huang Qi, Dang Shen, Bai Zhu, Fu Ling,* and mix-fried *Gan Cao* fortify the spleen and boost the qi. Also *Fu Ling* and *Bai Zhu* prevent the accumulation of dampness due to the moist nature of yin-supplementing medicinals. *Han Lian Cao, Nu Zhen Zi, Bei Jia,* and *Niu Xi* supplement the kidneys and enrich yin also without engendering damp accumulation. *Zhi Mu* and *Huang Bai* clear vacuity heat.

ADDITIONS & SUBTRACTIONS: If there is wind causing dizziness and vertigo, add nine grams each of Radix Angelicae Sinensis (*Dang Gui*), Rhizoma Gastrodiae Elatae (*Tian Ma*), and Ramulus Uncariae Cum Uncis (*Gou Teng*). For wind causing spasticity, add 15 grams of Bombyx Batryticatus (*Jiang Can*) and 30 grams of Radix Albus Paeoniae Lactiflorae (*Bai Shao*). If there is liver depression qi stagnation, add six grams each of Fructus Meliae Toosendan (*Chuan Lian Zi*) and Radix Auklandiae Lappae (*Mu Xiang*). If there is low back pain, add nine grams each of Ramulus Loranthi Seu Visci (*Sang Ji Sheng*) and Cortex Eucommiae Ulmoidis (*Du Zhong*). If there is numbness and tingling, add 18 grams of Caulis Milletiae Seu Spatholobi (*Ji Xue Teng*) and nine grams each of Radix Angelicae Sinensis (*Dang Gui*), Periostracum Cicadae (*Chan Tui*), and Bombyx Batryticatus (*Jiang Can*). For concomitant damp heat diarrhea, add six grams each of Rhizoma Coptidis Chinensis (*Huang Lian*) and Radix Scutellariae Baicalensis (*Huang Qin*) and delete *Zhi Mu*. For concomitant blood stasis, add 12 grams each of Radix Angelicae Sinensis (*Dang Gui*) and Radix Salviae Miltiorrhizae (*Dan Shen*). For nausea due to spleen dampness, add nine grams each of Rhizoma Pinelliae Ternatae

(*Ban Xia*) and Pericarpium Citri Reticulatae (*Chen Pi*). Please also see the additions and subtractions of patterns # 3 and 4 above.

ACUPUNCTURE & MOXIBUSTION: 1. Please see pattern #1 above. 2. *Pi Shu* (Bl 20), *Shen Shu* (Bl 23), *Zu San Li* (St 36), *Fu Liu* (Ki 7). 3. Please see pattern #1 above.

ANALYSIS OF FORMULA: *Pi Shu, Shen Shu, Zu San Li,* and *Fu Liu* fortify the spleen and boost the qi, supplement the kidneys and enrich yin.

ADDITIONS & SUBTRACTIONS: Please see pattern #1 above.

6. KIDNEY YANG INSUFFICIENCY PATTERN

MAIN SYMPTOMS: Poor vision, bilateral lower limb lack of strength, lack of warmth in the four extremities, especially in the lower limbs, loose stools, diarrhea, or possible constipation, frequent urination or incontinence, a pale tongue with thin, white fur, and a deep, fine pulse

NOTE: In Western MS patients, this pattern rarely presents in its pure form. Kidney yang vacuity mostly appears in those where spleen qi vacuity has reached kidney yang. Now there is both spleen qi and kidney yang vacuity plus at least one or two other disease mechanisms or patterns.

TREATMENT PRINCIPLES: Warm yang and supplement the kidneys assisted by boosting the qi and freeing the flow of the network vessels. These last two principles imply concomitant spleen vacuity and blood stasis.

RX: *You Gui Yin Jia Jian* (Restore the Right [Kidney] Drink with Additions & Subtractions)

INGREDIENTS: Cooked Radix Rehmanniae (*Shu Di*), Herba Leonuri Heterophylli (*Yi Mu Cao*), and Radix Astragali Membranacei (*Huang Qi*), 30g each, Semen Cuscutae Chinensis (*Tu Si Zi*), 20g, Cortex Eucommiae Ulmoidis (*Du Zhong*) and Radix Angelicae Sinensis (*Dang Gui*), 15g each, Radix Lateralis Praeparatus Aconiti Carmichaeli (*Fu Zi*), 9g, and Cortex Cinnamomi Cassiae (*Rou Gui*) and mixs-fried Radix Glycyrrhizae (*Gan Cao*), 6g each

ANALYSIS OF FORMULA: *Shu Di, Fu Zi, Rou Gui, Du Zhong,* and *Tu Si Zi* together supplement the kidneys and invigorate yang. *Huang Qi* and mix-fried *Gan Cao* fortify the spleen and boost the qi. *Dang Gui* and *Yi Mu Cao* quicken the blood and free the flow of the network vessels.

ADDITIONS & SUBTRACTIONS: If there is constipation, one can add nine grams each of Herba Cistanchis Deserticolae (*Rou Cong Rong*) and Herba Cynomorii Songarici (*Suo Yang*). For poor vision, add 12 grams each of Semen Astragali Complanati (*Sha Yuan Zi*) and Fructus Rubi Chingii (*Fu Pen Zi*). For bilateral lower limb lack of strength, add 12 grams each of Cortex Radicis Acanthopanacis Gracilistylis (*Wu Jia Pi*), Radix Dipsaci (*Xu Duan*), and Radix Morindae Officinalis (*Ba Ji Tian*). For lack of warmth in the four extremities, add six grams of dry Rhizoma Zingiberis (*Gan Jiang*) and three grams of Herba Asari Cum Radice (*Xi Xin*). For loose stools or diarrhea, add nine grams of Fructus Psoraleae Corylifoliae (*Bu Gu Zhi*) and six grams each of Fructus Schisandrae Chinensis (*Wu Wei Zi*) and Semen Myristicae Fragrantis (*Rou Dou Kou*). For frequent urination or incontinence, add nine grams each of Fructus Alpiniae Oxyphyllae (*Yi Zhi Ren*), Fructus Rosae Laevigatae (*Jin Ying Zi*), and Fructus Rubi Chingii (*Fu Pen Zi*). For marked qi vacuity, add 12 grams each of Radix Codonopsitis Pilosulae (*Dang Shen*), Sclerotium Poriae Cocos (*Fu Ling*), and Rhizoma Atractylodis Macrocephalae (*Bai Zhu*).

ACUPUNCTURE & MOXIBUSTION: 1. Please see pattern #1 above. 2. *Ming Men* (GV 4), *Guan Yuan* (CV 4), *Shen Shu* (Bl 23). 3. Please see pattern #1 above.

ANALYSIS OF FORMULA: *Ming Men, Guan Yuan,* and *Shen Shu* warm yang and supplement the kidneys.

ADDITIONS & SUBTRACTIONS: Please see pattern #1 above.

REMARKS

1. In our experience, the single most commonly seen pattern of MS in real-life Western patients is qi and yin dual vacuity, meaning spleen qi and liver-kidney yin vacuity. However, this pattern is always complicated by liver depression, and it is often complicated by any combination of the following: A) damp heat, B) blood stasis, C) internal stirring of wind, D) kidney qi vacuity not securing, and E) kidney yang vacuity. In our experience, it is the rule rather than the exception that there will be five or more concomitant patterns in cases of MS. Whenever there are such complicated patterns, one should first identify all patterns present in order of predominance; two, state the requisite treatment principles for each of those patterns in the same order; and three, compose on an *ad hoc* basis a treatment plan that addresses all those patterns in the same proportions and with the same priorities.

2. Because spleen qi vacuity and dampness play a central role in most Western MS patients' disease mechanisms, Chinese dietary therapy must also play a correspondingly central role in any comprehensive treatment plan. This generally means eating a clear, bland, hypoallergenic, yeast-free diet. The more marked spleen qi and dampness or damp heat are in a patient's over-all pattern, the more important is proper diet in the prevention of acute attacks and long-term maintenance.

3. Although Western physicians say that attacks and remis-

sions of MS are spontaneous, our clinical experience as Chinese doctors suggests that precipitating factors for both acute attacks and remissions can be identified by Chinese medicine. For instance, many female MS patients experience worsening of wind, liver, and/or spleen related symptoms premenstrually. If there is insufficient blood, when the blood descends to the uterus prior to menstruation, this may result in the arising or aggravation of internally stirring wind and/or liver depression. If liver depression is aggravated, then the spleen will tend to become more vacuous due to the liver counterflowing horizontally with wood assailing earth. Other acute attacks can be traced to unusual fatigue, emotional stress, and/or unregulated diet. Therefore, when MS patients experience acute aggravations, it is very important for their Chinese medical care-giver to identify the precipitating factor(s) and to explain these to the patient so that the patient may prevent such exacerbations in the future. For instance, if an MS patient's symptoms worsen on exposure to heat, they should consider moving to a cooler climate in the summer or installing air-conditioning in their home.

4. Chinese sources do not typically list blood stasis as a pattern of MS. However, blood stasis often does complicate MS based on the statement that, "Enduring diseases enter the network vessels." The clinical meaning of this statement is that blood stasis is commonly engendered within the network vessels of chronically ill patients. In such cases, one should add appropriate blood-quickening, network vessel-freeing medicinals to any other guiding formula, however remembering that blood vacuity may cause or aggravate blood stasis and that blood stasis may cause or aggravate blood vacuity. Therefore, in most cases, blood-quickening medicinals should be combined with blood-nourishing medicinals or medicinals should be chosen which inherently both quicken and nourish the blood, such as Radix Angelicae Sinensis (*Dang Gui*) and Radix Salviae Miltiorrhizae (*Dan Shen*). Further, because blood stasis in the network vessels and wind often exist simultaneously, one should not overlook those wind-extinguishing medicinals which also quicken and free the flow of the network vessels, such as Buthus Martensis (*Quan Xie*) and Scolopendra Subspinipes (*Wu Gong*).

5. Chinese research has shown that Chinese medicine can keep MS patients in remission longer and slow this condition's progress.[3]

6. Stress reduction and a low fat diet yet high in essential fatty acids are important adjunctive therapies in most cases of MS. When stress plays a part in the activation or aggravation of MS, Chinese medical practitioners should consider the use of appropriate spirit-quieting medicinals based on the patient's overall pattern discrimination.

ENDNOTES

[1] Agranoff, B.W. & Goldberg, D., "Diet and the Geographical Distribution of Multiple Sclerosis," *Lancet*, #7888, Nov., 1974, p. 1061-1066

[2] Vimy, M.J. *et al.*, "Glomerular Filtration Impairment by Mercury from Dental 'Silver' Fillings in Sheep," *The Physiologist*, #33, Aug., 1990, p. 94

[3] Lu Xi *et al.*, "A Study of the Chinese Medicine Prevention of Relapse of Multiple Sclerosis," *Zhong Yi Za Zhi (Journal of Chinese Medicine)*, #7, 1995, p. 417-418

47

MYASTHENIA GRAVIS

Myasthenia gravis literally means a "heavy weakness of the muscles." In Western medicine, it is classified as an autoimmune disease and is caused by an antibody attack on acetylcholine receptors at the post-synaptic neuromuscular junction. The original factor initiating this antibody attack is unknown. However, this loss then hinders efficient neuromuscular transmission. Although this disease is most commonly found in 20-40 year old females, it may occur at any age and in either sex.

The most common symptoms of myasthenia gravis are drooping eyelids, double vision, and abnormal muscle fatigue after exertion. Typically, the eye muscles are the first to be affected and eventually affect 85% of patients with this disease. Joint conditions, problems swallowing, and proximal limb weakness are common. The signs and symptoms of this condition tend to fluctuate, sometimes changing in intensity in the course of hours. Severe generalized paralysis may develop, especially during relapses. In addition, there may be alterations in voice, nasal regurgitation, and choking. Life-threatening respiratory muscle involvement is present in approximately 10% of patients.

Western medical diagnosis is made on the basis of the presence or history of the above signs and symptoms and is confirmed by improvement with anticholesterinase drugs, most commonly edrophonium. In addition, electrophysiologic and serologic tests may help substantiate the diagnosis. Western medical treatment of this disease primarily consists of cholinesterase inhibitors, thymectomy, corticosteriods, and immuno-suppressive agents. Within Western medicine, myasthenia gravis is considered a difficult problem to manage well, requiring treatment by an experienced specialist.

CHINESE DISEASE CATEGORIZATION: The main clinical symptoms of this condition are categorized as *wei zheng*, wilting condition, *shen zhong*, bodily heaviness, *pi juan fa li*, fatigue and lack of strength, *shi yin wei er*, double vision, and *shang bao xia chui*, drooping upper eyelids. Wilting refers to weakness and limpness of the sinews which, in severe cases, can prevent lifting of the arms and legs. Bodily heaviness means a subjective feeling as if the body were abnormally heavy. Fatigue and lack of strength in Chinese medicine mean exactly what they do in everyday English, and double vision and drooping upper eyelids are also self-explanatory.

DISEASE CAUSES: Taxation fatigue and unregulated eating and drinking which damage the spleen and eventually reach the kidneys, or former heaven natural endowment insufficiency with spleen-kidney depletion and vacuity

DISEASE MECHANISMS: Due to spleen vacuity, the central qi falls downward, qi and blood are insufficient, the four limbs lose their nourishment, and, therefore, there is lack of strength. If spleen yang is insufficient, this may reach and damage kidney yang. If there is yang vacuity, there is inability to warm and nourish. Hence the whole body lacks strength and the essence spirit becomes listless. If spleen yin is vacuous, this may reach and damage kidney yin. Yin vacuity leads to essence and blood depletion detriment. In that case, liver and kidney consumption damage may cause the sinews and flesh to lose their nourishment and thus result in the onset of wilting condition. It is also possible that, due to former heaven kidney qi insufficiency, the original qi is depleted and vacuous. In that case, the spleen and stomach will lose their warming and steaming which then leads to the onset of this disease. It is also possible for malnourishment of the sinew vessels and muscles and flesh to be due to obstruction of the network vessels by either phlegm dampness and/or blood stasis.

TREATMENT BASED ON PATTERN DISCRIMINATION:

1. QI VACUITY FALLING DOWNWARD PATTERN

MAIN SYMPTOMS: Drooping eyelids, double vision, a bright white, lusterless facial complexion, decreased eating, loose stools, fatigue, lassitude of the spirit, scanty qi, disinclination to speak, a weak voice, a slight degree of lack of strength and warmth in the extremities, symptoms better in the morning and worse in the afternoon, a pale tongue with white fur, and a fine, weak pulse. This pattern is mostly seen in patients with ptosis of the eyelids.

TREATMENT PRINCIPLES: Supplement the center and boost the qi, upbear yang and lift the fallen

RX: *Bu Zhong Yi Qi Tang Jia Jian* (Supplement the Center & Boost the Qi Decoction with Additions & Subtractions)

INGREDIENTS: Radix Codonopsitis Pilosulae (*Dang Shen*), Radix Dioscoreae Oppositae (*Shan Yao*), and Radix Astragali Membranacei (*Huang Qi*), 30g each, mix-fried Radix Glycyrrhizae (*Gan Cao*), Rhizoma Atractylodis Macrocephalae (*Bai Zhu*), Radix Angelicae Sinensis (*Dang Gui*), Semen Dolichoris Lablab (*Bian Dou*), Rhizoma Polygonati (*Huang Jing*), Placenta Hominis (*Zi He Che*), and Pericarpium Citri Reticulatae (*Chen Pi*), 9g each, and Rhizoma Cimicifugae (*Sheng Ma*) and Radix Bupleuri (*Chai Hu*), 5g each

ANALYSIS OF FORMULA: *Dang Shen*, *Huang Qi*, mix-fried *Gan Cao*, *Bai Zhu*, *Shan Yao*, *Bai Bian Dou*, and *Huang Jing*, all supplement the center and boost the qi. In addition, *Bai Bian Dou* and *Bai Zhu* with the help of *Chen Pi* transform dampness, *Huang Jing* and *Shan Yao* supplement the kidneys, and *Huang Qi* with the help of *Chai Hu* and *Sheng Ma* upbears yang and lifts the fallen. *Dang Gui* regulates the blood, while *Chen Pi* regulates the qi. *Zi He Che* supplements the qi, blood, yin, and yang and treats weakness and wilting condition.

ADDITIONS & SUBTRACTIONS: If there is chest oppression and venter glomus with slimy tongue fur, add nine grams each of Rhizoma Atractylodis (*Cang Zhu*) and Herba Eupatorii Fortunei (*Pei Lan*). If eating and drinking are devitalized, add 15 grams each of Fructus Crataegi (*Shan Zha*), Fructus Germinatus Hordei Vulgaris (*Mai Ya*), and Fructus Germinatus Oryzae Sativae (*Gu Ya*). If there is simultaneous emission of coolness of the four extremities, add 15 grams each of Semen Cuscutae Chinensis (*Tu Si Zi*), Radix Morindae Officinalis (*Ba Ji Tian*), and cooked Radix Rehmanniae (*Shu Di*). If there is a severe qi vacuity with severe fatigue, increase the dosage of *Huang Qi* and *Dang Shen* up to 50 grams and that of *Chai Hu* and *Sheng Ma* up to nine grams.

An alternative treatment to *Bu Zhong Yi Qi Tang* is *Sheng Xian Tang* (Upbear the Fallen Decoction) which is another famous formula for the treatment of the qi vacuity falling downward pattern: rice stir-fried Radix Codonopsitis Pilosulae (*Dang Shen*) and honey stir-fried Radix Astragali Membranacei (*Huang Qi*), 30g each, Radix Angelicae Sinensis (*Gang Gui*), Rhizoma Cimicifugae (*Sheng Ma*), and Radix Bupleuri (*Chai Hu*), 9g each, mix-fried Radix Glycyrrhizae (*Gan Cao*), 5g, Ramulus Cinnamomi Cassiae (*Gui Zhi*) and Radix Platycodi Grandiflori (*Jie Geng*), 3g each.

ACUPUNCTURE & MOXIBUSTION: For any pattern of myasthenia gravis, one can select points from the three following groups: 1) local points according to which limbs are weak, 2) distant points according to the pattern discrimination, and 3) symptomatic points according to the main manifestations of the patient

1. Local points: A) For weakness of the upper arm: *Da Zhui* (GV 14), *Jia Ji* (EX-B-2) T1-T8. Select 2-3 points per treatment. B) For weakness in the forearm: *Jian Yu* (LI 15), *Bi Nao* (LI 14), *Qu Chi* (LI 11), *Shou San Li* (LI 10), *He Gu* (LI 4), *Wai Guan* (TB 5). Select 2-3 points per treatment. C) For weakness in the buttocks and thighs: *Ci Liao* (Bl 32), *Zhi Bian* (Bl 34), *Yao Yang Guan* (GV 3), *Jia Ji* (EX-B-2) T10-L5. Select 2-3 points per treatment. D) For weakness in the lower legs: *Bi Guan* (St 31), *Fu Tu* (St 32), *Liang Qiu* (St 34), *Zu San Li* (St 36), *Shang Ju Xu* (St 37), *Jie Xi* (St 41). Select 2-3 points per treatment.

2. Distant points: *Qi Hai* (CV 6), *Zu San Li* (St 36), *Bai Hui* (GV 20)

3. Symptomatic points: For drooping eyelids, add *Zan Zhu* (Bl 2), *Si Zhu Kong* (TB 3), and *Yu Yao* (M-HN-6), or needle from *Zan Zhu* through to *Yu Yao* or *Si Zhu Kong* through to *Yu Yao* or *Yang Bai* (GB 14) through to *Yu Yao*. For weakness of the wrist, add *Yang Chi* (TB 4) and *Yang Xi* (LI 5). For weakness of the hands, add *He Gu* (LI 4) through to *Hou Xi* (SI 3) using penetrating needle method. For weakness or numbness of the fingers, add *Ba Xie* (M-UE-22). For weakness of the knees, add *Wei Zhong* (Bl 40) and *Qu Quan* (Liv 8). For weakness of the feet or numbness of the toes, add *Ba Feng* (M-LE-8). For talipes equinus due to weakness of the sinew vessels of the foot yang ming, foot shao yang, and foot jue yin, add *Shang Ju Xu* (St 37), *Jie Xi* (St 41), *Qiu Xu* (GB 40), *Zhong Feng* (Liv 4), and *Yang Ling Quan* (GB 34). For talipes varus due to weakness of the sinew vessels of the foot tai yang and foot shao yang, add *Kun Lun* (Bl 60), *Shen Mai* (Bl 62), *Xuan Zhong* (GB 39), and *Qiu Xu* (GB 40). For talipes valgus due to weakness of the sinew vessels of the foot tai yin and foot shao yin, add *Gong Sun* (Sp 4), *San Yin Jiao* (Sp 6), *Tai Xi* (Ki 3), and *Zhao Hai* (Ki 6).

ANALYSIS OF FORMULA: All the local or symptomatic points supplement vacuity and harmonize the network vessels. *Qi Hai, Zu San Li,* and *Bai Hui* supplement the center, boost the original qi, and upbear the clear. *Qi Hai* supplements the qi of the former heaven, while *Zu San Li* supplements the qi of the latter heaven. *Bai Hui,* being on the top of the body, draws the qi up to the top of the head. Moxibustion on these three points promotes the upward movement of qi due to the flaming upward nature of heat.

ADDITIONS & SUBTRACTIONS: Please see the symptomatic points above.

2. QI & YIN DUAL VACUITY PATTERN

MAIN SYMPTOMS: Drooping eyelids, double vision, lack of strength in the four extremities, scanty qi, disinclination to speak, spontaneous perspiration or night sweats, dry mouth and parched throat, heart vexation, dry stools, a red tongue with scanty fur, and a bowstring, fine or fine, rapid pulse. This pattern is mostly seen in patients with double vision.

TREATMENT PRINCIPLES: Boost the qi and nourish yin

RX: *Liu Wei Di Huang Tang* (Six Flavors Rehmannia Decoction) & *Sheng Mai San* (Engender the Pulse Powder) with additions and subtractions

INGREDIENTS: Radix Dioscoreae Oppositae (*Huai Shan Yao*) and Radix Astragali Membranacei (*Huang Qi*), 30g each, Radix Pseudostellariae (*Tai Zi Shen*), 25g, or Radix Quinquefoliii (*Xi Yang Shen*), 6g, uncooked & cooked Radix Rehmanniae (*Sheng Shu Di*), Fructus Corni Officinalis (*Shan Yu Rou*), Sclerotium Poriae Cocos (*Fu Ling*), and Tuber Ophiopogonis Japonici (*Mai Dong*), 15g each, Fructus Schisandrae Chinensis (*Wu Wei Zi*), Radix Albus Paeoniae Lactiflorae (*Bai Shao*), Rhizoma Polygonati (*Huang Jing*), and Radix Angelicae Sinensis (*Dang Gui*), 9g each, powdered Placenta Hominis (*Zi He Che*), washed down with the other medicinals, and mix-fried Radix Glycyrrhizae (*Gan Cao*), 6g each

ANALYSIS OF FORMULA: *Sheng Di, Shu Di, Shan Zhu Yu, Shan Yao, Mai Men Dong, Wu Wei Zi,* and *Zi He Che* supplement the kidneys and enrich yin. *Dang Gui, Zi He Che,* and *Bai Shao* also nourish the blood and supplement the liver. *Tai Zi Shen* or *Xi Yang Shen, Fu Ling, Huang Qi, Huang Jing, Shan Yao,* and mix-fried *Gan Cao* supplement the spleen and boost the qi. In addition, both *Tai Zi Shen* and *Xi Yang Shen* engender fluids, and *Huang Jing* and *Shan Yao* supplement the kidneys.

ADDITIONS & SUBTRACTIONS: If there is spontaneous perspiration, add 30 grams of Fructus Levis Tritici Aestivi (*Fu Xiao Mai*). If there are night sweats, add nine grams of Cortex Radicis Lycii Chinensis (*Di Gu Pi*) and six grams of Cortex Phellodendri (*Huang Bai*). If there are drooping eyelids, add six grams each of Rhizoma Cimicifugae (*Sheng Ma*) and Radix Bupleuri (*Chai Hu*) and 15 grams of Radix Puerariae (*Ge Gen*). If the stools are dry and bound, add 20 grams of Radix Scrophulariae Ningpoensis (*Xuan Shen*).

ACUPUNCTURE & MOXIBUSTION: 1. Please see pattern #1 above. 2. *Fu Liu* (Ki 7), *San Yin Jiao* (Sp 6), *Zu San Li* (St 36). 3. Please see pattern #1 above.

ANALYSIS OF FORMULA: All the local and symptomatic points supplement vacuity and harmonize the network vessels. *Fu Liu* is the metal point on the kidney channel. It nourishes yin and engenders fluids. It also stops perspiration or night sweats. *Zu San Li* supplements both qi and yin. *San Yin Jiao* helps *Fu Liu* to nourish kidney yin and *Zu San Li* to boost the qi. At the same time, it nourishes liver blood and secures the essence.

ADDITIONS & SUBTRACTIONS: Please see the symptomatic points in pattern #1 above. For double vision, one can use the same points as for drooping eyelids alternated with *Yi Ming* (M-HN-13), *Jing Ming* (Bl 1), and *Tai Yang* (M-HN-9). Clinical experience suggests that the distant points *Feng Chi* (GB 20) and *Guang Ming* (GB 37) have a better effect than purely local points.

3. SPLEEN-KIDNEY YANG VACUITY PATTERN

MAIN SYMPTOMS: Drooping eyelids, restricted ocular movement, lack of strength of the four limbs and lack of warmth, dread of cold, fear of chill, spontaneous perspiration, aphasia, difficulty swallowing, loose stools, low back and knee limpness and weakness, a pale tongue with white, wet fur, and a deep, fine pulse. This pattern is mostly seen in those with generalized symptoms affecting their whole body accompanied by double vision.

TREATMENT PRINCIPLES: Warm and supplement the spleen and kidneys

RX: *You Gui Yi* (Restore the Right Drink) & *Li Zhong Tang* (Rectify the Center Decoction) with additions and subtractions

INGREDIENTS: Cooked Radix Rehmanniae (*Shu Di*), Radix Morindae Officinalis (*Ba Ji Tian*), Radix Dioscoreae Oppositae (*Shan Yao*), and Radix Astragali Membranacei (*Huang Qi*), 30g each, Radix Lateralis Praeparatus Aconiti Carmichaeli (*Fu Zi*), dry Rhizoma Zingiberis (*Gan Jiang*), Rhizoma Atractylodis Macrocephalae (*Bai Zhu*), Fructus Corni Officinalis (*Shan Yu Rou*), and mix-fried Radix Glycyrrhizae (*Gan Cao*), 9g each, and Radix Rubrus Panacis Ginseng (*Hong Shen*), 6g

ANALYSIS OF FORMULA: *Shu Di, Shan Yao, Shan Zhu Yu, Fu Zi,* and *Ba Ji Tian* together warm and supplement the kidneys. *Shan Yao, Ren Shen, Huang Qi, Bai Zhu,* mix-fried *Gan Cao, Fu Zi,* and *Gan Jiang* together boost the qi, warm and supplement the spleen.

ADDITIONS & SUBTRACTIONS: If there are loose stools, add nine grams of Fructus Psoraleae Corylifoliae (*Bu Gu Zhi*) and replace *Gan Jiang* with six grams of blast-fried Rhizoma Zingiberis (*Pao Jiang*). If the disease course is either long or the disease's nature is relatively heavy, add six grams of powdered Placenta Hominis (*Zi He Che*) washed down with the decoction, and 15 grams of Gelatinum Cornu Cervi (*Lu Jiao Jiao*).

ACUPUNCTURE & MOXIBUSTION: 1. Please see pattern #1 above. 2. *Shen Shu* (Bl 23), *Tai Xi* (Ki 3), *Guan Yuan* (CV 4), *San Yin Jiao* (Sp 6). 3. Please see pattern #1 above.

ANALYSIS OF FORMULA: *Shen Shu* is the back transport point of the kidneys. It boosts the qi and essence of the kidneys and reinforces the low back. *Tai Xi* is the source point of the kidney channel. It boosts the qi and marrow. *Guan Yuan* is an abdominal intersection point with the spleen, liver, and kidney channels. It invigorates yang and supplements the source qi at the same time as it boosts yin essence. *San Yin Jiao* is the foot intersection point of the spleen, liver, and kidney channels. It nourishes liver blood and enriches kidney yin, supplements the spleen and boosts the essence. Together, these points warm and supplement spleen and kidney yang, boost the essence and nourish the blood.

ADDITIONS & SUBTRACTIONS: Please see the symptomatic points in pattern #1 above.

4. PHLEGM DAMPNESS OBSTRUCTING THE NETWORK VESSELS PATTERN

MAIN SYMPTOMS: Drooping eyelids, lack of strength in the extremities, symptoms better in the morning and worse in the afternoon, fatigue, chest and diaphragmatic distention and oppression, cough with profuse phlegm, dizziness, heart palpitations, nausea, vomiting, a pale tongue with white fur, and a slippery pulse

NOTE: This pattern is a complication of spleen qi vacuity.

TREATMENT PRINCIPLES: Transform phlegm and free the flow of the network vessels

RX: *Dao Tan Tang Jia Wei* (Abduct Phlegm Decoction with Added Flavors)

INGREDIENTS: Honey mix-fried Radix Astragali Membranacei (*Huang Qi*), 30g, Rhizoma Atractylodis Macrocephalae (*Bai Zhu*), 15g, Sclerotium Poriae Cocos (*Fu Ling*), clear Rhizoma Pinelliae Ternatae (*Ban Xia*), processed Rhizoma Arsiaematis (*Tian Nan Xing*), and Fructus Immaturus Citri Aurantii (*Zhi Shi*), 9g each, Pericarpium Citri Reticulatae (*Chen Pi*), Radix Bupleuri (*Chai Hu*), and Rhizoma Cimicifugae (*Sheng Ma*), 6g each, and mix-fried Radix Glycyrrhizae (*Gan Cao*), 4.5g

ANALYSIS OF FORMULA: *Dao Tan Tang* is a modification of *Er Chen Tang* (Two Aged [Ingredients] Decoction) plus *Tian Nan Xing* and *Zhi Shi*. *Er Chen Tang* is the main Chinese medicinal formula for the treatment of phlegm dampness. *Tian Nan Xing* is added to reinforce the phlegm-transforming function of *Ban Xia* and to increase the qi-moving function of *Chen Pi*. *Zhi Shi* is added based on the saying, "To treat phlegm, first treat the qi." In addition, *Bai Zhu* and *Huang Qi* supplement the center and boost the qi because the main cause of dampness and phlegm is a spleen qi vacuity. *Chai Hu* and *Sheng Ma* with *Huang Qi* lift the fallen, here shown by the drooping eyelids.

ADDITIONS & SUBTRACTIONS: Please see the additions and subtractions of patterns #1, 2, and 3 above. Sometimes, when recalcitrant phlegm does not respond to treatment because phlegm is well-known as difficult to treat, one can add two grams of Lapis Micae Seu Chloriti (*Meng Shi*). For enduring disease complicated by blood stasis, add 20 grams of Caulis Milletiae Seu Spatholobi (*Ji Xue Teng*).

ACUPUNCTURE & MOXIBUSTION: 1. Please see pattern #1 above. 2. *Feng Long* (St 40), *Yin Ling Quan* (Sp 9), *Zu San Li* (St 36). 3. Please see pattern #1 above.

ANALYSIS OF FORMULA: *Feng Long* is the main point for the treatment of phlegm with acupuncture, while *Yin Ling Quan* is the master point of dampness. Together, they are a key combination for treating phlegm dampness. They treat the branch manifestations of this condition. *Zu San Li* supplements the spleen and boosts the qi. It treats the root of the disease. Drain the two former points and supplement the latter.

ADDITIONS & SUBTRACTIONS: Please see the symptomatic points in pattern #1 above.

5. BLOOD STASIS OBSTRUCTING THE NETWORK VESSELS PATTERN

MAIN SYMPTOMS: Drooping eyelids, general weakness of the muscles, lack of strength in the lower limbs, chest and diaphragmatic fullness and oppression, rapid breathing, a dark red tongue, and a choppy pulse

NOTE: Although bloods stasis can be the consequence of any of the preceding patterns, it is also typical of thymoma causing myasthenia gravis.

TREATMENT PRINCIPLES: Transform stasis and free the flow of the network vessels

RX: *Xiong Long Tang* (Ligusticum & Lumbricus Decoction)

INGREDIENTS: Radix Puerariae (*Ge Gen*), Rhizoma Corydalis Yanhusuo (*Yan Hu Suo*), Rhizoma Sparganii (*San Leng*), and Rhizoma Curcumae Zedoariae (*E Zhu*), 30g each, wine stir-fried Radix Ligustici Wallichii (*Chuan Xiong*), Radix Codonopsitis Pilosulae (*Dang Shen*), and Lumbricus (*Di Long*), 15g each, and Fructus Citri Aurantii (*Zhi Ke*), 12g

ANALYSIS OF FORMULA: Blood stasis in the chest causes unsmooth circulation of qi and blood in the whole body since the chest center is the mansion of the gathering or ancestral qi which is responsible for both the respiration and blood circulation. If the circulation of the qi and blood is unsmooth, the muscles and flesh are not correctly nourished, thus leading to drooping eyelids and general weakness. Therefore, large doses of *Chuan Xiong, Yan Hu Suo, E Zhu,* and *San Leng* are used to strongly quicken the blood and transform stasis. *Di Long* frees the flow of the network vessels to treat blood stasis at an even deeper level. *Ge Gen* transports fluids to the surface to nourish and moisten the sinews and stimulate the muscles. *Zhi Ke* moves the qi based on the saying, "When the qi moves, the blood moves." *Dang Shen* supplements the spleen and boosts the qi.

ACUPUNCTURE & MOXIBUSTION: 1. Please see pattern #1 above. 2. *He Gu* (LI 4), *San Yin Jiao* (Sp 6), *Dan Zhong* (CV 17). 3. Please see pattern #1 above.

ANALYSIS OF FORMULAS: *He Gu* and *San Yin Jiao* are a special combination for the treatment of qi and blood stasis and stagnation. The former moves the qi, while the latter quickens the blood. *Dan Zhong* focuses the two preceding points' action on the chest which is the site of the source of this disease.

ADDITIONS & SUBTRACTIONS: Please see the symptomatic points in pattern #1 above.

REMARKS

1. Because of the relationship between the qi and blood, patients with this condition may also exhibit the complicating patterns of qi and blood dual vacuity, liver depression qi stagnation, and blood stasis. As in all chronic, enduring diseases, there will be an element of liver depression due to nothing other, than the frustration of being ill. Because this disease tends to be an enduring one, static blood commonly enters the network vessels over time. If there is concomitant blood vacuity signs and symptoms, it is appropriate to add blood supplementing and nourishing medicinals. If there is concomitant liver depression qi stagnation, one should add appropriate qi-rectifying medicinals. And if there is blood stasis, then one should add medicinals which either quicken the blood and transform stasis or quicken the blood and free the flow of the network vessels.

Bu Qi Zeng Li Tang (Supplement the Qi & Increase the Force Decoction) is an alternative treatment to *Bu Zhong Yi Qi Tang* for spleen qi vacuity complicated by blood vacuity, blood stasis, and liver depression: Radix Astragali Membranacei (*Huang Qi*), 60g, Caulis Milletiae Seu Spatholobi (*Ji Xue Teng*), 24g, Radix Angelicae Sinensis (*Dang Gui*) and Radix Puerariae (*Ge Gen*), 18g each, Radix Dioscoreae Oppositae (*Shan Yao*), 15g, Radix Codonopsitis Pilosulae (*Dang Shen*), Rhizoma Atractylodis Macrocephalae (*Bai Zhu*), and Sclerotium Poriae Cocos (*Fu Ling*), 15g each, Pericarpium Citri Reticulatae (*Chen Pi*), Radix Ligustici Wallichii (*Chuan Xiong*), Radix Rubrus Paeoniae Lactiflorae (*Chi Shao*), Radix Albus Paeoniae Lactiflorae (*Bai Shao*), Radix Bupleuri (*Chai Hu*), and Ramulus Cinnamomi Cassiae (*Gui Zhi*), 9g each.

2. As with most autoimmune diseases, proper diet is extremely important. Since all three major patterns of this disease involve a spleen qi vacuity, one should eat a spleen-supporting diet. This means little if any sugars and sweets, little if any uncooked and chilled foods and drinks, and care when eating foods which strongly engender fluids. Foods which engender fluids are typically those which have a lot of *wei* or "flavor." This includes many foods which enrich yin and fill the essence, such as dairy and animal products. When complicated by blood and/or yin vacuity, some yin-enriching foods are necessary. However, so many of these should not be eaten so as to damage the spleen. In general, it is always safer in terms of diet to foster essence via the spleen's engenderment and transformation of qi and blood than to eat a lot of slimy, enriching, flavor-laden, yin-supplementing foods.

3. Like most other autoimmune diseases, this condition's severity fluctuates, and there are often periods of relative remission. In general, Chinese medical treatment should mainly be used for the long-term prevention of future reoccurrences and the progression of this disease, while during acute attacks, a combination of Chinese medicine, including acupuncture and moxibustion, and modern Western medicine may be most effective. In particular, many patients with myasthenia gravis may be prescribed corticosteriods during acute exacerbations, and Chinese medicine can be used to treat the side effects of medicines like Prednisone. In that case, one simply treats the patient's presenting pattern.

48

Oral Leukoplakia

Oral leukoplakia refers to a thickened area on the mucosal lining of the mouth or tongue which looks like a white patch and hence its name – *leuko*, white, *plakia*, patch. Such lesions may be tiny or as large as a quarter and feel firm, rough, or stiff. There may be no subjective symptoms in their early stage. However, there may be sensitivity to hot, spicy foods. Oral leukoplakia are potentially precancerous lesions that develop on the tongue or the inside of the cheek as a response to chronic irritation. This irritation may be due to rough edges on the teeth, dentures, fillings, or crowns, repeated trauma to the oral region, such as from biting the inside cheek or lip, smoking or chewing tobacco, especially pipe smoking, eating hot, spicy food, and drinking alcohol. Although this condition may occur in all ages, it is most common in adults over 60. According to Chinese sources, it is more common in men than women,[1] although this is not corroborated in the Western medical literature. Possible contributing factors include viatmin A and/or B deficiency, deficiencies of either male or female hormones, and syphilis. Untreated lesions are cancerous in approximately 5% of patients.[2] Lesions are commonly removed by cryosurgery similar to actinic keratoses on the skin which are also considered precancerous. However, new lesions may develop after surgical treatment.

Western medical treatment includes the elimination of any recognizable irritation, including removal or repair of any irritating dental appliances. In terms of diet and lifestyle, it means elimination of hot, spicy foods and alcohol from the diet and cessation of all tobacco products. If lesions persist after elimination of all irritants, a biopsy may be performed. As mentioned above, lesions may be removed by cryosurgery.

Hairy leukoplakia is a specific, unusual form of this condition found only in patients with AIDS and ARC or HIV positive patients. It consists of fuzzy or hairy white patches on the tongue and, less frequently, elsewhere in the mouth. These lesions may resemble thrush or oral candidiasis. Hairy leukoplakia is typically one of the first signs of HIV infection.

Chinese disease categorization: This condition is called *kou kong bai ban bing* in Chinese, oral cavity white patch disease. It is only rarely mentioned in the premodern Chinese medical literature.[3]

Disease causes: Bodily weakness due to aging, externally contracted evils, unregulated eating and drinking.

Disease mechanisms: Due to debility and decline of spleen and kidney yang due to aging, the membranes in the oral cavity are not warmed and nourished. If cold evils take advantage of this vacuity, enter, accumulate, and are not scattered, they may obstruct the free flow of qi and blood to the area and give rise to this condition. It is also possible for addiction to smoking, alcohol, and hot, spicy food to give rise to dampness and heat internally. If damp heat brews and steams, it may attack the oral cavity above. If damp heat lingers and is retained, damp heat may damage both the spleen qi and yin fluids. Thus enduring damp heat may lead to qi and yin dual vacuity. Of course, qi and yin vacuity may also be due simply to the process of aging. It is also possible for local malnourishment of the tissues inside the mouth to be due to qi stagnation and blood stasis. The qi does not flow freely to the tissues of the mouth and thus neither does the blood. Hence the tissues become hard, white, and malnourished.

Treatment based on pattern discrimination:

1. Spleen-kidney yang vacuity pattern

Main symptoms: White patches on the oral mucosa which are stiff and hard with white borders, a relatively long disease course, a bland taste within the mouth, no thirst, a cold body and fear of chill, lack of warmth in the four extremities, a pale tongue with white fur, and a moderate (*i.e.*, slightly slow) pulse

TREATMENT PRINCIPLES: Warm and supplement spleen and kidney yang and scatter cold

RX: *Shen Qi Wan Jia Jian* (Kidney Qi Pills with Additions & Subtractions)

INGREDIENTS: Cooked Radix Rehmanniae (*Shu Di*), 20g, Radix Dioscoreae Oppositae (*Shan Yao*), Fructus Lycii Chinensis (*Gou Qi Zi*), and Fructus Corni Officinalis (*Shan Zhu Yu*), 15g each, Herba Epimedii (*Xian Ling Pi*) and Radix Angelicae Sinensis (*Dang Gui*), 12g each, Cortex Eucommiae Ulmoidis (*Du Zhong*) and Cortex Cinnamomi Cassiae (*Rou Gui*), 9g each, and Radix Lateralis Praeparatus Aconiti Carmichaeli (*Fu Zi*), 6g

ANALYSIS OF FORMULA: *Shu Di* supplements the kidneys and enriches yin based on the sayings that, "Yin and yang are mutually rooted," and, "Yang is engendered from yin." *Shan Yao* and *Shan Zhu Yu* supplement the kidney qi, while *Xian Ling Pi* and *Du Zhong* supplement kidney yang. *Dang Gui* and *Gou Qi Zi* supplement the liver and nourish the blood. "Blood and essence share a common source," and, "The liver and kidneys share a common source." *Rou Gui* and *Fu Zi* warm and supplement spleen and kidney yang, while *Shan Yao* also supplements the spleen.

ADDITIONS & SUBTRACTIONS: If spleen vacuity is more marked, add 15 grams of Radix Astragali Membranacei (*Huang Qi*), 12 grams of Radix Codonopsitis Pilosulae (*Dang Shen*), and nine grams of Rhizoma Atractylodis Macrocephalae (*Bai Zhu*). If dampness has accumulated, add nine grams each of Sclerotium Poriae Cocos (*Fu Ling*) and Rhizoma Atractylodis Macrocephalae (*Bai Zhu*). If there is concomitant liver depression, add nine grams each of Radix Bupleuri (*Chai Hu*) and Radix Albus Paeoniae Lactiflorae (*Bai Shao*). If there is concomitant blood stasis, add nine grams each of Cortex Radicis Moutan (*Dan Pi*) and Radix Rubrus Paeoniae Lactiflorae (*Chi Shao*).

ACUPUNCTURE & MOXIBUSTION: *Zu San Li* (St 36), *San Yin Jiao* (Sp 6), *Pi Shu* (Bl 20), *Wei Shu* (Bl 21), *Shen Shu* (Bl 23), *Ming Men* (GV 4)

ANALYSIS OF FORMULA: Supplementing *Zu San Li, San Yin Jiao, Pi Shu,* and *Wei Shu* supplements the spleen. Supplementing *San Yin Jiao, Shen Shu,* and *Ming Men* supplements the kidneys and invigorates yang. Also moxa *Pi Shu, Wei Shu,* and *Shen Shu.*

ADDITIONS & SUBTRACTIONS: For more marked spleen vacuity, add *Tai Bai* (Sp 3). For liver depression, add *Tai Chong* (Liv 3) and *He Gu* (LI 4). For concomitant blood stasis, add *He Gu* (LI 4) and *Xue Hai* (Sp 10) and use even supplementing-even draining technique at *San Yin Jiao.*

2. DAMP HEAT DEPRESSION & BINDING PATTERN

MAIN SYMPTOMS: White patches on the oral mucosa with red margins, dirty colored, brownish, or mixed red and white patches, possible ulceration, possible burning pain, a dry mouth with a bitter taste, a red tongue with slimy fur, and a slippery, rapid pulse

TREATMENT PRINCIPLES: Clear heat and transform dampness

RX: *Long Dan Xie Gan Tang Jia Jian* (Gentiana Drain the Liver Decoction with Additions & Subtractions)

INGREDIENTS: Semen Coicis Lachryma-jobi (*Yi Yi Ren*) and Sclerotium Poriae Cocos (*Fu Ling*), 15g each, Rhizoma Alismatis (*Ze Xie*) and Semen Plantaginis (*Che Qian Zi*), 12g each, Radix Gentianae Scabrae (*Long Dan Cao*), Radix Bupleuri (*Chai Hu*), and Cortex Magnoliae Officinalis (*Hou Po*), 9g each, and Radix Scutellariae Baicalensis (*Huang Qin*), Caulis Akebiae (*Mu Tong*), and Radix Glycyrrhizae (*Gan Cao*), 6g each

ANALYSIS OF FORMULA: *Long Dan Cao* and *Huang Qin* clear heat and eliminate dampness. *Yi Yi Ren, Fu Ling, Ze Xie, Che Qian Zi,* and *Mu Tong* all seep dampness. *Hou Po* transforms dampness and downbears turbidity, while *Chai Hu* courses the liver, resolves depression, and upbears the clear. *Gan Cao* harmonizes the other medicinals in this formula.

ADDITIONS & SUBTRACTIONS: If there is marked spleen vacuity, add nine grams each of Radix Codonopsitis Pilosulae (*Dang Shen*) and Rhizoma Atractylodis Macrocephalae (*Bai Zhu*). If there is concomitant blood stasis, add nine grams each of Extremitas Radicis Angelicae Sinensis (*Dang Gui Wei*) and uncooked Radix Rehmanniae (*Sheng Di*).

If there is spleen vacuity with liver depression and damp heat, replace *Long Dan Xie Gan Tang Jia Jian* with *Xiao Chai Hu Tang Jia Jian* (Minor Bupleurum Decoction with Additions & Subtractions): Radix Astragali Membranacei (*Huang Qi*), 12g, Radix Codonopsitis Pilosulae (*Dang Shen*), Rhizoma Pinelliae Ternatae (*Ban Xia*), and Radix Scutellariae Baicalensis (*Huang Qin*), 9g each, dry Rhizoma Zingiberis (*Gan Jiang*) and mix-fried Radix Glycyrrhizae (*Gan Cao*), 6g each, Rhizoma Coptidis Chinensis (*Huang Lian*), 3-6g, and Fructus Zizyphi Jujubae (*Da Zao*), 3 pieces. If enduring heat has damaged stomach fluids, add 12 grams of Tuber Ophiopogonis Japonici (*Mai Men Dong*) and nine grams of Fructus Pruni

Mume (*Wu Mei*). If there are marked cold extremities, add 6-9 grams of Ramulus Cinnamomi Cassiae (*Gui Zhi*).

Acupuncture & moxibustion: *Yang Ling Quan* (GB 34), *Yin Ling Quan* (Sp 9), *Xing Jian* (Liv 2), *He Gu* (LI 4)

Analysis of formula: Draining *Yang Ling Quan* and *Yin Ling Quan* strongly clears heat and eliminates dampness. Draining *Xing Jian* clears heat from the liver-gallbladder and resolves depression. Draining *He Gu* clears heat from the entire body based on the saying, "The yang ming has lots of qi and lots of blood." In addition, *He Gu* is the master point of the head and face and treats all diseases of the face and mouth.

Additions & subtractions: If there are ulcers in the mouth, add *Di Cang* (St 4) and/or *Jia Che* (St 6). If there is stomach heat, add *Jie Xi* (St 41) and/or *Nei Ting* (St 44). If heat is exuberant and replete, add *Qu Chi* (LI 11). If heat is ascending and harassing the heart spirit, add *Lao Gong* (Per 8) and *Shao Fu* (Ht 8).

3. Qi & yin dual vacuity pattern

Main symptoms: Dry, white or sticky patches on the oral mucosa, enduring disease which does not heal, pale colored oral mucosa, a sallow yellow facial complexion or pale white facial complexion with flushed cheeks, fatigue, lack of strength, possible insomnia, profuse dreams, vexation and agitation, restlessness, a dry mouth but no particular desire to drink, dry stools, a pale, enlarged tongue with possibly a red tip and white fur, and a fine, forceless pulse

Treatment principles: Supplement the spleen and boost the qi, nourish yin and engender fluids

Rx: *Yi Wei Tang Jia Jian* (Boost the Stomach Decoction with Additions & Subtractions)

Ingredients: Radix Glehniae Littoralis (*Sha Shen*), Herba Dendrobii (*Shi Hu*), Radix Puerariae (*Ge Gen*), Radix Astragali Membranacei (*Huang Qi*), and Fructus Lycii Chinensis (*Gou Qi Zi*), 15g each, Tuber Ophiopogonis Japonici (*Mai Men Dong*), Radix Codonopsitis Pilosulae (*Dang Shen*), and Rhizoma Polygonati (*Huang Jing*), 12g each, Rhizoma Atractylodis Macrocephalae (*Bai Zhu*), 9g, and Radix Glycyrrhizae (*Gan Cao*), 6g

Analysis of formula: *Sha Shen, Shi Hu, Ge Gen, Gou Qi Zi, Mai Men Dong,* and *Huang Jing* all supplement yin and engender fluids. *Huang Jing* also supplements the spleen and boosts the qi. *Huang Qi, Dang Shen,* and *Bai Zhu* fortify the spleen and supplement the qi. In addition, *Bai Zhu*'s drying nature prevents the yin-enriching medicinals' enriching, slimy nature from engendering evil dampness. *Gan Cao* harmonizes the other medicinals in this formula as well as assists in fortifying the spleen and supplementing the qi.

Additions & subtractions: If there is liver depression qi stagnation, add 12 grams of Fructus Meliae Toosendan (*Chuan Lian Zi*). If there are lingering heat evils, add nine grams each of Rhizoma Anemarrhenae Aspheloidis (*Zhi Mu*) and Cortex Phellodendri (*Huang Bai*). If there are profuse dreams, insomnia, and restlessness due to nonconstruction and malnourishment of the heart spirit, add 12 grams each of Semen Biotae Orientalis (*Bai Zi Ren*) and Semen Zizyphi Spinosae (*Suan Zao Ren*).

If there is yin fluid dryness with concomitant liver depression and damp heat, replace *Yi Wei Tang Jia Jian* with *Gan Lu Yin* (Sweet Dew Drink): uncooked Radix Rehmanniae (*Sheng Di*), 15g, Tuber Ophiopogonis Japonici (*Mai Men Dong*), Tuber Asparagi Cochinensis (*Tian Men Dong*), and Herba Dendrobii (*Shi Hu*), 12g each, Folium Eriobotryae Japonicae (*Pi Pa Ye*), Radix Scutellariae Baicalensis (*Huang Qin*), and Herba Artemisiae Capillaris (*Yin Chen Hao*), 9g each, and Fructus Immaturus Citri Aurantii (*Zhi Shi*) and Radix Glycyrrhizae (*Gan Cao*), 6g each. If there is concomitant qi vacuity, add 15 grams of Radix Astragali Membranacei (*Huang Qi*) and 12 grams of Radix Pseudostellariae Heterophyllae (*Tai Zi Shen*).

Acupuncture & moxibustion: *Zu San Li* (St 36), *San Yin Jiao* (Sp 6), *Fu Liu* (Ki 7), *He Gu* (LI 4)

Analysis of formula: Supplementing *Zu San Li* and *San Yin Jiao* supplements the spleen and boosts the qi. Supplementing *San Yin Jiao* and *Fu Liu* supplements the kidneys and enriches yin. Supplementing *He Gu* helps treat the mouth based on the fact that *He Gu* is the master point of the head and face.

Additions & subtractions: If spleen qi vacuity is severe, add *Tai Bai* (Sp 3). If the heart spirit is restless due to nonconstruction and malnourishment, add *Shen Men* (Ht 7). If the heart spirit is harassed by heat evils, add *Da Ling* (Per 7) and *Shao Fu* (Ht 8). For liver depression qi stagnation, add *Ge Shu* (Bl 17) and *Gan Shu* (Bl 18) to emolliate and harmonize the liver. If there are lingering damp heat evils, drain *He Gu* and add *Yin Ling Quan* (Sp 9). To more forcefully enrich yin and engender fluids, replace *Fu Liu* with *Zhao Hai* (Ki 6) and add *Lie Que* (Lu 7).

4. Qi stagnation & blood stasis pattern

Main symptoms: White patches on the oral mucosa which are lumpy and raised or whose surface is uneven and which are hard and stiff, possible pain or itching, dry skin on the entire body, ductal and abdominal fullness and distention, a dark tongue with thin fur, and a bowstring pulse

NOTE: This pattern does not typically present in this pure form. However, qi stagnation and blood stasis may complicate any of the preceding patterns.

TREATMENT PRINCIPLES: Quicken the blood and move the qi, transform stasis and rectify the qi

RX: *Shi Xiao San Jia Wei* (Loose a Smile Powder with Added Flavors)

INGREDIENTS: Semen Pruni Persicae (*Tao Ren*), Flos Carthami Tinctorii (*Hong Hua*), and Radix Rubrus Paeoniae Lactiflorae (*Chi Shao*), 15g each, Radix Angelicae Sinensis (*Dang Gui*), 12g, Pollen Typhae (*Pu Huang*), Feces Trogopterori Seu Pteromi (*Wu Ling Zhi*), Radix Bupleuri (*Chai Hu*), and Fructus Citri Aurantii (*Zhi Ke*), 9g each, and Radix Glycyrrhizae (*Gan Cao*), 6g

ANALYSIS OF FORMULA: *Tao Ren, Hong Hua, Chi Shao, Pu Huang, Dang Gui,* and *Wu Ling Zhi* all quicken the blood and dispel stasis. *Dang Gui* also nourishes the blood. *Chai Hu* and *Zhi Ke* move and rectify the qi. *Gan Cao* harmonizes the other medicinals in this formula.

ADDITIONS & SUBTRACTIONS: If there is concomitant spleen qi vacuity, add nine grams each of Radix Astragali Membranacei (*Huang Qi*), Radix Codonopsitis Pilosulae (*Dang Shen*), and Rhizoma Atractylodis Macrocephalae (*Bai Zhu*). If there is concomitant blood vacuity, add 18 grams of Caulis Milletiae Seu Spatholobi (*Ji Xue Teng*) and 12 grams of uncooked Radix Rehmanniae (*Sheng Di*). If there is concomitant yin vacuity, add 12 grams each of Radix Polygoni Multiflori (*He Shou Wu*) and Fructus Lycii Chinensis (*Gou Qi Zi*).

ACUPUNCTURE & MOXIBUSTION: *San Yin Jiao* (Sp 6), *He Gu* (LI 4), *Tai Chong* (Liv 3), *Di Cang* (St 4), *Jia Che* (St 6)

ANALYSIS OF FORMULA: *San Yin Jiao* and *He Gu* together quicken the blood and transform stasis throughout the body. *Tai Chong* and *He Gu* regulate and rectify the qi of the entire body. In addition, *He Gu* treats all diseases of the head and face. *Di Cang* and *Jia Che* free the flow of the network vessels locally. All these points should be drained.

ADDITIONS & SUBTRACTIONS: If there is concomitant blood vacuity, add *Ge Shu* (Bl 17) and *Gan Shu* (Bl 18). If there is marked spleen vacuity, add *Tai Bai* (Sp 3) and/or *Zu San Li* (St 36).

REMARKS

1. In real-life practice, most cases of oral leukoplakia display multipattern presentations. For instance, spleen vacuity and liver depression are common factors in the causation of damp heat in addition to hot, spicy and greasy, fatty foods and alcohol. Since most cases of leukoplakia occur in those over 60, most patients have qi and yin, qi and yang, or yin and yang vacuities which are then complicated by dampness, heat, qi stagnation, and/or blood stasis. Therefore, the above protocols will usually have to be combined and modified to fit each individual patient.

2. Since an element of damp heat typically does complicate many, if not most, cases of oral leukoplakia, Chinese dietary therapy supports the necessity of eliminating hot, spicy foods from the diet as well as alcohol. In addition, if dampness is engendered internally due to spleen vacuity, sugars and sweets should also be avoided or minimized.

3. If there are damp heat lesions with ulcerations and pain, one can spray the Chinese ready-made medicine *Xi Gua Shuang* (Watermelon Frost) onto the affected area.

4. Most oral leukoplakia occurs on the rear edges of the tongue where the tongue rubs up against the crowns of the teeth. However, unless the tongue is enlarged, it should not rub up against the crowns of the teeth. An enlarged tongue suggests internal accumulation of water dampness in turn due to spleen vacuity. Therefore, we consider spleen vacuity to be an important component of this condition and reducing the enlargement of the tongue as an important component of its treatment.

5. Chewing on the inner surface of the cheeks or lips is a type of restless stirring or agitation, and, if there is no heat, there is no agitation. All stirring is an expression of yang activity. Commonly such restless stirring is associated with liver depression transforming heat or yin vacuity with vacuity heat. However, if spleen vacuity has engendered phlegm, then it may also be due to phlegm heat.

ENDNOTES

[1] Wu Jun-xi, *Lao Nian Chang Xian Bing Zheng Fang Zhi Fa (The Prevention & Treatment of Commonly Seen Geriatric Diseases)*, Chinese National Chinese Medicine & Medicinal Press, Beijing, 1998, p. 380

[2] The University of Illinois at Chicago Medical Center, "Leukoplakia," www.healthgate.com/choice/uic/cons/mdx-books/sym/sym278.html

[3] Wu Jun-xi, *op. cit.*, p. 381

49

OSTEOARTHRITIS

Also called degenerative joint disease, osteoarthrosis, and hypertrophic osteoarthritis, osteoarthritis (OA) is a joint disease characterized by loss of articular cartilage and hypertrophy of the bone producing osteophytes or bone spurs. It is the most common articular disorder. Osteoarthritis typically begins asymptomatically in the 20s and 30s and is extremely common by age 70. Almost all persons by age 40 have some pathological changes in weight-bearing joints, although relatively few have symptoms. Although men and women are equally affected by this disease, onset tends to be earlier in males.

Osteoarthritis is divided into two broad categories: primary (*i.e.*, idiopathic) and secondary. Primary generalized OA typically involves the distal and proximal interphalangeal joints, the first carpo-metacarpal joint, the intervertebral disks and zygapophyseal joints in the cervical and lumbar vertebrae, the first metatarso-phalangeal joint, hip, and knee. Secondary OA appears to result from conditions changing the microenvironment of the chondrocytes. These include congenital joint abnormalities, genetic defects, infectious, metabolic, endocrine, and neuropathic diseases, diseases that alter normal structure and function of the hyaline cartilage, and trauma to the hyaline cartilage or surrounding tissue. This trauma also include micro-trauma due to prolonged repetition of specific movements and overuse.

Pain is the earliest symptom of this disease. It is usually worsened by exercise and relieved by rest. Morning stiffness follows inactivity but lasts less than 15-30 minutes and lessens with movement. As OA progresses, joint mobility diminishes, tenderness and crepitus appear, and flexion contractures may develop. Proliferation of cartilage, bone, ligament, tendon, capsules, and synovium, along with varying amounts of joint effusion, ultimately produces the joint enlargement characteristic of this disease.

The Western medical diagnosis of osteoarthritis is based on signs and symptoms and on x-ray. X-ray generally reveals narrowing of the joint space, increased density of the subchondral bone, osteophyte formation at the periphery of the joints, and pseudocysts in the subchondral marrow. ESR is normal or only moderately increased. Blood studies help rule out other diseases with similar symptoms, such as rheumatoid arthritis and gout. The Western medical treatment of OA involves lifestyle and activity counseling, such as the avoidance of soft, deep chairs by those with osteoarthritis of the hip, exercise and stretching, and the symptomatic use of analgesics, such as NSAIDs. Muscle relaxants may be temporarily prescribed to relieve pain arising from muscle strained attempting to support OA joints. However, drug therapy comprises only 15% of a total treatment program and is the least important aspect of optimum management. Adjunctive treatments include transcutaneous electrical stimulation (TENS) and local rubs such as with capsaicin, a capsicum derivative. Surgery, including laminectomy, osteotomy, and total joint replacement, may be used when conservative therapy fails.

CHINESE DISEASE CATEGORIZATION: Osteoarthritis falls within the general category of *bi zheng*, impediment conditions, in Chinese medicine. It is also called *feng shi bing*, literally, wind dampness disease but often translated as rheumatic disease, and *li jie feng*, wind visiting the joints.

DISEASE CAUSES: External contraction of wind, cold, damp evils and bodily weakness due to former heaven natural endowment insufficiency and/or aging

DISEASE MECHANISMS: Due to habitual bodily vacuity weakness, the defensive exterior may fail in its duty. If wind, cold, and/or damp evils take advantage of this vacuity to invade the body and flow to the joints, they may impede and obstruct the qi and blood in the local area, thus causing joint aching and pain, swelling and distention, and inhibition in flexing and extending. If these external evils block the yang qi, enduring depression of wind, cold, and dampness may transform into heat. In that case, there will be burning heat, redness, and swelling in the affected area. If wind is the main evil, the pain will be migratory and not fixed in location. If cold is predominant, there will be severe, chilly pain which may feel like being cut by a knife. If dampness is predominant, the aching and pain will be heavy and fixed. In the early stage of this disease when evils are still lodged in the muscle or fleshy exterior and are causing disharmony of the defensive and constructive, there may be aversion to wind, sweating, and emission of heat.

Because impediment implies lack of free flow of the qi and blood, enduring impediment may be associated with qi stagnation and blood stasis. Because fluids flow with the blood, enduring dampness may congeal into phlegm nodulations. In addition, habitual bodily yin and blood may fail to nourish the sinews and engender the marrow, while habitual bodily yang vacuity may aggravate externally contracted cold with vacuity cold. Since cold's nature is constricting and contracting, such vacuity cold only worsens impediment pain.

TREATMENT BASED ON PATTERN DISCRIMINATION:

1. MOVING IMPEDIMENT PATTERN

MAIN SYMPTOMS: Migratory joint aching, pain, and soreness which is not fixed in location, aggravation of pain with the weather, *i.e.*, low pressure systems, possible accompanying aversion to wind and fever, thin, white tongue fur, and a floating, moderate (*i.e.*, slightly slow) pulse

NOTE: This pattern is also called predominant wind pattern.

TREATMENT PRINCIPLES: Dispel wind and free the flow of the network vessels assisted by scattering cold and dispelling dampness

NOTE: In actual fact, the three evils of wind, dampness, and cold are almost always combined together in the case of wind cold damp impediment. When wind is predominant, we call this moving impediment. When cold is predominant, we call this painful impediment, and when the dampness is predominant, we call this fixed impediment. Thus, and especially in textbook presentations such as this, we distinguish three types of impediment and give specific treatment principles for each. However, in real-life practice, in the majority of cases of impediment, we course wind, scatter cold, and eliminate dampness at the same time. Then, according to the disease mechanisms, one should clear depressive heat, supplement vacuity, dispel the stasis, and transform phlegm as necessary.

RX: *Fang Feng Tang Jia Jian* (Ledebouriella Decoction with Additions & Subtractions)

INGREDIENTS: Ramulus Mori Albi (*Sang Zhi*), 30g, Sclerotium Poriae Cocos (*Fu Ling*), Radix Puerariae (*Ge Gen*), Radix Clematidis Chinensis (*Wei Ling Xian*), and Herba Aristolochiae (*Xun Gu Feng*), 12g each, Radix Ledebouriellae Divaricatae (*Fang Feng*), Radix Et Rhizoma Notopterygii (*Qiang Huo*), Radix Gentianae Macrophyllae (*Qin Jiao*), and Radix Angelicae Sinensis (*Dang Gui*), 9g each, and Radix Ligustici Wallichii (*Chuan Xiong*) and Radix Glycyrrhizae (*Gan Cao*), 6g each

ANALYSIS OF FORMULA: *Fang Feng, Sang Zhi, Ge Gen, Wei Ling Xian, Xun Gu Feng, Qiang Huo*, and *Qin Jiao* all course wind and treat impediment. In addition, *Fang Feng* eliminates dampness, *Sang Zhi* frees the flow of the network vessels and works on the upper limbs, and *Xun Gu Feng* eliminates dampness and stops pain. *Qin Jiao* eliminates dampness and works on the trunk and four limbs, *Ge Gen* relaxes spasms and resolves the muscles, and *Wei Ling Xian* eliminates dampness and works on the whole body, while *Qiang Huo* eliminates dampness and works on the upper part of the body. *Dang Gui* and *Chuan Xiong* move the qi and quicken the blood in the network vessels to stop pain. Also, *Dang Gui* nourishes the blood to fill the channels and network vessels to avoid further invasion of evils. *Fu Ling* seeps dampness, and *Gan Cao* harmonizes the other medicinals in this formula.

ADDITIONS & SUBTRACTIONS: If there is pain in the upper limbs, add nine grams of Ramulus Cinnamomi Cassiae (*Gui Zhi*). If there is pain in the lower limbs, add nine grams of Radix Angelicae Pubescentis (*Du Huo*). If there is knee pain, add nine grams of Radix Achyranthis Bidentatae (*Niu Xi*). If pain is in the shoulder, add nine grams of Rhizoma Curcumae Longae (*Jiang Huang*). If pain is in the spinal column, add nine grams of Ramulus Loranthi Seu Visci (*Sang Ji Sheng*). If pain is in the low back, add nine grams of Cortex Eucommiae Ulmoidis (*Du Zhong*). If there is a more marked cold sensation in the limbs, add nine grams of Ramulus Cinnamomi Cassiae (*Gui Zhi*) and three grams of Herba Asari Cum Radice (*Xi Xin*). In case of enduring disease with qi and blood vacuity, add 15 grams of Radix Astragali Membranacei (*Huang Qi*) and nine grams of Radix Codonopsitis Pilosulae (*Dang Shen*). In case of enduring disease with liver-kidney vacuity, add nine grams each of Radix Dipsaci (*Xu Duan*), Cortex Eucommiae Ulmoidis (*Du Zhong*), and Radix Achyranthis Bidentatae (*Niu Xi*).

ACUPUNCTURE & MOXIBUSTION: *Feng Chi* (GB 20), *Ge Shu* (Bl 17), *Xue Hai* (Sp 10), *Tai Chong* (Liv 3), appropriate local points

ANALYSIS OF FORMULA: Draining *Feng Chi* resolves the

exterior and courses wind. Draining *Xue Hai* and *Ge Shu* quickens the blood based on the statement, "To treat wind, first treat the blood." And draining *Tai Chong* rectifies the qi in order to increase the strength of quickening the blood. The local points free the flow of the network vessels in the affected area.

ADDITIONS & SUBTRACTIONS: For jaw impediment, add *Xia Guan* (St 7), *Yin Feng* (TB 17), and *He Gu* (LI 4). For cervical impediment, add *Feng Chi* (GB 20), *Wan Gu* (GB 12), and *Tian Zhu* (Bl 10). For thoracic vertebral impediment, add *Hua Tuo Jia Ji* (M-BW-35l) points at the level of involvement. For sacrococcygeal impediment, add *Da Chang Shu* (Bl 25), *Ming Men* (GV 4), *Ba Liao* (Bl 31-34), and *Wei Zhong* (Bl 40). For shoulder impediment, add *Jian Yu* (LI 15), *Tian Zong* (SI 11), and *Ji Quan* (Ht 1). For elbow impediment, add *Qu Chi* (LI 11), *Xiao Hai* (SI 8), *Zhou Liao* (LI 12), and *Shou San Li* (LI 10). For wrist impediment, add *Wai Guan* (TB 5), *Yang Chi* (TB 4), and *Wan Gu* (SI 4). For upper extremity phalageal and metacarpal impediment, add *Bai Xie* (M-UE-22), *He Gu* (LI 4), and *Hou Xi* (SI 3). For sacroiliac impediment, add *Guan Yuan Shu* (Bl 26), *Xiao Chang Shu* (Bl 27), *Bai Huan Shu* (Bl 30), *Huan Tiao* (GB 30), *Zhi Bian* (Bl 54), and *Ju Liao* (GB 29). For hip impediment, add *Huan Tiao* (GB 30) and *Yang Ling Quan* (GB 34). For knee impediment, add *Du Bi* (St 35), *Xi Yan* (M-LE-16a), *Qu Quan* (Liv 8), and *Wei Zhong* (Bl 40). For ankle impediment, choose between *Jie Xi* (St 41), *Shang Qiu* (Sp 5), *Qiu Xu* (GB 40), *Kun Lun* (Bl 60), *Tai Xi* (Ki 3), *Shen Mai* (Bl 62), and *Zhao Hai* (Ki 6). For metatarsal and lower extremity phalangeal impediment, add *Jie Xi* (St 41), *Gong Sun* (Sp 4), *Tai Chong* (Liv 3), *Zu Lin Qi* (GB 41), and *Ba Feng* (M-LE-8).

2. PAINFUL IMPEDIMENT PATTERN

MAIN SYMPTOMS: Severe joint aching and pain which may feel like being cut with a knife, spasms and contractures, aggravation on exposure to cold, relief on obtaint of warmth, pain which is relatively fixed in location, pain which is better during the day and worse at night, inhibited flexion and extension of the joint, emission of coolness of the skin in the affected area and no redness or hotness, a pale tongue with white or glossy, white fur, and a deep, tight or bowstring, tight pulse

NOTE: This pattern is also called predominant cold pattern.

TREATMENT PRINCIPLES: Scatter cold and stop pain assisted by dispelling wind and eliminating dampness

RX: *Wu Tou Tang Jia Wei* (Aconite Decoction with Added Flavors)

INGREDIENTS: Mel (*Feng Mi*), 50g, Caulis Milletiae Seu Spatholobi (*Ji Xue Teng*), 30g, Radix Astragali Membranacei (*Huang Qi*) and Radix Albus Paeoniae Lactiflorae (*Bai Shao*), 15g each, processed Radix Aconiti Carmichaeli (*Chuan Wu*), mix-fried Radix Glycyrrhizae (*Gan Cao*), and Rhizoma Atractylodis Macrocephalae (*Bai Zhu*), 9g each, and Herba Ephedrae (*Ma Huang*), 6g

ANALYSIS OF FORMULA: *Chuan Wu* strongly scatters cold, courses wind, and stops impediment pain. *Ma Huang* courses wind and scatters cold. With *Chuan Wu,* it expels wind cold from the bones. *Huang Qi, Bai Zhu, Bai Shao,* and mix-fried *Gan Cao* supplement vacuity to avoid further invasion of wind, cold, and damp evils in the channels. In addition, *Bai Zhu* dries dampness. *Ji Xue Teng* frees the flow of the network vessels and quicken the blood based on the statement, "To treat wind, first treat the blood." *Feng Mi* and *Gan Cao* check the toxicity of *Chuan Wu.*

ADDITIONS & SUBTRACTIONS: If there are accompanying signs of dampness, add 18 grams of Semen Coicis Lachryma-jobi (*Yi Yi Ren*) and nine grams of Rhizoma Atractylodis (*Cang Zhu*). If there is a severe cold sensation in the limbs, add three grams of Herba Asari Cum Radice (*Xi Xin*). If there is blood stasis with pricking pain, add six grams each of Resina Olibani (*Ru Xiang*) and Resina Myrrhae (*Mo Yao*). If there is pain in the upper limbs, add nine grams of Ramulus Cinnamomi Cassiae (*Gui Zhi*). If there is pain in the lower limbs, add nine grams of Radix Angelicae Pubescentis (*Du Huo*). If there is knee pain, add nine grams of Radix Achyranthis Bidentatae (*Niu Xi*). If there is shoulder pain, add nine grams of Rhizoma Curcumae Longae (*Jiang Huang*). If there is pain in the spinal column, add nine grams of Radix Gentianae Macrophyllae (*Qin Jiao*). If there is low back pain, add nine grams of Cortex Eucommiae Ulmoidis (*Du Zhong*). In case of enduring disease with liver-kidney vacuity, add nine grams each of Radix Dipsaci (*Xu Duan*), Cortex Eucommiae Ulmoidis (*Du Zhong*), and Radix Achyranthis Bidentatae (*Niu Xi*).

If pain is less severe, replace *Wu Tou Tang* with *Gui Zhi Fu Zi Tang* (Cinnamon Twig & Aconite Decoction): Ramulus Cinnamomi Cassiae (*Gui Zhi*), Radix Lateralis Praeparatus Aconiti Carmichaeli (*Fu Zi*), and Radix Glycyrrhizae (*Gan Cao*), 9g each, uncooked Rhizoma Zingiberis (*Sheng Jiang*), 3 slices, and Fructus Zizyphi Jujubae (*Da Zao*), 5 pieces.

ACUPUNCTURE & MOXIBUSTION: *Shen Shu* (Bl 23), *Guan Yuan* (CV 4), the same local points as described under the additions and subtractions of the previous pattern

ANALYSIS OF FORMULA: Needling *Shen Shu* and *Guan Yuan* with even supplementing-even draining technique followed by moxibustion stimulates the source yang in order to free the flow of yang so it can scatter cold and warm the channels. Draining the local points frees the flow of the network vessels in the affected area.

Additions & subtractions: Please see pattern #1 above.

3. Fixed impediment pattern

Main symptoms: Joint aching, pain, soreness, numbness, and heaviness which is fixed in location, marked swelling of the affected area, difficulty flexing and extending the joint, worse pain in damp environments or rainy weather, worse pain in the lower half of the body, a pale tongue with slimy, white fur, and a soggy, moderate (*i.e.*, slightly slow) pulse

Note: This pattern is also called predominant dampness pattern.

Treatment principles: Eliminate dampness and free the flow of impediment assisted by dispelling wind and scattering cold

Rx: *Yi Yi Ren Tang Jia Jian* (Coix Decoction with Additions & Subtractions)

Ingredients: Uncooked Semen Coicis Lachyrma-jobi (*Yi Yi Ren*), 30g, Caulis Milletiae Seu Spatholobi (*Ji Xue Teng*) and Cortex Erythinae (*Hai Tong Pi*), 15g each, Radix Stephaniae Tetrandrae (*Fang Ji*) and Herba Siegesbeckiae (*Xi Xian Cao*), 12g each, Radix Angelicae Sinensis (*Dang Gui*), Radix Angelicae Pubescentis (*Du Huo*), Radix Et Rhizoma Notopterygii (*Qiang Huo*), Ramulus Cinnamomi Cassiae (*Gui Zhi*), Rhizoma Atractylodis Macrocephalae (*Bai Zhu*), and Rhizoma Atractylodis (*Cang Zhu*), 9g each, and Radix Ligustici Wallichii (*Chuan Xiong*) and Radix Ledebouriellae Divaricatae (*Fang Feng*), 6g each

Analysis of formula: *Yi Yi Ren, Hai Tong Pi, Fang Ji, Xi Xian Cao, Du Huo, Qiang Huo, Cang Zhu, Chuan Xiong,* and *Fang Feng* all eliminate wind damp evils and disinhibit impediment. In addition, *Yi Yi Ren* treats muscle spasms and tension, *Hai Tong Pi* clears and eliminates dampness and heat, *Xi Xian Cao* clears heat, and *Fang Ji* and *Du Huo* especially treat impediment in the lower limbs, while *Qiang Huo* especially treats impediment in the upper limbs. *Cang Zhu* strongly dries dampness, *Chuan Xiong* quickens the blood, and *Fang Feng* strongly courses wind. *Ji Xue Teng, Dang Gui,* and *Chuan Xiong* quicken the blood and free the flow of the network vessels. *Gui Zhi* courses wind, scatters cold, and treats painful impediment, especially in the upper part of the body. *Bai Zhu* boosts the qi and dries dampness, with *Dang Gui,* it supports the righteous or correct qi to prevent further invasion of evils.

Additions & subtractions: If wind dampness transforms into heat, please see the next pattern. If there is pain in the upper limbs, add nine grams of Ramulus Mori Albi (*Sang Zhi*). If there is pain in the lower limbs, add nine grams of Fructus Chaenomelis Lagenariae (*Mu Gua*). If there is knee pain, add nine grams of Radix Achyranthis Bidentatae (*Niu Xi*). If there is shoulder pain, add nine grams of Rhizoma Curcumae Longae (*Jiang Huang*). If there is pain in the spinal column, add nine grams of Ramulus Loranthi Seu Visci (*Sang Ji Sheng*). If there is low back pain, add nine grams of Cortex Eucommiae Ulmoidis (*Du Zhong*). If there is a more marked cold sensation in the limbs, add three grams of Herba Asari Cum Radice (*Xi Xin*). In case of enduring disease with qi and blood vacuity, add 15 grams of Radix Astragali Membranacei (*Huang Qi*) and nine grams of Radix Codonopsitis Pilosulae (*Dang Shen*). In case of enduring disease with liver-kidney vacuity, add nine grams each of Radix Dipsaci (*Xu Duan*), Cortex Eucommiae Ulmoidis (*Du Zhong*), and Radix Achyranthis Bidentatae (*Niu Xi*).

Acupuncture & moxibustion: *Yin Ling Quan* (Sp 9), *Zu San Li* (St 36), the local points described under the additions and subtractions in pattern #1 above with draining technique

Analysis of formula: *Zu San Li* supplements the spleen, and the spleen governs the movement and transformation of water fluids in the body. *Yin Ling Quan* seeps dampness. The local points free the flow of the network vessels in the affected area. Needle the first two points with lifting and thrusting technique and drain the rest.

Additions & subtractions: Please see pattern #1 above.

4. Heat impediment pattern

Main symptoms: Joint aching and pain which is burning hot, swollen and distended, and/or erythematous in the affected area, severe pain, possibly difficulty flexing and extending the joint, possible fever, oral thirst with a desire to drink, heart vexation, a predilection for chilled things and fear of heat, torpid intake, fatigue, a red tongue with yellow or slimy, yellow fur, and a slippery, rapid or soggy, rapid pulse

Treatment principles: Clear heat and free the flow of the network vessels assisted by coursing wind and eliminating dampness

Rx: *Bai Hu Jia Cang Zhu Tang* (White Tiger Plus Atractylodes Decoction) & *San Miao San* (Three Wonders Powder) with additions and subtractions

Ingredients: Caulis Lonicerae Japonicae (*Ren Dong Teng*), 60g, Gyspum Fibrosum (*Shi Gao*), 50g, Rhizoma Anemarrhenae Aspheloidis (*Zhi Mu*), Rhizoma Atractylodis

(*Cang Zhu*), Cortex Phellodendri (*Huang Bai*), Radix Cyathulae (*Chuan Niu Xi*), and Radix Ledebouriellae Divaricatae (*Fang Feng*), 9g each, and Radix Glycyrrhizae (*Gan Cao*), 6g

ANALYSIS OF FORMULA: *Ren Dong Teng* clears heat and frees the flow of the network vessels. *Shi Gao* and *Zhi Mu* clear heat and discharge fire. *Huang Bai* and *Cang Zhu* together clear and eliminate dampness and heat. *Fang Feng* courses wind, eliminates dampness, and disinhibits impediment. *Chuan Niu Xi* quickens and cools the blood. *Gan Cao* harmonizes the other medicinals in this formula, protecting the stomach from the cold nature of the other medicinals.

ADDITIONS & SUBTRACTIONS: If there is damp heat impediment with generalized fever which is not relieved by sweating, oral thirst and profuse drinking, and slimy, yellow tongue fur, replace *Bai Hu Jia Cang Zhu Tang* and *San Miao San* with *Mu Fang Ji Tang Jia Jian* (Cocculus Decoction with Additions & Subtractions): Gypsum Fibrosum (*Shi Gao*), 25g, Semen Coicis Lachyrma-jobi (*Yi Yi Ren*), 20g, Radix Stephaniae Tetrandrae (*Han Fang Ji*), 18g, Semen Pruni Armeniacae (*Xing Ren*) and Talcum (*Hua Shi*), 12g each, Ramulus Cinnamomi Cassiae (*Gui Zhi*), 9g, and Medulla Papyriferi Tetrapanacis (*Tong Cao*), 6g. If there is severe pain and a hot sensation in the joints of the limbs, add nine grams each of Herba Siegesbeckiae (*Xi Xian Cao*) and Caulis Sargentodoxae (*Hong Teng*). If there is swelling of the joints of the limbs, add nine grams of Radix Stephaniae Tetrandrae (*Han Fang Ji*) and five grams of Caulis Akebiae (*Mu Tong*).

If there is heat impediment and yin vacuity with pain which is worse at night, tidal fever, night sweats, dryness of the mouth and throat, muscle wilting, red tongue with scanty fur, and a fine, rapid pulse, replace *Bai Hu Jia Cang Zhu Tang* and *San Miao San* with *Qing Hao Bie Jia Tang Jia Wei* (Artemisia Apiacea & Carapax Amydae Decoction with Added Flavors): uncooked Radix Rehmanniae (*Sheng Di*), 30g, Carapax Amydae Sinensis (*Bie Jia*), Herba Artemisiae Apiacae (*Qing Hao*), Caulis Milletiae Seu Spatholobi (*Ji Xue Teng*), and Semen Coicis Lachryma-jobi (*Yi Yi Ren*), 15g each, Cortex Radicis Moutan (*Dan Pi*), Radix Scrophulariae Ningpoensis (*Xuan Shen*), Radix Gentianae Macrophyllae (*Qin Jiao*), and Radix Stephaniae Tetrandrae (*Han Fang Ji*), 12g each, Radix Angelicae Sinensis (*Dang Gui*), Radix Rubrus Paeoniae Lactiflorae (*Chi Shao*), Rhizoma Atractylodis (*Cang Zhu*), and Zaocys Dhumnades (*Wu Shao She*), 9g each. For alternating cold and heat (*i.e.*, fever and chills), add nine grams each of Radix Bupleuri (*Chai Hu*) and Radix Scutellariae Baicalensis (*Huang Qin*). For heat damaging yin fluids, add nine grams each of Herba Dendrobii (*Shi Hu*) and Radix Trichosanthis Kirlowii (*Tian Hua Fen*). If there is pain in the upper limbs, add nine grams of Ramulus Mori Albi (*Sang Zhi*). If there is pain in the lower limbs, add nine grams of Fructus Chaenomelis Lagenariae (*Mu Gua*). If there is pain in the shoulder, add nine grams of Rhizoma Curcumae Longae (*Jiang Huang*). In case of enduring disease with qi and blood vacuity, add 15 grams of Radix Astragali Membranacei (*Huang Qi*) and nine grams each of Radix Codonopsitis Pilosulae (*Dang Shen*) and Radix Angelicae Sinensis (*Dang Gui*). In case of enduring disease with liver-kidney vacuity, add nine grams each of Cortex Eucommiae Ulmoidis (*Du Zhong*) and Radix Achyranthis Bidentatae (*Niu Xi*).

ACUPUNCTURE & MOXIBUSTION: *Da Zhui* (GV 14), *Qu Chi* (LI 11), *He Gu* (LI 4), the local points described under the additions and subtractions of pattern #1 above

ANALYSIS OF FORMULA: Bleeding *Da Zhui* clears heat and dispels wind. Draining *Qu Chi* and *He Gu* with lifting and thrusting technique clears heat, since the yang ming channel has lots of qi and lots of blood. Draining the local points frees the flow of the network vessels in the affected area.

ADDITIONS & SUBTRACTIONS: Please see pattern #1 above.

5. PHLEGM & STASIS OBSTRUCTING THE NETWORK VESSELS PATTERN

MAIN SYMPTOMS: A long course of disease, stiffness of the joints with inhibited flexion and extension, deformation of the joint, severe fixed, stabbing pain which becomes worse on pressure, possible numbness, possible swollen joints, thickening and hardening of the tendons of the articulation, possible darkness or discoloration of the affected joint, muscular atrophy around the articulation, possible subcutaneous nodules on or surrounding the joint, a purple dark tongue with static spots or macules and slimy, white fur, and a soft, choppy, fine or bowstring and slippery pulse

TREATMENT PRINCIPLES: Quicken the blood and transform stasis, dispel phlegm and free the flow of the network vessels

RX: *Sou Feng Yin Jia Jian* (Track Down Wind Drink with Additions & Subtractions)

INGREDIENTS: Zaocys Dhumnades (*Wu Shao She*), processed Radix Aconiti Carmichaeli (*Chuan Wu*), and processed Radix Aconiti Kusnezofii (*Cao Wu Tou*), 12g each, Semen Sinapis Albae (*Bai Jie Zi*), Eupolyphaga Seu Opisthoplatia (*Tu Bie Chong*), Flos Carthami Tinctorii (*Hong Hua*), Rhizoma Drynariae (*Gu Sui Bu*), Radix Et Rhizoma Notopterygii (*Qiang Huo*), and Lumbricus (*Di Long*), 9g each, Resina Olibani (*Ru Xiang*), 6g, and Scolopendra Subspinipes (*Wu Gong*), 0.5g (powdered and taken with the strained decoction)

ANALYSIS OF FORMULA: *Wu Shao She*, *Tu Bie Chong*, *Di*

Long, and *Wu Gong* together free the flow of the network vessels, dispel phlegm, and strongly stop pain. *Chuan Wu* and *Cao Wu* track down wind in the vessels and bones, dispel evils and strongly stop pain. *Bai Jie Zi* transforms phlegm and treats impediment associated with phlegm. *Hong Hua* and *Ru Xiang* quicken the blood, transform stasis, and stop pain. *Gu Sui Bu* quickens the blood and transforms stasis, connects the sinews and knits the bones. *Qiang Huo* dispels wind dampness and treats impediment.

NOTE: *Cao Wu* and *Chuan Wu* should only be used in their processed form and should be decocted for a long time. The amounts used above are very strong. Therefore, one must attentively supervise the reactions of the patient and observe the six precautions when using Aconite (see *Dui Yao: The Art of Combining Chinese Medicinals* available from Blue Poppy Press).

ADDITIONS & SUBTRACTIONS: If there is concomitant qi vacuity, add 18 grams of Radix Astragali Membranacei (*Huang Qi*) and 15 grams of Radix Codonopsitis Pilosulae (*Dang Shen*). If there is concomitant kidney yang vacuity, add nine grams each of Herba Epimedii (*Yin Yang Huo*) and Rhizoma Curculiginis Orchioidis (*Xian Mao*). If there is concomitant kidney yin vacuity, subtract *Cao Wu* and *Chuan Wu* and add 15 grams each of uncooked Radix Rehmanniae (*Sheng Di*), Radix Achyranthis Bidentatae (*Niu Xi*), and Ramulus Loranthi Seu Visci (*Sang Ji Sheng*). If there is concomitant blood vacuity, decrease the dosage of *Chuan Wu* and *Cao Wu* down to six grams and add 12 grams of Radix Angelicae Sinensis (*Dang Gui*). If there are subcutaneous nodulations, add 18 grams of Semen Vaccariae Segetalis (*Wang Bu Liu Xing*). If there is severe numbness, add 18 grams of Caulis Milletiae Seu Spatholobi (*Ji Xue Teng*). If there is concomitant damp heat, subtract *Cao Wu*, *Chuan Wu*, and *Qiang Huo*, and add 12 grams each of Radix Stephaniae Tetrandrae (*Han Fang Ji*) and Radix Gentianae Macrophyllae (*Qin Jiao*). For slimy tongue fur with chest and abdominal oppression, add nine grams each of Pericarpium Citri Reticulatae (*Chen Pi*), Sclerotium Poriae Cocos (*Fu Ling*), and Rhizoma Pinelliae Ternatae (*Ban Xia*).

If there are no nodulations, deformation of the joint, or slimy tongue fur, *i.e.,* there is no phlegm but only stasis, replace *Su Feng Yin Jia Jian* with *Shen Tong Zhu Yu Tang Jia Jian* (Body Pain Expel Stasis Decoction with Additions & Subtractions): Semen Pruni Persicae (*Tao Ren*), Flos Carthami Tinctorii (*Hong Hua*), Radix Achyranthis Bidentatae (*Niu Xi*), Feces Trogopterori Seu Pteromi (*Wu Ling Zhi*), and Radix Angelicae Sinensis (*Dang Gui*), 12g each, and Rhizoma Cyperi Rotundi (*Xiang Fu*), Radix Gentianae Macrophyllae (*Qin Jiao*), Radix Et Rhizoma Notopterygii (*Qiang Huo*), Lumbricus (*Di Long*), and Radix Ligustici Wallichii (*Chuan Xiong*), 9g each.

ACUPUNCTURE & MOXIBUSTION: *Feng Long* (St 40), *Zu San Li* (St 36), *Ge Shu* (Bl 17), *Xue Hai* (Sp 10), the local points described under the additions and subtractions in pattern #1 above

ANALYSIS OF FORMULA: Supplementing *Zu San Li* supplements the spleen to prevent further phlegm accumulation. It also boosts the qi to move the phlegm and blood. Draining *Feng Long* transforms phlegm. Draining *Ge Shu* and *Xue Hai* quickens the blood and this helps to also transform phlegm. Draining the local points frees the flow of the network vessels in the affected area. For this pattern, the systemic points are not very powerful. Needling just the local points with internally administered Chinese medicinals is more effective.

6. QI & BLOOD DUAL VACUITY PATTERN

MAIN SYMPTOMS: Enduring joint pain with swelling and possible slight deformation, worsening of pain when carrying weight and walking, difficulty walking or seizing objects, inhibited flexion and extension of the affected joints, alternating periods of improvement and aggravation, possible muscular tics, a pale facial complexion, heart palpitations, dizziness, torpid intake, weakness, fatigue, a pale, swollen tongue with thin, white fur, and a deep, fine, bowstring pulse

TREATMENT PRINCIPLES: Supplement qi and nourish the blood assisted as needed by dispelling evils

RX: *Dang Gui Bu Xue Tang* (Dang Gui Supplement the Blood Decoction) plus *Si Jun Zi Tang* (Four Gentlemen Decoction) with additions & subtractions

INGREDIENTS: Radix Astragali Membranacei (*Huang Qi*), Rhizoma Atractylodis Macrocephalae (*Bai Zhu*), Sclerotium Poriae Cocos (*Fu Ling*), and Caulis Milletiae Seu Spatholobi (*Ji Xue Teng*), 20g each, Radix Angelicae Sinensis (*Dang Gui*), cooked Radix Rehmanniae (*Shu Di*), Radix Et Rhizoma Notopterygii (*Qiang Huo*), and Radix Angelicae Pubescentis (*Du Huo*), 15g each, and Radix Codonopsitis Pilosulae (*Dang Shen*) and Ramulus Cinnamomi Cassiae (*Gui Zhi*), 9g each

ANALYSIS OF FORMULA: *Huang Qi*, *Dang Shen*, *Fu Ling*, and *Bai Zhu* fortify the spleen and boost the qi. In addition, *Bai Zhu* and *Fu Ling* dry and disinhibit dampness. *Ji Xue Teng*, *Shu Di*, and *Dang Gui* nourish the blood. *Ji Xue Teng*, and *Dang Gui* also quicken the blood and transform stasis. *Qiang Huo* and *Du Huo* dispel wind dampness in the upper and lower parts of the body which has penetrated the network vessel due to vacuity. *Gui Zhi* warms and quickens the network vessels to stop pain.

ADDITIONS & SUBTRACTIONS: For heart palpitations, add nine grams of Radix Polygalae Tenuifoliae (*Yuan Zhi*) and 15 grams of Arillus Euphoriae Longanae (*Long Yan Rou*). For severe joint pain, add six grams each of Resina Olibani (*Ru Xiang*) and Resina Myrrhae (*Mo Yao*). If there is coolness of the joint, add nine grams of Radix Lateralis Praeparatus Aconiti Carmichaeli (*Fu Zi*). For joint pain in the upper limbs, add 15 grams of Rhizoma Curcumae Longae (*Jiang Huang*). For joint pain in the lower limbs, add 15 grams of Radix Cyathulae (*Chuan Niu Xi*). If there is concomitant yin vacuity, add 15 grams of uncooked Radix Rehmanniae (*Sheng Di*). For swollen joints, add 15 grams of Semen Coicis Lachryma-jobi (*Yi Yi Ren*) and nine grams of Rhizoma Atractylodis (*Cang Zhu*).

If wind damp evils are marked, replace *Dang Gui Bu Xue Tang* plus *Si Jun Zi Tang* with *Juan Bi Tang Jia Jian* (Alleviate Impediment Decoction with Additions & Subtractions): Radix Astragali Membranacei (*Huang Qi*), 30g, Caulis Trachelospermi Jasminoidis (*Luo Shi Teng*), Semen Coicis Lachryma-jobi (*Yi Yi Ren*), Radix Angelicae Sinensis (*Dang Gui*), Caulis Milletiae Seu Spatholobi (*Ji Xue Teng*), and Radix Codonopsitis Pilosulae (*Dang Shen*), 12g each, Radix Et Rhizoma Notopterygii (*Qiang Huo*), Radix Angelicae Pubescentis (*Du Huo*), Radix Ledebouriellae Divaricatae (*Fang Feng*), Ramulus Cinnamomi Cassiae (*Gui Zhi*), Radix Lateralis Praeparatus Aconiti Carmichaeli (*Fu Zi*), Rhizoma Atractylodis (*Cang Zhu*), Radix Ligustici Wallichii (*Chuan Xiong*), Radix Albus Paeoniae Lactiflorae (*Bai Shao*), and Radix Achyranthis Bidentatae (*Niu Xi*), 9g each, and mix-fried Radix Glycyrrhizae (*Gan Cao*), 6g.

ACUPUNCTURE & MOXIBUSTION: *San Yin Jiao* (Sp 6), *Zu San Li* (St 36), the local points described under the additions and subtractions in pattern #1 above

ANALYSIS OF FORMULA: Supplementing *San Yin Jiao* and *Zu San Li* supplements the qi and blood, while draining the local points frees the flow of the network vessels in the affected area. For this pattern, the systemic points are not very powerful. Using just the local points with the internal administration of Chinese medicinals is more effective.

7. KIDNEY YIN VACUITY PATTERN

MAIN SYMPTOMS: Enduring disease which does not cure, joint pain with stiffness of the sinews, a slight burning sensation, redness, and swelling in the affected area, worse pain at night, possible slightly inhibited flexion and extension of the affected joints, a tendency towards a thin body, dizziness, vertigo, tinnitus, a dry throat, heart vexation, insomnia, night sweats, low back and knee soreness and weakness, vexatious heat in the five centers, a red tongue with scanty fluids, and a fine, rapid pulse

TREATMENT PRINCIPLES: Supplement the liver and kidneys, enrich yin, harmonize the blood, and free the flow of the network vessels

RX: *Du Huo Ji Sheng Tang Jia Jian* (Angelica Pubescens & Loranthus Decoction with Additions & Subtractions)

INGREDIENTS: Ramulus Loranthi Seu Visci (*Sang Ji Sheng*), Cortex Eucommiae Ulmoidis (*Du Zhong*), and cooked Radix Rehmanniae (*Shu Di*), 15g each, Gentianae Macrophyllae (*Qin Jiao*), Sclerotium Poriae Cocos (*Fu Ling*), and Radix Angelicae Pubescentis (*Du Huo*), 12g each, Radix Angelicae Sinensis (*Dang Gui*), Radix Albus Paeoniae Lactiflorae (*Bai Shao*), and Radix Achyranthis Bidentatae (*Niu Xi*), 9g each, Radix Ledebouriellae Divaricatae (*Fang Feng*), Radix Ligustici Wallichii (*Chuan Xiong*), and mix-fried Radix Glycyrrhizae (*Gan Cao*), 6g each, and Herba Asari Cum Radice (*Xi Xin*), 3g

ANALYSIS OF FORMULA: *Sang Ji Sheng*, *Shu Di*, and *Niu Xi* supplement the liver and kidneys, enrich yin, boost the marrow, and reinforce the bones. *Shu Di*, *Dang Gui*, and *Bai Shao* nourish liver blood in order to strengthens the sinews and help supplement yin. *Du Zhong* gently supplements both kidney yin and yang, strengthens the sinews and reinforces the bones. *Sang Ji Sheng*, *Du Huo*, *Qin Jiao*, *Fang Feng*, *Xi Xin*, and *Chuan Xiong* dispel wind and eliminate dampness which have taken advantage of vacuity to enter, diffuse impediment and free the flow of the network vessels. *Fu Ling* and mix-fried *Gan Cao* boost the latter heaven to engender acquired essence and replenish the former heaven. In addition, *Fu Ling* helps to eliminate dampness.

ADDITIONS & SUBTRACTIONS: If there is concomitant kidney yang vacuity, add 12 grams each of Herba Epimedii (*Yin Yang Huo*) and Rhizoma Curculiginis Orchioidis (*Xian Mao*) and three grams of Cortex Cinnamomi Cassiae (*Rou Gui*), powdered and taken with the strained decoction. For concomitant qi vacuity, add 12 grams each of Radix Astragali Membranacei (*Huang Qi*) and Radix Codonopsitis Pilosulae (*Dang Shen*). If there is yin vacuity fire effulgence, add nine grams each of Cortex Phellodendri (*Huang Bai*) and Rhizoma Anemarrhenae Asphodeloidis (*Zhi Mu*). If there is severe stiffness of the sinews and inhibited flexion and extension of the joints, add 20 grams of Caulis Milletiae Seu Spatholobi (*Ji Xue Teng*), 15 grams of Caulis Trachelospermi Jasminoidis (*Luo Shi Teng*), and three grams of Lumbricus (*Di Long*), powdered and taken with the strained decoction. If there is concomitant wind damp heat with a burning sensation, redness, and swelling in the affected area, subtract *Xi Xin*, *Fang Feng*, and *Du Zhong*, and add 12 grams each of Caulis Lonicerae Japonicae (*Ren Dong Teng*), Ramulus Mori Albi (*Sang Zhi*), Radix Stephaniae Tetrandrae (*Han Fang Ji*), and Herba Siegesbeckiae (*Xi Xian Cao*).

ACUPUNCTURE & MOXIBUSTION: *Fu Liu* (Ki 7), *Da Zhu* (Bl 11), *Xuan Zhong* (GB 39), the local points described under the additions and subtractions in pattern #1 above

ANALYSIS OF FORMULA: *Fu Liu* is the supplementing point

of the kidney channel. Supplementing it supplements both the yin and yang of the kidneys as well as former heaven essence, *Xuan Zhong* is the meeting point of the marrow. Supplementing it boosts the marrow, *Da Zhu* is the meeting point of the bones. Supplementing it reinforces the bones. Draining the local points frees the flow of the network vessels in the affected area.

8. Spleen-kidney yang vacuity pattern

Main symptoms: Enduring disease which does not cure, slight joint pain with stiffness of the sinews which prevents walking, sometimes deformation of the joint with inhibited flexion and extension of the joint, possible coolness of the joints, a pale facial complexion, lassitude of the spirit, fatigue, reduced food intake, loose stools, aversion to cold, cold limbs, low back and knee soreness and weakness, frequent copious urine, nocturia, a pale tongue, and a deep, thin, weak pulse

Treatment principles: Warm and supplement the spleen and kidneys, course the vessels and free the flow of the network vessels

Rx: *Zhen Wu Tang Jia Jian* (True Warrior Decoction with Additions & Subtractions)

Ingredients: Radix Astragali Membranacei (*Huang Qi*), Ramulus Cinnamomi Cassiae (*Gui Zhi*), Ramulus Mori Albi (*Sang Zhi*), and Radix Achyranthis Bidentatae (*Niu Xi*), 20g each, processed Radix Aconiti Carmichaeli (*Chuan Wu*), Rhizoma Atractylodis Macrocephalae (*Bai Zhu*), and Radix Albus Paeoniae Lactiflorae (*Bai Shao*), 12g each, and Herba Epimedii (*Yin Yang Huo*), Sclerotium Poriae Cocos (*Fu Ling*), and mix-fried Radix Glycyrrhizae (*Gan Cao*), 9g each

Analysis of formula: *Gui Zhi*, *Chuan Wu*, *Niu Xi*, and *Yin Yang Huo* together warm and supplement kidney yang and diffuse impediment. In addition, *Gui Zhi* warms the vessels, *Chuan Wu* frees the flow of the 12 vessels, and *Yin Yang Huo* courses wind dampness. Thus the combination of these medicinals stop pain due to cold. *Niu Xi* strengthens the sinews and reinforces the bones, while *Sang Zhi* frees the flow of the network vessels. The former works on the lower part of the body, while the latter works on the upper part of the body. *Huang Qi*, *Bai Zhu*, *Fu Ling*, and mix-fried *Gan Cao*, with the help of *Gui Zhi*, warm and supplement spleen yang. *Bai Shao* and *Gui Zhi* harmonize the constructive and defensive, qi and blood to treat vacuity impediment.

Additions & subtractions: If there are loose stools, add nine grams each of Radix Codonopsitis Pilosulae (*Dang Shen*) and Fructus Psoraleae Corylifoliae (*Bu Gu Zhi*). For swelling in the joints, add 15 grams of Rhizoma Atractylodis (*Cang Zhu*) and Semen Coicis Lachryma-jobi (*Yi Yi Ren*). If there is severe pain or a cold sensation in the joints, add three grams of Herba Asari Cum Radice (*Xi Xin*).

Acupuncture & moxibustion: *Guan Yuan* (CV 4), *Ming Men* (GV 4), *Da Zhu* (Bl 11), *Xuan Zhong* (GB 39), the local points described under the additions and subtractions in pattern #1 above

Analysis of formula: Supplementing *Guan Yuan* and *Ming Men* with moxibustion warms and supplements spleen and kidney yang and also boosts the former heaven essence. Supplementing *Xuan Zhong*, the meeting point of the marrow, boosts the marrow, while supplementing *Da Zhu*, the meeting point of the bones, reinforces the bones. Draining the local points free the flow of the network vessels in the affected area.

Remarks

1. Because osteoarthritis occurs mainly in older patients, it usually manifests as a mixed vacuity and repletion pattern. Therefore, there may be pronounced qi, blood, yin, or yang vacuities. In that case, guiding formulas should be picked based on the patient's predominant pattern and modified to treat accompanying patterns and branch symptoms. When impediment is complicated by either kidney yin or yang vacuity, this is called recalcitrant impediment. Recalcitrant impediment is then divided into heat recalcitrant impediment if there is yin vacuity and cold recalcitrant impediment if there is yang vacuity. Of course, yin and yang vacuities may exist simultaneously.

Most patients with OA will also present at least some symptoms of qi stagnation and blood stasis. When these occur, qi-rectifying and blood-quickening medicinals should be added to the formula. Appropriate blood-quickening medicinals include Caulis Milletiae Seu Spatholobi (*Ji Xue Teng*), Radix Salviae Miltiorrhizae (*Dan Shen*), Radix Angelicae Sinensis (*Dang Gui*), Radix Ligustici Wallichii (*Chuan Xiong*), Radix Rubrus Paeoniae Lactiflorae (*Chi Shao*), Resina Olibani (*Ru Xiang*), Resina Myrrhae (*Mo Yao*), and Radix Pseudoginseng (*Tian San Qi*).

Du Huo Ji Sheng Tang (Angelica Pubescens & Loranthus Decoction) is designed to treat wind cold damp impediment complicated by spleen qi, liver blood and kidney yang vacuities (but without damp or vacuity heat). It is comprised of: cooked Radix Rehmanniae (*Shu Di*), Sclerotium Poriae Cocos (*Fu Ling*), and Ramulus Loranthi Seu Visci (*Sang Ji Sheng*), 12g each, Radix Angelicae Pubescentis (*Du Huo*), Cortex Eucommiae Ulmoidis (*Du Zhong*), Radix Angelicae Sinensis (*Dang Gui*), Radix Albus Paeoniae Lactiflorae (*Bai Shao*), and Radix Achyranthis Bidentatae (*Niu Xi*), 9g each, Radix Gentianae Macrophyllae (*Qin Jiao*), Radix Ledebouriellae Divaricatae (*Fang Feng*), Radix Panacis

Ginseng (*Ren Shen*), and mix-fried Radix Glycyrrhizae (*Gan Cao*), 6g each, and Cortex Cinnamomi Cassiae (*Rou Gui*) and Herba Asari Cum Radice (*Xi Xin*), 3g each. If pain is severs, add six grams of Radix Aconiti Carmichaeli (*Chuan Wu*). If there is concomitant blood stasis, add nine grams each of Semen Pruni Persicae (*Tao Ren*) and Flos Carthami Tinctorii (*Hong Hua*). Other formulas for recalcitrant impediment include *San Bi Tang* (Three Impediments Decoction), *Da Qin Jiao Tang* (Major Gentiana Macrophylla Decoction), and *Da Fang Feng Tang* (Major Ledebouriella Decoction).

For liver-spleen-kidney qi and blood, yin and yang vacuity with wind, damp, cold evils, and qi stagnation and blood stasis, a common complex pattern in the elderly, one can use *Fu Yuan Juan Bi Tang* (Restore the Origin & Alleviate Impediment Decoction): Radix Angelicae Sinensis (*Dang Gui*) and Ramulus Loranthi Seu Visci (*Sang Ji Sheng*), 20g each, Herba Epimedii (*Yin Yang Huo*), Rhizoma Homalomenae Occultae (*Qian Nian Jian*), Radix Et Rhizoma Notopterygii (*Qiang Huo*), Rhizoma Corydalis Yanhusuo (*Yan Hu Suo*), Ramulus Cinnamomi Cassiae (*Gui Zhi*), and Radix Astragali Membranacei (*Huang Qi*), 15g each, and Radix Ligustici Wallichii (*Chuan Xiong*), Radix Glycyrrhizae (*Gan Cao*), Herba Asari Cum Radice (*Xi Xin*), and Scolopendra Subspinipes (*Wu Gong*), 3g each. If there is concomitant liver depression, one can add nine grams each of Radix Bupleuri (*Chai Hu*) and Radix Albus Paeoniae Lactiflorae (*Bai Shao*) to this formula. If there is depressive heat, one can also add nine grams each of Fructus Gardeniae Jasminoidis (*Zhi Zi*) and Cortex Radicis Moutan (*Dan Pi*).

2. Joint deformation and periarticular nodules are usually seen as phlegm nodulation in Chinese medicine. In that case, medicinals for softening the hard and scattering nodulation, such as Herba Sargassii (*Hai Zao*), Thallus Algae (*Kun Bu*), Herba Laminariae (*Hai Dai*), Concha Ostreae (*Mu Li*), and Os Draconis (*Long Gu*), should be added to any other formulas being used. While these medicinals will not reverse deformation or eliminate nodulations, they will help relieve pain and prevent further deformation.

3. If one cannot distinguish between predominant wind, damp, or cold, one may use *Juan Bi Tang* (Alleviate Impediment Decoction) and modify it accordingly. This formula consists of: Caulis Piperis Futokadsurae (*Hai Feng Teng*) and Ramulus Mori Albi (*Sang Zhi*), 15g each, Resina Olibani (*Ru Xiang*), 12g, Radix Et Rhizoma Notopterygii (*Qiang Huo*), Radix Angelicae Pubescentis (*Du Huo*), Ramulus Cinnamomi Cassiae (*Gui Zhi*), Radix Gentianae Macrophyllae (*Qin Jiao*), Radix Angelicae Sinensis (*Dang Gui*), and Radix Ligustici Wallichii (*Chuan Xiong*), 9g each, and Radix Auklandiae Lappae (*Mu Xiang*) and Radix Glycyrrhizae (*Gan Cao*), 6g each.

4. In cases of active disease, elevated sedimentation rate, and elevated anti-O factor, if there is heat impediment, one should add one or more blood-cooling, toxin-resolving medicinals to the formula, such as uncooked Radix Rehmanniae (*Sheng Di*), Cortex Radicis Moutan (*Dan Pi*), Radix Rubrus Paeoniae Lactiflorae (*Chi Shao*), Radix Lithospermi Seu Arnebiae (*Zi Cao*), Herba Taraxaci Mongolici Cum Radice (*Pu Gong Ying*), and Caulis Lonicerae Japonicae (*Ren Dong Teng*). In case of cold impediment, one should add one or more qi-boosting, blood-quickening medicinals to the formula, such as Radix Astragali Membranacei (*Huang Qi*), Radix Codonopsitis Pilosulae (*Dang Shen*), Rhizoma Atractylodis Macrocephalae (*Bai Zhu*), and Caulis Milletiae Seu Spatholobi (*Ji Xue Teng*).

5. When acupuncture is accompanied by the internal administration of Chinese medicinals appropriate to the patient's pattern(s), one can use only the local points as described under the additions and subtractions of pattern #1 above without the other points described in the acupuncture and moxibustion sections under each pattern.

6. Uncooked Fructus Xanthii Sibirici (*Cang Er Zi*), Semen Strychnotis (*Ma Qian Zi*), Herba Asari Cum Radice (*Xi Xin*), and Herba Tripterygii Wilfordii (*Lei Gong Teng*) are all effective for the treatment of impediment pain. However, due to the risk of nephrotoxicity, these medicinals should not be used long-term. Most, if not all, of the toxins in *Cang Er Zi* are destroyed by decoction at high heat. However, *Lei Gong Teng*, an extremely effective impediment-assuaging medicinal is so toxic it is currently prohibited for sale in the People's Republic of China. Likewise, Radix Stephaniae Tetrandrae (*Han Fang Ji*) and Caulis Akebiae (*Mu Tong*) are also effective medicinals for the treatment of impediment pain. If one chooses to use these, it is important to verify that they have not been substituted by the Aristolochia species.

50

Osteoporosis

Osteoporosis is a generalized, progressive diminution of bone density causing skeletal weakness event though the ratio of mineral to organic elements remains unchanged. In women, osteoclast activity is increased over osteoblast activity due to decreased estrogen postmenopausaly. Therefore, virtually all women lose 5-10% of bone mass during the first five years after menopause with another one percent loss per year after that. However, osteoblast activity decreases in both men and women after age 60. Therefore, osteoporosis may occur in either men or women. If men do develop osteoporosis, it can be severe. Late menarche, early menopause, nulliparity, caffeine ingestion, alcohol use, and cigarette smoking may all increase the risk of osteoporosis. Because African Americans and Hispanics have higher bone mass than whites and Asians, African Americans and Hispanics tend to develop osteoporosis at a later age than whites and Asians. Other factors associated with the development of osteoporosis include immobilization or insufficient exercise, lower weight and muscle mass, dietary factors, such as insufficient intake of calcium, potassium, and vitamin D, and a bodily acid-base balance that is more acidic due to consumption of sugar, salt, excessive protein, carbonated soft drinks, caffeine, and processed foods. Another possible cause for modern people's bodies being more acidic is acid rain which causes drinking water to be more acidic. Other risk factors may include use of broad spectrum antibiotics and glucocorticoid medications, such as Prednisone, fluoride, and excess thyroxin.

Patients with uncomplicated osteoporosis may either be asymptomatic or may complain of muscle-bone pain, particularly in their back. Vertebral crush fractures may develop with minimal or no trauma. In fact, each year in the United States, 1.3 million people over 45 years of age experience bone fractures associated with osteoporosis. These usually occur in the weight-bearing vertebrae, T8 and below. When symptomatic, the pain is of acute onset, usually does not radiate, is aggravated by weight-bearing, may be associated with local tenderness, and typically begins to subside in one week. However, residual pain may last three months or more. Multiple compression fractures may result in dorsal kyphosis with exaggerated cervical lordosis. Abnormal stress on the spinal muscles and ligaments may cause, dull, aching pain which is particularly prominent in the lower thoracic and lumbar regions. Fractures at other sites, most commonly the hip and distal radius, usually are the result of falls. Twelve to 20% of older people with hip fractures die within a year of fracture. The resulting immobility of hip fractures becomes debilitating in and of itself and causes a downward spiral with rapid loss of muscle, bone, endurance, strength, and appetite.

The Western medical diagnosis of osteoporosis is mainly based on X-ray of the vertebrae and other bones showing decreased radiodensity. However, osteoporosis cannot be diagnosed via X-ray until more than 30% of bone mass has been lost. Single and dual photon absorptiometry, dual X-ray absorptiometry, and quantitative CT scan can also measure bone density in the lumbar spine, hip, and distal radius and are also useful in diagnosis and assessing treatment response. About 20% of postmenopausal osteoporotic women have significant hypercalciuria which may lead to elevated serum parathyroid hormone. In addition, indicators of bone turnover, such as urinary excretion of hydroxyproline-containing peptides, urinary pyridium peptide, or serum osteocalcin, may be increased.

The Western medical prevention of osteoporosis consists of maintaining adequate body weight, increased walking and weight-bearing exercise, avoidance of long-acting benzodiazepines, minimal caffeine and alcohol intake, and decreased smoking. The Western medical treatment of osteoporosis consists of pharmaceutical agents to minimize further bone loss, dietary calcium supplementation, and hormone replacement therapy for women. Treatment with growth factors and parathyroid hormone are currently under investigation. Acute back pain from vertebral crush fracture is typically treated by orthopedic support, analgesics, heat, and massage. Chronic back pain is treated by an orthopedic garment and exercises to strengthen the paravertebral muscles. Short-term androgen administration is used in women with severe, uncontrolled fractures. Men with osteoporosis also may be given exogenous androgens if there is an androgen deficiency.

CHINESE DISEASE CATEGORIZATION: The clinical symptoms of early symptomatic osteoporosis fall under the categories of *yao tong*, lumbar pain, and *bei tong*, upper back pain. Bone fractures are referred to as *gu zhe*. Bone pain is called *gu bi*, bone impediment.

DISEASE CAUSES: Former heaven natural endowment insufficiency, aging, unregulated eating and drinking, unregulated stirring and stillness (*i.e.*, too little weight-bearing exercise)

DISEASE MECHANISMS: The kidneys rule the bones and engender both the bones and marrow. When the kidneys are full, the marrow is replete and the bones are strong. The lumbus is the mansion of the kidneys, and the upper back is reached by the pathways of the kidneys. Therefore, osteoporosis is mainly due to vacuity decline of the kidneys, both yin and yang. Kidney yang vacuity typically evolves out of spleen qi vacuity, while liver blood-kidney yin vacuity is due to the aging process, habitual bodily vacuity, and enduring heat. For instance, alcohol damages the spleen and engenders damp heat, while cigarette-smoking damages the lungs and consumes yin fluids.

TREATMENT BASED ON PATTERN DISCRIMINATION:

1. SPLEEN-KIDNEY YANG VACUITY PATTERN

MAIN SYMPTOMS: Lower and upper back soreness and pain, fatigue, lassitude of the spirit, lack of strength, cold hands and feet, poor appetite, loose stools, a pale, enlarged tongue with thin, white fur, and a fine, weak, possibly slow pulse

TREATMENT PRINCIPLES: Fortify the spleen and boost the qi, supplement the kidneys and invigorate yang, strengthen the low back and bones

RX: *You Gui Yin Jia Wei* (Restore the Right [Kidney] Drink with Added Flavors)

INGREDIENTS: Cooked Radix Rehmanniae (*Shu Di*), 30g, Fructus Lycii Chinensis (*Gou Qi Zi*), 15g, Fructus Corni Officinalis (*Shan Zhu Yu*) and Radix Dioscoreae Oppositae (*Shan Yao*), 12g each, Radix Lateralis Praeparatus Aconiti Carmichaeli (*Fu Zi*), Cortex Eucommiae Ulmoidis (*Du Zhong*), Radix Dipsaci (*Xu Duan*), Fructus Psoraleae Corylifoliae (*Bu Gu Zhi*), and Rhizoma Atractylodis Macrocephalae (*Bai Zhu*), 9g each, and Radix Panacis Ginseng (*Ren Shen*), Cortex Cinnamomi Cassiae (*Rou Gui*), and mix-fried Radix Glycyrrhizae (*Gan Cao*), 6g each

ANALYSIS OF FORMULA: *Shu Di*, *Shan Yao*, and *Shan Zhu Yu* are the three supplementing medicinals of *Liu Wei Di Huang Wan* (Six Flavors Rehmannia Pills) which supplement and enrich the kidney yin. With *Gou Qi Zi*, they nourish yin to supplement yang based on the sayings, "Yin and yang are rooted in each other," and, "Yang is engendered from yin." *Bu Gu Zhi*, *Du Zhong*, *Xu Duan*, *Rou Gui*, and *Fu Zi* all warm and supplement kidney yang and all reinforce the low back. In addition, *Xu Duan* quickens the blood, strengthens the bones, and knits fractures. *Du Zhong* is the master medicinal for low back pain. *Bu Gu Zhi* strengthens the bones. *Fu Zi* warms the 14 channels and stops pain. *Ren Shen*, *Bai Zhu*, and mix-fried *Gan Cao* supplement latter heaven to support former heaven.

ADDITIONS & SUBTRACTIONS: If there is diarrhea, add nine grams of Semen Myristicae Fragrantis (*Rou Dou Kou*). If there is blood vacuity, add nine grams of Radix Angelicae Sinensis (*Dang Gui*). If there is pain in the lower back, add nine grams of Cortex Radicis Acanthopanacis (*Wu Jia Pi*). If there is pain in the mid back, add nine grams of Ramulus Loranthi Seu Visci (*Sang Ji Sheng*). If there is pain in the upper back, add nine grams of Radix Puerariae (*Ge Gen*). If the pain is accompanied by a cold sensation in the spine, add nine grams of Rhizoma Cibotii Barometsis (*Gou Ji*). If there is severe osteoporosis, add nine grams each of Rhizoma Drynariae (*Gu Sui Bu*) and Plastrum Testudinis (*Gui Ban*). For fixed, piercing, or severe pain due to blood stasis, add 12 grams of Radix Rubrus Paeoniae Lactiflorae (*Chi Shao*) and six grams each of Resina Olibani (*Ru Xiang*) and Resina Myrrhae (*Mo Yao*).

ACUPUNCTURE & MOXIBUSTION: *Fu Liu* (Ki 7), *Da Zhu* (Bl 11), *Xuan Zhong* (GB 39) plus a choice from the following local points depending on the location of pain: *Jia Ji* (M-BW-35), *a shi* points, *Da Zhui* (GV 14), *Ji Zhong* (GV 6), *Xuan Shu* (GV 5), *Ming Men* (GV 4), *Yao Yang Guan* (GV 3), *San Jiao Shu* (Bl 22), *Shen Shu* (Bl 23), *Qi Hai Shu* (Bl 24), *Da Chang Shu* (Bl 25), *Guan Yuan Shu* (Bl 26), *Yao Yan* (M-BW-24)

ANALYSIS OF FORMULA: The kidneys store the essence, the essence engenders the marrow, and the marrow nourishes the bones. Therefore, if the kidneys are effulgent, the essence is abundant, the marrow is prosperous, and hence the bones are firm. Conversely, in case of weakness of the bones, one should supplement the kidneys, boost the marrow, and strengthen the bones. Supplementing *Fu Liu* with moxibustion supplements both the yin and yang of the kidneys as well as the former heaven essence. Supplementing *Xuan Zhong*, the meeting point of the marrow, boosts the marrow. Supplementing *Da Zhu*, the meeting point of the bones, strengthens the bones. These three points are the key combination for bone troubles due to kidney vacuity when the spinal column is mainly affected. Supplementing and moxaing local points supplements vacuity and strengthen the low back and bones.

ADDITIONS & SUBTRACTIONS: For osteoporosis of the neck, please refer to the chapter on cervical vertebrae disease. For severe spleen vacuity, add *Zu San Li* (St 36). For low back pain with concomitant digestive troubles, add *Gong Sun* (Sp 4). For buttock pain, add *Zhi Bian* (Bl 54). For cold pain in the low back, buttocks, and lower limbs, moxa *Zhi Bian* (Bl 54), *Cheng Fu* (Bl 36), and *Cheng Shan* (Bl 57). For lumbosacral and coccygeal pain, add *Ci Liao* (Bl 32) and/or other *Ba Liao* points.

2. LIVER BLOOD-KIDNEY YIN VACUITY PATTERN

MAIN SYMPTOMS: Lower and upper back pain, knee and lower leg soreness and weakness, tinnitus, dizziness, insomnia, a pale facial complexion but possible malar flushing in the afternoon, a red tongue with scanty fur, and a fine, bowstring, rapid pulse

TREATMENT PRINCIPLES: Supplement the kidneys and nourish the liver, strengthen the low back and bones

RX: *Zuo Gui Yin Jia Wei* (Restore the Left [Kidney] Drink with Added Flavors)

INGREDIENTS: Cooked Radix Rehmanniae (*Shu Di*), 30g, Fructus Lycii Chinensis (*Gou Qi Zi*) and Ramulus Loranthi Seu Visci (*Sang Ji Sheng*), 15g each, Radix Dioscoreae Oppositae (*Shan Yao*), 12g, Sclerotium Poriae Cocos (*Fu Ling*), Fructus Corni Officinalis (*Shan Zhu Yu*), and Fructus Psoraleae Corylifoliae (*Bu Gu Zhi*), 9g each, and mix-fried Radix Glycyrrhizae (*Gan Cao*), 6g

ANALYSIS OF FORMULA: *Shu Di*, *Shan Yao*, and *Shan Zhu Yu* are the three supplementing medicinals of *Liu Wei Di Huang Wan* (Six Flavors Rehmannia Pills) which supplement the liver and kidneys and nourish and enrich yin essence. *Gou Qi Zi*, *Shan Zhu Yu*, and *Sang Ji Sheng* nourish liver blood. *Fu Ling*, *Shan Yao*, and mix-fried *Gan Cao* supplement the latter heaven to support the former heaven. If yin, blood, and essence are effulgent and the marrow is filled, then the bones are strong. Finally, *Bu Gu Zhi* warms the kidneys, strengthens the low back, and reinforces the bones, while *Sang Ji Sheng* is well-known for diffusing wind damp impediment as well as for reinforcing the spinal column.

ADDITIONS & SUBTRACTIONS: For osteoporosis of the neck, please refer to the chapter on cervical spondylosis. If there is heat in the lungs and stomach damaging yin fluids, add 12 grams of Tuber Ophiopogonis Japonici (*Mai Men Dong*) and nine grams of Herba Dendrobii (*Shi Hu*). If there is heat in the heart, add 15 grams of Radix Scrophulariae Ningpoensis (*Xuan Shen*). If there is heat in the spleen with rapid hungering after meals, add 15 grams of Radix Albus Paeoniae Lactiflorae (*Bai Shao*). If vacuity heat is marked, add nine grams each of Rhizoma Anemarrhena Aspheloidis (*Zhi Mu*) and Cortex Phellodendri (*Huang Bai*). If there is bleeding due to heat entering the blood division, add 15 grams of uncooked Radix Rehmanniae (*Sheng Di*) and Herba Ecliptae Prostratae (*Han Lian Cao*). If there is blood vacuity, add nine grams of Radix Angelicae Sinensis (*Dang Gui*). If there is severe osteoporosis, add nine grams each of Rhizoma Drynariae (*Gu Sui Bu*) and Plastrum Testudinis (*Gui Ban*). For fixed, piercing, or severe pain due to blood stasis, add 12 grams of Radix Rubrus Paeoniae Lactiflorae (*Chi Shao*) and six grams each of Resina Olibani (*Ru Xiang*) and Resina Myrrhae (*Mo Yao*).

ACUPUNCTURE & MOXIBUSTION: Please see pattern #1 above but without moxibustion.

ADDITIONS & SUBTRACTIONS: Please see pattern #1 above.

3. SPLEEN QI AND KIDNEY YIN & YANG VACUITY PATTERN

MAIN SYMPTOMS: Lower and upper back soreness and limpness, fatigue, lassitude of the spirit, lack of strength, malar flushing, cold lower half of the body, dizziness, tinnitus, nocturia, decreased sexual desire, poor appetite, loose stools, a fat, red tongue with scanty fur, and a surging pulse in the inch positions, a soggy pulse in the right bar, a fine, bowstring pulse in the left bar, and a deep or fine, floating pulse in one or both cubit positions

TREATMENT PRINCIPLES: Fortify the spleen and boost the qi, supplement both yin and yang, clear vacuity heat as necessary, strengthen the low back and bones

RX: *Bu Yin Tang* (Supplement Yin Decoction)

INGREDIENTS: Cooked Radix Rehmanniae (*Shu Di*) and uncooked Radix Rehmanniae (*Sheng Di*), 15g each, Radix Achyranthis Bidentatae (*Niu Xi*) and Fructus Psoraleae Corylifoliae (*Bu Gu Zhi*), 12g each, Radix Angelicae Sinensis (*Dang Gui*), Radix Albus Paeoniae Lactiflorae (*Bai Shao*), Rhizoma Anemarrhenae Aspheloidis (*Zhi Mu*), Cortex Phellodendri (*Huang Bai*), Cortex Eucommiae Ulmoidis (*Du Zhong*), and Sclerotium Poriae Cocos (*Fu Ling*), 9g each, and Fructus Foeniculi Vulgaris (*Xiao Hui Xiang*), Pericarpium Citri Reticulatae (*Chen Pi*), Radix Panacis

Ginseng (*Ren Shen*), and mix-fried Radix Glycyrrhizae (*Gan Cao*), 6g each

ANALYSIS OF FORMULA: *Shu Di, Sheng Di, Niu Xi, Dang Gui,* and *Bai Shao* nourish both liver blood and kidney yin and so strengthen the sinews and reinforce the bones. *Bu Gu Zhi* and *Du Zhong* warm and supplement kidney yang, strengthen the low back and reinforce the bones. *Zhi Mu* and *Huang Bai* clear vacuity heat and downbear ministerial fire. In addition, *Huang Bai* clears and eliminates dampness and heat in the lower burner, while *Zhi Mu* nourishes yin. *Fu Ling, Ren Shen,* and mix-fried *Gan Cao* supplement the center and boost the qi to support the former heaven. *Chen Pi* and *Xiao Hui Xiang* move the qi and help the qi transformation.

ADDITIONS & SUBTRACTIONS: For osteoporosis of the neck, please refer to the chapter on cervical spondylosis. If there is severe osteoporosis, add nine grams each of Rhizoma Drynariae (*Gu Sui Bu*) and Plastrum Testudinis (*Gui Ban*). If there is fixed, piercing, or severe pain due to blood stasis, add 12 grams of Radix Rubrus Paeoniae Lactiflorae (*Chi Shao*) and six grams each of Resina Olibani (*Ru Xiang*) and Resina Myrrhae (*Mo Yao*). If there is pain in the lower back, add nine grams of Cortex Radicis Acanthopanacis Gracilistylis (*Wu Jia Pi*). If there is pain in the mid back, add nine grams of Ramulus Loranthi Seu Visci (*Sang Ji Sheng*). If there is pain in the upper back, add nine grams of Radix Puerariae (*Ge Gen*).

ACUPUNCTURE & MOXIBUSTION: Please see pattern #1 above plus *San Yin Jiao* (Sp 6).

ANALYSIS OF FORMULA: *San Yin Jiao* is the intersection point of the three foot yin of the spleen, liver, and kidneys. Supplementing it supplements the qi, blood, and essence.

ADDITIONS & SUBTRACTIONS: Please see pattern #1 above.

4. QI STAGNATION & BLOOD STASIS PATTERN

MAIN SYMPTOMS: Enduring bodily pain which may be fixed in location or severe in intensity, a dark, sooty facial complexion, age spots, varicosities, cherry hemagiomas, and spider nevi, purple tongue and lips, possible static macules or spots on the tongue, and a bowstring, choppy pulse

NOTE: This disease mechanism does not typically cause osteoporosis all by itself. However, most patients with osteoporosis will have elements in their overall pattern discrimination of both qi stagnation and blood stasis. This is based on the statements, "If there is pain, there is no free flow," and, "Enduring diseases enter the network vessels," this latter statement implying that enduring diseases are typically complicated by blood stasis.

TREATMENT PRINCIPLES: Quicken the blood, free the flow of the network vessels, and stop pain

RX: *Shen Tong Zhu Yu Tang* (Body Pain Dispel Stasis Decoction)

INGREDIENTS: Semen Pruni Persicae (*Tao Ren*), Flos Carthami Tinctorii (*Hong Hua*), Radix Angelicae Sinensis (*Dang Gui*), and Radix Cyathulae (*Chuan Niu Xi*), 9g each, Radix Ligustici Wallichii (*Chuan Xiong*), Radix Glycyrrhizae (*Gan Cao*), Resina Myrrhae (*Mo Yao*), Feces Trogopterori Seu Pteromi (*Wu Ling Zhi*), and Lumbricus (*Di Long*), 6g each, and Radix Gentianae Macrophyllae (*Qin Jiao*), Radix Et Rhizoma Notopterygii (*Qiang Huo*), and Rhizoma Cyperi Rotundi (*Xiang Fu*), 3g each

ANALYSIS OF FORMULA: *Tao Ren, Hong Hua, Dang Gui, Chuan Xiong, Mo Yao, Wu Ling Zhi,* and *Chuan Niu Xi* quicken the blood, dispel stasis, and stop pain. *Xiang Fu* moves the qi to quicken the blood. *Qiang Huo, Chuan Xiong,* and *Qin Jiao* diffuse and eliminate wind damp impediment and stop pain. *Di Long* quickens the network vessels to stop pain, and *Gan Cao* harmonizes the other medicinals in this formula.

ADDITIONS & SUBTRACTIONS: For osteoporosis of the neck, please refer to the chapter on cervical spondylosis. If there is severe blood stasis with stubborn pain, add six grams of Eupolyphaga Seu Opisthoplatia (*Tu Bie Chong*) and three grams each of Scolopendra Subspinipes (*Wu Gong*) and Buthus Martensis (*Quan Xie*). If there is qi stagnation and blood stasis due to wind damp impediment, add nine grams each of Radix Angelicae Pubescentis (*Du Huo*), Radix Clematidis Chinensis (*Wei Ling Xian*), and Rhizoma Atractylodis (*Cang Zhu*). If there has been traumatic injury to the low back, add three grams of Radix Pseudoginseng (*San Qi*), powdered and swallowed with the decoction, plus nine grams each of Resina Olibani (*Ru Xiang*) and Lignum Sappan (*Su Mu*). If there is concomitant spleen vacuity, add 15 grams of Radix Astragali Membranacei (*Huang Qi*) and nine grams each of Rhizoma Atractylodis Macrocephalae (*Bai Zhu*) and Sclerotium Poriae Cocos (*Fu Ling*). If there is concomitant kidney yin vacuity, add nine grams each of Ramulus Loranthi Seu Visci (*Sang Ji Sheng*) and Plastrum Testudinis (*Gui Ban*) and replace *Chuan Niu Xi* with Radix Achyranthis Bidentatae (*Niu Xi*). If there is concomitant kidney yang vacuity, add nine grams each of Cortex Radicis Acanthopanacis Gracilistylis (*Wu Jia Pi*), Herba Epimedii (*Yin Yang Huo*), and Radix Dipsaci (*Xu Duan*). If there is severe osteoporosis, add nine grams each of Rhizoma Drynariae (*Gu Sui Bu*), Radix Dipsaci (*Xu Duan*), and Plastrum Testudinis (*Gui Ban*).

ACUPUNCTURE & MOXIBUSTION: *Shui Gou* (GV 26), *Hou Xi* (SI 3) plus local points chosen based on the site of pain and selected from: *Jia Ji* (M-BW-35), *a shi* points, *Da Zhui* (GV 14), *Ji Zhong* (GV 6), *Xuan Shu* (GV 5), *Ming Men* (GV 4), *Yao Yang Guan* (GV 3), *San Jiao Shu* (Bl 22), *Shen Shu* (Bl 23), *Qi Hai Shu* (Bl 24), *Da Chang Shu* (Bl 25), *Guan Yuan Shu* (Bl 26), *Yao Yan* (M-BW-24)

NOTE: Needle the *a shi* points moderately with even supplementing-even draining technique for 20 minutes and then withdraw the needles. Next, needle *Shui Gou* and *Hou Xi* with draining method and ask the patient to do some movement for five minutes or so, such as turning, bending, and stretching, until the pain is relieved. Alternate needle stimulation and mobilization three times. If three successive treatments fail to achieve an effect, add *San Yin Jiao* (Sp 6) and *He Gu* (LI 4), while subtracting *Shui Gou* and *Hou Xi*.

ANALYSIS OF FORMULA: All the local points as well as *Shui Gou* and *Hou Xi* free the flow of the governing vessels and foot tai yang bladder channel to transform stasis and stop pain.

ADDITIONS & SUBTRACTIONS: Please see pattern #1 above.

REMARKS

1. Most patients with osteoporosis do not have discrete spleen-kidney or liver-kidney patterns. Rather, they tend to have spleen, liver, and kidney vacuities, with the kidney vacuity being a yin and yang dual vacuity. In this case, the choice of guiding formula is based on the relative proportions between yin and yang vacuities.

2. Avoidance of sugars and sweets as well as minimization or avoidance of caffeine, tobacco, and alcohol are important in order to get a good effect on this condition with Chinese medicine. In addition, increases in weight-bearing exercise and stretching are important adjuncts to successful treatment.

3. The best form of supplemental dietary calcium in order to increase bone density is that made out of bone matrix as opposed to that made from fossilized sea shells, *i.e.*, dolomite. Excessive intake of calcium carbonate may damage the spleen, and most patients with senile osteoporosis do have at least some spleen qi vacuity. This latter assumption is based on the saying, "In the elderly, blame the spleen."

4. While modifications of *Er Xian Tang* (Two Immortals Decoction) are the most commonly prescribed formulas for the treatment of menopausal syndrome, because of the presence of toxins in Rhizoma Curculiginis Orchioidis (*Xian Mao*), the ingredients in that formula are not appropriate for long-term administration. Since the treatment of senile osteoporosis requires such long-term administration, we prefer Gong Ding-xian's safer and more balanced formula, *Bu Yin Tang*, for treating a dual yin and yang vacuity. In addition, this latter formula also does address spleen qi vacuity and liver depression as well as an element of blood stasis.

The ingredients in *Bu Yin Tang* are: Radix Angelicae Sinensis (*Dang Gui*) and Sclerotium Poriae Cocos (*Fu Ling*), 15g each, cooked and uncooked Radix Rehmanniae (*Sheng Shu Di*), 12g each, Radix Panacis Ginseng (*Ren Shen*), Radix Achyranthis Bidentatae (*Niu Xi*), Radix Albus Paeoniae Lactiflorae (*Bai Shao*), Fructus Psoraleae Corylifoliae (*Bu Gu Zhi*), Cortex Eucommiae Ulmoidis (*Du Zhong*), Pericarpium Citri Reticulatae (*Chen Pi*), Rhizoma Anemarrhenae Aspheloidis (*Zhi Mu*), and Cortex Phellodendri (*Huang Bai*), 9g each, and Fructus Foeniculi Vulgaris (*Xiao Hui Xiang*) and Radix Glycyrrhizae (*Gan Cao*), 6g each.

5. Chinese and Japanese research has shown that Chinese medicinals are effective in preventing and reversing osteoporosis.[1]

ENDNOTES

[1] Shen Lin *et al.*, "Experiences in the Treatment of 52 Cases of Senile Osteoporosis with *Qing E Wan Jia Wei* (Young Pretty Girl Pills with Added Flavors), *Hu Bei Zhong Yi Za Zhi* (Hubei Journal of Chinese Medicine), #3, 1994, p. 16-18

51

Parkinson's Disease

Parkinson's disease (PD) is an idiopathic, slowly progressive, degenerative disorder of the central nervous system characterized by four main features: 1) slowness and poverty of movement, 2) muscular rigidity, 3) resting tremor, and 4) postural instability. The first symptom of this disease in 50-80% of patients is a resting "pill-rolling" tremor of one hand. This tremor is most pronounced during rest and diminishes during movement. It is absent during sleep. The hands, arms, and legs are usually the most affected body parts in that order. Jaw, tongue, forehead, and eyelids may also be involved. Another early sign is a severe decrease in eye-blinking. Many patients only exhibit rigidity and never manifest tremor. Rigidity and hypokinesia may contribute to muscular aches and a subjective sensation of fatigue. Eventually the face becomes mask-like and open-mouthed, while the posture becomes stooped. Dementia occurs in approximately 50% of patients, and depression is common. Onset generally occurs after age 40 with increasing incidence with age. In the United States, 50,000 new cases of Parkinson's disease are diagnosed in the geriatric population per year. This is a rate of one in 200 of the elderly. Men are more susceptible than women. Pathophysiologically, this condition is due to loss of pigmented neurons of the substantia nigra, locus ceruleus, and other brain stem cell groups.

The Western medical diagnosis of Parkinson's disease is based on the clinical symptoms. Early clues include infrequent blinking, lack of facial expression, poverty of movement, impaired postural reflexes, and a characteristic gait abnormality. Western medical treatment consists of internal administration of levodopa. While on this medication, mildly affected patients may return to nearly normal, while bedridden patients may become ambulatory. Unfortunately, more than 50% of patients begin to experience fluctuations in their response to levodopa after 2-5 years. Other medications may also be used, such as amantadine and bromocriptine. However, none are entirely effective and all have a high incidence of side effects. Tricyclic antidepressants are also sometimes used in low doses at night as sedatives and to treat depression. If left untreated, this disease progresses over 15 years to severe incapacitation.

Although the cause of this disease is currently unknown, a deficiency of dopamine in the brain may be due to underlying nutritional deficiencies, cerebral vascular disease resulting in blockage of the blood vessels in the brain, the side effects of natipsychotic drugs, carbon monoxide poisoning, abuse of certain so-called designer drugs, and a rare form of infectious encephalitis called encephalitis lethargica.

Chinese disease categorization: Parkinson's disease is mainly categorized as *zhen chan*, tremors, *ma mu*, numbness, and *si zhi ruan ruo*, limpness and weakness of the four limbs. This last condition is considered a species of *wei zheng* or wilting condition.

Disease causes: Former heaven natural endowment insufficiency, aging, enduring disease, taxation fatigue, internal damage by the seven affects, and faulty diet

Disease mechanisms: The main disease mechanism of Parkinson's disease is aging resulting in consumption and damage of liver blood and kidney yin. Thus the blood fails to nourish and construct the sinews and vessels, and spasms and contractures, and stiffness and rigidity occur. If yin vacuity leads to yang hyperactivity, this may cause liver wind to stir internally. Especially if wind mixes with phlegm and dampness, these may congest and obstruct the channels and network vessels resulting in tremors and shaking.

It is also possible for unfulfilled desires and anger and frustration to damage the liver. The liver loses its control over coursing and discharge and the qi becomes stagnant. Because the qi moves the blood, over time, the blood may thus become static. On the one hand, static blood blocks the flow of nourishment to the sinew vessels. On the other, it inhibits the engenderment of new or fresh blood. Thus for both these two reasons, blood stasis may result in malnourishment of the sinew vessels with consequent spasms and contractures, stiffness and rigidity.

Due to a combination of faulty diet, aging, worry and anxiety, and taxation fatigue, spleen vacuity may reach the kidneys, thus resulting in kidney yang vacuity. In that case, spleen and kidney vacuity and debility cannot move and transform fluids in the body. Instead, these collect and transform first into dampness and subsequently congeal into phlegm. Phlegm dampness may then obstruct the network vessels, therefore depriving the sinew vessels of nourishment and moistening and causing numbness and blockage. If phlegm becomes mixed with depressive heat or fire, it may also stir wind, leading to tremors and shaking.

TREATMENT BASED ON PATTERN DISCRIMINATION:

1. LIVER YIN INSUFFICIENCY, VACUITY WIND INTERNALLY STIRRING PATTERN

MAIN SYMPTOMS: Muscular stiffness, hand and foot or lower jaw trembling, aching, pain, and numbness of the four limbs which is worse after rest and better after movement, instability walking, blurred vision, spiritless eyes or dark circles under the eyes, possible difficulty swallowing, constipation, a red, possibly quivering tongue with scanty fur, and a bowstring, fine pulse

TREATMENT PRINCIPLES: Enrich and supplement the liver and kidneys, nourish yin and extinguish wind

RX: *Yi Guan Jian* (One Link Decoction) & *Ling Yan Gou Teng Tang* (Antelope Horn & Uncaria Decoction) with additions and subtractions

INGREDIENTS: Ramulus Loranthi Seu Visci (*Sang Ji Sheng*) and Concha Ostreae (*Mu Li*), 20g each, cooked Radix Rehmanniae (*Shu Di*), uncooked Radix Rehmanniae (*Sheng Di*), Radix Albus Paeoniae Lactiflorae (*Bai Shao*), and Concha Haliotidis (*Shi Jue Ming*), 15g each, Fructus Corni Officinalis (*Shan Zhu Yu*), Bombyx Batryticatus (*Jiang Can*), Rhizoma Gastrodiae Elatae (*Tian Ma*), Radix Achyranthis Bidentatae (*Niu Xi*), and Radix Angelicae Sinensis (*Dang Gui*), 9g each, and Radix Glycyrrhizae (*Gan Cao*), 6g

ANALYSIS OF FORMULA: *Sang Ji Sheng, Shu Di, Sheng Di, Bai Shao, Shan Zhu Yu, Niu Xi,* and *Dang Gui* nourish liver blood and enrich kidney yin. *Mu Li, Shi Jue Ming, Jiang Can, Tian Ma,* and *Niu Xi* level the liver and subdue yang, extinguish wind and settle tremors. *Gan Cao* harmonizes the other medicinals in this formula.

ADDITIONS & SUBTRACTIONS: If there is concomitant qi vacuity with slow, difficult movement, lassitude of the spirit, and fatigue, add 15 grams of Radix Astragali Membranacei (*Huang Qi*) and nine grams each of Radix Panacis Ginseng (*Ren Shen*) and Radix Dioscoreae Oppositae (*Shan Yao*). If there is simultaneous liver depression, add 12 grams of Fructus Meliae Toosendan (*Chuan Lian Zi*). If there is simultaneous blood stasis, add nine grams each of Semen Pruni Persicae (*Tao Ren*) and Radix Salviae Miltiorrhizae (*Dan Shen*). For headache and dizziness, add nine grams each of Ramulus Uncariae Cum Uncis (*Gou Teng*) and Flos Chrysanthemi Morifolii (*Ju Hua*). For dry, rough eyes, photophobia, and blurred vision, add 20 grams of Fructus Lycii Chinensis (*Gou Qi*) and nine grams each of Fructus Ligustri Lucidi (*Nu Zhen Zi*) and Semen Cassiae Torae (*Jue Ming Zi*). For numbness, add 20 grams of Caulis Milletiae Seu Spatholobi (*Ji Xue Teng*) and nine grams of Fasciculus Vascularis Luffae Cylindricae (*Si Gua Luo*). For easy anger and irritability due to depressive heat, add nine grams each of Radix Scutellariae Baicalensis (*Huang Qin*) and Fructus Gardeniae Jasminoidis (*Zhi Zi*). For profuse urination due to kidney qi vacuity, add 15 grams each of Fructus Rosae Laevigatae (*Jin Ying Zi*), Fructus Rubi Chingii (*Fu Pen Zi*), and Semen Nelumbinis Nuciferae (*Lian Zi*). For concomitant kidney yang vacuity, add nine grams each of Herba Epimedii (*Yin Yang Huo*) and Semen Cuscutae Chinensis (*Tu Si Zi*) and one gram of Cortex Cinnamomi Cassiae (*Rou Gui*), powdered and taken with the strained decoction. For dry mouth and thirst, add 15 grams of Radix Trichosanthis Kirlowii (*Tian Hua Fen*) and nine grams of Tuber Ophiopogonis Japonici (*Mai Men Dong*).

ACUPUNCTURE & MOXIBUSTION: *Tai Xi* (Ki 3), *San Yin Jiao* (Sp 6), *Tai Chong* (Liv 3), *He Gu* (LI 4)

ANALYSIS OF FORMULA: Supplementing *Tai Xi* and *San Yin Jiao* nourishes liver blood and enriches kidney yin, while draining *Tai Chong* and *He Gu*, the four gates or bars, levels the liver and subdues yang, extinguishes wind and settles tremors.

ADDITIONS & SUBTRACTIONS: For muscular stiffness, add *Da Zhui* (GV 14) and *Yang Ling Quan* (GB 34). For severe trembling, add *Feng Chi* (GB 20). For numbness of the four limbs, add *Wai Guan* (TB 5) and *Cheng Shan* (Bl 57). For instability walking, add *Shen Mai* (Bl 62) and *Zhao Hai* (Ki 6). For spiritless eyes, impaired memory, and mental slowness, add *Si Shen Cong* (M-HN-1). For blurred vision, add *Guang Ming* (GB 37). For difficulty swallowing, add *Liang Quan* (CV 23). For constipation, add *Zhi Gou* (TB 6). For headache, add *Tai Yang* (M-HN-9) and *Tong Tian* (Bl 7).

For dizziness, add *Bai Hui* (GV 20) and *Feng Chi* (GB 20). For tinnitus, add *Ting Hui* (GB 2). For insomnia, profuse dreams, and restlessness, add *Da Ling* (Per 7). For concomitant qi vacuity, add *Zu San Li* (St 36). For concomitant liver depression, add *Nei Guan* (Per 6). For concomitant kidney yang vacuity, add *Guan Yuan* (CV 4). For easy anger and irritability due to depressive heat, add *Yang Ling Quan* (GB 34) and *Zhi Gou* (TB 6). For profuse urination, add *Zhi Shi* (Bl 52).

2. LIVER QI DEPRESSION & BINDING, QI STAGNATION & BLOOD STASIS PATTERN

MAIN SYMPTOMS: Head, lower jaw, hand and foot shaking, especially at rest and at night, inhibited bending and stretching, fixed pain and numbness in the body and/or limbs, irritability, a purplish, dark tongue or possible static macules or spots, and a fine, bowstring, choppy pulse

NOTE: Static blood may also complicate liver-kidney yin vacuity, spleen-kidney yang vacuity, and phlegm fire patterns.

TREATMENT PRINCIPLES: Settle the liver and extinguish wind, quicken the blood and free the flow of the network vessels

RX: *Zhen Gan Xi Feng Tang* (Settle the Liver & Extinguish Wind Decoction) & *Tong Qiao Huo Xue Tang* (Free the Flow of the Orifices & Quicken the Blood Decoction) with additions and subtractions

INGREDIENTS: Ramulus Loranthi Seu Visci (*Sang Ji Sheng*), 20g, Radix Salviae Miltiorrhizae (*Dan Shen*), uncooked Haemititum (*Dai Zhe Shi*), Concha Haliotidis (*Shi Jue Ming*), and Radix Albus Paeoniae Lactiflorae (*Bai Shao*), 15g each, Fructus Meliae Toosendan (*Chuan Lian Zi*) and Rhizoma Cyperi Rotundi (*Xiang Fu*), 12g each, Rhizoma Gastrodiae Elatae (*Tian Ma*), Ramulus Uncariae Cum Uncis (*Gou Teng*), Radix Achyranthis Bidentatae (*Niu Xi*), Radix Angelicae Sinensis (*Dang Gui*), Semen Pruni Persicae (*Tao Ren*), Flos Carthami Tinctorii (*Hong Hua*), Tuber Curcumae (*Yu Jin*), and Rhizoma Acori Graminei (*Shi Chang Pu*), 9g each, and Resina Olibani (*Ru Xiang*), Resina Myrrhae (*Mo Yao*), and Radix Glycyrrhizae (*Gan Cao*), 6g each

ANALYSIS OF FORMULA: *Bai Shao, Chuan Lian Zi, Xiang Fu,* and *Yu Jin* course the liver, rectify the qi, and resolve depression. *Dai Zhe Shi, Shi Jue Ming, Tian Ma, Gou Teng,* and *Niu Xi* level the liver and subdue yang, extinguish wind and settle tremors. *Dan Shen, Dang Gui, Tao Ren, Hong Hua, Yu Jin, Ru Xiang,* and *Mo Yao* quicken the blood and free the flow of the network vessels. *Sang Ji Sheng, Dang Gui,* and *Niu Xi* nourish liver blood and enrich kidney yin to check yang. *Shi Chang Pu* transforms phlegm and opens the orifices, and *Gan Cao* harmonizes the other medicinals in this formula.

ADDITIONS & SUBTRACTIONS: For liver depression transforming heat with restlessness, dryness and bitterness in the mouth, easy anger, constipation with dry bound stools, scanty, reddish urine, and yellow tongue fur, add 15 grams of Cortex Radicis Moutan (*Dan Pi*) and nine grams each of Fructus Gardeniae Jasminoidis (*Zhi Zi*) and Radix Scutellariae Baicalensis (*Huang Qin*). For concomitant blood vacuity, add nine grams of Gelatinum Corii Asini (*E Jiao*) and increase the dosage of *Bai Shao* up to 30 grams. For liver-spleen disharmony with borborygmus and/or painful diarrhea, add 20 grams each of Rhizoma Atractylodis Macrocephalae (*Bai Zhu*) and Sclerotium Poriae Cocos (*Fu Ling*). For liver-stomach disharmony with nausea and vomiting, add nine grams each of uncooked Rhizoma Zingiberis (*Sheng Jiang*), Rhizoma Pinelliae Ternatae (*Ban Xia*), and Flos Inulae Racemosae (*Xuan Fu Hua*). For severe fixed pain, add 15 grams each of Radix Salviae Miltiorrhizae (*Dan Shen*) and Caulis Milletiae Seu Spatholobi (*Ji Xue Teng*). For twitching sinews and flesh or severe tremors, add 12 grams of Fructus Tribuli Terrestris (*Bai Ji Li*) and three grams each of Buthus Martensis (*Quan Xie*) and Scolopendra Subspinipes (*Wu Gong*), powdered and taken with the strained decoction, and increase the dosage of *Bai Shao* up to 30 grams. For inhibited bending and stretching, add 15 grams each of Lumbricus (*Di Long*) and Radix Puerariae (*Ge Gen*) and two grams of Agkistrodon Seu Bungarus (*Bai Hua She*), powdered and taken with the strained decoction. For pain and numbness in the upper limbs, add nine grams of Rhizoma Curcumae Longae (*Jiang Huang*). For pain and numbness in the lower limbs, add nine grams of Fructus Chaenomelis Lagenariae (*Mu Gua*). For generalized joint pain, add 12 grams of Radix Clematidis Chinensis (*Wei Ling Xian*).

For qi stagnation and phlegm binding with trembling of the four limbs which does not get better with movement, clumsy movement, stiffness of both hands, ataxia, difficult or impossible writing, headache, insomnia, inhibited throat, chest and rib-side bitterness and fullness, slimy tongue fur, and a slippery, bowstring pulse, replace *Zhen Gan Xi Feng Tang* and *Tong Qiao Huo Xue Tang* with *Ban Xia Hou Po Tang Jia Jian* (Pinellia & Magnolia Decoction with Additions & Subtractions): Rhizoma Pinelliae Ternatae (*Ban Xia*), Cortex Magnoliae Officinalis (*Hou Po*), Sclerotium Poriae Cocos (*Fu Ling*), Radix Bupleuri (*Chai Hu*), Radix Albus Paeoniae Lactiflorae (*Bai Shao*), Fructus Citri Aurantii (*Zhi Ke*), Radix Ligustici Wallichii (*Chuan Xiong*), Rhizoma Atractylodis Macrocephalae (*Bai Zhu*), Bombyx Batryticatus (*Jiang Can*), bile-processed Rhizoma Arisaematis (*Dan Nan Xing*), and Periostracum Cicadae (*Chan Tui*), 9g each, and Radix Glycyrrhizae (*Gan Cao*), 5g.

ACUPUNCTURE & MOXIBUSTION: *Tai Chong* (Liv 3), *He Gu* (LI 4), *Yang Ling Quan* (GB 34), *San Yin Jiao* (Sp 6)

ANALYSIS OF FORMULA: Draining *Tai Chong* and *He Gu*, the four gates or bars, courses the liver and resolves depression, extinguishes wind and settles tremors. *Yang Ling Quan*, the meeting point of the sinews, courses the liver and settles tremor, while *San Yin Jiao* quickens the blood and transforms stasis.

ADDITIONS & SUBTRACTIONS: For concomitant blood vacuity, add *Ge Shu* (Bl 17) and *Pi Shu* (Bl 20). For liver-spleen disharmony, add *Zu San Li* (St 36). For liver-stomach disharmony, add *Zhong Wan* (CV 12). For concomitant kidney yang vacuity, add *Guan Yuan* (CV 4). For concomitant liver-kidney yin vacuity, add *Gan Shu* (Bl 18) and *Shen Shu* (Bl 23). For twitching sinews and flesh or severe trembling, add *Feng Chi* (GB 20) and *Da Zhui* (GV 14). For inhibited bending and stretching, add *Da Zhui* (GV 14), *Shui Gou* (GV 26), and *Cheng Jiang* (CV 24). For pain and numbness in the upper limbs, add *Wai Guan* (TB 5). For pain and numbness in the lower limbs, add *Cheng Shan* (Bl 57). For generalized joint pain, add *Qu Chi* (LI 11), *Yin Ling Quan* (Sp 9), and *a shi* points. For instability walking, add *Shen Mai* (Bl 62) and *Zhao Hai* (Ki 6). For headache, add *Tai Yang* (M-HN-9) and *Tong Tian* (Bl 7). For dizziness, add *Bai Hui* (GV 20) and *Feng Chi* (GB 20). For easy anger and irritability, add *Hun Men* (Bl 47).

3. QI & BLOOD DUAL VACUITY, SINEW VESSEL LOSS OF NOURISHMENT, VESSEL & NETWORK VESSELS STASIS & OBSTRUCTION PATTERN

MAIN SYMPTOMS: A somber white facial complexion, fatigue, lassitude of the spirit, lack of strength, fear of cold, disinclination to speak, spasms and contractures of the extremities, trembling of the limbs and stiffness of the neck and back, difficulty moving, spontaneous cool perspiration, dizziness, a tendency to loose stools, possible edema, a fat, pale tongue with thin fur and possible static spots, and a deep, fine pulse

TREATMENT PRINCIPLES: Supplement the qi and nourish the blood, extinguish wind and free the flow of the network vessels

RX: *Gui Pi Tang* (Restore the Spleen Decoction), *Bu Yang Huan Wu Tang* (Supplement Yang & Restore the Five [Viscera] Decoction) & *Tian Ma Gou Teng Yin* (Gastrodia & Uncaria Drink) with additions and subtractions

INGREDIENTS: Radix Salviae Miltiorrhizae (*Dan Shen*), Sclerotium Poriae Cocos (*Fu Ling*), and Radix Astragali Membranacei (*Huang Qi*), 20g each, cooked Radix Rehmanniae (*Shu Di*), Radix Albus Paeoniae Lactiflorae (*Bai Shao*), and Fructus Schisandrae Chinensis (*Wu Wei Zi*), 15g each, Ramulus Uncariae Cum Uncis (*Gou Teng*), 12g, and Radix Panacis Ginseng (*Ren Shen*), Rhizoma Atractylodis Macrocephalae (*Bai Zhu*), Rhizoma Gastrodiae Elatae (*Tian Ma*), Radix Ligustici Wallichii (*Chuan Xiong*), Lumbricus (*Di Long*), and Buthus Martensis (*Quan Xie*), 9g each

ANALYSIS OF FORMULA: *Huang Qi*, *Fu Ling*, *Ren Shen*, and *Bai Zhu* fortify the spleen and boost the qi. *Wu Wei Zi* supplements heart, lungs, and kidneys and stops both diarrhea and perspiration. *Shu Di* and *Bai Shao* nourish the blood. *Dan Shen*, *Chuan Xiong*, and *Di Long* quicken the blood and free the flow of the network vessels. *Bai Shao*, *Gou Teng*, *Tian Ma*, *Di Long*, and *Quan Xie* together level the liver and subdue yang, extinguish wind and settle tremors.

ADDITIONS & SUBTRACTIONS: For spleen yang vacuity, add six grams each of Radix Lateralis Praeparatus Aconiti Carmichaeli (*Fu Zi*) and dry Rhizoma Zingiberis (*Gan Jiang*). For concomitant kidney yang vacuity, add 15 grams of Fructus Psoraleae Corylifoliae (*Bu Gu Zhi*), nine grams of Semen Myristicae Fragrantis (*Rou Dou Kou*), and three grams of Fructus Evodiae Rutecarpae (*Wu Zhu Yu*). For more severe blood vacuity, add 15 grams of Caulis Milletiae Seu Spatholobi (*Ji Xue Teng*) and nine grams of Radix Angelicae Sinensis (*Dang Gui*). For concomitant blood stasis, add 15 grams each of Radix Salviae Miltiorrhizae (*Dan Shen*) and Caulis Milletiae Seu Spatholobi (*Ji Xue Teng*). For severe fatigue and lack of strength, increase the dosage of *Huang Qi* up to 30-50 grams. For edema, add nine grams each of Sclerotium Polypori Umbellati (*Zhu Ling*), Rhizoma Alismatis (*Ze Xie*), and Ramulus Cinnamomi Cassiae (*Gui Zhi*). For twitching sinews and flesh or severe tremors, add 12 grams each of Fructus Tribuli Terrestris (*Bai Ji Li*) and Periostracum Cicadae (*Chan Tui*). For inhibited bending and stretching, add 20 grams of Radix Puerariae (*Ge Gen*) and two grams of Agkistrodon Seu Bungarus (*Bai Hua She*), powdered and taken with the strained decoction. For pain and numbness in the upper limbs, add nine grams of Rhizoma Curcumae Longae (*Jiang Huang*). For pain and numbness in the lower limbs, add nine grams of Fructus Chaenomelis Lagenariae (*Mu Gua*).

ACUPUNCTURE & MOXIBUSTION: *Ge Shu* (Bl 17), *Gan Shu* (Bl 18), *Pi Shu* (Bl 20), *Wei Shu* (Bl 21), *Tai Chong* (Liv 3), *He Gu* (LI 4)

ANALYSIS OF FORMULA: Supplementing *Ge Shu* and *Gan Shu* nourishes liver blood. Supplementing *Pi Shu* and *Wei Shu* fortifies the spleen and boosts the qi. Draining *Tai Chong* and *He Gu*, the four gates or bars, levels the liver and extinguishes wind, frees the flow of the network vessels and settles tremors.

ADDITIONS & SUBTRACTIONS: For spleen yang vacuity,

moxa *Guan Yuan* (CV 4) as well as *Pi Shu* and *Wei Shu*. For concomitant kidney yang vacuity, add *Shen Shu* (Bl 23) and *Ming Men* (GV 4). For more severe blood vacuity, add *Xin Shu* (Bl 15). For concomitant blood stasis, add *San Yin Jiao* (Sp 6). For severe fatigue and lack of strength, add *Zu San Li* (St 36). For edema, add *Yin Ling Quan* (Sp 9) and *Shui Fen* (CV 9). For twitching sinews and flesh or severe tremors, add *Feng Chi* (GB 20) and *Yang Ling Quan* (GB 34). For inhibited bending and stretching, add *Da Zhui* (GV 14), *Shui Gou* (GV 26), and *Cheng Jiang* (CV 24). For pain and numbness in the upper limbs, add *Wai Guan* (TB 5). For pain and numbness in the lower limbs, add *Cheng Shan* (Bl 57). For instability walking, add *Shen Mai* (Bl 62) and *Zhao Hai* (Ki 6).

4. SPLEEN VACUITY WITH DAMP HEAVINESS, PHLEGM FIRE STIRRING WIND PATTERN

MAIN SYMPTOMS: Heavy-headedness, fear of cold, chilled limbs, vexatious heat in the five hearts, reduced food intake, loose stools, inhibited movement of the hands and feet or restless shaking, a fat tongue with red tip and slimy, white fur, and a bowstring, slippery pulse

NOTE: In this pattern, spleen vacuity with damp heaviness is the main thing, and phlegm fire stirring wind is secondary. That is why the signs and symptoms are relatively minor.

TREATMENT PRINCIPLES: Extinguish wind and subdue yang, transform phlegm and disinhibit dampness, free the flow of the channels and quicken the network vessels

RX: *Tian Ma Gou Teng Yin Jia Jian* (Gastrodia & Uncaria Drink with Additions & Subtractions)

INGREDIENTS: Ramulus Loranthi Seu Visci (*Sang Ji Sheng*), 20g, Concha Haliotidis (*Shi Jue Ming*) and Sclerotium Poriae Cocos, 15g each, Rhizoma Pinelliae Ternatae (*Ban Xia*), bile-processed Rhizoma Arisaematis (*Dan Nan Xing*), Fructus Immaturus Citri Aurantii (*Zhi Shi*), Pericarpium Citri Reticulatae (*Chen Pi*), Rhizoma Gastrodiae Elatae (*Tian Ma*), Ramulus Uncariae Cum Uncis (*Gou Teng*), Radix Achyranthis Bidentatae (*Niu Xi*), Radix Scutellariae Baicalensis (*Huang Qin*), and Bombyx Batryticatus (*Jiang Can*), Succus Bambusae (*Zhu Li*), 9g each, and Radix Glycyrrhizae (*Gan Cao*), 6g

ANALYSIS OF FORMULA: *Shi Jue Ming, Tian Ma, Gou Teng, Niu Xi,* and *Jiang Can* extinguish wind and subdue yang. *Sang Ji Sheng* and *Niu Xi* nourish and enrich liver-kidney yin to check yang. *Ban Xia, Dan Nan Xing, Zhi Shi, Chen Pi, Huang Qin,* and *Zhu Li* together clear and transform phlegm heat and transform and extinguish phlegm wind. *Gan Cao* harmonizes the other medicinals in this formula.

ADDITIONS & SUBTRACTIONS: For twitching sinews and flesh or severe tremors, add 12 grams each of Fructus Tribuli Terrestris (*Bai Ji Li*) and Periostracum Cicadae (*Chan Tui*). For inhibited bending and stretching, add 20 grams of Radix Puerariae (*Ge Gen*) and two grams of Agkistrodon Seu Bungarus (*Bai Hua She*), powdered and taken with the strained decoction. For pain and numbness in the upper limbs, add nine grams of Rhizoma Curcumae Longae (*Jiang Huang*). For pain and numbness in the lower limbs, add nine grams of Fructus Chaenomelis Lagenariae (*Mu Gua*).

For more marked spleen qi vacuity, replace *Tian Ma Gou Teng Yin Jia Jian* with *Dao Tan Tang Jia Jian* (Abduct Phlegm Decoction with Additions & Subtractions): Radix Astragali Membranacei (*Huang Qi*) and Rhizoma Pinelliae Ternatae (*Ban Xia*), 20g each, Sclerotium Poriae Cocos (*Fu Ling*) and Rhizoma Atractylodis Macrocephalae (*Bai Zhu*), 15g each, Pericarpium Citri Reticulatae (*Chen Pi*), Rhizoma Cyperi Rotundi (*Xiang Fu*), Fructus Amomi (*Sha Ren*), Radix Ligustici Wallichii (*Chuan Xiong*), Fructus Citri Aurantii (*Zhi Ke*), bile-processed Rhizoma Arisaematis (*Dan Nan Xing*), Ramulus Cinnamomi Cassiae (*Gui Zhi*), and Rhizoma Gastrodiae Elatae (*Tian Ma*), 9g each, and Buthus Martensis (*Quan Xie*) and Scolopendra Subspinipes (*Wu Gong*), 3g each, powdered and taken with the strained decoction.

ACUPUNCTURE & MOXIBUSTION: *Tai Chong* (Liv 3), *He Gu* (LI 4), *Feng Chi* (GB 20), *Feng Long* (St 40)

ANALYSIS OF FORMULA: Draining *Tai Chong* and *He Gu*, the four gates or bars, as well as *Feng Chi* levels the liver and subdues yang, extinguishes wind and settles tremors. Draining *Feng Long* transforms phlegm and disinhibits dampness.

ADDITIONS & SUBTRACTIONS: For more marked spleen qi vacuity, add *Zu San Li* (St 36) and *Yin Ling Quan* (Sp 9). For twitching sinews and flesh or severe tremors, add *Yang Ling Quan* (GB 34). For inhibited bending and stretching, add *Da Zhui* (GV 14), *Shui Gou* (GV 26), and *Cheng Jiang* (CV 24). For pain and numbness in the upper limbs, add *Wai Guan* (TB 5). For pain and numbness in the lower limbs, add *Cheng Shan* (Bl 57). For instability walking, add *Shen Mai* (Bl 62) and *Zhao Hai* (Ki 6).

REMARKS

1. During the early stage of this disease, the above treatments may slow its progression and thus delay the use of Western medicinals, such as levodopa, which only tend to work for several years. The longer the patient can avoid using these drugs, the longer they will work for them when they do. In addition, these protocols may help the Western medicines achieve a more satisfactory and longer lasting effect with fewer side effects. Although not a Chinese medicinal, when

Herba Passiflorae Incarnatae (Passion Flower) is administered in tandem with levodopa, the reduction in passive tremor is greater than that when using levodopa alone.[1] We believe this fact helps substantiate the hypothesis that Chinese medicinals used in tandem with Western pharmaceuticals may achieve a better result in this condition than Western medicines used alone.

2. Yin vacuity is often complicated by qi vacuity, qi stagnation, and blood stasis. In those cases, one should add appropriate medicinals to supplement the qi, rectify the qi, and quicken the blood.

3. Chinese research suggests that Flos Daturae (*Yang Jin Hua*) is effective for the treatment of Parkinson's disease. However, this medicinal is very toxic. The dosage is 0.3-0.6g per day. If one chooses to use this medicinal, the patient should be kept under close observation.

4. Other acupuncture methods which achieve good results for Parkinson's disease include the following:

A. Electoacupuncture on *Qian Ding* (GV 21), *Bai Hui* (GV 20), *Cheng Ling* (GB 18), and *Xuan Lu* (GB 5). One treatment per day for two weeks equals one course. Allow five days rest between successive courses.

B. Scalp acupuncture on the chorea and tremor area, motor area, and sensory area and possibly on the vertigo and hearing area and leg motor area. One treatment every other day for 10 treatments equals one course. Allow five days rest between successive courses.

5. Supplementation with vitamin C may help treat some of the side effects of levodopa and prolong this medication's duration of effectiveness.

6. Vitamin B_6 may be just as effective in some patients as taking levodopa. Paradoxically, vitamin B_6 cannot be taken with some forms of levodopa. Happily, Sinemet (a combination of levodopa and carbidopa) can be taken along with supplemental vitamin B_6 and/or a diet high in vitamin B_6. Foods high in this nutrient include grains, especially oats, raw nuts, especially peanuts, bananas, potatoes, liver, and fish.

ENDNOTES

[1] The Burton Goldberg Group, *Alternative Medicine, The Definitive Guide*, Future Medicine Publishing, Inc., Puyallup, WA, 1993, p. 958

52

Peptic Ulcers

Peptic ulcers are a chronic inflammatory condition of the stomach and duodenum resulting in circumscribed ulceration of the mucous membranes penetrating through to the muscularis mucosa and occuring in areas exposed to stomach acid and pepsin. Because there must be exposure to stomach acid and pepsin, these ulcers are called peptic ulcers. If such ulcerations occur in the stomach, they are called gastric ulcers. If they occur in the duodenum of the small intestine, they are called duodenal ulcers. Approximately 25 million or one in every 10 Americans suffer from peptic ulcers some time in their life. While, according to the U.S. Center for Disease Control, infection by the *Heliobacter pylori* bacterium is the proximal cause of 90% of this disease, not all persons infected with this bacterium develop this disease. For instance, half of all Americans over 60 years of age are infected with this bacterium. Depending on other identified and unidentified factors, this bacterium appears to weaken the stomach and duodenal lining's resistance to acid and pepsin. While this disease may occur in anyone of any sex or age, it is predominantly found in middle-aged and older males. Risk or cofactors of this condition include stress, anxiety, irregular meals or skipping meals, smoking, heavy alcohol use, NSAID use, caffeine use, a family history, and type O blood. Although mortality from this condition is low, the suffering it produces is high, not to mention that it accounts for one million hospitalizations per year in the U.S. alone.

The main symptom of peptic ulcer is burning, gnawing, or pinching pain in the upper abdomen between the tip of the breast bone and navel which may last for minutes or hours. Duodenal ulcer pain is typically absent on awakening but appears mid-morning. It is relieved by eating but recurs 2-3 hours after meals. Pain may also awaken the patient between 1-2 AM each night. Frequently, the pain occurs once or more each day for one to several weeks and then may disappear without treatment. However, the pain commonly recurs within the next two to several years. The symptoms of gastric ulcer do not follow the preceding pattern of duodenal ulcers, and eating may actually worsen the pain. Other symptoms include anorexia, nausea, and vomiting. If ulceration results in hemorrhage, there may be either coffee ground like vomiting of blood or black, tarry defecation of blood. Bleeding may then result in anemia, fatigue, and weakness.

The Western medical diagnosis of this disease is based on the patient's history and presenting signs and symptoms, barium x-ray of the upper gastro-intestinal tract, and endoscopy. Diagnosis of *Heliobacter pylori* infection is made via blood test, urea breath test, and endoscopy with tissue biopsy. Until recently, this disease was treated by antacids and histamine H_2 receptor blocking agents, such as cimetidine. Now, when *Heliobacter pylori* are found, this condition is commonly treated by what is referred to as "triple therapy." This means two antibiotics plus either an acid-suppressor or stomach lining shield. The course of treatment lasts two weeks and requires taking up to 20 pills per day. When two antibiotics and both acid-suppressors and stomach lining shields are used, this is called "bismuth triple therapy." If bleeding is severe or recurrent, surgery is sometimes necessary. However, with advances in drug therapy, the number of patients requiring surgery has declined significantly.

Chinese disease categorization: This condition is mainly categorized as *wei wan tong*, stomach venter pain, and *cao za*, clamoring stomach. If there is vomiting of blood, this is called *tu xue*, while *bian xue* refers to hemafecia. In addition, torpid intake is *na dai*, fatigue is *juan pi*, lack of strength is *fa li*, and weight loss is *xing ti xiao xue*, bodily dispersion and whittling.

Disease causes: Internal damage by the seven affects, unregulated eating and drinking, and habitual bodily vacuity due to aging

DISEASE MECHANISMS: The disease mechanisms of peptic ulcers are essentially the same as for reflux gastritis. The root mechanism in the overwhelming majority of cases is a liver-stomach disharmony which may then be complicated by depressive heat, spleen vacuity, phlegm dampness, cold dampness, food stagnation, yin vacuity, and/or blood stasis.

TREATMENT BASED ON PATTERN DISCRIMINATION:

1. LIVER-STOMACH DISHARMONY PATTERN

MAIN SYMPTOMS: Stomach duct distention and pain possibly worsened by emotional stress and upset, bilateral rib-side distention and oppression, belching and burping, torpid intake, reduced food intake, possible tendency to sighing, a dark tongue with thin, white fur, and a bowstring pulse

TREATMENT PRINCIPLES: Course the liver and rectify the qi, harmonize the stomach and stop pain

RX: *Si Ni San* (Four Counterflows Powder) & *Jin Ling Zi San* (Melia Powder) with additions and subtractions

INGREDIENTS: Concha Arcae Inflatae (*Wa Leng Zi*), 30g, Rhizoma Cyperi Rotundi (*Xiang Fu*), Fructus Meliae Toosendan (*Chuan Lian Zi*), Caulis Perillae Frutescentis (*Su Geng*), and Rhizoma Corydalis Yanhusuo (*Yan Hu Suo*), 12g each, Radix Bupleuri (*Chai Hu*), Radix Albus Paeoniae Lactiflorae (*Bai Shao*), Fructus Citri Aurantii (*Zhi Ke*), Pericarpium Citri Reticulatae (*Chen Pi*), Radix Auklandiae Lappae (*Mu Xiang*), and Fructus Citri Sacrodactylis (*Fo Shou*), 9g each, and mix-fried Radix Glycyrrhizae (*Gan Cao*), 6g

ANALYSIS OF FORMULA: *Chai Hu, Bai Shao, Xiang Fu, Fo Shou,* and *Chuan Lian Zi* course the liver and rectify the qi, resolve depression and stop pain. In addition, *Bai Shao* nourishes liver blood to prevent further liver depression and relaxes spasms. When *Chuan Lian Zi* is combined with *Yan Hu Suo,* this moves the qi and quickens the blood strongly stopping pain. *Su Geng, Zhi Ke, Mu Xiang,* and *Chen Pi* harmonize the stomach and loosen the center. *Wa Leng Zi* controls acidity and stops pain, and *Gan Cao* harmonizes the other medicinals in this formula as well as relaxes spasms.

ADDITIONS & SUBTRACTIONS: For a cold sensation in the stomach and a liking for hot beverages, add three grams of Fructus Evodiae Rutecarpae (*Wu Zhu Yu*) and six grams of dry Rhizoma Zingiberis (*Gan Jiang*). For occasional severe fixed pain, add 15 grams of Radix Salviae Miltiorrhizae (*Dan Shen*). For severe stomach distention, add nine grams of Pericarpium Citri Reticulatae Viride (*Qing Pi*). For spasmodic pain, increase the dosage of *Bai Shao* and *Gan Cao* up to 12 grams. For food stagnation or if drinking the above decoction reduces food intake and causes stomach distention, add nine grams each of Massa Medica Fermentata (*Shen Qu*) and Fructus Germinatus Hordei Vulgaris (*Mai Ya*). For concomitant liver blood vacuity, add nine grams each of Radix Angelicae Sinensis (*Dang Gui*) and cooked Radix Rehmanniae (*Shu Di*). For concomitant spleen qi vacuity, add nine grams each of Rhizoma Atractylodis Macrocephalae (*Bai Zhu*), Sclerotium Poriae Cocos (*Fu Ling*), and Radix Codonopsitis Pilosulae (*Dang Shen*). For frequent belching, add nine grams of Flos Inulae Racemosae (*Xuan Fu Hua*).

ACUPUNCTURE & MOXIBUSTION: *Zhong Wan* (CV 12), *Nei Guan* (Per 6), *Gong Sun* (Sp 4), *Zu San Li* (St 36), *Tai Chong* (Liv 3)

ANALYSIS OF FORMULA: Draining *Nei Guan* courses the liver and harmonizes the stomach, while draining *Gong Sun* harmonizes the stomach and rectifies the qi. Together, they harmonize upbearing and downbearing and stop pain. *Zu San Li* is the master point of the abdomen. Draining it harmonizes the stomach and stops pain. *Zhong Wan* is the front *mu* or alarm point of the stomach. Draining it loosens the center and downbears counterflow, harmonizes the stomach and stops pain.

ADDITIONS & SUBTRACTIONS: For vomiting, frequent belching, gastric spasm, or acid stomach, add *Liang Qiu* (St 34). For irregular bowel movements, add *Zhi Gou* (TB 6). For food stagnation, add *Xuan Ji* (CV 21) or *Liang Men* (St 21). For enduring, recurrent stomach distention and pain, lassitude of the spirit, and lack of strength due to concomitant spleen vacuity, add *Pi Shu* (Bl 20) and *Wei Shu* (Bl 21) and supplement *Zu San Li.* For pain, heaviness, or tension in the solar plexus or diaphragmatic area, add *Jiu Wei* (CV 15). For rib-side and stomach pain, add *Qi Men* (Liv 14). For acid regurgitation, add *Ri Yue* (GB 24). For hiccup, add *Ge Shu* (Bl 17).

2. DEPRESSIVE HEAT PATTERN

MAIN SYMPTOMS: Intermittent clamoring of the stomach which occurs or is worse with emotional stress, possible acid regurgitation, a bitter taste in the mouth, chest oppression, stomach distention, frequent belching, nausea, possible rib-side distention and pain, premenstrual breast distention and pain in women, a red tongue, red tongue edges, or swollen edges and thin, white or yellow tongue fur, and a bowstring, slippery, rapid pulse

NOTE: Although liver-stomach disharmony is the root of this condition, most Western patients do not just have a liver-stomach disharmony but depressive heat as well. In addition, it is also very common to find heat and cold mixed together. Clamoring stomach refers to a sensation of emptiness and burning in the stomach duct or heart region which is described as like hunger but is not hunger, like pain but is not pain.

TREATMENT PRINCIPLES: Course the liver and rectify the qi, clear heat and harmonize the stomach

RX: *Xiao Yao San* (Rambling Powder) & *Zuo Jin Wan* (Left Metal Pills)

INGREDIENTS: Radix Angelicae Sinensis (*Dang Gui*), 12g, Radix Bupleuri (*Chai Hu*), Radix Albus Paeoniae Lactiflorae (*Bai Shao*), and Sclerotium Poriae Cocos (*Fu Ling*), 9g each, mix-fried Radix Glycyrrhizae (*Gan Cao*), Rhizoma Atractylodis Macrocephalae (*Bai Zhu*), and Rhizoma Coptidis Chinensis (*Huang Lian*), 6g each, Herba Menthae Haplocalycis (*Bo He*), 3g, Fructus Evodiae Rutecarpae (*Wu Zhu Yu*), 1g, and uncooked Rhizoma Zingiberis (*Sheng Jiang*), 2 slices

ANALYSIS OF FORMULA: *Chai Hu* and *Bo He* course the liver and resolve depression. *Bai Shao* and *Dang Gui* nourish liver blood to prevent further liver depression. *Fu Ling*, mix-fried *Gan Cao*, and *Bai Zhu* fortify the spleen and boost the qi. Also, mix-fried *Gan Cao* and *Bai Shao* relax spasms and stop pain. *Huang Lian* plus *Wu Zhu Yu* is a specific combination for the treatment of acid regurgitation in peptic ulcer or in reflux esophagitis. When a small amount of *Wu Zhu Yu* is used as a messenger, it leads *Huang Lian* to the jue yin liver. *Huang Lian* clears depressive heat from both the stomach and liver. *Sheng Jiang* and *Chen Pi* harmonize the stomach and stop vomiting.

ADDITIONS & SUBTRACTIONS: For stabbing pain in the stomach due to blood stasis, add nine grams each of Radix Salviae Miltiorrhizae (*Dan Shen*) and Radix Rubrus Paeoniae Lactiflorae (*Chi Shao*). For severe acid regurgitation, add 12 grams each of Os Sepiae Seu Sepiellae (*Hai Piao Xiao*) and Concha Arcae Inflatae (*Wa Leng Zi*). For rib-side pain, add nine grams each of Fructus Meliae Toosendan (*Chuan Lian Zi*) and Rhizoma Corydalis Yanhusuo (*Yan Hu Suo*). For rib-side and/or severe pain, add nine grams each of Fructus Meliae Toosendan (*Chuan Lian Zi*) and Rhizoma Corydalis Yanhusuo (*Yan Hu Suo*). For thirst, add nine grams each of Radix Trichosanthis Kirlowii (*Tian Hua Fen*) and Rhizoma Phragmitis Communis (*Lu Gen*). For constipation, add six grams of uncooked Radix Et Rhizoma Rhei (*Da Huang*).

For less liver depression and more dampness, replace *Xiao Yao San* plus *Zuo Jin Wan* with *Qi Yu Tang* (Qi Depression Decoction): Rhizoma Pinelliae Ternatae (*Ban Xia*), Bulbus Fritillariae Thunbergii (*Zhe Bei Mu*), Radix Glycyrrhizae (*Gan Cao*), Fructus Gardeniae Jasminoidis (*Zhi Zi*), Radix Auklandiae Lappae (*Mu Xiang*), and Semen Arecae Catechu (*Bing Lang*), 9g each, Rhizoma Cyperi Rotundi (*Xiang Fu*), Rhizoma Atractylodis (*Cang Zhu*), Pericarpium Citri Reticulatae (*Chen Pi*), Folium Perillae Frutescentis (*Zi Su Ye*), and Sclerotium Poriae Cocos (*Fu Ling*), 6g each, and Radix Ligustici Wallichii (*Chuan Xiong*), 3g.

For more pronounced stomach heat, replace *Xiao Yao San* and *Zuo Jin Wan* with *Wen Dan Tang* (Warm the Gallbladder Decoction) and *Qing Wei San* (Clear the Stomach Powder) with additions and subtractions: uncooked Radix Rehmanniae (*Sheng Di*), 12g, Sclerotium Poriae Cocos (*Fu Ling*), 9g, Rhizoma Pinelliae Ternatae (*Ban Xia*), Caulis Bambusae In Taeniis (*Zhu Ru*), Fructus Immaturus Citri Aurantii (*Zhi Shi*), Pericarpium Citri Reticulatae (*Chen Pi*), and Cortex Radicis Moutan (*Dan Pi*), 6g each, and mix-fried Radix Glycyrrhizae (*Gan Cao*) and Rhizoma Coptidis Chinensis (*Huang Lian*), 3g each. For even more severe stomach heat with possible vomiting of blood, add nine grams of Fructus Gardeniae Jasminoidis (*Zhi Zi*). For stabbing pain in the stomach, add nine grams each of Radix Salviae Miltiorrhizae (*Dan Shen*) and Radix Rubrus Paeoniae Lactiflorae (*Chi Shao*). For severe acid regurgitation, add nine grams each of Os Sepiae Seu Sepiellae (*Hai Piao Xiao*) and Concha Arcae Inflatae (*Wa Leng Zi*). For severe thirst, add nine grams each of Rhizoma Phragmitis Communis (*Lu Gen*) and Radix Trichosanthis Kirlowii (*Tian Hua Fen*).

For enduring heat damaging yin and consuming fluids, replace *Xiao Yao San* and *Zuo Jin Wan* with *Sha Shen Mai Dong Tang Jia Jian* (Glehnia & Ophiopogon Decoction with Additions & Subtractions): Radix Glehniae Littoralis (*Sha Shen*) and Tuber Ophiopogonis Japonicae (*Mai Men Dong*), 12g each, Rhizoma Polygonati Odorati (*Yu Zhu*), Herba Dendrobii (*Shi Hu*), Semen Dolichoris Lablab (*Bai Bian Dou*), and Fructus Citri Sacrodactylis (*Fo Shou*), 9g each, and mix-fried Radix Glycyrrhizae (*Gan Cao*), 6g. If liver depression is marked, add nine grams of Fructus Meliae Toosendan (*Chuan Lian Zi*). If there is simultaneous qi vacuity, add nine grams of Radix Codonopositis Pilosulae (*Dang Shen*) and Radix Dioscoreae Oppositae (*Shan Yao*). If there is simultaneous blood stagnation, add 15 grams of Radix Salviae Miltiorrhizae (*Dan Shen*).

ACUPUNCTURE & MOXIBUSTION: *Zhong Wan* (CV 12), *Nei Guan* (Per 6), *Gong Sun* (Sp 4), *Zu San Li* (St 36), *Liang Qiu* (St 34)

ANALYSIS OF FORMULA: Draining *Nei Guan* courses the liver and harmonizes the stomach. Draining *Gong Sun* harmonizes the stomach and rectifies the qi. Together, they harmonize upbearing and downbearing and stop pain. *Zu San Li* is the master point of the abdomen. Draining it harmonizes the stomach, drains the yang ming, and stops pain. *Zhong Wan* is the front *mu* or alarm point of the stomach. Draining it loosens the center and downbears counterflow, clears and harmonizes the stomach and stops pain.

ADDITIONS & SUBTRACTIONS: For severe heat in the liver and stomach, add *Yang Ling Quan* (GB 34) and *Nei Ting* (St 44). For burning pain in the stomach, add *Xia Ju Xu* (St 37). For bleeding gums, add *San Jian* (LI 3). For swift digestion with rapid hungering, add *San Yin Jiao* (Sp 6). For torpid intake, stomach glomus, vexatious heat in the chest, a bitter taste and sliminess in the mouth, thin, slimy, yellow tongue fur, and a slippery, rapid pulse, add *Feng Long* (St 40) and *Xia Xi* (GB 43). For constipation, add *Zhi Gou* (TB 6). For food stagnation, add *Xuan Ji* (CV 21) or *Liang Men* (St 21). For enduring, recurrent stomach distention and pain, lassitude of the spirit, and lack of strength due to concomitant spleen vacuity, add *Pi Shu* (Bl 20) and *Wei Shu* (Bl 21) and supplement *Zu San Li*. For pain, heaviness, or tension in the solar plexus or diaphragmatic area, add *Jiu Wei* (CV 15). For rib-side and stomach pain, add *Qi Men* (Liv 14). For acid regurgitation or a sour taste in the mouth, add *Ri Yue* (GB 24). For a bitter taste in the mouth, add *Yang Fu* (GB 38). For frequent belching or hiccup add *Ge Shu* (Bl 17). For torpid intake, stomach glomus, vexatious heat in the chest, a bitter taste and sliminess in the mouth, thin, slimy, yellow tongue fur, and a slippery, rapid pulse, add *Feng Long* (St 40) and *Xia Xi* (GB 43) to clear and transform phlegm heat in the stomach and gallbladder.

3. SPLEEN-STOMACH VACUITY WEAKNESS PATTERN

MAIN SYMPTOMS: Slight clamoring in the stomach which usually occurs when the stomach is empty and is better after eating, especially warm things, but is worse after eating uncooked, chilled foods, possible vomiting of clear water with a sour taste which also gets worse after eating uncooked, chilled foods, abdominal distention after eating, reduced appetite, a bland taste in the mouth or lack of taste, fatigued limbs and lack of strength, possible cold hands and feet, a white facial complexion, loose stools, a pale tongue with thin, white fur, and a vacuous or weak pulse

NOTE: This pattern often complicates a liver-stomach pattern, in which case, the stomach is hot and possibly dry, while the spleen is cold and typically damp. However, it is possible to see this as the main pattern in the elderly with peptic ulcers.

TREATMENT PRINCIPLES: Fortify the spleen and boost the qi, warm the center and scatter cold

RX: *Xiang Sha Liu Jun Zi Tang Jia Jian* (Aucklandia & Amomum Six Gentlemen Decoction with Additions & Subtractions)

INGREDIENTS: Radix Codonopsitis Pilosulae (*Dang Shen*), Rhizoma Atractylodis Macrocephalae (*Bai Zhu*), and Sclerotium Poriae Cocos (*Fu Ling*), 9g each, mix-fried Radix Glycyrrhizae (*Gan Cao*), Pericarpium Citri Reticulatae (*Chen Pi*), and Radix Auklandiae Lappae (*Mu Xiang*), 6g each, and Fructus Amomi (*Sha Ren*), 3g

ANALYSIS OF FORMULA: *Dang Shen, Bai Zhu, Fu Ling,* and mix-fried *Gan Cao* are the four gentlemen of *Si Jun Zi Tang* (Four Gentlemen Decoction). They fortify the spleen and boost the qi. *Mu Xiang* and *Sha Ren* mainly move the qi and harmonize the stomach. In addition, *Sha Ren* warms the center and scatters cold. *Chen Pi* helps the latter to move the qi and to loosen the center. Also, it disperses food and improves appetite.

ADDITIONS & SUBTRACTIONS: For severe vacuity cold, add six grams each of dry Rhizoma Zingiberis (*Gan Jiang*) and Ramulus Cinnamomi Cassiae (*Gui Zhi*). For damp accumulation, add nine grams each of Herba Agastachis Seu Pogostemi (*Huo Xiang*) and Cortex Magnoliae Officinalis (*Hou Po*). For phlegm, add nine grams of Rhizoma Pinelliae Ternatae (*Ban Xia*). For phlegm or vomiting of clear fluids, add nine grams each of Rhizoma Pinelliae Ternatae (*Ban Xia*) and uncooked Rhizoma Zingiberis (*Sheng Jiang*). For acid regurgitation, take Os Sepiae Seu Sepiellae (*Hai Piao Xiao*) and Bulbus Fritillariae Thunbergii (*Zhe Bei Mu*) at a 4:1 ratio. Grind these two medicinals into a fine powder and take 3-5 grams of this powder after each meal in addition to the above decoction. If there are some digestive side effects, such as abdominal distention and reduced appetite, add one gram each of Massa Medica Fermentata (*Shen Qu*) and Fructus Germinatus Hordei Vulgaris (*Mai Ya*) to the preceding powder. For black stools, add 20 grams of Terra Flava Usta (*Fu Long Gan*) and three grams of Rhizoma Bletillae Striatae (*Bai Ji*), powdered and taken with the strained decoction. If melena is severe, add an additional 30 grams of Herba Agrimoniae Pilosae (*Xian He Cao*) and nine grams of Radix Sanguisorbae Officinalis (*Di Yu*). For fatigue and weakness, add 15 grams of Radix Astragali Membranacei (*Huang Qi*). For severe pain, add *Liang Fu Wan* (Alpinia & Cyperus Pills), *i.e.*, Rhizoma Alpiniae Officinari (*Gao Liang Jiang*), 9g, and Rhizoma Cyperi Rotundi (*Xiang Fu*), 6g.

ACUPUNCTURE & MOXIBUSTION: *Liang Men* (St 21), *Zhong Wan* (CV 12), *Pi Shu* (Bl 20), *Wei Shu* (Bl 21), *Zu San Li* (St 36)

ANALYSIS OF FORMULA: *Liang Men* and *Zhong Wan* warm the center and scatter cold when needled with moxibustion on the heads of the needles, while *Pi Shu, Wei Shu,* and *Zu San Li* supplement the spleen and boost the stomach when needled with supplementing technique.

ADDITIONS & SUBTRACTIONS: For cold pain in the stomach, add *Liang Qiu* (St 34). For acid regurgitation and vomiting of clear water, add *Li Nei Ting* (M-LE-1). For stomach and abdominal glomus and fullness, add *Gong Sun* (Sp 4) and *Nei Guan* (Per 6).

4. CONSTRUCTIVE & BLOOD INSUFFICIENCY PATTERN

MAIN SYMPTOMS: Clamoring in the stomach, especially when the stomach is empty, which gets better on food intake, a lusterless facial complexion, pale lips, dizziness, heart palpitations, spontaneous perspiration, lassitude of the spirit, lack of strength, a pale red and thin tongue, and a fine, weak pulse

NOTE: This pattern describes a qi and blood dual vacuity due to prolonged or massive hemorrhaging.

TREATMENT PRINCIPLES: Supplement the qi and nourish the blood

RX: *Gui Pi Tang Jia Jian* (Return the Spleen Decoction with Additions & Subtractions)

INGREDIENTS: Radix Astragali Membranacei (*Huang Qi*) and Rhizoma Atractylodis Macrocephalae (*Bai Zhu*), 12g each, Radix Angelicae Sinensis (*Dang Gui*), Arillus Euphoriae Longanae (*Long Yan Rou*), Sclerotium Poriae Cocos (*Fu Ling*), Radix Codonopsitis Pilosulae (*Dang Shen*), and Radix Albus Paeoniae Lactiflorae (*Bai Shao*), 9g each, Semen Zizyphi Spinosae (*Suan Zao Ren*) and Radix Auklandiae Lappae (*Mu Xiang*), 6g each, and mix-fried Radix Glycyrrhizae (*Gan Cao*), 3g

ANALYSIS OF FORMULA: *Huang Qi, Bai Zhu, Fu Ling, Dang Shen,* and mix-fried *Gan Cao* supplement the center and boost the qi. *Dang Gui, Long Yan Rou, Bai Shao,* and *Suan Zao Ren* nourish the blood. *Mu Xiang* moves the qi and harmonizes the stomach. *Bai Shao* and *Gan Cao* relax spasms and stop pain.

ADDITIONS & SUBTRACTIONS: If there is concomitant liver depression, add six grams of Radix Bupleuri (*Chai Hu*) and nine grams each of Fructus Meliae Toosendan (*Chuan Lian Zi*) and Rhizoma Corydalis Yanhusuo (*Yan Hu Suo*). If there is concomitant food stagnation, add nine grams each of Massa Medica Fermentata (*Shen Qu*), Fructus Crataegi (*Shan Zha*), and Fructus Germinatus Hordei Vulgaris (*Mai Ya*). If there is concomitant hematemsis, add three grams each of Rhizoma Bletillae Striatae (*Bai Ji*) and Radix Pseudoginseng (*San Qi*), powdered and taken with the strained decoction. If there is concomitant hemafecia, add 20 grams of Terra Flava Usta (*Fu Long Gan*) and three grams of Rhizoma Bletillae Striatae (*Bai Ji*), powdered and taken with the strained decoction. If blood in either the vomitus or stools is severe, also add 30 grams of Herba Agrimoniae Pilosae (*Xian He Cao*) and nine grams of Radix Sanguisorbae Officinalis (*Di Yu*).

ACUPUNCTURE & MOXIBUSTION: *Ge Shu* (Bl 17), *Pi Shu* (Bl 20), *Wei Shu* (Bl 21), *Zhong Wan* (CV 12), *Zu San Li* (St 36)

ANALYSIS OF FORMULA: *Ge Shu, Pi Shu,* and *Wei Shu* fortify the spleen and nourish the blood when needled with supplementing technique. *Zhong Wan* and *Zu San Li* boost the stomach and harmonize the center when needled with supplementing technique.

ADDITIONS & SUBTRACTIONS: For retching, add *Nei Guan* (Per 6). For hiccup, add *Ju Que* (CV 14). For dull pain in the stomach, add *San Yin Jiao* (Sp 6). For hunger with no desire to eat, add *Tai Xi* (Ki 3). For dry stool and constipation, add *Zhi Gou* (TB 6). For vomiting of blood, add *Yin Xi* (Ht 6), *San Yin Jiao* (Sp 6), and *Yin Bai* (Sp 1). For black stools, add *Xi Men* (Per 4), *San Yin Jiao* (Sp 6), and *Yin Bai* (Sp 1).

5. FOOD STAGNATION PATTERN

MAIN SYMPTOMS: Clamoring stomach which gets better after vomiting, acid, putrid regurgitation, nausea, dislike of the smell of food, stomach duct distention and fullness, bad breath, possible sour, foul-smelling stools, slimy or normal tongue fur, and a normal or slippery pulse

NOTE: This pattern really only complicates other patterns of peptic ulcer.

TREATMENT PRINCIPLES: Disperse food and abduct stagnation

RX: *Bao He Wan* (Preserve Harmony Pills)

INGREDIENTS: Stir-fried Fructus Crataegi (*Shan Zha*), 18g, Sclerotium Poriae Cocos (*Fu Ling*), Fructus Forsythiae Suspensae (*Lian Qiao*), and Semen Raphani Sativi (*Lai Fu Zi*), 9g each, and Pinellia Massa Medica Fermentata (*Ban Xia Qu*) and Pericarpium Citri Reticulatae (*Chen Pi*), 6g each

ANALYSIS OF FORMULA: *Shan Zha, Shen Qu, Lai Fu Zi,* and *Ban Xia Qu* disperse food and abduct stagnation. *Lian Qiao* prevents the transformation of stagnation into heat. *Fu Ling, Chen Pi,* and *Ban Xia* seep and transform dampness and transform phlegm due to food stagnation. Also, *Chen Pi* moves the qi to help disperse food and transform dampness.

ADDITIONS & SUBTRACTIONS: For severe food stagnation, add nine grams each of Fructus Germinatus Hordei Vulgaris (*Mai Ya*) and Endothelium Corneum Gigeriae Galli (*Ji Nei Jin*). For food stagnation transforming into heat with constipation, a bitter taste in the mouth, and thirst, add six grams each of Radix Scutellariae Baicalensis (*Huang Qin*) and Rhizoma Coptidis Chinensis (*Huang Lian*). For constipation, add six grams of Radix Et Rhizoma Rhei (*Da Huang*) and nine grams of Fructus Immaturus Citri Aurantii (*Zhi Shi*).

For stomach duct distention, fullness, and pain, replace *Bao He Wan* with *Yue Ju Bao He Wan* (Escape Restraint &

Preserve Harmony Pills): Fructus Crataegi (*Shan Zha*), Rhizoma Pinelliae Ternatae (*Ban Xia*), Sclerotium Poriae Cocos (*Fu Ling*), Fructus Forsythiae Suspensae (*Lian Qiao*), and Rhizoma Cyperi Rotundi (*Xiang Fu*), 9g each, Massa Medica Fermentata (*Shen Qu*), Pericarpium Citri Reticulatae (*Chen Pi*), Semen Raphani Sativi (*Lai Fu Zi*), Rhizoma Atractylodis (*Cang Zhu*), and Fructus Gardeniae Jasminoidis (*Zhi Zi*), 6g each, and Radix Ligustici Wallichii (*Chuan Xiong*), 3g.

ACUPUNCTURE & MOXIBUSTION: *Zhong Wan* (CV 12), *Liang Men* (St 21), *Xuan Ji* (CV 21), *Zu San Li* (St 36), *Li Nei Ting* (M-LE-1)

ANALYSIS OF FORMULA: Draining *Zhong Wan, Liang Men*, and *Xuan Ji* disperses food and harmonizes the center. Draining *Zu San Li* and *Li Nei Ting* disperses food and abducts stagnation.

ADDITIONS & SUBTRACTIONS: For abdominal pain, add *Tian Shu* (St 25). For stomachache, add *Liang Qiu* (St 34). For diarrhea, add *Gong Sun* (Sp 4). For yellow tongue fur and constipation, add *Jie Xi* (St 41) and *Shang Ju Xu* (St 37). For fatty, meaty food accumulation, replace *Liang Men* (St 21) with *Hua Rou Men* (St 24).

6. PHLEGM DAMPNESS OBSTRUCTING THE CENTER PATTERN

MAIN SYMPTOMS: Clamoring stomach, chest and abdominal glomus and oppression, reduced appetite, profuse phlegm, nausea, possible vomiting of thin, clear fluids, head distention, fatigue and somnolence, especially after eating, encumbered limbs, thick, white, slimy tongue fur, and a bowstring or slippery pulse

NOTE: Once again, this pattern mostly complicates other patterns of peptic ulcers.

TREATMENT PRINCIPLES: Harmonize the stomach and transform phlegm, upbear the clear and downbear the turbid

RX: *Bai Zhu Wan Jia Jian* (Atractylodes Pills with Additions & Subtractions)

INGREDIENTS: Rhizoma Atractylodis Macrocephalae (*Bai Zhu*), Rhizoma Pinelliae Ternatae (*Ban Xia*), and Sclerotium Poriae Cocos (*Fu Ling*), 9g each, processed Rhizoma Arsiaematis (*Tian Nan Xing*), Pericarpium Citri Reticulatae (*Chen Pi*), and Massa Medica Fermentata (*Shen Qu*), 6g each, and mix-fried Radix Glycyrrhizae (*Gan Cao*), 3g

ANALYSIS OF FORMULA: *Ban Xia, Tian Nan Xing, Fu Ling*, and *Chen Pi* seep and transform dampness and transform phlegm. In addition, *Chen Pi* and *Ban Xia* harmonize the stomach. Also, this group, with the help of *Shen Qu* which disperses food, downbears turbidity. *Bai Zhu, Fu Ling*, and mix-fried *Gan Cao* supplement the center and boost the qi. Also, this group upbears the clear and prevents further damp accumulation and phlegm engenderment.

ADDITIONS & SUBTRACTIONS: For vomiting of clear fluids, add three slices of uncooked Rhizoma Zingiberis (*Sheng Jiang*) and nine grams of Flos Inulae Racemosae (*Xuan Fu Hua*). For phlegm heat, add nine grams of Radix Scutellariae Baicalensis (*Huang Qin*) and six grams of Rhizoma Coptidis Chinensis (*Huang Lian*).

ACUPUNCTURE & MOXIBUSTION: *Shang Wan* (CV 13), *Zhong Wan* (CV 12), *Xia Wan* (CV 10), *Zu San Li* (St 36), *Feng Long* (St 40)

ANALYSIS OF FORMULA: Draining *Shang Wan, Zhong Wan*, and *Xia Wan* harmonizes the stomach, upbearing the clear and downbearing the turbid. Supplementing *Zu San Li* supplements the center, while draining *Feng Long* transforms phlegm.

ADDITIONS & SUBTRACTIONS: For vomiting, frequent belching, gastric spasm, or acid stomach, add *Liang Qiu* (St 34). For irregular bowel movements, add *Zhi Gou* (TB 6). For enduring, recurrent stomach distention and pain, lassitude of the spirit, and lack of strength due to concomitant spleen vacuity, add *Pi Shu* (Bl 20) and *Wei Shu* (Bl 21). For hiccup, add *Ge Shu* (Bl 17). For a bitter taste in the mouth, add *Yang Fu* (GB 38).

7. BLOOD STASIS OBSTRUCTING THE NETWORK VESSELS PATTERN

MAIN SYMPTOMS: Severe stomach duct pain which is lancinating in character and fixed in location, dark, purplish, black blood or clots within any hemorrhagic blood, a dark, purplish tongue or possible static macules or spots, and a bowstring, choppy pulse

NOTE: This pattern may complicate other, typically enduring disease mechanisms or may be the main presenting pattern which is itself modified by other patterns and mechanisms.

TREATMENT PRINCIPLES: Quicken the blood and transform stasis, free the flow of the network vessels and stop pain

RX: *Dan Shen Yin* (Salvia Drink), *Jin Ling Zi San* (Melia Powder) & *Shi Xiao San* (Loose a Smile Powder) with additions and subtractions

INGREDIENTS: Radix Salviae Miltiorrhizae (*Dan Shen*), 20g,

Fructus Meliae Toosendan (*Chuan Lian Zi*), Radix Angelicae Sinensis (*Dang Gui*), and Rhizoma Corydalis Yanhusuo (*Yan Hu Suo*), 12g each, Fructus Amomi (*Sha Ren*), Pollen Typhae (*Pu Huang*), Feces Trogopterori Seu Pteromi (*Wu Ling Zhi*), and Radix Rubrus Paeoniae Lactiflorae (*Chi Shao*), 9g each, and mix-fried Radix Glycyrrhizae (*Gan Cao*), 6g

ANALYSIS OF FORMULA: *Dan Shen*, *Dang Gui*, *Yan Hu Suo*, *Pu Huang*, *Wu Ling Zhi*, and *Chi Shao* quicken the blood, transform stasis, and stop pain. In addition, *Shi Xiao San* (Loose a Smile Powder), *i.e.*, *Wu Ling Zhi* and *Pu Huang*, stops bleeding. *Chuan Lian Zi*, with the help of *Yan Hu Suo* and *Sha Ren*, moves the qi to stop pain. *Gan Cao* harmonizes the other medicinals in this formula and relaxes spasms.

ADDITIONS & SUBTRACTIONS: For vomiting of blood, add three grams each of Rhizoma Bletillae Striatae (*Bai Ji*) and Radix Pseudoginseng (*San Qi*), both powdered and taken with the strained decoction. For bloody stool, add nine grams of Radix Rubiae Cordifoliae (*Qian Cao Gen*) and three grams of Radix Pseudoginseng (*San Qi*), powdered and taken with the strained decoction. For concomitant qi vacuity, add 15 grams of Radix Astragali Membranacei (*Huang Qi*) and nine grams of Rhizoma Atractylodis Macrocephalae (*Bai Zhu*). For severe distention, add nine grams of Radix Auklandiae Lappae (*Mu Xiang*).

ACUPUNCTURE & MOXIBUSTION: *Zhong Wan* (CV 12), *Wei Shu* (Bl 21), *Ge Shu* (Bl 17), *Shang Wan* (CV 13), *Xia Wan* (CV 10)

ANALYSIS OF FORMULA: *Zhong Wan* is the front *mu* or alarm point of the stomach, while *Wei Shu* is its back transport point. Together, when needled with draining method, they are a basic combination to drain repletion of the stomach. Here, they quicken the blood, transform stasis, and stop stomach pain. *Ge Shu* is the meeting point of the blood. Draining it moves the blood and also stops bleeding due to blood stasis. *Shang Wan* is the upper duct, while *Xia Wan* is the lower duct. When needled with the central duct, *i.e.*, *Zhong Wan*, and draining technique, they harmonize the stomach and regulate and rectify upbearing and downbearing, abduct stagnation, free the flow of the network vessels, and stop stomach pain.

ADDITIONS & SUBTRACTIONS: For vomiting of blood, add *Yin Xi* (Ht 6), *San Yin Jiao* (Sp 6), and *Yin Bai* (Sp 1). For black stools, add *Xi Men* (Per 4), *San Yin Jiao* (Sp 6), and *Yin Bai* (Sp 1). For retching, hiccup, or nausea, add *Nei Guan* (Per 6). For dry stools and constipation, add *Zhi Gou* (TB 6). For vomiting, frequent belching, gastric spasm, or acid stomach, add *Liang Qiu* (St 34). For enduring, recurrent stomach distention and pain, lassitude of the spirit, and lack of strength due to concomitant spleen vacuity, add *Pi Shu* (Bl 20) and supplement *Wei Shu* (Bl 21).

8. STOMACH YIN VACUITY PATTERN

MAIN SYMPTOMS: Dry lips and mouth, difficulty swallowing, acid regurgitation, hiccup, vomiting, dry heaves, clamoring stomach, a burning feeling in the epigastrium, hunger but inability to eat much, constipation with dry stools, a red tongue with scanty fur or glossy, mirror-like fur, and a fine, rapid pulse

NOTE: Stomach yin vacuity is often seen in the elderly either in its pure form or as a complication of one or more other patterns. "Enduring heat consumes fluids."

TREATMENT PRINCIPLES: Nourish stomach yin with sweet and cool, rectify the qi and harmonize the stomach

RX: *Mai Men Dong Tang* (Ophiopogon Decoction)

INGREDIENTS: Semen Oryzae Sativae (*Geng Mi*), 30g, Tuber Ophiopogonis Japonici (*Mai Men Dong*), 15g, Rhizoma Pinelliae Ternatae (*Ban Xia*), 9g, Radix Panacis Ginseng (*Ren Shen*) and Radix Glycyrrhizae (*Gan Cao*), 6g each, and Fructus Zizyphi Jujubae (*Da Zao*), 5 pieces

ANALYSIS OF FORMULA: *Mai Men Dong* engenders fluids and enriches yin. *Ren Shen* and *Geng Mi* fortify the spleen, boost the qi, and engender fluids. *Gan Cao* cools and clears the stomach at the same time as supplementing the spleen. *Ban Xia* harmonizes the stomach and downbears counterflow. *Da Zao* fortifies the spleen and supplements the qi, nourishes the blood and, therefore, helps engender fluids, since, "Blood and fluids share a common source."

ADDITIONS & SUBTRACTIONS: For severe hiccups, add nine grams each of Calyx Kaki Diospyros (*Shi Di*) and Flos Caryophylli (*Ding Xiang*). For vomiting due to depressive heat, add three grams of Rhizoma Coptidis Chinensis (*Huang Lian*) and nine grams of Caulis Bambusae In Taeniis (*Zhu Ru*). For constipation, add 12 grams each of Radix Scrophulariae Ningpoensis (*Xuan Shen*) and uncooked Radix Rehmanniae (*Sheng Di*).

ACUPUNCTURE & MOXIBUSTION: *Nei Ting* (St 44), *Zhong Wan* (CV 12), *Qi Hai* (CV 6), *San Yin Jiao* (Sp 6), *Nei Guan* (Per 6)

ANALYSIS OF FORMULA: *Nei Ting* is the water point on the stomach channel. Therefore, supplementing it enriches yin and engenders fluids within the stomach. *Zhong Wan* is the front *mu* or alarm point of the stomach. Draining it harmonizes the stomach, regulating and rectifying upbearing and downbearing. *Qi Hai* is the sea of qi. Needling it with supplementing technique can help descend the qi as well as supplement the righteous or correct qi of the body. *San Yin Jiao* is the intersection point of the three foot yin of the spleen, liver, and kidneys. Therefore, needling it with even supplementing-even draining technique harmonize the liver and spleen at the same time as it enriches yin and engenders fluids. *Nei Guan* is the network point on the hand jue yin. When needled with draining technique combined with *Zhong Wan*, it strongly harmonizes the liver and stomach.

ADDITIONS & SUBTRACTIONS: For vomiting of blood, add *Yin Xi* (Ht 6) and *Yin Bai* (Sp 1). For black stools, add *Xi Men* (Per 4) and *Yin Bai* (Sp 1). For dry stools and constipation, add *Zhi Gou* (TB 6). For vomiting, frequent belching, gastric spasm, or acid stomach, add *Liang Qiu* (St 34). For enduring, recurrent stomach distention and pain, lassitude of the spirit, and lack of strength due to concomitant spleen vacuity, add *Pi Shu* (Bl 20) and *Wei Shu* (Bl 21)

REMARKS

1. Since most Western patients with peptic ulcers will have some sort of evil heat, clearing heat will typically play a part in most peptic ulcer patient's over-all Chinese medical treatment plan, and heat-clearing medicinals tend to be bacteriocidal.

2. In modern China, most practitioners routinely add calcium-based medicinals, such as Concha Arcae Inflatae (*Wa Leng Zi*), Concha Ostreae (*Mu Li*), and Os Sepiae Seu Sepiellae (*Wu Zei Gu*) to peptic ulcer patients' Chinese medicinal prescriptions based on the principle of lowering or reducing or neutralizing acid. However, because these heavy, mineral medicinals can damage the spleen and stomach, they should be used with care in patients with spleen-stomach vacuity. In some case, combining these medicinals with food-dispersing, center-harmonizing medicinals can help prevent their damaging the spleen and stomach.

3. Although modern Western medicine has de-emphasized the role of diet in the treatment of peptic ulcers, in Chinese medicine, diet is still considered very important. Alcohol, hot, spicy, and greasy fatty foods should be avoided and, in general, a clear, bland diet should be adopted.

4. Although the current Western medical treatment of peptic ulcers with antibiotics typically gets good results in a relatively short period of time, it may still create unwanted side effects. Therefore, Chinese medicine can be used in combination with modern Western medicine in order to A) eliminate or minimize those side effects, and B) make the Western medical treatment even more effective by treating the whole pattern and, therefore, the whole person.

53

Periarthritis of the Shoulder

Also referred to as scapulohumoral periarthritis, periarthritis of the shoulder refers to inflammation of the tissues surrounding the shoulder joint causing pain and restriction of movement. Typically, pain is the earliest symptom of this condition. It is usually made worse by exercise. However, there is also morning stiffness following inactivity which lasts 15-30 minutes or less and is improved by activity. As the disease progresses, joint motion becomes diminished, flexion contractures occur, and tenderness and crepitus or grating sensations appear. Periarthritis of the shoulder is more common in the elderly than the young and in women than in men. Its Western medical diagnosis is based on the above signs and symptoms and x-ray of the shoulder. Besides educating patients regarding proper rest and exercise, NSAIDs are used for pain relief along with muscle relaxants, such as diazepam (*i.e.*, Valium).

Chinese disease categorization: In general, this condition is classified as a species of *bi zheng* or impediment condition, especially when joint pain is its main symptom. However, when inhibition of movement is its main symptom, it is also referred to as *jian ning*, congealed shoulder, and *dong jie jian*, frozen shoulder. Because wind taking advantage of vacuity is often the Chinese medical cause of this condition, it is also called *lou jian feng*, leaky shoulder wind. Because this condition commonly occurs in the elderly or in those around 50 years of age, it is also often referred to as *lao nian jian*, elderly shoulder, and *wu shi jian*, 50 (years) shoulder. Other names include *jian bei tong*, shoulder and upper back pain, and simply *jian tong*, shoulder pain.

Disease causes: External contraction of wind, cold, and/or damp evils and/or bodily vacuity due to age or taxation fatigue

Disease mechanisms: Commonly due to a righteous qi vacuity, external wind, cold, and/or damp evils may take advantage of this vacuity to invade and enter the body. If wind, cold, and/or dampness remain in the muscles and skin surrounding the shoulder, they may obstruct the free flow of qi and blood. Because there is a lack of free flow in the channels and network vessels of the shoulder and its adjacent tissue, there is shoulder pain and lack of movement, since movement is a function of the flow of qi. In addition, cold congelation, qi stagnation, qi vacuity, blood vacuity, and/or trauma severing the channels and vessels may all cause blood stasis. And further, yang vacuity of the spleen and kidneys may give rise to accumulation of water dampness which, over time, may transform into phlegm rheum. This phlegm rheum may overflow from the interior and lodge in the space between the skin and the muscles, thus also obstructing the free flow of qi and blood. It is also possible for phlegm to be formed due to any other long-term cause obstructing the free flow of the qi and blood. This is because the blood and fluids flow together, and enduring dampness transforms into phlegm. Although periarthritis of the shoulder frequently involves at least some evil qi, it may also be due to malnourishment of the sinews due to either qi and blood vacuity or liver-kidney essence debility.

Treatment based on pattern discrimination:

1. External contraction of wind cold pattern

Main symptoms: The pain in the shoulder is comparatively minor and possibly accompanied by local numbness. The disease course is typically short, and the pain is dull or vague. This pain is limited to the shoulder or, in some cases, may involve the upper back if the pain is mainly in the posterior part of the shoulder. It may also involve the upper arm if the pain is mainly in the anterior part of the shoulder. Very often the back of the neck and upper back or the upper arm feel tight. A cold sensation in the shoulder is present and this is relieved by warmth or local massage, while it may be worsened by cold. There is no or very slight restriction of joint mobility. The tongue fur is white, while the pulse may be floating or appear normal.

TREATMENT PRINCIPLES: Dispel wind, scatter cold, and free the flow of the network vessels

RX: *Wu Tou Tang Jia Jian* (Aconite Decoction with Additions & Subtractions)

INGREDIENTS: Radix Albus Paeoniae Lactiflorae (*Bai Shao*) and Radix Astragali Membranacei (*Huang Qi*), 9g each, Ramulus Cinnamomi Cassiae (*Gui Zhi*), Rhizoma Curcumae Longae (*Jiang Huang*), and Radix Aconiti Carmichaeli (*Chuan Wu*), 6g each, and Herba Ephedrae (*Ma Huang*) and Radix Glycyrrhizae (*Gan Cao*), 3g each

ANALYSIS OF FORMULA: *Ma Huang* and *Gui Zhi* strongly dispel wind, scatter cold, and resolve the muscles. In addition, *Gui Zhi* is well-known to warm the channels, free the flow of the network vessels, and treat impediment pain, especially in the upper limbs. When *Ma Huang* is combined with *Chuan Wu,* it dispels cold in the bones. By itself, *Chuan Wu* strongly scatters cold and stops pain. *Jiang Huang* is the main medicinal ambassador or messenger to the shoulder. This means that it leads other ingredients to the region of the shoulder. At the same time, *Jiang Huang* expels wind, frees the flow of the network vessels, and stops pain. *Bai Shao* with *Gui Zhi* regulate and rectify the qi and blood, yin and yang, and interior and exterior as well as harmonize the constructive and defensive. With *Huang Qi,* they boost the qi and secure the exterior, thus preventing further penetration of evils into the channels and muscles. *Gan Cao* supplements the qi and harmonizes the other ingredients in this formula.

ADDITIONS & SUBTRACTIONS: In case of chronic disease with qi and blood vacuity, subtract *Chuan Wu* and add nine grams each of Radix Et Rhizoma Notopterygii (*Qiang Huo*), wine mix-fried Radix Angelicae Sinensis (*Dang Gui*), and uncooked Radix Codonopsitis Pilosulae (*Dang Shen*).

In case of chronic disease with liver-kidney vacuity, replace *Wu Tou Tang* with *San Bi Tang Jia Jian* (Three Impediments Decoction with Additions & Subtractions): Radix Astragali Membranacei (*Huang Qi*), 12g, Radix Ledebouriellae Divaricatae (*Fang Feng*), Radix Gentianae Macrophyllae (*Qin Jiao*), and Radix Et Rhizoma Notopterygii (*Qiang Huo*) 9g each, Radix Dipsaci (*Xu Duan*), Cortex Eucommiae Ulmoidis (*Du Zhong*), Sclerotium Poriae Cocos (*Fu Ling*), Radix Ligustici Wallichii (*Chuan Xiong*), Rhizoma Curcumae Longae (*Jiang Huang*), and Radix Achyranthis Bidentatae (*Niu Xi*), 6g each, Herba Asari Cum Radice (*Xi Xin*), Radix Codonopsitis Pilosulae (*Dang Shen*), Radix Angelicae Sinensis (*Dang Gui*), Radix Albus Paeoniae Lactiflorae (*Bai Shao*), and Radix Glycyrrhizae (*Gan Cao*), 3g each, and Cortex Cinnamomi Cassiae (*Rou Gui*), 1g.

ACUPUNCTURE & MOXIBUSTION: *Jian Yu* (LI 15), *Jian Liao* (TB 14), *Jian Zhen* (SI 9), *Qu Chi* (LI 11), *Wai Guan (TB5)*

ANALYSIS OF FORMULA: *Jian Yu, Jian Liao,* and *Jian Zhen* are yang channel points located around the shoulder and, when drained, are able to course wind and quicken the network vessels to stop pain. When *Qu Chi* and *Wai Guan* are combined with draining technique, they upbear and emit yang qi to expel wind cold. *Wai Guan* is also a key point for stopping pain in the arms. Needle all the points with draining method plus moxibustion.

ADDITIONS & SUBTRACTIONS: Add *Hou Xi* (SI 3) and *Xiao Hai* (SI 8) if the pain is in the posterior part of the shoulder and along the pathway of the small intestine channel. Add *Bi Nao* (LI 14) and *Qu Chi* (LI 11) if the pain is in the posterior part of the shoulder and along the pathway of the large intestine channel. Add *Tian Jing* (TB 10) and *Zhong Zhu* (TB 3) if the pain is in the posterior part of the shoulder and along the pathway of the triple burner. Add *He Gu* (LI 4) and *Lie Que* (Lu 7) if the pain is in the anterior part of the shoulder. If the pain radiates to the upper back and back of the neck, add *Nao Shu* (SI 10), *Tian Zong* (SI 11), *Jian Wai Shu* (SI 14), and/or *Jian Zhong Shu* (SI 15). Add *Da Zhui* (GV 14) and *He Gu* (LI 4) if there is qi vacuity and insecurity of the defensive yang. If the pain is accompanied by numbness of the middle, ring, and little fingers, add *Zhong Zhu* (TB 3). Also, needle every *a shi* point in the shoulder and the upper back or arm. Please also see remarks #4 and 5 below.

2. INVASION OF WIND DAMP EVILS PATTERN

MAIN SYMPTOMS: The disease course is usually long and the pain in and around the shoulder is severe. There is a cold sensation and aversion to cold in the shoulder. The pain and this cold sensation can be relieved by warmth, although this relief does not last long. If severe, the pain can cause sweating and even disturb working, sleeping, and eating. Restriction of joint mobility may be present in enduring cases. Other symptoms may include a pale tongue with white fur, and a bowstring or bowstring, fine pulse.

TREATMENT PRINCIPLES: Dispel wind, overcome dampness, and free the flow of the network vessels

RX: *Qiang Huo Sheng Shi Tang Jia Wei* (Notopterygium Overcome Dampness Decoction with Added Flavors)

INGREDIENTS: Radix Et Rhizoma Notopterygii (*Qiang Huo*) and Radix Angelicae Pubescentis (*Du Huo*), 9g each, Radix Et Rhizoma Ligustici Chinensis (*Gao Ben*), Radix

Ledebouriellae Divaricatae (*Fang Feng*), Radix Ligustici Wallichii (*Chuan Xiong*), Fructus Viticis (*Man Jing Zi*), and Rhizoma Curcumae Longae (*Jiang Huang*), 6g each, and Radix Glycyrrhizae (*Gan Cao*), 3g

ANALYSIS OF FORMULA: *Qiang Huo, Du Huo, Fang Feng, Chuan Xiong, Gao Ben,* and *Man Jing Zi* dispel wind and overcome dampness. *Qiang Huo* overcomes dampness and treats impediment pain in the upper part of the body, while *Du Huo* treats impediment pain in the lower part. Together, they treat wind damp impediment all over the whole body. *Fang Feng* expels the wind hidden in the bones. *Chuan Xiong, Man Jing Zi,* and *Gao Ben* treat impediment pain in the upper part of the body. *Jiang Huang* is the main medicinal ambassador or messenger to the shoulder. It leads other ingredients to the region of the shoulder. At the same time, *Jiang Huang* moves the qi and quickens the blood, expels wind, frees the flow of the network vessels, and stops pain.

ADDITIONS & SUBTRACTIONS: For severe restriction of joint mobility, add nine grams each of Herba Lycopodii (*Shen Jin Cao*) and Caulis Trachelospermi Jasminoidis (*Luo Shi Teng*). For a severe cold sensation in the shoulder, subtract *Man Jing Zi* and add nine grams of Ramulus Cinnamomi Cassiae (*Gui Zhi*) and six grams of processed Radix Aconiti Carmichaeli (*Chuan Wu*).

If wind and damp transform into heat, heat impediment will appear. This is characterized by severe pain, swelling, and a sensation of heat in the shoulder which is made better by cold and worsened by heat. There is severe restriction of movement and sometimes fever, vexatious heat, thirst, red urine, constipation, a red tongue, dry, yellow fur, and a slippery, rapid pulse. In that case, replace *Qiang Huo Sheng Shi Tang* with *Bai Hu Jia Gui Zhi Tang Jia Wei* (White Tiger Plus Cinnamon Twig Decoction with Added Flavors): Gypsum Fibrosum (*Shi Gao*), 20g, Semen Oryzae Sativae (*Geng Mi*), 12g, Rhizoma Anemarrhenae Asphodeloidis (*Zhi Mu*), Ramulus Mori Albi (*Sang Zhi*), Ramus Lonicerae Japonicae (*Ren Dong Teng*), Rhizoma Curcumae Longae (*Jiang Huang*), and Cortex Phellodendri (*Huang Bai*), 9g each, and Caulis Sargentodoxae (*Hong Teng*), Ramulus Cinnamomi Cassiae (*Gui Zhi*), and Radix Glycyrrhizae (*Gan Cao*), 6g each.

ACUPUNCTURE & MOXIBUSTION: Please see pattern #1 above but use moxibustion on the heads of the needles.

ADDITIONS & SUBTRACTIONS: Add *He Gu* (LI 4) and *Ge Shu* (Bl 17) if the case is enduring and the pain becomes pricking or piercing due to blood stasis. Add *Da Zhui* (GV 14) if there is concomitant yang vacuity. Add *Qi Hai* (CV 6) with acupuncture plus moxibustion and *He Gu* (LI 4), acupuncture only, if there is qi vacuity with spontaneous perspiration, shortness of breath, susceptibility to common cold, and fatigue.

NOTE: In clinical practice, heat impediment is often seen as an acute crisis or exacerbation of a more chronic wind damp impediment.

3. STATIC BLOOD BLOCKING THE NETWORK VESSELS PATTERN

MAIN SYMPTOMS: The pain in the shoulder is severe and sharp or pricking and can lead to slight restriction of movement of the shoulder. In this pattern, the methods of warming the channels and scattering cold or dispelling wind dampness and stopping pain get only slight effect. If blood stasis is due to other than trauma, there will not be any swelling or obvious *a shi* points. If blood stasis is due to traumatic injury, then an *a shi* point can be located and localized swelling may be present. Likewise, the tongue and pulse may be normal or there may be a dark tongue and choppy pulse. Usually there are no generalized symptoms.

TREATMENT PRINCIPLES: Quicken the blood, transform stasis, and stop pain

RX: *Shen Tong Zhu Yu Tang Jia Jian* (Body Pain Dispel Stasis Decoction with Additions & Subtractions)

INGREDIENTS: Radix Gentianae Macrophyllae (*Qin Jiao*), Semen Pruni Persicae (*Tao Ren*), Flos Carthami Tinctorii (*Hong Hua*), Radix Et Rhizoma Notopterygii (*Qiang Huo*), Resina Olibani (*Ru Xiang*), Radix Angelicae Sinensis (*Dang Gui*), Radix Cyathulae (*Chuan Niu Xi*), and Lumbricus (*Di Long*), 9g each, Rhizoma Curcumae Longae (*Jiang Huang*), Radix Ligustici Wallichii (*Chuan Xiong*), and Rhizoma Cyperi Rotundi (*Xiang Fu*), 6g each, and Radix Glycyrrhizae (*Gan Cao*), 3g

ANALYSIS OF FORMULA: *Tao Ren, Hong Hua, Ru Xiang, Dang Gui, Chuan Niu Xi, Chuan Xiong,* and *Jiang Huang* quicken the blood, transform stasis, and stop pain. *Xiang Fu* moves the qi to quicken the blood. *Qin Jiao, Qiang Huo, Jiang Huang,* and *Chuan Xiong* dispel the wind and overcome dampness. *Ru Xiang, Di Long,* and *Jiang Huang* free the flow of the network vessels to stop pain, and *Gan Cao* harmonizes the other ingredients in this formula.

ADDITIONS & SUBTRACTIONS: For blood stasis due to enduring impediment with restricted movement, add 12 grams each of Herba Pyrolae (*Lu Ti Cao*) and Herba Lycopodii (*Shen Jin Cao*) and nine grams of Radix Et Rhizoma Notopterygii (*Qiang Huo*). For concomitant qi vacuity, add 15 grams of Radix Astragali Membranacei (*Huang Qi*) and nine grams of Radix Codonopsitis Pilosulae (*Dang Shen*). For concomitant kidney yin vacuity, add nine grams each of Ramulus Loranthi Seu Visci (*Sang Ji Sheng*) and Plastrum Testudinis (*Gui Ban*) and replace *Chuan Niu Xi* with Radix Achyranthis Bidentatae (*Niu Xi*). For concomitant kidney yang vacuity, add nine grams each of Cortex Radicis Acanthopanacis Gracilistylis (*Wu Jia Pi*), Herba Epimedii (*Yin Yang Huo*), and Radix Dipsaci (*Xu Duan*).

ACUPUNCTURE & MOXIBUSTION: Same as for pattern #1 above but prick any *a shi* points and then use cupping over these *a shi* points in order to promote bleeding.

ADDITIONS & SUBTRACTIONS: Please see pattern #1 above.

4. PHLEGM DAMPNESS OBSTRUCTING THE NETWORK VESSELS PATTERN

MAIN SYMPTOMS: In this pattern, the disease course is long and the condition often seems incurable. In fact, classic wind cold damp impediment treatment seems to aggravate the condition or do nothing. There is severe pain in the sinews and muscles of the shoulder area. Restriction of mobility is ameliorated for a short time by movement and warmth but is worsened by cold and dampness. In addition, there is a pale tongue with slimy, white fur and a slippery pulse.

TREATMENT PRINCIPLES: Fortify the spleen and dispel wind dampness, transform phlegm and free the flow of the network vessels

RX: *Ban Xia Fu Ling Wan Jia Wei* (Pinellia & Poria Pills with Added Flavors)

INGREDIENTS: Rhizoma Pinelliae Ternatae (*Ban Xia*), Sclerotium Poriae Cocos (*Fu Ling*), Rhizoma Alismatis (*Ze Xie*), Radix Stephaniae Tetrandrae (*Han Fang Ji*), and Caulis Trachelospermi Jasminoidis (*Luo Shi Teng*), 9g each, and Fructus Citri Aurantii (*Zhi Ke*), Rhizoma Atractylodis Macrocephalae (*Bai Zhu*), and Rhizoma Curcumae Longae (*Jiang Huang*), 6g each

ANALYSIS OF FORMULA: *Ban Xia* and *Fu Ling* transform phlegm. *Bai Zhu* and *Fu Ling* fortify the spleen. *Zhi Ke* moves the qi to help transform phlegm. *Han Fang Ji* and *Jiang Huang* dispel wind dampness and treat impediment. *Ze Xie* helps *Ban Xia* to transform phlegm dampness and *Han Fang Ji* to overcome dampness. *Luo Shi Teng* and *Jiang Huang* free the flow of the network vessels to stop pain.

ADDITIONS & SUBTRACTIONS: For severely restricted movement, add 12 grams each of Herba Pyrolae (*Lu Ti Cao*) and Herba Lycopodii (*Shen Jin Cao*). For nodulations in the shoulder area, add 15 grams of Semen Sinapis Albae (*Bai Jie Zi*) and nine grams of Herba Ephedrae (*Ma Huang*). If qi vacuity is severe, add 15 grams of Radix Astragali Membranacei (*Huang Qi*) and nine grams of Radix Codonopsitis Pilosulae (*Dang Shen*).

If phlegm dampness causes blood stasis with localized, fixed pain, severe restriction of movement, and numbness of the hands and feet, replace *Ban Xia Fu Ling Wan* with *Xiao Huo Luo Dan* (Minor Quicken the Network Vessels Elixir): processed Radix Aconiti Kusnezofii (*Cao Wu Tou*), processed Radix Aconiti Carmichaeli (*Chuan Wu Tou*), and processed Rhizoma Arsiaematis (*Tian Nan Xing*), 60g each, and Resina Myrrhae (*Mo Yao*) and Resina Olibani (*Ru Xiang*), 20g each. Grind into powder and mix the medicinals. Boil six grams of this powder in 250cc of plain water for 15 minutes. Take the resulting infusion (liquid *and* dregs) in two divided doses.

ACUPUNCTURE & MOXIBUSTION: *Jian Yu* (LI 15), *Jian Liao* (TB 14), *Jian Zhen* (SI 9), *Feng Long* (St 40), *Yin Ling Quan* (Sp 9), *Zu San Li* (St 36)

ANALYSIS OF FORMULA: *Jian Yu, Jian Liao,* and *Jian Zhen* are all yang channel points located around the shoulder which can quicken the network vessels and stop pain when needled with draining technique. When *Feng Long, Yin Ling Quan,* and *Zu San Li* are used together, they fortify the spleen, transform phlegm, and disinhibit dampness. In that case, drain *Feng Long* and *Yin Ling Quan* and supplement *Zu San Li.* Use moxa on the handles of the needles in the shoulder.

ADDITIONS & SUBTRACTIONS: Please see pattern #1 above.

5. QI & BLOOD DUAL VACUITY PATTERN

MAIN SYMPTOMS: Aching and pain around the shoulder, inhibited bending and stretching, pain which is worse on waking up in the morning or after prolonged inactivity but better after use, pain also worse after taxation, possible muscle whittling and weakness in the shoulder area, a lusterless facial complexion, shortness of breath, fatigue, lack of strength, lassitude of the spirit, sinew vessel spasms and contractions, insensitivity of the skin, an enduring condition which does not heal, a pale tongue with possible teeth-marks on its edges, and a deep, fine, forceless pulse

TREATMENT PRINCIPLES: Supplement the qi and nourish the blood, harmonize the constructive and stop pain

RX: *Huang Qi Gui Zhi Wu Wu Tang Jia Jian* (Astragalus & Cinnamon Twig Five Materials Decoction with Additions & Subtractions)

INGREDIENTS: Radix Astragali Membranacei (*Huang Qi*) and uncooked Rhizoma Zingiberis (*Sheng Jiang*), 15g each, Radix Salviae Miltiorrhizae (*Dan Shen*) and Caulis Milletiae Seu Spatholobi (*Ji Xue Teng*), 12g each, Radix Albus Paeoniae Lactiflorae (*Bai Shao*) and Ramulus Cinnamomi Cassiae (*Gui Zhi*), 9g each, and Fructus Zizyphi Jujubae (*Da Zao*), 12 pieces

ANALYSIS OF FORMULA: *Huang Qi* and *Da Zao* supplement

the qi. *Bai Shao, Ji Xue Teng,* and *Dan Shen* nourish the blood. *Gui Zhi* and *Bai Shao* plus *Sheng Jiang* and *Da Zao* harmonize the constructive. *Dan Shen, Ji Xue Teng,* and *Gui Zhi* quicken the blood, free the flow of the network vessels, and stop pain.

ADDITIONS & SUBTRACTIONS: For restricted movement, add nine grams each of Herba Pyrolae (*Lu Ti Cao*), Herba Lycopodii (*Shen Jin Cao*), and Caulis Trachelospermi Jasminoidis (*Luo Shi Teng*). For severe qi vacuity, add nine grams each of Radix Codonopsitis Pilosulae (*Dang Shen*) and Sclerotium Poriae Cocos (*Fu Ling*). For concomitant kidney vacuity with bone weakness, add nine grams each of Cortex Radicis Acanthopanacis Gracilistylis (*Wu Jia Pi*), Radix Dipsaci (*Xu Duan*), and Radix Achyranthis Bidentatae (*Niu Xi*).

For predominant blood vacuity, replace *Huang Qi Gui Zhi Wu Wu Tang* with *Dang Gui Ji Xue Teng Tang Jia Jian* (Dang Gui & Milletia Decoction with Additions & Subtractions): Radix Angelicae Sinensis (*Dang Gui*), cooked Radix Rehmanniae (*Shu Di*), and Caulis Milletiae Seu Spatholobi (*Ji Xue Teng*), 15g each, Radix Albus Paeoniae Lactiflorae (*Bai Shao*), Radix Salviae Miltiorrhizae (*Dan Shen*), Rhizoma Curcumae Longae (*Jiang Huang*), and Resina Olibani (*Ru Xiang*), 9g each, and Ramulus Cinnamomi Cassiae (*Gui Zhi*), 6g.

ACUPUNCTURE & MOXIBUSTION: Please see pattern #1 above plus *Ge Shu* (Bl 17), *Pi Shu* (Bl 20), *Wei Shu* (Bl 21)

ANALYSIS OF FORMULA: *Ge Shu* is the meeting point of the blood. Supplementing it nourishes the blood. *Pi Shu* and *Wei Shu* are the back transport points of the spleen and stomach, the latter heaven roots of qi and blood engenderment and transformation. They should also be supplemented. The local points free the flow of the channel qi and quicken the blood. Drain them.

ADDITIONS & SUBTRACTIONS: Please see pattern #1 above.

6. LIVER-KIDNEY ESSENCE DEBILITY PATTERN

MAIN SYMPTOMS: Marked limitation of the range of movement of the shoulder, not very severe aching or pain, dizziness and vertigo, tinnitus, low back and knee soreness and limpness, lack of strength when lifting and/or walking, loss of teeth if extreme, scanty qi, disinclination to speak, a red tongue with thin fur, and a fine, weak pulse

TREATMENT PRINCIPLES: Supplement the liver and boost the kidneys, boost the qi and nourish the blood

RX: *Du Huo Ji Sheng Tang Jia Jian* (Angelica Pubescens & Loranthus Decoction with Additions & Subtractions)

INGREDIENTS: Ramulus Loranthi Seu Visci (*Sang Ji Sheng*) and cooked Radix Rehmanniae (*Shu Di*), 12g each, Radix Angelicae Pubescentis (*Du Huo*), Radix Gentianae Macrophyllae (*Qin Jiao*), Radix Ledebouriellae Divaricatae (*Fang Feng*), Radix Angelicae Sinensis (*Dang Gui*), Radix Albus Paeoniae Lactiflorae (*Bai Shao*), and Sclerotium Poriae Cocos (*Fu Ling*), 9g each, Cortex Eucommiae Ulmoidis (*Du Zhong*), Radix Achyranthis Bidentatae (*Niu Xi*), Ramulus Cinnamomi Cassiae (*Gui Zhi*), Radix Ligustici Wallichii (*Chuan Xiong*), Radix Panacis Ginseng (*Ren Shen*), and mix-fried Radix Glycyrrhizae (*Gan Cao*), 6g each, and Herba Asari Cum Radice (*Xi Xin*), 3g

ANALYSIS OF FORMULA: *Sang Ji Sheng, Shu Di,* and *Niu Xi* supplement the liver and kidneys, boost the marrow and reinforce the bones. In addition, *Sang Ji Sheng* eliminates wind damp impediment. *Shu Di, Dang Gui,* and *Bai Shao* nourish liver blood so as to strengthen the sinews. *Du Zhong* gently supplements both kidney yin and yang, strengthens the sinews and reinforces the bones. *Ren Shen, Fu Ling,* and mix-fried *Gan Cao* boost the latter heaven to engender acquired essence and thus replenish the former heaven. *Du Huo, Qin Jiao, Fang Feng, Gui Zhi, Xi Xin,* and *Chuan Xiong* dispel wind dampness, stop pain, and treat impediment.

ADDITIONS & SUBTRACTIONS: For restriction of movement, add nine grams each of Herba Pyrolae (*Lu Ti Cao*), Herba Lycopodii (*Shen Jin Cao*), and Caulis Trachelospermi Jasminoidis (*Luo Shi Teng*). For weakness of the bones, add nine grams each of Radix Dipsaci (*Xu Duan*) and Rhizoma Drynariae (*Gu Sui Bu*). For severe kidney yin vacuity, add 15 grams of Plastrum Testudinis (*Gui Ban*). For concomitant kidney yang vacuity, add nine grams each of Cortex Radicis Acanthopanacis Gracilistylis (*Wu Jia Pi*), Herba Epimedii (*Yin Yang Huo*), and Radix Morindae Officinalis (*Ba Ji Tian*). For severe qi vacuity, add 15 grams of Radix Astragali Membranacei (*Huang Qi*).

ACUPUNCTURE & MOXIBUSTION: Please see pattern #1 above plus *Tai Xi* (Ki 3), *Da Zhu* (Bl 11), *Xuan Zhong* (GB 39)

ANALYSIS OF FORMULA: The kidneys store the essence, the essence engenders the marrow, and the marrow nourishes the bones. Therefore, if the kidneys are strong, the essence is effulgent, and the marrow is prosperous, then the bones are firm. Conversely, in case of weakness of the bones, one should supplement the kidneys, boost the marrow, and reinforce the bones. *Tai Xi* is the source point of the kidney channel. Supplementing it supplements both the yin and yang of the kidneys and also the former heaven essence. *Xuan Zhong* is the meeting point of the marrow. Supplementing it, therefore, boosts the marrow. *Da Zhu* is the meeting point of the bones. Supplementing it reinforces the bones. This is the key combination for bone troubles due to kidney vacuity.

ADDITIONS & SUBTRACTIONS: Please see pattern #1 above.

7. FROZEN SHOULDER PATTERN

MAIN SYMPTOMS: In this pattern, pain typically follows restriction of movement of the shoulder and is triggered by such movement. This restriction of mobility develops slowly, and the inability to raise the shoulder gradually worsens over a period of days or months. In the daytime, the pain is better, while it worsens at night, disturbing sleep. In severe cases, even a light touch on the shoulder can trigger pain severe enough to cause tears. In most cases, the pain radiates to the upper arm, elbow, and hand. In enduring cases, the muscles around the shoulder may wilt and the sinews may become inflexible, thus eventually leading to complete restriction of shoulder movement. Hence, the patient may have difficulty combing their hair and putting on and off their clothes or cap. Other symptoms may include a cold feeling in the shoulder, spontaneous sweating in the palms, and a fine pulse. The tongue often remains normal.

NOTE: This pattern describes a combination of wind cold impediment, qi and blood vacuity, and blood stasis.

TREATMENT PRINCIPLES: Eliminate wind, overcome dampness, and scatter cold, quicken the blood, supplement vacuity, and free the flow of the network vessels

RX: *Juan Bi Tang Jia Jian* (Alleviate Impediment Decoction with Additions & Subtractions)

INGREDIENTS: Radix Astragali Membranacei (*Huang Qi*), 12g, Radix Angelicae Sinensis (*Dang Gui*), Radix Ligustici Wallichii (*Chuan Xiong*), and Caulis Trachelospermi Jasminoidis (*Luo Shi Teng*), 9g each, and Radix Et Rhizoma Notopterygii (*Qiang Huo*), Radix Angelicae Pubescentis (*Du Huo*), Ramulus Cinnamomi Cassiae (*Gui Zhi*), Radix Gentianae Macrophyllae (*Qin Jiao*), Caulis Piperis Futokadsurae (*Hai Feng Teng*), Ramulus Mori Albi (*Sang Zhi*), Resina Olibani (*Ru Xiang*), and Rhizoma Curcumae Longae (*Jiang Huang*), 6g each

ANALYSIS OF FORMULA: *Huang Qi* supplements the qi, while *Dang Gui* nourishes the blood. *Chuan Xiong, Dang Gui,* and *Ru Xiang* quicken the blood and free the flow of the network vessels to stop pain. *Luo Shi Teng, Chuan Xiong, Qiang Huo, Du Huo, Gui Zhi, Hai Feng Teng, Qin Jiao, Jiang Huang,* and *Sang Zhi* eliminate wind, overcome dampness, and treat impediment pain. *Chuan Xiong, Qiang Huo, Gui Zhi, Qin Jiao,* and *Sang Zhi* all act especially in the upper part of the body or on the upper limbs, while *Jiang Huang* is the main medicinal ambassador or messenger to the shoulder. It leads the other ingredients to the region of the shoulder. At the same time, *Jiang Huang* moves the qi and quickens the blood, expels wind, frees the flow of the network vessels, and stops pain.

ADDITIONS & SUBTRACTIONS: For restricted movement, add 12 grams each of Herba Pyrolae (*Lu Ti Cao*) and Herba Lycopodii (*Shen Jin Cao*). For kidney vacuity with bone weakness, add 12 grams each of Rhizoma Drynariae (*Gu Sui Bu*) and Radix Dipsaci (*Xu Duan*). If there is marked qi and blood vacuity, subtract *Qiang Huo* and *Hai Feng Teng* and add six grams each of Radix Albus Paeoniae Lactiflorae (*Bai Shao*) and Radix Codonopsitis Pilosulae (*Dang Shen*) and increase the dosage of *Huang Qi* up to 18 grams. If there is kidney yin vacuity, subtract *Qiang Huo* and *Hai Feng Teng* and add nine grams each of Radix Achyranthis Bidentatae (*Niu Xi*), Ramulus Loranthi Seu Visci (*Sang Ji Sheng*), and Plastrum Testudinis (*Gui Ban*). For kidney yang vacuity, subtract *Qin Jiao* and add nine grams each of Cortex Eucommiae Ulmoidis (*Du Zhong*), Rhizoma Cibotii Barometsis (*Gou Ji*), and Cortex Radicis Acanthopanacis Gracilistylis (*Wu Jia Pi*). If the patient is menopausal, subtract *Qiang Huo* and *Hai Feng Teng* and add nine grams each of Cortex Phellodendri (*Huang Bai*) and Rhizoma Anemarrhenae Asphodeloidis (*Zhi Mu*) and three grams each of Rhizoma Curculiginis Orchioidis (*Xian Mao*) and Herba Epimedii (*Yin Yang Huo*). These four medicinals with *Dang Gui* are the main medicinals of *Er Xian Tang* (Two Immortals Decoction), a famous formula for perimenopausal complaints due to kidney yin and yang vacuity. *Xian Mao* and *Yin Yang Huo* not only treat menopausal syndrome by supplementing liver blood and kidney yang vacuity, they are also two important medicinals to quicken the network vessels, dispel wind dampness, and treat impediment. If there is phlegm dampness, add nine grams each of processed Rhizoma Arsiaematis (*Tian Nan Xing*) and Sclerotium Poriae Cocos (*Fu Ling*). If there is severe blood stasis, add 15 grams of Caulis Milletiae Seu Spatholobi (*Ji Xue Teng*) and six grams of Resina Myrrhae (*Mo Yao*). If there is liver depression, add nine grams each of Fructus Meliae Toosendan (*Chuan Lian Zi*), Rhizoma Cyperi Rotundi (*Xiang Fu*), and Radix Bupleuri (*Chai Hu*).

ACUPUNCTURE & MOXIBUSTION: Please see pattern #1 above.

ADDITIONS & SUBTRACTIONS: Please see pattern #1 above.

REMARKS

1. Most cases of periarthritis of the shoulder in Western patients involve both wind cold damp impediment and vacuity. However, some cases, especially in older patients, only involve malnourishment of the sinews. Therefore, it is important to distinguish whether or not there are really evils present. It is also common in the elderly to see malnourishment of the sinews complicated by blood stasis.

2. Passive motion of the shoulder is extremely helpful, especially when there is frozen shoulder. Although this may be painful, it makes a large difference in the outcome of treatment.

3. Various Chinese medicinal tinctures and plasters may be helpful as adjunctive treatments of this disease. These can be self-administered on a daily basis by patients in their own homes.

4. Several extra-channel points have proven especially effective in clinical practice for the treatment of periarthritis of the shoulder. *Zhong Ping,* also named *Jian Zhou,* is located one *cun* under *Zu San Li* (St 36) and two *cun* above *Shang Ju Xu* (St 37). *Jian Ling* is located approximately 8-9 *fen* under *Yin Ling Quan* (Sp 9). This point should be painful to palpation before being needled. *Yang Ling Quan Xia* is located 2 centimeters under *Yang Ling Quan* (GB 34), and the *Jia Ji* (M-BW-35) point of the fifth cervical vertebrae. When using these points, the patient should mobilize their shoulder while the needles are in place.

5. There are two famous points for shoulder pain which can be used according to one needle method. *Yang Ling Quan* (GB 34) is especially good if the pain is located in the triple burner channel or when the patient suffers from liver depression/depressive heat. *Tiao Kou* (St 38) is especially effective when the pain is located on the large intestine channel. *Yang Ling Quan* is the meeting point of the sinews. It should be needled with draining method and relatively strong stimulation. After manipulation, the patient should gently move the affected shoulder for 10 minutes. Every 10 minutes, repeat the needle manipulation followed by mobilization of the shoulder. *Tiao Kou* should be needled through to *Cheng Shan* (Bl 57) with a long needle. This method is efficient but sometimes painful. Acupuncture with mobilization of the affected joint should then be carried out the same for *Yang Ling Quan.* Further, both *Er Jian* (LI 2) and *San Jian* (LI 3) also are very effective when used according to one needle method.

6. It is interesting to note that two points in the neck, *Fu Tu* (LI 18) and *Tian Chuang* (SI 16), also get good results in the treatment of periarthritis of the shoulder. However, when using these two points, deep needling and retention should be avoided.

7. For very severe pain or obstinate impediment, one should add "worm" medicinals, such as Eupolyphaga Seu Opisthoplatia (*Tu Bie Chong*), Buthus Martensis (*Quan Xie*), Scolopendra Subspinipes (*Wu Gong*), and/or Lumbricus (*Di Long*) to quicken the blood and free the flow of the network vessels.

8. The following two formulas treat enduring periarthritis of the shoulder with qi and blood, liver and kidney vacuity with wind, damp, and cold evils and blood stasis:

Juan Bi Jie Ning Tang (Assuage Impediment & Resolve the Congealed Decoction): Radix Astragali Membranacei (*Huang Qi*) and Radix Puerariae (*Ge Gen*), 20g each, Radix Gentianae Macrophyllae (*Qin Jiao*), 15g, Radix Angelicae Sinensis (*Dang Gui*) and Radix Ledebouriellae Divaricatae (*Fang Feng*), 12g each, Fructus Corni Officinalis (*Shan Zhu Yu*), Herba Lycopodii (*Shen Jin Cao*), Rhizoma Curcumae Longae (*Jiang Huang*), and Ramulus Cinnamomi Cassiae (*Gui Zhi*), 9g each, and Radix Pseudoginseng (*San Qi*), powdered and swallowed with the strained decoction, and Radix Glycyrrhizae (*Gan Cao*), 5g each

Jian Ning Tang (Congealed Shoulder Decoction): Radix Astragali Membranacei (*Huang Qi*), 12g, Cortex Eucommiae Ulmoidis (*Du Zhong*), Radix Angelicae Sinensis (*Dang Gui*), Radix Codonopsitis Pilosulae (*Dang Shen*), Radix Dipsaci (*Xu Duan*), Semen Cuscutae Chinensis (*Tu Si Zi*), Radix Et Rhizoma Notopterygii (*Qiang Huo*), Cornu Degelatinum Cervi (*Lu Jiao Shuang*), Fructus Lycii Chinensis (*Gou Qi*), Radix Polygoni Multiflori (*He Shou Wu*), Radix Ligustici Wallichii (*Chuan Xiong*), Fructus Crataegi (*Shan Zha*), Fructus Germinatus Oryzae Sativae (*Gu Ya*), and Herba Lycopodii (*Shen Jin Cao*), 9g each, and Radix Glycyrrhizae (*Gan Cao*), 3g

54

PERIODONTAL DISEASE

Periodontal disease refers to inflammation or degeneration of the tissues surrounding and supporting the teeth. It most commonly begins as gingivitis and progresses to periodontitis. While the greatest single cause of gingivitis is poor oral hygiene, because it is commonly noted at puberty and during pregnancy, it is also probably related to endocrine factors. Therefore, gingivitis may be the first sign of a systemic disorder with lowered tissue resistance, such as hypovitaminosis, leukopenic disorders, allergic reactions, or endocrine disorders (*e.g.*, diabetes mellitus). This condition is actually an autoimmune disease. The inflammation and tissue destruction that follows it is due to the immune system's attack on bacterial plaque. Therefore, it should come as no surprise that people with periodontal disease may have other systemic conditions. Other factors involved in the occurrence of this disease include malocclusion, breathing through the mouth, nutritional deficiencies, especially folic acid and vitamin B complex, calcium insufficiency (whether due to insufficient intake or stressor foods that rob it from the system), and a diet low in fiber, and hydrocholoric acid deficiency. Birth control pills tend to increase the body's requirements for folic acid, and, if this is not met, there may be an increased risk of gingivitis. In addition, smokers are 2-4 times more likely to suffer periodontal disease than nonsmokers.

The main symptoms of this condition are red, inflamed gum tissue surrounding the bases of the teeth, edematous swelling of the interdermal papillae, and bleeding on minimal injury, such as when brushing the teeth. Pain is usually absent. If gingivitis progresses to the point of periodontitis, there are deepening pockets between the gingivae and the teeth, enlarged calcium deposits, loss of attachment of the gums to the teeth, and loss of supporting bone. This may then lead to bone loss, and, in fact, periodontal disease is the leading cause of tooth loss in adults.

Within Western medicine, the diagnosis and treatment of this condition is mainly carried out by dentists. Its treatment relies mainly on daily brushing and flossing of the teeth combined with daily massage of the surrounding gum tissue. When this condition is associated with another systemic disease, treatment of that systemic disease is obviously necessary. However, only the gingivitis of diabetes and leukemia are usually given much consideration, and patients with less recognizable endrocrine dyscrasias, lowered immunity, and allergies usually are not treated systemically. If periodontal disease becomes severe, surgery may be necessary to remove the chronically inflamed tissue.

CHINESE DISEASE CATEGORIZATION: Periodontal disease is mainly categorized as *ya xuan*, gaping gums, *ya lou*, leaking gums, and *ya nu*, bleeding gums.

DISEASE CAUSES: External contraction of wind heat toxins, habitual bodily yang exuberance, unregulated eating and drinking, enduring disease, and bodily weakness due to aging

DISEASE MECHANISMS: If external wind heat toxins invade the body and enter the yang ming, heat may follow the channels upward to the mouth, thus causing redness, swelling, pain, ulcerations, and bleeding. However, it is also possible for habitual bodily yang exuberance and over-eating hot, spicy, oily, sweet, thick-flavored foods, and alcohol to engender heat internally within the stomach and intestines. This internally engendered heat may also follow the channels upward causing similar redness, pain, swelling, heat, and bleeding. Enduring heat may damage and consume yin or yin may simply be consumed by aging. In either case, vacuity heat may likewise flare upward to harass the upper orifices. In this case, there may be redness, swelling, pain, and bleeding, but all less severe though more enduring. If heat not only consumes yin but eats the qi, spleen vacuity may eventually reach the kidneys, thus giving rise to kidney yang vacuity. Spleen-kidney yang vacuity may also be due to the debility and decline of aging. Spleen vacuity may fail to contain the blood within its channels, while kidney vacuity may result in loose or falling teeth.

TREATMENT BASED ON PATTERN DISCRIMINATION:

1. HEAT TOXINS FLAMING & EXUBERANT PATTERN

MAIN SYMPTOMS: Commonly seen in those with habitual spleen-stomach accumulation heat who have been invaded by wind heat toxic evils as evidenced by gingival redness, swelling, heat, and pain, spillage of pus and blood, bad breath, possible fever and aversion to cold, oral thirst, a red tongue tip with dry, white fur, and a floating, rapid pulse

NOTE: This pattern corresponds to acute attacks of purulent, swollen gingivitis.

TREATMENT PRINCIPLES: Course wind and clear heat, resolve toxins and disperse swelling

RX: *Wu Wei Xiao Du Yin Jia Wei* (Five Flavors Disperse Toxins Drink with Added Flavors)

INGREDIENTS: Flos Lonicerae Japonicae (*Jin Yin Hua*), 15g, Flos Chrysanthemi Indici (*Ye Ju Hua*), Herba Taraxaci Mongolici Cum Radice (*Pu Gong Ying*), and Herba Violae Yedoensitis Cum Radice (*Zi Hua Di Ding*), 12g each, Radix Semiaquilegiae (*Tian Kui Zi*), Radix Scutellariae Baicalensis (*Huang Qin*), Radix Ledebouriellae Divaricatae (*Fang Feng*), and Fructus Forsythiae Suspensae (*Lian Qiao*), 9g each, and Herba Menthae Haplocalycis (*Bo He*), 3g

ANALYSIS OF FORMULA: *Jin Yin Hua, Fang Feng,* and *Bo He* course wind and clear heat. *Ye Ju Hua, Pu Gong Ying, Zi Hua Di Ding, Tian Kui Zi, Huang Qin, Lian Qiao,* and *Jin Yin Hua* clear heat, resolve toxins, and disperse swelling, especially in the skin.

ADDITIONS & SUBTRACTIONS: If there is fever or other signs of heat are marked, add six grams of Rhizoma Coptidis Chinensis (*Huang Lian*).

ACUPUNCTURE & MOXIBUSTION: *Jiao Sun* (TB 20), *Xiao Hai* (SI 8), *He Gu* (LI 4), *Wen Liu* (LI 7)

ANALYSIS OF FORMULA: The combination of *Jiao Sun* and *Xiao Hai* is a classic formula for painful, swollen gums. Together, with the draining method, these points clear heat, disperse swelling, and stop pain. Draining *He Gu* and *Wen Liu* courses wind, clears heat, and resolves toxins. In addition, *He Gu* is the master point of the face and mouth.

ADDITIONS & SUBTRACTIONS: If the upper gums are affected, add *Nei Ting* (St 44). For frontal headache, add *Tou Wei* (St 8). For occipital headache, add *Feng Chi* (GB 20). For severe gingival redness, swelling, heat, and pain, add *Jia Che* (St 6) and *Xia Guan* (St 7). If there is fever, add *Guan Chong* (TB 1) and *Zhong Chong* (Per 9).

2. STOMACH & INTESTINE FIRE & HEAT PATTERN

MAIN SYMPTOMS: Gingival redness, swelling, heat, and pain, bleeding gums, fresh red colored blood, possible discharge of pussy, bloody secretions, bad breath, oral dryness and thirst with a predilection for chilled drinks, reddish urine, constipation, a red tongue with scanty fluids and thick, yellow fur, and a surging, large or slippery, rapid pulse

NOTE: This pattern is commonly seen in those with acute gingivitis or recurrent gingival swelling and purulence.

TREATMENT PRINCIPLES: Clear the stomach and drain fire

RX: *Qing Wei San Jia Jian* (Clear the Stomach Powder with Additions & Subtractions)

INGREDIENTS: Uncooked Gypsum Fibrosum (*Shi Gao*), 24g, uncooked Radix Rehmanniae (*Sheng Di*), 12g, Radix Scutellariae Baicalensis (*Huang Qin*) and Cortex Radicis Moutan (*Dan Pi*), 9g each, Rhizoma Coptidis Chinensis (*Huang Lian*) and Rhizoma Cimicifugae (*Sheng Ma*), 6g each, and Radix Glycyrrhizae (*Gan Cao*), 3g

ANALYSIS OF FORMULA: *Shi Gao, Huang Qin, Huang Lian,* and *Sheng Ma* clear the stomach and drain fire. *Sheng Di* and *Dan Pi* cool the blood. In addition, *Sheng Di* engenders fluids which tend to be damaged by heat. *Huang Qin* and *Huang Lian* also resolve toxins, while *Gan Cao* harmonizes the other medicinals in this formula.

ADDITIONS & SUBTRACTIONS: If there is depressive heat in the liver and stomach but simultaneous spleen vacuity and dampness, replace *Qing Wei San* with *Xiao Chai Hu Tang Jia Wei* (Minor Bupleurum Decoction with Added Flavors): Radix Scutellariae Baicalensis (*Huang Qin*), 12g, Radix Bupleuri (*Chai Hu*), Rhizoma Cimicifugae (*Sheng Ma*), Radix Codonopsitis Pilosulae (*Dang Shen*), and Rhizoma Pinelliae Ternatae (*Ban Xia*), 9g each, mix-fried Radix Glycyrrhizae (*Gan Cao*) and Rhizoma Coptidis Chinensis (*Huang Lian*), 6g each, Fructus Zizyphi Jujubae (*Da Zao*), and uncooked Rhizoma Zingiberis (*Sheng Jiang*), 2 slices. For bleeding gums, add 12 grams of Rhizoma Imperatae Cylindricae (*Bai Mao Gen*). For a bitter taste in the mouth, add six grams of Fructus Gardeniae Jasminoidis (*Zhi Zi*). For dry mouth and oral thirst, add 12 grams of Tuber Ophiopogonis Japonici (*Mai Men Dong*). For simultaneous internal cold, replace *Sheng Jiang* with six grams of dry Rhizoma Zingiberis (*Gan Jiang*).

Acupuncture & moxibustion: *He Gu* (LI 4), *Qu Chi* (LI 11), *Nei Ting* (St 44), *Jia Che* (St 6), *Xia Guan* (St 7)

Analysis of formula: Draining *He Gu* and *Qu Chi* clears large intestine heat, while draining *Nei Ting* clears stomach heat. Draining *Jia Che* and *Xia Guan* clears heat from the affected area, frees the flow of the network vessels, and stops pain.

Additions & subtractions: For persistent bad breath, add *Da Ling* (Per 7) or *Lao Gong* (Per 8). For constipation, add *Shang Ju Xu* (St 37) and *Tian Shu* (St 25). For a bitter taste in the mouth, add *Yang Ling Quan* (GB 34).

3. Liver-kidney yin vacuity pattern

Main symptoms: Loose teeth, receding, atrophic gums, lost teeth, possible gum swelling with slight pain, low back and knee soreness and limpness, tinnitus, dizziness, vexatious heat in the five hearts, a red tongue with scanty fur or flowery peeling, and a fine, rapid or floating, rapid pulse

Treatment principles: Nourish yin and engender essence, strengthen the bones and harden the teeth

Rx: *Liu Wei Di Huang Wan Jia Wei* (Six Flavors Rehmanniae Pills with Added Flavors)

Ingredients: Cooked Radix Rehmanniae (*Shu Di*), 18g, Fructus Corni Officinalis (*Shan Zhu Yu*), 12g, Radix Dioscoreae Oppositae (*Shan Yao*), Sclerotium Poriae Cocos (*Fu Ling*), Rhizoma Drynariae (*Gu Sui Bu*), Radix Dipsaci (*Xu Duan*), Radix Achyranthis Bidentatae (*Niu Xi*), and Fructus Lycii Chinensis (*Gou Qi Zi*), 9g each, and Rhizoma Alismatis (*Ze Xie*) and Cortex Radicis Moutan (*Dan Pi*), 6g each

Analysis of formula: *Shu Di, Shan Zhu Yu, Shan Yao, Fu Ling, Ze Xie,* and *Dan Pi* are the six ingredients of *Liu Wei Di Huang Wan* (Six Flavors Rehmannia Pills), a key formula for nourishing yin and engendering essence, which also clears or, at least, prevents vacuity heat. *Gou Qi Zi* and *Niu Xi* reinforce the yin-supplementing action of *Liu Wei Di Huang Wan.* In addition, *Gou Qi Zi* is fosters the essence and *Niu Xi* strengthens the bones and, therefore, the teeth which are the surplus of the bones. *Gu Sui Bu* and *Xu Duan* supplement the kidneys, strengthen the bones, and reinforce the teeth.

Additions & subtractions: For effulgent fire, delete *Xu Duan* and *Gou Qi Zi* and add nine grams each of Rhizoma Anemarrhenae Aspheloidis (*Zhi Mu*), Cortex Phellodendri (*Huang Bai*), and Cortex Radicis Lycii Chinensis (*Di Gu Pi*).

Acupuncture & moxibustion: *San Yin Jiao* (Sp 6), *Tai Xi* (Ki 3), *Da Ying* (St 5), *Jia Che* (St 6), *Xia Guan* (St 7)

Analysis of formula: Supplementing *San Yin Jiao* and *Tai Xi* strengthens the bones, enriches yin, and boosts the essence to secure the teeth. *Da Ying, Jia Che,* and *Xia Guan,* with the even supplementing-even draining method, free the flow of the network vessels, strengthen the bones, and harden the teeth.

Additions & subtractions: For seminal emission, add *Zhi Shi* (Bl 52). For sore throat, add *Zhao Hai* (Ki 6). For constipation, add *Zhao Hai* (Ki 6) and *Zhi Gou* (TB 6). For marked vacuity heat, add *Fu Liu* (Ki 7) and *Yin Xi* (Ht 6).

4. Mixed vacuity & repletion pattern

Main symptoms: Loose teeth, gingival swelling and pain, bleeding and spilling over of pus, bad breath, dizziness, tinnitus, low back pain, seminal emission, vexatious heat in the five hearts, a dry mouth with a liking to drink, clamoring stomach, abdominal distention after meals, hiccup, a red tongue with scanty fur, and a fine, rapid pulse

Note: This pattern describes a combination of kidney vacuity and stomach heat. It is often seen in diabetic, hypertensives, and those suffering from tuberculosis and menstrual irregularity. Diabetes may itself be an autoimmune disease, and ovarian dysfunction resulting in endometriosis, infertility, and menstrual irregularities may also be due to an autoimmune ovaritis.

Treatment principles: Nourish yin and clear heat

Rx: *Yu Nu Jian Jia Wei* (Jade Maiden Decoction with Added Flavors)

Ingredients: Uncooked Gypsum Fibrosum (*Shi Gao*) and cooked Radix Rehmanniae (*Shu Di*), 18g each, Tuber Ophiopogonis Japonici (*Mai Dong*), 12g, and Rhizoma Anemarrhenae Aspheloidis (*Zhi Mu*), Cortex Phellodendri (*Huang Bai*), Radix Achyranthis Bidentatae (*Niu Xi*), and Herba Dendrobii (*Shi Hu*), 9g each

Analysis of formula: *Shu Di, Mai Men Dong, Niu Xi,* and *Shi Hu* supplement the kidneys and enrich yin, boost the essence and secure the teeth. *Shi Gao* and *Huang Bai* clear and drain replete heat, while *Zhi Mu* and *Huang Bai* clear and descend vacuity heat.

Additions & subtractions: For severe loose teeth, add nine grams of Rhizoma Drynariae (*Gu Sui Bu*). For severe bleeding and spilling over of pus, add six grams of Rhizoma Coptidis Chinensis (*Huang Lian*) and 12 grams each of Herba Violae Yedoensitis Cum Radice (*Zi Hua Di Ding*) and Herba Taraxaci Mongolici Cum Radice (*Pu Gong Ying*). For bad breath, add nine grams each of Fructus Gardeniae

Jasminoidis (*Zhi Zi*) and Herba Eupatorei Fortunii (*Pei Lan*). For dizziness, add nine grams each of Fructus Tribuli Terrestris (*Bai Ji Li*) and Rhizoma Gastrodiae Elatae (*Tian Ma*). For tinnitus, add nine grams of Rhizoma Acori Graminei (*Shi Chang Pu*). For low back pain, add 12 grams of Cortex Eucommiae Ulmoidis (*Du Zhong*). For clamoring stomach and abdominal distention after meals, add nine grams each of Rhizoma Acori Graminei (*Shi Chang Pu*), Radix Auklandiae Lappae (*Mu Xiang*), and Rhizoma Atractylodis Macrocephalae (*Bai Zhu*).

ACUPUNCTURE & MOXIBUSTION: *Zhao Hai* (Ki 6), *San Yin Jiao* (Sp 6), *He Gu* (LI 4), *Nei Ting* (St 44), *Jia Che* (St 6), *Xia Guan* (St 7)

ANALYSIS OF FORMULA: *Zhao Hai* and *San Yin Jiao* together enrich yin and downbear vacuity heat when needled with supplementing technique. Draining *He Gu* clears large intestine heat and treats the teeth and gums of the lower jaw. Draining *Nei Ting* clears stomach heat and treats the teeth and gums of the upper jaw. Draining *Jia Che* and *Xia Guan* clears heat in the affected area, frees the flow of the network vessels, and stops pain.

ADDITIONS & SUBTRACTIONS: For bad breath, add *Da Ling* (Per 7). For dizziness, add *Feng Chi* (GB 20) and *Bai Hui* (GV 20). For tinnitus, add *Ting Hui* (GB 2). For low back pain, add *Gong Sun* (Sp 4) and replace *Zhao Hai* with *Fu Liu* (Ki 7). For clamoring stomach and abdominal distention after meals, add *Zu San Li* (St 36) and *Zhong Wan* (CV 12). For marked vacuity heat with vexatious heat in the five hearts and night sweats, add *Yin Xi* (Ht 6) and *Da Zhui* (GV 14).

5. SPLEEN VACUITY NOT CONTAINING THE BLOOD PATTERN

MAIN SYMPTOMS: Bleeding gums on slight stimulation, blood possibly profuse in amount, bleeding worse when fatigued, pale gums, easy bruising, fatigue, lassitude of the spirit, lack of strength, shortness of breath, disinclination to speak, a weak voice, a somber white or sallow yellow facial complexion, heart palpitations, insomnia, a pale, fat tongue with teeth-marks on its edges, and a fine, weak pulse

TREATMENT PRINCIPLES: Fortify the spleen and boost the qi, contain the blood and stop bleeding

RX: *Gui Pi Tang Jia Jian* (Return the Spleen Decoction with Additions & Subtractions)

INGREDIENTS: Radix Astragali Membranacei (*Huang Qi*), 18g, Radix Codonopsitis Pilosulae (*Dang Shen*), 15g, Semen Zizyphi Spinosae (*Suan Zao Ren*), 12g, Herba Agrimoniae Pilosae (*Xian He Cao*), Rhizoma Bletillae Striatae (*Bai Ji*), Cacumen Biotae Orientalis (*Ce Bai Ye*), Rhizoma Atractylodis Macrocephalae (*Bai Zhu*), Radix Angelicae Sinensis (*Dang Gui*), Arillus Euphoriae Longanae (*Long Yan Rou*), and Sclerotium Poriae Cocos (*Fu Ling*), 9g each, and Radix Auklandiae Lappae (*Mu Xiang*) and mix-fried Radix Glycyrrhizae (*Gan Cao*), 6g each

ANALYSIS OF FORMULA: *Huang Qi, Dang Shen, Bai Zhu, Long Yan Rou, Fu Ling,* and mix-fried *Gan Cao* fortify the spleen and boost the qi to contain the blood and stop bleeding. *Dang Gui* harmonizes the blood, while *Mu Xiang* rectifies the qi, thus respectively promoting the stopping of bleeding and spleen transformation. *Xian He Cao, Bai Ji,* and *Ce Bai Ye* astringe, secure, and stop bleeding. In addition, *Suan Zao Ren* and *Long Yan Rou* supplement and nourish heart blood, calm the spirit and settle palpitations.

ADDITIONS & SUBTRACTIONS: For atrophic, pale, receding gums with less bleeding due to qi and blood dual vacuity, replace *Gui Pi Tang Jia Jian* with *Ba Zhen Tang Jia Wei* (Eight Pearls Decoction with Added Flavors): cooked Radix Rehmanniae (*Shu Di*), 12g, Radix Angelicae Sinensis (*Dang Gui*), Radix Albus Paeoniae Lactiflorae (*Bai Shao*), Radix Codonopsitis Pilosulae (*Dang Shen*), Rhizoma Atractylodis Macrocephalae (*Bai Zhu*), Sclerotium Poriae Cocos (*Fu Ling*), Radix Achyranthis Bidentatae (*Niu Xi*), and Radix Drynariae (*Gu Sui Bu*), 9g each, and mix-fried Radix Glycyrrhizae (*Gan Cao*) and Radix Ligustici Wallichii (*Chuan Xiong*), 6g each.

For painful, swollen gums and fissuring which occasionally discharges pus accompanied by qi and blood vacuity, replace *Gui Pi Tang Jia Jian* with *Tuo Li Xiao Du San* (Support the Interior & Disperse Toxins Powder): Radix Astragali Membranacei (*Huang Qi*), 15g, Radix Codonopsitis Pilosulae (*Dang Shen*), Rhizoma Atractylodis Macrocephalae (*Bai Zhu*), Radix Angelicae Sinensis (*Dang Gui*), Radix Ligustici Wallichii (*Chuan Xiong*), and Spina Gleditschiae Chinensis (*Zao Jiao Ci*), 9g each, Radix Angelicae Dahuricae (*Bai Zhi*), Squama Manitis Pentadactylis (*Chuan Shan Jia*), and mix-fried Radix Glycyrrhizae (*Gan Cao*), 6g each, and Rhizoma Cimicifugae (*Sheng Ma*), 3g.

ACUPUNCTURE & MOXIBUSTION: *Yin Bai* (Sp 1), *Tai Bai* (Sp 3), *Zu San Li* (St 36), *Jia Che* (St 6), *Xia Guan* (St 7)

ANALYSIS OF FORMULA: Moxaing *Yin Bai* fortifies the spleen and stops bleeding. Supplementing *Tai Bai* and *Zu San Li* fortifies the spleen and boosts the qi. Supplementing *Jia Che* and *Xia Guan* harmonizes the network vessels and stops bleeding.

ADDITIONS & SUBTRACTIONS: For concomitant blood vacuity add *San Yin Jiao* (Sp 6) and *Ge Shu* (Bl 17). For lassitude of the spirit, lack of strength, shortness of breath, disinclination to speak, and a weak voice, add *Pi Shu* (Bl 20) and *Wei Shu* (Bl 21). For heart palpitations and insomnia, add *Shen Men* (Ht 7). For dampness, add *Yin Ling Quan* (Sp 9).

6. SPLEEN-KIDNEY YANG VACUITY PATTERN

MAIN SYMPTOMS: Receding gums, loose teeth, a thin secretion from cracks in the gums, somber white colored gums, no marked inflammation or hyperemia, listlessness of the essence spirit, scanty qi, lack of strength, chilled limbs, fear of cold, torpid intake, loose stools, a fat, pale tongue with teeth-marks on its edges and thin, white fur, and a deep, fine, weak pulse

TREATMENT PRINCIPLES: Warm and supplement the spleen and kidneys

RX: *Jin Gui Shen Qi Wan Jia Wei* (*Golden Cabinet* Kidney Qi Pills with Added Flavors)

INGREDIENTS: Radix Astragali Membranacei (*Huang Qi*), 15g, cooked Radix Rehmanniae (*Shu Di*), 12g, Radix Dioscoreae Oppositae (*Shan Yao*), Fructus Corni Officinalis (*Shan Zhu Yu*), Sclerotium Poriae Cocos (*Fu Ling*), Radix Drynariae (*Gu Sui Bu*), Radix Achyranthis Bidentatae (*Niu Xi*), Ramulus Cinnamomi Cassiae (*Gui Zhi*), and Radix Codonopsitis Pilosulae (*Dang Shen*), 9g each, and Rhizoma Alismatis (*Ze Xie*), Cortex Radicis Moutan (*Dan Pi*), and mix-fried Radix Glycyrrhizae (*Gan Cao*), 6g each

ANALYSIS OF FORMULA: *Huang Qi* boosts the qi and secures the exterior. *Shu Di, Shan Yao, Shan Zhu Yu, Fu Ling, Ze Xie*, and *Dan Pi* are the six flavors of *Liu Wei Di Huang Wan* (Six Flavors Rehmannia Pills), a basic formula for nourishing liver and kidney yin. Here, they are used to nourish yin to supplement yang, since, "Yin and yang are mutually rooted," and, "Yang is engendered from yin." *Niu Xi* and *Gu Sui Bu* supplement the liver and kidneys, strengthen the sinews and bones, and harden the teeth. *Gui Zhi* and *Gu Sui Bu* warm and supplement spleen and kidney yang, while *Gan Cao* harmonizes the other medicinals in this formula.

ADDITIONS & SUBTRACTIONS: For severe spleen qi vacuity, with scanty qi and lack of strength, add 12 grams of Radix Codonopsitis Pilosulae (*Dang Shen*). For severe yang vacuity with chilled limbs and fear of cold, add three grams of Herba Asari Cum Radice (*Xi Xin*). For torpid intake and loose stools, add nine grams each of Rhizoma Acori Graminei (*Shi Chang Pu*) and Rhizoma Atractylodis Macrocephalae (*Bai Zhu*).

ACUPUNCTURE & MOXIBUSTION: *Yin Bai* (Sp 1), *Tai Bai* (Sp 3), *Guan Yuan* (CV 4), *Qi Hai* (CV 6), *Jia Che* (St 6), *Xia Guan* (St 7)

ANALYSIS OF FORMULA: Moxaing *Yin Bai* fortifies the spleen and stops bleeding. Supplementing *Tai Bai* fortifies the spleen and boosts the qi. Supplementing *Guan Yuan* and *Qi Hai* with moxibustion warms and supplements spleen and kidney yang. Supplementing *Jia Che* and *Xia Guan* harmonizes the network vessels and supplements vacuity.

ADDITIONS & SUBTRACTIONS: For severe spleen qi vacuity with scanty qi and lack of strength, add *Zu San Li* (St 36). For severe yang vacuity with chilled limbs and fear of cold, add *Ming Men* (GV 4). For torpid intake and loose stools, add *Zhong Wan* (CV 12) and *Yin Ling Quan* (Sp 9).

REMARKS

1. While good oral and dental hygiene are vitally important to treat the proximal causes of periodontal disease, Chinese medical treatment seeks to treat the underlying imbalance. When dentists and oral hygienists are asked why some people are more prone to this condition than others, they simply say constitution or genes. In fact, up to 30% of the population may be genetically predisposed to this condition. However, Chinese medicine can discriminate the internal patterns causing this condition. By redressing those conditions, one not only treats the root of this condition but also helps improve one's total health and well-being. For instance, early internal treatment of gingivitis may help prevent diabetes. It is also our experience that many patients with gingivitis and pyorrhea have a history of allergies and/or intestinal dysbiosis. Allergies may lead to both immune insufficiency and autoimmune diseases, and this disease is actually a form of autoimmune disease.

2. It is very common to see periodontal disease due to a liver-spleen disharmony plus depressive heat. In that case, there is depressive heat in the liver and stomach plus spleen qi vacuity failing to contain the blood.

3. Because middle-aged and older patients with periodontal disease often have other diseases, such as diabetes and hypertension, they also typically have other patterns or disease mechanisms as well which do not play a direct part in gingivitis or periodontitis but do play a part in the patient's total, inter-related pattern. In particular, we are thinking of blood stasis and phlegm dampness. When these disease mechanisms complicate any of the above patterns, they should be taken into account in the total treatment plan even though they may not directly result in the periodontal signs and symptoms.

55

Peripheral Neuropathy

Peripheral neuropathy (PN), a.k.a. polyneuritis, is a syndrome composed of sensory, motor, and vasomotor symptoms which may occur singly or in combination caused by simultaneous disease of a number of different nerves. This condition is usually secondary to collagen vascular conditions, such as polyarteritis nodosa, SLE, scleroderma, and RA, metabolic diseases, such as diabetes mellitus and hypothyroidism, infectious agents, such as Lyme disease and HIV, or poisoning by such things as heavy metals, carbon monoxide, many solvents, and various drugs. The symptoms of this syndrome include bilateral numbness and insensitivity, tingling, burning pain, muscle weakness, and atrophy. Pain is frequently worse at night and may be aggravated by touch and temperature changes.

Because peripheral neuropathy is a symptom complex rather than a disease in its own right, the Western medical diagnosis and treatment of PN primarily revolve around that of the primary disease. However, electromyography and nerve conduction velocity tests may be used to help confirm neuropathy. Treatment of the underlying systemic disorder may halt the progression of this condition and even improve symptoms, but recovery tends to be slow at best. Various experimental drug therapies, such as the antidepressant amytriptilline (Elavil), have shown mixed results in clinical trials.

Chinese disease categorization: Peripheral neuropathy is categorized as *wei zheng*, wilting condition, in Chinese medicine. Numbness and tingling are referred to as *ma mu*, tingling and woodenness. Insensitivity is *bu ren*, no feeling. Since PN associated with systemic disease tends to affect the lower extremities first, this condition may also be referred to as *xia zhi ma mu*, lower extremity numbness and tingling, or *xia zhi teng tong*, lower extremity aching and pain.

Disease causes: The six environmental excesses, the seven affects, unregulated eating and drinking, taxation fatigue, enduring disease, aging, poisoning, and iatrogenesis

Disease mechanisms: The disease mechanisms of PN are nothing other than the disease mechanisms of wilting, pain, and numbness and tingling. Any evil qi, whether externally invading or internally engendered may lodge in the channels and network vessels, thus obstructing the flow of qi and blood. On the one hand, lack of free flow may cause pain. On the other hand, malnourishment may result in insensitivity and wilting. Lack of nourishment may also be due to A) anything which damages the spleen, the latter heaven root of qi and blood engenderment and transformation, B) enduring evil heat damaging and consuming blood and fluids, C) over or erroneous use of windy, dispersing medicines and recreational drugs, and D) the debility and decline of aging.

Treatment based on pattern discrimination:

1. Damp heat invasion & excessiveness pattern

Main symptoms: Soreness, heaviness, and lack of strength of the four extremities or two lower extremities, possible progressive paralysis or atrophy, insensitivity, numbness, and tingling of the four extremities, limb aching and pain, burning heat which is ameliorated by coolness, generalized fever which is not easily emitted, possible deviation of the face, mouth, and eyes, ductal oppression, torpid intake, thirst but no desire to drink, nausea and vomiting, abnormal vaginal discharge in females, red, hot, rough, painful urination, loose stools, a red tongue with slimy, yellow fur, and a rapid or slippery and rapid pulse

Treatment principles: Clear heat and disinhibit dampness

RX: *Si Miao San Jia Wei* (Four Wonders Powder with Added Flavors)

INGREDIENTS: Radix Salviae Miltiorrhizae (*Dan Shen*), Caulis Milletiae Seu Spatholobi (*Ji Xue Teng*), and Ramulus Mori Albi (*Sang Zhi*), 30g each, Sclerotium Poriae Cocos (*Fu Ling*) and Radix Achyranthis Bidentatae (*Niu Xi*), 15g each, Rhizoma Atractylodis (*Cang Zhu*), Semen Coicis Lachryma-jobi (*Yi Yi Ren*), Radix Angelicae Pubescentis (*Du Huo*), Fructus Chaenomelis Lagenariae (*Mu Gua*), and Radix Clematidis Chinensis (*Wei Ling Xian*), 12g each, and Cortex Phellodendri (*Huang Bai*) and Rhizoma Dioscoreae Hypoglaucae (*Bei Xie*), 9g each

ANALYSIS OF FORMULA: *Bei Xie, Huang Bai, Yi Yi Ren, Fu Ling,* and *Cang Zhu* together clear heat and dry or seep dampness. *Sang Zhi, Mu Gua, Du Huo, Wei Ling Xian* and also *Cang Zhu, Yi Yi Ren,* and *Bei Xie* disinhibit dampness and free the flow of impediment. *Dan Shen, Niu Xi,* and *Ji Xue Teng* quicken the blood and transform stasis.

ADDITIONS & SUBTRACTIONS: For muscle and flesh aching and pain, add nine grams each of Resina Olibani (*Ru Xiang*) and Resina Myrrhae (*Mo Yao*). For chest fullness, glomus, and oppression, add 12 grams each of Cortex Magnoliae Officinalis (*Hou Po*) and Fructus Citri Aurantii (*Zhi Ke*) and nine grams of Pericarpium Citri Reticulatae Viride (*Qing Pi*). For deviation of the face, mouth, or eyes, add 15 grams of Bombyx Batryticatus (*Jiang Can*), 12 grams of Rhizoma Typhonii Gigantei (*Bai Fu Zi*), and six grams of Buthus Martensis (*Quan Xie*). For severe heaviness and swelling of the limbs, add nine grams of Rhizoma Alismatis (*Ze Xie*).

ACUPUNCTURE & MOXIBUSTION: *Xue Hai* (Sp 10), *Yin Ling Quan* (Sp 9), *San Yin Jiao* (Sp 6), *Zu San Li* (St 36), local points depending on the area of pain or discomfort

ANALYSIS OF FORMULA: *Xue Hai* is the meeting point of the blood. Draining it quickens the blood and dispels stasis. Draining *Yin Ling Quan* clears heat and eliminates dampness, especially from the lower half of the body. When *San Yin Jiao* is combined with *Yin Ling Quan,* it strengthens the function of clearing and eliminating dampness and heat from the lower limbs. *Zu San Li* is a main point for treating all diseases of the lower limbs.

ADDITIONS & SUBTRACTIONS: If there is pain in the heel, needle *Kun Lun* (Bl 60). If there is tingling or burning on the sole of the foot, add *Yong Quan* (Ki 1). If there is pain, tingling, or numbness of the toes, needle the *Ba Feng* (M-LE-8).

2. LUNG-STOMACH FLUID DAMAGE PATTERN

MAIN SYMPTOMS: Either during or after the fever associated with an external contraction there is upper or lower limb weakness and loss of strength, inability of the hands to graps or the feet to stand and walk, if severe, paralysis, progressive emaciation, dry, withered skin, abnormal sensations, dry throat and parched lips, heart vexation, hoarse voice, oral thirst, short, reddish, hot, painful urination, constipation, a red tongue with thin fur and scanty fluids, and a fine, rapid or surging, vacuous, rapid pulse.

TREATMENT PRINCIPLES: Clear heat, engender fluids, and moisten dryness

RX: *Qing Zao Jiu Fei Tang* (Clear Dryness & Rescue the Lungs Decoction) & *Yi Wei Tang* (Boost the Stomach Decoction)

INGREDIENTS: Gypsum Fibrosum (*Shi Gao*), 30g, Tuber Ophiopogonis Japonicae (*Mai Dong*), Radix Glehniae Littoralis (*Sha Shen*), and uncooked Radix Rehmanniae (*Sheng Di*), 15g each, Folium Mori Albi (*Sang Ye*), Folium Eriobotryae Japonicae (*Pi Pa Ye*), Radix Pseudostellariae (*Tai Zi Shen*), and Radix Dioscoreae Oppositae (*Shan Yao*), 12g each, and Semen Cannabis Sativae (*Huo Ma Ren*) and Radix Glycyrrhize (*Gan Cao*), 9g each

ANALYSIS OF FORMULA: *Shi Gao* clears heat and drains fire, while *Sheng Di* clears heat and cools the blood. *Mai Men Dong, Sha Shen,* and *Sheng Di* enrich yin, engender fluids, and moisten dryness. *Sang Ye* clears heat from the lungs, while *Pi Pa Ye* clears heat from the stomach. *Huo Ma Ren* moistens the intestines and frees the flow of the stools. *Shan Yao, Tai Zi Shen,* and *Gan Cao* boost the qi and engender fluids.

ADDITIONS & SUBTRACTIONS: If stomach fluid damage is severe, add nine grams each of Herba Dendrobii (*Shi Hu*), Rhizoma Polygoni Odorati (*Yu Zhu*), and Radix Trichosanthis Kirlowii (*Tian Hua Fen*). If heat evils are severe, add 12 grams each of Folium Bambusae (*Zhu Ye*) and Rhizoma Phragmitis Communis (*Lu Gen*).

If oral thirst leads to drinking and there's a surging, large, vacuous, or scallion-stalk pulse due to summerheat heat damaging qi and yin, replace *Qing Zao Jiu Fei Tang* and *Yi Wei Tang* with *Bai Hu Jia Ren Shen Tang* (White Tiger Plus Ginseng Decoction): Gypsum Fibrosum (*Shi Gao*), 30g, Semen Oryzae Sativae (*Jing Mi*), 20g, Rhizoma Anemarrhenae Aspheloidis (*Zhi Mu*), 12g, and Radix Panacis Ginseng (*Ren Shen*) and mix-fried Radix Glycyrrhizae (*Gan Cao*), 6g each.

ACUPUNCTURE & MOXIBUSTION: *Nei Ting* (St 44), *Zu San Li* (St 36), *Zhi Gou* (TB 6), *Zhao Hai* (Ki 6), *Da Zhui* (GV 14), local points according to the affected areas

ANALYSIS OF FORMULA: Draining *Nei Ting* clears heat and engenders fluids. Draining *Zu San Li* frees the flow of the qi and blood in the lower extremities as well as frees the flow of the stools. Draining *Zhi Gou* clears heat from the three burners and frees the flow of the stools. Supplementing *Zhao Hai* supplements the kidneys and engenders fluids. The kidneys are the water viscus and, therefore, control the fluids and humors of the entire body. *Da Zhui* is the intersection point of the six yang channels and the governing vessel. Draining it clears heat from the entire body and recedes or abates fever.

ADDITIONS & SUBTRACTIONS: Add the *Ba Feng* (M-LE-8) if there is numbess and tingling in the toes. Add *Yong Quan* (Ki 1) if there is burning pain on the sole of the foot. If there is heel pain, add *Tai Xi* (Ki 3) needled through to *Kun Lun* (Bl 60). Add *Tian Shu* (St 25), *Da Chang Shu* (Bl 25), and *He Gu* (LI 4) if there is constipation. Add *Lie Que* (Lu 7) if there is marked lung dryness. Add the *Ba Xie* (M-UE-22), *He Gu* (LI 4), and *Qu Chi* (LI 11) if there is numbness and tingling of the fingers. Add *He Gu* (LI 4) and *Qu Chi* (LI 11) if there is fever.

3. SPLEEN-STOMACH VACUITY WEAKNESS PATTERN

MAIN SYMPTOMS: Paralysis of the four extremities which is most severe in the lower limbs, swelling and distention of the hands and feet, reduced food intake, abdominal distention, muscular cramping and pain, possible emaciation, a sallow yellow, lusterless facial complexion, loose stools, a pale tongue with thin, white fur, and a fine, forceless pulse

TREATMENT PRINCIPLES: Fortify the spleen and boost the qi

RX: *Shen Ling Bai Zhu San Jia Jian* (Ginseng, Poria & Atractylodes Powder with Additions & Subtractions)

INGREDIENTS: Radix Salviae Miltiorrhizae (*Dan Shen*), 30g, Radix Codonopsitis Pilosulae (*Dang Shen*), 15g, Sclerotium Poriae Cocos (*Fu Ling*), Radix Dioscoreae Oppositae (*Shan Yao*), Radix Et Rhizoma Notopterygii (*Qiang Huo*), Radix Dipsaci (*Xu Duan*), and Fructus Chaenomelis Lagenariae (*Mu Gua*), 12g each, and Pericarpium Citri Reticulatae (*Chen Pi*) and Ramulus Cinnamomi Cassiae (*Gui Zhi*), 9g each

ANALYSIS OF FORMULA: *Dang Shen, Fu Ling*, and *Shan Yao* supplement the spleen and boost the qi. *Chen Pi* transforms dampness and rectifies and regulates upbearing and downbearing. *Gui Zhi* warms the spleen at the same time as it quickens the blood and frees the flow in the extremities. In particular it leads yang qi to move back downwards. *Qiang Huo* frees the flow of impediment and stops pain by moving the qi. *Mu Gua* soothes the sinews and frees the flow of the channels as well as guides the other medicinals to the lower legs. *Dan Shen* quickens the blood and transforms stasis. In addition, *Shan Yao* and *Xu Duan* supplement the kidney qi and yang respectively. These last three medicinals are included in this formula because enduring disease typically includes blood stasis and enduring spleen disease reaches the kidneys.

ADDITIONS & SUBTRACTIONS: If there is muscular cramping and pain, add nine grams each of Resina Olibani (*Ru Xiang*) and Resina Myrrhae (*Mo Yao*) and three grams of Herba Asari Cum Radice (*Xi Xin*). If there is swelling and distention of the hands and feet, add 12 grams of Rhizoma Trachelospermi Jasminoidis (*Luo Shi Teng*) and Rhizoma Dioscoreae Hypoglaucae (*Bi Xie*). If the tongue is red with scanty fur or the fur is dry and yellow with oral thirst, delete *Chen Pi, Gui Zhi*, and *Qiang Huo* and add 30 grams each of uncooked Radix Rehmanniae (*Sheng Di*), Ramulus Mori Albi (*Sang Zhi*), and Gypsum Fibrosum (*Shi Gao*), 12 grams each of Tuber Ophiopogonis Japonici (*Mai Men Dong*) and Radix Glehniae Littoralis (*Sha Shen*), and nine grams of Radix Gentianae Macrophyllae (*Qin Jiao*).

ACUPUNCTURE & MOXIBUSTION: *San Yin Jiao* (Sp 6), *Xue Hai* (Sp 10), *Zu San Li* (St 36), *Pi Shu* (Bl 20), *Wei Shu* (Bl 21), local points depending on the area of pain or discomfort

ANALYSIS OF FORMULA: *San Yin Jiao, Zu San Li, Pi Shu,* and *Wei Shu* together supplement the spleen and boost the qi. *Xue Hai* quickens the blood and dispels stasis. In addition, *Zu San Li* frees the flow of the qi and blood in the lower extremities.

ADDITIONS & SUBTRACTIONS: If there is pain in the heel, needle *Kun Lun* (Bl 60). If there is tingling or burning on the sole of the foot, add *Yong Quan* (Ki 1). If there is pain, tingling, or numbness of the toes, needle the *Ba Feng* (M-LE-8). If there is downward falling of the central qi with dizziness, fatigue, and lack of strength, moxa *Bai Hui* (GV 20).

4. LIVER-KIDNEY INSUFFICIENCY PATTERN

MAIN SYMPTOMS: A long, slow disease course with gradual but progressive atrophy, weakness, and loss of use of the upper or lower limbs, low back and knee soreness and limpness, emaciation, numbness and tingling of the hands and feet, dizziness, tinnitus, blurred vision, tidal heat, night sweats, a dry mouth and a parched throat, hoarse voice, a red crimson tongue with scanty fluids and teeth-marks on its edges with possible cracks and fissures, and a fine, rapid or fine, bowstring, and rapid pulse

NOTE: In actuality, this is a qi and yin vacuity pattern.

TREATMENT PRINCIPLES: Supplement and boost the liver and kidneys, foster yin and clear heat

RX: *Hu Qian Wan Jia Jian* (Hidden Tiger Pills with Additions & Subtractions)

INGREDIENTS: Radix Astragali Membranacei (*Huang Qi*),

Plastrum Testudinis (*Gui Ban*), cooked Radix Rehmanniae (*Shu Di*), and Ramulus Mori Albi (*Sang Zhi*), 30g each, Radix Cyathulae (*Chuan Niu Xi*), 15g, Radix Angelicae Sinensis (*Dang Gui*), processed Radix Polygoni Multiflori (*He Shou Wu*), Radix Rubrus Paeoniae Lactiflorae (*Chi Shao*), and Radix Et Rhizoma Notopterygii (*Qiang Huo*), 12g each, and Cortex Phellodendri (*Huang Bai*), Rhizoma Anemarrhenae Aspheloidis (*Zhi Mu*), and Gelatinum Corii Asini (*E Jiao*), 9g each

ANALYSIS OF FORMULA: *Gui Ban, Shu Di, He Shou Wu, Dang Gui*, and *E Jiao* nourish liver blood and enrich kidney yin. In addition, *Gui Ban* strengthens the sinews and reinforces the bones. *Huang Bai* and *Zhi Mu* clear and descend vacuity heat. *Huang Qi* fortifies the spleen and boosts the qi. *Sang Zhi* and *Qiang Huo* dispel wind, eliminate dampness, and free the flow of impediment. *Chuan Niu Xi, Dang Gui*, and *Chi Shao* quicken the blood and free the flow of the network vessels.

ADDITIONS & SUBTRACTIONS: If yin vacuity has reached yang with chilled limbs, a pale tongue, and a deep, fine pulse, add nine grams each of Gelatinum Cornu Cervi (*Lu Jiao Jiao*), Fructus Psoraleae Corylifoliae (*Bu Gu Zhi*), Cortex Cinnamomi Cassiae (*Rou Gui*), and Radix Lateralis Praeparatus Aconiti Carmichaeli (*Fu Zi*).

ACUPUNCTURE & MOXIBUSTION: *San Yin Jiao* (Sp 6), *Tai Xi* (Ki 3), *Fu Liu* (Ki 7), *Zu San Li* (St 36), *Xue Hai* (Sp 10), local points depending on the site of pain or discomfort

ANALYSIS OF FORMULA: Supplementing *San Yin Jiao, Tai Xi*, and *Fu Liu* supplements the kidneys and enriches yin. Supplementing *San Yin Jiao* and *Zu San Li* supplements the spleen and boosts the qi. *Zu San Li* frees the flow of qi and blood in the lower extremities. Draining *Xue Hai* quickens the blood and dispels stasis.

ADDITIONS & SUBTRACTIONS: For more marked spleen qi vacuity, add *Pi Shu* (Bl 20) and *Wei Shu* (Bl 21). For marked kidney vacuity, add *Shen Shu* (Bl 23). If there is concomitant yang vacuity, moxa *Shen Shu* (Bl 23) and *Ming Men* (GV 4). If there is tingling or burning on the sole of the foot, add *Yong Quan* (Ki 1). If there is pain, tingling, or numbness of the toes, needle the *Ba Feng* (M-LE-8).

5. SPLEEN-KIDNEY INSUFFICIENCY WITH COLD DAMPNESS POURING DOWN PATTERN

MAIN SYMPTOMS: Lower limb paralysis or paralysis and heaviness, numbness, tingling, and insensitivity of the four limbs, coolness emitting from the hands and feet, if severe, chilled body and limbs with frequent sweating, a stagnant feeling in the chest which may progress to difficulty swallowing, stagnating and lingering phlegm fluids, cough, distressed, hasty breathing, greenish-purple, *i.e.*, cyanotic, nails, a pale tongue with thin, white or slimy, white fur, and a deep, slow, or deep, hidden pulse

TREATMENT PRINCIPLES: Scatter cold and dispel dampness, warm both the spleen and kidneys

RX: *Ma Huang Fu Zi Xi Xin Tang* (Ephedra, Aconite & Asarum Decoction) & *Shen Zhu Tang* (Ginseng & Atractylodes Decoction) with additions and subtractions

INGREDIENTS: Radix Panacis Ginseng (*Ren Shen*) and Radix Lateralis Praeparatus Aconiti Carmichaeli (*Fu Zi*), 30g each, Rhizoma Atractylodis Macrocephalae (*Bai Zhu*) and Herba Ephedrae (*Ma Huang*), 9g each, and Herba Asari Cum Radice (*Xi Xin*), 3g

ANALYSIS OF FORMULA: *Ma Huang* and *Xi Xin* scatter cold, while *Fu Zi* warms and supplements spleen and kidney yang. *Bai Zhu* fortifes the spleen and dries dampness. *Ren Shen* fortifies the spleen and boosts the qi.

ADDITIONS & SUBTRACTIONS: If cold and dampness are heavy, add 12 grams of Rhizoma Atractylodis (*Cang Zhu*) to fortify the spleen and dry dampness. If there are chilled limbs and sweating, delete *Ma Huang* and add 30 grams of Radix Astragali Membranacei (*Huang Qi*).

If there are no cold and dampness above but there is source vacuity below resulting in wilting, replace *Ma Huang Fu Zi Xi Xin Tang* and *Shen Zhu Tang* with *Er Xian Tang* (Two Immortals Decoction) and *Si Wu Tang* (Four Materials Decoction): cooked Radix Rehmanniae (*Shu Di*), 12g, Rhizoma Curculiginis Orchioidis (*Xian Mao*), Herba Epimedii (*Xian Ling Pi*), Radix Morindae Officinalis (*Ba Ji Tian*), Radix Angelicae Sinensis (*Dang Gui*), Radix Albus Paeoniae Lactiflorae (*Bai Shao*), Radix Ligustici Wallichii (*Chuan Xiong*), Rhizoma Anemarrhenae Aspheloidis (*Zhi Mu*), and Cortex Phellodendri (*Huang Bai*), 9g each.

ACUPUNCTURE & MOXIBUSTION: *San Yin Jiao* (Sp 6), *Tai Xi* (Ki 3), *Pi Shu* (Bl 20), *Wei Shu* (Bl 21), *Shen Shu* (Bl 23), *Ming Men* (GV 4), local points depending on the site of pain or discomfort

ANALYSIS OF FORMULA: *San Yin Jiao* is the intersection point of the three foot yin. Therefore, supplementing it supplements both the spleen and the kidneys. *Tai Xi* is the source point of the kidneys. Supplementing *Pi Shu, Wei Shu, Shen Shu*, and *Ming Men* with moxibustion warms and supplements spleen and kidney yang.

ADDITIONS & SUBTRACTIONS: If there is tingling or burning on the sole of the foot, add *Yong Quan* (Ki 1). If there is pain, tingling, or numbness of the toes, needle the *Ba Feng*

(M-LE-8). If there is marked dampness pouring downward or even concomitant damp heat, add *Yin Ling Quan* (Sp 9). If there is simultaneous blood stasis, add *Xue Hai* (Sp 10).

REMARKS

1. Because PN is usually seen in enduring, chronic diseases, there will be liver depression qi stagnation even though none of the above patterns mention it. One can also count on fatigue due to spleen vacuity. Further, as the majority of the above formulas imply, there will also be concomitant blood stasis. Qi and yin vacuity with damp heat and qi and blood stasis and stagnation is a commonly seen combination of patterns in patients with PN due to diabetes, SLE, RA, and AIDS. If yin vacuity reaches yang, there may also be concomitant yang vacuity.

2. If blood stasis has entered the network vessels, worm and insect ingredients should be used, such as Lumbricus (*Di Long*), Bombyx Batryticatus (*Jiang Can*), Buthus Martensis (*Quan Xie*), Scolopendra Subspinipes (*Wu Gong*), Hirudo (*Shui Zhi*), and Eupolyphaga Seu Ophisthoplatia (*Zhe Chong*). Most of these medicinals also track down and extinguish wind, thus relieving tingling and itching.

3. When needling either the *Ba Feng* (M-LE-8) or *Ba Xie* (M-UE-22) points, it is necessary to needle deeply into the interosseous spaces, taking care not to needle into the periostreum on either side. By deep needling, we mean at least 1-1.5 cun. In order to do this, one should spread the fingers or toes apart manually while inserting and guiding the needle to its right depth and position.

4. The majority of published research from China on PN is on the oral administration of Chinese medicinals, not acupuncture. Since PN tends to be a root vacuity (commonly qi and yin vacuity) with a branch repletion (blood stasis and/or damp heat impediment), acupuncture alone is not generally considered the standard of care for this condition. Nevertheless, it may be an effective adjunctive therapy.

5. In order to treat blood stasis and damp heat impediment locally more effectively, it is possible to use Chinese medicinal hot foot soaks. One such formula consists of: Herba Siegesbeckiae (*Xi Xian Cao*), 100g, Caulis Milletiae Seu Spatholobi (*Ji Xue Teng*), Caulis Lonicerae Japonicae (*Ren Dong Teng*), and Folium Artemisiae Argyii (*Ai Ye*), 60g each, Cortex Radicis Acanthopanacis Gracilistylis (*Wu Jia Pi*) and Herba Impatientis Balsaminae (*Tou Gu Cao*), 30g each, and Flos Carthami Tinctorii (*Hong Hua*), Radix Sophorae Falvescentis (*Ku Shen*) and Resina Myrrhae (*Mo Yao*), 20g each. These medicinals are boiled twice–the first time in seven times more water than the medicinals for 1.5 hours, the second time in five times as much water for one hour. The resulting two batches of medicinal liquid are combined. This should result in aproximately one liter of medicinal liquid. Bottle and reserve for use. Each time, use 30ml of this liquid in three liters of hot water (40-50° C), soaking both feet for 30 minutes each time, four times per day if possible.

6. Restless leg syndrome, which is also seen in diabetics and hypertensives, is treated according to basically the same pattern discrimination as above with an emphasis on qi and yin vacuity, dampness or damp heat, wind, and blood stasis.

56

Piriformis Syndrome

Piriformis syndrome refers to sciatic nerve pain caused by entrapment or pinching of the sciatic nerve as it exits the greater sciatic notch in the gluteal region. Entrapment in this area is due to myospasm or contracture of either the piriformis or gemellus muscles. The main symptoms of this condition are deep, chronic, nagging aching and pain in the buttock and thigh on the involved side, pain aggravated by sitting, squatting, or walking, possible low back pain, and occasional pain, numbness, and tingling below the knee and into the foot. Many weekend athletes and people who spend long hours sitting are prone to this syndrome. In the athlete's case, it is due to improper stretching and inadequate warm-up exercises as well as over-use during activity. In the case of those who sit for prolonged periods of time, inappropriate posture causes contracture of the piriformis muscle. Females are more prone to this syndrome by a 6:1 ratio.

The Western medical diagnosis of this condition consists of first ruling out lumbar disk herniation. The affected leg is often externally rotated when relaxed, such as when lying face down with one's feet hanging over the edge of the bed or examination table. Various physical examination maneuvers confirm the diagnosis (*e.g.*, Freiberg's maneuver, Pace's maneuver, Beatty's maneuver, and the Mirkin test). The Western medical treatment of this condition mainly consists of stopping any offending exercises or activities. While many clinicians prescribe stretching exercises, the authors of *The Merck Manual* say such exercises are "rarely beneficial."[1] Corticosteroids are sometimes injected into the site where the piriformis muscle crosses the sciatic nerve, presumably reducing fat around the muscle.

Chinese disease categorization: Piriformis syndrome is categorized as *bi feng*, thigh wind, *gu tong*, thigh pain, and *yao tui tong*, low back and leg pain, in Chinese medicine.

Disease causes: External injury and over-taxation combined with former heaven natural endowment insufficiency and aging

Disease mechanisms: Traumatic injury may sever the channels and vessels causing blood stasis and qi stagnation, thus resulting in pain. It is also possible for over-taxation, natural endowment insufficiency, and aging to result in malnourishment of the sinews and vessels, also causing pain. In addition, some Chinese sources also say that piriformis syndrome may be due to wind damp cold impediment hindering and obstructing the free flow of qi and blood, resulting in pain.

Treatment based on pattern discrimination:

1. Qi stagnation & blood stasis pattern

Main symptoms: A history of traumatic injury to the low back and/or hip region, severe pain, enduring pain, pain which is fixed in location, pain which is worse at night, pain extending from the low back to the thigh, possible pain which radiates from the buttock area to the lower part of the thigh and lateral part of the leg, pressure pain, possible pain due to coughing or if the patient strains on his or her thigh, possible palpable cords or hardness in the buttock area, possible restricted movement of the lower limbs, possible systemic symptoms of qi stagnation and blood stasis, such as irritability, premenstrual breast distention and pain, painful menstruation, a dark, sooty facial complexion, a dark, purplish tongue with possible static macules or spots, and a bowstring, choppy pulse

Treatment principles: Quicken the blood and dispel stasis, move the qi and abduct stagnation

Rx: *Shun Qi Huo Xue Tang* (Normalize the Flow of Qi & Quicken the Blood Decoction)

INGREDIENTS: Caulis Perillae Frutescentis (*Su Geng*), 18g, Lingum Sappan (*Su Mu*), 15g, Extremitas Radicis Angelicae Sinensis (*Dang Gui Wei*), 12g, Radix Rubrus Paeoniae Lactiflorae (*Chi Shao*), Semen Pruni Persicae (*Tao Ren*), Fructus Citri Aurantii (*Zhi Ke*), Cortex Magnoliae Officinalis (*Hou Po*), Rhizoma Cyperi Rotundi (*Xiang Fu*), Radix Auklandiae Lappae (*Mu Xiang*), and Fructus Amomi (*Sha Ren*), 9g each, and Flos Carthami Tinctorii (*Hong Hua*), 6g

ANALYSIS OF FORMULA: *Su Geng, Zhi Ke, Hou Po, Xiang Fu, Mu Xiang*, and *Sha Ren* all move the qi and abduct stagnation. When the qi moves, the blood moves. *Dang Gui Wei, Su Mu, Chi Shao, Tao Ren,* and *Hong Hua* all quicken the blood, dispel stasis, and stop pain. In addition, *Dang Gui Wei* and *Su Mu* free the flow of the network vessels and are empirically specific medicinals for traumatic injury.

ADDITIONS & SUBTRACTIONS: For severe pain, especially at night, subtract *Zhi Ke* and *Sha Ren* and add three grams each of Buthus Martensis (*Quan Xie*) and Scolopendra Subspinipes (*Wu Gong*), six grams of Eupolyphaga Seu Opisthoplatia (*Tu Bie Chong*), and nine grams each of Pollen Typhae (*Pu Huang*) and Feces Trogopterori Seu Pteromi (*Wu Ling Zhi*). For pain which is worse with cold and better with warmth, add 12 grams each of Ramulus Cinnamomi Cassiae (*Gui Zhi*) and Radix Angelicae Pubescentis (*Du Huo*) and three grams of Herba Asari Cum Radice (*Xi Xin*). For concomitant kidney vacuity, add nine grams of Cortex Eucommiae Ulmoidis (*Du Zhong*), Radix Dipsaci (*Xu Duan*), and Ramulus Loranthi Seu Visci (*Sang Ji Sheng*). For concomitant qi vacuity, add 15 grams of Radix Astragali Membranacei (*Huang Qi*) and nine grams of Radix Codonopsitis Pilosulae (*Dang Shen*). If there is spasmodic pain, add 18 grams of Radix Albus Paeoniae Lactiflorae (*Bai Shao*).

ACUPUNCTURE & MOXIBUSTION: Bilateral *Xue Hai* (Sp 10), *Zhi Bian* (Bl 54) on the affected side, *a shi* points in the affected area. If there is a visible purple vein in the area of *Wei Zhong* (Bl40), bleed this.

ANALYSIS OF FORMULA: Draining *Xue Hai* quickens the blood and dispels stasis. Draining *Zhi Bian* and *Wei Zhong* moves the qi and frees the flow of the network vessels in the affected area as do any local *a shi* points.

ADDITIONS & SUBTRACTIONS: For low back pain, add *Shen Shu* (Bl 23) and/or *Yao Yang Guan* (GV 3). For pain radiating to the lateral part of the leg, add *Yang Ling Quan* (GB 34) and *Xuan Zhong* (GB 39). For pain radiating to the calf, add *Cheng Shan* (Bl 57). For pain in the lateral part of the feet, add *Kun Lun* (Bl 60) and *Ba Feng* (M-LE-8).

2. LIVER DEPRESSION QI STAGNATION WITH BLOOD VACUITY PATTERN

MAIN SYMPTOMS: Hip and thigh pain which is worse premenstrually or after prolonged inactivity but which is better with exercise, premenstrual breast distention and pain, irritability, fatigue, loose stools, constipation, or alternating diarrhea and constipation, abdominal distention, possible painful menstruation, a pale but dark tongue, and a bowstring, fine pulse

TREATMENT PRINCIPLES: Course the liver and resolve depression, supplement the qi and nourish the blood

Rx: *Xiao Yao San Jia Jian* (Rambling Powder with Additions & Subtractions)

INGREDIENTS: Caulis Milletiae Seu Spatholobi (*Ji Xue Teng*) and Radix Albus Paeoniae Lactiflorae (*Bai Shao*), 18g each, Radix Angelicae Sinensis (*Dang Gui*) and Radix Achyranthis Bidentatae (*Niu Xi*), 12g each, Radix Bupleuri (*Chai Hu*), Cortex Eucommiae Ulmoidis (*Du Zhong*), Rhizoma Atractylodis Macrocephalae (*Bai Zhu*), and Sclerotium Poriae Cocos (*Fu Ling*), 9g each, mix-fried Radix Glycyrrhizae (*Gan Cao*), 6g, and uncooked Rhizoma Zingiberis (*Sheng Jiang*), 3 slices

ANALYSIS OF FORMULA: Within this formula, *Ji Xue Teng, Bai Shao, Dang Gui, Du Zhong*, and *Niu Xi* all supplement the blood and nourish the sinews. In addition, when the liver obtains sufficient blood, it can do its duty of coursing and discharging. *Dang Gui, Ji Xue Teng*, and *Niu Xi* also quicken the blood and transform stasis. *Chai Hu* courses the liver and rectifies the qi. *Bai Zhu, Fu Ling*, and mix-fried *Gan Cao* fortify the spleen and supplement the qi. *Sheng Jiang* helps rectify the qi and harmonize the center as well as harmonizes all the other medicinals in this formula. It assists *Gan Cao* in this latter function.

ADDITIONS & SUBTRACTIONS: If there is marked fatigue, add 15 grams of Radix Astragali Membranacei (*Huang Qi*) and nine grams of Radix Codonopsitis Pilosulae (*Dang Shen*). If there is depressive heat, add nine grams each of Fructus Gardeniae Jasminoidis (*Zhi Zi*) and Cortex Radicis Moutan (*Dan Pi*). If there is damp heat, add nine grams of Radix Scutellariae Baicalensis (*Huang Qin*) and three grams of Rhizoma Coptidis Chinensis (*Huang Lian*) and replace *Sheng Jiang* with six grams of dry Rhizoma Zingiberis (*Gan Jiang*). If there are cold hands and feet, add nine grams of Ramulus Cinnamomi Cassiae (*Gui Zhi*). If there is constipation, add six grams of Radix Et Rhizoma Rhei (*Da Huang*).

ACUPUNCTURE & MOXIBUSTION: Bilateral *Tai Chong* (Liv 3), *Ge Shu* (Bl 17), and *Gan Shu* (Bl 18), *Zhi Bian* (Bl 54), and *Wei Zhong* (Bl40) on the affected side, any *a shi* points in the affected area. If there is a visible purple vein in the area of *Wei Zhong*, bleed this.

ANALYSIS OF FORMULA: When needled with even supplementing-even draining technique, *Tai Chong, Ge Shu,* and *Gan Shu* together course the liver and nourish the blood. Draining *Zhi Bian, Wei Zhong,* and any *a shi* points moves the qi and frees the flow of the network vessels in the affected area.

ADDITIONS & SUBTRACTIONS: If spleen vacuity is marked, add *Pi Shu* (Bl 20) and *Zu San Li* (St 36) with supplementing method to fortify the spleen and supplement the qi. If there is depressive heat, drain *Xing Jian* (Liv 2) either instead of or in addition to *Tai Chong.* If there is heat in the yang ming, drain *Nei Ting* (St 44). For low back pain, add *Shen Shu* (Bl 23) and/or *Yao Yang Guan* (GV 3). For pain radiating to the lateral part of the leg, add *Yang Ling Quan* (GB 34) and *Xuan Zhong* (GB 39). For pain radiating to the calf, add *Cheng Shan* (Bl 57). For pain in the lateral part of the feet, add *Kun Lun* (Bl 60) and *Ba Feng* (M-LE-8).

3. LIVER-KIDNEY YIN VACUITY WITH BLOOD STASIS PATTERN

MAIN SYMPTOMS: Enduring disease in an older, commonly ectomorphic patient, enduring but less severe pain, pain which is worse in the evening and after prolonged inactivity but which is better after moderate exercise, however, pain which is also worse with excessive activity, a liking for pressure or massage in the affected area, dizziness, tinnitus, insomnia, heart palpitations, age spots, dry, scaly skin, low back and knee soreness and weakness, muscle whittling and weakness of the lower limbs, possible dry mouth and throat, possible red tongue with scanty fur or fluids, and a bowstring, fine, possibly rapid pulse

TREATMENT PRINCIPLES: Supplement and nourish the liver and kidneys, quicken the blood and strengthen the low back

RX: *Bu Shen Huo Xue Tang Jia Jian* (Supplement the Kidneys & Quicken the Blood Decoction with Additions & Subtractions)

INGREDIENTS: Cooked Radix Rehmanniae (*Shu Di*), 18g, Radix Angelicae Sinensis (*Dang Gui*) and Semen Cuscutae Chinensis (*Tu Si Zi*), 15g each, Fructus Lycii Chinensis (*Gou Qi Zi*), Radix Achyranthis Bidentatae (*Niu Xi*), and Fructus Psoraleae Corylifoliae (*Bu Gu Zhi*), 12g each, and Fructus Corni Officinalis (*Shan Zhu Yu*), Herba Cistanchis Deserticolae (*Rou Cong Rong*), Resina Myrrhae (*Mo Yao*), Flos Carthami Tinctorii (*Hong Hua*), Radix Gentianae Macrophyllae (*Qin Jiao*), and Cortex Eucommiae Ulmoidis (*Du Zhong*), 9g each

ANALYSIS OF FORMULA: *Shu Di, Niu Xi,* and *Gou Qi Zi* enrich kidney yin and strengthen the bones. *Dang Gui, Shu Di, Gou Qi Zi,* and *Shan Zhu Yu* nourish liver blood and strengthen the sinews. *Tu Si Zi, Bu Gu Zhi, Du Zhong,* and *Rou Cong Rong* warm the kidneys and strengthen the low back. In addition, *Du Zhong* leads the action of the other medicinals to the low back region. *Mo Yao, Hong Hua,* and *Dang Gui* quicken the blood and stop pain. *Qin Jiao* dispels wind dampness and treats impediment pain. Also, *Qin Jiao* leads the action of the other medicinals to the spinal column and limbs.

ADDITIONS & SUBTRACTIONS: If there is marked liver depression qi stagnation, add nine grams of Fructus Meliae Toosendan (*Chuan Lian Zi*) and six grams of Fructus Immaturus Citri Aurantii (*Zhi Shi*). If there is more pronounced blood vacuity, add 15 grams of Caulis Milletiae Seu Spatholobi (*Ji Xue Teng*) and nine grams of Radix Polygoni Multiflori (*He Shou Wu*). If there is concomitant qi vacuity, add 15 grams of Radix Astragali Membranacei (*Huang Qi*) and nine grams each of Radix Codonopsitis Pilosulae (*Dang Shen*) and Radix Dioscoreae Oppositae (*Shan Yao*). If there is fluid dryness constipation, add nine grams each of Semen Cannabis Sativae (*Huo Ma Ren*) and Semen Pruni Persicae (*Tao Ren*). If there is concomitant yang vacuity, add nine grams each of Radix Morindae Officinalis (*Ba Ji Tian*) and Herba Cynomorii Songarici (*Suo Yang*). If there is internal heat, add 9-12 grams of Radix Scutellariae Baicalensis (*Huang Qin*). If there is qi vacuity with muscle whittling and weakness in the lower limbs, add 15 grams of Radix Astragali Membranacei (*Huang Qi*) and nine grams each of Rhizoma Atractylodis Macrocephalae (*Bai Zhu*) and Radix Codonopsitis Pilosulae (*Dang Shen*). If there is spasmodic pain, add 18 grams of Radix Albus Paeoniae Lactiflorae (*Bai Shao*).

ACUPUNCTURE & MOXIBUSTION: Bilateral *Xue Hai* (Sp 10), *San Yin Jiao* (Sp 6), and *Fu Liu* (Ki 7), *Zhi Bian* (Bl 54), *Wei Zhong* (Bl 40), and any locally tender *a shi* points on the affected side

ANALYSIS OF FORMULA: Supplementing *San Yin Jiao* and *Fu Liu* supplements and nourishes the liver and kidneys. Even supplementing-even draining *Xue Hai* quickens the blood and dispels stasis, while the rest of the points move the qi and free the flow of the network vessels in the affected area.

ADDITIONS & SUBTRACTIONS: For pain radiating to the lateral part of the leg, add *Yang Ling Quan* (GB 34) and *Xuan Zhong* (GB 39). For pain radiating to the calf, add *Cheng Shan* (Bl 57). For pain in the lateral part of the feet, add *Kun Lun* (Bl 60) and *Ba Feng* (M-LE-8).

4. WIND COLD DAMP IMPEDIMENT PATTERN

MAIN SYMPTOMS: A cool sensation, heaviness, and pain in

the low back and buttock area, difficulty turning the waist due to this pain, impaired walking, worsening of pain due to damp, cold, or simply changing weather, possible slimy tongue fur, and a deep, slow pulse

TREATMENT PRINCIPLES: Course wind and scatter cold, eliminate dampness and stop pain

RX: *Juan Bi Tang Jia Jian* (Alleviate Impediment Decoction with Additions & Subtractions)

INGREDIENTS: Ramulus Mori Albi (*Sang Zhi*), 15g, Caulis Piperis Futokadsurae (*Hai Feng Teng*), Radix Gentianae Macrophyllae (*Qin Jiao*), Radix Angelicae Sinensis (*Dang Gui*), and Cortex Eucommiae Ulmoidis (*Du Zhong*), 12g each, Radix Et Rhizoma Notopterygii (*Qiang Huo*), Radix Angelicae Pubescentis (*Du Huo*), Radix Ligustici Wallichii (*Chuan Xiong*), Resina Olibani (*Ru Xiang*), and Radix Cyathulae (*Chuan Niu Xi*), 9g each, Ramulus Cinnamomi Cassiae (*Gui Zhi*) and Radix Auklandiae Lappae (*Mu Xiang*), 6g each, and mix-fried Radix Glycyrrhizae (*Gan Cao*), 3g

ANALYSIS OF FORMULA: *Sang Zhi, Hai Feng Teng, Qin Jiao, Qiang Huo, Du Huo, Chuan Xiong,* and *Gui Zhi* together course wind and scatter cold, eliminate dampness and stop pain. *Du Zhong* courses and eliminates wind dampness and stregnthens the low back and reinforces the thigh area. *Dang Gui, Chuan Xiong, Chuan Niu Xi,* and *Ru Xiang* quicken the blood and transform stasis, free the flow of the network vessels and stop pain. *Mu Xiang* moves the qi to help quicken the blood and stops pain. In addition, *Du Huo* and *Chuan Niu Xi* lead the other medicinals to the lower part of the body.

ADDITIONS & SUBTRACTIONS: If there is a severe cold sensation in the affected area, add nine grams each of Radix Lateralis Praeparatus Aconiti Carmichaeli (*Fu Zi*) and Herba Ephedrae (*Ma Huang*). If there is restricted movement of the lower limbs, add 12 grams each of Cortex Erythiniae (*Hai Tong Pi*) and Herba Siegesbeckiae (*Xi Xian Cao*). For concomitant qi vacuity, add 15 grams of Radix Astragali Membranacei (*Huang Qi*) and 12 grams of Radix Codonopsitis Pilosulae (*Dang Shen*). If there is concomitant blood vacuity, add 12 grams each of Radix Albus Paeoniae Lactiflorae (*Bai Shao*) and cooked Radix Rehmanniae (*Shu Di*). For concomitant liver blood-kidney yang vacuity, add nine grams each of Cortex Radicis Acanthopanacis Gracilistylis (*Wu Jia Pi*), Herba Epimedii (*Yin Yang Huo*), and Radix Morindae Officinalis (*Ba Ji Tian*). For concomitant liver blood-kidney yin vacuity, add 12 grams each of Ramulus Loranthi Seu Visci (*Sang Ji Sheng*) and cooked Radix Rehmanniae (*Shu Di*) and replace *Chuan Niu Xi* with Radix Achyranthis Bidentatae (*Niu Xi*).

ACUPUNCTURE & MOXIBUSTION: Bilateral *Qu Chi* (LI 11) and *Yin Ling Quan* (Sp 9), *Zhi Bian* (Bl 54), *Wei Zhong* (Bl 40), and any locally tender *a shi* points on the affected side

ANALYSIS OF FORMULA: Draining *Qu Chi* and *Yin Ling Quan* is a special combination for coursing wind, scattering cold, eliminating dampness, and stopping pain wherever there is impediment pain. Draining *Zhi Bian* and *Wei Zhong* courses and eliminates wind and dampness, diffuses impediment and frees the flow of the network vessels in the affected area as do any local *a shi* points. Draining method and moxibustion should be used for all points.

ADDITIONS & SUBTRACTIONS: For pain radiating to the lateral part of the leg, add *Yang Ling Quan* (GB 34) and *Xuan Zhong* (GB 39). For pain radiating to the posterior part of the calf, add *Cheng Shan* (Bl 57). For pain in the lateral part of the foot, add *Kun Lun* (Bl 60) and *Ba Feng* (M-LE-8).

REMARKS

1. Piriformis syndrome in females is usually due to a combination of liver depression, blood not nourishing the sinews, and blood stasis, with blood vacuity in females mostly being associated with concomitant spleen vacuity. In women in their late 30s and 40s, this combination of patterns is commonly complicated by yin or yin and yang vacuity.

ENDNOTES

[1] Beers, Mark H. & Berkow, Robert, eds., *The Merck Manual*, 17th edition, Merck Research Laboratories, Whitehouse Station, NJ, 1999, p. 503

57

PNEUMONIA

Pneumonia or pneumonitis refers to an acute infection of the lung parenchyma, including the alveolar spaces (bronchopneumonia) and interstitial tissues (interstitial pneumonia). It may also affect an entire lobe (lobar pneumonia) or a segment of a lobe (segemental or lobular pneumonia). Approximately two million Americans develop pneumonia per year and 40-70,000 of these die from this disease. It is the most common hospital-acquired infection and the sixth most common cause of death in the U.S. of all disease categories. Infectious agents causing pneumonia include bacteria, such as *Streptococcus pneumoniae, Staphylococcus aureus, Haemophilus influenzae,* and *Chlamydia pneumoniae, Mycoplasma pneumoniae,* a bacteria-like organism, mycobacteria, such as *Mycobacterium tuberculosis,* fungi, such as *Pneumocystis carinii,* and rickettsiae, such as *Coxiella burnetii.* Parainfluenza virus and influenza viruses A and B may also cause pneumonia. Less frequently, varicella-zoster virus, Epstein-Barr virus, Coxsackie virus, and Hanta virus may be at fault. These are all air-borne, inhaled pathogens. Predisposing factors include upper respiratory viral infections, alcoholism, institutionalization, cigarette-smoking, heart failure, chronic obstructive airway disease, age extremes (in either direction), debility, immuno-compromise, as in diabetes mellitus, compromised consciousness, dysphagia, and exposure to transmissable agents.

The symptoms of pneumonia include cough, fever, and mucus production usually developing over days and possibly accompanied by pleurisy. Physical examination may detect tachypnea and crackles with the bronchial breath sounds. The Western medical diagnosis of pneumonia is based on these characteristic symptoms plus the presence of infiltrates on chest X-ray. Pathogens are identified by culturing expectorated sputum. However, 30-50% of patients have no identifiable pathogen. Western medical treatment consists of respiratory support, including oxygen if indicated, plus antibiotics selected on the basis of Gram stain results, the patient's age, epidemiology, host risk factors, and the severity of the illness.

CHINESE DISEASE CATEGORIZATION: In Chinese medicine, this disease is discussed under *chuan ke,* panting and cough, *fei zhang,* lung distention, *fei yong,* lung abscess (when there is pus production), *shang han,* damage due to cold, and *wen bing,* warm disease.

DISEASE CAUSES: External contraction of evils

DISEASE MECHANISMS: Wind warm evils may enter the mouth and nose, invade the region of the lungs, and develop into this disease. This is what is meant by the saying, "Warm evils contracted above first invade the lungs." However, external invasion by wind cold may also cause this disease. In that case, depression transforms into heat. This heat then congests in the lungs. After external evils invade, they pass from the exterior to the interior and from the superficial part to the deep region. This generally develops according to the warm disease theory of defensive, qi, constructive, and blood. At first, evils are in the lung defensive and an exterior pattern and lung symptoms appear. Then they enter the qi division and there is great heat. At this stage, symptoms of phlegm heat congesting in the lungs appear. If the disease develops further, evils enter and burn the constructive. If these evils are severe, the righteous may not vanquish these evils. Evil heat may thus damage true yin and true yang. In that case, yin fluids are consumed and exhausted or yang qi may become vacuous and desert.

TREATMENT BASED ON PATTERN DISCRIMINATION:

1. WIND HEAT EXTERNAL CONTRACTION PATTERN

MAIN SYMPTOMS: During the initial stage of pneumonia,

there is slight aversion to cold, emission of heat (*i.e.*, fever), slight sweating, cough with white phlegm, possible rapid breathing, chest and rib-side pain, headache, possible nasal congestion, dry mouth leading to drinking, sides of the tongue inflamed and red, thin, white or thin, slightly yellow tongue fur, and a floating, rapid pulse

TREATMENT PRINCIPLES: Resolve the exterior, clear heat, and disperse phlegm

RX: *Ma Xing Shi Gan Tang Jia Wei* (Ephedra, Armeniaca, Gyspum & Licorice Decoction with Added Flavors)

INGREDIENTS: Uncooked Gypsum Fibrosum (*Shi Gao*) and Radix Isatidis Seu Baphicanthi (*Ban Lan Gen*), 15g each, Fructus Forsythiae Suspensae (*Lian Qiao*) and Radix Scutellariae Baicalensis (*Huang Qin*), 12g each, Herba Ephedrae (*Ma Huang*), Semen Pruni Armeniacae (*Xing Ren*), Fructus Trichosanthis Kirlowii (*Gua Lou*), and Cortex Radicis Mori Albi (*Sang Bai Pi*), 9g each, Radix Platycodi Grandiflori (*Jie Geng*), 6g, and Radix Glycyrrhizae (*Gan Cao*), 3g

ANALYSIS OF FORMULA: *Shi Gao* clears lung heat and drains fire, resolves the muscles and engenders fluids. *Ma Huang* diffuses the lungs and resolves the exterior. *Huang Qin, Jie Geng, Gan Cao,* and *Sang Bai Pi* clear the lungs. *Gua Lou* and *Jie Geng* loosen the chest. *Ma Huang, Xing Ren,* and *Sang Bai Pi* diffuse and downbear the lung qi. *Xing Ren, Gua Lou,* and *Jie Geng* disperse phlegm. *Lian Qiao* and *Ban Lan Gen* clear heat both in the defensive and qi divisions. With *Huang Qin*, they also resolve toxins. *Gan Cao* also harmonizes all the other medicinals in the formula.

ADDITIONS & SUBTRACTIONS: If there is severe cough with profuse, thick phlegm, add 30 grams of Herba Houttuyniae Cordatae Cum Radice (*Yu Xing Cao*) and 12 grams each of Pulvis Indigonis (*Qing Dai*) and Concha Cyclinae Meretricis (*Hai Ge Ke*). If oral thirst is severe, add nine grams of Radix Trichosanthis Kirlowii (*Tian Hua Fen*). If there are vexation, agitation, and restlessness, double the *Shi Gao* and add nine grams of Fructus Gardeniae Jasminoidis (*Zhi Zi*). If there is a dry, red tongue with dry lips, add 15 grams of Radix Scrophulariae Ningpoensis (*Xuan Shen*) and 12 grams of uncooked Radix Rehmanniae (*Sheng Di*).

ACUPUNCTURE & MOXIBUSTION: *He Gu* (LI 4), *Qu Chi* (LI 11), *Wai Guan* (TB 5), *Chi Ze* (Lu 5)

ANALYSIS OF FORMULA: Together, draining *He Gu, Qu Chi,* and *Wai Guan* courses wind and clears heat while draining *Chi Ze* clears heat from the lungs.

NOTE: For the treatment of pneumonia, acupuncture must be combined with internally administered medicinals.

ADDITIONS & SUBTRACTIONS: For phlegm, add *Nei Guan* (Per 6) and *Feng Long* (St 40). For chest pain, add *Dan Zhong* (CV 17) and *Nei Guan* (Per 6). For high fever, add *Da Zhui* (GV 14). For severe cough, add *Yu Ji* (Lu 10).

2. WIND COLD EXTERNAL CONTRACTION PATTERN

MAIN SYMPTOMS: Slight fever with no perspiration, aversion to cold, cough, shortness of breath, no particular thirst, thin, white phlegm, thin, white or white, slimy tongue fur, and a floating, tight pulse

TREATMENT PRINCIPLES: Resolve the exterior with acrid, warm medicinals, diffuse the lungs and transform phlegm

RX: *San Ao Tang Jia Jian* (Three [Ingredients] for Twisting Decoction with Additions & Subtractions)

INGREDIENTS: Herba Ephedrae (*Ma Huang*), 12g, Rhizoma Pinelliae Ternatae (*Ban Xia*), 9g, Semen Pruni Armeniacae (*Xing Ren*), Fructus Perillae Frutescentis (*Zi Su Zi*), Semen Raphani Sativi (*Lai Fu Zi*), Semen Sinapis Albae (*Bai Jie Zi*), 9g each, and Pericarpium Citri Reticulatae (*Chen Pi*), 6g

ANALYSIS OF FORMULA: *Ma Huang* courses wind and scatters cold, resolves the exterior and diffuses the lungs. *Ban Xia* transforms phlegm. *Xing Ren, Zi Su Zi, Lai Fu Zi,* and *Bai Jie Zi* disperse phlegm. *Xing Ren, Zi Su Zi,* and *Bai Jie Zi* also diffuse and downbear the lung qi and stop coughing. *Chen Pi* moves the qi to help phlegm transformation.

ADDITIONS & SUBTRACTIONS: If there is counterflow chilling of the four limbs and white, slimy tongue fur, add six grams of Radix Lateralis Praeparatus Aconiti Carmichaeli (*Fu Zi*) and three grams of Herba Asari Cum Radice (*Xi Xin*).

ACUPUNCTURE & MOXIBUSTION: *He Gu* (LI 4), *Wai Guan* (TB 5), *Feng Men* (Bl 12), *Fei Shu* (Bl 13)

ANALYSIS OF FORMULA: Draining *Feng Men* and *Fei Shu* resolves the exterior and diffuses the lungs, disperses phlegm and stops cough. Draining *He Gu* and *Wai Guan* courses wind and scatters cold, promotes sweating and resolves the exterior.

ADDITIONS & SUBTRACTIONS: For absence of sweating, add *Fu Liu* (Ki 7) with supplementing method. For phlegm, add *Nei Guan* (Per 6) and *Feng Long* (St 40). For chest pain, add *Dan Zhong* (CV 17) and *Nei Guan* (Per 6). For severe emission of heat (*i.e.*, fever), add *Da Zhui* (GV 14).

3. PHLEGM HEAT CONGESTING THE LUNGS PATTERN

MAIN SYMPTOMS: Emission of heat (*i.e.*, fever), possibly

high, but no cold or possible cold shivering, possible incessant sweating, oral thirst, cough, chest pain, thick, yellow, pasty phlegm which may contain threads of blood or possibly be an iron-rust color, flaring nostrils, hard breathing, yellow urine, a dry tongue with yellow fur, and a surging, large or slippery, rapid pulse

TREATMENT PRINCIPLES: Clear heat, diffuse the lungs, and transform phlegm

RX: *Ma Xing Shi Gan Tang* (Ephedra, Armeniaca, Gypsum & Licorice Decoction) & *Ting Li Da Zao Xie Fei Tang* (Descurainia & Red Date Drain the Lung Decoction) with additions and subtractions

INGREDIENTS: Gypsum Fibrosum (*Shi Gao*) and Herba Houttuyniae Cordatae Cum Radice (*Yu Xing Cao*), 30g each, Herba Ephedrae (*Ma Huang*), Semen Pruni Armeniacae (*Xing Ren*), Semen Descurainiae Seu Lepidii (*Ting Li Zi*), Cortex Radicis Lycii Chinensis (*Di Gu Pi*), Radix Scutellariae Baicalensis (*Huang Qin*), Cortex Radicis Mori Albi (*Sang Bai Pi*), and *Dai Ge San* (Indigo & Clam Shell Powder),[1] 9g each, and uncooked Radix Glycyrrhizae (*Gan Cao*), 3g

ANALYSIS OF FORMULA: *Shi Gao, Yu Xing Cao, Huang Qin, Sang Bai Pi, Qing Dai, Di Gu Pi,* and *Gan Cao* clear the lungs. *Hai Ge Ke, Xing Ren,* and *Ting Li Zi* disperse phlegm, while *Yu Xing Cao* disperses pus. *Ma Huang, Xing Ren,* and *Sang Bai Pi* diffuse and downbear the lung qi, and *Gan Cao* harmonizes all the other medicinals in the formula.

ADDITIONS & SUBTRACTIONS: If there is concomitant constipation and abdominal distention, add six grams each of Radix Et Rhizoma Rhei (*Da Huang*) and Fructus Immaturus Citri Aurantii (*Zhi Shi*). If the face and lips are cyanotic, add 15 grams of Radix Salviae Miltiorrhizae (*Dan Shen*) and nine grams each of Flos Carthami Tinctorii (*Hong Hua*), Semen Pruni Persicae (*Tao Ren*), and Radix Rubrus Paeoniae Lactiflorae (*Chi Shao*). If there is profuse, thick, yellow phlegm, add six grams of bile-processed Rhizoma Arsiaematis (*Dan Nan Xing*) and nine grams of Bulbus Fritillariae Thunbergii (*Zhe Bei Mu*). If heat toxins are severe, add 12 grams each of Radix Et Rhizoma Polygoni Cuspidati (*Hu Zhang*) and Herba Oldenlandiae Diffusae Cum Radice (*Bai Hua She She Cao*).

ACUPUNCTURE & MOXIBUSTION: *He Gu* (LI 4), *Chi Ze* (Lu 5), *Yu Ji* (Lu 10), *Feng Long* (St 40), *Nei Ting* (St 44)

ANALYSIS OF FORMULA: Draining *Chi Ze* and *Yu Ji* clears heat from the lungs. Draining *He Gu* clears both exterior and interior heat. It also moves the qi to help disperse phlegm. *Nei Ting* is a key point for clearing interior heat, while *Feng Long* is a main point for transforming phlegm. Used together with draining technique, these two points clear and transform phlegm heat.

ADDITIONS & SUBTRACTIONS: For phlegm which is difficult to expectorate, add *Nei Guan* (Per 6). For chest pain, add *Dan Zhong* (CV 17) and *Nei Guan* (Per 6). For high emission of heat (*i.e.*, fever), add *Da Zhui* (GV 14).

4. QI & YIN DUAL VACUITY, PHLEGM & HEAT JOINING & CONTENDING PATTERN

MAIN SYMPTOMS: Cough, low-grade fever, lassitude of the spirit, fatigue, poor appetite, spontaneous perspiration, heart vexation, a fat or tender, red tongue with thin fur, and a fine, rapid pulse

TREATMENT PRINCIPLES: Boost the qi and nourish yin, transform phlegm and dispel stasis

RX: *Sha Shen Mai Dong Tang Jia Jian* (Glehnia & Ophiopogon Decoction with Additions & Subtractions)

INGREDIENTS: Rhizoma Phragmitis Communis (*Lu Gen*), 30g, Semen Coicis Lachryma-jobi (*Yi Yi Ren*) and Concha Arcae Inflatae (*Wa Leng Zi*), 15g each, Radix Adenophorae Strictae (*Nan Sha Shen*), Radix Glehniae Littoralis (*Bei Sha Shen*), and Tuber Ophiopogonis Japonicae (*Mai Dong*), 12g each, and Semen Benincasae Hispidae (*Dong Gua Zi*), Semen Pruni Persicae (*Tao Ren*), Folium Bambusae (*Zhu Ye*), Cortex Radicis Moutan (*Dan Pi*), and Cortex Radicis Lycii Chinensis (*Di Gu Pi*), 9g each

ANALYSIS OF FORMULA: *Nan Sha Shen* and *Bei Sha Shen* both supplement the lung qi. In addition, they and *Mai Men Dong* nourish lung yin. *Lu Gen* and *Zhu Ye* engender fluids. *Lu Gen, Yi Yi Ren, Dong Gua Zi,* and *Tao Ren* all disperse pus and treat lung abscess. *Wa Leng Zi* transforms phlegm. *Di Gu Pi* and *Dan Pi* clear vacuity heat. *Lu Gen* and *Di Gu Pi* clear lung heat. *Dan Pi* also dispels stasis.

ADDITIONS & SUBTRACTIONS: For severe cough, add nine grams each of Radix Stemonae (*Bai Bu*), Folium Eriobotryae Japonicae (*Pi Pa Ye*), and Bulbus Fritillariae Cirrhosae (*Chuan Bei Mu*). For even more marked signs of heat, add nine grams of Pulvis Indigonis (*Qing Dai*). For blood-streaked phlegm, add 12 grams each of Cacumen Biotae Orientalis (*Ce Bai Ye*) and uncooked Radix Rehmanniae (*Sheng Di*).

ACUPUNCTURE & MOXIBUSTION: *Fei Shu* (Bl 13), *Gao Huang Shu* (Bl 43), *He Gu* (LI 4), *Chi Ze* (Lu 5)

ANALYSIS OF FORMULA: Supplementing *Fei Shu* and *Gao Huang Shu* boosts the qi and nourishes lung yin. Draining *He Gu* and *Chi Ze* clears lung heat and disperses phlegm.

ADDITIONS & SUBTRACTIONS: For phlegm, add *Nei Guan* (Per 6) and *Feng Long* (St 40). For chest pain, add *Dan Zhong* (CV 17) and *Nei Guan* (Per 6). For severe emission of heat (*i.e.*, fever), add *Da Zhui* (GV 14).

5. ORIGINAL QI VACUITY DESERTION, YIN & YANG NOT INTERACTING PATTERN

MAIN SYMPTOMS: A somber white facial complexion, cyanotic lips, great perspiration dribbling and dripping, inversion chill of the four limbs, a fine, minute or bound, regularly interrupted pulse

NOTE: This is a critical pattern denoting that evil toxins have fallen inward damaging heart yang.

TREATMENT PRINCIPLES: Secure yang and stem counterflow, quicken the blood and transform stasis

RX: *Shen Fu Tang Jia Wei* (Ginseng & Aconite Decoction with Added Flavors)

INGREDIENTS: Radix Codonopsis Pilosulae (*Dang Shen*), calcined Os Draconis (*Long Gu*), and calcined Concha Ostreae (*Mu Li*), 30g each, Radix Salviae Miltiorrhizae (*Dan Shen*), 15g, Radix Lateralis Praeparatus Aconiti Carmichaeli (*Fu Zi*), Tuber Ophiopogonis Japonici (*Mai Dong*), Fructus Schizandrae Chinensis (*Wu Wei Zi*), Flos Carthami Tinctorii (*Hong Hua*), and Radix Rubrus Paeoniae Lactiflorae (*Chi Shao*), 9g each, and mix-fried Radix Glycyrrhizae (*Gan Cao*) and Ramulus Cinnamomi (*Gui Zhi*), 4.5g each

ANALYSIS OF FORMULA: Within this formula, *Fu Zi* secures yang and stems counterflow. *Dang Shen* and *Gui Zhi* help *Fu Zi* secure both qi and yang. *Long Gu* and *Mu Li* constrain, secure, and stop sweating to avoid further qi desertion. *Wu Wei Zi* helps these latter two stop spontaneous perspiration. In addition, with *Mai Men Dong*, it engenders fluids to engender the pulse. *Dan Shen, Chi Shao, Hong Hua*, and *Gui Zhi* quicken the blood and transform stasis, especially heat stasis. Mix-fried *Gan Cao* boosts and harmonizes the qi.

ACUPUNCTURE & MOXIBUSTION: *Qi Hai* (CV 6), *Guan Yuan* (CV 4), *Nei Guan* (Per 6), *He Gu* (LI 4)

ANALYSIS OF FORMULA: Supplementing *Qi Hai* and *Guan Yuan* with moxibustion secures yang and stems counterflow. *He Gu* secures the qi and the exterior and, therefore, also stops sweating when needled with supplementing method. Draining *Nei Guan* quickens the blood and transforms stasis in order to protect the heart.

REMARKS

1. Although many Chinese clinical manuals also give yin vacuity with lung heat and lung-spleen qi vacuity patterns, strong heat typically consumes both qi and yin. Therefore, these two patterns are rarely seen in their pure forms. In addition, even after righteous qi and yin have become vacuous and weak, there is still usually lingering evil heat and phlegm.

2. If high fever in pneumonia does not recede, in addition to the above decoctions, also administer the Chinese ready-made medicine *Zi Xue Dan* (Purple Snow Elixir), 1g each time, 2-3 times per day.

3. Because the lungs rule the qi of the entire body and the qi moves the blood, serious impairment of the lungs' diffusion and downbearing is often complicated by blood stasis. This is especially so in those who have already been ill a long time, as in so-called walking pneumonia, and the elderly.

4. Most Chinese sources agree that *Ma Xing Shi Gan Tang* is the main formula for use in wind heat and phlegm heat patterns of this disease. In addition, Herba Houttuyniae Cordatae Cum Radice (*Yu Xing Cao*) is regarded as an empirically specific medicinal for most forms of pneumonia, in which case, it is usually administered in relatively large doses. Other empirically effective Chinese medicinals for pneumonia include Radix Et Rhizoma Polygoni Cuspidati (*Hu Zhang*), Radix Isatidis Seu Baphicacanthi (*Ban Lan Gen*), and Herba Taraxaci Mongolici Cum Radice (*Pu Gong Ying*).

5. Pneumonia is usually seen in immune-compromised persons, including drug and alcohol abusers. People with HIV are especially vulnerable to this disease.

ENDNOTES

[1] This is a patent medicine composed of: calcined Concha Cyclinae Meretricis (*Hai Ge Ke*), 180g, and Pulvis Indigonis (*Qing Dai*), 18g.

58

POLYMYOSITIS/DERMATOMYOSITIS

Polymyositis is a systemic connective tissue disease characterized by inflammatory and degenerative changes in the muscles. If these inflammatory and degenerative changes also affect the skin, then it is called dermatomyositis. The etiology of this condition is unknown, and it is a condition that shares many of the same clinical symptoms with scleroderma and SLE. It is less common than these two diseases, but it is not rare. If affects twice as many women as men. Although it can appear at any age, it most commonly occurs in adults from 40-60 and in children from 5-15.

The onset of this condition may be either acute or insidious. Acute infections may precede or incite the initial symptoms which may consist of proximal muscle weakness, muscle pain, rashes, polyarthralgias, Raynaud's phenomenon, dysphagia, fever, and weight loss. Muscle weakness may appear suddenly and progress over weeks and months. Patients may have trouble raising their arms over their heads, climbing stairs, or getting up from a sitting position, eventually becoming wheelchair-bound or bedridden. Typically, the muscles in the hands, feet, and face are not involved. In the late chronic stage, there may be contractures of the limbs.

If there are cutaneous lesions, these are dusky and erythematous. In addition, there may be a butterfly mask on the face similar to SLE. The skin rash may be slightly elevated and either smooth or scaly. Such rash commonly occurs on the forehead, the vee of the neck and shoulders, chest and back, forearms and lower legs, elbows and knees, medial malleoli, and dorsum of the proximal interphalangeal and matecarpophalangeal joints. In addition, the base and sides of the fingernails may be hyperemic. Muscular pain, tenderness, and induration are associated with the rash. Visceral involvement is relatively rare.

In terms of Western medical diagnosis, ESR is frequently elevated. Antinuclear antibodies are found in a few patients, most often in those with another simultaneous connective tissue disease. Serum muscle enzymes, such as the transaminases, creatine kinase, and aldolase are usually elevated. Corticosteriods are the treatment of choice in Western medicine coupled with rest. In terms of prognosis, this varies from long remissions and even apparent recovery to potential death if the viscera are involved.

DISEASE CATEGORIZATION: In general, polymyositis and dermatomyositis are categorized as *wei zheng*, wilting condition, and *bi zheng*, impediment condition in Chinese medicine. Polymyositis is also more particularly referred to traditionally as *ji bi*, flesh impediment, while dermatomyositis is referred to as *pi bi*, skin impediment.

DISEASE CAUSES: Constructive and defensive insecurity with invasion of wind, cold, damp external evils or liver-kidney yin depletion with damp heat

DISEASE MECHANISMS: Due to the constructive and defensive not securing, wind, cold, and/or damp evils may invade externally and lodge internally within the lungs and spleen where they become depressed. This depression may transform into heat brewing within the skin and muscles and flesh where it causes skin redness and muscular pain. If this endures, it may consume the qi and damage the blood, in which case, the qi becomes vacuous and the blood becomes depleted. If heat is severe, it may brew toxins. It is also possible for there to be liver-kidney yin depletion with either externally invading or internally engendered damp heat. This damp heat then congests in the network vessels. Hence the qi and blood become depressed and stagnant and the sinew vessels and muscles lose their nourishment. This can then lead to hand and foot wasting, wilting, and inutility.

TREATMENT BASED ON PATTERN DISCRIMINATION:

1. LUNG HEAT DAMAGING FLUIDS PATTERN

MAIN SYMPTOMS: The disease either arises with the emission of heat (*i.e.*, fever) or limb limpness, weakness, and lack of strength or numbness and insensitivity arise after the fever recedes. The preceding symptoms are accompanied by heart vexation, oral thirst, dry throat, irritated throat, possible cough, scanty, yellow urination, a tendency to dry stools, a red tongue with yellow fur, and a rapid pulse.

TREATMENT PRINCIPLES: Clear heat and moisten dryness, nourish the lungs and engender fluids

RX: *Qing Zao Jiu Fei Tang Jia Jian* (Clear Dryness & Rescue the Lungs Decoction with Additions & Subtractions)

INGREDIENTS: Radix Codonopsitis Pilosulae (*Dang Shen*) and Tuber Ophiopogonis Japonici (*Mai Dong*), 15g each, Gypsum Fibrosum (*Shi Gao*), 30g, decocted first, and Folium Mori Albi (*Sang Ye*), Semen Pruni Armeniacae (*Xing Ren*), Semen Cannabis Sativae (*Ma Ren*), Ramulus Mori Albi (*Sang Zhi*), Radix Angelicae Pubescentis (*Du Huo*), and Radix Achyranthis Bidentatae (*Niu Xi*), 9g each

ANALYSIS OF FORMULA: *Shi Gao* clears the lungs, discharges fire, and engenders fluids. *Dang Shen* boosts the qi and engenders fluids. *Mai Men Dong* clears heat and nourishes yin. *Sang Ye* clears and moistens the lungs and stops cough. *Xing Ren* diffuses the lungs and, with *Huo Ma Ren,* moistens the intestines and frees the flow of the stools. *Sang Zhi* and *Du Huo* free the flow of the network vessels in the upper and lower part of the body. *Niu Xi* quickens the blood, strengthens the sinews, and reinforces the bones.

ADDITIONS & SUBTRACTIONS: If there is high fever, oral thirst, and sweating, increase the amount of *Shi Gao* up to 60 grams and add nine grams each of Rhizoma Anemarrhenae Aspheloidis (*Zhi Mu*), Radix Puerariae (*Ge Gen*), and Fructus Forsythiae Suspensae (*Lian Qiao*). If there's coughing with scanty phlegm, add 15 grams of Fructus Trichosanthis Kirlowii (*Quan Gua Lou*) and nine grams each of Cortex Radicis Mori Albi (*Sang Bai Pi*) and Folium Eriobotryae Japonicae (*Pi Pa Ye*). If there is limb numbness and insensitivity, add nine grams each of Rhizoma Atractylodis (*Cang Zhu*) and Radix Clematidis Chinensis (*Wei Ling Xian*) and 30 grams of Caulis Milletiae Seu Spatholobi (*Ji Xue Teng*).

Once generalized heat has receded completely, if there is decreased eating and drinking, a dry mouth and parched throat, muscle and flesh limpness, weakness, and lack of strength, and a red tongue with scanty fluids, one should use *Yi Wei Tang Jia Wei* (Boost the Stomach Decoction with Added Flavors): Semen Coicis Lachryma-jobi (*Yi Yi Ren*), 21g, Tuber Ophiopogonis Japonici (*Mai Men Dong*) and uncooked Radix Rehmanniae (*Sheng Di*), 15g each, Radix Glehniae Littoralis (*Sha Shen*), 12g, Radix Dioscoreae Oppositae (*Shan Yao*) and Fructus Germinatus Oryzae Sativae (*Gu Ya*), 9g each.

ACUPUNCTURE & MOXIBUSTION: *Chi Ze* (Lu 5), *He Gu* (LI 4), *Fu Liu* (Ki 7), *Zhi Gou* (TB 6), *Yang Ling Quan* (GB 34), *Da Zhu* (Bl 11)

ANALYSIS OF FORMULA: Draining *He Gu* clears heat and moves the qi. Draining *Chi Ze* specifically clears heat from the lungs. Supplementing *Fu Liu* enriches yin and engenders fluids. Draining *Zhi Gou* clears heat from the three burners and frees the flow of the stools. Supplementing *Yang Ling Quan,* the meeting point of the sinews, strengthens the sinews, while supplementing *Da Zhu,* the meeting point of the bones, reinforces the bones.

ADDITIONS & SUBTRACTIONS: For high fever, add *Da Zhui* (GV 14) and *Qu Chi* (LI 11). For fatigue, add *Zu San Li* (St 36).

2. HEAT TOXINS BLAZING & EXUBERANT PATTERN

MAIN SYMPTOMS: The acute stage of dermatomyositis or a whole body condition which is relatively heavy and accompanied by strong fever, dry throat and mouth with a desire to drink, tidal redness and burning heat of the skin of the eyelids and face, dark red macules, burning joint and muscle pain, torpid intake, spirit clouding and vexation and agitation if severe, dry stools, reddish yellow urine, dry, yellow tongue fur, and a bowstring, slippery, rapid pulse

TREATMENT PRINCIPLES: Clear heat, cool the constructive, and resolve toxins

RX: *Qing Wen Bai Du Yin Jia Jian* (Clear the Scourge & Vanquish Toxins Drink with Additions & Subtractions)

INGREDIENTS: Gypsum Fibrosum (*Shi Gao*), 30g, uncooked Radix Rehmanniae (*Sheng Di*), 15g, Rhizoma Anemarrhenae Aspheloidis (*Zhi Mu*), Fructus Forsythiae Suspensae (*Lian Qiao*), Radix Scrophulariae Ningpoensis (*Xuan Shen*), and Cornu Bubali (*Shu Niu Jiao*), 12g each, Radix Rubrus Paeoniae Lactiflorae (*Chi Shao*), Cortex Radicis Moutan (*Dan Pi*), Radix Scutellariae Baicalensis (*Huang Qin*), Fructus Gardeniae Jasminoidis (*Zhi Zi*), and Cortex Phellodendri (*Huang Bai*), 9g each, Caulis Akebiae (*Mu Tong*) and Radix Platycodi Grandiflori (*Jie Geng*), 6g each, and Rhizoma Coptidis Chinensis (*Huang Lian*) and Radix Glycyrrhizae (*Gan Cao*), 3g each

ANALYSIS OF FORMULA: *Shi Gao* and *Zhi Mu* clear heat

from the qi division or aspect, while *Sheng Di, Xuan Shen, Shui Niu Jiao, Chi Shao,* and *Dan Pi* clear heat from the constructive. *Lian Qiao, Huang Lian, Huang Qin, Huang Bai,* and *Zhi Zi* clear heat and resolve toxins. *Jie Geng* guides the other medicinals to the lungs, and *Mu Tong* clears and disinhibits dampness and heat.

ADDITIONS & SUBTRACTIONS: If there is spirit clouding, add the ready-made Chinese medicine *An Gong Niu Huang Wan* (Quiet the Palace Cow Bezoar Pills). If there is constipation, add 3-6 grams each of Radix Et Rhizoma Rhei (*Da Huang*) and Mirabilitum (*Mang Xiao*). For very high fever, add 12-15 grams each of Folium Daqingye (*Da Qing Ye*) and Radix Isatidis Seu Baphicacanthi (*Ban Lan Gen*). For dark, purple skin lesions, add 15 grams of Radix Lithospermi Seu Arnebiae (*Zi Cao*) and nine grams each of Flos Carthami Tinctorii (*Hong Hua*), Semen Pruni Persicae (*Tao Ren*), and Radix Angelicae Sinensis (*Dang Gui*).

ACUPUNCTURE & MOXIBUSTION: *Shi Xuan* (M-UE-1), *He Gu* (LI 4), *Wei Zhong* (Bl 40), *Qu Ze* (Per 3), *Ling Tai* (GV 10)

ANALYSIS OF FORMULA: When pricked to exit 7-10 drops of the blood at each point, the *Shi Xuan* points discharge fire and abate fever. Draining *He Gu* clears heat from the qi division or aspect. When pricked to bleed, *Wei Zhong* and *Qu Ze* clear heat from the constructive aspect and treat skin disease. Draining *Ling Tai* is an empirical treatment for skin diseases due to heat.

ADDITIONS & SUBTRACTIONS: If there is spirit clouding, add *Shui Gou* (GV 26). If there is constipation, add *Zhi Gou* (TB 6). For very high fever, add *Qu Chi* (LI 11), *Da Zhui* (GV 14), and *Wai Guan* (TB 5). For dark, purple skin lesions, add *Xue Hai* (Sp 10) and *Qu Chi* (LI 11).

3. DAMP HEAT SOAKING & SPREADING PATTERN

MAIN SYMPTOMS: Heavy, encumbered extremities, wilting, limpness, and lack of strength, possible simultaneous minor swelling and numbness, condition worse in the lower extremities, possible emission of heat or fever, chest and venter glomus and oppression, short, reddish urination, a red tongue with slimy, yellow or slimy, yellow and white fur, and a soggy, rapid or slippery, rapid pulse

TREATMENT PRINCIPLES: Clear heat and disinhibit dampness, soothe the sinews and quicken the network vessels

RX: *Jia Wei Si Miao San* (Added Flavors Four Wonders Powder)

INGREDIENTS: Semen Coicis Lachryma-jobi (*Yi Yi Ren*), 30g, Rhizoma Dioscoreae Hypoglaucae (*Bei Xie*) and Fructus Chaenomelis Lagenariae (*Mu Gua*), 15g each, and Cortex Phellodendri (*Huang Bai*), Rhizoma Atractylodis (*Cang Zhu*), Radix Achyranthis Bidentatae (*Niu Xi*), Radix Stephaniae Tetrandrae (*HanFang Ji*), Caulis Akebiae (*Mu Tong*), and Excrementum Bombycis Mori (*Can Sha*), 9g each

ANALYSIS OF FORMULA: *Huang Bai, Cang Zhu, Han Fang Ji, Mu Tong,* and *Bei Xie* together clear and disinhibit dampness and heat. *Niu Xi* quickens the blood and strengthens the sinews. In addition, it leads the other medicinals towards the lower limbs. *Can Sha, Mu Gua,* and *Yi Yi Ren* course and eliminate wind and dampness and soothe the sinews.

ADDITIONS & SUBTRACTIONS: If dampness is predominant and there is chest and ductal glomus and oppression, heavy, swollen limbs, glossy, slimy tongue fur, and a soggy pulse, one can add nine grams each of Cortex Magnoliae Officinalis (*Hou Po*), Sclerotium Poriae Cocos (*Fu Ling*), Rhizoma Alismatis (*Ze Xie*), Herba Agastachis Seu Pogostemi (*Huo Xiang*), and Herba Eupatorii Fortunei (*Pei Lan*). If there is numbness and insensitivity of the limbs, inhibited bending and extending, and a purple tongue or static macules and/or spots, add nine grams each of Semen Pruni Persicae (*Tao Ren*), Flos Carthami Tinctorii (*Hong Hua*), Radix Rubrus Paeoniae Lactiflorae (*Chi Shao*), and Radix Salviae Miltiorrhizae (*Dan Shen*). If the limbs are numb and insensitive but also chilly feeling, then omit *Huang Bai* and add nine grams of Ramulus Cinnamomi Cassiae (*Gui Zhi*).

ACUPUNCTURE & MOXIBUSTION: *Nei Ting* (St 44), *Yin Ling Quan* (Sp 9), *Zhong Ji* (CV 3), *Zu San Li* (St 36), local points in the affected area

ANALYSIS OF FORMULA: Together, draining *Nei Ting* and *Yin Ling Quan* clears and disinhibits dampness and heat. Draining *Zhong Ji,* the front *mu* or alarm point of the bladder, helps seep dampness and, therefore, clear heat. Supplementing *Zu San Li* fortifies the spleen and boosts the qi, and spleen vacuity is the main mechanism for the internal engenderment of damp heat. Draining local points regulates and rectifies the qi and blood in the affected area.

ADDITIONS & SUBTRACTIONS: If dampness is predominant and there is chest and venter glomus and oppression with heavy, swollen limbs, add *Zhong Wan* (CV 12) and *San Yin Jiao* (Sp 6). If there is numbness and insensitivity of the limbs, inhibited bending and extending, and a purple tongue or static macules and/or spots, add *Xue Hai* (Sp 10) and *Qu Chi* (LI 11). If the limbs are numb and insensitive but also chilly feeling, add *Guan Yuan* (CV 4) with moxibustion.

4. WIND DAMP HEAT DAMAGING THE BLOOD PATTERN

MAIN SYMPTOMS: Dark red, swollen skin lesions which

may be itchy, generalized pain and weakness which tends to be worse in hot weather, possible hot, swollen, red, painful joints, aggravation of symptoms in women before and during menstruation, a red or pale tongue with red tip and dry or scanty, possibly also slimy at the root, yellow fur, and a fine, slippery, rapid pulse

NOTE: If enduring damp heat fumes and steams and, therefore, consumes and damages yin and blood, it may give rise to the above pattern in which damp heat evils are still exuberant and pronounced.

TREATMENT PRINCIPLES: Disperse wind, clear heat, and dry dampness, nourish and quicken the blood

RX: *Yang Xue Xiao Feng Zao Shi Fang* (Nourish the Blood, Disperse Wind & Dry Dampness Formula)

INGREDIENTS: Cooked Radix Rehmanniae (*Shu Di*), Cortex Radicis Dictamni Dasycarpi (*Bai Xian Pi*), and Fructus Forsythiae Suspensae (*Lian Qiao*), 25g each, Radix Angelicae Sinensis (*Dang Gui*), Radix Rubrus Paeoniae Lactiflorae (*Chi Shao*), Periostracum Cicadae (*Chan Tui*), Cortex Phellodendri (*Huang Bai*), Rhizoma Atractylodis (*Cang Zhu*), Fructus Tribuli Terrestris (*Bai Ji Li*), and Radix Polygoni Multiflori (*He Shou Wu*), 15g each, and Radix Ligustici Wallichii (*Chuan Xiong*), Bombyx Batryticatus (*Jiang Can*), and Radix Glycyrrhizae (*Gan Cao*), 9g each

ANALYSIS OF FORMULA: *Bai Xian Pi, Chan Tui, Bai Ji Li,* and *Jiang Can* course wind and stop itching. *Bai Xian Pi, Lian Qiao, Huang Bai,* and *Cang Zhu* together clear and dry dampness and heat. *Dang Gui, Chi Shao,* and *Chuan Xiong* quicken the blood and transform stasis. *Gan Cao* harmonizes the other medicinals in this formula, while *Shu Di, Dang Gui,* and *He Shou Wu* nourish the blood.

ADDITIONS & SUBTRACTIONS: If there is concomitant blood stasis, add nine grams of Radix Salviae Miltiorrhizae (*Dan Shen*) and 20 grams of Caulis Milletiae Seu Spatholobi (*Ji Xue Teng*). For severe itching, add nine grams each of Zaocys Dhumnades (*Wu Shao She*) and Herba Pycnostelmae (*Xu Chang Qing*). For hot, swollen, red, painful joints, add 12 grams each of Caulis Lonicerae Japonicae (*Ren Dong Teng*), Caulis Sargentodoxae (*Hong Teng*), and Cortex Erythiniae (*Hai Tong Pi*).

ACUPUNCTURE & MOXIBUSTION: *Xue Hai* (Sp 10), *Qu Chi* (LI 11), *Ling Tai* (GV 10), *San Yin Jiao* (Sp 6), local points in the affected area

ANALYSIS OF FORMULA: Draining *Xue Hai* and *Qu Chi* is a special formula for treating skin disorders with itching due to wind and/or damp heat. *Ling Tai* is an empirical point for treating skin diseases due to heat. It should also be drained. Supplementing *San Yin Jiao* nourishes the blood and regulates menstruation. Draining local points in the affected area moves the qi and quickens the blood, thus stopping pain.

ADDITIONS & SUBTRACTIONS: In case of hot, swollen, red, painful joints, add *a shi* points or points selected according to the location of pain. For severe blood vacuity, add *Zu San Li* (St 36) and *Ge Shu* (Bl 17). For concomitant blood stasis, also add *Ge Shu* (Bl 17). For severe itching, add *Feng Shi* (GB 30).

5. SPLEEN-STOMACH VACUITY WEAKNESS PATTERN

MAIN SYMPTOMS: Limb wilting, limpness, and lack of strength which gradually gets worse accompanied by scanty eating, loose stools, facial edema and lack of luster, lassitude of the spirit, a pale, tongue with thin, white fur, and a fine, weak pulse

NOTE: This pattern does not typically manifest by itself in Western patients. Usually, it is complicated by wind cold damp or wind damp heat evils. In fact, it is spleen qi vacuity which causes the defensive qi which allows these evils to invade and enter the body. In addition, when there is spleen vacuity in Western patients, there will essentially always be concomitant liver depression qi stagnation.

TREATMENT PRINCIPLES: Fortify the spleen and boost the qi, nourish the blood and strengthen the sinews

RX: *Shen Ling Bai Zhu San Jia Jian* (Ginseng, Poria & Atractylodes Powder with Additions & Subtractions)

INGREDIENTS: Radix Codonopsitis Pilosulae (*Dang Shen*), 15g, Rhizoma Atractylodis Macrocephalae (*Bai Zhu*), Semen Dolichoris Lablab (*Bai Bian Dou*), Sclerotium Poriae Cocos (*Fu Ling*), Fructus Amomi (*Sha Ren*), decocted later, and Pericarpium Citri Reticulatae (*Chen Pi*), 10g each, Radix Dioscoreae Oppositae (*Shan Yao*) and Semen Coicis Lachryma-jobi (*Yi Yi Ren*), 30g each, and Semen Nelumbinis Nuciferae (*Lian Rou*), Ramulus Loranthi Seu Visci (*Sang Ji Sheng*), and Radix Achyranthis Bidentatae (*Huai Niu Xi*), 15g each

ANALYSIS OF FORMULA: *Dang Shen, Bai Zhu, Bai Bian Dou, Fu Ling, Shan Yao,* and *Lian Zi* together fortify the spleen and boost the qi. *Bai Zhu, Bai Bian Dou, Fu Ling, Yi Yi Ren, Chen Pi,* and *Sha Ren* dry, seep, disinhibit, and/or transform dampness. In addition, *Sha Ren* warms the spleen and *Chen Pi* rectifies the qi. *Sang Ji Sheng* and *Niu Xi* nourish the blood and strengthen the sinews.

ADDITIONS & SUBTRACTIONS: If there is dread of cold and chilled limbs, add 6-9 grams of Radix Lateralis Praeparatus Aconiti Carmichaeli (*Fu Zi*) and nine grams of dry Rhizoma Zingiberis (*Gan Jiang*). If the disease is enduring and the body is weak with qi and blood dual vacuity, one can double the amounts of *Dang Shen*, *Bai Zhu*, and *Shan Yao* and add 15 grams each of Radix Astragali Membranacei (*Huang Qi*) and cooked Radix Rehmanniae (*Shu Di*) and nine grams of Radix Angelicae Sinensis (*Dang Gui*). If there are simultaneous wind cold damp evils, add nine grams each of Radix Clematidis Chinensis (*Wei Ling Xian*), Radix Et Rhizoma Notopterygii (*Qiang Huo*), and Radix Angelicae Pubescentis (*Du Huo*). If there are simultaneous wind damp heat evils, add nine grams each of Radix Gentianae Macrophyllae (*Qin Jiao*), Rhizoma Atractylodis (*Cang Zhu*), and Cortex Phellodendri (*Huang Bai*). If pain is experienced primarily in the upper body, add nine grams each of Rhizoma Curcumae Longae (*Jiang Huang*) and Ramulus Mori Albi (*Sang Zhi*). If pain is primarily experienced in the lower body, add nine grams each of Fructus Chaenomelis Lagenariae (*Mu Gua*) and Radix Angelicae Pubescentis (*Du Huo*). For simultaneous liver depression qi stagnation, add nine grams of Radix Bupleuri (*Chai Hu*) and/or other such qi-rectifying medicinals depending on the main symptoms and locations of qi stagnation. For instance, if there is chest and abdominal oppression and distention, add nine grams of Fructus Citri Aurantii (*Zhi Ke*). If there is breast and rib-side pain, add nine grams of Pericarpium Citri Reticulatae Viride (*Qing Pi*). If there is lower abdominal or menstrual pain, add nine grams of Radix Linderae Strychnifoliae (*Wu Yao*).

ACUPUNCTURE & MOXIBUSTION: *Zu San Li* (St 36), *San Yin Jiao* (Sp 6), *Ge Shu* (Bl 17), *Gan Shu* (Bl 18), *Pi Shu* (Bl 20), *Wei Shu* (Bl 21), *Yang Ling Quan* (GB 34)

ANALYSIS OF FORMULA: Together, supplementing *Zu San Li*, *San Yin Jiao*, *Ge Shu*, *Gan Shu*, *Pi Shu*, and *Wei Shu* fortifies the spleen and boosts the qi, supplements the liver and nourishes the blood. Supplementing *Yang Ling Quan*, the meeting point of the sinews, strengthens the sinews.

ADDITIONS & SUBTRACTIONS: If there is dread of cold and chilled limbs, add *Guan Yuan* (CV 4) with moxibustion. If there are simultaneous wind cold damp evils, add *Qu Chi* (LI 11) and *Yin Ling Quan* (Sp 9). If there are simultaneous wind damp heat evils, add *Yin Ling Quan* (Sp 9), *Qu Chi* (LI 11), and *Nei Ting* (St 44). For simultaneous liver depression qi stagnation, add *Tai Chong* (Liv 3).

6. SPLEEN-KIDNEY YANG VACUITY PATTERN

MAIN SYMPTOMS: Dark red or crimson skin lesions, muscular atrophy, joint pain, cyanosis of the fingertips and toes, emaciation, reduced food intake, fatigue, lassitude of the spirit, lack of strength, abdominal chill, loose stools or daybreak diarrhea if severe, aversion to cold, chilled extremities, low back and knee soreness and weakness, a fat, pale tongue with thin, white fur, and a deep, weak, possibly slow pulse

NOTE: As with the above pattern, this pattern does not usually present in its pure form in Western patients with this condition. It is always accompanied by liver depression, is commonly accompanied by blood stasis (*viz.* the dark red skin lesions and cyanotic fingertips), and there may even be signs and symptoms of lingering wind cold damp or wind damp heat evils.

TREATMENT PRINCIPLES: Supplement the kidneys and invigorate yang, fortify the spleen and boost the qi

RX: *Jin Gui Shen Qi Wan Jia Jian* (*Golden Cabinet* Kidney Qi Pills with Additions & Subtractions)

INGREDIENTS: Rhizoma Alismatis (*Ze Xie*), Herba Epimedii (*Xian Ling Pi*), Radix Morindae Officinalis (*Ba Ji Tian*), and Semen Trigonellae Foeni-graeci (*Hu Lu Ba*), 15g each, cooked Radix Rehmanniae (*Shu Di*), Fructus Corni Officinalis (*Shan Zhu Yu*), Radix Dioscoreae Oppositae (*Shan Yao*), Radix Codonopsitis Pilosulae (*Dang Shen*), and Rhizoma Atractylodis Macrocephalae (*Bai Zhu*), 12g each, Radix Astragali Membranacei (*Huang Qi*) and mix-fried Radix Glycyrrhizae (*Gan Cao*), 9g each, and stir-fried Cortex Radicis Moutan (*Dan Pi*), 6g

ANALYSIS OF FORMULA: *Shu Di*, *Shan Zhu Yu*, *Shan Yao*, *Ze Xie*, and *Dan Pi* are five of the six ingredients of *Liu Wei Di Huang Wan* (Six Flavors Rehmannia Pills), a key formula for enriching kidney yin to grow kidney yang. *Yin Yang Huo*, *Ba Ji Tian*, and *Hu Lu Ba* warm and supplement kidney yang. *Dang Shen*, *Shan Yao*, *Bai Zhu*, *Huang Qi*, and mix-fried *Gan Cao* fortify the spleen and boost the qi.

ADDITIONS & SUBTRACTIONS: For pain primarily in the upper body, add nine grams of Ramulus Cinnamomi Cassiae (*Gui Zhi*). For pain primarily in the lower body, add nine grams of Radix Achyranthis Bidentatae (*Niu Xi*). If there is liver depression qi stagnation, add nine grams each of Radix Bupleuri (*Chai Hu*) and Radix Albus Paeoniae Lactiflorae (*Bai Shao*). If there is concomitant blood stasis, add nine grams of Radix Salviae Miltiorrhizae (*Dan Shen*) and 20 grams of Caulis Milletiae Seu Spatholobi (*Ji Xue Teng*).

ACUPUNCTURE & MOXIBUSTION: *Zu San Li* (St 36), *Shen Que* (CV 8), *Guan Yuan* (CV 4), *Ming Men* (GV 4)

ANALYSIS OF FORMULA: Supplementing *Zu San Li* fortifies the spleen and boosts the qi. Moxaing *Shen Que* warms and supplements spleen yang. With moxibustion and supplementing method, *Guan Yuan* (CV 4) and *Ming Men* (GV 4) warm and supplement kidney yang.

ADDITIONS & SUBTRACTIONS: For cyanosis of the fingertips and toes, add *Ba Xie* (M-UE-22) or *Ba Feng* (M-LE-8). If there is liver depression qi stagnation, add *Tai Chong* (Liv

3). If there is concomitant blood stasis, add *Xue Hai* (Sp 10) and *He Gu* (LI 4).

7. LIVER BLOOD-KIDNEY YIN VACUITY PATTERN

MAIN SYMPTOMS: A relatively long disease course, wilting, limpness, and lack of strength of the four extremities which is especially severe in the lower extremities and which may be accompanied by spasms and cramps and/or numbness of the limbs, low and upper back soreness and weakness, dizziness and tinnitus, seminal emission or menstrual irregularity, a red tongue with scanty fur, and a fine, rapid pulse

TREATMENT PRINCIPLES: Supplement and boost the liver and kidneys, enrich yin and clear heat

RX: *Hu Qian Wan Jia Jian* (Hidden Tiger Pills with Additions & Subtractions)

INGREDIENTS: Os Canis (*Gou Gu*), 30g, cooked Radix Rehmanniae (*Shu Di*) and Plastrum Testudinis (*Gui Ban*), 15g each, and Radix Achyranthis Bidentatae (*Niu Xi*), Herba Cynomorii Songarici (*Suo Yang*), Radix Angelicae Sinensis (*Dang Gui*), Radix Albus Paeoniae Lactiflorae (*Bai Shao*), Radix Dipsaci (*Xu Duan*), Ramulus Loranthi Seu Visci (*Sang Ji Sheng*), Cortex Phellodendri (*Huang Bai*), and Rhizoma Anemarrhenae Aspheloidis (*Zhi Mu*), 9g each

ANALYSIS OF FORMULA: *Shu Di, Niu Xi,* and *Sang Ji Sheng* enrich kidney yin. *Shu Di, Gui Ban, Dang Gui, Bai Shao,* and *Sang Ji Sheng* nourish liver blood. *Suo Yang* and *Xu Duan* supplement kidney yang. *Niu Xi, Sang Ji Sheng, Gui Ban, Xu Duan,* and *Gou Gu* strengthen the sinews and reinforce the bones. *Huang Bai* and *Zhi Mu* clear and downbear vacuity heat.

ADDITIONS & SUBTRACTIONS: If heat is severe, omit *Suo Yang.* If there is simultaneous qi and blood vacuity with a sallow yellow facial complexion, heart palpitations, and insomnia, add 15 grams of Radix Astragali Membranacei (*Huang Qi*), nine grams each of Radix Codonopsitis Pilosulae (*Dang Shen*) and Radix Angelicae Sinensis (*Dang Gui*), and 30 grams of Caulis Milletiae Seu Spatholobi (*Ji Xue Teng*). If, due to enduring disease, yin vacuity has reached yang with dread of cold and chilled limbs, impotence, a pale tongue, and a deep pulse, omit *Zhi Mu* and *Huang Bai* and add nine grams each of Cornu Cervi (*Lu Jiao Pian*), Fructus Psoraleae Corylifoliae (*Bu Gu Zhi*), Herba Epimedii (*Xian Ling Pi*), Radix Morindae Officinalis (*Ba Ji Tian*), Radix Lateralis Praeparatus Aconiti Carmichaeli (*Fu Zi*), and/or Cortex Cinnamomi Cassiae (*Rou Gui*).

ACUPUNCTURE & MOXIBUSTION: *Fu Liu* (Ki 7), *Gan Shu* (Bl 18), *Pi Shu* (Bl 20), *Shen Shu* (Bl 23)

ANALYSIS OF FORMULA: Supplementing *Fu Liu,* the metal-mother point of the kidney channel, supplements the kidneys, enriches yin, and engenders fluids. Supplementing *Gan Shu,* the back transport point of the liver, nourishes the blood and yin of the liver. Supplementing *Pi Shu,* the back transport point of the spleen, boosts the latter heaven to support the former heaven. Supplementing *Shen Shu,* the back transport point of the kidneys, nourishes and enriches the yin essence of the kidneys.

ADDITIONS & SUBTRACTIONS: If vacuity heat is severe, add *Ran Gu* (Ki 2). If there is simultaneous qi and blood vacuity with a sallow yellow facial complexion, heart palpitations, and insomnia, add *Ge Shu* (Bl 17) and *Xin Shu* (Bl 15). If, due to enduring disease, yin vacuity has reached yang with dread of cold and chilled limbs, impotence, a pale tongue, and a deep pulse, add *Ming Men* (GV 4) with moxibustion.

8. STATIC BLOOD OBSTRUCTING THE NETWORK VESSELS PATTERN

MAIN SYMPTOMS: Enduring polymyositis/dermatomyositis with marked Raynaud's phenomenon or skin and flesh sclerosis, possible accompanying tumors or static lumps within the abdomen, wilting and weakness of the four extremities, numbness and insensitivity of the hands and feet, spasmodic pain in the body and limbs, purplish red macules, a purple tongue or possible static macules or spots, and a fine, choppy pulse

NOTE: This pattern does not typically present in the pure form described above. Rather, blood stasis tends to complicate most chronic, enduring patterns of this disease.

TREATMENT PRINCIPLES: Boost the qi and nourish the constructive, quicken the blood and free the flow of the network vessels

NOTE: The principles of boosting the qi and nourishing the constructive are added to this pattern because static blood impedes the engenderment of fresh or new blood and the blood is the mother of the qi.

RX: *Sheng Yu Tang Jia Wei* (Sagely Healing Decoction with Added Flavors)

INGREDIENTS: Cooked Radix Rehmanniae (*Shu Di*) and uncooked Radix Rehmanniae (*Sheng Di*), 12g each, Semen Pruni Persicae (*Tao Ren*), Flos Carthami Tinctorii (*Hong Hua*), Radix Achyranthis Bidentatae (*Niu Xi*), Radix Panacis Ginseng (*Ren Shen*), and Radix Ligustici Wallichii (*Chuan Xiong*), 9g each, and Radix Angelicae Sinensis (*Dang Gui*) and Radix Astragali Membranacei (*Huang Qi*), 1.5g each

ANALYSIS OF FORMULA: *Tao Ren, Hong Hua, Chuan Xiong, Sheng Di,* and *Dang Gui* quicken the blood and transform stasis. *Shu Di*, *Sheng Di*, *Niu Xi*, and *Dang Gui* nourish the blood. *Ren Shen* and *Huang Qi* boost the qi.

ACUPUNCTURE & MOXIBUSTION: *Ge Shu* (Bl 17), *Xue Hai* (Sp 10), *San Yin Jiao* (Sp 6), *Zu San Li* (St 36)

ANALYSIS OF FORMULA: *Ge Shu* is the meeting point of the blood, and *Xue Hai* is the "sea of the blood." Therefore, draining these two points quickens the blood and transforms stasis. *San Yin Jiao* nourishes the blood, while *Zu San Li* supplements the spleen and boosts the qi.

ADDITIONS & SUBTRACTIONS: For cyanosis of the fingertips and toes, add *Ba Xie* (M-UE-22) or *Ba Feng* (M-LE-8). If there is liver depression qi stagnation, add *Tai Chong* (Liv 3).

REMARKS

1. As with most other autoimmune diseases, polymyositis/dermatomyositis is most commonly found in females, and females, due to menstruation, gestation, and lactation, are more apt to exhibit spleen vacuity than men. Such spleen vacuity tends to become more pronounced at around 35 years of age in women. Because the spleen becomes vacuous and weak and, therefore, does not engender and transform blood as abundantly as before, the liver tends to become or become more depressed. If spleen qi vacuity reaches the kidneys, spleen qi vacuity will evolve into spleen-kidney yang vacuity. If liver blood vacuity reaches the kidneys, liver blood vacuity will evolve into kidney yin vacuity. As it is said, "Yin is automatically half at 40 years of age." Because yin and yang are mutually rooted, vacuity of one will commonly involve at least some element or lead to vacuity of the other. Thus, in real-life clinical practice, it is not uncommon to see Western women in their 40s with autoimmune diseases who display liver depression qi stagnation and spleen qi, liver blood, and kidney yin and yang vacuities. Because of the interrelationships between the qi, blood, and fluids and humors, these five patterns may also be complicated by blood stasis, damp accumulation, phlegm obstruction, and/or some kind of evil heat. In such complicated, multi-pattern scenarios, which are the rule rather than the exception, one must treat all of these disease mechanisms at the same time since they are all mutually engendering.

2. Whenever enduring disease has caused blood stasis in the network vessels, one must use medicinals which quicken the blood and free the flow of the network vessels. Such medicinals generally belong to one of three categories: 1) worm and insect medicinals, *e.g.*, Buthus Martensis (*Quan Xie*), Scolopendra Subspinipes (*Wu Gong*), and Zaocys Dhumnades (*Wu Shao She*), 2) tree saps and resins, *e.g.*, Resina Olibani (*Ru Xiang*), Resina Myrrhae (*Mo Yao*), and Sanguis Draconis (*Xue Jie*), and 3) medicinals which are network-like in form, *e.g.*, Fasciculus Vascularis Luffae Cylindricae (*Si Gua Luo*) and Fasciculus Vascularis Citri Reticulatae (*Ju Luo*). When dealing with rheumatic complaints, the worm and insect medicinals are usually the most effective of these three categories.

3. During the initial stage of skin lesions, one can make a wash out of 30 grams of Herba Impatientis Balsaminae (*Tou Gu Cao*), 25 grams of Ramulus Cinnamomi Cassiae (*Gui Zhi*), and nine grams of Flos Carthami Tinctorii (*Hong Hua*). Decoct these three medicinals in water and use the resulting medicinal liquid as an external wash applied warm one time per day.

4. *Er Shen Er Teng Tang* (Two Roots & Two Vines Decoction) treats dermatomyositis presenting as qi, blood, and yin vacuity with blood stasis and heat toxins: Caulis Milletiae Seu Spatholobi (*Ji Xue Teng*) and Caulis Trachelospermi Jasminoidis (*Luo Shi Teng*), 30g each, Radix Astragali Membranacei (*Huang Qi*), 20g, Radix Codonopsitis Pilosulae (*Dang Shen*), Radix Glehniae Littoralis (*Sha Shen*), and uncooked Radix Rehmanniae (*Sheng Di*), 15g each, and Cortex Radicis Moutan (*Dan Pi*) and Radix Lithospermi Seu Arnebiae (*Zi Cao*), 12g each. During the initial stage with fever, throat pain, red macules, and red tongue, add 12 grams each of Folium Daqingye (*Da Qing Ye*) and Flos Lonicerae Japonicae (*Jin Yin Hua*) and 18-30 grams of Herba Taraxaci Mongolici Cum Radice (*Pu Gong Ying*). For muscle pain and aversion to cold due to concomitant yang vacuity with wind damp evils, add nine grams each of Radix Lateralis Praeparatus Aconiti Carmichaeli (*Fu Zi*), Herba Epimedii (*Yin Yang Huo*), and Radix Et Rhizoma Notopterygii (*Qiang Huo*). For enduring disease leading to blood stasis, add nine grams each of Radix Salviae Miltiorrhizae (*Dan Shen*) and Flos Carthami Tinctorii (*Hong Hua*).

59

POSTCONCUSSION SYNDROME

Postconcussion syndrome is made up of a wide variety of symptoms, such as headache and impaired memory, even though no defect can be demonstrated objectively. After a mild head injury, there is headache, dizziness, difficulty concentrating, depression, apathy, and anxiety. These symptoms can cause considerable disability and tend to be worse than after severe head injury. The part of the brain damaged is unclear, and this syndrome is more common in those with a premorbid neurotic disposition. The results of treatment with Western drugs and psychotherapy vary.

CHINESE DISEASE CATEGORIZATION: The symptoms of postconcussion syndrome fall under the Chinese medical disease categories of *tou tong*, headache, *tou xuan*, dizziness, *jian wang*, forgetfulness, *yu zheng*, depression, *nan si*, difficulty thinking, *shen si huang hu*, abstraction of the spirit, and *you*, anxiety.

DISEASE CAUSES: External injury to the region of the head

DISEASE MECHANISMS: External injury to the head results in severing the channels and vessels in the local region. Since the vessels promote the movement of the blood, extravasated blood becomes static. This static blood may obstruct the clear orifices of the head, thus resulting in unclear thinking and speech, headache, dizziness, etc. Since the qi moves the blood and qi and blood travel together, static blood impedes the free flow of the qi. Hence blood stasis may be complicated by the symptoms of qi stagnation, such as irritability and depression. Qi stagnation may then lead to ascendant hyperactivity of liver yang, thus giving rise to dizziness, emotional rashness, vexation and agitation, and a pounding headache. Qi stagnation may also lead to spleen vacuity if a replete liver assails spleen earth, while spleen qi vacuity may lead to heart blood vacuity. In that case, there will be heart palpitations, anxiety, forgetfulness, and difficulty thinking. Static blood may also block kidney essence from filling the sea of marrow, *i.e.*, the brain. In that case, there will be difficulty thinking, dizziness, tinnitus, deafness, etc.

TREATMENT BASED ON PATTERN DISCRIMINATION:

1. STASIS OBSTRUCTING THE ORIFICES OF THE BRAIN PATTERN

MAIN SYMPTOMS: After an acute traumatic head injury, there is unclear thinking, spirit mind haziness and clouding, unclear speech, vexation, agitation, and restlessness, headache, dizziness, a dark facial complexion, a dark, purplish tongue, and a bowstring, choppy or fine, choppy pulse. These symptoms may be worse at night.

TREATMENT PRINCIPLES: Free the flow of the orifices and quicken the blood, arouse the spirit and open the orifices

RX: *Tong Qiao Huo Xue Tang Jia Wei* (Free the Flow of the Orifices & Quicken the Blood Decoction with Added Flavors)

INGREDIENTS: Radix Ligustici Wallichii (*Chuan Xiong*), Bulbus Allii Fistulosi (*Cong Bai*), and Semen Pruni Persicae (*Tao Ren*), 15g each, Flos Carthami Tinctorii (*Hong Hua*), 12g, Radix Rubrus Paeoniae Lactiflorae (*Chi Shao*), Feces Trogopterori Seu Pteromi (*Wu Ling Zhi*), and Fructus Viticis (*Man Jing Zi*), 9g each, uncooked Rhizoma Zingiberis (*Sheng Jiang*), 3 slices, Fructus Zizyphi Jujubae (*Da Zao*), 7 pieces, and Secretio Moschi Moschiferi (*She Xiang*), 0.15g

ANALYSIS OF FORMULA: Within this formula, *Chi Shao, Chuan Xiong, Tao Ren*, and *Hong Hua* are the main medicinals which quicken the blood and transform stasis. *Sheng Jiang, Cong Bai*, and *She Xiang* move, scatter, run, and scurry. Hence they strengthen the effects of the blood-quickening medicinals. *Wu Ling Zhi* and *Man Jing Zi* move the qi and stop pain, especially in the area of the head. *Da Zao* harmonizes the blood and nourishes yin. When all these medicinals are used together, they have the effect of quickening the blood and freeing the flow of the orifices, moving stasis and freeing the flow of the channels.

ADDITIONS & SUBTRACTIONS: One can substitute 15 grams each of Radix Angelicae Dahuricae (*Bai Zhi*) and Lumbricus (*Di Long*) for *Cong Bai* and *She Xiang*. For headache and dizziness complicated by dry, bound stools, add 12 grams of Concha Haliotidis (*Shi Jue Ming*), nine grams each of Rhizoma Gastrodiae Elatae (*Tian Ma*), Rhizoma Acori Graminei (*Shi Chang Pu*), and Ramulus Uncariae Cum Uncis (*Gou Teng*), and six grams of Radix Et Rhizoma Rhei (*Da Huang*). For insomnia, add 12 grams each of Radix Polygalae Tenuifoliae (*Yuan Zhi*) and Semen Zizyphi Spinosae (*Suan Zao Ren*). For severe headache and unclear thinking and speech, add three grams each of Buthus Martensis (*Quan Xie*), Scolopendra Subspinipes (*Wu Gong*), and Eupolyphaga Seu Opisthoplatia (*Tu Bie Chong*), powdered and taken with the strained decoction. For enduring disease which has damaged the righteous, add 15 grams of Radix Astragali Membranacei (*Huang Qi*) and nine grams of Radix Angelicae Sinensis (*Dang Gui*).

ACUPUNCTURE & MOXIBUSTION: *Feng Chi* (GB 20), *Feng Fu* (GV 16), *Bai Hui* (GV 20), *Si Shen Cong* (M-HN-1), *He Gu* (LI 4), *San Yin Jiao* (Sp 6)

ANALYSIS OF FORMULA: Draining *Feng Chi*, *Feng Fu*, *Bai Hui*, and *Si Shen Cong* quickens the blood and frees the flow of the network vessels in the brain, arouses the spirit and opens the orifices. Draining *He Gu*, the master point of the face and head, moves the qi, while *San Yin Jiao* quickens the blood. Together, they transform stasis throughout the whole body.

ADDITIONS & SUBTRACTIONS: For insomnia, impaired memory, and unclear speech, add *Shen Ting* (GV 24) and *Ben Shen* (GB 13). For vexation, agitation, and restlessness, add *Yong Quan* (Ki 1) and *Da Dun* (Liv 1). For severe blood stasis, add *Ge Shu* (Bl 17).

2. QI & BLOOD STASIS & STAGNATION PATTERN

MAIN SYMPTOMS: Emotional lability, spirit mind torpor and stagnation, emotional depression, scanty speech or no speech, difficulty thinking or slow thinking, decreased memory power, and piercing headache following a traumatic injury to the head, accompanied by chest and rib-side distention and pain, a dark red tongue with possible static macules or spots and thin, white or yellow fur, and a bowstring, choppy pulse

TREATMENT PRINCIPLES: Rectify the qi and resolve depression, quicken the blood and transform stasis

RX: *Xiao Yao San Jia Wei* (Rambling Powder with Added Flavors)

INGREDIENTS: Herba Eupatorii Fortunei (*Pei Lan*), 15g, Radix Bupleuri (*Chai Hu*), Radix Angelicae Sinensis (*Dang Gui*), Radix Rubrus Paeoniae Lactiflorae (*Chi Shao*), Rhizoma Atractylodis Macrocephalae (*Bai Zhu*), Sclerotium Poriae Cocos (*Fu Ling*), Flos Carthami Tinctorii (*Hong Hua*), Semen Pruni Persicae (*Tao Ren*), and blast-fried Rhizoma Zingiberis (*Pao Jiang*), 9g each, and Herba Menthae Haplocalycis (*Bo He*) and mix-fried Radix Glycyrrhizae (*Gan Cao*), 6g each

ANALYSIS OF FORMULA: Within this formula, *Dang Gui* and *Chi Shao* quicken the blood and transform stasis, nourish the blood and soften the liver. *Chai Hu* courses the liver and resolves depression. *Fu Ling*, *Bai Zhu*, and mix-fried *Gan Cao* fortify the spleen and seep dampness. *Pao Jiang*, when combined with *Dang Gui* and *Chi Shao*, regulates and harmonizes the qi and blood. When combined with *Bo He*, it lessens that medicinal's coursing, scattering, outthrusting nature. *Pei Lan*, *Hong Hua*, and *Tao Ren* quicken the blood and transform stasis, arouse the brain and open the orifices.

ADDITIONS & SUBTRACTIONS: If headache is severe, add six grams each of Buthus Martensis (*Quan Xie*) and Bombyx Batryticatus (*Jiang Can*) to quicken the blood and free the flow of the network vessels. If dizziness and heavy-headedness are marked, add nine grams each of Rhizoma Curcumae (*Yu Jin*) and Rhizoma Acori Graminei (*Shi Chang Pu*). If there is a bitter taste in the mouth, vexation and agitation, and emotional lability, add three grams of Rhizoma Coptidis Chinensis (*Huang Lian*) and nine grams of Folium Bambusae (*Zhu Ye*). If spleen vacuity is pronounced with fatigue and bodily weakness, add 15 grams of Radix Astragali Membranacei (*Huang Qi*) and nine grams of Radix Codonopsitis Pilosulae (*Dang Shen*). If there is more pronounced yin and blood vacuity, add 12 grams each of cooked Radix Rehmanniae (*Shu Di*) and Radix Polygoni Multiflori (*He Shou Wu*). If there are marked cold hands and feet, add nine grams of Ramulus Cinnamomi Cassiae (*Gui Zhi*).

ACUPUNCTURE & MOXIBUSTION: *Feng Chi* (GB 20), *Feng Fu* (GV 16), *Bai Hui* (GV 20), *Si Shen Cong* (M-HN-1), *Jian Shi* (Per 5), *Tai Chong* (Liv 3)

ANALYSIS OF FORMULA: Draining *Feng Chi*, *Feng Fu*, *Bai Hui*, and *Si Shen Cong* quickens the blood and frees the flow of the network vessels in the brain, arouses the spirit and opens the orifices. Draining *Jian Shi* and *Tai Chong* rectifies the qi and resolves depression.

ADDITIONS & SUBTRACTIONS: If there is a bitter taste in the mouth, vexation and agitation, and emotional lability, add *Gan Shu* (Bl 18) and *Hun Men* (Bl 47). If spleen vacuity is pronounced with fatigue and bodily weakness, add *Zu San Li* (St 36). If there is more pronounced yin and blood vacuity, add *San Yin Jiao* (Sp 6). If there are marked cold hands and feet, add *Guan Yuan* (CV 4) with moxibustion. For insomnia, impaired memory, and unclear speech, add *Shen Ting* (GV 24) and *Ben Shen* (GB 13). For vexation, agitation, and restlessness, add *Yong Quan* (Ki 1) and *Da Dun* (Liv 1). For severe blood stasis, add *Ge Shu* (Bl 17).

3. ASCENDANT LIVER YANG HYPERACTIVITY PATTERN

MAIN SYMPTOMS: Emotional impetuosity and rashness, vexation, agitation, and restlessness, easy anger and irritability, pounding headache, and possible vomiting of white foam or bitter bile following a traumatic injury to the head, plus a dark red tongue with yellow fur, and a bowstring, rapid pulse

TREATMENT PRINCIPLES: Level the liver and subdue yang, quicken the blood and transform stasis

RX: *Ling Jiao Gou Teng Tang Jia Jian* (Antelope Horn & Uncaria Decoction with Additions & Subtractions)

INGREDIENTS: Ramulus Uncariae Cum Uncis (*Gou Teng*), uncooked Radix Rehmanniae (*Sheng Di*), and Radix Albus Paeoniae Lactiflorae (*Bai Shao*), 30g each, Folium Mori Albi (*Sang Ye*), Flos Chrysanthemi Morifolii (*Ju Hua*), and Sclerotium Pararadicis Poriae Cocos (*Fu Shen*), 15g each, Caulis Bambusae In Taeniis (*Zhu Ru*), 12g, Semen Pruni Persicae (*Tao Ren*), Flos Carthami Tinctorii (*Hong Hua*), Bulbus Fritillariae Thunbergii (*Zhe Bei Mu*), Cornu Caprae (*Shan Yang Jiao*), and Radix Salviae Miltiorrhizae (*Dan Shen*), 9g each, and Radix Glycyrrhizae (*Gan Cao*), 6g

ANALYSIS OF FORMULA: Within this formula, *Shan Yang Jiao* levels the liver, extinguishes wind, and clears heat. *Gou Teng* clears heat and levels the liver, extinguishes wind and stabilizes fright. When these two medicinals are combined together, they have a strong effect for clearing heat and cooling the liver, extinguishing wind and stopping tetany. They are the ruling medicinals in this formula. *Sang Ye* and *Ju Hua* assist the main medicinals in clearing heat and extinguishing wind. When yang becomes hyperactive, it engenders fire, and, when fire becomes effulgent, it engenders wind. When wind and fire combine, they damage and consume yin fluids. Therefore, *Bai Shao*, *Sheng Di*, and *Gan Cao* enrich and nourish yin fluids. When yang heat becomes hyperactive and exuberant, it easily burns the fluids and engenders phlegm. Hence *Zhu Ru* and *Zhe Bei Mu* clear heat and transform phlegm. If heat becomes internally depressed and exuberant, it may ascend to harass the spirit. Thus *Fu Shen* calms the heart and quiets the spirit. *Hong Hua*, *Tao Ren*, and *Dan Shen* quicken the blood and transform stasis to treat retained and stagnating vanquished blood.

ADDITIONS & SUBTRACTIONS: If there is vexation, agitation, and restlessness, add 12 grams each of uncooked Frusta Ferri (*Tie Luo*), Os Draconis (*Long Gu*), and Concha Ostreae (*Mu Li*) to heavily settle and quiet the spirit. If there is nausea, vomiting, and constipation, add nine grams of Haemititum (*Dai Zhe Shi*) and six grams of Radix Et Rhizoma Rhei (*Da Huang*). If there are epileptiform symptoms, add nine grams each of Buthus Martensis (*Quan Xie*), Bombyx Batryticatus (*Jiang Can*), Lumbricus (*Di Long*), and Rhizoma Gastrodiae Elatae (*Tian Ma*). For severe headache, add 12 grams each of Radix Angelicae Dahuricae (*Bai Zhi*) and Tuber Curcumae (*Yu Jin*) and nine grams of Spica Prunellae Vulgaris (*Xia Ku Cao*). For insomnia and restlessness, add 12 grams each of Caulis Polygoni Multiflori (*Ye Jiao Teng*), Flos Albizziae Julibrissinis (*He Huan Hua*), and Semen Zizyphi Spinosae (*Suan Zao Ren*). For mental depression, anger without reason, and frequent worry, add 15 grams each of Fructus Zizyphi Jujubae (*Da Zao*), Semen Levis Tritici Aestivi (*Xiao Mai*), Cortex Albizziae Julibrissinis (*He Huan Pi*), and Rhizoma Acori Graminei (*Shi Chang Pu*) and nine grams of Herba Menthae Haplocalysis (*Bo He*).

ACUPUNCTURE & MOXIBUSTION: *Feng Chi* (GB 20), *Feng Fu* (GV 16), *Bai Hui* (GV 20), *Si Shen Cong* (M-HN-1), *Tai Chong* (Liv 3), *Yong Quan* (Ki 1)

ANALYSIS OF FORMULA: Draining *Feng Chi*, *Feng Fu*, *Bai Hui*, and *Si Shen Cong* quickens the blood and frees the flow of the network vessels in the brain, quiets the spirit and opens the orifices. Draining *Yong Quan*, *Feng Chi*, and *Tai Chong* levels the liver and subdues yang.

ADDITIONS & SUBTRACTIONS: If there is vexation, agitation, and restlessness, add *Gan Shu* (Bl 18) and *Hun Men* (Bl 47). If there is nausea, vomiting, and constipation, add *Nei Guan* (Per 6) and *Zhi Gou* (TB 6). If there are epileptiform symptoms, add *He Gu* (LI 4) and *Da Zhui* (GV 14). For insomnia, impaired memory, and unclear speech, add *Shen Ting* (GV 24) and *Ben Shen* (GB 13).

4. HEART-SPLEEN DEPRESSION PATTERN

MAIN SYMPTOMS: Fatigue, forgetfulness, heart palpitations, worry and anxiety, depression, irritability, possible headaches, and dizziness following a traumatic head injury accompanied by insomnia, a pale white or sallow yellow facial complexion, pale lips and fingernails, cold hands and feet, possible loose stools, a pale but slightly dark, enlarged tongue with possible centerline crease and thin fur, and a bowstring, fine, moderate (*i.e.*, slightly slow) pulse

NOTE: This pattern describes a heart blood-spleen qi vacuity complicated by liver depression qi stagnation.

TREATMENT PRINCIPLES: Nourish the heart and fortify the spleen, rectify the qi and resolve depression

RX: *Gui Pi Tang Jia Wei* (Restore the Spleen Decoction with Added Flavors)

INGREDIENTS: Radix Astragali Membranacei (*Huang Qi*), 15g, Semen Zizyphi Spinosae (*Suan Zao Ren*), 12g, Radix Codonopsitis Pilosulae (*Dang Shen*), Radix Angelicae Sinensis (*Dang Gui*), Arillus Euphoriae Longanae (*Long Yan Rou*), Rhizoma Atractylodis Macrocephalae (*Bai Zhu*), Sclerotium Poriae Cocos (*Fu Ling*), Fructus Alpiniae Oxyphyllae (*Yi Zhi Ren*), and Radix Polygalae Tenuifoliae (*Yuan Zhi*), 9g each, Rhizoma Acori Graminei (*Shi Chang Pu*), Radix Auklandiae Lappae (*Mu Xiang*), and mix-fried Radix Glycyrrhizae (*Gan Cao*), 6g each, uncooked Rhizoma Zingiberis (*Sheng Jiang*), 2 slices, and Fructus Zizyphi Jujubae (*Da Zao*), 3-5 pieces

ANALYSIS OF FORMULA: Within this formula, *Huang Qi*, *Dang Shen*, *Bai Zhu*, *Fu Ling*, and mix-fried *Gan Cao* all fortify the spleen and supplement the qi. *Dang Gui*, *Da Zao*, *Suan Zao Ren*, and *Long Yan Rou* supplement the heart and nourish the blood. *Yuan Zhi* and *Mu Xiang* rectify the qi and resolve depression. *Yuan Zhi* also supplements the heart, promotes the interaction between the heart and kidneys, and transforms phlegm, while *Mu Xiang* harmonizes the liver and spleen. *Shi Chang Pu* arouses the brain and opens the orifices. *Yi Zhi Ren* warms the spleen and kidneys as well as boosts the intelligence. *Sheng Jiang*, *Gan Cao*, and *Da Zao* harmonize all the medicinals in the formula. In addition, *Sheng Jiang* moves the qi and transforms dampness.

ADDITIONS & SUBTRACTIONS: If there is concomitant blood stasis, add nine grams each of Semen Pruni Persicae (*Tao Ren*), Flos Carthami Tinctorii (*Hong Hua*), and Radix Salviae Miltiorrhizae (*Dan Shen*). If liver depression is pronounced, add nine grams of Radix Bupleuri (*Chai Hu*). If there is depressive heat in the stomach and heart, add 3-6 grams of Rhizoma Coptidis Chinensis (*Huang Lian*). If there is depressive heat in the lungs, stomach, and intestines, add nine grams of Radix Scutellariae Baicalensis (*Huang Qin*). If there is depressive heat in the liver causing a bitter taste in the mouth and irritability, add nine grams each of Fructus Gardeniae Jasminoidis (*Zhi Zi*) and Cortex Radicis Moutan (*Dan Pi*). If there is a bland taste in the mouth and thick, white tongue fur, add nine grams of Herba Eupatorii Fortunei (*Pei Lan*).

ACUPUNCTURE & MOXIBUSTION: *Feng Fu* (GV 16), *Bai Hui* (GV 20), *San Yin Jiao* (Sp 6), *Shen Men* (Ht 7), *Tai Chong* (Liv 3)

ANALYSIS OF FORMULA: According to the *Ling Shu (Spiritual Pivot)*, *Feng Fu* below and *Bai Hui* above govern the flow of qi and blood in the head. When *Feng Fu* is needled with even supplementing-even draining method and *Bai Hui* is moxaed, they nourish the sea of marrow and free the flow of the orifices. Supplementing *San Yin Jiao* fortifies the spleen, boosts the qi, and nourishes the blood. Supplementing *Shen Men* nourishes the blood and supplements the heart. Draining *Tai Chong* courses the liver and rectifies the qi.

ADDITIONS & SUBTRACTIONS: For severe impaired memory and unclear speech, add *Si Shen Cong* (M-HN-1). If there is concomitant blood stasis, add *Ge Shu* (Bl 17) and *Gan Shu* (Bl 18). If there is depressive heat in the stomach and heart, add *Da Ling* (Per 7) and *Nei Ting* (St 44). If there is depressive heat in the liver causing a bitter taste in the mouth and irritability, add *Gan Shu* (Bl 18) and *Hun Men* (Bl 47). If there is a bland taste in the mouth and thick, white tongue fur, add *Yin Ling Quan* (Sp 9). If there are epileptiform symptoms, add *He Gu* (LI 4) and *Da Zhui* (GV 14).

5. KIDNEY QI DEBILITY & VACUITY PATTERN

MAIN SYMPTOMS: A history of traumatic injury to the head plus essence spirit listlessness, slow, difficult thinking, decreased visual acuity, markedly decreased memory power, dizziness, vertigo, tinnitus, deafness, low back and lower leg soreness and limpness, a pale tongue with thin fur, and a fine, weak pulse

TREATMENT PRINCIPLES: Supplement the kidneys and fortify the brain, boost the marrow and engender essence

RX: *Zi Yin Da Bu Wan* (Enrich Yin Greatly Supplementing Pills)

INGREDIENTS: Cooked Radix Rehmanniae (*Shu Di*), 60g, Radix Achyranthis Bidentatae (*Niu Xi*) and Radix Dioscoreae Oppositae (*Shan Yao*), 45g each, Fructus Corni Officinalis (*Shan Zhu Yu*), Cortex Eucommiae Ulmoidis (*Du Zhong*), Sclerotium Poriae Cocos (*Fu Ling*), Radix Morindae Officinalis (*Ba Ji Tian*), Fructus Schisandrae Chinensis (*Wu Wei Zi*), Fructus Foeniculi Vulgaris (*Xiao Hui Xiang*), Herba Cistanchis Deserticolae (*Rou Cong Rong*), and Radix Polygalae Tenuifoliae (*Yuan Zhi*), 30g each, and Rhizoma Acori Graminei (*Shi Chang Pu*) and Fructus Lycii Chinensis (*Gou Qi Zi*), 20g each

ANALYSIS OF FORMULA: Within this formula, a heavy dose of *Shu Di* enriches yin and fills the essence. *Niu Xi*, *Shan Zhu Yu*, *Du Zhong*, *Ba Ji Tian*, *Gou Qi Zi*, and *Rou Cong Rong* all supplement the kidneys, fill the essence, and boost the marrow, hence revitalizing the essence spirit. *Shan Yao* and *Fu Ling* fortify the spleen and seep dampness, thus supplying a source for engenderment and transformation. *Wu Wei Zi* and *Yuan Zhi* nourish the heart and quiet the spirit, while *Xiao Hui Xiang* and *Shi Chang Pu* acridly scatter and free the flow of the orifices. When all these medicinals are combined together, their effect is to supplement the kidneys and engender essence, boost the marrow and fortify the brain.

ADDITIONS & SUBTRACTIONS: If there is bone-steaming or tidal fever with aching and heat in the feet or knees, and a red tongue with a rapid pulse, add nine grams each of Cortex Radicis Lycii Chinensis (*Di Gu Pi*), Rhizoma Anemarrhenae Aspheloidis (*Zhi Mu*), and Cortex Phellodendri (*Huang Bai*) to enrich yin and clear heat. If there are heart palpitations, fright and fear, vexation, agitation, and restlessness, add 12 grams each of Semen Zizyphi Spinosae (*Suan Zao Ren*), Os Draconis (*Long Gu*), and Concha Ostreae (*Mu Li*) to quiet the spirit and settle fright. If there is piercing headache due to retained and stagnant vanquished blood, add nine grams each of Flos Carthami Tinctorii (*Hong Hua*), Semen Pruni Persicae (*Tao Ren*), Bombyx Batryticatus (*Jiang Can*), and Buthus Martensis (*Quan Xie*) to quicken the blood and transform stasis, stop tetany, and stop pain.

ACUPUNCTURE & MOXIBUSTION: *Bai Hui* (GV 20), *Feng Fu* (GV 16), *Tai Xi* (Ki 3), *Xuan Zhong* (GB 39), *Shen Shu* (Bl 23), *Zhi Shi* (Bl 52)

ANALYSIS OF FORMULA: As explained above, *Feng Fu* and *Bai Hui* nourish the sea of marrow and free the flow of the orifices. Even supplementing-even draining *Xuan Zhong*, the meeting point of the marrow, boosts the sea of marrow, drains the brain, and treats the sequelae of postconcussion syndrome. Supplementing *Tai Xi*, *Shen Shu*, and *Zhi Shi* supplements the kidneys and boosts the intelligence, nourishes the sea of marrow and increases memory power.

ADDITIONS & SUBTRACTIONS: If there is bone-steaming or tidal fever with aching and heat in the feet or knees, a red tongue, and a rapid pulse, add *Da Zhui* (GV 14) and *Yin Xi* (Ht 6). If there are heart palpitations, fright and fear, vexation, agitation, and restlessness, add *Da Ling* (Per 7). If there is piercing headache due to retained and stagnant vanquished blood, add *Si Shen Cong* (M-HN-1). For severely impaired memory and unclear speech, add *Si Shen Cong* (M-HN-1). If there are epileptiform symptoms, add *Tai Chong* (Liv 3), *He Gu* (LI 4), and *Da Zhui* (GV 14).

REMARKS

1. In general, Chinese medicine is quite effective for treating postconcussion syndrome. As always, the key is doing an accurate, personalized pattern discrimination and then designing a customized treatment plan to address every element of that pattern. In most cases of postconcussion syndrome, there is an underlying or pre-existing liver-spleen disharmony which is then aggravated by blood stasis or the complications of blood stasis, such as phlegm obstruction.

2. When treating blood stasis in postconcussion syndrome, the use of so-called worm or insect medicinals is usually important for freeing the flow of the network vessels. These include Buthus Martensis (*Quan Xie*), Hirudo Seu Whitmania (*Shui Zhi*), Eupolyphaga Seu Opisthoplatia (*Tu Bie Chong*), Lumbricus (*Di Long*), and Carapax Amydae Sinensis (*Bie Jia*).

3. The following two contemporary empirical formulas both treat the typically complex sorts of patterns seen in real-life patients with postconcussion syndrome. The first is *Xiao Yi Tang* (Disperse Sequelae Decoction): Radix Codonopsitis Pilosulae (*Dang Shen*), 15-30g, Radix Albus Paeoniae Lactiflorae (*Bai Shao*), Fructus Lycii Chinensis (*Gou Qi Zi*), Magnetitum (*Ci Shi*), and Dens Draconis (*Long Chi*), 15g each, Pericarpium Arecae Catechu (*Da Fu Pi*), Cortex Radicis Mori Albi (*Sang Bai Pi*), and Semen Pruni Persicae (*Tao Ren*), 12g each, Radix Rubrus Paeoniae Lactiflorae (*Chi Shao*), 9g, Herba Schizonepetae Tenuifoliae (*Jing Jie*), Radix Bupleuri (*Chai Hu*), and Rhizoma Cyperi Rotundi (*Xiang Fu*), 6g each, and Succinum (*Hu Po*) and Cinnabar (*Zhu Sha*), 3g each. This formula settles the heart and quiets the spirit, upbears the clear and downbears the turbid, quickens the blood and transforms stasis, rectifies the qi and courses the liver, supplements the kidneys and boosts the spleen.

San Bian Di Huang Tang (Scatter the Inclined Rehmannia Decoction): cooked Radix Rehmanniae (*Shu Di*) and Radix Albus Paeoniae Lactiflorae (*Bai Shao*), 15-30g each, Fructus Corni Officinalis (*Shan Zhu Yu*), 10-30g, Radix Ligustici Wallichii (*Chuan Xiong*), 15-20g, Radix Dioscoreae Oppositae (*Shan Yao*), 10-15g, Radix Angelicae Dahuricae (*Bai Zhi*), Rhizoma Cyperi Rotundi (*Xiang Fu*), Semen Sinapis Albae (*Bai Jie Zi*), and Cortex Radicis Moutan (*Dan Pi*), 6-12g each, and Radix Glycyrrhizae (*Gan Cao*), 3-10g. This formula quickens the blood and transforms stasis, courses the liver and boosts the spleen, enriches the kidneys and boosts the essence. In comparison to the preceding formula, it more strongly boosts the essence and fills the marrow. For severe headache, add nine grams each of Flos Carthami Tinctorii (*Hong Hua*), Radix Salviae Miltiorrhizae (*Dan Shen*), and Radix Rubrus Paeoniae Lactiflorae (*Chi Shao*). For dizziness, add nine grams each of Rhizoma Gastrodiae Elatae (*Tian Ma*), Ramulus Uncariae Cum Uncis (*Gou Teng*), and Flos Chrysanthemi Morifolii (*Ju Hua*). For insomnia, add 15 grams of Semen Zizyphi Spinosae (*Suan Zao Ren*), nine grams of Cortex Albizziae Julibrissinis (*He Huan Pi*) and Sclerotium Pararadicis Poriae Cocos (*Fu Shen*), and three grams of Succinum (*Hu Po*). For vomiting, add nine grams each of Pericarpium Citri Reticulatae (*Chen Pi*) and Rhizoma Pinelliae Ternatae (*Ban Xia*). For concomitant qi and blood vacuity, add 15 grams each of Radix Pseudostellariae Heterophyllae (*Tai Zi Shen*) and Radix Astragali Membranacei (*Huang Qi*) and nine grams of Radix Angelicae Sinensis (*Dang Gui*). For severe liver-kidney vacuity, add nine grams each of Fructus Lycii Chinensis (*Gou Qi Zi*), Semen Juglandis Regiae (*Hu Tao Ren*), Cortex Eucommiae Ulmoidis (*Du Zhong*), Gelatinum Cornu Cervi (*Lu Jiao Jiao*), and Gelatinum Plastri Testudinis (*Gui Ban Jiao*).

60

PULMONARY TUBERCULOSIS

Tuberculosis is a chronic, recurrent infection primarily caused by *Mycobacterium tuberculosis* which most commonly affects the lungs. Clinical symptoms may develop within months or only after years or even decades after infection. Rates of infection vary by country, age, race, sex, and socioeconomic status. In the United States, TB is responsible for 1,800 deaths per year, and 20,000 new cases are reported each year. The incidence of TB has increased alarmingly among persons infected with HIV, particularly African American and Hispanic drug users, and, in the United States, this disease is most commonly seen in city-dwelling men 25-44 years old. Although TB has been almost eliminated in some segments of society, signs of a potentially dangerous epidemic have appeared, with drug resistant strains especially being transmitted to the West from the former Soviet republics of Eastern Europe and Siberia. The stages of TB are primary or initial infection, latent or dormant infection, and recrudescence or adult-type TB. Primary TB may become active at any age. Often it becomes active after years or decades of latency due to decreased immune competence associated with such diseases as diabetes mellitus and HIV infection or due to immunosuppression by corticosteroids or other immunosuppressant drugs.

Pulmonary TB is often nearly asymptomatic, at least in its beginning stages. Patients may only report a vague sense of malaise or fatigue. Cough is the first symptom. At first, it is minimally productive of yellow or green mucus, especially on rising in the morning. As the disease progresses, phlegm tends to become more profuse. Hemoptysis usually does not occur till the latter stages of TB. The course of disease varies greatly from individual to individual and from ethnic or racial group to group. Whites more commonly have chronic fibrotic disease without obvious symptoms for a longer period of time, while the disease progresses more rapidly in blacks and American Indians.

The Western medical diagnosis of pulmonary TB consists of chest x-ray, sputum culture, and transbronchial biopsy. The tubercullin skin test, while being far from definitive, is still an important adjunctive diagnostic method. However, patients who are quite ill with TB may show no reaction to this skin test due to inhibiting antibodies or extreme mobilization of T cells to the lesion. This test may also be negative in persons with HIV infection. The Western medical treatment of pulmonary TB consists of administration of a combination of bactericidal and bacteriostatic medicines over a relatively long course (6-9 months). While such chemotherapy is usually effective, many patients fail to comply with the full course, and, therefore, more and more worrisome drug-resistant strains of this mycobacterium are emerging.

CHINESE DISEASE CATEGORIZATION: Pulmonary TB is known by a number of names in traditional Chinese medicine. These include *fei lao*, lung consumption, *lao zhai*, consumption, *lao zhu*, consumptive infixation,[1] *lao ke*, consumptive cough, *lao re*, consumptive fever, *lao zhai gu zheng*, consumptive steaming bones, *chong zhu*, worm infixation, *chuan shi*, corpse transmission, *fei shi*, flying corpse, *shi zhu*, corpse influx, and *gui zhu*, demonic influx.

DISEASE CAUSES: External contraction of evils and bodily vacuity due to enduring disease, age, bedroom taxation, drug use and iatrogenesis

DISEASE MECHANISMS: Ge Hong, author of the *Zhou Hou Bei Ji Fang (Emergency Formulas [to Keep Tucked] Behind One's Elbow)*, understood the infectious nature of this disease as early as the Western Jin dynasty (265-316 CE). In the Song dynasty (960-1279 CE), it was posited to be caused by *zhai chong* or *lao chong*, consumptive worms. However, it is a righteous qi vacuity weakness which is the predisposing factor allowing for this worm infixation or influx or this worm influx transforming from hidden to apparent. Such bodily weakness may be due to former heaven natural endowment insufficiency, unregulated eating and drinking, bedroom taxation, and taxation fatigue due to excessive thinking and worrying as well as poverty and poor living conditions. Evils within the lungs obstruct and hinder the lungs' depurative downbearing. Therefore, lung fluids gather and accumulate, transforming into phlegm. Depressed phlegm and dampness may then transform heat, and heat evils within the lungs may further steam and stew lung fluids, yet again congealing them into phlegm. If these heat evils endure, they will also eventually eat the qi and consume yin. Because the spleen is the mother of the lungs, enduring lung qi vacuity may reach the spleen. Because the spleen and kidneys support and bolster one another, spleen qi vacuity may eventually damage kidney yang. Qi vacuity results in fatigue, spontaneous perspiration, and loss of strength. Since it is the qi which moves the blood, qi vacuity may also become complicated by blood stasis. If yin becomes damaged and insufficient to control yang, effulgent fire may be engendered internally. Because the kidneys are the child of the lungs, lung yin vacuity may also reach kidney yin. If vacuous yin fails to control yang, there will be low-grade fevers and night sweats. If heat damages the network vessels in the lungs, there will be hacking or coughing of blood. If both yin and yang become damaged, there will be yin and yang dual vacuity. However, according to the author of the *Yi Men Fa Lu (The Laws of Medicine),* in eight out of 10 cases, it is yin which is damaged first.

TREATMENT BASED ON PATTERN DISCRIMINATION:

1. LUNG YIN DEBILITY & DETRIMENT PATTERN

MAIN SYMPTOMS: Dry cough, scanty phlegm, possible phlegm mixed with blood, chest pain, tidal fever, malar flushing, a dry mouth and parched throat, a red tongue with thin, yellow fur and scanty fluids, and a fine, rapid pulse

TREATMENT PRINCIPLES: Nourish yin and moisten the lungs, clear heat and stop coughing

RX: *Bai He Gu Jin Tang Jia Jian* (Lily Secure Metal Decoction with Additions & Subtractions)

INGREDIENTS: Radix Salviae Miltiorrhizae (*Dan Shen*), 15g, Bulbus Lilii (*Bai He*), Tuber Ophiopogonis Japonici (*Mai Dong*), Radix Scrophulariae Ningpoensis (*Xuan Shen*), uncooked Radix Rehmanniae (*Sheng Di*), cooked Radix Rehmanniae (*Shu Di*), Radix Stemonae (*Bai Bu*), Radix Scutellariae Baicalensis (*Huang Qin*), and Folium Mahoniae (*Gong Lao Ye*), 12g each, Radix Albus Paeoniae Lactiflorae (*Bai Shao*), 9g, Radix Platycodi Grandiflori (*Jie Geng*) and Bulbus Fritillariae Cirrhosae (*Chuan Bei Mu*), 6g each, and Radix Glycyrrhizae (*Gan Cao*), 3g

ANALYSIS OF FORMULA: *Bai He, Mai Men Dong, Sheng Di, Shu Di, Xuan Shen,* and *Gong Lao Ye* all nourish yin and moisten the lungs. In addition, *Sheng Di* and *Xuan Shen* clear vacuity heat, while *Huang Qin* clears lung heat. *Bai Bu, Gong Lao Ye, Chuan Bei Mu,* and *Jie Geng* stop cough. *Chuan Bei Mu* and *Jie Geng* transform and disperse phlegm. In addition, *Jie Geng* is a messenger which leads the other medicinals to the lungs. *Bai Shao* nourishes the blood and, therefore, helps enrich yin, constrains yin and stops night sweats.

ADDITIONS & SUBTRACTIONS: For severe lung dryness, add 12 grams each of Radix Glehniae Littoralis (*Sha Shen*) and Herba Dendrobii (*Shi Hu*) and nine grams of Rhizoma Polygonati Odorati (*Yu Zhu*). For hacking of blood, add 30 grams of Herba Agrimoniae Pilosae (*Xian He Cao*), 12 grams of Dolomitum (*Hua Rui Shi*), and nine grams of Rhizoma Bletillae Striatae (*Bai Ji*). For tidal fever and malar flushing, add 15 grams of Carapax Amydae Sinensis (*Bei Jia*), 12 grams of Cortex Radicis Lycii Chinensis (*Di Gu Pi*), and nine grams of Radix Cynanchi Atrati (*Bai Wei*). For thick, yellow phlegm which is difficult to expectorate, add nine grams each of Pumice (*Hai Fu Shi*) and Pericarpium Trichosanthis Kirlowii (*Gua Lou Pi*).

ACUPUNCTURE & MOXIBUSTION: *Fei Shu* (Bl 13), *Gao Huang Shu* (Bl 43), *Fu Liu* (Ki 7)

ANALYSIS OF FORMULA: Supplementing *Fei Shu* and *Gao Huang Shu* nourish yin and moisten the lungs, clear vacuity heat from the lungs and stop coughing. Supplementing *Fu Liu,* the mother-metal point of the foot water channel, engenders fluids and nourishes yin not only of the kidneys but also of the lungs.

ADDITIONS & SUBTRACTIONS: For night sweats, add *Yin Xi* (Ht 6). For severe cough, add *Chi Ze* (Lu 5). For phlegm mixed with blood or hacking of blood, add *Ge Shu* (Bl 17) and *Yu Ji* (Lu 10) or *Kong Zui* (Lu 6). For tidal fever, add *Da Zhui* (GV 14) and *San Yin Jiao* (Sp 6). For chest pain or oppression, add *Nei Guan* (Per 6) and *Dan Zhong* (CV 17). For concomitant qi vacuity, add *Tai Yuan* (Lu 9) and *Zu San Li* (St 36).

2. YIN VACUITY WITH FIRE EFFULGENCE PATTERN

MAIN SYMPTOMS: Bone-steaming, tidal fever, night sweats, vexatious heat in the five hearts, insomnia, profuse dreams, easy agitation, easy anger, cough with no, scanty, or yellow, sticky, thick phlegm, recurrent episodes of hacking blood which is excessive in amount and fresh in color, cramping pain in the chest and rib-side, emaciation, dry skin, throat, mouth, and nose, red lips, malar flushing, a crimson red tongue, and a fine, rapid pulse

NOTE: The difference between this pattern and the preceding is that, in pattern #1, there is marked lung dryness but little evidence of heat, while, in this pattern, there are the signs and symptoms not only of yin vacuity but fire effulgence.

TREATMENT PRINCIPLES: Enrich yin and downbear fire, transform phlegm and stop cough, cool the blood and stop bleeding

RX: *Qin Jiao Bei Jia He Yue Hua Wan Jia Jian* (Gentiana Macrophylla & Carapax Amydae Plus Moonshine Pills with Additions & Subtractions)

INGREDIENTS: Carapax Amydae Sinensis (*Bei Jia*), 15g, Cortex Radicis Lycii Chinensis (*Di Gu Pi*), uncooked Radix Rehmanniae (*Sheng Di*), Radix Glehniae Littoralis (*Bei Sha Shen*), Radix Adenophorae Strictae (*Nan Sha Shen*), and Radix Stemonae (*Bai Bu*), 12g each, Herba Artemisiae Apiaceae (*Qing Hao*), Rhizoma Anemarrhenae Aspheloidis (*Zhi Mu*), Tuber Ophiopogonis Japonici (*Mai Dong*), Tuber Asparagi Cochinensis (*Tian Men Dong*), and Gelatinum Corii Asini (*E Jiao*), 9g each, and Radix Gentianae Macrophyllae (*Qin Jiao*), Radix Stellariae Dichotomae (*Yin Chai Hu*), and Bulbus Fritillariae Cirrhosae (*Chuan Bei Mu*), 6g each

ANALYSIS OF FORMULA: *Bei Jia, Sheng Di, Bei Sha Shen, Nan Sha Shen, Zhi Mu, Mai Men Dong, Tian Men Dong,* and *E Jiao* all enrich yin, engender fluids, and moisten the lungs. *Bei Jia, Di Gu Pi, Qing Hao, Qin Jiao, Zhi Mu,* and *Yin Chai Hu* downbear fire and clear vacuity heat. *Sheng Di* and *Di Gu Pi* cool the blood and, with *E Jiao,* stop bleeding. *Chuan Bei Mu* engenders fluids and transforms phlegm.

ADDITIONS & SUBTRACTIONS: If night sweats are severe, remove *Qing Hao* and add 30 grams of Fructus Levis Tritici Aestivi (*Fu Xiao Mai*), 15-30 grams of Concha Ostreae (*Mu Li*) and Os Draconis (*Long Gu*), and nine grams of Fructus Schisandrae Chinensis (*Wu Wei Zi*). For seminal emission, add 15 grams of Plastrum Testudinis (*Gui Ban*) and nine grams of Cortex Phellodendri (*Huang Bai*). For vexation and agitation and insomnia, add 30 grams of Caulis Polygoni Multiflori (*Ye Jiao Teng*), 12 grams of Semen Zizyphi Spinosae (*Suan Zao Ren*), and nine grams of scorched Fructus Gardeniae Jasminoidis (*Zhi Zi*). For thick, sticky, yellow phlegm, add 12 grams of Concha Cyclinae Meretricis (*Hai Ge Ke*), nine grams of Semen Trichosanthis Kirlowii (*Gua Lou Ren*), and six grams of Fructus Aristolochiae (*Ma Dou Ling*). For hacking of blood, add 15 grams each of Rhizoma Imperatae Cyclindricae (*Bai Mao Gen*) and Radix Bletillae Striatae (*Bai Ji*).

ACUPUNCTURE & MOXIBUSTION: *Fei Shu* (Bl 13), *Gao Huang Shu* (Bl 43), *Fu Liu* (Ki 7), *Da Zhui* (GV 14), *Kong Zui* (Lu 6)

ANALYSIS OF FORMULA: Supplementing *Fei Shu* and *Gao Huang Shu* nourishes yin and moistens the lungs, clears vacuity heat from the lungs and stops coughing. Supplementing *Fu Liu*, the mother-metal point of the foot water channel, engenders fluids and nourishes yin not only of the kidneys but also of the lungs. Draining *Da Zhui* downbears fire and clears vacuity heat. Draining *Kong Zui* transforms phlegm and stops cough, cools the blood and stops bleeding.

ADDITIONS & SUBTRACTIONS: For night sweats, add *Yin Xi* (Ht 6). For severe cough, add *Chi Ze* (Lu 5). For severe hacking of blood, add *Ge Shu* (Bl 17) and *Yu Ji* (Lu 10). For tidal fever, add *Ran Gu* (Ki 2). For chest pain or oppression, add *Nei Guan* (Per 6) and *Dan Zhong* (CV 17). For concomitant qi vacuity, add *Tai Yuan* (Lu 9) and *Zu San Li* (St 36). For insomnia, add *Shen Men* (Ht 7) and *Zhao Hai* (Ki 6).

3. QI & YIN DUAL VACUITY PATTERN

MAIN SYMPTOMS: Cough with possible blood-streaked phlegm, forceless cough provoked by talking, movement, or exertion, possible incessant or recurrent low-grade fever, tidal fever, a lusterless white facial complexion with malar flushing, especially in the afternoon, possible aversion to wind and cold, spontaneous perspiration and night sweats, fatigue, lassitude of the spirit, shortness of breath, timid voice, devitalized eating and drinking, abdominal distention, loose stools, a shiny red tongue with thin or peeled fur, and a fine, rapid, forceless pulse

TREATMENT PRINCIPLES: Boost the qi and nourish yin, transform phlegm and stop cough, cool the blood and stop bleeding

RX: *Sheng Mai San* (Engender the Pulse Powder) & *Yue Hua Wan* (Moonshine Pills) with additions and subtractions

INGREDIENTS: Tuber Ophiopogonis Japonici (*Mai Dong*), Tuber Asparagi Cochinensis (*Tian Men Dong*), uncooked Radix Rehmanniae (*Sheng Di*), cooked Radix Rehmanniae (*Shu Di*), Radix Glehniae Littoralis (*Bei Sha Shen*), and Radix Adenophorae Strictae (*Nan Sha Shen*), 12g each, Radix Panacis Ginseng (*Ren Shen*), Radix Dioscoreae Oppositae (*Shan Yao*), Radix Stemonae (*Bai Bu*), Gelatinum Corii Asini (*E Jiao*), Flos Chrysanthemi Morifolii (*Ju Hua*), and Folium Mori Albi (*Sang Ye*), 9g each, Fructus Schisandrae Chinensis (*Wu Wei Zi*) and Bulbus Fritillariae Cirrhosae (*Chuan Bei Mu*), 6g each, and powdered Radix Pseudoginseng (*Tian San Qi*), 3g, swallowed with the decoction

ANALYSIS OF FORMULA: *Mai Men Dong, Tian Men Dong, Sheng Di, Shu Di, Bei Sha Shen, Nan Sha Shen, E Jiao,* and *Wu Wei Zi* all nourish yin, engender fluids, and moisten the lungs. *Ren Shen, Shan Yao,* and *Wu Wei Zi* supplement the spleen and boost the qi. *Bai Bu, Sang Ye,* and *Wu Wei Zi* stop cough. In addition, *Chuan Bei Mu* engenders fluids and transforms phlegm, while *E Jiao*, *Sang Ye*, and *San Qi* stop bleeding.

ADDITIONS & SUBTRACTIONS: For decreased eating and loose stools, add 15 grams of Semen Coicis Lachryma-jobi (*Yi Yi Ren*), 12 grams of Semen Dolichoris Lablab (*Bai Bian Dou*), and three grams of Fructus Amomi (*Sha Ren*). For severe spontaneous perspiration, add 15-30 grams each of Concha Ostreae (*Mu Li*) and Os Draconis (*Long Gu*) and 15 grams of Radix Astragali Membranacei (*Huang Qi*). For coughing and panting, add 12 grams of Flos Tussilaginis Farfarae (*Kuan Dong Hua*) and 10 pieces of Semen Ginkgonis Bilobae (*Bai Guo*). For hacking of blood, add 30 grams of Herba Agrimoniae Pilosae (*Xian He Cao*) and 15-30 grams of Nodus Rhizomatis Nelumbinis Nuciferae (*Ou Jie*).

ACUPUNCTURE & MOXIBUSTION: *Fei Shu* (Bl 13), *Gao Huang Shu* (Bl 43), *Fu Liu* (Ki 7), *Zu San Li* (St 36)

ANALYSIS OF FORMULA: Supplementing *Fei Shu* and *Gao Huang Shu* nourishes yin and moistens the lungs, clears vacuity heat from the lungs and stops coughing. Supplementing *Fu Liu*, the mother-metal point of the foot water channel, engenders fluids and nourishes yin not only of the kidneys but also of the lungs. Supplementing *Zu San Li*, the earth uniting point of the stomach channel, fortifies the spleen and boosts the qi, thus indirectly preventing the accumulation of phlegm.

ADDITIONS & SUBTRACTIONS: For night sweats, add *Yin Xi* (Ht 6). For severe cough, add *Chi Ze* (Lu 5). For phlegm mixed with blood or hacking of blood, add *Ge Shu* (Bl 17) and *Yu Ji* (Lu 10) or *Kong Zui* (Lu 6). For tidal fever, add *Da Zhui* (GV 14) and *San Yin Jiao* (Sp 6). For chest pain or oppression, add *Nei Guan* (Per 6) and *Dan Zhong* (CV 17). For severe qi vacuity, add *Tai Bai* (Sp 3). For insomnia, add *Shen Men* (Ht 7) and *Zhao Hai* (Ki 6).

4. VACUITY COLD PATTERN

MAIN SYMPTOMS: No cough but spitting of drool and foam which is clear, watery, and profuse in nature, no oral thirst, dizziness, frequent, numerous urination or urinary incontinence, a pale tongue, and a vacuous, weak pulse

NOTE: This pattern describes the small percentage of patients whose disease evolves from lung-spleen qi vacuity to spleen-kidney yang vacuity.

TREATMENT PRINCIPLES: Warm the lungs and boost the qi

RX: *Gan Cao Gan Jiang Tang Jia Wei* (Licorice & Dry Ginger Decoction with Added Flavors)

INGREDIENTS: Sclerotium Poriae Cocos (*Fu Ling*), 12g, Semen Pruni Armeniacae (*Xing Ren*), processed Rhizoma Pinelliae Ternatae (*Ban Xia*), and mix-fried Radix Glycyrrhizae (*Gan Cao*), 9g each, and dry Rhizoma Zingiberis (*Gan Jiang*), 6g

ANALYSIS OF FORMULA: *Gan Jiang* warms the lungs. Mix-fried *Gan Cao* and *Fu Ling* supplement the spleen and boost the qi, *Fu Ling* and *Ban Xia* transform phlegm, *Xing Ren* disperses phlegm and diffuses the lungs.

ADDITIONS & SUBTRACTIONS: In order to increase the strength of the treatment by fortifying the spleen and boosting the qi, add 15 grams of Radix Astragali Membranacei (*Huang Qi*) and nine grams each of Radix Codonopsitis Pilosulae (*Dang Shen*) and Rhizoma Atractylodis Macrocephalae (*Bai Zhu*). If dizziness is severe, add nine grams of Rhizoma Acori Graminei (*Shi Chang Pu*).

ACUPUNCTURE & MOXIBUSTION: *Fei Shu* (Bl 13), *Shen Shu* (Bl 23), *Zu San Li* (St 36), *Tai Bai* (Sp 3)

ANALYSIS OF FORMULA: With moxibustion and supplementing method, *Fei Shu*, *Shen Shu*, *Zu San Li*, and *Tai Bai* warm and supplement respectively the lungs, kidneys, stomach, and spleen. Since phlegm is congealed from water dampness and the lungs, spleen, and kidneys are the three viscera which control water fluids in the body, they also transform phlegm.

ADDITIONS & SUBTRACTIONS: For severe spleen vacuity, add *Pi Shu* (Bl 20) and *Wei Shu* (Bl 21). For profuse phlegm, add *Feng Long* (St 40) and *Zhong Wan* (CV 12). For insomnia, add *Shen Men* (Ht 7) and *Zhao Hai* (Ki 6).

5. YIN & YANG DUAL VACUITY PATTERN

MAIN SYMPTOMS: Coughing and hacking of blood, incessant tidal fever, spontaneous perspiration and/or night sweats, low back soreness, impotence in men, amenorrhea in women, cold body, chilled limbs, panting breathing, shortness of breath, perspiration on slight exertion, facial edema, swollen limbs, bodily emaciation, lassitude of the spirit, loose stools, decreased eating and drinking, mouth and tongue sores, dark, purplish lips, a shiny tongue with scanty fluids or a possibly pale, fat tongue, and a faint, fine pulse

TREATMENT PRINCIPLES: Foster and supplement the essence and blood, warm and supplement the spleen and kidneys, clear heat, transform phlegm, and stop bleeding

RX: *Pao Zhen Tang* (Protect the True Decoction) & *Cheng Yang Li Lao Tang* (Save Yang & Rectify Taxation Decoction) with additions and subtractions

INGREDIENTS: Herba Agrimoniae Pilosae (*Xian He Cao*), 30g, Radix Astragali Membranacei (*Huang Qi*) and Radix Pseudostellariae (*Tai Zi Shen*), 15g each, uncooked Radix Rehmanniae (*Sheng Di*), cooked Radix Rehmanniae (*Shu Di*), Tuber Ophiopogonis Japonici (*Mai Dong*), Tuber Asparagi Cochinensis (*Tian Men Dong*), and Cortex Radicis Lycii Chinensis (*Di Gu Pi*), 12g each, Radix Angelicae Sinensis (*Dang Gui*), Radix Albus Paeoniae Lactiflorae (*Bai Shao*), and Rhizoma Atractylodis Macrocephalae (*Bai Zhu*), 9g each, and Pericarpium Citri Reticulatae (*Chen Pi*), Fructus Schisandrae Chinensis (*Wu Wei Zi*), and Radix Stellariae Dichotomae (*Yin Chai Hu*), 6g each

ANALYSIS OF FORMULA: *Sheng Di, Shu Di, Mai Men Dong, Tian Men Dong,* and *Wu Wei Zi* foster and supplement essence and yin. *Shu Di, Sheng Di, Dang Gui,* and *Bai Shao* nourish the blood. *Huang Qi, Tai Zi Shen, Bai Zhu,* and *Wu Wei Zi* fortify the spleen and boost the qi. *Tai Zi Shen, Shu Di,* and *Wu Wei Zi* supplement the kidneys. *Di Gu Pi* and *Yin Chai Hu* clear vacuity heat. *Wu Wei Zi* astringes and secures the lung qi. *Chen Pi* moves the qi to help transform the phlegm. *Xian He Cao* cools the blood and stops bleeding.

ADDITIONS & SUBTRACTIONS: For severe essence and blood debility, add 3-6 grams of Cordyceps Chinensis (*Dong Chong Xia Cao*), 3-9 grams each of Gelatinum Cornu Cervi (*Lu Jiao Jiao*) and Gelatinum Plastri Testudinis (*Gui Ban Jiao*), and three grams of Placenta Hominis (*Zi He Che*), powdered and swallowed with the decoction. For chilled limbs and a deep, slow pulse, add 1.5 grams of Cortex Cinnamomi Cassiae (*Rou Gui*). For cockcrow diarrhea, add nine grams each of Fructus Psoraleae Corylifoliae (*Bu Gu Zhi*) and Fructus Evodiae Rutecarpae (*Wu Zhu Yu*) and six grams of Semen Myristicae Fragrantis (*Rou Dou Kou*). For severe cough with or without hacking of blood, add 12 grams each of Radix Asteris Tatarici (*Zi Wan*) and Flos Tussilaginis Farfarae (*Kuan Dong Hua*). For tidal heat, add 15 grams of Carapax Amydae Sinensis (*Bie Jia*) and 12 grams of Cortex Radicis Lycii Chinensis (*Di Gu Pi*). For night sweats, add 30 grams of Semen Levis Tritici Aestivi (*Fu Xiao Mai*).

ACUPUNCTURE & MOXIBUSTION: *Fei Shu* (Bl 13), *Gao Huang Shu* (Bl 43), *Shen Shu* (Bl 23), *Zu San Li* (St 36)

ANALYSIS OF FORMULA: Supplementing *Fei Shu* and *Gao Huang Shu* nourishes yin and moistens the lungs, clears vacuity heat from the lungs and stops coughing. With moxibustion and supplementing method, *Shen Shu* and *Zu San Li* warm and supplement the spleen and kidneys. *Zu San* also fortifies the spleen and boosts the qi and, thus, indirectly, prevents phlegm accumulation.

ADDITIONS & SUBTRACTIONS: For night sweats, add *Yin Xi* (Ht 6). For tidal fever, add *Da Zhui* (GV 14) or *Ran Gu* (Ki 2). For severe cough, add *Chi Ze* (Lu 5). For severe hacking of blood, add *Ge Shu* (Bl 17) and *Yu Ji* (Lu 10). For severe spleen vacuity, add *Pi Shu* (Bl 20) and *Wei Shu* (Bl 21). For profuse phlegm, add *Feng Long* (St 40) and *Zhong Wan* (CV 12). For severe kidney yang vacuity with impotence, seminal emission, etc., add *Zhi Shi* (Bl 52). For insomnia, add *Shen Men* (Ht 7) and *Zhao Hai* (Ki 6). For chest pain or oppression, add *Nei Guan* (Per 6) and *Dan Zhong* (CV 17).

REMARKS

1. TB should be treated with a combination of Chinese and Western medicines. One should not attempt to treat this disease with Chinese medicine alone. Two or more Western drugs are typically administered at a time to avoid bacterial resistance. Unfortunately, these drugs are hard on the liver and, therefore, lab test monitoring of liver functions must be carried out on a regular basis during the course of treatment. When Chinese medicine is used in tandem with Western drug therapy, Chinese medicinals and/or acupuncture can be used to help relieve any adverse reactions. In that case, treatment should be based on the patient's total pattern discrimination, including the symptoms of such adverse reactions.

2. Traditionally within Chinese medicine, there are four major symptoms of lung consumption: cough, hacking blood, tidal fever, and night sweats. It is also said that lung consumption has three natures: infectious nature, chronic nature, and vacuity nature. Based on these three natures, Li Shou-xin *et al.* say that one should kill the worms to severe the root and then supplement vacuity to recover the source.[2] However, in clinical practice, both root and source are typically treated simultaneously. The types of worm-killing medicinals given as examples are Cordyceps Chinensis (*Dong Chong Xia Cao*) and Scolopendra Subspinipes (*Wu Gong*). Neither of these medicinals is normally thought of as a worm-killing medicinal in standard contemporary Chinese medicine. Here, Li *et al.* are basing their use of the concept of killing worms on the principle of using worm or insect medicinals to hunt down and kill other, pathogenic worms.

3. External application of Chinese medicinal plasters over the site of foci in the lungs or over acupuncture points associated with lung diseases may be used as adjunctive treatments. One such formula is comprised of equal amounts of Radix Euphorbiae Kansui (*Gan Sui*), Radix Euphorbiae Seu Knoxiae (*Da Ji*), Herba Euphorbiae Helioscopiae (*Ze Qi*), Nidus Vespae (*Lu Feng Fang*), and Rhizoma Podophylli (*Ba Jiao Lian*) and 1/4-1/2 amount of Huechys (*Hong Niang Zi*). These medicinals are boiled in a suitable amount of sesame oil until the medicinals turn black. Strain the oil and add bee's wax to thicken. However, before this mixture hardens to the desired consistency, mix in smaller but equal amounts of Resina Olibani (*Ru Xiang*), Resina Myrrhae (*Mo Yao*), Pasta Acaciae Seu Uncariae (*Er Cha*), and powdered

Lapis Chloriti Seu Micae (*Meng Shi*) plus a very small amount of Secretio Moschi Moschiferi (*She Xiang*) if available. Spread on paper or cotton pads and apply warm. Five days equal one course of treatment with this plaster.

A simpler poultice consists of: Semen Sinapis Albae (*Bai Jie Zi*) and Bulbus Allii Sativi (*Da Suan*), 15g, and Radix Glycyrrhizae (*Gan Cao*), 6g. Powder the *Bai Jie Zi* and uncooked *Gan Cao* and mix together in a mashed paste of the garlic. Add a suitable amount of vinegar and spread on a cotton pad. Apply over the spine from the neck to the lumbar vertebrae in a strip approximately one inch wide. Leave in place for 1-2 hours until the skin feels a burning hot sensation. This should be done once per day, with seven days equaling one course of treatment.

Another adjunctive treatment is to place the juice made from 30-35 grams of mashed Bulbus Allii Sativi (*Da Suan*) in an atomizer or humidifier. Then inhale the resulting steam or mist for 30-60 minutes each time, two times per week. In this case, three months equal one course.

4. There are a number of other types of TB besides pulmonary TB. These include genitourinary tuberculosis, tuberculous meningitis, miliary tuberculosis, tuberculous peritonitis, tuberculous pericarditis, tuberculour lymphadenitis, tuberculosis of the bones and joints, gastrointestinal tuberculosis, and tuberculosis of the liver. In fact, this mycobacterium can infect and cause disease in any organ and tissue of the body. Tuberculous lymphadenitis is categorized as *luo li*, scrofula. However, no matter where this mycobacterium strikes, as Han Pei-rong suggests,[3] the single most important principle in its treatment is basing treatment on the patient's personal pattern.

5. If the only symptoms are cough and a dry mouth with desire to drink, the disease nature is simple and, therefore, easy to cure. If the mouth is opened wide when breathing like a fish out of water gasping for air and there is shortness of breath and distressed rapid breathing, the disease nature is relatively heavy. If the voice sounds hoarse and there is emaciation, hacking of blood, dry, scaly skin, shortness of breath, obstructed breathing, sweat pouring like water, facial and pedal edema, a greenish-blue, dark facial complexion, and a fine, rapid, racing, spiritless pulse, the prognosis is even worse. According to the author of the *Ming Yi Za Zhu (Ming Doctors' Miscellaneous Writings)*:

> If this disease is treated early, it is easy [to cure]. If one waits till the muscles and flesh are wasted and burnt, [the limbs are] heavy and encumbered, [the patient is] bedridden, and the pulse is deep, hidden, fine, and rapid, then treatment is difficult.

6. In yin vacuity patterns of lung consumption, one should eat a clear bland diet and avoid acrid, aromatic, hot, and drying foods. In yang vacuity patterns of lung consumption, one should eat warming and nourishing foods and stay away from anything greatly bitter or greatly cold.

7. The following Chinese medicinals have all been shown to empirically treat *Mycobacterium tuberculosis*: Radix Stemonae (*Bai Bu*), Rhizoma Bletillae Striatae (*Bai Ji*), Bulbus Allii Sativi (*Da Suan*), Herba Agrimoniae Pilosae (*Xian He Cao*), Radix Salviae Miltiorrhizae (*Dan Shen*), Herba Houttuyniae Cordatae Cum Radice (*Yu Xing Cao*), Radix Asteris Tatarici (*Zi Wan*), Cortex Radicis Lycii Chinensis (*Di Gu Pi*), Flos Tussilaginis Farfarae (*Kuan Dong Hua*), Radix Scutellariae Baicalensis (*Huang Qin*), Spica Prunellae Vulgaris (*Xia Ku Cao*), Flos Lonicerae Japonicae (*Jin Yin Hua*), and Fructus Forsythiae Suspensae (*Lian Qiao*).

ENDNOTES

1 The term infixation and its synonym influx refer to external contraction of evils which then become permanently lodged in the body.

2 Li Shou-xin *et al.*, "A Survey of the Treatment Effects of *Kang Lao San* (Combatting Consumption Powder) as the Main Treatment in 2,139 Cases of Tuberculosis," *Zhong Yi Za Zhi (Journal of Chinese Medicine)*, #10, 1994, p. 606-607

3 Han Pei-rong, "Experiences in the Treatment of Two Cases of Severe Pulmonary Tuberculosis," *Zhong Yi Za Zhi (Journal of Chinese Medicine)*, #9, 1995, p. 526

61

RAYNAUD'S PHENOMENON & DISEASE

Raynaud's disease refers to idiopathic spasming of the arterioles, usually in the fingers and toes, with intermittent pallor or cyanosis of the skin. When such spasming is secondary to other diseases, such as scleroderma, RA, or SLE, it is referred to as Raynaud's phenomenon. Sixty to 90% of reported cases of Raynaud's occur in females. The attacks of vasospasm may last from minutes to hours but are rarely serious enough to cause gross tissue loss. With long-standing Raynaud's disease, the skin of the digits may become smooth, shiny, and tight with loss of subcutaneous tissue. Pain is uncommon, but paresthesias are frequent during attacks. Color changes may be either triphasic (*i.e.*, white to cyanotic to red on rewarming) or biphasic (cyanotic, then red). Western medical treatment of Raynaud's depends on whether this condition is primary or secondary. If secondary, treatment is mainly aimed at the underlying disease condition, such as RA or SLE, believed responsible. If primary, biofeedback training may be recommended and/or mild sedatives may be prescribed. Obviously, anything which is a vasoconstrictor should be avoided, such as nicotine and exposure to cold. In addition, emotional upset is often a precipitating factor for iniatiting an acute Raynaud's event.

CHINESE DISEASE CATEGORIZATION: Raynaud's is mainly categorized as *xue bi*, blood impediment in Chinese medicine. However, it may also be categorized based on its main symptoms. Cold hands and feet are known in Chinese medicine as *shou zu leng*, chilly hands and feet, while pale white and cyanotic fingertips are referred to as *shou zhi dan bai* and *zhi jian fa gan* respectively.

DISEASE CAUSES: Bodily vacuity and/or repeated contraction of external evils, internal damage by the seven affects, and faulty diet

DISEASE MECHANISMS: The warmth and healthy pink color of the fingers and toes is dependent on the extremities receiving sufficient yang qi to warm them and sufficient blood to nourish them. Therefore, if for any reason, there is qi vacuity, blood vacuity, or yang vacuity, pallor and chilling of the fingers and toes may occur. In addition, wind, cold, damp, and even, paradoxically, heat evils may either take advantage of this vacuity and invade or be internally engendered, thus further obstructing the free flow of the channels and network vessels. The finger and toes are the beginning or ends of the 12 channels. If wind, cold, damp, or heat evils hinder and obstruct the free flow of qi and blood within the channels and vessels, the fingers and toes may be even further deprived of warming and nourishing. If this disease continues for a long time, these yin cold evils may transform into heat, thus giving rise to damp heat brewing and binding. However, it is also possible for internally engendered damp heat due to over-eating spicy, hot and/or fatty sweet foods or drinking too much alcohol to pour into the limbs and obstruct the free flow of channels and vessels in the hands and feet. In either case, damp heat evils may block the flow of yang qi and result in chilling of the fingers and toes.

Another mechanism of this disease is counterflow chilling due to liver depression qi stagnation. Due to emotional stress, unfulfilled desires, or anger, the liver may be damaged and fail in its duty of coursing and discharging. In this case, the qi mechanism is inhibited and the qi and, therefore, blood and body fluids are not able to flow freely to the extremities. In addition, the replete liver may counterflow horizontally to invade spleen earth, resulting in spleen qi vacuity. In that case, there is a combination of both qi stagnation and lack of qi and blood to warm and nourish the extremities. If spleen qi vacuity endures for some time, it may eventually reach the kidneys, damaging kidney yang. This is because the spleen qi and kidney yang are mutually promoting, one being the latter heaven and the other being the former heaven source. *Vice versa*, spleen qi vacuity resulting in failing to engender sufficient blood and kidney yang vacuity may both cause or aggravate liver depression.

If evils obstruct the flow of qi and blood over a long time or if there is either qi vacuity failing to move the blood, blood vacuity failing to nourish the vessels, or yang vacuity failing to warm and move, static blood may be engendered which may also block and obstruct the flow of qi and blood.

TREATMENT BASED ON PATTERN DISCRIMINATION:

1. YIN COLD PATTERN

MAIN SYMPTOMS: A preference for warmth and dread of chill, chilling of the fingers or toes leading to their skin becoming somber white or greenish purple (*i.e.*, cyanotic), emission of coolness and numbness in the affected area, possible slight pain, obtaint of warmth restoring the normal skin color and temperature, exposure to cold worsening the event, thin, white tongue fur, and a deep, fine, possibly slow pulse

TREATMENT PRINCIPLES: Warm yang and scatter cold, quicken the blood and free the flow of the vessels

RX: *Yang He Tang Jia Jian* (Yang Harmonizing Decoction with Additions & Subtractions)

INGREDIENTS: Cooked Radix Rehmanniae (*Shu Di*), Radix Astragali Membranacei (*Huang Qi*), and Radix Salviae Miltiorrhizae (*Dan Shen*), 30g each, Radix Angelicae Sinensis (*Dang Gui*) and Caulis Milletiae Seu Spatholobi (*Ji Xue Teng*), 15g each, Cortex Cinnamomi Cassiae (*Rou Gui*), dry Rhizoma Zingiberis (*Gan Jiang*), and Lumbricus (*Di Long*), 9g each, and Herba Ephedrae (*Ma Huang*) and Radix Glycyrrhizae (*Gan Cao*), 6g each

ANALYSIS OF FORMULA: *Rou Gui* and *Gan Jiang* warm yang, while *Ma Huang* scatters cold. Because evils may take advantage of vacuity to invade the channels, *Shu Di* and *Huang Qi* supplement the qi and blood and fill the channels to avoid further invasion. *Dan Shen, Dang Gui, Ji Xue Teng,* and *Di Long* quicken the blood and free the flow of the vessels. *Gan Cao* harmonizes the other medicinals in this formula.

ADDITIONS & SUBTRACTIONS: If there is spleen-kidney yang vacuity with cold congealing in the network vessels, replace *Yang He Tang* with the following unnamed formula: uncooked Radix Astragali Membranacei (*Huang Qi*) and Caulis Milletiae Seu Spatholobi (*Ji Xue Teng*), 30g each, Radix Salviae Miltiorrhizae (*Dan Shen*), 20g, Radix Codonopsitis Pilosulae (*Dang Shen*), Semen Cuscutae Chinensis (*Tu Si Zi*), Lignum Sappan (*Su Mu*), Fructus Ligustri Lucidi (*Nu Zhen Zi*), and Extremitas Radicis Angelicae Sinensis (*Dang Gui*), 15g each, and Cortex Cinnamomi Cassiae (*Rou Gui*) and Flos Carthami Tinctorii (*Hong Hua*), 9g each. If there is low back pain, add nine grams each of Ramulus Loranthi Seu Visci (*Sang Ji Sheng*) and Radix Dipsaci (*Xu Duan*). If aching and pain are marked, add nine grams of Fructus Meliae Toosendan (*Chuan Lian Zi*) and 15 grams of Rhizoma Corydalis Yanhusuo (*Yan Hu Suo*). If the fingertips become swollen, add nine grams each of Sclerotium Poriae Cocos (*Fu Ling*) and Rhizoma Atractylodis Macrocephalae (*Bai Zhu*). If the extremities become ulcerated, delete *Rou Gui* and add 20 grams each of Herba Taraxaci Mongolici Cum Radice (*Pu Gong Ying*) and Flos Lonicerae Japonicae (*Jin Yin Hua*) and nine grams of Radix Angelicae Dahuricae (*Bai Zhi*). For numbness and pain of the fingers or toes, add 12 grams each of Ramulus Cinnamomi Cassiae (*Gui Zhi*) and Ramulus Mori Albi (*Sang Zhi*). For even more marked cold symptoms, add three grams of Herba Asari Cum Radice (*Xi Xin*) and six grams of Radix Lateralis Praeparatus Aconiti Carmichaeli (*Fu Zi*). For concomitant qi vacuity, add 12 grams each of Radix Codonopsitis Pilosulae (*Dang Shen*) and Rhizoma Atractylodis Macrocephalae (*Bai Zhu*). For concomitant blood vacuity, add 12 grams of Gelatinum Corii Asini (*E Jiao*). For stomach and abdominal fullness and loose stools, add nine grams each of Rhizoma Atractylodis Macrocephalae (*Bai Zhu*) and Radix Auklandiae Lappae (*Mu Xiang*).

ACUPUNCTURE & MOXIBUSTION: *Guan Yuan* (CV 4), *Zu San Li* (St 36); for cold fingers, *Que Pen* (St 12), *Nei Guan* (Per 6), *Ba Xie* (M-UE-22); for cold toes, *Huan Tiao* (GB 30), *Cheng Shan* (Bl 57), *Ba Feng* (M-LE-8)

ANALYSIS OF FORMULA: Supplementing *Guan Yuan* and *Zu San Li* with moxibustion warms and supplements spleen and kidney yang. Draining *Que Pen* and *Nei Guan* or *Huan Tiao* and *Cheng Shan* quickens the blood and frees the flow of the vessels in the upper and lower extremities respectively. Moxaing either the *Ba Xie* or *Ba Feng* warms yang and scatters cold locally.

ADDITIONS & SUBTRACTIONS: For more marked purplish color, numbness, cold, and pain in the thumb and forefinger, add *Shou San Li* (LI 10). In the middle finger, add *Da Ling* (Per 7). In the ring finger and little finger, add *Shao Hai* (Ht 3). For more marked purplish color, numbness, cold, and pain in the first toe, add *Di Ji* (Sp 8). In the second and third toes, add *Feng Long* (St 40). In the fourth toe, add *Yang Ling Quan* (GB 34), and in the fifth toe, add *Kun Lun* (Bl 60). For severe purplish fingers or toes with pain, also bleed *Shi Xuan* (M-UE-1). For a cold sensation in the buttocks, add *Zhi Bian* (Bl 54). For a cold sensation or numbness in the upper arm, add *Ji Quan* (Ht 1). For spasmodic pain or for Raynaud's as a stress reaction, add *He Gu* (LI 4) and *Tai Chong* (Liv 3). For severe yang vacuity, moxa *Da Zhui* (GV 14) and *Shen Que* (CV 8).

2. LIVER DEPRESSION QI STAGNATION PATTERN

MAIN SYMPTOMS: Counterflow chilling of the hands caused and aggravated by stress, irritability, emotional depression, chest oppression, frequent sighing, breast, rib-side, and/or abdominal distention and pain, menstrual irregularities in females, a normal or darkish tongue with white fur, and a bowstring pulse

TREATMENT PRINCIPLES: Course the liver and rectify the qi, move the qi and normalize counterflow

RX: *Si Ni San* (Four Counterflows Powder)

INGREDIENTS: Radix Albus Paeoniae Lactiflorae (*Bai Shao*), 12g, Radix Bupleuri (*Chai Hu*), 9g, Fructus Immaturus Citri Aurantii (*Zhi Shi*), 6g, and Radix Glycyrrhizae (*Gan Cao*), 4.5g

ANALYSIS OF FORMULA: *Chai Hu* and *Zhi Shi* course the liver and rectify the qi, move the qi and normalize counterflow. *Bai Shao* and *Gan Cao* emolliate the liver and relax spasm.

ADDITIONS & SUBTRACTIONS: If there is chest, breast, and/or rib-side pain, add 9 grams each of Rhizoma Corydalis Yanhusuo (*Yan Hu Suo*) and Tuber Curcumae (*Yu Jin*). If there is concomitant blood vacuity with menstrual irregularities, delete *Zhi Shi* and add nine grams each of Rhizoma Atractylodis Macrocephalae (*Bai Zhu*), Sclerotium Poriae Cocos (*Fu Ling*), and Radix Angelicae Sinensis (*Dang Gui*). If there is concomitant food stagnation, add nine grams each of Fructus Crataegi (*Shan Zha*), Fructus Germinatus Hordei Vulgaris (*Mai Ya*), and Endothelium Corneum Gigeriae Galli (*Ji Nei Jin*). If there is painful menstruation, add nine grams each of Radix Angelicae Sinensis (*Dang Gui*), Radix Linderae Strychnifoliae (*Wu Yao*), Rhizoma Cyperi Rotundi (*Xiang Fu*), and Rhizoma Corydalis Yanhusuo (*Yan Hu Suo*). For intercostal neuralgia, add nine grams each of Pericarpium Trichosanthis Kirlowii (*Gua Lou Pi*), Bulbus Allii (*Xie Bai*), and Tuber Curcumae (*Yu Jin*). If there is constipation, add 3-6 grams of Radix Et Rhizoma Rhei (*Da Huang*).

If there is counterflow chilling of the hands and feet due to liver depression and blood stasis, replace *Si Ni San* with the following unnamed formula: Caulis Milletiae Seu Spatholobi (*Ji Xue Teng*), Radix Astragali Membranacei (*Huang Qi*), and Radix Albus Paeoniae Lactiflorae (*Bai Shao*), 30g each, Tuber Curcumae (*Yu Jin*), 15g, Ramulus Cinnamomi Cassiae (*Gui Zhi*), Radix Bupleuri (*Chai Hu*), Extremitas Radicis Angelicae Sinensis (*Dang Gui Wei*), Radix Rubrus Paeoniae Lactiflorae (*Chi Shao*), and Radix Glycyrrhizae (*Gan Cao*), 9g each, and Herba Asari Cum Radice (*Xi Xin*), 3g.

If liver depression has transformed internal heat with a dark red tongue and possibly bowstring, rapid pulse despite chilled hands and fingers, replace *Si Ni San* with *Dan Zhi Xiao Yao San* (Moutan & Gardenia Rambling Powder): Radix Albus Paeoniae Lactiflorae (*Bai Shao*), 12g, Radix Bupleuri (*Chai Hu*), Radix Angelicae Sinensis (*Dang Gui*), Rhizoma Atractylodis Macrocephalae (*Bai Zhu*), Sclerotium Poriae Cocos (*Fu Ling*), Cortex Radicis Moutan (*Dan Pi*), and Fructus Gardeniae Jasminoidis (*Zhi Zi*), 9g each, and mix-fried Radix Glycyrrhizae (*Gan Cao*), 6g.

ACUPUNCTURE & MOXIBUSTION: *Tai Chong* (Liv 3), *He Gu* (LI 4); for the fingers, *Nei Guan* (Per 6), *Ba Xie* (M-UE-22); for the toes, *Huan Tiao* (GB 30), *Cheng Shan* (Bl 57), *Ba Feng* (M-LE-8)

ANALYSIS OF FORMULA: Draining *Tai Chong* and *He Gu* courses the liver and rectifies the qi of the entire body. Draining *Nei Guan* and *Ba Xie* or *Huan Tiao, Cheng Shan*, and *Ba Feng* quickens the blood and frees the flow of the vessels in the upper and lower extremities respectively.

ADDITIONS & SUBTRACTIONS: Add *Pi Shu* (Bl 20) and *Wei Shu* (Bl 21) and/or *Zu San Li* (St 36) and *San Yin Jiao* (Sp 6) for concomitant spleen vacuity. Add *San Yin Jiao* (Sp 6) for menstrual irregularities and for concomitant blood stasis. Add *Dan Zhong* (CV 17) for chest oppression and breast distention.

3. BLOOD STASIS PATTERN

MAIN SYMPTOMS: Continuously greenish purple or purplish red fingers and toes which emit coolness accompanied by numbness and tingling, distention and pain with exposure to warmth making these symptoms more pronounced, possible deformation of the nails, a purple, dark tongue and/or static macules or spots, and a deep, fine or deep, choppy pulse

TREATMENT PRINCIPLES: Quicken the blood and transform stasis, warm yang and free the flow of the vessels

RX: *Huo Xue Wen Yang Tang* (Quicken the Blood & Warm Yang Decoction)

INGREDIENTS: Radix Astragali Membranacei (*Huang Qi*), 20g, Radix Salviae Miltiorrhizae (*Dan Shen*) and Radix Angelicae Sinensis (*Dang Gui*), 15g each, and Semen Pruni Persicae (*Tao Ren*), Flos Carthami Tinctorii (*Hong Hua*),

Lumbricus (*Di Long*), Ramulus Cinnamomi Cassiae (*Gui Zhi*), and dry Rhizoma Zingiberis (*Gan Jiang*), 9g each

ANALYSIS OF FORMULA: *Dan Shen, Dang Gui, Tao Ren, Hong Hua,* and *Di Long* together quicken the blood and transform stasis, free the flow of the vessels and stop pain. In addition, *Di Long* extinguishes wind and settles spasms, and *Dang Gui* nourishes the blood to avoid further external damage due to vacuity. *Huang Qi, Gui Zhi,* and *Gan Jiang* boost the qi and warm yang, scatter cold and stop pain.

ADDITIONS & SUBTRACTIONS: For swollen, painful joints, add nine grams each of Radix Stephaniae Tetrandrae (*Han Fang Ji*) and Radix Clematidis Chinensis (*Wei Ling Xian*). For severe blood stasis, add six grams of Hirudo Seu Whitmania (*Shui Zhi*). For severe cold, add three grams of Herba Asari Cum Radice (*Xi Xin*). For constipation, add nine grams each of Semen Pruni (*Yu Li Ren*) and Semen Trichosanthis Kirlowii (*Gua Lou Ren*). For numbness, add 30 grams of Caulis Milletiae Seu Spatholobi (*Ji Xue Teng*). For severe pain, add 15 grams of Rhizoma Corydalis Yanhusuo (*Yan Hu Suo*) and three grams of Buthus Martensis (*Quan Xie*), powdered and taken with the strained decoction. For more marked trouble in the upper limbs, add 12 grams of Ramulus Mori Albi (*Sang Zhi*). For more marked trouble in the lower limbs, add 15 grams of Herba Lycopi Lucidi (*Ze Lan*).

For blood stasis due to qi vacuity, replace *Huo Xue Wen Yang Tang* with *Huang Qi Gui Zhi Wu Wu Tang Jia Wei* (Astragalus & Cinnamon Five Materials Decoction with Added Flavors): Radix Astragali Membranacei (*Huang Qi*), 30g, Radix Codonopsitis Pilosulae (*Dang Shen*) and Fructus Zizyphi Jujubae (*Da Zao*), 20g each, Rhizoma Atractylodis Macrocephalae (*Bai Zhu*), Radix Albus Paeoniae Lactiflorae (*Bai Shao*), and Sclerotium Poriae Cocos (*Fu Ling*), 15g each, Ramulus Cinnamomi Cassiae (*Gui Zhi*), uncooked Rhizoma Zingiberis (*Sheng Jiang*), Rhizoma Corydalis Yanhusuo (*Yan Hu Suo*), and Radix Rubrus Paeoniae Lactiflorae (*Chi Shao*), 12g each, Lumbricus (*Di Long*), 9g, and mix-fried Radix Glycyrrhizae (*Gan Cao*), 6g.

For blood stasis due to liver depression, replace *Huo Xue Wen Yang Tang* with *Chai Hu Shu Gan San Jia Wei* (Bupleurum Course the Liver Powder with Added Flavors): Radix Albus Paeoniae Lactiflorae (*Bai Shao*) and Radix Salviae Miltiorrhizae (*Dan Shen*), 15g each, Rhizoma Cyperi Rotundi (*Xiang Fu*), Semen Pruni Persicae (*Tao Ren*), Radix Angelicae Sinensis (*Dang Gui*), and Radix Cyathulae (*Chuan Niu Xi*), 12g each, Radix Bupleuri (*Chai Hu*), Fructus Citri Aurantii (*Zhi Ke*), and Feces Trogopterori Seu Pteromi (*Wu Ling Zhi*), 9g each, Radix Ligustici Wallichii (*Chuan Xiong*), 6g, and Radix Glycyrrhizae (*Gan Cao*), 3g. For more severe liver depression, add nine grams of Fructus Meliae Toosendan (*Chuan Lian Zi*) and 15 grams of Rhizoma Corydalis Yanhusuo (*Yan Hu Suo*).

ACUPUNCTURE & MOXIBUSTION: *Guan Yuan* (CV 4), *San Yin Jiao* (Sp 6), *He Gu* (LI 4); for the fingers, *Que Pen* (St 12), *Nei Guan* (Per 6), *Ba Xie* (M-UE-22); for the toes, *Huan Tiao* (GB 30), *Cheng Shan* (Bl 57), *Ba Feng* (M-LE-8)

ANALYSIS OF FORMULA: Supplementing *Guan Yuan* with moxibustion warms and supplements spleen and kidney yang and scatters cold. Draining *San Yin Jiao* and *He Gu* moves the qi, quickens the blood, and transforms stasis in the whole body. Draining *Que Pen* and *Nei Guan* or *Huan Tiao* and *Cheng Shan* quickens the blood and frees the flow of the vessels in the upper and lower extremities respectively. Moxaing the *Ba Xie* or *Ba Feng* warms yang and scatters cold, frees the flow of the vessels and stops pain locally.

ADDITIONS & SUBTRACTIONS: For a more marked purplish color, numbness, cold, or pain in the thumb and forefinger, add *Shou San Li* (LI 10). In the middle finger, add *Da Ling* (Per 7). In the ring and little finger, add *Shao Hai* (Ht 3). For more marked purplish color, numbness, cold, or pain in the first toe, add *Di Ji* (Sp 8). In the second and third toes, add *Feng Long* (St 40). In the fourth toe, add *Yang Ling Quan* (GB 34). In the fifth toe, add *Kun Lun* (Bl 60). For severe purplish fingers or toes with pain, also bleed *Shi Xuan* (M-UE-1). For a cold sensation in the buttocks, add *Zhi Bian* (Bl 54). For a cold sensation or numbness in the upper arm, add *Ji Quan* (Ht 1). For spasmodic pain or Raynaud's as a stress reaction, add *Tai Chong* (Liv 3). For severe yang vacuity, moxa *Da Zhui* (GV 14) and *Shen Que* (CV 8).

4. DAMP HEAT PATTERN

MAIN SYMPTOMS: Swelling, distention, aching, and pain of the affected fingers or toes with benign sores or peripheral obstruction, a red tongue with slimy, yellow fur, and a bowstring, slippery, and rapid pulse

TREATMENT PRINCIPLES: Clear heat and dry dampness, transform stasis and stop pain

RX: *Qing Re Zao Shi Tang* (Clear Heat & Dry Dampness Decoction)

INGREDIENTS: Flos Lonicerae Japonicae (*Jin Yin Hua*), 20g, Herba Violae Yedoensitis (*Zi Hua Di Ding*), Radix Angelicae Sinensis (*Dang Gui*), and Radix Salviae Miltiorrhizae (*Dan Shen*), 15g each, and Radix Scutellariae Baicalensis (*Huang Qin*), Radix Scrophulariae Ningpoensis (*Xuan Shen*), Rhizoma Atractylodis (*Cang Zhu*), Tuber Curcumae Longae (*Jiang Huang*), Rhizoma Corydalis Yanhusuo (*Yan Hu Suo*), and Radix Glycyrrhizae (*Gan Cao*), 9g each

ANALYSIS OF FORMULA: *Jin Yin Hua, Zi Hua Di Ding, Huang Qin,* and *Xuan Shen* clear heat and resolve toxins. *Huang Qin, Cang Zhu,* and *Jiang Huang* together clear heat and dry dampness. *Dang Gui, Dan Shen,* and *Yan Hu Suo* quicken the blood, transform stasis, and stop pain. *Gan Cao* harmonizes the other medicinals in this formula.

ADDITIONS & SUBTRACTIONS: For damp heat toxins with severe ulceration, add 12 grams each of Cortex Phellodendri (*Huang Bai*), Herba Taraxaci Mongolici Cum Radice (*Pu Gong Ying*), and Radix Lithospermi Seu Arnebiae (*Zi Cao*). For predominantly an upper limb disorder, add 12 grams of Ramulus Mori Albi (*Sang Zhi*). For predominantly a lower limb disorder, add 12 grams of Radix Cyathulae (*Chuan Niu Xi*). For severe pain, add six grams each of Resina Olibani (*Ru Xiang*) and Resina Myrrhae (*Mo Yao*). For concomitant liver depression, add 12 grams each of Radix Bupleuri (*Chai Hu*) and Radix Albus Paeoniae Lactiflorae (*Bai Shao*).

ACUPUNCTURE & MOXIBUSTION: *Nei Ting* (St 44), *Yin Ling Quan* (Sp 9), *Shi Xuan* (M-UE-1); for the fingers, *Que Pen* (St 12), *Nei Guan* (Per 6), *Ba Xie* (M-UE-22); for the toes, *Huan Tiao* (GB 30), *Cheng Shan* (Bl 57), *Ba Feng* (M-LE-8)

ANALYSIS OF FORMULA: Draining *Nei Ting* and *Yin Ling Quan* and bleeding the *Shi Xuan* together clear heat and disinhibit dampness, disperse swelling, transform stasis, and stop pain. Draining *Que Pen* and *Nei Guan* or *Huan Tiao* and *Cheng Shan* quickens the blood and frees the flow of the vessels in the upper and lower extremities respectively. Draining the *Ba Xie* and *Ba Feng* clears heat and disperses swelling, frees the flow of the vessels and stops pain locally.

ADDITIONS & SUBTRACTIONS: For more swelling, numbness, or pain in the thumb and forefinger, add *Shou San Li* (LI 10). In the middle finger, add *Da Ling* (Per 7). In the ring and little finger, add *Shao Hai* (Ht 3). For more swelling, numbness, or pain in the first toe, add *Di Ji* (Sp 8). In the second and third toes, add *Feng Long* (St 40). In the fourth toe, add *Yang Ling Quan* (GB 34). In the fifth toe, add *Kun Lun* (Bl 60). For spasmodic pain or Raynaud's due to a stress reaction, add *Tai Chong* (Liv 3).

REMARKS

1. As in modern Western medicine, when Raynaud's phenomenon is merely a symptom of some other disease, Chinese medical treatment should be primarily addressed to the patterns corresponding to the patient's entire presentation. Since the disease mechanisms of Raynaud's phenomenon in that case are part and parcel of the pathomechanisms of the main disease, the symptoms of Raynaud's phenomenon will automatically disappear if those pathomechanisms are treated comprehensively.

2. If the fingertips or toes are markedly cold, numb, and/or painful, one can make a decoction of uncooked Rhizoma Zingiberis (*Sheng Jiang*), Herba Asari Cum Radice (*Xi Xin*), and Ramulus Cinnamomi Cassiae (*Gui Zhi*) as a warm soak. It is also possible to sprinkle a small amount ofcayenne pepper (*La Jiao*) into the gloves or socks during the wintertime or when working or playing outdoors.

3. Because Raynaud's disease refers to idiopathic spasming of the arterioles, some modern Chinese formulas use wind-extinguishing, network vessel freeing medicinals for their antispasmodic effect for the treatment of this condition. A representative modern Chinese formula using this idea is *Jie Jing Zhi Tong San* (Resolve Spasm & Stop Pain Powder): dry Rhizoma Zingiberis (*Gan Jiang*) and Radix Lateralis Praeparatus Aconiti Carmichaeli (*Fu Zi*), 60g each, Scolopendra Subspinipes (*Wu Gong*), Buthus Martensis (*Quan Xie*), Eupolyphaga Seu Opisthoplatia (*Tu Bie Chong*), Hirudo Seu Whitmania (*Shui Zhi*), Cornu Cervi (*Lu Jiao*), and Succinum (*Hu Po*), 45g each, and Flos Daturae (*Yang Jin Hua*), 20g. These medicinals are ground into powder and five grams are taken orally two times per day. This formula warms yang and scatters cold, quickens the blood and transforms stasis, frees the flow of the network vessels and stops pain.

4. According to Chinese practice, Radix Angelicae Sinensis (*Dang Gui*) and Ramulus Cinnamomi Cassiae (*Gui Zhi*) are the two most frequently prescribed medicinals for Raynaud's disease. For instance, this combination is found in *Dang Gui Si Ni Tang* (Dang Gui Four Counterflows Decoction). *Dang Gui* is acrid and warm, and it mainly treats disease of the blood division or aspect. It is a "holy medicinal among the [medicinals which treat] the blood." *Dang Gui* both supplements and quickens the blood. In other words, it harmonizes the blood of the whole body. It is a main medicinal for the treatment of counterflow chilling of the four limbs. *Gui Zhi* is sweet, acrid, and warm. It travels channels and network vessels, moves blood division or aspect, warms the channels and frees the flow of the vessels. It is a main medicinal for harmonizing the constructive and defensive. *Gui Zhi* is also a key ingredient for treating cold evils in the channels and network vessels.

5. Because cold, stasis, and vacuity are the main patterns of this disorder, other important medicinals for Raynaud's disease according to clinical experience are Radix Astragali Membranacei (*Huang Qi*) when there is yang qi vacuity, Radix Lateralis Praeparatus Aconiti Carmichaeli (*Fu Zi*) and Herba Asari Cum Radice (*Xi Xin*) when there is severe cold, Radix Albus Paeoniae Lactiflorae (*Bai Shao*) when thereis blood vacuity, and Radix Salviae Miltiorrhizae (*Dan Shen*) and Flos Carthami Tinctorii (*Hong Hua*) when there is blood stasis.

6. Some Chinese doctors prescribe Radix Astragali Membranacei (*Huang Qi*) for Raynaud's disease in a large dose of up to 60g. Similarly large doses of Radix Angelicae Sinensis (*Dang Gui*) are also sometimes used for this disease.

However, such large doses of *Dang Gui* may provoke the side effects of abdominal fullness, loose stools, and reduced appetite.

7. Since smoking tobacco results in constricting of the arterioles, cessation of smoking is a must if real improvement is to be expected.

8. Western drugs which trigger Raynaud's symptoms include beta-blockers used to treat hypertension and ergotamine used in the treatment of migraines.

9. When the symptoms of Raynaud's are due to a stress reaction, biofeedback is especially useful.

62

REFLUX ESOPHAGITIS

Reflux esophagitis refers to inflammation of the gastro-esophageal tract due to reflux of the gastric contents into the esophagus. Its main symptom is heartburn with or without regurgitation of the gastric contents into the mouth, and it mostly commonly occurs in middle-aged adults. The complications of esophagitis may cause tooth pain when eating and possibly massive but usually limited hemorrhage. Peptic stricture may cause gradual, progressive dysphagia of solid foods. The Western medical diagnosis of this condition is based on the patient's history, their presenting signs and symptoms, x-ray, endoscopy, esophageal manometry, pH monitoring, and the Bernstein acid perfusion test. Western medical treatment consists of A) elevating the head while sleeping, B) avoiding foods and beverages which stimulate acid secretion, such as coffee and alcohol, anticholingergic drugs, certain specific foods, such as fats and chocolate, and smoking, and C) administering antacids after meals and at bedtime. If these measures are not sufficient, cholingergic agonists, such as bethanechol or metoclopramide, and H_2 agonists, such as cimetidine, may be prescribed to increase sphincter pressure and reduce stomach acidity. If esophageal hemorrhage is massive or recurrent, it may require surgery. Esophageal strictures are treated by repeated dilation.

CHINESE DISEASE CATEGORIZATION: Reflux esophagitis is categorized as *tun suan*, swallowing acid, *i.e.*, acid regurgitation, *ou dan*, vomiting bile, *ou ku*, vomiting bitter, *fu pi*, abdominal glomus, and *wei wan tong*, stomach venter pain. Dysphagia is *ye ge*, dysphagia occlusion, and esophageal hemorrhage is *ou xue*, retching of blood.

DISEASE CAUSES: Internal damage by the seven affects, unregulated eating and drinking, and habitual bodily vacuity due to aging

DISEASE MECHANISMS: The primary disease mechanism of this disease is liver wood invading spleen and/or stomach earth, and the main mechanisms for the liver becoming replete are unfulfilled desires and/or anger, both of which may damage the liver. If the liver becomes damaged, it may lose control over coursing and discharge. The qi becomes stagnant and accumulates. Eventually it must counterflow somewhere. Typically it counterflows horizontally to assail either or both the spleen and stomach. If the liver invades the stomach, the stomach qi loses its harmony and counterflows upward. If the liver invades the spleen, the spleen becomes vacuous and weak. If the spleen becomes weak, it will fail to upbear the clear. If the spleen fails to upbear the clear, the stomach qi is less likely to downbear the turbid. Therefore, spleen qi vacuity makes upward counterflow of the stomach all the more likely. In addition, if the spleen loses control over the movement and transformation of liquids, these will collect and accumulate, transforming into dampness. If dampness obstructs the middle, it results in feelings of glomus and distention. In addition, vacuity cold due to spleen vacuity or cold due to over-eating chilled foods may lead to contraction and constricture resulting in pain.

If liver depression endures for some time or is extreme, it may transform into heat. Such transformative heat is all the more likely if the patient eats or drinks foods or beverages which also engender heat internally. Depressive heat may then mutually engender stomach heat. If heat is severe, it may force the blood to move frenetically outside its channels, thus resulting in retching of blood. If heat is complicated by spleen qi vacuity not containing the blood, this may also contribute to bleeding. If heat endures for some time, it may damage and consume stomach fluids. If heat combines with dampness, it may transform into damp heat. If qi stagnation endures for some time, it may eventually result in blood stasis. Likewise, since food is moved and transformed by the qi, if qi becomes stagnant so may food. Because the liver's functioning depends on that viscus receiving proper nourishment by the blood, the spleen is the root of blood engenderment, and the spleen typically becomes vacuous and weak as part of the aging process, liver depression tends to get worse in late middle age, especially since this is a time when most adults are stressed with work and family.

TREATMENT BASED ON PATTERN DISCRIMINATION:

1. WOOD-EARTH DISHARMONY MIXED WITH COLD DAMPNESS PATTERN

MAIN SYMPTOMS: Stomach duct distention and fullness, borborygmus, watery, loose stools, dull pain in the stomach relieved by warmth and pressure, moderate pain when eating, occasional vomiting of bitter water, a dry mouth but no desire to drink, a pale tongue with white fur, and a deep, fine, bowstring pulse

TREATMENT PRINCIPLES: Course the liver and rectify the qi, disinhibit the qi mechanism and harmonize upbearing and downbearing

RX: *Chai Hu Shu Gan San* (Bupleurum Course the Liver Powder) & *Er Chen Tang* (Two Aged [Ingredients] Decoction) with additions and subtractions

INGREDIENTS: Rhizoma Pinelliae Ternatae (*Ban Xia*), 12g, Radix Bupleuri (*Chai Hu*), Herba Artemisiae Capillaris (*Yin Chen Hao*), Radix Albus Paeoniae Lactiflorae (*Bai Shao*), Rhizoma Cyperi Rotundi (*Xiang Fu*), and Sclerotium Poriae Cocos (*Fu Ling*), 9g each, Fructus Evodiae Rutecarpae (*Wu Zhu Yu*), Fructus Cardamomi (*Bai Dou Kou*), Fructus Immaturus Citri Aurantii (*Zhi Shi*), and Pericarpium Citri Reticulatae (*Chen Pi*), 6g each, mix-fried Radix Glycyrrhizae (*Gan Cao*), 3g, and uncooked Rhizoma Zingiberis (*Sheng Jiang*), 3 slices

ANALYSIS OF FORMULA: *Ban Xia*, *Fu Ling*, and *Bai Dou Kou* dry, disinhibit, and transform dampness. In addition, *Ban Xia* with *Chen Pi* and *Sheng Jiang* harmonize the stomach and stop vomiting. *Chen Pi* and *Zhi Shi* move the qi to eliminate accumulated dampness. *Chai Hu* and *Xiang Fu* course the liver and resolve the depression. *Bai Shao* nourishes the blood and emolliates the liver. *Yin Chen Hao* clears and eliminates dampness and heat and stops vomiting of bitter fluids. *Wu Zhu Yu* warms the center and scatters cold, downbears counterflow and stops vomiting, especially of sour fluids. *Gan Cao* harmonizes the other medicinals in this formula and also treats acid regurgitation.

ADDITIONS & SUBTRACTIONS: If spleen vacuity is pronounced, add nine grams each of Radix Codonopsitis Pilosulae (*Dang Shen*) and Rhizoma Atractylodis Macrocephalae (*Bai Zhu*). For severe stomach distention, add six grams of Fructus Amomi (*Sha Ren*) and nine grams each of Herba Agastachis Seu Pogostemi (*Huo Xiang*) and Caulis Perillae Frutescentis (*Su Geng*). For aversion to cold, cold limbs, and a cold sensation in the stomach, add six grams each of Rhizoma Alpiniae Officinari (*Gao Liang Jiang*) and dry Rhizoma Zingiberis (*Gan Jiang*). For vomiting of phlegm, add 12 grams of Flos Inulae (*Xuan Fu Hua*). For rib-side and stomach pain, add nine grams each of Fructus Meliae Toosendan (*Chuan Lian Zi*) and Rhizoma Corydalis Yanhusuo (*Yan Hu Suo*).

ACUPUNCTURE & MOXIBUSTION: *Zu San Li* (St 36), *Shang Wan* (CV 13), *Zhong Wan* (CV 12), *Nei Guan* (Per 6), *Gong Sun* (Sp 4)

ANALYSIS OF FORMULA: Draining *Nei Guan* courses the liver and harmonizes the stomach. Draining *Gong Sun* harmonizes the stomach and rectifies the qi. Together, they disinhibit the qi mechanism and harmonize upbearing and downbearing. Draining *Zu San Li*, *Shang Wan*, and *Zhong Wan* disinhibits dampness and downbears counterflow, harmonizes the stomach and stops vomiting.

ADDITIONS & SUBTRACTIONS: For cold symptoms, add moxibustion on *Zu San Li*, *Shang Wan*, and *Zhong Wan*. For severe liver depression, add *Tai Chong* (Liv 3). For rib-side and stomach pain, add *Qi Men* (Liv 14). For acid regurgitation, add *Ri Yue* (GB 24). For hiccup or belching, add *Ge Shu* (Bl 17). For food stagnation, add *Liang Men* (St 21).

2. WOOD-EARTH DISHARMONY MIXED WITH DEPRESSIVE HEAT PATTERN

MAIN SYMPTOMS: Burning pain, clamoring stomach, bitter-tasting vomit, acid regurgitation, vexation and agitation, irascibility, a bitter taste in the mouth, a dry mouth and thirst with a predilection for chilled drinks, a red tongue with yellow fur, and a bowstring, rapid pulse

TREATMENT PRINCIPLES: Course the liver and clear heat, disinhibit the qi mechanism and harmonize upbearing and downbearing

RX: *Chai Hu Shu Gan San* (Bupleurum Course the Liver Powder) & *Er Chen Tang* (Two Aged [Ingredients] Decoction) with additions and subtractions

INGREDIENTS: Rhizoma Pinelliae Ternatae (*Ban Xia*) and Caulis Bambusae In Taeniis (*Zhu Ru*), 12g each, Radix Bupleuri (*Chai Hu*), Herba Artemisiae Capillaris (*Yin Chen Hao*), Radix Scutellariae Baicalensis (*Huang Qin*), Radix Albus Paeoniae Lactiflorae (*Bai Shao*), Rhizoma Cyperi Rotundi (*Xiang Fu*), and Sclerotium Poriae Cocos (*Fu Ling*), 9g each, Fructus Immaturus Citri Aurantii (*Zhi Shi*), and Pericarpium Citri Reticulatae (*Chen Pi*), 6g each, mix-fried Radix Glycyrrhizae (*Gan Cao*) and Rhizoma Coptidis

Chinensis (*Huang Lian*), 3g each, and uncooked Rhizoma Zingiberis (*Sheng Jiang*), 3 slices

ANALYSIS OF FORMULA: *Chai Hu, Bai Shao, Zhi Shi,* and *Xiang Fu* course the liver and resolve depression. *Huang Qin* and *Huang Lian* clear depressive heat from the liver, gallbladder, and stomach. *Sheng Jiang, Ban Xia, Zhu Ru,* and *Chen Pi* harmonize the stomach and stop vomiting. In addition, *Zhu Ru* clears the stomach and *Chen Pi* with *Fu Ling* eliminates dampness. *Yin Chen Hao* clears and disinhibits dampness and heat and treats a bitter taste in the mouth. *Gan Cao* harmonizes the other medicinals in this formula and also treats acid regurgitation.

ADDITIONS & SUBTRACTIONS: If heat is causing retching of blood, add 15 grams of Rhizoma Imperatae Cylindricae (*Bai Mao Gen*) and nine grams each of Fructus Gardeniae Jasminoidis (*Zhi Zi*) and Radix Rubiae Cordifoliae (*Qian Cao Gen*). If spleen vacuity is pronounced, add nine grams each of Radix Codonopsitis Pilosulae (*Dang Shen*) and Rhizoma Atractylodis Macrocephalae (*Bai Zhu*). For severe counterflow of the stomach, add 12 grams each of Folium Eriobotryae Japonicae (*Pi Pa Ye*) and Rhizoma Imperatae Cylindricae (*Bai Mao Gen*). For concomitant food stagnation, add nine grams each of Fructus Crataegi (*Shan Zha*) and Fructus Germinatus Hordei Vulgaris (*Mai Ya*). For severe rib-side distention and pain, add nine grams each of Fructus Meliae Toosendan (*Chuan Lian Zi*) and Tuber Curcumae (*Yu Jin*). For fixed, stabbing pain in the stomach, add 12 grams each of Rhizoma Corydalis Yanhusuo (*Yan Hu Suo*) and Radix Salviae Miltiorrhizae (*Dan Shen*).

ACUPUNCTURE & MOXIBUSTION: *Yang Ling Quan* (GB 34), *Nei Ting* (St 44), *Shang Wan* (CV 13), *Zhong Wan* (CV 12), *Nei Guan* (Per 6), *Gong Sun* (Sp 4)

ANALYSIS OF FORMULA: Draining *Nei Guan* courses the liver and harmonizes the stomach. Draining *Gong Sun* harmonizes the stomach and rectifies the qi. Together, they disinhibit the qi mechanism and harmonize upbearing and downbearing. Draining *Yang Ling Quan* courses and clears the liver and gallbladder and treats a bitter or sour taste in the mouth. Draining *Nei Ting* clears the stomach and discharges depressive heat of the yang ming. Draining *Shang Wan* and *Zhong Wan* clears and harmonizes the stomach, downbears counterflow, and stops vomiting.

ADDITIONS & SUBTRACTIONS: For concomitant spleen qi vacuity, add *Zu San Li* (St 36). For constipation or irregular defecation, add *Zhi Gou* (TB 6). For severe liver depression, add *Tai Chong* (Liv 3). For rib-side and stomach pain, add *Qi Men* (Liv 14). For acid regurgitation, add *Ri Yue* (GB 24). For acid stomach, add *Liang Qiu* (St 34). For hiccup or belching, add *Ge Shu* (Bl 17).

3. WOOD-EARTH DISHARMONY MIXED WITH VACUITY PATTERN

MAIN SYMPTOMS: Stomach duct pain which is tolerable and which lessens with eating, torpid intake, reduced food intake, abdominal distention after meals, fatigue, lassitude of the spirit, lack of strength, clear, watery vomit, a pale, fat tongue with teeth-marks on its edges and thin, white fur, and a fine, bowstring or soggy, bowstring pulse

TREATMENT PRINCIPLES: Course the liver and fortify the spleen, disinhibit the qi mechanism and harmonize upbearing and downbearing

RX: *Chai Hu Shu Gan San* (Bupleurum Course the Liver Powder) & *Er Chen Tang* (Two Aged [Ingredients] Decoction) with additions and subtractions

INGREDIENTS: Radix Astragali Membranacei (*Huang Qi*), 15g, Rhizoma Pinelliae Ternatae (*Ban Xia*), 12g, Radix Bupleuri (*Chai Hu*), Herba Artemisiae Capillaris (*Yin Chen Hao*), Radix Albus Paeoniae Lactiflorae (*Bai Shao*), Rhizoma Cyperi Rotundi (*Xiang Fu*), and Sclerotium Poriae Cocos (*Fu Ling*), 9g each, Fructus Immaturus Citri Aurantii (*Zhi Shi*) and Pericarpium Citri Reticulatae (*Chen Pi*), 6g each, mix-fried Radix Glycyrrhizae (*Gan Cao*), 3g, uncooked Rhizoma Zingiberis (*Sheng Jiang*), 3 slices, and Fructus Zizyphi Jujubae (*Da Zao*), 3 pieces

ANALYSIS OF FORMULA: *Chai Hu, Bai Shao, Zhi Shi,* and *Xiang Fu* course the liver and resolve depression. *Huang Qi, Fu Ling,* mix-fried *Gan Cao,* and *Da Zao* fortify the spleen and boost the qi. *Sheng Jiang, Ban Xia,* and *Chen Pi* harmonize the stomach and stop vomiting. In addition, *Chen Pi* with *Fu Ling* eliminates dampness. *Yin Chen Hao* clears and disinhibits dampness and heat and treats a bitter taste in the mouth. *Gan Cao* harmonizes the other medicinals in this formula and also treats acid regurgitation.

ADDITIONS & SUBTRACTIONS: If complicated by heat, add nine grams of Radix Scutellariae Baicalensis (*Huang Qin*). If heat is even more severe, add three grams of Rhizoma Coptidis Chinensis (*Huang Lian*). If complicated by food stagnation, add six grams each of Massa Medica Fermentatae (*Shen Qu*). If complicated by cold, replace *Sheng Jiang* with six grams of dry Rhizoma Zingiberis (*Gan Jiang*). If there is a qi and yin dual vacuity, add 12 grams each of Radix Glehniae Littoralis (*Sha Shen*) and Tuber Ophiopogonis Japonici (*Mai Dong*) and nine grams of Herba Dendrobii (*Shi Hu*). If there is concomitant blood stasis, add 15 grams of Radix Salviae Miltiorrhizae (*Dan Shen*). If there is hemorrhaging due to qi vacuity, add 12 grams of Terra Flava Usta (*Fu Long Gan*) and 15 grams of Rhizoma Bletillae Striatae (*Bai Ji*).

ACUPUNCTURE & MOXIBUSTION: *Zu San Li* (St 36), *Tai Bai* (Sp 3), *Shang Wan* (CV 13), *Nei Guan* (Per 6), *Gong Sun* (Sp 4)

ANALYSIS OF FORMULA: Draining *Nei Guan* courses the liver and harmonizes the stomach. Draining *Gong Sun* harmonizes the stomach and rectifies the qi. Together, they disinhibit the qi mechanism and harmonize upbearing and downbearing. Supplementing *Zu San Li* and *Tai Bai* bank the earth and boost the qi. Draining *Shang Wan* harmonizes the stomach and stops vomiting.

ADDITIONS & SUBTRACTIONS: For severe vomiting, add *Zhong Wan* (CV 12). For cold symptoms, add moxibustion on *Zu San Li* (St 36), *Tai Bai* (Sp 3), and *Shang Wan* (CV 13). For heat symptoms, add *Nei Ting* (St 44). For food stagnation, add *Liang Men* (St 21). For severe liver depression, add *Tai Chong* (Liv 3). For rib-side and stomach pain, add *Qi Men* (Liv 14). For acid regurgitation, add *Ri Yue* (GB 24). For hiccup and belching, add *Ge Shu* (Bl 17)

4. WOOD-EARTH DISHARMONY MIXED WITH YANG MING REPLETION PATTERN

MAIN SYMPTOMS: Stomach duct distention and fullness, severe pain, retching and bitter flooding vomiting worsened by eating, a bitter taste in the mouth, bad breath, dry, bound stools, a red tongue with yellow fur, and a bowstring, rapid, slippery, forceful pulse

NOTE: The yang ming repletion in this pattern's name is both heat and food stagnation.

TREATMENT PRINCIPLES: Clear heat and abduct stagnation, disinhibit the qi mechanism and harmonize upbearing and downbearing

RX: *Chai Hu Shu Gan San* (Bupleurum Course the Liver Powder) & *Er Chen Tang* (Two Aged [Ingredients] Decoction) with additions and subtractions

INGREDIENTS: Rhizoma Pinelliae Ternatae (*Ban Xia*) and Fructus Germinatus Hordei Vulgaris (*Mai Ya*), 12g each, Radix Bupleuri (*Chai Hu*), Herba Artemisiae Capillaris (*Yin Chen Hao*), Radix Albus Paeoniae Lactiflorae (*Bai Shao*), Rhizoma Cyperi Rotundi (*Xiang Fu*), Massa Medica Fermentata (*Shen Qu*), Fructus Crataegi (*Shan Zha*), and Sclerotium Poriae Cocos (*Fu Ling*), 9g each, Fructus Immaturus Citri Aurantii (*Zhi Shi*), Radix Et Rhizoma Rhei (*Da Huang*), and Pericarpium Citri Reticulatae (*Chen Pi*), 6g each, and mix-fried Radix Glycyrrhizae (*Gan Cao*), 3g

ANALYSIS OF FORMULA: *Chai Hu, Bai Shao, Zhi Shi,* and *Xiang Fu* course the liver and resolve depression. *Mai Ya, Shen Qu,* and *Shan Zha,* with the help of *Zhi Shi* and *Chen Pi,* disperse food and abduct stagnation. *Da Huang* discharges heat from the yang ming and, with the help of *Zhi Shi,* frees the flow of the stools. *Ban Xia* and *Chen Pi* harmonize the stomach and stop vomiting. In addition, *Chen Pi* with *Fu Ling* eliminates dampness. *Yin Chen Hao* clears and disinhibits dampness and heat and treats a bitter taste in the mouth. *Gan Cao* harmonizes the other medicinals in this formula and also treats acid regurgitation.

ADDITIONS & SUBTRACTIONS: For bitter tasting vomiting, add three grams of Rhizoma Coptidis Chinensis (*Huang Lian*) and six grams of Fructus Evodiae Rutecarpae (*Wu Zhu Yu*). For belching and hiccup, add nine grams each of Caulis Bambusae In Taeniis (*Zhu Ru*) and Folium Eriobotryae Japonicae (*Pi Pa Ye*). For pain, add 15 grams of Rhizoma Corydalis Yanhusuo (*Yan Hu Suo*) and nine grams each of Radix Angelicae Dahuricae (*Bai Zhi*) and Tuber Curcumae (*Yu Jin*). For more pronounced distention and fullness, add nine grams each of Semen Raphani Sativi (*Lai Fu Zi*) and Caulis Perillae Frutescentis (*Su Geng*).

ACUPUNCTURE & MOXIBUSTION: *He Gu* (LI 4), *Zhi Gou* (TB 6), *Shang Wan* (CV 13), *Zhong Wan* (CV 12), *Nei Guan* (Per 6), *Gong Sun* (Sp 4)

ANALYSIS OF FORMULA: Draining *Nei Guan* courses the liver and harmonizes the stomach. Draining *Gong Sun* harmonizes the stomach and rectifies the qi. Together, they disinhibit the qi mechanism and harmonize upbearing and downbearing. Draining *He Gu* clears the stomach and discharges depressive heat of the yang ming. Draining *Zhi Gou* clears the three burners. Together, they free the flow of the stools and treat constipation. Draining *Shang Wan* and *Zhong Wan* clear the stomach and disperse food, abduct stagnation and stop vomiting.

ADDITIONS & SUBTRACTIONS: For acid stomach, add *Liang Qiu* (St 34). For severe constipation, add *Tian Shu* (St 25) and *Xia Wan* (CV 10). For severe food stagnation, add *Liang Men* (St 21). For concomitant liver fire, add *Yang Ling Quan* (GB 34). For severe heat in the yang ming, add *Nei Ting* (St 44). For rib-side and stomach pain, add *Qi Men* (Liv 14). For acid regurgitation, add *Ri Yue* (GB 24). For hiccup or belching, add *Ge Shu* (Bl 17).

REMARKS

1. Liver invading earth is the main disease mechanism of this condition. Depending on the patient's constitution, age, diet, and lifestyle, this is then complicated by more or less stomach disharmony, spleen vacuity, cold, dampness, food stagnation, damp heat, depressive heat, yin vacuity, and/or blood stasis. In most Western patients with this condition, there will be depressive heat. When there is bile reflux, there is always either damp or depressive heat.

2. The disease mechanisms and patterns of hiatal hernia are essentially the same as for reflux esophagitis. Its root is a wood-earth disharmony causing stomach venter or chest pain. However, although depressive heat may be seen in hiatal hernia, its presence is not as common as in reflux esophagitis where one can mostly assume its presence in Western patients.

3. If pH monitoring shows that stomach acid is elevated, one can add 12 grams of Concha Arecae Inflatae (*Wa Leng Zi*) and/or Concha Ostreae (*Mu Li*) to the above formulas based on the modern Chinese treatment principles of lowering acid. In this case, these formulas should be taken after meals.

4. The main Chinese medicinals for treating acid regurgitation are Radix Glycyrrhizae (*Gan Cao*), Concha Ostreae (*Duan Mu Li*), Concha Cyclinae Sinensis (*Hai Ge Ke*), Os Sepiae Seu Sepiellae (*Hai Piao Xiao*), calcined Concha Arcae Inflatae (*Wa Leng Zi*), Concha Margaritiferae (*Zhen Zhu Mu*) and the pairs: Rhizoma Coptidis Chinensis (*Huang Lian*) and Fructus Evodiae Rutecarpae (*Wu Zhu Yu*) and Os Sepiae Seu Sepiellae (*Hai Piao Xiao*) and Bulbus Fritillariae Thunbergii (*Zhe Bei Mu*).

63

Rheumatoid Arthritis

Rheumatoid arthritis (RA) refers to a chronic syndrome whose main manifestation is nonspecific, usually symmetrical inflammation of the peripheral joints. This inflammation may potentially lead to progressive destruction of the articular and periarticular structures. In Western medicine, RA is usually considered an autoimmune disease, although, like so many autoimmune diseases, its etiology is unknown. Popular suspects include food allergies due to leaky gut, genetic susceptibility, lifestyle factors, and microorganisms. there may also be an association between RA and abnormal bowel function.[1] Rheumatoid arthritis affects approximately 2.1 million people in the United States, most often women. This condition usually starts between 20-50 years of age.[2]

The onset of this disease may be either abrupt or, more commonly, insidious. Its first signs and symptoms are usually simultaneous inflammation of several joints, especially the proximal interphalangeal and metacarpophalangeal joints. Other joints commonly affected include the small joints of the feet, wrists, elbows, and ankles. Those joints which are affected are typically tender to palpation, and there is eventual synovial thickening in most of the affected joints. In addition, there is stiffness lasting more than 30 minutes initially on arising in the morning after sleep or after prolonged inactivity. Early afternoon fatigue and malaise may also occur. If joint tissue degeneration continues, the affected joints may become deformed. However, the subcutaneous rheumatoid nodules which are characteristic of this disease usually only develop in advanced disease. If there is accompanying fever, it is typically low-grade. Other accompanying conditions may include visceral nodules, leg ulcers, pleural or pericardial effusions, lymphadenopathy, and Sjögren's syndrome.

In terms of Western medical diagnosis, rheumatoid factors (RFs) are present in 70% of cases, while ESR is elevated in 90% of cases. Synovial fluid is always abnormal during active joint inflammation, being cloudy, sterile, reduced in viscosity, and containing 3000-50,000WBCs/cu mm. Radiologically, only soft tissue swelling is seen in the first months of this disease. However, as the disease continues, X-rays may show periarticular osteoporosis, joint space narrowing, and marginal erosion. Western physicians treat RA with a combination of rest, nonsteriodal anti-inflammatory drugs (NSAIDs), such as salicylates, indomethacin, and ibuprofen, gold compounds, hydroxychloroquine, corticosteriods, immuno-suppressive drugs, exercise, physical therapy, and surgery.

Disease categorization: Rheumatoid arthritis is mainly categorized as *bi zheng*, impediment condition, in Chinese medicine. If there is fatigue, this is categorized as *pi juan*, fatigue, while low-grade fever is a species of *fa re*, emission of heat.

Disease causes: Habitual bodily righteous vacuity with external invasion of evils; long living in a damp environment and contraction of wind, cold, damp, and/or heat evils

Disease mechanisms: Due to habitual righteous qi vacuity, the interstices may be coursed and slack and the constructive and defensive may be disharmonious. In that case external evils may take advantage of this vacuity and assail and enter where they impede and obstruct the qi and blood. Hence the movement of the joints is inhibited. It is also possible that prolonged living in a damp environment or exposure to rain and cold, damp, chilly weather may lead to contraction of wind, cold, and damp evils. If evil qi lodges in the sinews, bones, and joints, it may congeal there and produce impediment. And finally, habitual bodily yang exuberance may transform these evils into heat which may course and pour into the joints where it obstructs and stagnates the qi and blood, thus producing this disease. If enduring heat damages and consumes yin fluids, this may give rise to liver-kidney yin vacuity. If either spleen qi vacuity reaches the kidneys or yin vacuity affects yang, there may be concomitant kidney yang vacuity. If impediment endures and is not treated, it may engender blood stasis which enters the network vessels. Because blood and fluids flow together, blood stasis may further become complicated phlegm obstruction and nodulation.

TREATMENT BASED ON PATTERN DISCRIMINATION:

1. WIND COLD DAMP IMPEDIMENT PATTERN

MAIN SYMPTOMS: This pattern typically presents at the initial stage or when this disease's course has not gone on too long. Either one or many joints are swollen and painful. However, the affected area is not hot or red and may, in fact, feel cool or cold. There is early morning stiffness, heaviness, numbness, and/or restricted movement. When the pain obtains cold, it gets worse; when it obtains heat, it gets better. Therefore, the pain typically follows changes in weather. Other symptoms include possible aversion to cold, loose stools, and clear, long urination. In the initial stage, fever, chills, and absence of sweating are possibly accompanied by severe pain in the joints. The tongue is pale with thin, white fur, and the pulse is deep and bowstring or deep and tight.

NOTE: This pattern is not commonly seen in its pure form in Western patients who tend to have spleen vacuity and liver depression in addition to wind cold damp impediment. In fact, it is a defensive qi vacuity due, in turn, to spleen qi vacuity which allows wind, cold, and/or damp evils to invade, resulting in impediment.

TREATMENT PRINCIPLES: Expel wind and dispel dampness, warm the channels and scatter cold

RX: *Wen Jing Juan Bi Tang Jia Jian* (Warm the Channels & Alleviate Impediment Decoction with Additions & Subtractions)

INGREDIENTS: Radix Angelicae Sinensis (*Dang Gui*), 20g, Ramulus Cinnamomi Cassiae (*Gui Zhi*), Herba Epimedii (*Yin Yang Huo*), and ginger-processed Rhizoma Pinelliae Ternatae (*Ban Xia*), 15g each, Herba Pyrolae (*Lu Xian Cao*), processed Radix Aconiti Carmichaeli (*Chuan Wu*), processed Radix Aconiti Kusnezoffi (*Cao Wu*), Eupolyphaga Seu Ophistoplatia (*Tu Bei Chong*), Zaocys Dhumnades (*Wu Shao She*), and Nidus Vespae (*Feng Fang*), 9g each, and Radix Glyycrrhizae (*Gan Cao*), 5g

ANALYSIS OF FORMULA: *Gui Zhi* courses wind, warms the channels, and scatters cold. *Lu Xian Cao* courses wind, eliminates dampness, and supplements the kidneys. *Lu Feng Fang* courses wind and stops pain. *Wu Shao She* courses wind, frees the flow of the network vessels, and stops pain. *Ban Xia* dries dampness. *Yin Yang Huo*, *Chuan Wu*, and *Cao Wu* course and eliminate wind and dampness, scatter cold and stop pain. *Dang Gui* and *Tu Bie Chong* quicken the blood and transform stasis, free the flow of the network vessels and stop pain. *Gan Cao* harmonizes the other medicinals in this formula and checks the toxicity of *Cao Wu* and *Chuan Wu*.

ADDITIONS & SUBTRACTIONS: If *Lu Xian Cao* is difficult to find, it can be substituted by nine grams of Radix Clematidis Chinensis (*Wei Ling Xian*). If *Feng Fang* is difficult to find, it can be substituted by three grams of Herba Asari Cum Radice (*Xi Xin*). If pain is movable and not localized, this is called movable impediment. In that case, add nine grams each of Cortex Radicis Schizophragmatis (*Zuan Di Feng*), Radix Et Rhizoma Notopterygii (*Qiang Huo*), and/or Radix Angelicae Pubescentis (*Du Huo*). If joint pain is severe with superficial edema, add nine grams of Rhizoma Atractylodis (*Cang Zhu*), 18-21 grams of uncooked Semen Coicis Lachryma-jobi (*Yi Yi Ren*), and 6-9 grams of stir-fried Semen Sinapis Albae (*Bai Jie Zi*). If there is a predilection for heat and dread of cold and when the pain obtains heat it is soothed but, when it obtains cold, it gets worse, this is cold impediment. In that case, one can add 3-6 grams each of Radix Lateralis Praeparatus Aconiti Carmichaeli (*Fu Zi*), Scolopendra Subspinipes (*Wu Gong*), and Buthus Martensis (*Quan Xie*). If joint pain is severe and feels lancinating, this is called painful impediment. For this, one can add Radix Pseudoginseng (*Tian San Qi*), Resina Myrrhae (*Mo Yao*), Rhizoma Corydalis Yanhusuo (*Yan Hu Suo*), Semen Pruni Persicae (*Tao Ren*), Flos Carthami Tinctorii (*Hong Hua*), Caulis Milletiae Seu Spatholobi (*Ji Xue Teng*), and/or other such medicinals to quicken the blood and transform stasis. If there is concomitant spleen qi vacuity, add 15 grams of Radix Astragali Membranacei (*Huang Qi*) and nine grams of Rhizoma Atractylodis Macrocephalae (*Bai Zhu*). If there is concomitant liver depression, add nine grams each of Radix Bupleuri (*Chai Hu*) and Radix Albus Paeoniae Lactiflorae (*Bai Shao*). For upper limb pain, add nine grams each of Radix Et Rhizoma Notopterygii (*Qiang Huo*) and Ramulus Mori Albi (*Sang Zhi*). If there is lower limb pain, add nine grams each of Radix Achyranthis Bidentatae (*Niu Xi*) and Radix Angelicae Pubescentis (*Du Huo*). For severe swelling, add nine grams of Rhizoma Alismatis (*Ze Xie*) and five grams of Caulis Akebiae (*Mu Tong*). For severe pain, add three grams of Buthus Martensis (*Quan Xie*), powdered and taken with the strained decoction.

ACUPUNCTURE & MOXIBUSTION: *Feng Chi* (GB 20), *Ge Shu* (Bl 17), *Shen Shu* (Bl 23), *Guan Yuan* (CV 4), appropriate local points

ANALYSIS OF FORMULA: Draining *Feng Chi* resolves the exterior and courses wind, while draining *Ge Shu* quickens the blood. This combination is based on the statement, "To treat wind, first treat the blood." Supplementing *Shen Shu* and *Guan Yuan* with moxibustion warms and supplements source yang so it can scatter cold and warm the channels. Draining the local points frees the flow of the network vessels in the affected area.

ADDITIONS & SUBTRACTIONS: For jaw impediment, add *Xia Guan* (St 7), *Yin Feng* (TB 17), and *He Gu* (LI 4). For cervical impediment, add *Feng Chi* (GB 20), *Wan Gu* (GB 12), and *Tian Zhu* (Bl 10). For thoracic vertebral impediment, add *Jia Ji* (M-BW-35) at the level of involvement. For sacrococcygeal impediment, add *Da Chang Shu* (Bl 25), *Ming Men* (GV 4), *Ba Liao* (Bl 31-34), and *Wei Zhong* (Bl 40). For shoulder impediment, add *Jian Yu* (LI 15), *Tian Zong* (SI 11), and *Ji Quan* (Ht 1). For elbow impediment, add *Qu Chi* (LI 11), *Xiao Hai* (SI 8), *Zhou Liao* (LI 12), and *Shou San Li* (LI 10). For wrist impediment, add *Wai Guan* (TB 5), *Yang Chi* (TB 4), and *Wan Gu* (SI 4). For upper extremity phalageal and metacarpal impediment, add *Bai Xie* (M-UE-22), *He Gu* (LI 4), and *Hou Xi* (SI 3). For sacroiliac impediment, add *Guan Yuan Shu* (Bl 26), *Xiao Chang Shu* (Bl 27), *Bai Huan Shu* (Bl 30), *Huan Tiao* (GB 30), *Zhi Bian* (Bl 54), and *Ju Liao* (GB 29). For hip impediment, add *Huan Tiao* (GB 30) and *Yang Ling Quan* (GB 34). For knee impediment, add *Du Bi* (St 35), *Xi Yan* (M-LE-16a), *Qu Quan* (Liv 8), and *Wei Zhong* (Bl 40). For ankle impediment, choose between *Jie Xi* (St 41), *Shang Qiu* (Sp 5), *Qiu Xu* (GB 40), *Kun Lun* (Bl 60), *Tai Xi* (Ki 3), *Shen Mai* (Bl 62), and *Zhao Hai* (Ki 6) depending upon what channels are involved with the site of pain. For metatarsal and lower extremity phalangeal impediment, add *Jie Xi* (St 41), *Gong Sun* (Sp 4), *Tai Chong* (Liv 3), *Zu Lin Qi* (GB 41), and *Ba Feng* (M-LE-8).

2. WIND DAMP HEAT IMPEDIMENT PATTERN

MAIN SYMPTOMS: This pattern is seen in those with the acute, active stage of rheumatoid arthritis. There is joint swelling, pain, heaviness, and restricted movement. The affected areas are burning hot to the touch and red to inspection. Coolness makes the pain less. Other accompanying symptoms include fever, sweating, aversion to wind, oral thirst but sometimes no desire to drink, possible vomiting, short, reddish urination, a red tongue with thin, yellow fur, and a slippery, rapid or soggy, rapid pulse.

NOTE: This pattern is not commonly seen in Western clinical practice in its pure form. Commonly, wind, damp, and heat evils complicate spleen vacuity and liver depression patterns where the damp evils are internally engendered as opposed to externally invading and the heat is due to depression transforming heat.

TREATMENT PRINCIPLES: Clear heat and disinhibit dampness, dispel wind and free the flow of the network vessels

RX: *Bai Hu Jia Gui Zhi Tang Jia Wei* (White Tiger Plus Cinnamon Twig Decoction with Added Flavors)

INGREDIENTS: Gypsum Fibrosum (*Shi Gao*), 30g, Rhizoma Anemarrhenae Aspheloidis (*Zhi Mu*), 9g, mix-fried Radix Glycyrrhizae (*Gan Cao*), 3g, Fructus Oryzae Sativae (*Geng Mi*), 9-15g, Ramulus Cinnamomi Cassiae (*Gui Zhi*), 9g, Cortex Phellodendri (*Huang Bai*), 9g, Rhizoma Atractylodis (*Cang Zhu*), 9g, and Rhizoma Arisaematis (*Nan Xing*), 6g

ANALYSIS OF FORMULA: *Shi Gao* and *Zhi Mu* clear heat and discharge fire. *Huang Bai* and *Cang Zhu* together eliminate dampness and heat. *Tian Nan Xing* dries dampness, disperses swelling, and stops pain. *Gui Zhi* frees the flow of the network vessels and stops pain. *Gan Cao* and *Geng Mi* harmonize the other medicinals in this formula and protect the stomach from the cold nature of the other ingredients.

ADDITIONS & SUBTRACTIONS: For persistent high fever with constipation, add nine grams each of Radix Et Rhizoma Rhei (*Da Huang*) and Mirabilitum (*Mang Xiao*). For persistent high fever without severe constipation, add 15 grams each of Caulis Lonicerae Japonicae (*Ren Dong Teng*), Herba Taraxaci Mongolici Cum Radice (*Pu Gong Ying*), and Herba Violae Yedoensitis Cum Radice (*Zi Hua Di Ding*). For alternating fever and chills, add nine grams each of Radix Bupleuri (*Chai Hu*) and Radix Scutellariae Baicalensis (*Huang Qin*). For severe swelling of the joints, add nine grams each of Rhizoma Alismatis (*Ze Xie*) and Radix Stephaniae Tetrandrae (*Han Fang Ji*) and five grams of Caulis Akebiae (*Mu Tong*). For red macules on the affected joints, add 12 grams each of uncooked Radix Rehmanniae (*Sheng Di*), Radix Rubrus Paeoniae Lactiflorae (*Chi Shao*), Radix Salviae Miltiorrhizae (*Dan Shen*), and Cortex Radicis Moutan (*Dan Pi*). For severe pain, add nine grams of Lumbricus (*Di Long*) and 15 grams each of Cortex Erythiniae (*Hai Tong Pi*) and Caulis Sargentodoxae (*Hong Teng*). For severe thirst, add 12 grams each of Rhizoma Phragmitis Communis (*Lu Gen*) and Radix Trichosanthis Kirlowii (*Tian Hua Fen*). For pain in the upper limbs, add nine grams of Ramulus Mori Albi (*Sang Zhi*). For pain in the lower limbs, add nine grams of Fructus Chaenomelis Lagenariae (*Mu Gua*). For concomitant qi and blood vacuity, add 15 grams of Radix Astragali Membranacei (*Huang Qi*) and nine grams each of Radix Codonopsitis Pilosulae (*Dang Shen*) and Radix Angelicae Sinensis (*Dang Gui*). For concomitant liver depression, add nine grams each of Radix Bupleuri (*Chai Hu*) and Radix Albus Paeoniae Lactiflorae (*Bai Shao*). For liver depression transforming heat, add 12 grams of Fructus Gardeniae Jasminoidis (*Zhi Zi*) and nine grams of Cortex Radicis Moutan (*Dan Pi*).

ACUPUNCTURE & MOXIBUSTION: *Da Zhui* (GV 14), *Qu*

Chi (LI 11), *He Gu* (LI 4), *Wai Guan* (TB 5), appropriate local points

ANALYSIS OF FORMULA: Bleeding *Da Zhui* clears heat and dispels wind. Draining *Qu Chi* and *He Gu* clears heat from the entire body because, "The yang ming channel has lots of qi and lots of blood." Draining *Wai Guan* courses wind and clears heat. Draining the local points frees the flow of the network vessels in the affected area.

ADDITIONS & SUBTRACTIONS: Please see pattern #1 above.

3. ENDURING IMPEDIMENT TRANSFORMS HEAT & DAMAGES YIN PATTERN

MAIN SYMPTOMS: Joint redness, swelling, heat, and pain, stiffness and inflexibility. Initially, when the pain obtains coolness, it gradually soothes. However, after it has endured for some time, the sensation does not improve and when it obtains warmth it is soothed. There is a dry mouth with a bitter taste, a parched throat, insomnia, vexation and agitation, a red tongue with yellow or yellow, slimy fur, and a bowstring, fine, rapid pulse.

NOTE: This pattern is sometimes also called mixed cold and heat pattern.

TREATMENT PRINCIPLES: Scatter cold and eliminate dampness, clear heat and free the flow of the network vessels

RX: *Gui Zhi Shao Yao Zhi Mu Tang Jia Jian* (Cinnamon Twig, Peony & Anemarrhena Decoction with Additions & Subtractions)

INGREDIENTS: Ramulus Cinnamomi Cassiae (*Gui Zhi*), 30g, Radix Rubrus Paeoniae Lactiflorae (*Chi Shao*) and Radix Albus Paeoniae Lactiflorae (*Bai Shao*), 20g each, Rhizoma Anemarrhenae Aspheloidis (*Zhi Mu*), processed Radix Aconiti Carmichaeli (*Chuan Wu*), processed Radix Aconiti Kusnezoffi (*Cao Wu*), Radix Angelicae Sinensis (*Dang Gui*), and Zaocys Dhumnades (*Wu Shao She*), 15g each, and uncooked Radix Rehmanniae (*Sheng Di*), Bombyx Batryticatus (*Jiang Can*), Lumbricus (*Di Long*), and Radix Glycyrrhizae (*Gan Cao*), 9g each

ANALYSIS OF FORMULA: *Gui Zhi* courses wind and scatters cold, frees the flow of and warms the network vessels. In addition, with *Bai Shao*, it harmonizes the constructive and defensive. *Chuan Wu* and *Cao Wu*, course and eliminate wind and dampness, scatter cold and stop pain. *Chi Shao* and *Sheng Di* cool the blood. *Chi Shao* and *Dang Gui* quicken the blood and stop pain. *Zhi Mu* and *Di Long* clear heat. *Jiang Can* courses and clears wind heat. *Wu Shao She* courses wind, frees the flow of the network vessels, and stops pain. *Gan Cao* harmonizes the other medicinals in this formula and checks the toxicity of *Cao Wu* and *Chuan Wu*.

ADDITIONS & SUBTRACTIONS: If heat is predominant, reduce the amount of *Gui Zhi, Chuan Wu*, and *Cao Wu* and add nine grams each of Rhizoma Polygoni Cuspidati (*Hu Zhang*), Calcitum (*Han Shui Shi*), Herba Humuli Scandentis (*Lu Cao*), and Cortex Phellodendri (*Huang Bai*). If there is yin vacuity with internal heat, increase the amount of *Sheng Di* to 30-40 grams.

ACUPUNCTURE & MOXIBUSTION: *Qu Chi* (LI 11), *He Gu* (LI 4), *Guan Yuan* (CV 4), appropriate local points

ANALYSIS OF FORMULA: Needling *Qu Chi* and *He Gu* with lifting and thrusting draining technique clears heat from the entire body because, "The yang ming channel has lots of qi and lots of blood." Needling *Guan Yuan* with even supplementing-even draining technique leads yang back down to its lower source so that it can scatter cold, and warm the channels. Draining the local points frees the flow of the network vessels in the affected area.

ADDITIONS & SUBTRACTIONS: Please see pattern #1 above.

4. QI & BLOOD DUAL VACUITY, PHLEGM & STASIS MUTUALLY BINDING PATTERN

MAIN SYMPTOMS: This pattern is mostly seen in the later stages of RA where there is joint rigidity and deformation. The joints aching and painful, swollen, distended, and deformed, and their movement is inhibited. In addition, there is an accompanying somber white facial complexion, heart palpitations, shortness of breath, bodily fatigue, encumbrance, and lassitude, a pale tongue with white fur, and a deep, fine, bowstring, and/or tight pulse.

TREATMENT PRINCIPLES: Boost the qi and nourish the blood, transform phlegm and dispel stasis, free the flow of the channels and quicken the network vessels

RX: If there is predominant cold, use *Huang Qi Gui Zhi Wu Wu Tang* (Astragalus & Cinnamon Twig Five Materials Decoction)

INGREDIENTS: Uncooked Rhizoma Zingiberis (*Sheng Jiang*), 18g, Radix Astragali Membranacei (*Huang Qi*), Radix Albus Paeoniae Lactiflorae (*Bai Shao*), and Ramulus Cinnamomi Cassiae (*Gui Zhi*), 9g each, and Fructus Zizyphi Jujubae (*Da Zao*), 12 pieces

NOTE: Perhaps more than some other guiding formulas in this book, this formula definitely needs modification with the various additions described below if it is realistically going to be used to treat RA.

ANALYSIS OF FORMULA: *Huang Qi* and *Da Zao* boost the qi. *Bai Shao* nourishes the blood. *Gui Zhi* warms and frees the flow of the channels and quickens the network vessels. *Bai Shao* and *Gui Zhi* as well as *Sheng Jiang* and *Da Zao* harmonize the constructive and defensive. *Sheng Jiang* transforms phlegm at the same time as it helps *Huang Qi* and *Da Zao* supplement the center to engender and transform the qi and blood.

ADDITIONS & SUBTRACTIONS: For marked blood vacuity, add nine grams each of cooked Radix Rehmanniae (*Shu Di*) and Radix Angelicae Sinensis (*Dang Gui*) and six grams of Radix Ligustici Wallichii (*Chuan Xiong*). For marked qi vacuity, add nine grams each of Radix Codonopsitis Pilosulae (*Dang Shen*) and Rhizoma Atractylodis Macrocephalae (*Bai Zhu*) and increase the dosage of *Huang Qi* up to 20 grams. For inhibited movement, add nine grams each of Caulis Piperis Futokadsurae (*Hai Feng Teng*), Caulis Trachelospermi Jasminoidis (*Luo Shi Teng*), and Radix Clematidis Chinensis (*Wei Ling Xian*). For severe pain with a cool sensation in the affected area, add six grams of Radix Lateralis Praeparatus Aconiti Carmichaeli (*Fu Zi*) and three grams of Herba Asari Cum Radice (*Xi Xin*). For pain in the upper limbs, add nine grams of Ramulus Mori Albi (*Sang Zhi*). For pain in the lower limbs, add nine grams of Radix Achyranthis Bidentatae (*Niu Xi*). For joint rigidity and deformation, add three grams each of Buthus Martensis (*Quan Xie*), Scolopendra Subspinipes (*Wu Gong*), and Zaocys Dhumnades (*Wu Shao She*) and nine grams of Radix Dipsaci (*Xu Duan*). For severe joint swelling, add 20 grams of Semen Coicis Lachryma-jobi (*Yi Yi Ren*) and nine grams of Rhizoma Atractylodis (*Cang Zhu*). For severe pain, add six grams each of Resina Olibani (*Ru Xiang*) and Resina Myrrhae (*Mo Yao*).

If there is lingering wind damp heat, use *Dang Gui Nian Tong Tang* (Dang Gui Assuage Pain Decoction)

INGREDIENTS: Radix Angelicae Sinensis (*Dang Gui*), Rhizoma Atractylodis Macrocephalae (*Bai Zhu*), Rhizoma Atractylodis (*Cang Zhu*), Radix Scutellariae Baicalensis (*Huang Qin*), Rhizoma Anemarrhenae Aspheloidis (*Zhi Mu*), Herba Artemisiae Capillaris (*Yin Chen Hao*), Radix Puerariae (*Ge Gen*), Radix Et Rhizoma Notopterygii (*Qiang Huo*), Radix Ledebouriellae Divaricatae (*Fang Feng*), and Sclerotium Polyporus Umbellati (*Zhu Ling*), 9g each, Radix Panacis Ginseng (*Ren Shen*) and Radix Sophorae Flavescentis (*Ku Shen*), 6g each, Rhizoma Cimicifugae (*Sheng Ma*), 4.5g, and Radix Glycyrrhizae (*Gan Cao*), 3g

ANALYSIS OF FORMULA: *Ren Shen, Bai Zhu,* and *Gan Cao* fortify the spleen and boost the qi, while *Dang Gui* nourishes the blood. *Cang Zhu* and *Huang Qin* together clear and eliminate dampness and heat. *Huang Qin, Zhi Mu,* and *Sheng Ma* clear heat. *Ku Shen* and *Yin Chen Hao* clear and disinhibit dampness and heat. *Cang Zhu, Qiang Huo,* and *Fang Feng* treat wind damp impediment. *Ge Gen* courses wind and resolves muscles. *Zhu Ling* disinhibits dampness.

ADDITIONS & SUBTRACTIONS: Please see pattern #1 above.

ACUPUNCTURE & MOXIBUSTION: *Zu San Li* (St 36), *San Yin Jiao* (Sp 6), appropriate local points

ANALYSIS OF FORMULA: Supplementing *Zu San Li* with supplementing lifting and thrusting technique boosts the qi, while supplementing *San Yin Jiao* in the same way nourishes the blood. The local points free the flow of the network vessels in the affected area.

ADDITIONS & SUBTRACTIONS: Please see pattern #1 above.

5. LIVER BLOOD-KIDNEY YIN & YANG VACUITY WITH PHLEGM & STASIS MUTUALLY BINDING PATTERN

MAIN SYMPTOMS: In this case, the symptoms of kidney yang vacuity are even more pronounced. There is joint and muscular atrophy, joint stiffness, inflexibility, and deformation, unceasing aching and pain which is worse on exposure to cold and during the winter and better on obtaint of warmth and during the summer. Other signs and symptoms include dizziness and tinnitus, long, clear, frequent urination, nocturia, low back and knee pain and chill, a pale tongue with white fur, and a deep, weak, slow pulse, especially in the cubit position.

TREATMENT PRINCIPLES: Supplement the kidneys and invigorate yang, nourish the liver and soothe the sinews, scatter nodulation and quicken the network vessels

RX: *Shen Qi Wan Jia Wei* (Kidney Qi Pills with Added Flavors)

INGREDIENTS: Cooked Radix Rehmanniae (*Shu Di*), 12g, Radix Dioscoreae Oppositae (*Shan Yao*), Fructus Corni Officinalis (*Shan Zhu Yu*), Sclerotium Poriae Cocos (*Fu Ling*), Rhizoma Alismatis (*Ze Xie*), Cortex Radicis Moutan (*Dan Pi*), Ramulus Cinnamomi Cassiae (*Gui Zhi*), Fructus Drynariae (*Gu Sui Bu*), Zaocys Dhumnades (*Wu Shao She*), Buthus Martensis (*Quan Xie*), and Scolopendra Subspinipes (*Wu Gong*), 9g each, and Radix Lateralis Praeparatus Aconiti Carmichaeli (*Fu Zi*), 6g

ANALYSIS OF FORMULA: *Shu Di, Shan Zhu Yu, Shan Yao, Fu Ling, Ze Xie,* and *Dan Pi* are the six ingredients of *Liu Wei Di Huang Wan* (Six Flavors Rehmannia Pills), a key formula for nourishing and enriching liver blood-kidney yin. *Gui Zhi* and *Fu Zi* supplement the kidneys and invigorate yang, warm the channels and free the flow of the network vessels.

Gu Sui Bu warms and supplements kidney yang and knits and connects the sinews and bones. *Quan Xie*, *Wu Gong*, and *Wu Shao She* course wind, free the flow of the network vessels, and stop pain. *Quan Xie* and *Wu Gong* also scatter nodulation.

ADDITIONS & SUBTRACTIONS: If there is concomitant spleen qi vacuity with fatigue, poor appetite, undigested food in the stools, orthostatic hypotension, and easy bruising, add 15 grams of Radix Astragali Membranacei (*Huang Qi*) and nine grams of Radix Codonopsitis Pilosulae (*Dang Shen*). For concomitant blood vacuity, add nine grams of Radix Angelicae Sinensis (*Dang Gui*). For low back pain, add nine grams each of Cortex Eucommiae Ulmoidis (*Du Zhong*) and Radix Dipsaci (*Xu Duan*). For pain in the upper limbs, add nine grams of Ramulus Mori Albi (*Sang Zhi*). For pain in the lower limbs, add nine grams of Radix Achyranthis Bidentatae (*Niu Xi*). For severe coolness of the affected area, add three grams of Herba Asari Cum Radice (*Xi Xin*) and nine grams of Herba Epimedii (*Yin Yang Huo*). For fixed, piercing, stabbing pain, add six grams each of Resina Olibani (*Ru Xiang*) and Resina Myrrhae (*Mo Yao*). For inhibited movement add nine grams each of Caulis Piperis Futokadsurae (*Hai Feng Teng*), Caulis Trachelospermi Jasminoidis (*Luo Shi Teng*) and Radix Clematidis Chinensis (*Wei Ling Xian*).

ACUPUNCTURE & MOXIBUSTION: *Shen Shu* (Bl 23), *Ming Men* (GV 4), *Guan Yuan* (CV 4), appropriate local points

ANALYSIS OF FORMULA: Needling *Shen Shu*, *Ming Men*, and *Guan Yuan* with even supplementing-even draining technique followed by moxibustion warms and supplements source yang so it can scatter cold and warm the channels. The local points free the flow of the network vessels in the affected area.

ADDITIONS & SUBTRACTIONS: Please see pattern #1 above.

REMARKS

1. As in all chronic, enduring diseases, there will be an element of liver depression due, if nothing other than to the frustration of being ill. If there is concomitant liver depression qi stagnation, one should add appropriate qi-rectifying medicinals. However, it should also be remembered that wind-treating medicinals can also be used to rectify the qi. Therefore, if there are wind-treating medicinals in the formula already, one may not have to add other ingredients to rectify the qi. This depends on the symptoms of qi stagnation and whether or not those wind-treating medicinals address those qi stagnation symptoms. For instance, Radix Ledebouriellae Divaricatae (*Fang Feng*) treats wind at the same time as it alleviates qi stagnation intestinal cramping.

2. As with most autoimmune diseases, proper diet is extremely important. If a person is invaded by external evils, it means their righteous qi is vacuous and weak. The defensive qi issues from the middle burner and its source is the spleen. Therefore, whether in the active or remittent stages, most patients with RA do also have spleen vacuity. When there is spleen vacuity, one should eat a spleen-supporting diet. This means little if any sugars and sweets, little if any uncooked and chilled foods and drinks, and care when eating foods which strongly engender fluids. Foods which engender fluids are typically those which have a lot of *wei* or "flavor." This includes many foods which enrich yin and fill the essence, such as dairy and animal products. When complicated by blood and/or yin vacuity, some yin-enriching foods are necessary. However, so many of these should not be eaten so as to damage the spleen. In general, it is always safer in terms of diet to foster essence via the spleen's engenderment and transformation of qi and blood than to eat a lot of slimy, enriching, flavor-laden, yin-supplementing foods.

When damp heat complicates RA, then patients should stick to a clear, bland, hypoallergenic, yeast-free diet. This means eating little or nothing made through fermentation or which molds easily. This includes, in addition to sugars and sweets, bread and yeasted grain products, cheese, alcohol, and vinegar, tomatoes, oranges, peaches, strawberries, raspberries, cantaloupe, etc. Although acrid, hot foods are contraindicated in cases of damp heat, if there are gu worms, one should eat onions and garlic liberally.

3. Like most other autoimmune diseases, this condition's severity fluctuates, and there are often periods of relative remission. In general, Chinese medical treatment should mainly be used for the long-term prevention of future reoccurrences and the progression of this disease, while during acute attacks, a combination of Chinese medicine, including acupuncture and moxibustion, and modern Western medicine may be most effective. In particular, many patients with rheumatoid arthritis may be prescribed corticosteriods during acute attacks, and Chinese medicine can be used to treat the side effects of medicines like Prednisone. In that case, treatment should merely be given based on the patient's total pattern discrimination.

ENDNOTES

[1] Pizzorno, J.E. & Murray, M.T., *Encyclopedia of Natural Medicine*, Prima Publishing, Rocklin, CA, 1991

[2] The Burton Goldberg Group, *Alternative Medicine, The Definitive Guide*, Future Medicine Publishing Inc., Puyallup, WA, 1993, p. 530

64

SCLERODERMA

Also referred to as progressive systemic scleroderma (PSS), scleroderma is a chronic, progessive, autoimmune disease of unknown etiology which is characterized by diffuse fibrosis, degenerative changes, and vascular abnormalities in the skin, articular structures, and internal organs. The internal organs which may be affected by this fibrosis include the esophagus, intestinal tract, lungs, heart, and kidneys. PSS occurs in women four times more often than in men. It is comparatively rare in children. The severity and progression of this disease are highly variable, but, if it progresses to the internal organs, it may be fatal.

The initial symptoms are Raynaud's phenomenon and insidious thickening of the acral portions of the extremities with gradual thickening of the skin of the fingers. Polyarthralgia is another prominent early symptom. In a few cases, heartburn and difficulty swallowing or dyspnea may be the first manifestations of this disease. Induration of the skin is symmetrical and may be confined to the fingers or affect most or all of the body. As the disease progresses, the skin becomes taut, shiny, and hyperpigmented. The face becomes mask-like and telangiectases appear on the fingers, chest, face, lips, and tongue. Subcutaneous calcifications develop on the fingertips or over bony prominences. Friction rubs develop over the joints, tendon sheaths, and large bursae, and there may be flexion contractures of the fingers, wrists, and elbows. Trophic ulcers on the fingertips and finger joints are common.

Esophageal dysfunction is the most common visceral disturbance and eventually occurs in most patients. Dysphagia, acid reflux, and peptic esophagitis are all common. Exertional dyspnea is the most common early stage cardiorespiratory symptom. Pulmonary hypertension may develop as well as cardiac arrhythmias and other ECG abnormalities. This may eventually evolve into chronic cardiac failure. Accelerated or malignant hypertension may be due to severe renal disease which, if left untreated, may progress to irreversible renal insufficiency and death.

In terms of Western medical diagnosis, RFs are found in approximately 1/3 of PSS patients. Serum antinuclear and/or antinuclear antibodies are found in 90% of patients. No Western medication has shown significant effect on the treatment of PSS, and the course of this disease is variable and unpredictable. In some patients, it is only slowly progressive. However, prognosis is poor in those patients with early heart, lung, and/or kidney involvement.

DISEASE CATEGORIZATION: This disease is mainly categorized as *bi zheng*, impediment condition, *pi bi*, skin impediment, and *feng bi*, wind impediment. Dysphagia is categorized as *ye ge*, dysphagia occlusion, while acid regurgitation is categorized as *tun suan*, swallowing acid.

DISEASE CAUSES: Contraction of wind damp evils due to qi and blood vacuity

DISEASE MECHANISMS: Due to qi and blood vacuity, the defensive exterior is not secure. This allows external invasion of wind damp evils which obstruct in the skin, the muscles and flesh, and the sinews and bones. This leads to disharmony of the constructive and defensive and impediment and obstruction of the channels and vessels. The movement and transportation of the qi and blood become uneasy or not smooth. If severe, this impediment and congestion result in complete non-free flow to the affected area and loss of regulation of the viscera and bowels. If this endures, it damages yang and consumes the qi, with the spleen and kidneys both becoming vacuous.

Treatment based on pattern discrimination:

I. Acute occurrence stage

Yin vacuity with heat evils brewing & binding pattern

Main symptoms: During acute occurrences, one mostly sees the above pattern which is characterized by cough, rapid or hasty breathing, heart fluster, heart throbbing, jaundice, dizziness, finger and toe wet or dry gangrene, low-grade fever, bleeding gums, a red tongue with dry, yellow or scanty fur, and a rapid pulse

Note: This is a potentially fatal, emergency condition. It should not be treated by Chinese medicine alone. If Chinese medical treatment is given, it should be in combination with modern Western medicine.

Treatment principles: Clear heat and resolve toxins, cool the blood and nourish yin

Rx: *Qing Ying Tang Jia Jian* (Clear the Constructive Decoction with Additions & Subtractions)

Ingredients: Uncooked Radix Rehmanniae (*Sheng Di*), Cortex Radicis Moutan (*Dan Pi*), Radix Lithospermi Seu Arnebiae (*Zi Cao*), Radix Salviae Miltiorrhizae (*Dan Shen*), and Rhizoma Imperatae Cylindricae (*Bai Mao Gen*), 30g each, Radix Scrophulariae Ningpoensis (*Xuan Shen*), Radix Rubrus Paeoniae Lactiflorae (*Chi Shao*), Flos Lonicerae Japonicae (*Jin Yin Hua*), and Spica Prunellae Vulgaris (*Xia Ku Cao*), 15g each, and Tuber Ophiopogonis Japonici (*Mai Dong*), 12g

Analysis of formula: *Sheng Di, Xuan Shen, Chi Shao, Dan Pi, Zi Cao, Bai Mao Gen,* and *Dan Shen* all cool the blood. *Sheng Di* and *Mai Men Dong* nourish yin, while *Bai Mao Gen* engenders fluids. *Xuan Shen, Zi Cao,* and *Jin Yin Hua* clear heat and resolve toxins. *Xia Ku Cao* clears heat and scatters binding or nodulation.

Additions & subtractions: For cough and shortness of breath, add nine grams each of Semen Pruni Armeniacae (*Xing Ren*) and Radix Peucedani (*Qian Hu*). For muscular aching and pain or numbness and stiffness, add 30 grams each of Semen Coicis Lachryma-jobi (*Yi Yi Ren*) and Caulis Milletiae Seu Spatholobi (*Ji Xue Teng*) and nine grams of Radix Angelicae Sinensis (*Dang Gui*).

Acupuncture & moxibustion: This emergency condition does not respond to acupuncture.

II. Slow progression stage

1. Wind cold mixed with qi vacuity, liver depression & blood stasis pattern

Main symptoms: The skin detriment may be either light or heavy. The color of the cheeks is static and dark. The four limbs emit coolness and numbness. This is accompanied by lassitude of the spirit, lack of strength, dizziness, torpid intake, decreased body weight, muscle and flesh aching and pain, heart palpitations, shortness of breath, a pale, purplish, dark tongue with thin, white fur, and a fine, choppy pulse.

Treatment principles: Course wind and scatter cold, fortify the spleen and boost the qi, free the flow of the vessels and transform stasis

Rx: *Qin Jiao Tang* (Gentiana Macrocephala Decoction) combined with *Bu Zhong Yi Qi Tang* (Supplement the Center & Boost the Qi Decoction) with additions & subtractions

Ingredients: Radix Codonopsitis Pilosulae (*Dang Shen*), Radix Astragali Membranacei (*Huang Qi*), and cooked Radix Rehmanniae (*Shu Di*), 30g each, Radix Gentianae Macrophyllae (*Qin Jiao*), Radix Ledebouriellae Divaricatae (*Fang Feng*), Rhizoma Atractylodis Macrocephalae (*Bai Zhu*) and Radix Angelicae Sinensis (*Dang Gui*), 15g each, Pericarpium Citri Reticulatae (*Chen Pi*), Tuber Curcumae (*Chuan Yu Jin*), Flos Carthami Tinctorii (*Hong Hua*), Radix Salviae Miltiorrhizae (*Dan Shen*), Ramulus Cinnamomi Cassiae (*Gui Zhi*), Rhizoma Cyperi Rotundi (*Xiang Fu*), mix-fried Radix Glycyrrhizae (*Gan Cao*), and Caulis Milletiae Seu Spatholobi (*Ji Xue Teng*), 9g each, and Radix Bupleuri (*Chai Hu*), 6g

Analysis of formula: *Dang Shen, Huang Qi, Bai Zhu,* and mix-fried *Gan Cao* fortify the spleen and boost the qi. *Chai Hu, Xiang Fu,* and *Chen Pi* course the liver and resolve depression. *Qin Jiao, Fang Feng,* and *Gui Zhi* course wind and scatter cold. *Dang Gui, Hong Hua, Dan Shen, Chuan Yu Jin,* and *Ji Xue Teng* quicken the blood, free the flow of the vessels, and transform stasis. *Dang Gui* and *Shu Di* also nourish the blood, thus harmonizing and emolliating the liver and nourishing the vessels.

Additions & subtractions: For soreness and pain of the muscles and flesh which is mainly in the upper body, add 30 grams of Flos Lonicerae Japonicae (*Jin Yin Hua*) and nine grams of Rhizoma Curcumae Longae (*Jiang Huang*). If the disease is mostly in the lower body, add nine grams each of Radix Achyranthis Bidentatae (*Niu Xi*) and Radix Lateralis Praeparatus Aconiti Carmichaeli (*Fu Zi*). If there is no soreness and pain, delete *Qin Jiao* and *Fang Feng*. If the disease is widely spread throughout the body, add nine grams each of mix-fried Herba Ephedrae (*Ma Huang*) and Gelatinum Cornu Cervi (*Lu Jiao Jiao*).

ACUPUNCTURE & MOXIBUSTION: *He Gu* (LI 4), *Tai Chong* (Liv 3), *Zu San Li* (St 36), *San Yin Jiao* (Sp 6)

ANALYSIS OF FORMULA: Draining *He Gu* courses wind, scatters cold, and moves the qi. When combined with *San Yin Jiao,* these two points also quicken the blood and transform stasis. Draining *Tai Chong* courses the liver and resolves depression. Supplementing *Zu San Li* fortifies the spleen and boosts the qi.

ADDITIONS & SUBTRACTIONS: For marked spleen vacuity, moxa *Pi Shu* (Bl 20) and *Wei Shu* (Bl 21). If there is concomitant blood vacuity, add *Ge Shu* (Bl 17) and *Gan Shu* (Bl 18). If blood stasis is pronounced, add *Xue Hai* (Sp 10).

2. ALTERNATING COLD & HEAT, LIVER DEPRESSION & BLOOD STASIS PATTERN

MAIN SYMPTOMS: The affected skin area is delimited, there is diffuse sclerosis, or the eyelids, facial area, hands, and upper back are purple, swollen, and distended. The affected area may emit white, purple, coolness, or burning heat, and there may be itching. These are accompanied by easy emotional stimulation, menstrual irregularity, nausea, vomiting, bleeding gums, loose stools, or stools which are sometimes loose and sometimes dry. The tongue is pale but dark with thin, white fur, and the pulse is fine and bowstring or bowstring and choppy.

NOTE: In this pattern, cold is mostly vacuity cold due to spleen vacuity, while heat is depressive heat transforming from liver depression. Loose stools suggest spleen vacuity, while dry stools suggest depressive heat consuming stomach and intestinal fluids.

TREATMENT PRINCIPLES: Harmonize the liver and spleen, clear heat and resolve depression, quicken the blood and transform stasis

RX: *Dan Zhi Xiao Yao San Jia Jian* (Moutan & Gardenia Rambling Powder with Additions & Subtractions)

INGREDIENTS: Radix Salviae Miltiorrhizae (*Dan Shen*) and Caulis Milletiae Seu Spatholobi (*Ji Xue Teng*), 30g each, Rhizoma Atractylodis Macrocephalae (*Bai Zhu*), 15g, Sclerotium Poriae Cocos (*Fu Ling*), 12g, Cortex Radicis Moutan (*Dan Pi*), Fructus Gardeniae Jasminoidis (*Zhi Zi*), Radix Bupleuri (*Chai Hu*), Radix Angelicae Sinensis (*Dang Gui*), Radix Albus Paeoniae Lactiflorae (*Bai Shao*), Flos Carthami Tinctorii (*Hong Hua*), Tuber Curcumae (*Chuan Yu Jin*), dry Lumbricus (*Di Long*), and Sanguis Draconis (*Xue Jie*), 9g each, and Periostracum Cicadae (*Chan Tui*) and mix-fried Radix Glycyrrhizae (*Gan Cao*), 6g each

ANALYSIS OF FORMULA: *Chai Hu* and *Bai Shao* course and harmonize the liver and resolve the depression. *Bai Zhu, Fu Ling,* and mix-fried *Gan Cao* fortify the spleen and boost the qi. Thus these first two groups of medicinals together harmonize the liver and spleen. *Dan Pi* and *Zhi Zi* clear and resolve depressive heat. *Dan Pi, Dang Gui, Hong Hua, Xue Jie, Dan Shen,* and *Ji Xue Teng* quicken the blood and transform stasis. *Di Long* clears heat and frees the flow of the network vessels. *Chan Tui* courses wind and stops itching.

ADDITIONS & SUBTRACTIONS: If qi vacuity is more severe, add 30 grams each of Radix Astragali Membranacei (*Huang Qi*) and Radix Codonopsitis Pilosulae (*Dang Shen*). Delete *Bai Zhu* and *Fu Ling* if there is no damp stagnation and loose stools.

If there is low-grade fever with aversion to cold, body pain, muscular pain, cough with thin phlegm, no thirst, loose stools, diffuse or delimited sclerosis, scaley, bright skin, atrophy if severe, joint mobility problems, difficulty opening the mouth, no perspiration or profuse perspiration, a pale red tongue with thin, white fur, and a rapid pulse, treatment should diffuse the lungs and scatter cold, regulate and harmonize the constructive and defensive, free the flow of the network vessels and transform stasis. In that case, one can use *Jing Fang Bai Du San* (Schizonepeta & Ledebouriella Vanquish Toxins Powder) plus Ramulus Cinnamomi Cassiae (*Gui Zhi*), Radix Albus Paeoniae Lactiflorae (*Bai Shao*), Radix Angelicae Sinensis (*Dang Gui*), Flos Carthami Tinctorii (*Hong Hua*), Zaocys Dhumnades (*Wu Shao She*), Lumbricus (*Di Long*), Fructus Chaenomelis Lagenariae (*Mu Gua*), Radix Salviae Miltiorrhizae (*Dan Shen*), Semen Coicis Lachryma-jobi (*Yi Yi Ren*), etc.

ACUPUNCTURE & MOXIBUSTION: *Zu San Li* (St 36), *Tai Chong* (Liv 3), *Xia Xi* (GB 43), *He Gu* (LI 4), *San Yin Jiao* (Sp 6)

ANALYSIS OF FORMULA: Draining *Tai Chong* courses the liver and rectifies the qi, while supplementing *Zu San Li* fortifies the spleen and boosts the qi. Together, these two points harmonize the liver and spleen. Draining *Xia Xi* clears depressive heat. Draining *He Gu* clears heat and moves the qi. When combined with *San Yin Jiao,* it quickens the blood and transforms stasis.

ADDITIONS & SUBTRACTIONS: If there is profuse sweating, also supplement *Fu Liu* (Ki 7). If blood stasis is severe, also drain *Xue Hai* (Sp 10). For severe spleen vacuity with loose stools, add *Pi Shu* (Bl 20) and *Wei Shu* (Bl 21).

3. Spleen-kidney yang vacuity with cold congealing in the interstices pattern

Main symptoms: Emission of purple, swollen, and distended lesions on the eyelids, face, hands, and upper back, inability to make a tight fist, affected area hard and sclerotic, powdery red or interspersed black and white skin, dread of cold, chilled limbs, joint aching and pain, low back and knee soreness and weakness, decreased sexual desire, loose teeth, fatigue, lassitude of the spirit, lack of strength, torpid intake, no thirst, loose stools, a pale, enlarged, swollen or fat, moist tongue with greyish fur, and a deep, fine, weak pulse

Treatment principles: Warm the kidneys and scatter cold, fortify the spleen and boost the qi, quicken the blood and transform stasis

Rx: *Yang He Tang Jia Jian* (Yang Harmonizing Decoction with Additions & Subtractions)

Ingredients: Cooked Radix Rehmanniae (*Shu Di*), Radix Astragali Membranacei (*Huang Qi*), Radix Codonopsitis Pilosulae (*Dang Shen*), Caulis Milletiae Seu Spatholobi (*Ji Xue Teng*), and Herba Pyrolae (*Lu Xian Cao*), 30g each, Cornu Cervi Degelatinum (*Lu Jiao Shuang*), 20g, and stir-fried Semen Sinapis Albae (*Bai Jie Zi*), Cortex Cinnamomi Cassiae (*Rou Gui*), mix-fried Herba Ephedrae (*Ma Huang*), dry Rhizoma Zingiberis (*Gan Jiang*), Radix Angelicae Sinensis (*Dang Gui*), Flos Carthami Tinctorii (*Hong Hua*), and mix-fried Radix Glycyrrhizae (*Gan Cao*), 9g each

Analysis of formula: *Shu Di* enriches yin to engender yang. *Lu Jiao Jiao* and *Rou Gui* warm and supplement kidney yang, while *Huang Qi, Dang Shen*, mix-fried *Gan Cao,* and *Gan Jiang* together warm and supplement spleen yang. Also, *Rou Gui, Gan Jiang,* and *Ma Huang* scatter internal and external cold. *Dang Gui, Hong Hua*, and *Ji Xue Teng* quicken the blood and transform stasis. *Lu Xian Cao* supplements the kidneys and courses wind damp. *Bai Jie Zi* transforms phlegm, scatters binding or nodulations, and disperses swelling.

Additions & subtractions: For dread of cold and relatively severe chilled limbs, add 15 grams of Radix Lateralis Praeparatus Aconiti Carmichaeli (*Fu Zi*) and 20 grams of Semen Cuscutae Chinensis (*Tu Si Zi*). If there are loose stools and slimy tongue fur, add 30 grams of Semen Coicis Lachryma-jobi (*Yi Yi Ren*), nine grams of Rhizoma Atractylodis (*Cang Zhu*), and 15 grams of Fructus Chaenomelis Lagenariae (*Mu Gua*). If the affected area is hard and sclerotic, add 15 grams each of vinegar-processed Carapax Amydae Sinensis (*Bie Jia*), Thallus Algae (*Kun Bu*), and Herba Sargassii (*Hai Zao*). If there is marked joint aching and pain, add 15 grams each of Radix Gentianae Macrophyllae (*Qin Jiao*) and Ramulus Loranthi Seu Visci (*Sang Ji Sheng*) and six grams of Zaocys Dhumnades (*Wu Shao She*).

Acupuncture & moxibustion: *Zu San Li* (St 36), *Guan Yuan* (CV 4), *Ming Men* (GV 4), *He Gu* (LI 4), *San Yin Jiao* (Sp 6)

Analysis of formula: Supplementing *Zu San Li* with moxibuston warms and supplements spleen yang as well as boosts the qi. Moxaing *Guan Yuan* and *Ming Men* warms and supplements kidney yang. Draining *He Gu* moves the qi. When combined with draining *San Yin Jiao,* it also quickens the blood.

Additions & subtractions: For severe spleen-kidney yang vacuity, moxa *Pi Shu* (Bl 20), *Wei Shu* (Bl 21), and *Shen Shu* (Bl 23).

4. Lung-kidney dual vacuity with blood stasis pattern

Main symptoms: Exertional dyspnea, shortness of breath, possible panting and wheezing, chest oppression, a somber white facial complexion, aversion to cold, cold feet, low back and knee soreness and limpness, dizziness, tinnitus, frequent, long, clear urination, and a pale tongue with white fur, and a deep, weak, possibly slow pulse

Note: This pattern describes PSS with lung fibrosis.

Treatment principles: Supplement the lungs and boost the kidneys, warm yang and quicken the blood

Rx: *Yang He Tang* (Yang Harmonizing Decoction) & *Zuo Gui Yin* (Restore the Left [Kidney] Drink) with additions & subtractions

Ingredients: Cooked Radix Rehmanniae (*Shu Di*) and Caulis Milletiae Seu Spatholobi (*Ji Xue Teng*), 30g each, Gelatinum Cornu Cervi (*Lu Jiao Jiao*), Radix Dioscoreae Oppositae (*Shan Yao*), Sclerotium Poriae Cocos (*Fu Ling*), Fructus Corni Officinalis (*Shan Zhu Yu*), Cortex Radicis Moutan (*Dan Pi*), and Tuber Curcumae (*Yu Jin*), 9g each, Semen Sinapis Albae (*Bai Jie Zi*), 6g, Cortex Cinnamomi Cassiae (*Rou Gui*) and mix-fried Radix Glycyrrhizae (*Gan Cao*), 3g each, and blast-fried Rhizoma Zingiberis (*Pao Jiang*) and Herba Ephedrae (*Ma Huang*), 1.5g each

Analysis of formula: *Shu Di, Shan Zhu Yu, Shan Yao, Fu*

Ling, and *Dan Pi* are five of the six ingredients of *Liu Wei Di Huang Wan* (Six Flavors Rehmannia Pills) which enrich kidney yin to engender kidney yang. *Lu Jiao Jiao* and *Rou Gui* warm kidney yang, while *Pao Jiang* and *Ma Huang* warm lung yang. *Ji Xue Teng* and *Yu Jin* quicken the blood and free the flow of the network vessels. *Bai Jie Zi* transforms phlegm, scatters binding or nodulations, and disperses swelling. *Gan Cao* harmonizes the other medicinals in this formula.

ADDITIONS & SUBTRACTIONS: For severe qi vacuity, add 15 grams of Radix Astragali Membranacei (*Huang Qi*) and 6-9 grams of Radix Panacis Ginseng (*Ren Shen*). For more severe cold, add 3-6 grams of Radix Lateralis Praeparatus Aconiti Carmichaeli (*Fu Zi*). If there are heart palpitations, add nine grams of Radix Salviae Miltiorrhizae (*Dan Shen*). If there is concomitant blood vacuity, add nine grams of Radix Angelicae Sinensis (*Dang Gui*).

ACUPUNCTURE & MOXIBUSTION: *Fei Shu* (Bl 13), *Gao Huang Shu* (Bl 43), *Shen Shu* (Bl 23), *Zhi Shi* (Bl 52), *Ming Men* (GV 4), *He Gu* (LI 4), *San Yin Jiao* (Sp 6)

ANALYSIS OF FORMULA: Supplementing *Fei Shu* and *Gao Huang Shu* with moxibustion warms and supplements lung yang. Moxaing *Shen Shu*, *Zhi Shi*, and *Ming Men* warms and supplements kidney yang. Draining *He Gu* and *San Yin Jiao* moves the qi and quickens the blood.

ADDITIONS & SUBTRACTIONS: If there is concomitant blood vacuity, add *Ge Shu* (Bl 17) and *Gan Shu* (Bl 18). For heart palpitations, add *Shen Men* (Ht 7) and *Xin Shu* (Bl 15). For dizziness, moxa *Bai Hui* (GV 20).

REMARKS

1. Dampness and phlegm are both yin depressions which may hinder and obstruct the free flow of qi and blood, thus depriving the tissues of proper moistening and nourishing. Because qi moves and transforms body fluids, if the qi is too vacuous to move and transform these properly or if the qi is stagnant and thus not freely flowing, fluids may collect and transform into evil dampness. In addition, because blood and body fluids move together, static blood may also hinder the movement of fluids, thus resulting in evil dampness. If evil dampness lingers and endures or if it is congealed by cold or cooked by heat, dampness may transform into phlegm. Because A) the spleen is the root of phlegm engenderment and spleen qi vacuity plays a part in most patterns of this disease, and B) most patterns of this disease also include qi stagnation and blood stasis, phlegm and dampness commonly complicate the above patterns of scleroderma.

When dampness and phlegm complicate the above patterns, one should add the main ingredients of *Er Chen Tang* (Two Aged [Ingredients] Decoction to the above formulas: Rhizoma Pinelliae Ternatae (*Ban Xia*), Sclerotium Poriae Cocos (*Fu Ling*), and Pericarpium Citri Reticulatae (*Chen Pi*). In addition, one may also add Thallus Algae (*Kun Bu*) and Herba Sargassii (*Hai Zao*) to transform phlegm and soften the hard, Rhizoma Arisaematis (*Nan Xing*) to transform phlegm and free the flow of the channels, and Rhizoma Typhonii Gigantei (*Bai Fu Zi*) to transform phlegm and dispel wind.

2. When scleroderma affects the skin, local treatments should be combined with systemic treatments. These local treatments should primarily seek to quicken the blood and free the flow of the network vessels. For instance, one can seven star hammer each day all around the margins of any sclerotic areas. If stasis is complicated by cold, one can soak the affected areas, especially if they are located on the fingers, in warm decoctions of acrid and warm, quickening and moving medicinals, such as Herba Asari Cum Radice (*Xi Xin*), Ramulus Cinnamomi Cassiae (*Gui Zhi*), Lignum Sappan (*Su Mu*), Sanguis Draconis (*Xue Jie*), etc. A warm, moving tincture for external application can be made from 60g each of Radix Angelicae Sinensis (*Dang Gui*) and Cortex Cinnamomi Cassiae (*Rou Gui*), 30g each of Flos Carthami Tinctorii (*Hong Hua*), dry Rhizoma Zingiberis (*Gan Jiang*), and Fructus Zanthoxyli Bungeani (*Chuan Jiao*), and 15g each of Camphora (*Zang Nao*) and Herba Asari Cum Radice (*Xi Xin*). Soak these in one liter of 95% alcohol for one week. Then strain the dregs and bottle the resulting tincture. Apply several times per day. Combining massage of the affected area with this external application increases its effect.

3. *Er Wu Tong Bi Tang* (Two Wu's Free the Flow of Impediment Decoction) achieves good results for enduring scleroderma. It works especially well when skin abnormalities (*pi bi*, skin impediment) are accompanied by emaciation or muscular atrophy and restricted movement (*i.e.*, *jin bi*, sinew impediment), painful joints and bones (*gu bi*, bone impediment), and lesions of the internal organs (*wu zang bi*, five viscera impediment). Its ingredients are: uncooked Radix Astragali Membranacei (*Huang Qi*), Herba Lycopodii (*Shen Jin Cao*), and Fructus Forsythiae Suspensae (*Lian Qiao*), 12g each, processed Radix Aconiti Carmichaeli (*Chuan Wu*), processed Radix Aconiti Kusnezofii (*Cao Wu Tou*), Ramulus Cinnamomi Cassiae (*Gui Zhi*), Radix Stephaniae Tetrandrae (*Han Fang Ji*), Radix Angelicae Sinensis (*Dang Gui*), Ramulus Loranthi Seu Visci (*Sang Ji Sheng*), Radix Cyathulae (*Chuan Niu Xi*), and Radix Scrophulariae Ningpoensis (*Xuan Shen*), 9g each, Radix Gentianae Macrophyllae (*Qin Jiao*) and Radix Ledebouriellae Divaricatae (*Fang Feng*), 6g each, Radix Et Rhizoma Notopterygii (*Qiang Huo*) and Radix Angelicae Pubescentis (*Du Huo*), 4,5g each, and Semen Sinapis Albae

(*Bai Jie Zi*), 1,5g. In case of Raynaud's phenomenon, subtract *Xuan Shen* and add nine grams each of Radix Lateralis Praeparatus Aconiti Carmichaeli (*Fu Zi*), Radix Salviae Miltiorrhizae (*Dan Shen*), and Herba Lycopi Lucidi (*Ze Lan*). For painful skin and joints, add nine grams each of Herba Lycopi Lucidi (*Ze Lan*), Radix Salviae Miltiorrhizae (*Dan Shen*), and Radix Cynanchi Baiwai (*Bai Wai*). For cough, add nine grams each of Herba Ephedrae (*Ma Huang*), Radix Platycodi Grandiflori (*Jie Geng*), and Radix Peucedani (*Qian Hu*). For liver lesions, add nine grams each of Radix Scutellariae Baicalensis (*Huang Qin*), Cortex Radicis Moutan (*Dan Pi*), and Rhizoma Cyperi Rotundi (*Xiang Fu*). For proteinuria, add nine grams of Rhizoma Atractylodis Macrocephalae (*Bai Zhu*) and 12 grams each of Stylus Zeae Maydis (*Yu Mi Xu*) and Semen Plantaginis (*Che Qian Zi*).

65

SJÖGREN'S SYNDROME

Sjögren's syndrome (SS) is a chronic, systemic autoimmune disorder of unknown etiology which is characterized by dryness of the mouth, eyes, and other mucous membranes. It is often associated with rheumatic disorders, and shares certain features with RA, SLE, and PSS. This disease is more common than SLE but less common than RA. In some patients, SS affects only the eyes or mouth. This is referred to as primary SS. In other cases, there is associated generalized collagen vascular disease. This is referred to as secondary SS.

One third of SS patients develop enlarged parotid glands that are usually firm, smooth, fluctuate in size, and are mildly tender to palpation. Dry mouth and lips inhibit chewing and swallowing, and the faculties of taste and smell may be diminished. Desiccation may also develop in the skin and in the mucuous membranes of the nose, throat, larynx, bronchi, vulva, and vagina, and alopecia may occur. Dryness of the respiratory tract often leads to pulmonary infections and may result in fatal pneumonia. SS is often associated with chronic hepatobiliary disease as is pancreatitis. Sensory neuropathy is common, especially of the 2nd and 3rd divisions of the 5th cranial nerve. Interstitial nephritis is frequent, and the incidence of lymphoma is 44 times greater in SS patients.

The Western medical diagnosis of this syndrome involves various measurements of the tears and saliva. Blood analysis shows elevated levels of antibodies against certain globulins, nuclear protein, and many tissue constituents. In particular, SS-B antibodies are highly specific for primary SS, and rheumatoid factor is present and ESR is elevated in 70% or more cases. Western medicine has no drug treatment for the dry symptoms associated with this condition. When connective tissue involvement is severe, corticosteroids and immuno-suppressive agents may be prescribed. In terms of prognosis, this is commonly related to any associated connective tissue disorder.

DISEASE CATEGORIZATION: In Chinese medicine, Sjögren's syndrome is mostly categorized as *zao zheng*, dryness condition, or *zao du*, dry toxins. Dry, rough eyes are referred to as *mu se*, rough eyes; dry nose is called *bi gan*, dry nose; and dry throat is called *yan gan*, dry throat.

DISEASE CAUSES: Habitual bodily yin vacuity, enduring disease, possible invasion or engenderment by heat toxins

DISEASE MECHANISMS: Either habitual bodily yin vacuity or enduring disease internally damaging essence blood result in yin vacuity and internal dryness. Such enduring disease may involve wind, dampness, heat, dryness, phlegm, blood stasis, or a combination of these. For instance, damp heat may brew and steam, consuming yin fluids over time, or static blood may inhibit the production of new or fresh blood. In this case, by the time the yin is vacuous and depleted, the root is yin vacuity and any evil qi are the branch. Yin vacuity and the presence of such evils may also give rise to qi and yin dual vacuity. Or, yin vacuity may reach yang, resulting in yin and yang dual vacuity.

TREATMENT BASED ON PATTERN DISCRIMINATION:

1. WIND HEAT PATTERN

MAIN SYMPTOMS: Commonly seen in the initial stage of this disease, there are dry mouth, parched throat, sore throat, somewhat red, swollen eyes that are also dry, itchy, and/or painful, swollen parotid glands, aversion to wind, if severe, high fever, joint redness, swelling, and pain, especially of the small joints, a red tongue with thin, slightly yellow fur, and a floating, rapid pulse.

TREATMENT PRINCIPLES: Dispel wind and scatter heat assisted by nourishing yin and engendering fluids

RX: *Sang Xing Tang* (Morus & Armeniaca Decoction)

INGREDIENTS: Radix Glehniae Littoralis (*Sha Shen*), 12-15g, Folium Mori Albi (*Sang Ye*), Semen Pruni Armeniacae (*Xing Ren*), Semen Praeparatus Sojae (*Dan Dou Chi*), Fructus Gardeniae Jasminoidis (*Zhi Zi*), 9g each, Pear Skin, 6-9g, and Bulbus Fritillariae Cirrhosae (*Chuan Bei Mu*), 3-6g

ANALYSIS OF FORMULA: *Sang Ye* and *Dan Dou Chi* dispel wind and scatter heat. However, they dispel wind without damaging fluids. *Zhi Zi* clears heat. *Chuan Bei Mu* engenders fluids at the same time as it transforms phlegm. Therefore, it is especially good for the treatment of dry phlegm. *Xing Ren* diffuses the lungs and moistens the intestines. *Sha Shen* and pear skin nourish yin and engender fluids.

ADDITIONS & SUBTRACTIONS: For marked joint aching and pain, add nine grams each of Ramulus Mori Albi (*Sang Zhi*), Radix Et Rhizoma Notopterygii (*Qiang Huo*), and Radix Ledebouriellae Divaricatae (*Fang Feng*). For low back and knee soreness and weakness, add nine grams each of Fructus Lycii Chinensis (*Gou Qi Zi*) and Radix Achyranthis Bidentatae (*Huai Niu Xi*). For severe dryness with difficulty swallowing dry food, dry, crimson lips, dry stools, scanty urine, and dry eyes, add 15 grams of uncooked Radix Rehmanniae (*Sheng Di*), and nine grams each of Tuber Ophiopogonis Japonici (*Mai Men Dong*) and Radix Scrophulariae Ningpoensis (*Xuan Shen*). For swollen, enlarged parotid glands, add nine grams of Bubus Shancigu (*Shan Ci Gu*).

ACUPUNCTURE & MOXIBUSTION: *He Gu* (LI 4), *Chi Ze* (Lu 5), *Fu Liu* (Ki 7)

ANALYSIS OF FORMULA: Draining *He Gu* dispels wind and scatters heat. Draining *Chi Ze* diffuses and clears the lungs. Supplementing *Fu Liu* nourishes yin and engenders fluids.

ADDITIONS & SUBTRACTIONS: For fever, add *Qu Chi* (LI 11). For severe dry mouth, add *Cheng Jiang* (CV 24). For parched and sore throat, add *Lie Que* (Lu 7) and *Zhao Hai* (Ki 6). For red, dry, swollen eyes, add *Feng Chi* (GB 20). For itchy and/or painful, swollen parotid glands, add *Yi Feng* (TB 17). For marked joint aching and pain, add local *a shi* points. For low back and knee soreness and weakness, add *Shen Shu* (Bl 23).

2. DAMP HEAT PATTERN

MAIN SYMPTOMS: Usually seen in the beginning stages, there are a bitter taste in the mouth, dry, sticky mouth, slightly dry eyes which is worse in the canthi, possible swollen, painful parotids, swollen, painful gums, vexatious heat in the chest, torpid intake and scanty eating, bad breath, thirst but not much drinking, red, hot urination, stools either hard or loose, red, swollen, painful, heavy joints, a red tongue with yellow, slimy fur, and a slippery, rapid pulse.

NOTE: In this pattern, the disease is located in the spleen and stomach.

TREATMENT PRINCIPLES: Clear heat and disinhibit dampness, arouse the spleen and harmonize the stomach

RX: *Gan Lu Xiao Du Dan* (Sweet Dew Disperse Toxins Elixir)

INGREDIENTS: Talcum (*Hua Shi*), 15-20g, Herba Artemisiae Capillaris (*Yin Chen Hao*) and Radix Scutellariae Baicalensis (*Huang Qin*), 9-15g each, Fructus Forsythiae Suspensae (*Lian Qiao*), Rhizoma Belamcandae Chinensis (*She Gan*), Rhizoma Acori Graminei (*Shi Chang Pu*), Herba Agastachis Seu Pogostemi (*Huo Xiang*), Fructus Cardamomi (*Bai Dou Kou*), and Fritillariae Thunbergii (*Zhe Bei Mu*), 9g each, Caulis Akebiae (*Mu Tong*), 6g, and Herba Menthae Haplocalycis (*Bo He*), 3-6g

ANALYSIS OF FORMULA: *Hua Shi*, *Yin Chen Hao*, and *Mu Tong* clear heat and disinhibit dampness. *Huang Qin* dries dampness, clears heat, and resolves toxins. *Bo He* scatters heat. *Lian Qiao* and *She Gan* clear heat and resolve toxins. *Shi Chang Pu*, *Huo Xiang*, and *Bai Dou Kou* transform damp warmth, damp summerheat, and damp turbidity. *Zhe Bei Mu* transforms phlegm and clears heat. *Shi Chang Pu* and *Huo Xiang* harmonize the stomach.

ADDITIONS & SUBTRACTIONS: If dry throat is pronounced, add 12 grams each of Radix Glehniae Littoralis (*Sha Shen*) and Tuber Ophiopogonis Japonici (*Mai Dong*). If there is constipation, add nine grams of Fructus Trichosanthis Kirlowii (*Quan Gua Lou*). If there is joint swelling and pain, add 12 grams of Ramulus Loranthi Seu Visci (*Sang Ji Sheng*) and nine grams of Rhizoma Cibotii Barometsis (*Gou Ji*).

ACUPUNCTURE & MOXIBUSTION: *He Gu* (LI 4), *Qu Chi* (LI 11), *Yin Ling Quan* (Sp 9), *Zu San Li* (St 36)

ANALYSIS OF FORMULA: Draining *He Gu* and *Qu Chi* combined with *Yin Ling Quan* clears heat and disinhibits dampness. With even supplementing-even draining method, *Zu San Li* fortifies the spleen and harmonizes the stomach.

ADDITIONS & SUBTRACTIONS: For severe dryness, add *Fu Liu* (Ki 7). For a bitter taste in the mouth, add *Yang Ling Quan* (GB 34). For dry eyes which are worse in the corners, add *Zan Zhu* (Bl 2) and *Tong Zi Liao* (GB 1). For bad breath, add *Da Ling* (Per 7) and *Nei Ting* (St 44). For red, hot urination, add *Zhong Ji* (CV 3). For fever, add *Wai Guan* (TB 5). For severe dry mouth, add *Cheng Jiang* (CV 24). For itchy and/or painful, swollen parotid glands, add *Yi Feng* (TB 17). For marked joint aching and pain, add *a shi* points.

3. YIN VACUITY WITH INTERNAL DRYNESS PATTERN

MAIN SYMPTOMS: Due to natural endowment or prolonged use of steroids, there are dry mouth, parched throat, dry, astringent eyes, dizziness and pain, tinnitus, deafness, bodily emaciation, vexatious heat in the five hearts, red cheeks, night sweats, low back and knee joint aching and pain, seminal emission in men, menstrual irregularity in women, a red tongue with scanty fur or a bare, smooth, dry, peeled tongue, and a fine, rapid pulse.

NOTE: In this pattern the disease is located primarily in the liver and kidneys.

TREATMENT PRINCIPLES: Enrich yin and moisten dryness, supplement the liver and boost the kidneys

RX: *Yi Guan Jian Jia Jian* (One Link Decoction with Additions & Subtractions)

INGREDIENTS: Uncooked Radix Rehmanniae (*Sheng Di*), 9-15g, Radix Glehniae Littoralis (*Sha Shen*), Tuber Ophiopogonis Japonici (*Mai Dong*), and Tuber Asparagi Cochinensis (*Tian Dong*), 12g each, Radix Angelicae Sinensis (*Dang Gui*) and Fructus Lycii Chinensis (*Gou Qi Zi*), 9g each, and Fructus Meliae Toosendan (*Chuan Lian Zi*), 6g

ANALYSIS OF FORMULA: *Sheng Di, Tian Men Dong, Dang Gui,* and *Gou Qi Zi* nourish liver blood and enrich kidney yin. *Sha Shen, Mai Men Dong,* and *Sheng Di* enrich yin and moisten dryness. *Chuan Lian Zi* courses the liver and rectifies the qi without damaging yin.

ADDITIONS & SUBTRACTIONS: For fatigue and weakness of limbs, add 15 grams each of Radix Codonopsitis Pilosulae (*Dang Shen*) and Radix Astragali Membranacei (*Huang Qi*) and 20 grams of Rhizoma Polygonati (*Huang Jing*). For severe dryness, add nine grams each of Herba Dendrobii (*Shi Hu*) and Rhizoma Phragmitis Communis (*Lu Gen*). For vacuity heat with night sweats, tidal heat, bone steaming, and hot flashes in the face, add 12 grams each of Radix Scrophulariae Ningpoensis (*Xuan Shen*), Cortex Radicis Lycii Chinensis (*Di Gu Pi*), and Rhizoma Anemarrhenae Asphodeloidis (*Zhi Mu*). For swollen, enlarged parotid glands, add nine grams of Bubus Shancigu (*Shan Ci Gu*). For bleeding gums or nose, add 15 grams each of Herba Ecliptae Prostratae (*Han Lian Cao*), Nodus Rhizomatis Nelumbinis Nuciferae (*Ou Jie*), and Rhizoma Imperatae Cylindricae (*Bai Mao Gen*). For insomnia and restlessness, add 20 grams of Bulbus Lilii (*Bai He*) and nine grams of Fructus Schisandrae Chinensis (*Wu Wei Zi*).

If the main symptom is bilateral eye dryness and astringency, use *Qi Ju Di Huang Tang* (Lycium & Chrysanthemum Decoction) instead. This is comprised of: cooked Radix Rehmanniae (*Shu Di*), 10-15 grams, Fructus Corni Officinalis (*Shan Zhu Yu*), Fructus Lycii Chinensis (*Gou Qi Zi*), and Radix Dioscoreae Oppositae (*Shan Yao*), 12 grams each, Scleortium Poriae Cocos (*Fu Ling*), Rhizoma Alismatis (*Ze Xie*), Cortex Radicis Moutan (*Dan Pi*), and Flos Chrysanthemi Morifolii (*Ju Hua*), 9 grams each.

If there is marked joint aching and pain due to dryness mixed with impediment, then use *Da Qin Jiao Tang* (Great Gentiana Macrophylla Decoction) instead. This is composed of: Radix Gentianae Macrophyllae (*Qin Jiao*), 15 grams, uncooked & cooked Radix Rehmanniae (*Sheng Shu Di*), and Sclerotium Poriae Cocos (*Fu Ling*), 12 grams each, Radix Angelicae Sinensis (*Dang Gui*), Radix Albus Paeoniae Lactiflorae (*Bai Shao*), Radix Ligustici Wallichii (*Chuan Xiong*), Gypsum Fibrosum (*Shi Gao*), Radix Scutellariae Baicalensis (*Huang Qin*), Radix Angelicae Pubescentis (*Du Huo*), Radix Angelicae Dahuricae (*Bai Zhi*), Radix Et Rhizoma Notopterygii (*Qiang Huo*), and Radix Glycyrrhizae (*Gan Cao*), 9 grams each, Rhizoma Atractylodis Macrocephalae (*Bai Zhu*), 6 grams, and Herba Asari Cum Radice (*Xi Xin*), 3 grams.

ACUPUNCTURE & MOXIBUSTION: *Fu Liu* (Ki 7), *Gan Shu* (Bl 18), *Pi Shu* (Bl 20), *Shen Shu* (Bl 23)

ANALYSIS OF FORMULA: Supplementing *Fu Liu* enriches yin and moistens dryness, supplementing *Gan Shu* nourishes liver yin and blood, supplementing *Pi Shu* fortifies the latter heaven to support the former heaven, and supplementing *Shen Shu* supplements kidney yin.

ADDITIONS & SUBTRACTIONS: For dry mouth, add *Cheng Jiang* (CV 24). For parched throat, add *Zhao Hai* (Ki 6). For dry, astringent eyes, add *Guang Ming* (GB 37) and *Feng Chi* (GB 20). For dizziness, add *Bai Hui* (GV 20). For tinnitus or deafness, add *Ting Hui* (GB 2). For night sweats, add *Yin Xi* (Ht 6). For menstrual irregularity, add *San Yin Jiao* (Sp 6). For fatigue and weakness of the limbs, add *Zu San Li* (St 36). For vacuity heat with night sweats, tidal fever, bone steaming, and hot flashes in the face, add *Ran Gu* (Ki 2) and *Da Zhui* (GV 14). For insomnia and restlessness, add *Shen Men* (Ht 7). For enlarged, swollen parotid glands, add *Yi Feng* (TB 17). For marked joint aching and pain, add *a shi* points.

4. QI & YIN DUAL VACUITY PATTERN

MAIN SYMPTOMS: Due to enduring damage to the righteous, there are dry mouth and lips, hoarse voice, dry, itchy eyes, blurred vision, dry nose, difficulty distinguishing fragrance from fetor, a lusterless facial complexion, scanty qi, lack of strength, afternoon low-grade heat or emission of the heat from the hands, feet, and heart, a pale red tongue with scanty, dry fur, and a fine, rapid pulse.

NOTE: In this pattern, the disease is located in the liver, kidneys, lungs, and spleen.

TREATMENT PRINCIPLES: Boost the qi and nourish yin

RX: *Liu Wei Di Huang Wan* (Six Flavors Rehmannia Pills) & *Si Jun Zi Tang* (Four Gentlemen Decoction)

INGREDIENTS: Cooked Radix Rehmanniae (*Shu Di*), 15g, Radix Codonopsitis Pilosulae (*Dang Shen*), Dioscoreae Oppositae (*Huai Shan Yao*) and Fructus Corni Officinalis (*Shan Yu Rou*), 12g each, and Rhizoma Atractylodis Macrocephalae (*Bai Zhu*), Sclerotium Poriae Cocos (*Fu Ling*), Rhizoma Alismatis (*Ze Xie*), Cortex Radicis Moutan (*Dan Pi*), and mix-fried Radix Glycyrrhizae (*Gan Cao*), 9g each

ANALYSIS OF FORMULA: *Shu Di, Shan Yao, Shan Zhu Yu, Dan Pi, Ze Xie*, and *Fu Ling* are the six flavors of *Liu Wei Di Huang Wan* (Six Flavors Rehmannia Pills), a basic formula for supplementing the liver and kidneys and nourishing yin essence. *Dang Shen, Bai Zhu, Fu Ling,* and mix-fried *Gan Cao* are the four gentlemen of *Si Jun Zi Tang* (Four Gentlemen Decoction), a basic formula for supplementing lung and spleen qi. Together, these two formulas supplement the liver, kidneys, lungs, and spleen, boost the qi and nourish yin.

ADDITIONS & SUBTRACTIONS: If low-grade fever endures and does not recede, add nine grams each of Radix Stellariae Dichotomae (*Yin Chai Hu*), Carapax Amydae Chinensis (*Bie Jia*), and Herba Artemesiae Apiaceae (*Qing Hao*).

ACUPUNCTURE & MOXIBUSTION: *Fu Liu* (Ki 7), *Gan Shu* (Bl 18), *Pi Shu* (Bl 20), *Shen Shu* (Bl 23), *Zu San Li* (St 36)

ANALYSIS OF FORMULA: Supplementing *Fu Liu* enriches yin and moistens dryness, supplementing *Gan Shu* nourishes liver yin and blood, and supplementing *Shen Shu* supplements kidney yin. Supplementing *Zu San Li* and *Pi Shu* fortifies the spleen and boosts the qi.

ADDITIONS & SUBTRACTIONS: Please see pattern #3 above.

5. YIN & YANG DUAL VACUITY PATTERN

MAIN SYMPTOMS: Seen during the latter stages of this disease or due to steroid use, there are dry mouth and eyes, lassitude of the spirit, lack of strength, low back and knee aching and weakness, vexatious heat in the five hearts or lack of warmth in the four extremities, dry skin, frequent urination, especially frequent night-time urination, loose stools, impotence, premature ejaculation, or seminal emission in men, infertility in women, a pale red tongue with thin fur, and a deep, fine, forceless pulse.

NOTE: In this pattern, the disease is located in the liver and kidneys.

TREATMENT PRINCIPLES: Enrich the liver and supplement the kidneys, regulate and supplement yin and yang

RX: *Shen Qi Wan* (Kidney Qi Pills)

INGREDIENTS: Cooked Radix Rehmanniae (*Shu Di*), 15g, Radix Dioscoreae Oppositae (*Shan Yao*) and Fructus Corni Officinalis (*Shan Yu Rou*), 12g each, Sclerotium Poriae Cocos (*Fu Ling*), Rhizoma Alismatis (*Ze Xie*), Cortex Radicis Moutan (*Dan Pi*), and Cortex Cinnamomi Cassiae (*Rou Gui*), 9g each, and Radix Lateralis Praeparatus Aconiti Carmichaeli (*Fu Zi*), 6-9g

ANALYSIS OF FORMULA: *Shu Di, Shan Yao, Shan Zhu Yu, Dan Pi, Ze Xie*, and *Fu Ling* are the six flavors of *Liu Wei Di Huang Wan* (Six Flavors Rehmannia Pills), a basic formula for nourishing liver-kidney yin. They also supplement yin to engender yang based on the sayings, "Yin and yang are mutually rooted," and, "Yang is engendered from yin." *Fu Zi* and *Rou Gui* warm and supplement kidney yang.

ADDITIONS & SUBTRACTIONS: If yang is more vacuous than yin, add nine grams each of Gelatinum Cornu Cervi (*Lu Jiao Jiao*), Fructus Psoraleae Corylifoliae (*Bu Gu Zhi*), and Herba Cistanchis Deserticolae (*Rou Cong Rong*). For concomitant qi vacuity, add *Sheng Mai San* (Engender the Pulse Powder): Radix Panacis Ginseng (*Ren Shen*), 5g, Tuber Ophiopogonis Japonici (*Mai Men Dong*), 9g, and Fructus Schisandrae Chinensis (*Wu Wei Zi*), 6g. For low back and knee joint aching and pain, add nine grams each of Cortex Eucommiae Ulmoidis (*Du Zhong*), Ramulus Loranthi Seu Visci (*Sang Ji Sheng*), and Radix Achyranthis Bidentatae (*Niu Xi*).

ACUPUNCTURE & MOXIBUSTION: *Fu Liu* (Ki 7), *Tai Xi* (Ki 3), *Shen Shu* (Bl 23), *Zhi Shi* (Bl 52)

ANALYSIS OF FORMULA: Supplementing *Fu Liu, Tai Xi, Shen Shu,* and *Zhi Shi* enriches the liver and supplements the kidneys, regulates and supplements yin and yang.

ADDITIONS & SUBTRACTIONS: For marked lack of warmth in the four extremities, frequent urination, nocturia, and infertility in women, also moxa *Guan Yuan* (CV 4). For impotence and/or premature ejaculation, also moxa *Ming Men* (GV 4). Please also see pattern #3 above.

6. QI STAGNATION & BLOOD STASIS PATTERN

MAIN SYMPTOMS: Commonly seen during the latter stage when enduring disease has damaged the righteous and entered the network vessels, there are dry mouth, parched throat, an abnormal sensation in the eyes, swollen, distended parotid region and hard to disperse piercing pain, a dark, stagnant facial complexion, purple red maculopapular skin lesions whose color does not recede when pressed, joint aching and pain, numbness and insensitivity, abdominal concretions and accumulations, fixed pain, a pale red tongue with purple qi or static macules, and a fine, choppy pulse.

TREATMENT PRINCIPLES: Boost the qi and quicken the blood assisted by clearing heat, moistening dryness, and freeing the flow of the network vessels

RX: *Sheng Xue Run Pi Yin* (Engender the Blood & Moisten the Skin Drink)

INGREDIENTS: Uncooked & cooked Radix Rehmanniae (*Sheng Shu Di*) and Radix Astragali Membranacei (*Huang Qi*), 15g each, Tuber Asparagi Cochinensis (*Tian Dong*) and Tuber Ophiopogonis Japonici (*Mai Dong*), 12g each, Radix Angelicae Sinensis (*Dang Gui*), Fructus Schisandrae Chinensis (*Wu Wei Zi*), Radix Scutellariae Baicalensis (*Huang Qin*), Semen Trichosanthis Kirlowii (*Gua Lou Ren*), Semen Pruni Persicae (*Tao Ren*), and alcohol stir-fried Flos Carthami Tinctorii (*Hong Hua*), 9g each, and Rhizoma Cimicifugae (*Sheng Ma*), 1.5-4.5g

ANALYSIS OF FORMULA: *Sheng Di, Shu Di, Tian Men Dong, Mai Men Dong*, and *Wu Wei Zi* nourish yin and moisten dryness. *Dang Gui, Hong Hua,* and *Tao Ren* quicken the blood and transform stasis. In addition, *Dang Gui* and *Tao Ren* moisten dryness. *Huang Qi* boosts the qi. *Huang Qin* and *Sheng Ma* clear heat.

ADDITIONS & SUBTRACTIONS: If small joint pain is marked, add nine grams each of Radix Clematidis Chinensis (*Wei Ling Xian*), Rhizoma Smilacis Glabrae (*Tu Fu Ling*), Fructus Chaenomelis Lagenariae (*Mu Gua*), and Rhizoma Polygoni Cuspidati (*Hu Zhang*).

For abdominal concretions and accumulations which are hard in substance and aching and painful, use instead *Shao Fu Zhu Yu Tang Jia Wei* (Lower Abdomen Dispel Stasis Decoction with Added Flavors): Herba Oldenlandiae Diffusae (*Bai Hua She She Cao*) and Herba Scutellariae Barbatae (*Ban Zhi Lian*), 15g each, Radix Angelicae Sinensis (*Dang Gui*), Radix Ligustici Wallichii (*Chuan Xiong*), Radix Rubrus Paeoniae Lactiflorae (*Chi Shao*), Semen Abutili Seu Malvae (*Dong Kui Zi*), Ramulus Et Folium Sarcandrae (*Zhong Jie Feng*), Feces Trogopterori Seu Pteromi (*Wu Ling Zhi*), and Pollen Typhae (*Pu Huang*), 9g each, Fructus Foeniculi Vulgaris (*Xiao Hui Xiang*), Ramulus Cinnamomi Cassiae (*Gui Zhi*), Resina Olibani (*Ru Xiang*), and Resina Myrrhae (*Mo Yao*), 6g each, and dry Rhizoma Zingiberis (*Sheng Jiang*), 3g.

ACUPUNCTURE & MOXIBUSTION: *San Yin Jiao* (Sp 6), *He Gu* (LI 4), *Zu San Li* (St 36), *Fu Liu* (Ki 7)

ANALYSIS OF FORMULA: Draining *San Yin Jiao* and *He Gu* moves the qi, quickens the blood, and frees the flow of the network vessels. Supplementing *Zu San Li* boosts the qi, while supplementing *Fu Liu* enriches yin and engenders fluids.

ADDITIONS & SUBTRACTIONS: For dry mouth, add *Cheng Jiang* (CV 24). For parched throat, add *Zhao Hai* (Ki 6). For dry, astringent eyes or an abnormal sensation in the eyes, add *Guang Ming* (GB 37) and *Feng Chi* (GB 20). For fatigue, add *Tai Bai* (Sp 3). For swollen, distended parotid region, add *Yi Feng* (TB 17). For marked joint aching and pain, add *a shi* points. For abdominal concretions and accumulations and fixed abdominal pain, add *Tian Shu* (St 25), *Zhong Wan* (CV 12), *Qi Hai* (CV 6), and *Nei Guan* (Per 6).

7. PHLEGM TURBIDITY INTERNALLY BINDING PATTERN

MAIN SYMPTOMS: Slightly dry mouth and eyes, parotid region swollen and distended, gradual enlargement that does not disperse, swollen submaxillary nodules which are difficult to move, fixed, circumscribed lumps in the abdomen which are also immovable possibly accompanied by pain, cough, chest oppression, profuse phlegm, a pale tongue with white, slimy fur, and a bowstring, slippery pulse. This pattern is mostly seen in those where the disease course has been prolonged and in whom habitual bodily yin vacuity and dryness are severe. It may also be encountered in those who eat too much sweet, thick-flavored, fatty foods, or in those who are repeatedly invaded by damp heat evils. In any of these instances, phlegm and dampness may be engendered internally which then binds into nodules.

NOTE: In this pattern, the disease is located in the lungs, spleen, liver, and kidneys.

TREATMENT PRINCIPLES: Transform phlegm and soften the hard assisted by moistening dryness

RX: *Hai Zao Yu Hu Tang* (Sargassum Jade Flask Decoction)

INGREDIENTS: Herba Sargassii (*Hai Zao*), Herba Zosterae Marinae (*Hai Dai*), and Thallus Algae (*Kun Bu*), 12g each, Rhizoma Pinelliae Ternatae (*Ban Xia*), Bulbus Fritillariae Thunbergii (*Zhe Bei Mu*), Radix Angelicae Sinensis (*Dang Gui*), Radix Ligustici Wallichii (*Chuan Xiong*), Fructus Forsythiae Suspensae (*Lian Qiao*), and Radix Angelicae Pubescentis (*Du Huo*), 9g each, Pericarpium Citri Reticulatae (*Chen Pi*) and Pericarpium Citri Reticulatae Viride (*Qing Pi*), 6g each, and Radix Glycyrrhizae (*Gan Cao*), 3g

ANALYSIS OF FORMULA: *Hai Zao, Hai Dai, Kun Bu, Ban Xia*, and *Zhe Bei Mu* all transform phlegm and soften hardness. *Lian Qiao* also softens the hard, *Chen Pi* helps to transform phlegm, and *Qing Pi* breaks the qi and disperses binding. *Dang Gui* nourishes the blood and moistens dryness. With *Chuan Xiong*, it also quickens the blood. *Du Huo* is an example of using a wind medicinal to move the qi and scatter dampness and turbidity. According to the *Shen Nong Ben Cao Jing (The Divine Farmer's Materia Medica Classic)*, *Du Huo* treats women's mountings and concretions. According to the *Yi Xue Qi Yuan (Opening the Source of the Study of Medicine)*, it is able to dry dampness that otherwise cannot be eliminated, and according to the *Ben Cao Tong Xuan (Materia Medica Profound Communications)*, it treats red, itchy eyes. *Gan Cao* harmonizes the other medicinals

ADDITIONS & SUBTRACTIONS: If there is chest oppression and discomfort, add nine grams each of Tuber Curcumae (*Yu Jin*) and Fructus Trichosanthis Kirlowii (*Gua Lou*). If the nodulations are hard, add nine grams each of Rhizoma Dioscoreae Bulbiferae (*Huang Yao Zi*), Rhizoma Curcumae Zedoariae (*E Zhu*), and Radix Salviae Miltiorrhizae (*Dan Shen*). One may also add nine grams each of Bulbus Pleionis Cremastrae (*Shan Ci Gu*), Herba Oldenlandiae Diffusae Cum Radice (*Bai Hua She She Cao*), and/or Spica Prunellae Vulgaris (*Xia Ku Cao*).

ACUPUNCTURE & MOXIBUSTION: *Feng Long* (St 40), *Yin Ling Quan* (Sp 9), *Fu Liu* (Ki 7), *Bai Lao* (M-HN-30)

ANALYSIS OF FORMULA: Draining *Feng Long* and *Yin Ling Quan* transform phlegm. Draining *Bai Lao* softens the hard. Supplementing *Fu Liu* enriches yin and moistens dryness.

ADDITIONS & SUBTRACTIONS: For swollen submaxillary nodules which are difficult to move, add *Tian Ding* (LI 17), *Fu Tu* (LI 18), and *Ji Quan* (Ht 1). For fixed, circumscribed lumps in the abdomen, add *Tian Ding* (LI 17), *Fu Tu* (LI 18), *Zhong Wan* (CV 12), and *Tian Shu* (St 25). For dry mouth, add *Cheng Jiang* (CV 24). For swollen, distended parotid region, add *Yi Feng* (TB 17).

REMARKS

1. Recent Chinese research suggests that routine addition of heat-clearing, toxin-resolving medicinals which enter the blood division achieves a better clinical result no matter what the pattern of this disease.[1] Such medicinals include Radix Lithospermi Seu Arnebiae (*Zi Cao*), Radix Istadis Seu Baphicacanthi (*Ban Lan Gen*), Herba Taraxaci Mongolici Cum Radice (*Pu Gong Ying*), Cortex Radicis Moutan (*Dan Pi*), and Radix Cynanchi Atrati (*Bai Wei*).

ENDNOTES

1 Hong Qing-xiang, "A Clinical Survey of the Treatment of 12 Cases of Sjögren's Syndrome," *Shang Hai Zhong Yi Yao Za Zhi (Shanghai Journal of Chinese Medicine & Medicinals)*, #9, 1995, p. 16-17

66

Stress Incontinence

Stress incontinence refers to the involuntary loss of urine on coughing, straining, sneezing, lifting, or any maneuver that suddenly increases intra-abdominal pressure. While this condition may sometimes be seen in men after prostatectomy, it is the most common cause of involuntary loss of urine in women. It may be due to shortening of the urethra and loss of normal posterior urethrovesical angle resulting from pelvic relaxation secondary to aging or multiparity.

The Western medical diagnosis of this condition is based in the patient's history, pelvic examination, and demonstrating loss of urine with coughing or straining, which may be stopped by finger elevation of the paraurethral vaginal tissues at the neck of the bladder. Mild cases of this condition may respond to pubococcygeal muscle exercises (*i.e.*, Kegels) or to sympathomimetic drug therapy. Severe cases may require surgery.

Chinese disease categorization: Urinary incontinence is called *niao shi jin, xiao bian bu jin,* and *xiao bian shi jin* in Chinese.

Disease causes: Former heaven natural endowment insufficiency, aging, enduring diseases, multiparity, internal damage by the seven affects, and unregulated eating and drinking

Disease mechanisms: Because this condition is most commonly seen in the same age women as interstitial cystitis and both conditions have to do with abnormal discharge of urine, their disease causes and mechanisms are essentially the same. Although textbooks divide incontinence in general into lung-spleen qi vacuity, lower source vacuity cold (*i.e.*, kidney yang vacuity), and liver channel depressive fire types, according to most Chinese authorities, a spleen-kidney dual vacuity lies at the center of the overwhelming majority of cases of stress incontinence. However, because of the interrelationships between the spleen and liver, qi and blood, and yin and yang, this core pattern may be complicated by liver depression, blood stasis, and/or yin vacuity.

Treatment based on pattern discrimination:

Spleen-kidney yang vacuity pattern

Main symptoms: Female, mid-30s or older with involuntary loss of urine when coughing, hiccuping, straining, or laughing, frequent night-time urination, fatigue, lassitude of the spirit, lack of strength, cold hands and feet, dizziness standing up, possible chronic hemorrhoids, possible chronic vaginal tract discharge, low back and knee soreness and limpness, decreased sexual desire, a tendency to loose stools or diarrhea, a fat, pale tongue with thin, white fur, and a deep, weak pulse

Treatment principles: Fortify the spleen and boost the qi, supplement the kidneys and invigorate yang

Rx: *Bu Zhong Yi Qi Tang* (Supplement the Center & Boost the Qi Decoction) & *Suo Quan Wan* (Stream-reducing Pills)

Ingredients: Radix Astragali Membranacei (*Huang Qi*), 18g, Radix Codonopsitis Pilosulae (*Dang Shen*) and Radix Dioscoreae Oppositae (*Shan Yao*), 12g each, Fructus Alpiniae Oxyphyllae (*Yi Zhi Ren*), Radix Linderae Strychnifoliae (*Wu Yao*), and Rhizoma Atractylodis Macrocephalae (*Bai Zhu*), 9g each, Radix Angelicae Sinensis (*Dang Gui*), Pericarpium Citri Reticulatae (*Chen Pi*), and mix-fried Radix Glycyrrhizae (*Gan Cao*), 6g each, Rhizoma Cimicifugae (*Sheng Ma*), 4.5g, and Radix Bupleuri (*Chai Hu*), 3g

Analysis of formula: *Huang Qi, Dang Shen, Shan Yao,* and *Bai Zhu* fortify the spleen and boost the qi. With *Sheng*

Ma and *Chai Hu,* they upbear clear yang. *Dang Gui* harmonizes the blood, while *Chen Pi* rectifies the qi. *Wu Yao* warms the lower origin and secures the kidneys. *Shan Yao* and *Yi Zhi Ren,* together supplement and secure the kidneys and reduce urination.

ADDITIONS & SUBTRACTIONS: For more pronounced yang vacuity, add nine grams each of Radix Lateralis Praeparatus Aconiti Carmichaeli (*Fu Zi*) and Cortex Cinnamomi Cassiae (*Rou Gui*). If there is concomitant yin vacuity, add 12 grams of cooked Radix Rehmanniae (*Shu Di*). To increase the securing and astringing function of the above formula, add nine grams each of Fructus Schisandrae Chinensis (*Wu Wei Zi*) and Semen Cuscutae Chinensis (*Tu Si Zi*). If there is low back pain, add nine grams each of Radix Dipsaci (*Xu Duan*) and Cortex Eucommiae Ulmoidis (*Du Zhong*). For concomitant break down in interaction between the heart and kidneys, add nine grams each of Radix Polygalae Tenuifoliae (*Yuan Zhi*), Rhizoma Acori Graminei (*Shi Chang Pu*), Sclerotium Pararadicis Poriae Cocos (*Fu Shen*), and Semen Nelumbinis Nuciferae (*Lian Zi*). For liver depression, add nine grams each of Rhizoma Cyperi Rotundi (*Xiang Fu*) and Fructus Meliae Toosendan (*Chuan Lian Zi*). For nocturia, add nine grams each of Fructus Rubi Chingii (*Fu Pen Zi*) and Fructus Rosae Laevigatae (*Jin Ying Zi*).

ACUPUNCTURE & MOXIBUSTION: *Zu San Li* (St 36), *Bai Hui* (GV 20), *Guan Yuan* (CV 4), *Tai Xi* (Ki 3)

ANALYSIS OF FORMULA: Supplementing *Zu San Li, Bai Hui,* and *Guan Yuan* with moxibustion fortifies the spleen and boosts the qi, upbears yang and reduces urination. In addition, moxaing *Guan Yuan* and *Tai Xi* supplements yang and secures the kidneys.

ADDITIONS & SUBTRACTIONS: For more pronounced yang vacuity, add *Ming Men* (GV 4). If there is concomitant kidney yin vacuity, add *Fu Liu* (Ki 7). If there is marked qi vacuity, add *San Yin Jiao* (Sp 6). If there is low back pain, add *Gong Sun* (Sp 4) and *Fu Liu* (Ki 7). For concomitant break down in interaction between the heart and kidneys, add *Zhi Shi* (Bl 52) and *Shen Men* (Ht 7). For liver depression, add *Zhong Feng* (Liv 4). For nocturia, add *Zhi Shi* (Bl 52). For concomitant damp heat, replace *Guan Yuan* with *Qu Gu* (CV 2). For stress incontinence but dysuria or painful urination, add *Zhi Bian* (Bl 54).

REMARKS

1. Of course, in real-life, if there is spleen qi vacuity and kidney yang vacuity, there will be liver depression qi stagnation. In perimenopausal women there may also be both yin and yang vacuity. Although blood stasis may complicate any or all of these patterns, blood stasis *per se* does not play a direct part in the disease mechanisms associated with this condition.

2. Recently, a Western medical procedure has been developed for older female patients with stress incontinence due to atrophy of the tissues surrounding the urethra. This consists of injecting a bulking agent into the tissues surrounding the urethra, thus narrowing the urethral passageway. Although this procedure seems to have few side effects, it is not 100% effective in all patients and may need to be repeated. Chinese herbal medicine is relatively effective for stress incontinence. Therefore, Chinese medicine might be tried first before such injection therapy, or administered in tandem to make that injection therapy even more effective with fewer side effects.

3. A recent report from the U.S. Department of Health & Human Services analyzed 22 different studies and concluded that muscular re-education through biofeedback training has a success rate for treating urinary incontinence ranging from 54-95% depending on the patient group.[1]

4. Based on modern clinical experience, several acupoint combinations seem to achieve good results when treating stress incontinence. These include: *Tong Tian* (Bl 7) needled in the direction of *Luo Que* (Bl 8) and *Guan Yuan* (CV 4) treated with a moxa pole; *Tai Xi* (Ki 3) and *Guan Yuan* (CV 4) needled with the burning mountain fire method; *Zhi Bian* (Bl 54) and *San Yin Jiao* (Sp 6) with strong needle sensation at *Zhi Bian*; and *Jia Ji* (M-BW-35) at the levels of L1 to S2 needled in the direction of the spinal column.

ENDNOTES

[1] Urinary Incontinence Guideline Panel, "Urinary Incontinence in Adults: Clinical Practice Guideline," AHCPR Pub. No. 92-0038, Rockville, MD, March, 1992

67

Subarachnoid Hemorrhage

Subarachnoid hemorrhage refers to sudden bleeding into the subarachnoid space. This bleeding may be secondary to head trauma. However, spontaneous or primary subarachnoid hemorrhage may also result from rupture of a congenital intracranial aneurysm or mycotic or arteriosclerotic aneurysm. This may occur at any age but most commonly occurs between 25-50 years. Before the rupture, most aneurysms are asymptomatic. Following rupture, there is usually acute severe headache often followed or accompanied by at least brief syncope. This severe headache may also be accompanied by vomiting, dizziness, and alterations in the pulse and respiratory rates. Convulsions occasionally occur. Within 24 hours of the onset of the headache, there are usually marked stiffness of the neck, Kernig's sign, and bilateral Babinski's sign. Posthemorrhagic swelling of the brain may result in stroke. Therefore, in 25% of cases, there is hemiplegia. Mortality rates with first hemorrhage are approximately 35% with an additional 15% of patients dying from subsequent rupture within a few weeks. Prognosis is best when no lesion is found with arteriography, presumably meaning that the lesion was small and sealed itself.

Diagnosis of this condition is based on spinal puncture yielding bloody cerebrospinal fluid and arteriography or angiogram. Treatment includes strict bed rest, diazepam for restlessness, and codeine or meperidine for the headache. In addition, Prednisone may be used to relieve swelling and inflammation, thus preventing stroke. If arteriography reveals the presence of an aneurysm, surgery may be used to trap or obliterate such aneurysms.

Chinese disease categorization: Subarachnoid hemorrhage is mainly categorized as *zhen tou tong*, true head pain. As such, it has always been recognized as a potentially fatal occurrence. Accompanying dizziness is categorized as *xuan yun*, vomiting is *ou tu*, syncope is *jue zheng*, reversal condition, and hemiplegia is *ban shen bu sui*, half-body paralysis, or *zhong feng*, wind stroke.

Disease causes: Internal damage by the seven affects and faulty diet

Disease mechanisms: In Chinese medicine, mostly this disease is believed to be due to emotional discomfort resulting in liver qi depression and binding. This then causes spleen loss of regulation and spreading and depression transforming into fire. If liver yang suddenly and violently rises, the blood may follow the qi counterflow to ascend and harass the clear orifices. This then results in headache. If liver qi counterflows horizontally and invades and checks spleen earth, spleen earth may suffer detriment and lose its control over fortification and movement. Dampness may then gather and accumulate, engendering phlegm. If dampness and phlegm also become depressed, they may likewise transform fire. In that case, liver fire mixed with phlegm may ascend and harass. It is also possible for undisciplined or unregulated eating and drinking to damage the spleen and stomach. This may also give rise to the internal engenderment of phlegm dampness which may transform fire and ascend to assail the clear orifices. And finally, long-term or severe liver qi depression and binding may cause qi stagnation and blood stasis, hence resulting in this disease.

Treatment based on pattern discrimination:

1. Phlegm heat harassing above pattern

Main symptoms: Severe headache, nausea and vomiting, a dry mouth but no desire to drink, a bland, tasteless feeling in the mouth, abdominal distention, torpid intake, heart vexation, insomnia, no defecation for several days, a red tongue with thick, yellow, slimy fur, and a slippery, bowstring, rapid pulse

Treatment principles: Clear heat and dispel phlegm, free the flow of the network vessels and stop pain

RX: *Huang Lian Wen Dan Tang Jia Jian* (Coptis Warm the Gallbladder Decoction with Additions & Subtractions)

INGREDIENTS: Sclerotium Poriae Cocos (*Fu Ling*), 12g, and Rhizoma Coptidis Chinensis (*Huang Lian*), Caulis Bambusae In Taeniis (*Zhu Ru*), Rhizoma Pinelliae Ternatae (*Ban Xia*), Pericarpium Citri Reticulatae (*Chen Pi*), bile-processed Rhizoma Arisaematis (*Dan Nan Xing*), Fructus Immaturus Citri Aurantii (*Zhi Shi*), Semen Plantaginis (*Che Qian Zi*), uncooked Radix Et Rhizoma Rhei (*Da Huang*), Buthus Martensis (*Quan Xie*), Scolopendra Subspinipes (*Wu Gong*), and Rhizoma Atractylodis (*Cang Zhu*), 9g each

ANALYSIS OF FORMULA: *Dan Nan Xing, Fu Ling, Zhu Ru, Ban Xia, Chen Pi, Zhi Shi,* and *Che Qian Zi* together clear heat and transform phlegm. In addition, *Ban Xia, Chen Pi,* and *Zhu Ru* stop vomiting. *Huang Lian* specifically clears heat from the heart, liver, gallbladder, and stomach, while *Fu Ling, Cang Zhu,* and *Che Qian Zi* eliminate dampness and turbidity. *Da Huang* discharges fire and frees the flow of the stools. *Quan Xie* and *Wu Gong* free the flow of the network vessels and help stop the unbearable pain.

ADDITIONS & SUBTRACTIONS: If there is no constipation, either reduce or delete the *Da Huang*. If signs and symptoms of concomitant blood stasis are marked, add nine grams each of Semen Pruni Persicae (*Tao Ren*), Flos Carthami Tinctorii (*Hong Hua*), and Radix Rubrus Paeoniae Lactiflorae (*Chi Shao*).

ACUPUNCTURE & MOXIBUSTION: *Feng Long* (St 40), *Nei Ting* (St 44), *Zhong Wan* (CV 12), *a shi* point at the site of pain or *Nao Hu* (GV 7), *Hou Ding* (GV 19), *Si Shen Cong* (M-HN-1), *Qian Ding* (GV 21), *Shang Xing* (GV 23)

ANALYSIS OF FORMULA: Together, draining *Feng Long, Nei Ting,* and *Zhong Wan* clears and transforms phlegm and heat and stops vomiting. Draining the *a shi* point at the site of pain or *Nao Hu, Hou Ding, Si Shen Cong, Qian Ding,* and *Shang Xing* frees the flow of the network vessels and stops headache. One can also bleed these points after needling them. Select the *a shi* point directly over the site of the pain during the initial phase of this condition when the site of hemorrhage is small. Choose the points on the governing vessel when the area affected by the hemorrhage is large. It is also possible to use both the *a shi* point and governing vessel points.

ADDITIONS & SUBTRACTIONS: For a tasteless feeling in the mouth, abdominal distention, and torpid intake replace *Zhong Wan* with *Nei Guan* (Per 6) and *Gong Sun* (Sp 4). For severe unbearable headache, add *Zhong Zhu* (TB 3) and *Wai Guan* (TB 5). For concomitant fatigue, add *Zu San Li* (St 36).

2. BLOOD STASIS OBSTRUCTING THE NETWORK VESSELS PATTERN

MAIN SYMPTOMS: Enduring headache which does not heal, fixed location pain, emotional tension, easy anger, bilateral rib-side distention and fullness, possible history of traumatic injury to the head, a dark, purplish tongue or possible static macules or spots, and a bowstring, choppy pulse

TREATMENT PRINCIPLES: Quicken the blood and transforms stasis, free the flow of the network vessels and stop pain

RX: *Tong Qiao Huo Xue Tang Jia Jian* (Free the Flow of the Orifices & Quicken the Blood Decoction with Additions & Subtractions)

INGREDIENTS: Radix Cyathulae (*Chuan Niu Xi*) and Radix Angelicae Sinensis (*Dang Gui*), 15g each, Lumbricus (*Di Long*), 12g, Radix Ligustici Wallichii (*Chuan Xiong*), Semen Pruni Persicae (*Tao Ren*), Radix Rubrus Paeoniae Lactiflorae (*Chi Shao*), uncooked Radix Rehmanniae (*Sheng Di*), and Radix Et Rhizoma Notopterygii (*Qiang Huo*), 9g each, wine-fried Radix Et Rhizoma Rhei (*Da Huang*), 6g, and Bulbus Allii Fistulosi (*Cong Bai*), 2 bulbs

ANALYSIS OF FORMULA: *Chuan Niu Xi, Chuan Xiong, Tao Ren, Chi Shao, Sheng Di, Dang Gui* and *Da Huang* all quicken the blood and transform stasis to stop pain. *Di Long* frees the flow of the network vessels and stops pain. *Qiang Huo* leads the other medicinals to the upper part of the body and also treats headache. *Sheng Di* also nourishes the blood and stops bleeding. *Cong Bai* frees the flow of yang and, therefore, promotes the flow of the network vessels.

ADDITIONS & SUBTRACTIONS: For emotional tension, easy anger, and bilateral rib-side distention and fullness, add nine grams each of Radix Bupleuri (*Chai Hu*), Radix Albus Paeoniae Lactiflorae (*Bai Shao*), and Tuber Curcumae (*Yu Jin*). For vomiting, add nine grams each of Rhizoma Pinelliae Ternatae (*Ban Xia*), Pericarpium Citri Reticulatae (*Chen Pi*), and Caulis Bambusae In Taeniis (*Zhu Ru*). For severe headache, add six grams each of Resina Olibani (*Ru Xiang*) and Resina Myrrhae (*Mo Yao*).

ACUPUNCTURE & MOXIBUSTION: *Tai Chong* (Liv 3), *He Gu* (LI 4), *a shi* point or *Nao Hu* (GV 7), *Hou Ding* (GV 19), *Si Shen Cong* (M-HN-1), *Qian Ding* (GV 21), *Shang Xing* (GV 23)

ANALYSIS OF FORMULA: Together with draining method, *Tai Chong* and *He Gu* move the qi and quicken the blood, transform stasis and stop pain. In addition *Tai Chong* courses the liver and resolves the depression. Draining the *a shi* point and/or *Nao Hu*, *Hou Ding*, *Si Shen Cong*, *Qian Ding*, and *Shang Xing* quickens the blood, frees the flow of the network vessels, and stops headache. One can also bleed these points after needling them.

ADDITIONS & SUBTRACTIONS: For severe blood stasis with severe headache, add *San Yin Jiao* (Sp 6) and *Zhong Zhu* (TB 3). For nausea and vomiting, add *Nei Guan* (Per 6) and *Zhong Wan* (CV 12). For severe emotional tension, add *Jian Shi* (Per 5).

3. LIVER FIRE FLARING UPWARD PATTERN

MAIN SYMPTOMS: Severe headache mostly located at the vertex and back of the neck or starting at the vertex and eventually affecting the back of the neck, possible forehead, ocular, or generalized head pain, rashness and impatience, easy anger, nausea, vomiting, stiff neck, insomnia, restlessness, a red face and eyes, dry stools, yellow urine, a red tongue with thin, yellow or thick, yellow fur, and a bowstring, rapid pulse

TREATMENT PRINCIPLES: Clear the liver and drain fire, quicken the network vessels and stop pain

RX: *Long Dan Xie Gan Tang Jia Jian* (Gentiana Drain the Liver Decoction with Additions & Subtractions)

INGREDIENTS: Radix Puerariae (*Ge Gen*), 15g, Radix Scutellariae Baicalensis (*Huang Qin*), Radix Angelicae Sinensis (*Dang Gui*), and uncooked Radix Rehmanniae (*Sheng Di*), 12 each, and stir-fried Fructus Gardeniae Jasminoidis (*Zhi Zi*), Radix Gentianae Scabrae (*Long Dan Cao*), Spica Prunellae Vulgaris (*Xia Ku Cao*), Flos Chrysanthemi Morifolii (*Ju Hua*), Radix Bupleuri (*Chai Hu*), Cortex Radicis Moutan (*Dan Pi*), and Semen Plantaginis (*Che Qian Zi*), 9g each

ANALYSIS OF FORMULA: *Huang Qin*, *Zhi Zi*, *Long Dan Cao*, *Xia Ku Cao*, *Ju Hua*, and *Gou Teng* clear the liver and discharge fire. *Chai Hu* courses the liver and prevents depression from transforming into fire. *Dan Pi* cools and quickens the blood and transforms stasis. *Ge Gen* resolves the muscles and clears heat. It specifically relieves spasms and pain in the nape of the neck and occipital region. It also empirically lowers intracranial pressure.

ADDITIONS & SUBTRACTIONS: If there is marked somnolence, add nine grams each of Rhizoma Acori Graminei (*Shi Chang Pu*), Tuber Curcumae (*Yu Jin*), and Radix Polygalae Tenuifoliae (*Yuan Zhi*) to transform phlegm and open the orifices. If there is deranged speech, add nine grams of Rhizoma Coptidis Chinensis (*Huang Lian*) to clear heart fire. If there is paralysis of the limbs, add 30 grams of Ramulus Mori Albi (*Sang Zhi*), 15 grams of Radix Cyathulae (*Chuan Niu Xi*), and nine grams of Lumbricus (*Di Long*) to course wind and free the flow of the network vessels. If there are spasms and contractures, add nine grams each of Rhizoma Gastrodiae Elatae (*Tian Ma*), Bombyx Batryticatus (*Jiang Can*), and Ramulus Uncariae Cum Uncis (*Gou Teng*) and six grams of Buthus Martensis (*Quan Xie*) to extinguish wind and stop pain.

ACUPUNCTURE & MOXIBUSTION: *Tai Chong* (Liv 3), *Xuan Zhong* (GB 39), a *shi* point or *Nao Hu* (GV 7), *Hou Ding* (GV 19), *Si Shen Cong* (M-HN-1), *Qian Ding* (GV 21), *Shang Xing* (GV 23)

ANALYSIS OF FORMULA: Draining *Tai Chong* and *Xuan Zhong* clears the liver and drains fire. In addition, *Tai Chong* courses the liver and prevents liver depression from transforming into heat. *Xuan Zhong* is the meeting point of the marrow. Therefore, draining it drains the sea of the marrow. The *a shi* point and/or *Nao Hu*, *Hou Ding*, *Si Shen Cong*, *Qian Ding*, and *Shang Xing* all quicken the blood, free the flow of the network vessels, and stop headache. One can also bleed these points after needling them.

ADDITIONS & SUBTRACTIONS: If there is marked somnolence, add *San Jian* (LI 3). If there is deranged speech, add *Ya Men* (GV 15). If there is paralysis of the limbs, please see the additions and subtractions of cerebral vascular disease. If there are spasms and contractures, add *He Gu* (LI 4).

4. STOMACH FIRE FLARING UPWARD PATTERN

MAIN SYMPTOMS: Severe headache which is mainly located frontally but which may affect the entire head, nausea, vomiting, bad breath, dry mouth, sores on the tongue, thirst with a predilection for chilled drinks, insomnia, restlessness, constipation, reddish yellow urine, a red tongue with yellow fur, and a slippery, rapid, bowstring pulse

TREATMENT PRINCIPLES: Clear the stomach and drain fire, free the flow of the network vessels and stop pain

RX: *Xie Xin Tang Jia Wei* (Drain the Heart Decoction with Added Flavors)

INGREDIENTS: Uncooked Gypsum Fibrosum (*Shi Gao*), 30g, Radix Achyranthis Bidentatae (*Niu Xi*), 15g, Rhizoma Anemarrhenae Aspheloidis (*Zhi Mu*), 12g, and Rhizoma Coptidis Chinensis (*Huang Lian*), Radix Scutellariae Baicalensis (*Huang Qin*), Radix Et Rhizoma Rhei (*Da Huang*), Fructus Immaturus Citri Aurantii (*Zhi Shi*), Tuber Curcumae (*Yu Jin*), Radix Angelicae Sinensis (*Dang Gui*), and Caulis Bambusae In Taeniis (*Zhu Ru*), 9g each

ANALYSIS OF FORMULA: *Shi Gao*, *Zhi Mu*, *Huang Lian*,

Huang Qin, *Da Huang*, and *Zhu Ru* clear the stomach and drain fire. In addition, *Da Huang*, with the help of *Zhi Shi*, frees the flow of the stools and treats constipation, *Shi Gao* and *Zhi Mu* engender fluids damaged by heat, *Huang Lian* clears and drains heart fire and treats insomnia and restlessness due to heat harassing the spirit. *Zhu Ru* and *Huang Lian* stop vomiting. *Niu Xi* leads the blood to move downward. *Yu Jin*, *Niu Xi*, and *Dang Gui* quicken the blood, transform stasis, and stop pain.

ADDITIONS & SUBTRACTIONS: For unbearable headache, add 20 grams of Radix Angelicae Dahuricae (*Bai Zhi*) and three grams each of Buthus Martensis (*Quan Xie*) and Scolopendra Subspinipes (*Wu Gong*), powdered and taken with the strained decoction. If there is no constipation, either reduce or delete *Da Huang*.

ACUPUNCTURE & MOXIBUSTION: *He Gu* (LI 4), *Nei Ting* (St 44), *a shi* point or, *Xin Hui* (GV 22), *Shang Xing* (GV 23), *Shen Ting* (GV 24), *Yang Bai* (GB 14), *Tou Wei* (St 8)

ANALYSIS OF FORMULA: Draining *He Gu* and *Nei Ting* clears the stomach and drains fire in the yang ming. The *a shi* point and/or *Xin Hui*, *Shang Xing*, *Shen Ting*, *Yang Bai*, and *Tou Wei* all free the flow of the network vessels and stop headache. One can also bleed these points after needling them.

ADDITIONS & SUBTRACTIONS: If the pain in generalized, subtract *Tou Wei* (St 8) and *Shen Ting* (GV 24) and add *Nao Hu* (GV 7), *Hou Ding* (GV 19), *Si Shen Cong* (M-HN-1), and *Qian Ding* (GV 21). If there is deranged speech, add *Ya Men* (GV 15). If there are spasms and contractures, add *Tai Chong* (Liv 3).

REMARKS

1. The headache pain is so severe in this condition that patients will typically go to their local emergency room or call their Western physician. Therefore, Western practitioners of Chinese medicine will typically only see patients with subarachnoid hemorrhage after they have been hospitalized and, even more likely, after they have been discharged. While the combination of Chinese and Western medicine can make the Western medicine even more effective and help eliminate any negative side effects, Chinese medicine can also be used to prevent recurrences of bleeding in the future. In that case, one must determine what were the disease mechanisms that led to the bleeding and which of the patient's currently manifesting patterns might lead to such an occurrence again. Then one should treat those current patterns so that they do not have the opportunity to cause another hemorrhagic incident.

2. After the patient has been stabilized, many patients with subarachnoid hemorrhage display the pattern of qi vacuity and blood stasis. In that case, one may consider administering the following unnamed formula beginning anywhere from 48 hours to 15 days after first admittance to the hospital: Radix Astragali Membranacei (*Huang Qi*), 45g, Radix Codonopsitis Pilosulae (*Dang Shen*), 20g, Radix Angelicae Sinensis (*Dang Gui*) and Radix Ligustici Wallichii (*Chuan Xiong*), 15g each, Hirudo Seu Whitmania (*Shui Zhi*), Lumbricus (*Di Long*), Radix Rubrus Paeoniae Lactiflorae (*Chi Shao*), Fructus Immaturus Citri Aurantii (*Zhi Shi*), and Pericarpium Citri Reticulatae (*Chen Pi*), 9g each, and Flos Carthami Tinctorii (*Hong Hua*), 6g. This formula supplements the qi, quickens the blood, and transforms stasis. It treats headache, fatigue, lack of strength, and clouding of the spirit.

3. Although Western medicine understands that this condition is due to subarachnoid bleeding, practitioners of Chinese medicine should not attempt to treat this disorder with stop-bleeding medicinals alone. The traditional Chinese doctor does not know that there is bleeding in this situation based on the four examinations. In fact, in most cases, the single most evident Chinese pattern is blood stasis. However, no matter what pattern the patient presents, that should be the pattern that is treated, not some Western medical concept or idea.

4. It is also possible to have liver depression with stomach heat, heart blood and spleen qi vacuity, and blood stasis as well as phlegm. In this case, neither the liver nor stomach fire is as exuberant and replete as in the patterns above. In such complicated cases, one should simply tally all the patterns present in order of their predominance, state the necessary treatment principles for each pattern in the same order, and then compose an *ad hoc* treatment plan based on those principles. For instance, if heart-spleen dual vacuity predominates, one should begin with *Gui Pi Tang* (Restore the Spleen Decoction) and modify it with medicinals which clear heat from the yang ming, quicken the blood, and transform phlegm.

5. As stated above, due to the intense, localized nature of the pain, most patients with subarachnoid bleeding do have blood stasis as part of their overall pattern discrimination. Therefore, blood-quickening, network vessel freeing, pain-relieving medicinals should be used in virtually all cases. These include Buthus Martensis (*Quan Xie*), Scolopendra Subspinipes (*Wu Gong*), Hirudo Seu Whitmania (*Shui Zhi*), Lumbricus (*Di Long*), Resina Myrrhae (*Mo Yao*), and Resina Olibani (*Ru Xiang*).

6. Prednisone is commonly used to stop inflammation that would otherwise cause intracranial swelling. However, Prednisone itself has many side effects. If Prednisone use

causes side effects in the treatment of subarachnoid hemorrhage, please see the chapter on Cushing's syndrome in terms of the pattern discrimination treatment of such side effects.

7. Patients with a history of subarachnoid hemorrhage may consider taking Radix Pseudoginseng (*San Qi*) prophylactically to quicken the blood and transform stasis, free the flow of the network vessels and prevent bleeding. Other prophylactic treatments include *gua sha* of the nape of the neck and upper back and cupping the upper back.

68

SYSTEMIC LUPUS ERYTHMATOSUS

Also known as disseminated lupus erythmatosus, this is yet another autoimmune disease causing inflammation of the connective tissue. According to Western medicine, its etiology is unknown. Ninety percent of SLE patients are female. It predominantly affects young women, but it may also occur in children. Lupus may begin abruptly with fever or may develop insidiously over months and years. Although symptoms may manifest in any organ system, 90% of patients complain of articular symptoms ranging from intermittent arthralgias to acute polyarthritis. A past history of "growing pains" during childhood is not uncommon.

This condition is characterized by butterfly-shaped malar erythema. Other skin conditions may include discoid lesions and erythematous, firm, maculopapular lesions on the face, exposed areas of the neck, upper chest, and elbows. Oral ulcers are common, and generalized alopecia is frequent during active phases of this disease. Forty percent of lupus patients are also photosensitive. Generalized adenopathy is common, especially in children, young adults, and African Americans, and splenomegaly occurs in 10% of patients. CNS involvement can cause headache, personality changes, epilepsy, psychoses, and organic brain syndrome. Lupus patients frequently experience spontaneous abortions (probably due to autoimmune ovaritis), and postpartum flares are common.

In terms of the Western diagnosis of this condition, most patients have antinuclear antibodies (ANA) in their serum. In fact, 98% of SLE patients test positive for ANAs. When one tests positive for ANAs, then typically one is further tested for anti-DNA antibodies. High titers of anti-DNA antibodies are almost specific for lupus, while the ESR is elevated almost uniformly during active disease. Mild lupus is also diagnosed by the presence of fever, arthritis, pleurisy, pericarditis, headaches, and rashes, while severe lupus consists of potentially life-threatening hemolytic anemia, thrombocytopenic purpura, renal damage, and acute vasculitis of the gastro-intestinal tract and/or the extremities. In mild cases, arthralgias are usually controlled with NSAIDs. If both skin and joint manifestations are prominent, antimalarials are often used. Severe disease requires immediate corticosteroid therapy.

According to the American Rheumatoid Association, there must be four of the following eight symptoms present for lupus to be diagnosed: ANA antibodies in the blood, low white blood cell or platelet count or hemolytic anemia, joint pain in a number of joints, butterfly rash on the cheeks, abnormal cells in the urine, sensitivity to light, sores in the mouth, and seizures or psychosis. Some drugs give a false positive test, including hydralazine, procainamide, and beta blockers. Sometimes these drugs produce a lupus-like condition that goes away when the drug is stopped. In addition, birth control pills may cause flare-ups of lupus.

The Western prognosis of this disease varies widely depending on the organs involved and the intensity of the inflammatory reaction. The course of SLE is commonly chronic and relapsing, often with periods of remission lasting for years. Provided the initial acute phase is controlled, long-term prognosis is good with a better than 95% 10 year survival in most Western countries.

CHINESE DISEASE CATEGORIZATION: The skin lesions of lupus are variously called *hong mu die chuang*, red butterfly lesions, *zhu yu dan*, Evodia redness, *ri shai chuang*, sunshine lesions, *yin yang du*, yin yang toxins, *xue feng chuang*, blood wind lesions, *mian fa du*, face emission toxins, etc. Other symptoms of lupus fall under the categories of *shui zhong*, water swelling, *xu sun*, vacuity detriment, *chuan xi*, panting breath, *xue zheng*, bleeding conditions, *guan ge*, block and repulsion, *bi zheng*, impediment condition, etc.

DISEASE CAUSES: Former heaven natural endowment insufficiency, external contraction of the six environmental evils, both unregulated emotions and unregulated eating and drinking, over-taxation, and excessive sex

DISEASE MECHANISMS: Any of the above causes can result in loss of regulation of yin and yang, qi and blood depletion and vacuity, lack of ease or smoothness in movement and transportation, qi stagnation and blood stasis, and channel and network vessel obstruction which may then give rise to the multiplicity of signs and symptoms associated with this disease. Because this disease mostly occurs or worsens after exposure to sunshine, it is believed to be mostly due to external contraction of heat toxins evils. These heat toxins enter the interior where they scorch and burn yin and blood, impede and obstruct the channels and vessels, damage the viscera and bowels, and corrode the sinews and bones and the skin. In addition, allergic reactions to foods and medicinals, addiction to thick-flavored foods, living in damp environments, and contraction of the six environmental evils may all give rise to internal engenderment of heat toxins. If the former heaven natural endowment is insufficient and original yin or original yang are depleted and vacuous, then this can give rise to all the various symptoms of SLE. Joint pain associated with SLE is mainly due to wind damp heat impediment.

TREATMENT BASED ON PATTERN DISCRIMINATION:

1. HEAT EVILS BLAZING & EXUBERANT PATTERN

MAIN SYMPTOMS: A high fever or a continuous fever which will not recede, the emission of red macules or edematous red macules on the skin of the facial region, if severe, these lesions may be large or they may be blood blisters, generalized lack of strength, muscle and joint aching and pain, vexation and agitation, insomnia, emotional worry and anxiety, possible spirit clouding and delirious speech, spasms and contractures, dry, bound stools, short, reddish urination, oral thirst with a predilection for chilled drinks, red eyes, red lips, possible spitting of blood, spontaneous ejection of blood (*i.e.*, epistaxis), and/or hemafecia, possible sores inside the mouth, sore, swollen throat, a red, crimson, or purplish, dark tongue with yellow, slimy, yellow, dry, or yellow and white, slimy fur or a smooth bare tongue, and a bowstring, rapid pulse

NOTE: This pattern describes the signs and symptoms of the initial attack or a subsequent acute, active exacerbation of this disease. Such active episodes can be life-threatening and should be treated with a combination of modern Western and Chinese medicine.

TREATMENT PRINCIPLES: Clear heat and resolve toxins, cool the blood and nourish yin, transform stasis and disperse macules

RX: *Qing Wen Bai Du Yin Jia Jian* (Clear the Scourge & Vanquish Toxins Drink with Additions & Subtractions)

INGREDIENTS: Uncooked Gypsum Fibrosum (*Shi Gao*), 60g, Cornu Bubali (*Shui Niu Jiao*), 30g, Rhizoma Anemarrhenae Aspheloidis (*Zhi Mu*), Rhizoma Coptidis Chinensis (*Huang Lian*), Radix Scutellariae Baicalensis (*Huang Qin*), Fructus Gardeniae Jasminoidis (*Zhi Zi*), Fructus Forsythiae Suspensae (*Lian Qiao*), and Radix Scrophulariae Ningpoensis (*Xuan Shen*), 15g each, uncooked Radix Rehmanniae (*Sheng Di*), Cortex Radicis Moutan (*Dan Pi*), Radix Rubrus Paeoniae Lactiflorae (*Chi Shao*), and Radix Angelicae Sinensis (*Dang Gui*), 20g each, and Folium Bambusae (*Zhu Ye*), Radix Platycodi Grandiflori (*Jie Geng*), and Radix Glycyrrhizae (*Gan Cao*), 9g each

ANALYSIS OF FORMULA: *Shi Gao* and *Zhi Mu* clear heat from the qi division or aspect and engender fluids, while *Shui Niu Jiao*, *Xuan Shen*, *Sheng Di*, *Dan Pi*, and *Chi Shao* clear heat from the blood aspect, and *Zhu Ye* and *Lian Qiao* clear heat from the defensive aspect. *Huang Lian*, *Huang Qin*, *Zhi Zi*, and *Lian Qiao* clear heat and resolve toxins from the three burners. In addition, *Zhu Ye* engenders fluids, *Xuan Shen* resolves toxins, and *Dan Pi*, *Chi Shao*, and *Dang Gui* quicken the blood and transform stasis. *Jie Geng* is the messenger which leads the other medicinals to the lungs which are linked to the skin. *Sheng Di* nourishes yin, and *Gan Cao* harmonizes the other medicinals in this formula.

ADDITIONS & SUBTRACTIONS: For dry, bound stools, add nine grams of Radix Et Rhizoma Rhei (*Da Huang*), decocted later. For high fever which will not recede or essence will symptoms, add 0.3-0.5 grams of Cornu Antelopis Saigatatarici (*Ling Yang Jiao*), swallowed down with the decoction. For low-grade fever which will not recede, add 15 grams each of Radix Stellariae Dichotomae (*Yin Chai Hu*) and Cortex Radicis Lycii Chinensis (*Di Gu Pi*). For bleeding, add 9-20 grams each of Nodus Rhizomatis Nelumbinis Nuciferae (*Ou Jie*), Rhizoma Imperatae Cylindricae (*Bai Mao Gen*), Herba Agrimoniae Pilosae (*Xian He Cao*), and/or Cacumen Biotae Orientalis (*Ce Bai Ye*) depending on the site and cause of the bleeding. If damp heat is marked with thick, slimy tongue fur, add nine grams each of Rhizoma Atractylodis (*Cang Zhu*) and Rhizoma Acori Graminei (*Shi Chang Pu*) and delete the *Sheng Di*, *Xuan Shen*, and *Zhi Mu*. For arthralgia, add nine grams each of Radix Et Rhizoma Notopterygii (*Qiang Huo*), Radix Gentianae Macrophyllae (*Qin Jiao*), and Radix Angelicae Pubescentis (*Du Huo*). For severe thirst, add 12 grams each of Tuber Ophiopogonis Japonici (*Mai Men Dong*), Herba Dendrobii (*Shi Hu*), and Rhizoma Polygonati Odorati (*Yu Zhu*). For profuse erythema, petechiae, or purpurae, add 12 grams each of Radix Lithospermi Seu Arnebiae (*Zi Cao*), Flos Immaturus Sophorae Japonicae (*Huai Hua Mi*), and Flos Campsitis (*Ling Xiao Hua*).

ACUPUNCTURE & MOXIBUSTION: *Shi Xuan* (M-UE-1), *He Gu* (LI 4), *Wei Zhong* (Bl 40), *Qu Ze* (Per 3), *Ling Tai* (GV 10)

ANALYSIS OF FORMULA: For this pattern of SLE, acupuncture is only an adjunctive treatment. In that case, prick to bleed 7-10 drops of the blood at each of the 10 *Shi Xuan* points in order to discharge fire and abate fever. Draining *He Gu* clears heat from the qi aspect. Bleeding *Wei Zhong* and *Qu Ze* clear heat from the blood aspect and treats skin disease. Draining *Ling Tai* is an empirical treatment for skin disease due to heat.

ADDITIONS & SUBTRACTIONS: If there is spirit clouding, add *Shui Gou* (GV 26). If there is constipation, add *Zhi Gou* (TB 6). For very high fever, add *Qu Chi* (LI 11), *Da Zhui* (GV 14), and *Wai Guan* (TB 5). For dark, purple skin lesions, add *Xue Hai* (Sp 10) and *Qu Chi* (LI 11). For muscle and joint aching and pain, add *Yang Ling Quan* (GB 34) and *Xuan Zhong* (GB 39). For severe lack of strength, add *Zu San Li* (St 36). For vexation and agitation, add *Da Ling* (Per 7).

2. WIND DAMP HEAT IMPEDIMENT PATTERN

MAIN SYMPTOMS: Early stage disease with profuse, severe joint pain, especially in the fingers, toes, ankles, and wrists, migrating pain of several joints, fever, dry throat, oral thirst, sore, aching muscles, weakness of the limbs, possible joint swelling, a red tongue with yellow and/or slimy fur, and a bowstring, slippery pulse

TREATMENT PRINCIPLES: Dispel wind and eliminate dampness, clear heat and alleviate impediment

RX: *Du Huo Ji Sheng Tang Jia Jian* (Angelica Pubescens Decoction with Additions & Subtractions)

INGREDIENTS: Uncooked Gypsum Fibrosum (*Shi Gao*), 30g, Ramulus Loranthi Seu Visci (*Sang Ji Sheng*), 15-30g, Cortex Erythinae (*Hai Tong Pi*), 15g, and Radix Et Rhizoma Notopterygii (*Qiang Huo*), Radix Gentianae Macrophyllae (*Qin Jiao*), Radix Clematidis Chinensis (*Wei Ling Xian*), Radix Ledebouriellae Divaricatae (*Fang Feng*), Radix Stephaniae Tetrandrae (*Fang Ji*), and Rhizoma Anemarrhenae Aspheloidis (*Zhi Mu*), 9g each

ANALYSIS OF FORMULA: *Shi Gao* and *Zhi Mu* drain fire and clear heat, enrich yin and engender fluids. *Hai Tong Pi, Qiang Huo, Qin Jiao, Wei Ling Xian, Fang Feng,* and *Fang Ji* all dispel wind, eliminate dampness, and alleviate impediment. *Sang Ji Sheng* nourishes and supplements the liver and kidneys, strengthens the sinews and reinforces the bones. It also moistens the skin.

ADDITIONS & SUBTRACTIONS: If fever abates and only joint pain remains, *Shi Gao* and *Zhi Mu* should be replaced by Cortex Phellodendri (*Huang Bai*) and Rhizoma Atractylodis (*Cang Zhu*) and nine grams each of Radix Angelicae Sinensis (*Dang Gui*) and Radix Albus Paeoniae Lactiflorae (*Bai Shao*) should be added. If there is then marked fatigue, add 15 grams of Radix Astragali Membranacei (*Huang Qi*) and nine grams of Radix Codonopsitis Pilosulae (*Dang Shen*).

ACUPUNCTURE & MOXIBUSTION: *Qu Chi* (LI 11), *Da Zhui* (GV 14), *Yin Ling Quan* (Sp 9), local points depending on the affected joints (see chapter on osteoarthritis)

ANALYSIS OF FORMULA: Draining *Qu Chi* and *Da Zhui* clears heat and abates fever, while draining *Yin Ling Quan* clears heat and eliminates dampness. Draining the local points frees the flow of the network vessels and alleviates impediment.

ADDITIONS & SUBTRACTIONS: Also bleed *Wei Zhong* (Bl 40) and *Shi Xuan* (M-UE-1) if necessary to clear heat and abate fever. For dark, purple skin lesions, add *San Yin Jiao* (Sp 6) and *Xue Hai* (Sp 10). For vexation and agitation, add *Da Ling* (Per 7).

3. HEAT DAMAGING QI & YIN PATTERN

MAIN SYMPTOMS: Vexatious heat, spontaneous perspiration, heart palpitations, chest oppression, shortness of breath, cough, vacuity vexation insomnia. Vexation and agitation may be relatively severe and the lips may be greenish purple or the facial complexion may be somber white. There may also be counterflow chilling of the four extremities. The four extremities may lack strength and the essence spirit may be listless and fatigued. The pulse is fine and weak, bound, or regularly intermittent. The tongue is pale with thin, white fur. This pattern is mostly seen in those with accompanying cardiopulmonary damage or central nervous system damage.

TREATMENT PRINCIPLES: Clear heat and nourish yin, boost the qi and quiet the spirit

RX: *Zhi Gan Cao Tang* (Mix-fried Licorice Decoction) & *Xie Xin Tang* (Drain the Heart Decoction) with additions and subtractions

INGREDIENTS: Radix Panacis Ginseng (*Ren Shen*), 15g, Fructus Zizyphi Jujubae (*Da Zao*), 20 pieces, uncooked Radix Rehmanniae (*Sheng Di*), 50g, mix-fried Radix Glycyrrhizae (*Gan Cao*), 15g, Gelatinum Corii Asini (*E Jiao*), Tuber Ophiopogonis Japonici (*Mai Dong*), uncooked Rhizoma Zingiberis (*Sheng Jiang*), Ramulus Cinnamomi Cassiae (*Gui Zhi*), Semen Cannabis Sativae (*Huo Ma Ren*), Rhizoma Coptidis Chinensis (*Huang Lian*), Radix Scutellariae Baicalensis (*Huang Qin*), and Radix Et Rhizoma Rhei (*Da Huang*), 10g each

Analysis of formula: *Ren Shen*, *Da Zao*, and mix-fried *Gan Cao* fortify the spleen and boost the qi. *Sheng Di* and *Mai Men Dong* nourish yin, while *Sheng Di* and *E Jiao* nourish the blood. *Huo Ma Ren* moistens dryness. *Huang Lian*, *Huang Qin*, and *Da Huang* clear heat and resolve toxins. *Gui Zhi* scatters cold and frees the flow of the blood vessels. It especially treats counterflow chilling of the four extremities and heart palpitations. *Ren Shen* and *Da Zao* quiet the spirit.

Additions & subtractions: If qi vacuity is severe, add 30-100 grams of Radix Astragali Membranacei (*Huang Qi*), increasing the dosage gradually. If spleen vacuity is pronounced and resulting in loose stools and decreased eating, add nine grams each of Sclerotium Poriae Cocos (*Fu Ling*), Rhizoma Atractylodis Macrocephalae (*Bai Zhu*), and scorched Three Immortals (*San Xian*: Massa Medica Fermentata, *Shen Qu*, Fructus Crataegi, *Shan Zha*, and Fructus Germinatus Hordei Vulgaris, *Mai Ya*). If yin vacuity is marked with dry mouth, parched throat, and dry cough, add 20 grams of Radix Glehniae Littoralis (*Sha Shen*) and 12 grams each of Tuber Asparagi Cochinensis (*Tian Dong*) and Tuber Ophiopogonis Japonici (*Mai Men Dong*). If there is vacuity vexation with difficulty sleeping, add nine grams each of Cortex Albizziae Julibrissinis (*He Huan Pi*), Caulis Polygoni Multiflori (*Ye Jiao Teng*), and Semen Zizyphi Spinosae (*Suan Zao Ren*). If vexation and agitation are severe, add five grams of Folium Bambusae (*Zhu Ye*) and nine grams each of Fructus Forsythiae Suspensae (*Lian Qiao*) and Cortex Radicis Lycii Chinensis (*Di Gu Pi*). If there is hasty, rapid breathing, cough, and uneasy hacking out of phlegm, add nine grams each of Cortex Radicis Mori Albi (*Sang Bai Pi*), Herba Houttuyniae Cordatae Cum Radice (*Yu Xing Cao*), Radix Asteris Tatarici (*Zi Wan*), and Flos Tussilaginis Farfarae (*Kuan Dong Hua*) and 15 grams of Herba Oldenlandiae Diffusae (*Bai Hua She She Cao*). If the facial complexion is somber white and dread of cold and chilled extremities are pronounced, add nine grams each of Radix Lateralis Praeparatus Aconiti Carmichaeli (*Fu Zi*), Cortex Cinnamomi Cassiae (*Rou Gui*), and Herba Epimedii (*Yin Yang Huo*).

Acupuncture & moxibustion: *Tai Yuan* (Lu 9), *Fu Liu* (Ki 7), *Zu San Li* (St 36), *Nei Guan* (Per 6), *He Gu* (LI 4)

Analysis of formula: Supplementing *Tai Yuan* supplements the lung and heart qi, stops cough, and settles palpitations. Supplementing *Fu Liu* nourishes yin and engenders fluids. Supplementing *Zu San Li* fortifies the spleen and boosts the qi. Draining *He Gu* clears heat and, when combined with *Fu Liu,* stops sweating. Draining *Nei Guan* quiets the spirit, loosens the chest, and frees the flow of the network vessels of the heart, thus preventing cardiopulmonary damage.

Additions & subtractions: For night sweats, add *Yin Xi* (Ht 6). For insomnia and vexation and agitation, add *Shen Men* (Ht 7), *Shen Ting* (GV 24), and/or *Da Ling* (Per 7). For counterflow chilling of the four extremities, lack of strength, and fatigue, add *Guan Yuan* (CV 4) with moxibustion.

4. Liver channel depressive heat pattern

Main symptoms: Liver area aching and pain, possible chest, rib-side, duct, or abdominal glomus, fullness, distention, and/or pain, heart vexation, easy anger, emotional depression or dysphoria, red or purple, dark-colored skin lesions, dysmenorrhea or amenorrhea in females, and/or menstrual irregularity. It is not uncommon to also see (due to concomitant spleen vacuity) dread of cold but emission of heat, torpid intake, lack of strength, dizziness, and insomnia. The tongue is crimson and may have static macules and there is either thin, white or yellow, dry fur. The pulse is tight and fine or bowstring and rapid. This pattern is mostly seen in those who have used steroids for a prolonged period of time. Typically, the blood pressure is elevated and there is liver-spleen enlargement and functional impairment.

Note: The signs and symptoms given include some blood stasis symptoms even though the words "blood stasis" do not appear in the name of the pattern.

Treatment principles: Course the liver and clear heat, quicken the blood and transform stasis

Rx: *Yi Guan Jian* (One Link Decoction) & *Si Miao Yong An Tang* (Four Wonders Resting Hero Decoction) with additions and subtractions

Ingredients: Radix Angelicae Sinensis (*Dang Gui*) and uncooked Radix Rehmanniae (*Sheng Di*), 30g each, Radix Scrophulariae Ningpoensis (*Xuan Shen*) and Fructus Lycii Chinensis (*Gou Qi Zi*), 20g each, Flos Lonicerae Japonicae (*Jin Yin Hua*), 15g, Radix Glehniae Littoralis (*Sha Shen*), Tuber Ophiopogonis Japonici (*Mai Dong*), Fructus Meliae Toosendan (*Chuan Lian Zi*), and uncooked Radix Glycyrrhizae (*Gan Cao*), 9g each

Analysis of formula: *Yi Guan Jian* is typically a guiding prescription for liver blood-kidney yin vacuity with liver depression. *Dang Gui*, *Sheng Di*, *Gou Qi*, *Sha Shen*, and *Mai Men Dong* nourish yin blood, thus harmonizing and emolliating the liver. *Sheng Di* and *Xuan Shen* clear heat and cool the blood. *Dang Gui* and *Sheng Di* quicken the blood and transform stasis. *Jin Yin Hua* also clears heat, while *Chuan Lian Zi* clears and courses the liver, and *Gan Cao* harmonizes the other medicinals in the formula.

Additions & subtractions: For liver-spleen enlargement and liver area aching and pain, add 30 grams each of Plastrum Testudinis (*Gui Ban*) and Carapax Amydae

Chinensis (*Bie Jia*) and 15 grams each of Rhizoma Cyperi Rotundi (*Xiang Fu*) and Tuber Curcumae (*Yu Jin*). If blood stasis is severe, add 15 grams each of Rhizoma Sparganii (*Sang Leng*) and Rhizoma Curcumae Zedoariae (*E Zhu*) and nine grams each of Radix Rubrus Paeoniae Lactiflorae (*Chi Shao*) and Cortex Radicis Moutan (*Dan Pi*). If spleen vacuity is pronounced, add 20 grams of Sclerotium Poriae Cocos (*Fu Ling*) and nine grams each of Radix Panacis Ginseng (*Ren Shen*) and Rhizoma Atractylodis Macrocephalae (*Bai Zhu*). If heat toxins tend to be exuberant, add nine grams each of Radix Et Rhizoma Rhei (*Da Huang*), Radix Gentianae Scabrae (*Long Dan Cao*), Radix Bupleuri (*Chai Hu*), and Fructus Gardeniae Jasminoidis (*Zhi Zi*).

Acupuncture & moxibustion: *San Yin Jiao* (Sp 6), *He Gu* (LI 4), *Xing Jian* (Liv 2), *Yang Ling Quan* (GB 34)

Analysis of formula: Draining *Xing Jian* and *Yang Ling Quan* courses and clears the liver. Draining *He Gu* clears heat and, with *San Yin Jiao,* quickens the blood and transforms stasis.

Additions & subtractions: For liver-spleen enlargement and liver area aching and pain, add *Qi Men* (Liv 14) and *Zhang Men* (Liv 13). If blood stasis is severe, add *Ge Shu* (Bl 17). If spleen vacuity is pronounced, add *Zu San Li* (St 36). If heat toxins tend to be exuberant, add *Qu Chi* (LI 11) and *Xia Xi* (GB 43).

5. Yin vacuity with fire effulgence pattern

Main symptoms: Long-term low-grade fever which gets worse with taxation and stirring, vexatious heat in the five hearts, tidal redness of the facial region, red cheeks, night sweats, spontaneous perspiration, lack of strength, red or pale red skin lesions which begin in small number and gradually get more or larger, especially after stirring or activity, more skin lesions on the face, joint aching and pain, dizziness and vertigo, tinnitus, dry, lusterless or falling hair, dry mouth, parched throat, red urine, dry stools, menstrual irregularity in females, a red tongue with scanty fur, and a bowstring, fine, rapid pulse. This pattern is mostly seen in those with acute or subacute disease occurrence.

Treatment principles: Enrich the kidneys, nourish yin, and clear heat

Rx: *Da Bu Yin Wan* (Greatly Supplementing Yin Pills) & *Si Wu Tang* (Four Materials Decoction) with additions and subtractions

Ingredients: Plastrum Testudinis (*Gui Ban*) and Carapax Amydae Chinensis (*Bie Jia*), 30g each, uncooked Radix Rehmanniae (*Sheng Di*), Cortex Phellodendri (*Huang Bai*), Rhizoma Anemarrhenae Aspheloidis (*Zhi Mu*), and Radix Angelicae Sinensis (*Dang Gui*), 20g each, Radix Albus Paeoniae Lactiflorae (*Bai Shao*) and Radix Ligustici Wallichii (*Chuan Xiong*), 9g each

Analysis of formula: *Gui Ban, Bei Jia,* and *Sheng Di* supplement the kidneys and enrich yin, while *Dang Gui* and *Bai Shao* supplement the liver and nourish the blood. As it is said, "Blood and essence share a common source," and, "The liver and kidneys share a common source." *Gui Ban, Bei Jia, Zhi Mu,* and *Huang Bai* clear vacuity heat. Since vacuity heat has entered the blood division or aspect, the ingredients of *Si Wu Tang* are used even though the principles of nourishing and/or quickening the blood are not stated.

Additions & subtractions: If qi vacuity is severe, add 20 grams of Radix Astragali Membranacei (*Huang Qi*) and nine grams of Radix Panacis Quinquefolii (*Xi Yang Shen*). If nights sweats and/or spontaneous perspiration are pronounced, add nine grams each of Os Draconis (*Long Gu*) and Concha Ostreae (*Mu Li*). For spleen vacuity with scanty eating, add 20 grams each of Radix Dioscoreae Oppositae (*Shan Yao*) and Sclerotium Poriae Cocos (*Fu Ling*) and nine grams of Rhizoma Atractylodis Macrocephalae (*Bai Zhu*). For marked tidal heat and vexatious heat in the five hearts, add 20 grams each of Radix Dioscoreae Oppositae (*Shan Yao*) and Sclerotium Poriae Cocos (*Fu Ling*) and nine grams each of Cortex Radicis Moutan (*Dan Pi*), Fructus Corni Officinalis (*Shan Zhu Yu*), and Rhizoma Alismatis (*Ze Xie*). Or one can add 9-15 grams each of Cortex Radicis Lycii Chinensis (*Di Gu Pi*), Radix Scrophulariae Ningpoensis (*Xuan Shen*), Radix Trichosanthis Kirlowii (*Tian Hua Fen*), and Herba Artemensiae Apiaceae (*Qing Hao*). For static blood and marked skin lesions, add nine grams each of Semen Pruni Persicae (*Tao Ren*) and Flos Carthami Tinctorii (*Hong Hua*), 15 grams each of Radix Salviae Miltiorrhizae (*Dan Shen*) and Radix Rubrus Paeoniae Lactiflorae (*Chi Shao*), and 20 grams each of Rhizoma Imperatae Cylindricae (*Bai Mao Gen*) and Nodus Rhizomatis Nelumbinis Nuciferae (*Ou Jie*). If kidney depletion is marked with low back and knee soreness and weakness, dizziness, and tinnitus, add nine grams each of Fructus Lycii Chinensis (*Gou Qi Zi*), Semen Cuscutae Chinensis (*Tu Si Zi*), Fructus Rubi Chingii (*Fu Pen Zi*), Herba Cistanchis Deserticolae (*Rou Cong Rong*), Radix Achyranthis Bidentatae (*Huai Niu Xi*), and Radix Polygoni Multiflori (*He Shou Wu*).

Acupuncture & moxibustion: *Fu Liu* (Ki 7), *Yin Xi* (Ht 6), *Shen Shu* (Bl 23), *Ran Gu* (Ki 2)

Analysis of formula: Supplementing *Fu Liu* supplements the kidneys, enriches yin, and engenders fluids. Supplementing *Yin Xi* nourishes yin, quiets the spirit, and stops sweating. Supplementing *Shen Shu* supplements the kidneys and enriches yin, while draining *Ran Gu* clears vacuity heat.

ADDITIONS & SUBTRACTIONS: If qi vacuity is severe, add *Zu San Li* (St 36). For marked tidal heat and vexatious heat in the five hearts, add *Da Zhui* (GV 14). For static blood and marked skin lesions, add *Ge Shu* (Bl 17) and *Ling Tai* (GV 10). For joint aching and pain, add *Qu Chi* (LI 11) and *Yin Ling Quan* (Sp 9). For dizziness and vertigo, add *Feng Chi* (GB 20) and/or *Bai Hui* (GV 20). For menstrual irregularity, add *San Yin Jiao* (Sp 6).

6. QI STAGNATION & BLOOD STASIS PATTERN

MAIN SYMPTOMS: Cyanosis of the tips of the extremities or a mixture of somber white and greenish purple, purple-colored skin macules or disciform, deep or abnormally colored skin lesions, scaley, cracked skin, joint and muscle aching and pain, emotional depression in females with menstrual irregularity, dysmenorrhea, or amenorrhea, a purple red tongue, and static, purple, engorged sublingual veins. This pattern is mostly seen in those with accompanying serious Raynaud's disease or pronounced vasculitis.

NOTE: This pattern typically does not present in its pure form like this. Rather, blood stasis commonly complicates most, if not all, patterns of chronic, enduring disease.

TREATMENT PRINCIPLES: Quicken the blood and transform stasis, rectify the qi and free the flow of the network vessels

RX: *Xue Fu Zhu Yu Tang Jia Jian* (Blood Mansion Dispel Stasis Decoction with Additions & Subtractions)

INGREDIENTS: Uncooked Radix Rehmanniae (*Sheng Di*), Semen Pruni Persicae (*Tao Ren*), Flos Carthami Tinctorii (*Hong Hua*), Radix Rubrus Paeoniae Lactiflorae (*Chi Shao*), and Radix Achyranthis Bidentatae (*Niu Xi*), 20g each, Radix Bupleuri (*Chai Hu*) and Radix Ligustici Wallichii (*Chuan Xiong*), 15g each, and Fructus Immaturus Citri Aurantii (*Zhi Shi*), 9g

ANALYSIS OF FORMULA: *Tao Ren, Hong Hua, Chi Shao, Sheng Di, Niu Xi,* and *Chuan Xiong* quicken the blood and transform stasis. *Chai Hu* and *Zhi Shi* move and rectify the qi. *Sheng Di* and *Niu Xi* also nourish the blood. Blood vacuity leads to blood stasis, and blood stasis leads to blood vacuity.

ADDITIONS & SUBTRACTIONS: If there is emotional depression or dysphoria with chest and rib-side distention and pain, add nine grams each of Tuber Curcumae (*Yu Jin*), Rhizoma Cyperi Rotundi (*Xiang Fu*), Pericarpium Citri Reticulatae Viride (*Qing Pi*), and Fructus Citri Sacrodactylis (*Fo Shou*). For aching and pain of the tips of the extremities and/or joint aching and pain, add 9-15 grams each of Ramulus Mori Albi (*Sang Zhi*), Ramulus Cinnamomi Cassiae (*Gui Zhi*), Radix Gentianae Macrophyllae (*Qin Jiao*), Caulis Milletiae Seu Spatholobi (*Ji Xue Teng*), and Caulis Lonicerae Japonicae (*Ren Dong Teng*). If there is more blood stasis with cyanosis of the tips of the extremities and greenish purple of the skin with a relatively prolonged disease course, increase the *Chuan Xiong* up to 20 grams and add nine grams each of Rhizoma Sparganii (*San Leng*) and Rhizoma Curcumae Zedoariae (*E Zhu*), 15 grams each of Radix Pseudoginseng (*San Qi*) and Radix Angelicae Sinensis (*Dang Gui*), and six grams each of Resina Olibani (*Ru Xiang*) and Resina Myrrhae (*Mo Yao*). If there is more qi stagnation with inability of the yang qi to spread to the four limbs and, therefore, a somber white color of the tips of the four extremities and the skin with counterflow chilling over a continuously long time, then add nine grams each of Cortex Cinnamomi Cassiae (*Rou Gui*), Radix Lateralis Praeparatus Aconiti Carmichaeli (*Fu Zi*), Caulis Akebiae (*Mu Tong*), Radix Aconiti Kusnezoffi (*Cao Wu*), and Radix Aconiti Carmichaeli (*Chuan Wu*) and three grams of Herba Asari Cum Radice (*Xi Xin*). If joint and extremity aching and pain are pronounced, add nine grams each of Herba Oldenlandiae Diffusae Cum Radice (*Bai Hua She She Cao*), Buthus Martensis (*Quan Xie*), and Scolopendra Subspinipes (*Wu Gong*).

ACUPUNCTURE & MOXIBUSTION: *San Yin Jiao* (Sp 6), *He Gu* (LI 4), *Ge Shu* (Bl 17), *Ling Tai* (GV 10)

ANALYSIS OF FORMULA: Even supplementing-even draining *San Yin Jiao* nourishes and, with the draining of *He Gu,* quickens the blood and transforms stasis. Even supplementing-even draining *Ge Shu,* the meeting point of the blood, reinforces both these actions of the two first points. *Ling Tai* is an empirical point for the treatment of skin disease.

ADDITIONS & SUBTRACTIONS: For cyanosis or pain of the tips of the lower extremities, add *Ba Feng* (M-LE-8). For cyanosis of the tips of the upper extremities, add *Ba Xie* (M-UE-22). If there is marked liver depression, add *Tai Chong* (Liv 3) and *Nei Guan* (Per 6). If there is more qi stagnation with inability of the yang qi to spread to the four limbs and, therefore, a somber white color to the tips of the four extremities and the skin with counterflow chilling over a continuously long time, then add *Guan Yuan* (CV 4) with moxibustion. If joint and extremity aching and pain are pronounced, add *Qu Chi* (LI 11) and *Yin Ling Quan* (Sp 9).

7. SPLEEN-KIDNEY DUAL DEPLETION PATTERN

MAIN SYMPTOMS: Cold body, chilled limbs, low-grade fever or tidal heat, lassitude of the spirit, lack of strength, scanty qi, disinclination to speak, stirring leading to aggravation of these symptoms, torpid intake, abdominal distention, if severe, vomiting and diarrhea, a somber white or sallow yellow facial complexion, low back and knee soreness and weakness, joint swelling and pain, superficial edema, inhibited urination, skin lesions not marked or purple and dark in color, a pale, fat tongue or dark and pale tongue with teeth-marks on its edges and thin, white fur, and a soggy, fine or deep, fine pulse. This pattern is mostly seen in those with concomitant kidney disease, Raynaud's disease, or those who have undergone prolonged hormone (*i.e.*, steroid) therapy.

TREATMENT PRINCIPLES: Supplement the kidneys and fortify the spleen, warm yang and disinhibit water

RX: *Shen Qi Wan* (Kidney Qi Pills) & *Si Jun Zi Tang* (Four Gentlemen Decoction) with additions and subtractions

INGREDIENTS: Cortex Cinnamomi Cassiae (*Rou Gui*) and Radix Lateralis Praeparatus Aconiti Carmichaeli (*Fu Zi*), 15g each, Radix Dioscoreae Oppositae (*Shan Yao*), 20g, Sclerotium Poriae Cocos (*Fu Ling*), 30g, Rhizoma Atractylodis Macrocephalae (*Bai Zhu*), Rhizoma Alismatis (*Ze Xie*), Fructus Corni Officinalis (*Shan Zhu Yu*), and Cortex Radicis Moutan (*Dan Pi*), 12g each, and Radix Panacis Ginseng (*Ren Shen*) and mix-fried Radix Glycyrrhizae (*Gan Cao*), 6g each

ANALYSIS OF FORMULA: *Rou Gui, Fu Zi,* and *Shan Zhu Yu* warm and supplement kidney yang. *Shan Yao, Fu Ling, Ren Shen, Bai Zhu,* and mix-fried *Gan Cao* fortify the spleen and boost the qi. *Dan Pi* quickens the blood, and *Bai Zhu, Ze Xie,* and *Fu Ling* transform and disinhibit water.

ADDITIONS & SUBTRACTIONS: For severe nausea and vomiting, add 20 grams of uncooked Rhizoma Zingberis (*Sheng Jiang*), and nine grams each of Pericarpium Citri Reticulatae (*Chen Pi*), Rhizoma Pinelliae Ternatae (*Ban Xia*), Cortex Magnoliae Offiicinalis (*Hou Po*), and Rhizoma Acori Graminaei (*Shi Chang Pu*). For more kidney vacuity, add 9-15 grams each of Semen Cuscutae Chinensis (*Tu Si Zi*), Rhizoma Curculiginis Orchioidis (*Xian Mao*), Herba Epimedii (*Xian Ling Pi*), Ramulus Loranthi Seu Visci (*Sang Ji Sheng*), Radix Dipsaci (*Chuan Duan*), Fructus Lycii Chinensis (*Gou Qi Zi*), Cortex Eucommiae Ulmoidis (*Du Zhong*), Radix Polygoni Multiflori (*He Shou Wu*), and Herba Cistanchis Deserticolae (*Rou Cong Rong*). If urination is inhibited and water swelling is severe, add 9-15 grams each of Sclerotium Polypori Umbellati (*Zhu Ling*), Pericarpium Arecae Catechu (*Da Fu Pi*), Rhizoma Imperatae Cylindricae (*Bai Mao Gen*), and Semen Phaseoli Calcarati (*Chi Xiao Dou*). If there is diarrhea, increase the amount of *Shan Yao* up to 30 grams and add 20 grams of stir-fried Rhizoma Atractylodis Macrocephalae (*Bai Zhu*) and nine grams each of Semen Myristicae Fragrantis (*Rou Dou Kou*) and Fructus Amomi (*Sha Ren*).

ACUPUNCTURE & MOXIBUSTION: *Tai Xi* (Ki 3), *Guan Yuan* (CV 4), *Zu San Li* (St 36), *Yin Ling Quan* (Sp 9)

ANALYSIS OF FORMULA: Supplementing *Tai Xi* with moxibustion supplements the kidney qi and disinhibits water. Supplementing *Guan Yuan* with moxibustion warms and supplements kidney yang. Supplementing *Zu San Li* with moxibustion fortifies the spleen, boosts the qi, and downbears the turbid. Draining *Yin Ling Quan* disinhibits water and disperses swelling.

ADDITIONS & SUBTRACTIONS: For nausea and vomiting, add *Shang Wan* (CV 13) and *Nei Guan* (Per 6). For more marked kidney vacuity, add *Ming Men* (GV 4) and *Shen Shu* (Bl 23). If urination is inhibited and water swelling is severe, add *Zhong Ji* (CV 3) and *San Yin Jiao* (Sp 6). If there is diarrhea, add *Shen Que* (CV 8).

8. HEART-SPLEEN DUAL VACUITY PATTERN

MAIN SYMPTOMS: In the latter stages, if disease has damaged the heart, there may be heart palpitations, shortness of breath, chest oppression, profuse sweating, chilled limbs, insomnia, profuse dreams, low-grade fever, night sweats, fatigue, lack of strength, emaciation, disinclination to speak and/or weak voice, poor appetite, possible abdominal distention and loose stools, a pale white or sallow yellow facial complexion, a pale, enlarged tongue with white fur, and a fine, weak, possibly rapid, possibly bound or regularly intermittent pulse.

TREATMENT PRINCIPLES: Supplement and fortify the heart and spleen, nourish the blood and quiet the spirit

RX: *Gui Pi Tang* (Restore the Spleen Decoction) & *Tian Wang Bu Xin Dan* (Heavenly Emperor Supplement the Heart Elixir) with additions and subtractions

INGREDIENTS: Sclerotium Pararadicis Poriae Cocos (*Fu Shen*), 12g, and Radix Codonopsitis Pilosulae (*Dang Shen*), Radix Astragali Membranacei (*Huang Qi*), Radix Angelicae Sinensis (*Dang Gui*), Radix Scrophulariae Ningpoensis (*Xuan Shen*), Radix Salviae Miltiorrhizae (*Dan Shen*), Tuber Ophiopogonis Japonici (*Mai Men Dong*), Fructus Schisandrae Chinensis (*Wu Wei Zi*), Semen Biotae Orientalis (*Bai Zi Ren*), Semen Zizyphi Spinosae (*Suan Zao Ren*), Radix Polygalae Tenuifoliae (*Yuan Zhi*), and Arillus Euphoriae Longanae (*Long Yan Rou*), 9g each

ANALYSIS OF FORMULA: *Fu Shen, Suan Zao Ren, Bai Zi Ren, Wu Wei Zi,* and *Long Yan Rou* all supplement and nourish the heart. *Dang Shen* and *Huang Qi* fortify the spleen and boost the qi. *Dang Gui* and *Dan Shen* nourish and quicken the blood. *Mai Men Dong, Wu Wei Zi,* and *Xuan Shen* enrich yin and engender fluids. *Xuan Shen* also clears vacuity heat. *Fu Shen, Wu Wei Zi,* and *Yuan Zhi* quiet the spirit.

ADDITIONS & SUBTRACTIONS: During remission periods, *Gui Pi Wan* (Restore the Spleen Pills) or *Tian Wang Bu Xin*

Dan (Heavenly Emperor Supplement the Heart Elixir) may be administered in ready-made pill form to patients with mild heart vacuity symptoms.

If heart qi vacuity is marked with spontaneous perspiration, replace *Gui Pi Tang* and *Tian Wang Bu Xin Dan* with *Zhi Gan Cao Tang Jia Jian* (Mix-fried Licorice Decoction with Additions & Subtractions): uncooked Radix Rehmanniae (*Sheng Di*), 15-20g, mix-fried Radix Glycyrrhizae (*Gan Cao*), 12g, Tuber Ophiopogonis Japonici (*Mai Men Dong*), and Gelatinum Corii Asini (*E Jiao*), 9g each, Radix Panacis Ginseng (*Ren Shen*), and Ramulus Cinnamomi Cassiae (*Gui Zhi*), 6g each, uncooked Rhizoma Zingiberis (*Sheng Jiang*), 2 slices, and Fructus Zizyphi Jujubae (*Da Zao*), 3-5 pieces. If there are heart palpitations or arrhythmia, add 12 grams of Semen Zizyphi Spinosae (*Suan Zao Ren*) and nine grams of Magnetitum (*Ci Shi*). If there is constipation with dry, bound stools, add 9-12 grams of Semen Cannabis Sativae (*Huo Ma Ren*). For concomitant blood stasis with chest pain, add nine grams each of Semen Pruni Persicae (*Tao Ren*) and Radix Salviae Miltiorrhizae (*Dan Shen*).

If there is heart yang vacuity with spontaneous perspiration and chilled limbs, replace *Gui Pi Tang* and *Tian Wang Bu Xin Dan* with *Zhi Gan Cao Tang* (Mix-fried Licorice Decoction) and *Shen Fu Tang* (Ginseng & Aconite Decoction) with additions and subtractions: uncooked Radix Rehmanniae (*Sheng Di*), 15-20g, mix-fried Radix Glycyrrhizae (*Gan Cao*), 12g, Tuber Ophiopogonis Japonici (*Mai Men Dong*), and Gelatinum Corii Asini (*E Jiao*), 9g each, Radix Panacis Ginseng (*Ren Shen*), Radix Lateralis Praeparatus Aconiti Carmichaeli (*Fu Zi*), and Ramulus Cinnamomi Cassiae (*Gui Zhi*), 6g each, uncooked Rhizoma Zingiberis (*Sheng Jiang*), 2 slices, and Fructus Zizyphi Jujubae (*Da Zao*), 3-5 pieces. If there are fright palpitations, add 12 grams each of Os Draconis (*Long Gu*) and Concha Ostreae (*Mu Li*). If there is concomitant blood stasis with chest pain, add nine grams each of Radix Salviae Miltiorrhizae (*Dan Shen*) and Radix Rubrus Paeoniae Lactiflorae (*Chi Shao*).

ACUPUNCTURE & MOXIBUSTION: *Shen Men* (Ht 7), *Zu San Li* (St 36)

ANALYSIS OF FORMULA: Supplementing *Shen Men* supplements the heart and quiets the spirit. Supplementing *Zu San Li* fortifies the spleen and boosts the qi.

ADDITIONS & SUBTRACTIONS: If there is spontaneous perspiration, add *He Gu* (LI 4) and *Fu Liu* (Ki 7). If there are heart palpitations, add *Jian Shi* (Per 5). If there is chest pain, add *Nei Guan* (Per 6) and *He Gu* (LI 4).

9. LIVER-SPLEEN DISHARMONY PATTERN

MAIN SYMPTOMS: In the latter stages, if disease has damaged the liver and spleen, there may be chest and rib-side distention and pain, hypochondral accumulations (*i.e.*, hepatosplenomegaly), reduced food intake, nausea and vomiting, adbdominal pain and diarrhea, jaundice, dizziness, insomnia, menstrual irregularities or amenorrhea, a normal or darkish tongue with thin, slimy fur, and a bowstring, fine pulse.

NOTE: Although Chinese sources say that this pattern presents in the latter stages of this disease, it is our experience that most SLE sufferers present this pattern early on, even before an SLE diagnosis has been made, and often revert to this pattern during periods of remission. In that case, digestive symptoms may or may not be pronounced.

TREATMENT PRINCIPLES: Course the liver and rectify the qi, fortify the spleen and harmonize the stomach

RX: *Xiao Yao San Jia Jian* (Rambling Powder with Additions & Subtractions)

INGREDIENTS: Rhizoma Atractylodis Macrocephalae (*Bai Zhu*) and Sclerotium Poriae Cocos (*Fu Ling*), 12g each, Radix Bupleuri (*Chai Hu*), Radix Angelicae Sinensis (*Dang Gui*), Radix Albus Paeoniae Lactiflorae (*Bai Shao*), Radix Codonopsitis Pilosulae (*Dang Shen*), and Cortex Magnoliae Officinalis (*Hou Po*), 9g each, and Pericarpium Citri Reticulatae (*Chen Pi*), 6g

ANALYSIS OF FORMULA: *Bai Zhu, Fu Ling,* and *Dang Shen* fortify the spleen and supplement the qi. *Chai Hu, Hou Po,* and *Chen Pi* course the liver and rectify the qi. *Hou Po* and *Chen Pi* also downbear turbidity, thus freeing the flow of the qi mechanism. *Dang Gui* and *Bai Shao* nourish the blood, thus emolliating and harmonizing the liver.

ADDITIONS & SUBTRACTIONS: If there is chest and rib-side distention and pain, add nine grams each of Radix Rubrus Paeoniae Lactiflorae (*Chi Shao*), Radix Salviae Miltiorrhizae (*Dan Shen*), and Lignum Dalbergiae Odoriferae (*Jiang Xiang*). For poor appetite, add nine grams each of scorched Fructus Germinatus Hordei Vulgaris (*Mai Ya*), Massa Medica Fermentata (*Shen Qu*), and Fructus Crataegi (*Shan Zha*). For nausea and vomiting, add nine grams each of Rhizoma Pinelliae Ternatae (*Ban Xia*) and Caulis Bambusae In Taeniis (*Zhu Ru*). For abdominal pain and diarrhea, add nine grams each of Radix Auklandiae Lappae (*Mu Xiang*), Radix Puerariae (*Ge Gen*), and Fructus Terminaliae Chebulae (*He Zi*). For jaundice, add nine grams each of Herba Artemisiae Capillaris (*Yin Chen Hao*) and Fructus Gardeniae Jasminoidis (*Zhi Zi*) and three grams of Radix Et Rhizoma Rhei (*Da Huang*).

If there is chest and rib-side distention and pain and marked hepatosplenomegaly, replace *Xiao Yao San Jia Jian* with *Chai Hu Shu Gan San* (Bupleurum Course the Liver Powder) and *Ping Wei San* (Level the Stomach Powder) with additions and subtractions: Radix Bupleuri (*Chai Hu*), 12g, Radix Albus Paeoniae Lactiflorae (*Bai Shao*), Radix Ligustici Wallichii (*Chuan Xiong*), Rhizoma Cyperi Rotundi (*Xiang Fu*), Cortex Magnoliae Officinalis (*Hou Po*), Fructus Citri Aurantii (*Zhi Ke*), and Pericarpium Citri Reticulatae (*Chen Pi*), 9g each, and Radix Glycyrrhizae (*Gan Cao*), 3g. If there is severe abdominal pain, add 15 grams of Rhizoma Corydalis Yanhusuo (*Yan Hu Suo*) and 12 grams of Fructus Meliae Toosendan (*Chuan Lian Zi*). If depression has transformed heat with a bitter taste in the mouth, add nine grams of Radix Scutellariae Baicalensis (*Huang Qin*) and three grams of Rhizoma Coptidis Chinensis (*Huang Lian*).

Acupuncture & moxibustion: *Tai Chong* (Liv 3), *Zu San Li* (St 36), *San Yin Jiao* (Sp 6), *He Gu* (LI 4)

Analysis of formula: Draining *Tai Chong* and *He Gu* courses the liver and rectifies the qi, thus disinhibiting the qi mechanism. Supplementing *Zu San Li* and even supplementing-even draining *San Yin Jiao* supplements the spleen and boosts the qi. In addition, the combination of *San Yin Jiao* and *He Gu* quickens the blood and dispels stasis from the whole body if necessary.

Additions & subtractions: If there is marked chest oppression, add *Nei Guan* (Per 6) and *Dan Zhong* (CV 17). If blood stasis is severe, add *Ge Shu* (Bl 17) and *Xue Hai* (Sp 10). If there is abdominal distention, add *Shang Wan* (CV 13) and *Zhong Wan* (CV 12). If there is lack of appetite due to food stagnation, add *Liang Men* (St 21) and *Nei Ting* (St 44). If depression has tranformed heat, replace *Tai Chong* with *Xing Jian* (Liv 2) and consider adding *Yang Ling Quan* (GB 34). If there is marked diarrhea, add *Pi Shu* (Bl 20) and *Wei Shu* (Bl 21). If there is nausea and vomiting, add *Nei Guan* (Per 6) and *Zhong Wan* (CV 12). If there are menstrual irregularities, add *Qi Hai* (CV 6) and *Gui Lai* (St 29).

10. Liver wind internally stirring pattern

Main symptoms: During critical stages of this disease, there may be persistent high fever, vexation, agitation, and restlessness, deranged speech, crying and laughing without constancy, possible convulsions or seizures, possible spirit clouding, hemi- or paraplegia, urinary incontinence or retention, a red or dark tongue with no or scorched yellow fur, and a bowstring, rapid or bowstring and fine pulse.

Note: This stage of this disease should be treated with a combination of Chinese and Western medicines.

Treatment principles: Clear the liver and extinguish wind, quiet the spirit and settle tetany

Rx: *Ling Yang Gou Teng Tang Jia Jian* (Saiga Antelope & Uncaria Decoction with Additions & Subtractions)

Ingredients: Uncooked Radix Rehmanniae (*Sheng Di*) and uncooked Concha Haliotidis (*Shi Jue Ming*), 30g each, Bulbus Fritillariae Cirrhosae (*Chuan Bei Mu*), Caulis Bambusae In Taeniis (*Zhu Ru*), and Sclerotium Pararadicis Poriae Cocos (*Fu Shen*), 15g each, Flos Chrysanthemi Morifolii (*Ju Hua*), Radix Albus Paeoniae Lactiflorae (*Bai Shao*), and Ramulus Uncariae Cum Uncis (*Gou Teng*), 12g each, Folium Mori Albi (*Sang Ye*), 6g, and Cornu Caprae (*Shan Yang Jiao*), 3g

Analysis of formula: *Shan Yang Jiao* and *Gou Teng* settle the liver and extinguish wind. *Shi Jue Ming* heavily settles and subdues counterflow. *Sang Ye*, *Ju Hua*, and *Gou Teng* clear the liver. *Zhu Ru* also clears the liver, eliminates vexation, and downbears counterflow. *Fu Shen* quiets the spirit, while *Chuan Bei Mu* enriches yin at the same time as it transforms phlegm.

Additions & subtractions: If there is persistent high fever with convulsions, add 15 grams each of uncooked Gypsum Fibrosum (*Shi Gao*) and Radix Scrophulariae Ningpoensis (*Xuan Shen*) and nine grams each of Rhizoma Anemarrhenae Aspheloidis (*Zhi Mu*) and Tuber Ophiopogonis Japonici (*Mai Men Dong*). For heat harassing the spirit with deranged speech, add nine grams each of Fructus Forsythiae Suspensae (*Lian Qiao*) and Radix Polygalae Tenuifoliae (*Yuan Zhi*) and six grams each of Plumula Nelumbinis Nuciferae (*Lian Zi Xin*) and Rhizoma Copitidis Chinensis (*Huang Lian*). For tremors and convulsions, add 12 grams each of Concha Margaritiferae (*Zhen Zhu Mu*), Haemititum (*Dai Zhe Shi*), Os Draconis (*Long Gu*), and/or Concha Ostreae (*Mu Li*).

Acupuncture & moxibustion: *Tai Chong* (Liv 3), *Feng Chi* (GB 20), *Yang Ling Quan* (GB 34), *Qu Chi* (LI 11)

Analysis of formula: Draining *Yang Ling Quan* and *Tai Chong* clears and drains liver heat. Draining *Feng Chi* extinguishes wind and opens the orifices. Draining *Qu Chi* clears heat and abates fever.

Additions & subtractions: If there is dizziness, vertigo, agitation, and restlessness, add *Bai Hui* (GV 20) and *Yin Tang* (M-HN-3). For persistent high fever, also bleed *Da Zhui* (GV 14) and/or *Shi Xuan* (M-UE-1). For concomitant phlegm fire, add *Lao Gong* (Per 8) and *Feng Long* (St 40). For loss of consciousness, add *Ren Zhong* (GV 26).

Remarks

1. Most cases of lupus display the following combination of patterns: qi and yin vacuity; some sort of evil heat (whether

toxic, depressive, damp, or vacuity); and liver depression qi stagnation. If the condition has endured, there is often blood stasis as well. If the patient is a female 45-55 years old, spleen qi vacuity may also have evolved into kidney yang vacuity. Unlike rheumatoid arthritis, there is no cold damp impediment pattern of lupus.

2. Additional medicinals for specific symptoms may be chosen depending on the presenting pattern:

A. For low back and knee soreness & weakness, dizziness, tinnitus & kidney vacuity, one can choose from: Fructus Lycii Chinensis (*Gou Qi Zi*), Cortex Eucommiae Ulmoidis (*Du Zhong*), Herba Cistanchis Deserticolae (*Rou Cong Rong*), Semen Cuscutae Chinensis (*Tu Si Zi*), Rhizoma Cibotii Barometsis (*Gou Ji*), Rhizoma Polygoni Cuspidati (*Hu Zhang*), Radix Dipsaci (*Chuan Duan*), Ramulus Loranthi Seu Visci (*Sang Ji Sheng*), Ramulus Cinnamomi Cassiae (*Gui Zhi*), Cortex Cinnamomi Cassiae (*Rou Gui*), Rhizoma Curculiginis Orchioidis (*Xian Mao*), Herba Epimedii (*Xian Ling Pi*), Herba Cynomorii Songarici (*Suo Yang*), and Fructus Alpiniae Oxyphyllae (*Yi Zhi Ren*).

B. For superficial edema, one can choose from: Semen Plantaginis (*Che Qian Zi*), Herba Plantaginis (*Che Qian Cao*), Rhizoma Alismatis (*Ze Xie*), Seme Phaseoli Calcarati (*Chi Xiao Dou*), Pericarpium Arecae Catechu (*Da Fu Pi*), Semen Coicis Lachryma-jobi (*Yi Yi Ren*), Sclerotium Poriae Cocos (*Fu Ling*), Sclerotium Polypori Umbellati (*Zhu Ling*), Rhizoma Imperatae Cylindricae (*Bai Mao Gen*), Stylus Zeae Maydis (*Yu Mi Xu*), and Folium Pyrrosiae (*Shi Wei*).

C. For joint aching and pain, one can choose from: Radix Gentianae Macrophyllae (*Qin Jiao*), Ramulus Cinnamomi Cassiae (*Gui Zhi*), Ramulus Mori Albi (*Sang Zhi*), Ramulus Loranthi Seu Visci (*Sang Ji Sheng*), Radix Clematidis Chinensis (*Wei Ling Xian*), Radix Stephaniae Tetrandrae (*Fang Ji*), Radix Ledebouriellae Divaricatae (*Fang Feng*), Rhizoma Polygoni Cuspidati (*Hu Zhang*), Caulis Milletiae Seu Spatholobi (*Ji Xue Teng*), Caulis Lonicerae Japonicae (*Ren Dong Teng*), Radix Dipsaci (*Chuan Duan*), Rhizoma Corydalis Yanhusuo (*Yan Hu Suo*), Rhizoma Sinomenii Acuti (*Qing Feng Teng*), and Herba Pycnostelmae (*Xu Chang Jing*).

D. For rib-side distention and pain and emotional depression, one can choose from: Tuber Curcumae (*Yu Jin*), Rhizoma Cyperi Rotundi (*Xiang Fu*), Pericarpium Citri Reticulatae Viride (*Qing Pi*), Rhizoma Corydalis Yanhusuo (*Yan Hu Suo*), Fructus Citri Aurantii (*Zhi Ke*), Fructus Citri Sacrodactylis (*Fo Shou*), and Radix Bupleuri (*Chai Hu*).

E. For heart palpitations, one can choose from: Fructus Schisandrae Chinensis (*Wu Wei Zi*), Rhizoma Acori Graminei (*Shi Chang Pu*), Radix Polygalae Tenuifoliae (*Yuan Zhi*), Sclerotium Poriae Cocos (*Fu Ling*), Sclerotium Pararadicis Poriae Cocos (*Fu Shen*), Cortex Eucommiae Ulmoidis (*Du Zhong*), Radix Scrophulariae Ningpoensis (*Xuan Shen*), and Semen Biotae Orientalis (*Bai Zi Ren*).

F. For insomnia, one can choose from: Caulis Polygoni Multiflori (*Ye Jiao Teng*), Flos Albizziae Julibrissinis (*He Huan Hua*), Fructus Alpiniae Oxyphyllae (*Yi Zhi Ren*), Rhizoma Sinomenii Acuti (*Qing Feng Teng*), Rhizoma Acori Graminei (*Shi Chang Pu*), and Semen Zizyphi Spinosae (*Suan Zao Ren*).

G. For dry cough or yin vacuity cough, one can choose from: Tuber Asparagi Cochinensis (*Tian Dong*), Tuber Ophiopogonis Japonici (*Mai Dong*), Bulbus Lilii (*Bai He*), Radix Glehniae Littoralis (*Sha Shen*), Radix Rubiae Cordifoliae (*Qian Cao Gen*), Radix Platycodi Grandiflori (*Jie Geng*), Bulbus Fritillariae Cirrhosae (*Chuan Bei Mu*), and Folium Eriobotryae Japonicae (*Pi Pa Ye*).

H. For precordial pain and coronary artery insufficiency with heart viscus impairment, one can choose from: Radix Pseudoginseng (*San Qi*), Radix Ligustici Wallichii (*Chuan Xiong*), Radix Angelicae Sinensis (*Dang Gui*), Fructus Crataegi (*Shan Zha*), Radix Ilicis Pubescentis (*Mao Dong Qing*), Rhizoma Corydalis Yanhusuo (*Yan Hu Suo*), Fructus Trichosanthis Kirlowii (*Quan Gua Lou*), Herba Leonuri Heterophylli (*Yi Mu Cao*), Radix Salviae Miltiorrhizae (*Dan Shen*), Ramulus Cinnamomi Cassiae (*Gui Zhi*), and Radix Albus Paeoniae Lactiflorae (*Bai Shao*).

I. For liver area pain, liver-spleen enlargement, or liver viscus impairment, one can choose from:Tuber Curcumae (*Yu Jin*), Radix Bupleuri (*Chai Hu*), Rhizoma Atractylodis Macrocephalae (*Bai Zhu*), Herba Artemisiae Capillaris (*Yin Chen Hao*), Herba Taraxaci Mongolici Cum Radice (*Pu Gong Ying*), Plastrum Testudinis (*Gui Ban*), Carapax Amydae Chinensis (*Bie Jia*), Radix Salviae Miltiorrhizae (*Dan Shen*), Radix Ligustici Wallichii (*Chuan Xiong*), Radix Angelicae Sinensis (*Dang Gui*), Rhizoma Sparganii (*San Leng*), and Rhizoma Curcumae Zedoariae (*E Zhu*).

J. For kidney viscus impairment with albuminuria, one can choose from: Radix Codonopsitis Pilosulae (*Dang Shen*), Radix Astragali Membranacei (*Huang Qi*), Fructus Rosae Laevigatae (*Jin Ying Zi*), Fructus Schisandrae Chinensis (*Wu Wei Zi*), Fructus Crataegi (*Shan Zha*), Semen Euryalis Ferocis (*Qian Shi*), Fructus Germinatus Hordei Vulgaris (*Mai Ya*), Rhizoma Imperatae Cylindricae (*Bai Mao Gen*), Flos Lonicerae Japonicae (*Jin Yin Hua*), etc. For granular casts, choose from: Fructus Crataegi (*Shan Zha*), Radix Dioscoreae Oppositae (*Huai Shan Yao*), Herba Cynomorii Songarici (*Suo Yang*), and Radix Morindae Officinalis (*Ba Ji Tian*). For pus cells, choose from: Semen Abutilonis Seu Malvae (*Dong Kui Zi*), Semen Plantaginis (*Che Qian Zi*), Flos Lonicerae Japonicae (*Yin Hua*), and Herba Houttuyniae

Cordatae Cum Radice (*Yu Xing Cao*). For viral disease, choose from: *Shen Fu Tang* (Ginseng & Aconite Decoction), Rhizoma Anemarrhenae Aspheloidis (*Zhi Mu*), Cortex Phellodendri (*Huang Bai*), Cortex Cinnamomi Cassiae (*Rou Gui*), and Radix Et Rhizoma Rhei (*Da Huang*).

K. For bleeding or abnormal blood coagulation, one can choose from: Cacumen Biotae Orientalis (*Ce Bai Ye*), Radix Rubiae Cordifoliae (*Qian Cao Gen*), Pollen Typhae (*Pu Huang*), Cornu Bubali (*Shui Niu Jiao*), Herba Agrimoniae Pilosae (*Xian He Cao*), Rhizoma Imperatae Cylindricae (*Bai Mao Gen*), Gelatinum Corii Asini (*E Jiao*), carbonized Radix Sanguisorbae (*Di Yu*), and Nodus Rhizomatis Nelumbinis Nuciferae (*Ou Jie*).

L. For decreased white blood cells, one can choose from: Fructus Ligustri Lucidi (*Nu Zhen Zi*), Rhizoma Atractylodis Macrocephalae (*Bai Zhu*), Cortex Cinnamomi Cassiae (*Rou Gui*), Radix Sophorae Flavescentis (*Ku Shen*), and Herba Solani Nigri (*Long Kui*).

M. For decreased eating and drinking and torpid intake, one can choose from: Endothelium Corneum Gigeriae Galli (*Ji Nei Jin*), Radix Linderae Strychnifoliae (*Wu Yao*), uncooked Rhizoma Zingiberis (*Sheng Jiang*), Pericarpium Citri Reticulatae (*Chen Pi*), and Radix Gentianae Scabrae (*Long Dan Cao*).

N. For high blood pressure, one can choose from: Fructus Crataegi (*Shan Zha*), Fructus Schisandrae Chinensis (*Wu Wei Zi*), Radix Ilicis Pubescentis (*Mao Dong Qing*), Radix Salviae Miltiorrhizae (*Dan Shen*), Rhizoma Atractylodis Macrocephalae (*Bai Zhu*), Radix Scrophulariae Ningpoensis (*Xuan Shen*), Cortex Radicis Lycii Chinensis (*Di Gu Pi*), Cortex Eucommiae Ulmoidis (*Du Zhong*), Cortex Radicis Moutan (*Dan Pi*), Radix Puerariae (*Ge Gen*), and Rhizoma Sinomenii Acuti (*Qing Feng Teng*).

O. For central nervous system impairment with emotional and nervous disorders, one can choose from: Rhizoma Gastrodiae Elatae (*Tian Ma*), Ramulus Uncariae Cum Uncis (*Gou Teng*), Radix Stephaniae Tetrandrae (*Fang Ji*), Rhizoma Arisaematis (*Tian Nan Xing*), Rhizoma Acori Graminei (*Shi Chang Pu*), Radix Polygalae Tenuifoliae (*Yuan Zhi*), Bombyx Batryticatus (*Bai Jiang Can*), Sclerotium Poriae Cocos (*Fu Ling*), Succinum (*Hu Po*), Margarita (*Zhen Zhu*), and Cornu Antelopis Saiga-tatarici (*Ling Yang Jiao*).

P. For qi vacuity emission of heat (*i.e.*, fever), one can choose from: Radix Astragali Membranacei (*Huang Qi*), Rhizoma Atractylodis Macrocephalae (*Bai Zhu*), Radix Codonopsitis Pilosulae (*Dang Shen*), Fructus Zizyphi Jujubae (*Da Zao*), and Arillus Euphoriae Longanae (*Long Yan Rou*).

Q. For blood vacuity fever, one can choose from: Radix Angelicae Sinensis (*Dang Gui*), cooked Radix Rehmanniae (*Shu Di*), Gelatinum Corii Asini (*E Jiao*), Rhizoma Polygonati (*Huang Jing*), and Rhizoma Polygoni Odorati (*Yu Zhu*).

R. For yin vacuity fever, one can choose from: Herba Artemisiae Apiaceae (*Qing Hao*), Cortex Radicis Lycii Chinensis (*Di Gu Pi*), Radix Stellariae Dichotomae (*Yin Chai Hu*), Rhizoma Picrorrhizae (*Hu Huang Lian*), Gelatinum Corii Asini (*E Jiao*), Caulis Milletiae Seu Spatholobi (*Ji Xue Teng*), and Radix Scrophulariae Ningpoensis (*Xuan Shen*).

S. For allergic fever, one can choose from: Radix Scutellariae Baicalensis (*Huang Qin*), Radix Stephaniae Tetrandrae (*Fang Ji*), Pericarpium Citri Reticulatae (*Chen Pi*), Herba Ephedrae (*Ma Huang*), and Radix Glycyrrhizae (*Gan Cao*).

T. For bacterial fever, one can choose from: Fructus Forsythiae Suspensae (*Lian Qiao*), Herba Houttuyniae Cordatae Cum Radice (*Yu Xing Cao*), Rhizoma Coptidis Chinensis (*Huang Lian*), Flos Chrysanthemi Morifolii (*Ju Hua*), Flos Lonicerae Japonicae (*Jin Yin Hua*), Herba Taraxaci Mongolici Cum Radice (*Pu Gong Ying*), Radix Bupleuri (*Chai Hu*), Folium Daqingye (*Da Qing Ye*), Radix Pulsatillae Chinensis (*Bai Tou Weng*), and Cortex Radicis Lycii Chinensis (*Di Gu Pi*).

U. For viral fever, one can choose from: Folium Daqingye (*Da Qing Ye*), Radix Isatidis Seu Baphicacanthi (*Ban Lan Gen*), Radix Pulsatillae Chinensis (*Bai Tou Weng*), Herba Oldenlandiae Diffusae (*Bai Hua She She Cao*), Herba Scutellariae Barbatae (*Ban Zhi Lian*), Herba Lobeliae Chinensis (*Ban Bian Lian*), Radix Dianthi (*Qu Mai Gen*), Flos Lonicerae Japonicae (*Jin Yin Hua*), Herba Taraxaci Mongolici Cum Radice (*Pu Gong Ying*), Herba Violae Yedoensitis Cum Radice (*Zi Hua Di Ding*), Radix Albus Paeoniae Lactiflorae (*Bai Shao*), Cortex Radicis Lycii Chinensis (*Di Gu Pi*), Radix Bupleuri (*Chai Hu*), Folium Eriobotryae Japonicae (*Pi Pa Ye*), Fructus Rosae Laevigatae (*Jin Ying Zi*), Herba Artemisiae Capillaris (*Yin Chen Hao*), and Herba Artemisiae Apiaceae (*Qing Hao*).

3. According to the authors of *Alternative Medicine, The Definitive Guide* (Future Medicine Publishing, Inc., Puyallup, WA, 1993), 100% of SLE patients have food allergies and improve with appropriate identification and treatment. This suggests a combination of spleen vacuity and possible damp heat. Eighty percent of sufferers have extremely decreased secretion of hydrochloric acid in the stomach. This also suggests spleen vacuity. Over 50% of female SLE patients have lower than normal levels of testosterone and DHEA, suggesting spleen and/or kidney yang vacuity.

4. Five hundred milligrams of vitamin B_6 three times per day can be useful as an adjunctive therapy for reducing the severity of symptoms.

69

TEMPOROMANDIBULAR JOINT SYNDROME

Temporomandibular joint syndrome (TMJ) refers to pain in the temporomandibular joint region with possible swelling, limited range of motion, muscle spasms, earaches, bruxism, facial asymmetry, clicking or popping noises, and, occasionally, tinnitus. Common causes of TMJ pain include blows to the jaw, overstretching as a result of dental or surgical procedures, and excessive grinding or clenching of the teeth. Most forms of arthritis can involve the TMJ, and the TMJ is involved in more than 50% of cases of rheumatoid arthritis. Up to 25 million Americans experience some form of TMJ, with women seemingly at greater risk.

The current Western medical treatment of TMJ consists of a combination of dental and medical approaches. These include the use of anti-inflammatory drugs, a soft diet, hot compresses, and intra-oral splints. Permanent dental corrections and removable protheses may also be recommended. Surgical correction is necessary in 5-10% of patients. When TMJ is primarily related to muscular tension, biofeedback and other stress management techniques may be recommended.

CHINESE DISEASE CATEGORIZATION: Bruxism is called *nie chi*, gnashing of teeth, or *nie he*, clenching of teeth, while jaw pain is categorized as *mian tong*. Earaches are called *er tong*, tinnitus is *er ming*, and facial swelling is *mian fu*.

DISEASE CAUSES: External injury, external contraction of wind evils, internal damage by the seven affects, habitual bodily vacuity, and worms

DISEASE MECHANISMS: If external wind cold or wind heat evils invade the exterior and lodge in the channels and vessels of the face, the flow of qi and blood there will be inhibited. Because there is lack of free flow, there will be pain. Pain in the face is especially likely if wind evils combine with phlegm internally engendered due to spleen vacuity. In addition, spleen vacuity is the root of defensive qi insecurity which allows external evils to invade. If, due to faulty diet, over-thinking, worry and anxiety, too little exercise, loss or consumption of the blood due to menstruation, gestation, or lactation, or due to aging, the spleen becomes vacuous and weak, the spleen and lung qi may not move and transport fluids. Hence swelling in the face may occur. If the spleen fails to engender sufficient blood to nourish the sinews, the sinews may contract. In addition, blood may fail to mother the qi, with blood vacuity internally engendering liver wind. Either of these causes may result in spasms and contraction. Further, emotional stress and upset may cause depressive heat or fire. Because of the inter-relationships between the liver, stomach, and heart, depressive heat may manifest in the heart and/or stomach, especially if the stomach is hot due to over-eating hot, spicy, fatty foods or alcohol. Both the heart and stomach channels connect with the mouth. If this heat follows the channels upward to the face, it may cause burning pain. Liver blood-kidney yin vacuity either due to aging, enduring disease, drug use, or excessive taxation and stirring, may fail to nourish the sea of marrow, thus giving rise to tinnitus and dizziness. In addition, liver blood vacuity failing to adequately nourish the sinews may lead to difficulty opening and closing the mouth. Blood stasis may be engendered locally due to any of several factors. These include qi vacuity not stirring or propelling the blood, enduring qi stagnation due to liver depression, or enduring lodgment of evil qi in the channels and vessels of the face. Because spleen qi and liver depression typically go hand in hand, most cases of TMJ have at their root a liver-spleen disharmony. This is also easily complicated by food stagnation. Although it is possible for external injury to cause blood stasis locally in the region of the face, this is not such a common cause of TMJ in the Western patients who come for treatment by acupuncturists and practitioners of Chinese medicine.

TREATMENT BASED ON PATTERN DISCRIMINATION:

1. WIND, COLD & PHLEGM OBSTRUCTING THE NETWORK VESSELS PATTERN

MAIN SYMPTOMS: Paroxysmal, spasmodic, unbearable face pain worsened by cold and ameliorated by warmth, facial pallor at the time of pain, possible facial swelling, heavy-headedness or head distention, a pale, fat tongue with either thin, white or thick, white, slimy fur, and a floating and tight or soggy, slippery pulse depending on the relative proportions of wind, cold, and phlegm

TREATMENT PRINCIPLES: Dispel wind and scatter cold, wash away phlegm and free the flow of the network vessels

RX: *Mian Tong Fang Er Hao* (Face Pain Formula No. 2)

INGREDIENTS: Radix Ligustici Wallichii (*Chuan Xiong*), 15g, Radix Ledebouriellae Divaricatae (*Fang Feng*), Radix Et Rhizoma Notopterygii (*Qiang Huo*), Radix Angelicae Dahuricae (*Bai Zhi*), Radix Angelicae Sinensis (*Dang Gui*), and Radix Salviae Miltiorrhizae (*Dan Shen*), 9g each, Rhizoma Typhonii Gigantei (*Bai Fu Zi*), Rhizoma Pinelliae Terantae (*Ban Xia*), and Lumbricus (*Di Long*), 6g each, and Herba Asari Cum Radice (*Xi Xin*) and Radix Glycyrrhizae (*Gan Cao*), 3g each

ANALYSIS OF FORMULA: *Chuan Xiong, Bai Zhi, Qiang Huo, Fang Feng,* and *Xi Xin* dispel wind and scatter cold. *Chuan Xiong* and *Bai Zhi* is a famous combination for treating pain in the face, especially along the gallbladder and stomach channels. *Qiang Huo* and *Fang Feng* dispel wind dampness which causes impediment pain. *Qiang Huo,* with its floating upbearing nature, leads the other medicinals in this formula to the upper part of the body. *Xi Xin* strongly scatters cold and stops pain effectively. *Bai Fu Zi* and *Ban Xia* transform phlegm. *Ban Xia* is the master Chinese medicinal for phlegm, while *Bai Fu Zi* washes away phlegm, especially in the face and channels. *Di Long* frees the flow of the network vessels and helps to wash away phlegm and wind cold obstructing the channels. *Dan Shen* and *Dang Gui* quicken the blood and transform stasis due to evils obstructing the free flow of the network vessels.

ADDITIONS & SUBTRACTIONS: For uneasy opening and closing of the mouth, add 12 grams of Herba Lycopodii (*Shen Jin Cao*). For severe swelling, add nine grams each of Rhizoma Atractylodis (*Cang Zhu*) and Radix Stephaniae Tetrandrae (*Han Fang Ji*). For concomitant qi vacuity, add 12 grams of Radix Astragali Membranacei (*Huang Qi*) and nine grams of Rhizoma Atractylodis Macrocephalae (*Bai Zhu*). For concomitant blood vacuity, add 12 grams of cooked Radix Rehmanniae (*Shu Di*) and nine grams of Radix Albus Paeoniae Lactiflorae (*Bai Shao*).

For a simple wind cold damp impediment without phlegm but with pain, numbness, heaviness of the joint of the jaw and concomitant impediment pain in other places in the body, uneasy opening and closing of the mouth, absence of hotness or redness in the jaw area, pain worsened by cold and ameliorated by warmth, etc., replace *Mian Tong Fang Er Hao* with *Juan Bi Tang Jia Wei* (Alleviate Impediment Decoction with Added Flavors): Radix Et Rhizoma Notopterygii (*Qiang Huo*), Radix Angelicae Pubescentis (*Du Huo*), Radix Angelicae Dahuricae (*Bai Zhi*), Radix Gentianae Macrophyllae (*Qin Jiao*), Radix Angelicae Sinensis (*Dang Gui*), Radix Ligustici Wallichii (*Chuan Xiong*), Ramulus Mori Albi (*Sang Zhi*), and Radix Et Rhizoma Ligustici Chinensis (*Gao Ben*), 9g each, and Resina Olibani (*Ru Xiang*), Ramulus Cinnamomi Cassiae (*Gui Zhi*), and mix-fried Radix Glycyrrhizae (*Gan Cao*), 5g each.

ACUPUNCTURE & MOXIBUSTION: *He Gu* (LI 4), *Xia Guan* (St 7), *Wai Guan* (TB 5), *Feng Long* (St 40)

ANALYSIS OF FORMULA: *Xia Guan* is the key local point of the temporomandibular joint region. Draining it frees the flow of the network vessels locally and stops pain. *He Gu* is the master point of the face and mouth. It can treat all types of disease and pain of the face, including joint trouble. Draining it enhances the local action of *Xia Guan.* These two points can be used for all patterns of TMJ. Draining *Wai Guan* dispels wind, while draining *Feng Long* transforms phlegm. These two points treat the disease causes and mechanisms of this specific pattern of TMJ.

ADDITIONS & SUBTRACTIONS: For pain in the upper border of the zygomatic arch, add *Shang Guan* (GB 3). For pain in the lower part of the jaw, add *Jia Che* (St 6). For pain in the cheekbone, add *Quan Liao* (SI 18). For pain behind the ear, earache, or tinnitus, add *Yi Feng* (TB 17). For pain in front of the ear, earache, or tinnitus, add *Ting Hui* (GB 2). For pain in the temples, add *Tai Yang* (M-HN-9). For pain in the forehead, add *Yang Bai* (GB 14) and/or *Tou Wei* (St 8). For muscles spasms, add *Tai Chong* (Liv 3). For swelling, add *Yin Ling Quan* (Sp 9). For severe pain, add *Zhong Zhu* (TB 3) or *San Jian* (LI 3) which also free the flow of the network vessels locally and stop pain. For neck and shoulder tension, add *Jian Jing* (GB 21) and/or *Tian Zhu* (Bl 10). For insomnia or restlessness, add *Shen Men* (Ht 7), *Tong Li* (Ht 5), and/or *Shen Ting* (GV 24) to quiet the spirit.

2. WIND, HEAT & PHLEGM OBSTRUCTING THE NETWORK VESSELS PATTERN

MAIN SYMPTOMS: Severe paroxysmal, lancinating pain which is aggravated by heat and ameliorated by cold accompanied by a red facial complexion, fever, sweating, a dry mouth, dark-colored urine, a red tongue with dry, yellow or slimy, yellow fur, and a bowstring, slippery, rapid pulse

TREATMENT PRINCIPLES: Dispel wind and clear heat, flush phlegm and free the flow of the network vessels

RX: *Mian Tong Fang Yi Hao* (Face Pain Formula No. 1)

INGREDIENTS: Radix Ligustici Wallichii (*Chuan Xiong*), 15g, Flos Chrysanthemi Morifolii (*Ju Hua*), 12g, Herba Seu Flos Schizonepetae Tenuifoliae (*Jing Jie*), Radix Angelicae Sinensis (*Dang Gui*), Radix Salviae Miltiorrhizae (*Dan Shen*), Radix Rubrus Paeoniae Lactiflorae (*Chi Shao*), Periostracum Cicadae (*Chan Tui*), Cortex Radicis Moutan (*Dan Pi*), and Lumbricus (*Di Long*), 9g each, Rhizoma Pinelliae Ternatae (*Ban Xia*) and Pericarpium Citri Reticulatae (*Chen Pi*), 6g each, and Radix Glycyrrhizae (*Gan Cao*), 3g

ANALYSIS OF FORMULA: *Chuan Xiong, Ju Hua, Jing Jie*, and *Chan Tui* dispel wind and clear heat. *Chuan Xiong* dispels wind and stops pain, especially in the face and bones. *Ju Hua* dispels wind and clears heat, especially in the head. *Jing Jie* reinforces the dispelling function of the cool, exterior-resolving medicinals which are usually somewhat weak for effectively dispelling and clearing wind heat. Also, *Jing Jie* with *Chan Tui* relieves spasms and stops pain. Together *Chen Pi* and *Ban Xia* transform phlegm. *Di Long* frees the flow of the network vessels and helps to wash away phlegm and evils obstructing the channels. *Chi Shao, Dan Pi, Dan Shen,* and *Dang Gui* quicken the blood, transform stasis due to evils obstructing the free flow of the network vessels, and stop pain.

ADDITIONS & SUBTRACTIONS: For uneasy opening and closing of the mouth, add 12 grams of Herba Lycopodii (*Shen Jin Cao*). For severe swelling, add nine grams each of Rhizoma Atractylodis (*Cang Zhu*), Cortex Erythiniae (*Hai Tong Pi*), and Rhizoma Dioscoreae (*Bei Xie*). For concomitant qi vacuity, add 12 grams of Radix Astragali Membranacei (*Huang Qi*) and nine grams of Rhizoma Atractylodis Macrocephalae (*Bai Zhu*). For concomitant blood vacuity, add 12 grams of cooked Radix Rehmanniae (*Shu Di*) and nine grams of Radix Albus Paeoniae Lactiflorae (*Bai Shao*).

For simple wind damp heat impediment without phlegm, but with swelling, severe pain, hotness, and redness in the jaw area, uneasy opening and closing of the mouth, possible general effusion of heat, heart restlessness, aversion to heat, a liking for coolness, dry, yellow tongue fur, and a rapid, floating pulse, replace *Mian Tong Fang Yi Hao* with *Xuan Bi Tang Jia Jian* (Diffuse Impediment Decoction with Additions & Subtractions): Caulis Lonicerae Japonicae (*Ren Dong Teng*), 30g, Radix Stephaniae Tetrandrae (*Han Fang Ji*), Semen Pruni Armeniacae (*Xing Ren*), Talcum (*Hua Shi*), Ramulus Mori Albi (*Sang Zhi*), and Cortex Erythiniae (*Hai Tong Pi*), 15g each, and Fructus Gardeniae Jasminoidis (*Zhi Zi*), Excrementum Bombicis Batryticati (*Can Sha),* Fructus Forsythiae Suspensae (*Lian Qiao*), and Semen Phaseoli Calcarati (*Chi Xiao Dou*), 9g each.

ACUPUNCTURE & MOXIBUSTION: *Feng Long* (St 40), *Qu Chi* (LI 11), *He Gu* (LI 4), *Xia Guan* (St 7)

ANALYSIS OF FORMULA: Draining *Feng Long* transforms phlegm, while draining *Qu Chi* and *He Gu* dispels wind, clears heat, and treats impediment pain in the region of the face. Draining *Xia Guan* frees the flow of the network vessels locally and stops pain.

ADDITIONS & SUBTRACTIONS: Please see pattern #1 above.

3. LIVER FIRE HARASSING ABOVE PATTERN

MAIN SYMPTOMS: Burning facial pain commonly triggered by emotional upset and exacerbated by heat, a bitter taste in the mouth, dry throat, irritability, heart vexation, chest oppression, rib-side distention, vexatious heat in the five hearts, frequent sighing, profuse dreams, dark-colored urine, dry stools, a red tongue with yellow fur, and a bowstring, rapid pulse

TREATMENT PRINCIPLES: Clear the liver and discharge fire, free the flow of the network vessels and stop pain

RX: *Mian Tong Fang San Hao* (Face Pain Formula No. 3)

INGREDIENTS: Cortex Radicis Moutan (*Dan Pi*), Radix Angelicae Sinensis (*Dang Gui*), Radix Rubrus Paeoniae Lactiflorae (*Chi Shao*), Radix Ligustici Wallichii (*Chuan Xiong*), Tuber Curcumae (*Yu Jin*), and Radix Salviae Miltiorrhizae (*Dan Shen*), 9g each, Radix Bupleuri (*Chai Hu*), Fructus Gardeniae Jasminoidis (*Zhi Zi*), Pulvis Indigonis (*Qing Dai*), Lumbricus (*Di Long*), and Pericarpium Citri Reticulatae (*Chen Pi*), 6g each, and Radix Glycyrrhizae (*Gan Cao*), 4.5g

ANALYSIS OF FORMULA: *Dang Gui* nourishes liver blood and harmonizes liver yin. *Chai Hu* courses the liver, resolves depression, and harmonizes liver yang. Together, they harmonize and rectify the liver to prevent further depression which is the fundamental cause of liver fire. In addition, *Yu Jin* and *Chen Pi* help *Chai Hu* to course the liver and rectify the qi. *Dan Pi, Chi Shao, Zhi Zi, Di Long,* and *Qing Dai* strongly clear the liver and discharge fire. *Di Long* frees the flow of the network vessels and stops pain. Together, *Dan Pi, Dang Gui, Chi Shao, Chuan Xiong,* and *Dan Shen* cool and quicken the blood and transform stasis due to either heat burning the blood in the network vessels or liver depression transforming heat. With *Yu Jin* and *Chen Pi,* they also stop pain.

ADDITIONS & SUBTRACTIONS: If there is constipation,

add six grams of Radix Et Rhizoma Rhei (*Da Huang*) and 3 grams of Mirabilitum (*Mang Xiao*). For concomitant spleen qi vacuity, add nine grams each of Radix Codonopsitis Pilosulae (*Dang Shen*) and Rhizoma Atractylodis Macrocephalae (*Bai Zhu*). For severe blood vacuity, add nine grams each of Radix Albus Paeoniae Lactiflorae (*Bai Shao*) and uncooked Radix Rehmanniae (*Sheng Di*). For liver yin vacuity, add nine grams each of uncooked Radix Rehmanniae (*Sheng Di*), Ramulus Loranthi Seu Visci (*Sang Ji Sheng*), and Radix Achyranthis Bidentatae (*Niu Xi*). For concomitant damp heat, add nine grams each of Rhizoma Atractylodis (*Cang Zhu*) and Cortex Phellodendri (*Huang Bai*).

ACUPUNCTURE & MOXIBUSTION: *Xing Jian* (Liv 2), *Zhi Gou* (TB 6), *He Gu* (LI 4), *Xia Guan* (St 7)

ANALYSIS OF FORMULA: Draining *Xing Jian*, the fire point of the liver channel, clears the liver and discharges the fire, while draining *Zhi Gou* courses the liver and resolves depression, clears heat and stops pain. Draining *He Gu* and *Xia Guan* frees the flow of the network vessels in the region of the temporomandibular joint and stops pain.

ADDITIONS & SUBTRACTIONS: Please see pattern #1 above.

4. EXUBERANT FIRE OF THE HEART & STOMACH PATTERN

MAIN SYMPTOMS: Grinding of teeth, heart vexation, bad breath, thirst with a liking for chilled drinks, swift digestion with rapid hungering, vomiting, clamoring stomach, possible immediate vomiting of ingested food, a red tongue with dry, yellow fur, and a slippery, bowstring, rapid pulse

TREATMENT PRINCIPLES: Clear the stomach and drain fire

RX: *Qing Wei San Jia Jian* (Clear the Stomach Powder with Additions & Subtractions)

INGREDIENTS: Uncooked Gypsum Fibrosum (*Shi Gao*), 18g, uncooked Radix Rehmanniae (*Sheng Di*), 15g, Radix Angelicae Sinensis (*Dang Gui*), Cortex Radicis Moutan (*Dan Pi*), and Fructus Gardeniae Jasminoidis (*Zhi Zi*), 9g each, Rhizoma Coptidis Chinensis (*Huang Lian*), 6g, and Rhizoma Cimicifugae (*Sheng Ma*), Radix Glycyrrhizae (*Gan Cao*), and Plumula Nelumbinis Nuciferae (*Lian Xin*), 3g each

ANALYSIS OF FORMULA: *Shi Gao*, *Huang Lian*, and *Sheng Ma* clear heat from the stomach, while *Huang Lian*, *Zhi Zi*, and *Lian Xin* clear heat from the heart. *Sheng Di* also clears heart fire and nourishes stomach yin which has been damaged by heat. *Dan Pi* cools the blood and prevents blood stasis due to heat when combined with *Dang Gui*.

ADDITIONS & SUBTRACTIONS: With concomitant spleen qi vacuity, add nine grams each of Radix Codonopsitis Pilosulae (*Dang Shen*) and Radix Dioscoreae Oppositae (*Shan Yao*). For a severe thirst, add 12 grams of Radix Trichosanthis Kirlowii (*Tian Hua Fen*). For hot flashes in the face, add nine grams each of Cortex Phellodendri (*Huang Bai*), Rhizoma Anemarrhenae Asphodeloidis (*Zhi Mu*), and Radix Cyathulae (*Chuan Niu Xi*). For dark, hot urine, add five grams of Caulis Akebiae (*Mu Tong*) and nine grams of Herba Lophatheri Gracilis (*Dan Zhu Ye*).

ACUPUNCTURE & MOXIBUSTION: *Tong Li* (Ht 5), *Nei Ting* (St 44), *He Gu* (LI 4), *Xia Guan* (St 7)

ANALYSIS OF FORMULA: *Tong Li* and *Nei Ting* are both the fire points on their respective channels. The former is a master point for heart fire, while the latter is a ruling point for stomach fire. Draining them discharges and downbears fire which follows the channels upward to the face. Draining *He Gu* and *Xia Guan* frees the flow of the network vessels in the region of the temporomandibular joint and stops pain.

ADDITIONS & SUBTRACTIONS: Please see pattern #1 above.

5. LIVER WIND STIRRING INTERNALLY PATTERN

MAIN SYMPTOMS: Grinding of the teeth, tremors of the hands and feet, malar flushing, night sweats, vexatious heat in the five hearts, a dry mouth and throat, a red tongue with scanty fluids, and a fine, bowstring, rapid pulse

TREATMENT PRINCIPLES: Nourish the liver and enrich the kidneys, subdue yang and extinguish wind

RX: *Zhen Gan Xi Feng Tang* (Settle the Liver & Extinguish Wind Decoction)

INGREDIENTS: Haemititum (*Dai Zhe Shi*) and Radix Achyranthis Bidentatae (*Niu Xi*), 18g each, Os Draconis (*Long Gu*), Concha Ostreae (*Mu Li*), Radix Albus Paeoniae Lactiflorae (*Bai Shao*), and Plastrum Testudinis (*Gui Ban*), 15g each, Radix Scrophulariae Ningpoensis (*Xuan Shen*) and Tuber Asparagi Cochinensis (*Tian Men Dong*), 9g each, and Herba Artemisiae Capillaris (*Yin Chen Hao*), Fructus Meliae Toosendan (*Chuan Lian Zi*), Fructus Germinatus Hordei Vulgaris (*Mai Ya*), and Radix Glycyrrhizae (*Gan Cao*), 6g each

ANALYSIS OF FORMULA: *Niu Xi* and *Bai Shao* nourish liver yin and blood. *Gui Ban* and *Tian Men Dong* enrich kidney yin. These four medicinals treat the root of the disease. *Dai Zhe Shi*, *Niu Xi*, *Long Gu*, *Mu Li*, and *Gui Ban* subdue yang and extinguish wind. They treat the branches of this disease. *Xuan Shen* clears vacuity heat due to yin vacuity, especially hot flashes in the face, night sweats, and malar flushing. *Yin*

Chen Hao and *Chuan Lian Zi* clear and eliminate liver-gallbladder damp heat, while the latter also clears and courses the liver to prevent liver fire. *Mai Ya* promotes the digestion of heavy medicinals like *Mu Li, Long Gu, Gui Ban,* and *Dai Zhe Shi* and prevents food stagnation.

ADDITIONS & SUBTRACTIONS: For headache and vertigo, add 15 grams of Spica Prunellae Vulgaris (*Xia Ku Cao*) and nine grams of Flos Chrysanthemi Morifolii (*Ju Hua*). For phlegm obstructing the network vessels, add nine grams each of Bulbus Fritillariae Thunbergii (*Zhe Bei Mu*) and Rhizoma Arisaematis (*Tian Nan Xing*). For more pronounced liver-kidney yin vacuity, add 12 grams each of cooked Radix Rehmanniae (*Shu Di*) and Fructus Corni Officinalis (*Shan Zhu Yu*).

ACUPUNCTURE & MOXIBUSTION: *Feng Chi* (GB 20), *Fu Liu* (Ki 7), *San Yin Jiao* (Sp 6), *He Gu* (LI 4), *Xia Guan* (St 7)

ANALYSIS OF FORMULA: *Fu Liu* is the water point of the kidney channel, therefore, supplementing it enriches kidney yin. *San Yin Jiao* is the intersection point of the three yin channels of the feet. Supplementing it nourishes liver yin. Together, these two points treat the root of this disease, *i.e.,* yin vacuity. Draining *Feng Chi* levels the liver, subdues yang, and extinguishes wind, especially when its manifestations are in the head and face. Draining *He Gu* and *Xia Guan* frees the flow of the network vessels in the region of the temporomandibular joint and stops pain.

ADDITIONS & SUBTRACTIONS: Please see pattern #1 above.

6. QI & BLOOD VACUITY PATTERN

MAIN SYMPTOMS: Grinding of the teeth, possible facial swelling, a somber white or sallow yellow facial complexion, fatigue, lassitude of the spirit, lack of strength, reduced food intake, abdominal distention after meals, loose stools, cold hands and feet, dizziness, heart palpitations, pale lips and nails, a tender, pale tongue with teeth-marks on its edges and thin, white fur, and a fine, weak pulse

TREATMENT PRINCIPLES: Boost the qi and nourish the blood

RX: *Ba Zhen Tang Jia Wei* (Eight Pearls Decoction with Added Flavors)

INGREDIENTS: Radix Albus Paeoniae Lactiflorae (*Bai Shao*), 18g, cooked Radix Rehmanniae (*Shu Di*) and Caulis Milletiae Seu Spatholobi (*Ji Xue Teng*), 12g each, Radix Codonopsitis Pilosulae (*Dang Shen*), Rhizoma Atractylodis Macrocephalae (*Bai Zhu*), Sclerotium Poriae Cocos (*Fu Ling*), Radix Angelicae Sinensis (*Dang Gui*), and Radix Ligustici Wallichii (*Chuan Xiong*), 9g each, and mix-fried Radix Glycyrrhizae (*Gan Cao*), 6g

ANALYSIS OF FORMULA: *Dang Shen, Bai Zhu, Fu Ling,* and mix-fried *Gan Cao* are the four gentlemen of *Si Jun Zi Tang* (Four Gentlemen Decoction), one of the basic Chinese medicinal formulas for fortifying the spleen and boosting the qi. *Shu Di, Dang Gui, Bai Shao,* and *Chuan Xiong* are the four ingredients of *Si Wu Tang* (Four Materials Decoction), one of the basic Chinese medicinal formulas for nourishing the blood. Together, they form the eight pearls of *Ba Zhen Tang* (Eight Pearls Decoction) which is a key formula for the treatment of qi and blood dual vacuity. *Jie Xue Teng* is then added to reinforce the supplementation of the blood and free the flow of the network vessels.

ADDITIONS & SUBTRACTIONS: For uneasy opening and closing of the mouth with pain, add 15 grams of Lumbricus (*Di Long*) and nine grams of Bombyx Batryticatus (*Jiang Can*). For severe weakness in opening the mouth or in the four limbs, add 15 grams of Radix Astragali Membranacei (*Huang Qi*) and 12 grams of Rhizoma Polygonati (*Huang Jing*). For abdominal fullness and reduced food intake, add nine grams of Cortex Magnoliae Officinalis (*Hou Po*) and Fructus Germinatus Hordei Vulgaris (*Mai Ya*). For loose stools, add nine grams of Rhizoma Atractylodis (*Cang Zhu*) and five grams of Fructus Amomi (*Sha Ren*).

If there is primarily qi vacuity with more facial swelling than pain, replace *Ba Zhen Tang Jia Wei* with *Bu Zhong Yi Qi Tang Jia Wei* (Supplement the Center & Boost the Qi Decoction with Added Flavors): Radix Astragali Membranacei (*Huang Qi*), 15g, Radix Ligustici Wallichii (*Chuan Xiong*), Radix Codonopsitis Pilosulae (*Dang Shen*), Rhizoma Atractylodis Macrocephalae (*Bai Zhu*), and Sclerotium Poriae Cocos (*Fu Ling*), 9g each, Radix Angelicae Sinensis (*Dang Gui*), Pericarpium Citri Reticulatae (*Chen Pi*), Rhizoma Cimicifugae (*Sheng Ma*), and mix-fried Radix Glycyrrhizae (*Gan Cao*), 6g each, and Radix Bupleuri (*Chai Hu*), 3g. If there is marked liver depression, double or triple the dose of *Chai Hu*. If there is concomitant depressive heat, add nine grams of Radix Scutellariae Baicalensis (*Huang Qin*) and three grams of Rhizoma Coptidis Chinensis (*Huang Lian*). If there is concomitant blood stasis, increase the dose of *Dang Gui* to nine grams and add nine grams of Radix Salviae Miltiorrhizae (*Dan Shen*). If there is concomitant kidney yang vacuity, add nine grams of Radix Dioscoreae Oppositiae (*Shan Yao*) and three grams of Radix Lateralis Praeparatus Aconiti Carmichaeli (*Fu Zi*).

ACUPUNCTURE & MOXIBUSTION: *Zu San Li* (St 36), *San Yin Jiao* (Sp 6), *He Gu* (LI 4), *Xia Guan* (St 7)

ANALYSIS OF FORMULA: Together, supplementing *Zu San Li* and *San Yin Jiao* supplement the source of engenderment and transformation of the qi and blood. Draining *He Gu* and *Xia Guan* frees the flow of the network vessels in the region of the temporomandibular joint and stops pain.

ADDITIONS & SUBTRACTIONS: Please see pattern #1 above.

7. Qi vacuity & blood stasis pattern

MAIN SYMPTOMS: Chronic pain and enduring attacks, severe, lancinating, fixed pain, pain which is worse at night, possible spasms, a somber white facial complexion, scaly skin, aversion to wind, spontaneous perspiration, shortness of breath, disinclination to speak, fatigue, lassitude of the spirit, a pale tongue with possible static macules or spots, and a deep, choppy, weak pulse

TREATMENT PRINCIPLES: Supplement the qi and quicken the blood, transform stasis and free the flow of the network vessels

Rx: *Mian Tong Fang Si Hao* (Face Pain Formula No. 4)

INGREDIENTS: Radix Astragali Membranacei (*Huang Qi*) and Caulis Milletiae Seu Spatholobi (*Ji Xue Teng*), 15g each, Radix Ligustici Wallichii (*Chuan Xiong*), Radix Rubrus Paeoniae Lactiflorae (*Chi Shao*), Radix Angelicae Sinensis (*Dang Gui*), Radix Salviae Miltiorrhizae (*Dan Shen*), and Radix Cyathulae (*Chuan Niu Xi*), 9g each, Rhizoma Gastrodiae Elatae (*Tian Ma*), Flos Carthami Tinctorii (*Hong Hua*), Rhizoma Curcumae Longae (*Jiang Huang*), and Sclerotium Poriae Cocos (*Fu Ling*), 6g each, and mix-fried Radix Glycyrrhizae (*Gan Cao*), 3g

ANALYSIS OF FORMULA: *Huang Qi*, *Fu Ling*, and mix-fried *Gan Cao* supplement the qi to move the blood. Uncooked *Huang Qi* goes to the network vessels and channels to supplement the qi inside the blood. *Ji Xue Teng*, *Chuan Xiong*, *Chi Shao*, *Dang Gui*, *Dan Shen*, *Chuan Niu Xi*, and *Hong Hua* move the blood and transform stasis, free the flow of the network vessels and stop pain. *Dang Gui* and *Ji Xue Teng* also nourish the blood. *Tian Ma* and *Jiang Huang* free the flow of the network vessels and stop pain. *Tian Ma* also relieves spasms.

ADDITIONS & SUBTRACTIONS: For uneasy opening and closing of the mouth or severe pain, add 15 grams of Lumbricus (*Di Long*). For a severe qi vacuity, add nine grams each of Radix Codonopsitis Pilosulae (*Dang Shen*) and Rhizoma Atractylodis Macrocephalae (*Bai Zhu*). For reduced food intake, add nine grams each of Fructus Germinatus Hordei Vulgaris (*Mai Ya*) and Massa Medica Fermentata (*Shen Qu*). For abdominal fullness, add nine grams each of Cortex Magnoliae Officinalis (*Hou Po*) and Radix Auklandiae Lappae (*Mu Xiang*). For sliminess in the mouth, slimy tongue fur, and a heavy body or head, add nine grams each of Rhizoma Atractylodis (*Cang Zhu*) and Herba Agastachis Seu Pogostemi (*Huo Xiang*).

ACUPUNCTURE & MOXIBUSTION: *Zu San Li* (St 36), *San Yin Jiao* (Sp 6), *He Gu* (LI 4), *Xia Guan* (St 7)

ANALYSIS OF FORMULA: Using even supplementing-even draining technique on *Zu San Li* and *San Yin Jiao* fortifies the spleen and supplements the qi. Draining *He Gu* in combination with *San Yin Jiao* quickens the blood and transforms stasis. Draining *He Gu* also drains evils from the head and face region. Draining *Xia Guan* frees the flow of the network vessels in the region of the temporomandibular joint and stops pain.

ADDITIONS & SUBTRACTIONS: Please see pattern #1 above.

8. Food stagnation pattern

MAIN SYMPTOMS: Grinding of the teeth during sleep at night, insomnia, chest and ductal glomus and oppression, no thought of eating, indigestion, inhibited defecation, diarrhea with abdominal pain or constipation, dark-colored urine, slimy, slightly yellow tongue fur, and a slippery pulse

NOTE: This pattern does not commonly cause TMJ by itself, but it may complicate a number of other patterns, especially those having to do with the liver, stomach, and spleen.

TREATMENT PRINCIPLES: Disperse food and abduct stagnation

Rx: *Bao He Wan Jia Wei* (Protect Harmony Pills with Added Flavors)

INGREDIENTS: Semen Panici Miliacei (*Shu Mi*), Fructus Crataegi (*Shan Zha*), Fructus Germinatus Hordei Vulgaris (*Mai Ya*), Massa Medica Fermentata (*Shen Qu*), Pericarpium Citri Reticulatae (*Chen Pi*), Sclerotium Poriae Cocos (*Fu Ling*), Fructus Forsythiae Suspensae (*Lian Qiao*), Semen Raphani Sativi (*Lai Fu Zi*), and Rhizoma Pinelliae Ternatae (*Ban Xia*), 9g each, and Fructus Citri Aurantii (*Zhi Ke*), 6g

ANALYSIS OF FORMULA: *Shu Mi*, *Shan Zha*, *Mai Ya*, *Shen Qu*, and *Lai Fu Zi* disperse food and abduct stagnation. *Shu Mi* is an empirically specific medicinal for the treatment of insomnia due to food stagnation, especially when it is combined with *Ban Xia*. *Shan Zha* treats the stagnation of meaty, oily foods, *Mai Ya* treats the stagnation of grains, fruits, and vegetables, *Shen Qu* treats any type of food stagnation, and *Lai Fu Zi* disperses food and moves the qi. The latter, with *Zhi Ke* and *Chen Pi*, moves the qi to help the dispersion of food. *Chen Pi*, *Fu Ling*, and *Ban Xia* dry dampness and transform phlegm to prevent damp and phlegm accumulation due to food stagnation. *Ban Xia* and *Chen Pi* also harmonize stomach qi, and *Lian Qiao* prevents heat from transforming from food stagnation.

ADDITIONS & SUBTRACTIONS: For spleen vacuity, add nine grams each of Radix Codonopsitis Pilosulae (*Dang*

Shen) and Rhizoma Atractylodis Macrocephalae (*Bai Zhu*). For damp accumulation, add nine grams each of Rhizoma Atractylodis (*Cang Zhu*) and Cortex Magnoliae Officinalis (*Hou Po*). For severe qi stagnation, add nine grams each of Cortex Magnoliae Officinalis (*Hou Po*) and Pericarpium Citri Reticulatae Viride (*Qing Pi*) and replace *Zhi Ke* with Fructus Immaturus Citri Aurantii (*Zhi Shi*). For constipation, add nine grams of Fructus Immaturus Citri Aurantii (*Zhi Shi*) and three grams of Radix Et Rhizoma Rhei (*Da Huang*). For food stagnation transforming into heat, add nine grams of Fructus Gardeniae Jasminoidis (*Zhi Zi*) and six grams of Radix Scutellariae Baicalensis (*Huang Qin*).

Acupuncture & moxibustion: *Liang Men* (St 21), *Nei Ting* (St 44), *He Gu* (LI 4), *Xia Guan* (St 7)

Analysis of formula: Draining *Liang Men* and *Nei Ting* drains the stomach and abducts stagnation. Draining *He Gu* also helps to clear and transport the yang ming at the same time as it dispels evils in the head and face. Draining *Xia Guan* frees the flow of the network vessels in the temporomandibular region and stops pain.

Additions & subtractions: Please see pattern #1 above.

9. Roundworms harassing internally pattern

Main symptoms: Grinding of teeth during sleep, stomach glomus, intermittent abdominal pain, addiction to peculiar foods, a sallow facial complexion, cold hands and feet, fatigue, a tendency to loose stools, possible itching in the nostrils, blue macules or speckles in the white of the eyes, white-colored roundworm macules on the face, translucent milliary eruptions on the insides of the lips, bright red speckled eruptions on the tip of the tongue or on the sides of the middle of the tongue, a pale or red tongue with white, possibly flowery, peeled fur, and a deep, bowstring, slippery pulse

Note: While this pattern describes roundworm infestation, it may also be used to describe other types of *chong* or worm conditions where there is a combination of great spleen vacuity, liver depression, damp heat, and cold.

Treatment principles: Fortify the spleen and transform dampness, clear heat and expel worms

Rx: *Wu Mei Wan* (Mume Pills)

Ingredients: Fructus Pruni Mume (*Wu Mei*), Radix Angelicae Sinensis (*Dang Gui*), Radix Codonopsitis Pilosulae (*Dang Shen*), and Cortex Phellodendri (*Huang Bai*), 9g each, Rhizoma Coptidis Chinensis (*Huang Lian*), dry Rhizoma Zingiberis (*Gan Jiang*), and Ramulus Cinnamomi Cassiae (*Gui Zhi*), 6g each, Herba Asari Cum Radice (*Xi Xin*), Fructus Zanthoxyli Bungeani (*Chuan Jiao*), and Radix Lateralis Praeparatus Aconiti Carmichaeli (*Fu Zi*), 3g each

Analysis of formula: This formula is based on Ke Qin's statement: "When roundworms encounter sourness, they are quieted. When they encounter acridity, they are spent. When they encounter bitterness, they are discharged." The flavors in this formula are a combination of sour, acrid, and bitter. This formula treats a complex combination of heat and cold, vacuity and repletion complicated by the presence of *chong* or worms. *Dang Shen* and *Dang Gui* respectively supplement the qi and blood. In addition, *Dang Gui* quickens the blood and transforms stasis. *Wu Mei* expels roundworms. *Huang Bai* and *Huang Lian* clear heat, eliminate dampness, and attack worms. *Chuan Jiao* and *Xi Xin* expel worms and warm the viscera. *Gan Jiang*, *Gui Zhi*, and *Fu Zi* assist *Chuan Jiao* and *Xi Xin* in warming the interior and scattering cold. In addition, *Gui Zhi* and *Xi Xin* promote the movement of qi and blood and, therefore, help stop pain.

Additions & subtractions: For roundworm infestation, add nine grams each of Semen Arecae Catechu (*Bing Lang*) and Fructus Quisqualis Indicae (*Shi Jun Zi*). For constipation, add six grams of Radix Et Rhizoma Rhei (*Da Huang*) and nine grams of Fructus Immaturus Citri Aurantii (*Zhi Shi*). For spleen vacuity, add 12 grams of Rhizoma Atractylodis Macrocephalae (*Bai Zhu*) and nine grams of Sclerotium Poriae Cocos (*Fu Ling*). For blood vacuity, add 12 grams of Radix Albus Paeoniae Lactiflorae (*Bai Shao*). For damp heat, add nine grams each of Rhizoma Atractylodis (*Cang Zhu*) and Radix Scutellariae Baicalensis (*Huang Qin*). For food stagnation, add nine grams each of Fructus Germinatus Hordei Vulgaris (*Mai Ya*), Fructus Crataegi (*Shan Zha*), Massa Medica Fermentata (*Shen Qu*), and Semen Raphani Sativi (*Lai Fu Zi*).

Acupuncture & moxibustion: *Bai Chong Wo* (M-LE-34), *Zu San Li* (St 36), *Yin Ling Quan* (Sp 9), *Nei Ting* (St 44), *He Gu* (LI 4), *Xia Guan* (St 7)

Analysis of formula: Draining *Bai Chong Wo* is an empirical treatment for expelling roundworms. Supplementing *Zu San Li* fortifies the spleen and supplements the qi, while draining *Yin Ling Quan* and *Nei Ting* clears and eliminates dampness and heat. Draining *He Gu* and *Xia Guan* frees the flow of the network vessels in the temporomandibular joint region and stops pain.

Additions & subtractions: Please see pattern #1 above.

10. Liver-kidney yin vacuity pattern

Main symptoms: Pain in the temporomandibular joint region, uneasy opening and closing of the mouth, loose teeth, limited opening of the mouth, dizziness, tinnitus, low back and knee soreness and limpness, insomnia, profuse dreams, a pale red tongue with scanty fur, and a fine pulse

TREATMENT PRINCIPLES: Supplement and boost the liver and kidneys

RX: *Da Bu Yin Wan Jia Jian* (Greatly Supplementing Yin Pills with Additions & Subtractions)

INGREDIENTS: Radix Albus Paeoniae Lactiflorae (*Bai Shao*), 20g, Lumbricus (*Di Long*) and Cortex Eucommiae Ulmoidis (*Du Zhong*), 15g each, Radix Angelicae Sinensis (*Dang Gui*) and Radix Rubrus Paeoniae Lactiflorae (*Chi Shao*), 12g each, and cooked Radix Rehmanniae (*Shu Di*), Plastrum Testudinis (*Gui Ban*), Rhizoma Anemarrhenae Asphodeloidis (*Zhi Mu*), Bombyx Batryticatus (*Jiang Can*), and Rhizoma Gastrodiae Elatae (*Tian Ma*), 9g each

ANALYSIS OF FORMULA: *Shu Di* and *Gui Ban* nourish kidney yin, while *Dang Gui* and *Bai Shao* nourish liver blood. *Du Zhong* supplements both kidney yin and yang as well as strengthens the low back and reinforces the bones. *Zhi Mu* nourishes yin and downbears fire. In addition, *Gui Ban* reinforces the bones and *Bai Shao* relaxes spasm. *Di Long* frees the flow of the network vessels and, with *Tian Ma* and *Jiang Can,* dispels wind evils from the vessels. *Chi Shao* and *Dang Gui* quicken the blood and transform stasis to stop pain.

ADDITIONS & SUBTRACTIONS: For severe pain in the temporomandibular region or uneasy opening and closing of the mouth, add three grams each of Buthus Martensis (*Quan Xie*) and Scolopendra Subspinipes (*Wu Gong*), powdered and taken with the strained decoction. For loose teeth, add 12 grams of Rhizoma Drynariae (*Gu Sui Bu*). For dizziness and tinnitus, add 12 grams each of Fructus Lycii Chinensis (*Gou Qi Zi*) and Flos Chrysanthemi Morifolii (*Ju Hua*).

ACUPUNCTURE & MOXIBUSTION: *Fu Liu* (Ki 7), *Xuan Zhong* (GB 39), *Da Zhu* (Bl 11), *He Gu* (LI 4), *Xia Guan* (St 7)

ANALYSIS OF FORMULA: In this pattern, the pain comes from kidney vacuity. Therefore, supplementing *Fu Liu* supplements kidney yin and also the former heaven essence, while supplementing *Xuan Zhong,* the meeting point of the marrow, boosts the marrow. Likewise, supplementing *Da Zhu,* the meeting point of the bones, reinforces the bones. Draining *He Gu* and *Xia Guan* frees the flow of the network vessels locally and stops pain.

ADDITIONS & SUBTRACTIONS: Please see pattern #1 above.

REMARKS

1. As the majority of the formulas above imply, TMJ is usually associated with blood stasis. If stasis has endured and entered the network vessels, it is usually important to add worm or insect ingredients to the formula to specifically free the flow of the network vessels. These include Lumbricus (*Di Long*), Bombyx Batryticatus (*Jiang Can*), Buthus Martensis (*Quan Xie*), Scolopendra Subspinipes (*Wu Gong*), Hirudo (*Shui Zhi*), and Eupolyphaga Seu Ophithoplatia (*Zhe Chong*). Most of these medicinals also track down and extinguish wind, thus relieving spasms and contractures. To get the best action with these worm or insect ingredients, one should avoid decocting them but rather take them powdered with the strained decoction. This is especially so for relieving spasms and contractures.

2. Temporomandibular joint syndrome tends to be a yin fire disease where depressive, damp, or vacuity heat has shifted from the heart to the governing vessel and thence to the tai yang channels where it counterflows upward, congesting in the head and face. In our experience, most Western patients with TMJ have a liver-spleen disharmony with depressive heat in the liver, stomach, and/or heart complicated by blood stasis and possible blood vacuity. In addition, there is often phlegm and/or dampness and sometimes food stagnation. Depending on the patient's age, there may also be yin or yang vacuity. Therefore, in most cases, it is wise to chose a harmonizing formula such as *Xiao Chai Hu Tang* (Minor Bupleurum Decoction), *Xiao Yao San* (Rambling Powder), or *Ban Xia Xie Xin Tang* (Pinellia Drain the Heart Decoction) and modify one of these with additions and subtractions suggested by the ingredients in the simpler, more discreet formulas described above.

3. Although the Chinese medical literature does not discuss this, TMJ may also be due to clenching of the teeth as a stress response. In that case, there is most definitely liver depression qi stagnation. However, there may or may not be any heat evils. Since most cases of chronic or enduring liver depression involve a liver-spleen disharmony, *Xiao Chai Hu Tang* and *Xiao Yao San* are often the guiding formulas of choice. These should then be modified with medicinals that relax spasm, such as Radix Albus Paeoniae Lactiflorae (*Bai Shao*) and Radix Glycyrrhizae (*Gan Cao*), a.k.a. *Shao Yao Gan Cao Tang* (Peony & Licorice Decoction), and medicinals which move the qi and quicken the blood in the area of the jaw, such as Radix Ligustici Wallichii (*Chuan Xiong*) and Radix Et Rhizoma Notopterygii (*Qiang Huo*).

4. In terms of complicated mixed patterns, for wind cold damp impediment with liver-spleen disharmony and blood stasis, consider *He Bi Tang* (Jaw Impediment Decoction): Caulis Milletiae Seu Spatholobi (*Ji Xue Teng*), 18g, Ramulus Loranthi Seu Visci (*Sang Ji Sheng*), 15g, Radix Ledebouriellae Divaricatae (*Fang Feng*), Radix Et Rhizoma Notopterygii (*Qiang Huo*), Radix Gentianae Macrophyllae (*Qin Jiao*), Radix Angelicae Dahuricae (*Bai Zhi*), Radix Ligustici Wallichii (*Chuan Xiong*), Ramulus Cinnamomi

Cassiae (*Gui Zhi*), Rhizoma Cimicifugae (*Sheng Ma*), Rhizoma Atractylodis Macrocephalae (*Bai Zhu*), Sclerotium Poriae Cocos (*Fu Ling*), Radix Angelicae Sinensis (*Dang Gui*), Rhizoma Cyperi Rotundi (*Xiang Fu*), and Radix Achyranthis Bidentatae (*Niu Xi*), 9g each, and Herba Asari Cum Radice (*Xi Xin*), 4.5g.

For wind cold damp impediment with qi and blood stasis and stagnation, one can use *Qu Feng Huo Xue Tang* (Dispel Wind & Quicken the Blood Decoction): Herba Siegesbeckiae (*Xi Xian Cao*), 15g, Herba Lycopodii (*Shen Jin Cao*), Radix Angelicae Pubescentis (*Du Huo*), Ramulus Mori Albi (*Sang Zhi*), Radix Clematidis Chinensis (*Wei Ling Xian*), Caulis Trachelospermi Jasminoidis (*Luo Shi Teng*), Lignum Nodi Pini (*Song Jie*), Caulis Piperis Futokadsurae (*Hai Feng Teng*), Radix Angelicae Sinensis (*Dang Gui*), Radix Ligustici Wallichii (*Chuan Xiong*), 9g each, and Radix Gentianae Macrophyllae (*Qin Jiao*), 4.5g.

5. For temporomandibular joint syndrome from arthritis due to wind cold damp impediment, one can use warm needling method. Seven to nine moxa cones should be burnt on the heads of the needles at *Xia Guan* (St 7) and/or *Jia Che* (St 6) one time per day. For recalcitrant pain, electroacupuncture is sometimes also more effective than needling alone.

6. *Gua sha* of the nape of the neck and upper back can be useful as an adjunctive treatment in this condition in order to relieve counterflowing qi in the tai yang. If *gua sha* results in extreme erythema and petechiae, it should be repeated 1-3 times at 1-2 week intervals.

7. Biofeedback can also be useful as adjunctive therapy for TMJ as can craniosacral therapy.

70

TRIGEMINAL NEURALGIA

Trigeminal neuralgia is also called *tic douloreux*. It is a disorder of the sensory nucleus of the trigeminal nerve producing bouts of severe, seconds-long, lancinating pain along one or more of the divisions of the trigeminal nerve. Usually these bouts of pain affect the superior mandibular and maxillary branches of this nerve. According to Western medicine, trigeminal neuralgia's etiology is unknown, and this disease does not result in pathological changes. It usually affects older patients, and the pain is often set off by touching a trigger point or by such activities as chewing or brushing the teeth. Because the pain is intense even though brief, repeated bouts may incapacitate the patient. This condition mostly affects those over 40 years of age and more women than men.

In Western medicine, the diagnosis of this condition is based on its symptoms and history. It is treated with carbamazepine which is generally effective. However, during treatment with this drug, hemapoetic functions must be monitored since it can depress the bone marrow. Continual use on a regular schedule for three months is usually necessary to determine this drug's effectiveness in relieving the pain of trigeminal neuralgia. Phenytoin and baclofen are effective in some cases, and sometimes surgery is used to separate away structures that may be pressing on the nerve. Surgical section of the nerve may also be resorted to in cases of intractable pain.

CHINESE DISEASE CATEGORIZATION: Trigeminal neuralgia is categorized in Chinese medicine as *tou tong*, headache, *pian tou tong*, side head pain, *jue ni tou tong*, reverse flow headache, *mian tong*, face pain, and *tou feng*, head wind.

DISEASE CAUSES: External invasion by wind, cold, and heat evils, internal damage by the seven affects, faulty diet, as well as aging causing bodily vacuity

DISEASE MECHANISMS: If either wind cold or wind heat evils invade the body from outside, they may lodge in the channels and vessels on one side of the face where they impede and inhibit the free flow of qi and blood and thus result in pain. Commonly, it is a defensive qi vacuity due to aging that allows these external evils to enter the body. If these evils endure and are not out-thrust, they eventually result in blood stasis which causes severe, lancinating pain. It is also possible for unfulfilled desires and anger to damage the liver. The liver may lose its control over coursing and discharging with liver depression transforming into fire. Fire is yang and the liver is yin. Therefore, yang fire evils may shift into the liver's paired yang channel. If this fire ascends along the shao yang, it may harass and congest within the yang channels of the face.

By 40 years of age, yin is half consumed. If, due to aging, yin blood fails to nourish and moisten the liver, the liver may not be able to perform its function of coursing and discharge. Hence depression becomes more prevalent as we age. If yin fails to control yang, liver yang may become hyperactive and ascend. In addition, because the liver's function is also dependent on kidney yang's warming and steaming and this also weakens with age, that is yet another reason why liver depression tends to become aggravated with age. Both of these last two scenarios are especially common in women since women are often blood vacuous due to menstruation, gestation, and lactation. If spleen vacuity reaches the kidneys, as it commonly does premenopausally, qi vacuity evolves into yang vacuity. Further, either qi vacuity, qi stagnation, yin vacuity, or yang vacuity may result in blood stasis, while spleen qi vacuity, faulty diet, or qi stagnation may result in internal engenderment of dampness which may transform into phlegm and obstruct the channels and network vessels.

TREATMENT BASED ON PATTERN DISCRIMINATION:

1. WIND HEAT MIXED WITH PHLEGM OBSTRUCTING THE NETWORK VESSELS PATTERN

MAIN SYMPTOMS: Recurrent episodes of burning hot or cutting, piercing pain which is difficult to bear and mostly affects one side of the head and face, a red facial complexion and sweating during the pain, aggravation of the condition on exposure to heat and soothing on exposure to coolness, possible accompanying fever, dry mouth, reddish urine, a red tongue with dry, yellow fur, and a bowstring, rapid pulse. If phlegm fire obstructs the network vessels, there will be simultaneous dizziness, chest oppression, numbness of the limbs, a red tongue with slimy, yellow fur, and a bowstring, slippery, rapid pulse.

TREATMENT PRINCIPLES: Course wind and scatter heat, flush phlegm and quicken the network vessels

RX: *Xiong Zhi Shi Gao Tang Jia Wei* (Ligusticum, Angelica Dahurica & Gypsum Decoction with Added Flavors)

INGREDIENTS: Gypsum Fibrosum (*Shi Gao*), 20g, Radix Ligustici Wallichii (*Chuan Xiong*), Radix Puerariae (*Ge Gen*), and Radix Angelicae Dahuricae (*Bai Zhi*), 15g, and Radix Typhonii Gigantei (*Bai Fu Zi*), Rhizoma Arisaematis (*Nan Xing*), Rhizoma Pinelliae Ternatae (*Ban Xia*), Bombyx Batryticatus (*Jiang Can*), Herba Seu Flos Schizonepetae Tenuifoliae (*Jing Jie*), Flos Chrysanthemi Morifolii (*Ju Hua*), Radix Et Rhizoma Notopterygii (*Qiang Huo*), Radix Et Rhizoma Ligustici Chinensis (*Gao Ben*), and Flos Lonicerae Japonicae (*Jin Yin Hua*), 9g each

ANALYSIS OF FORMULA: The combination of *Chuan Xiong* and *Shi Gao* form a special pair for the treatment of pain in the head and face due to wind heat. By itself, *Chuan Xiong* dispels wind, quickens the blood, and stops pain. In addition, its ascending nature leads *Shi Gao* and the other medicinals to the head and face. By itself, *Shi Gao* drains heat and especially eliminates heat from the muscle division as well as from the exterior. This pair's action is reinforced with *Bai Zhi* which dispels wind in the face and especially in the large intestine and stomach channels. Some contemporary Chinese doctors think that *Bai Zhi* also opens the orifices and frees the flow of the network vessels. *Jing Jie, Jiang Can, Ju Hua, Qiang Huo,* and *Gao Ben* help these three main medicinals to dispel wind. In addition, *Jing Jie* stops spasms from external wind; *Jiang Can* transforms wind phlegm, resolves spasms, and treats stubborn pain; *Ju Hua* dispels wind heat in the face; *Qiang Huo* strongly treats wind in the upper part of the body and stops pain; and *Gao Ben* dispels wind damp and stops pain. *Jin Yin Hua* helps the preceding medicinals to dispel wind heat and prevents the transformation of heat into toxins. *Jiang Can, Bai Fu Zi, Ban Xia,* and *Nan Xing* all transform phlegm. In addition, *Bai Fu Zi* is well-known for eliminating wind phlegm in the head and face, while *Tian Nan Xing* transforms stubborn phlegm in the network vessels.

ADDITIONS & SUBTRACTIONS: For enduring disease or blood stasis with severe fixed and stabbing pain, add two grams of Euployphaga Seu Ophisthoplatia (*Tu Bie Chong*) and three grams of Radix Pseudoginseng (*San Qi*), powdered and taken with the strained decoction. For stubborn pain which is recalcitrant to treatment, add two grams each of Buthus Martensi (*Quan Xie*) with tail and Scolopendra Subspinipes (*Wu Gong*) and three grams of Bombyx Batryticatus (*Jiang Can*), all powdered and taken with the strained decoction. For a severely hot sensation in the face, add nine grams of Lumbricus (*Di Long*) and 12 grams of Rhizoma Cimicifugae (*Sheng Ma*). For poor appetite, indigestion, or nausea from taking this decoction, add nine grams each of Fructus Germinatus Hordei Vulgaris (*Mai Ya*) and Fructus Citri Aurantii (*Zhi Ke*).

ACUPUNCTURE & MOXIBUSTION: *He Gu* (LI 4), *Wai Guan* (TB 5), local points according to the location of the pain

First branch (eye, nose area/ocular nerve): *Zan Zhu* (Bl 2) through to *Yu Yao* (M-HN-6), *Si Zhu Kong* (TB 23) through to *Yu Yao* (M-HN-6), *Tai Yang* (M-HN-9), *Yang Bai* (GB 14), *Ying Xiang* (LI 20), *a shi* points. Use 2-3 points per treatment and alternate the points from treatment to treatment.

Second branch (upper jaw, nose, temporal area/maxillary nerve): *Si Bai* (St 2), *Ju Liao* (St 3), *Quan Liao* (SI 18), *Ying Xiang* (LI 20), *Xia Guan* (St 7), *a shi* points. Use 2-3 points per treatment and alternate the points from treatment to treatment.

Third branch (lower jaw, ear, parietal area/mandibular nerve): *Jia Che* (St 6), *Da Ying* (St 5), *Di Cang* (St 4), *Cheng Jiang* (CV 24), *Jia Cheng Jiang* (H-HN-18), *Xia Guan* (St 7), *a shi* points. Use 2-3 points per treatment and alternate the points from treatment to treatment.

Use draining method. Some Chinese acupuncturists use electro-acupuncture on all patterns of this disease.

ANALYSIS OF FORMULA: Draining *He Gu* and *Wai Guan* courses wind and scatters heat. *He Gu* is the main distant point because it is the ruling point for the face and mouth. Draining all the local points quickens the network vessels and stops pain according to the Chinese medical statement of fact, "If there is free flow, there is no pain."

ADDITIONS & SUBTRACTIONS: For severe pain or pain

which prevents sleep, add ear *Shen Men* and *Shen Ting* (GV 24). For a hot sensation in the face, add *Nei Ting* (St 44). For pain in the forehead, add *Tou Wei* (St 8) and *Yin Tang* (M-HN-3). For pain around the eyes, add *Tong Zi Liao* (GB 1) to *Zan Zhu*, *Yu Yao*, and *Si Zhu Kong*. For nose pain, add *Bi Tong* (M-HN-14), and *Su Liao* (GV 25) to *Ying Xiang*. For pain in front of the ear, add *Er Men* (TB 21), *Ting Gong* (SI 19), and *Ting Hui* (GB 2). For pain around the lips, add *Ren Zhong* (GV 26) to *Cheng Jiang* and *Di Cang*.

2. Wind cold mixed with phlegm & stasis pattern

Main symptoms: Recurrent episodes of cramping, spastic pain which, when severe, is difficult to bear, a somber white facial complexion during the pain, chilling worsening the pain and lessening with warmth, a pale tongue with thin, white fur, and a tight pulse. If cold and phlegm are obstructing the network vessels, there will be simultaneous facial vacuity puffiness, a pale, fat tongue with thick, white, slimy fur, and a soggy, slippery, or tight pulse.

Treatment principles: Course wind and scatter cold, flush phlegm and free the flow of the network vessels

Rx: *Chuan Xiong Cha Tiao San Jia Jian* (Ligusticum Mixed With Tea Powder with Additions & Subtractions)

Ingredients: Radix Ligustici Wallichii (*Chuan Xiong*) and Radix Angelicae Dahuricae (*Bai Zhi*), 15g each, Radix Et Rhizoma Notopterygii (*Qiang Huo*), Herba Seu Flos Schizonepetae Tenuifoliae (*Jing Jie*), and Radix Ledebouriellae Divaricatae (*Fang Feng*), 9g each, Buthus Martensis (*Quan Xie*), Scolopendra Subspinipes (*Wu Gong*), and Rhizoma Arisaematis (*Nan Xing*), 6g each, and Radix Glycyrrhizae (*Gan Cao*) and Herba Asari Cum Radice (*Xi Xin*), 3g each

Analysis of formula: *Chuan Xiong*, *Bai Zhi*, *Qiang Huo*, *Jing Jie*, and *Fang Feng* all course wind and scatter cold. In addition, *Chuan Xiong* dispels wind and moves the qi, quickens the blood and stops pain, especially in the head and face. *Bai Zhi* courses wind in the face, especially in the large intestine and stomach channels. As stated above, some contemporary Chinese doctors think that *Bai Zhi* also frees the flow of the network vessels. *Xi Xin* is very efficient for stopping pain, especially in the upper part of the body. *Jing Jie* and *Fang Feng* resolve the spasms. *Quan Xie* and *Wu Gong* free the flow of the network vessels and treat stubborn pain. And *Tian Nan Xing* transforms phlegm obstructing the network vessels.

Additions & subtractions: If cold is severe, add nine grams of Radix Lateralis Praeparatus Aconiti Carmichaeli (*Fu Zi*). If stasis is severe, add 12 grams each of Radix Rubrus Paeoniae Lactiflorae (*Chi Shao*), Radix Salviae Miltiorrhizae (*Dan Shen*), and Feces Trogopterori Seu Pteromi (*Wu Ling Zhi*). If exterior cold pattern signs and symptoms are marked, add nine grams of Herba Ephedrae (*Ma Huang*). If there is concomitant internal heat with thirst, constipation, and red, swollen, bleeding gums, add 25 grams of Gypsum Fibrosum (*Shi Gao*). For runny nose and nasal congestion, add nine grams each of Fructus Xanthii Sibirici (*Cang Er Zi*) and Flos Magnoliae Liliflorae (*Xin Yi Hua*). For poor appetite, indigestion, or nausea from taking this decoction, add nine grams each of Fructus Germinatus Hordei Vulgaris (*Mai Ya*) and Fructus Citri Aurantii (*Zhi Ke*).

Caution: It is not advisable to use *Fu Zi* and *Xi Xin* for a long time.

Acupuncture & moxibustion: *He Gu* (LI 4), *Lie Que* (Lu 7), local points according to the location of the pain. Please see pattern #1 above.

Analysis of formula: Draining *He Gu* and *Lie Que* courses wind and scatters cold. *He Gu* is the ruling point for diseases of the face and mouth, while *Lie Que* is the ruling point for diseases of the head and neck. Draining all the local points quickens the network vessels and stops pain.

Additions & subtractions: Please see pattern #1 above.

3. Liver depression transforming fire pattern

Main symptoms: In most cases, there is a tendency to impatience, irritability, violent anger, and emotional depression accompanied by one-sided head and face burning pain. This pain is aggravated by heat and emotional disturbance. Sometimes the pain causes headache. There is a red facial complexion and red eyes. In severe cases, there are muscular spasms or tics of the affected area in the face. Sometimes there are alternating periods of crisis and remission when the patient is completely normal. Further, there is a bitter taste in the mouth, dry throat, heart vexation, chest oppression, rib-side pain, great sighing, disquieted sleep at night, reddish yellow urine, dry, bound stools, a red tongue with dry, yellow fur, and a bowstring, rapid pulse.

Treatment principles: Clear the liver and discharge heat, free the flow of the channels and quicken the network vessels

Rx: *Zhi Zi Qing Gan San Jia Wei* (Gardenia Clear the Liver Powder with Added Flavors)

Ingredients: Gypsum Fibrosum (*Shi Gao*), 20g, Radix Ligustici Wallichii (*Chuan Xiong*), 15g, Fructus Arctii Lappae (*Niu Bang Zi*), Radix Bupleuri (*Chai Hu*), Radix

Albus Paeoniae Lactiflorae (*Bai Shao*), Radix Angelicae Sinensis (*Dang Gui*), Fructus Gardeniae Jasminoidis (*Zhi Zi*), Cortex Radicis Moutan (*Dan Pi*), Scolopendra Subspinipes (*Wu Gong*), Bombyx Batryticatus (*Jiang Can*), and Radix Scutellariae Baicalensis (*Huang Qin*), 9g each, and Rhizoma Coptidis Chinensis (*Huang Lian*), 3g

ANALYSIS OF FORMULA: Once again we meet the efficacious combination of *Chuan Xiong* and *Shi Gao* which here is mainly used to treat headache or face pain due to wind heat or replete heat, particularly in the shao yang, jue yin and yang ming channels. *Chuan Xiong* moves the qi, quickens the blood, and stops pain, while *Shi Gao* drains heat. The combination of *Bai Shao* and *Chai Hu* resolves liver depression via coursing and harmonizing. *Bai Shao* and *Dang Gui* nourish liver blood to prevent liver depression, while *Dang Gui* by itself quickens the blood. *Zhi Zi* and *Dan Pi* is also another famous combination for clearing heat transformed from liver depression. Their ability to clear heat is reinforced by *Huang Qin* and *Huang Lian* which clear and eliminate damp heat from the liver and also stomach heat. This latter is noteworthy because the pain in this pattern mainly manifests along the stomach channel. *Wu Gong* and *Jiang Can* free the flow of the channels, quicken the network vessels, and stop stubborn pain, and *Niu Bang Zi* is an empirical medicinal for the treatment of headache and facial pain due to heat.

ADDITIONS & SUBTRACTIONS: If there is concomitant yang ming stomach heat, add nine grams of Radix Puerariae (*Ge Gen*) and six grams of Radix Et Rhizoma Rhei (*Da Huang*). If heat has damaged stomach fluids, add nine grams each of Rhizoma Anemarrhenae Aspheloidis (*Zhi Mu*) and Tuber Ophiopogonis Japonici (*Mai Men Dong*). If there are red, tearing eyes, add 12 grams each of Flos Chrysanthemi Morifolii (*Ju Hua*) and Herba Equiseti Hiemalis (*Mu Zei Cao*). For severe pain, add three grams each of Lumbricus (*Di Long*) and Buthus Martensi (*Quan Xie*), powdered and taken with the strained decoction. For insomnia due to pain, add 12 grams of Semen Zizyphi Spinosae (*Suan Zao Ren*) and 18 grams of Caulis Polygoni Multiflori (*Ye Jiao Teng*). For chest oppression and/or rib-side pain, add nine grams each of Fructus Meliae Toosendan (*Chuan Lian Zi*) and Tuber Curcumae (*Yu Jin*). For poor appetite, indigestion, or nausea from taking this decoction, add nine grams each of Fructus Germinatus Hordei Vulgaris (*Mai Ya*) and Fructus Citri Aurantii (*Zhi Ke*).

If there is concomitant spleen qi vacuity, replace *Zhi Zi Qing Gan San* with *Dan Zhi Xiao Yao San Jia Wei* (Moutan & Gardenia Rambling Powder with Added Flavors): Radix Ligustici Wallichii (*Chuan Xiong*), 15g, Radix Scutellariae Baicalensis (*Huang Qin*), Fructus Gardeniae Jasminoidis (*Zhi Zi*), Cortex Radicis Moutan (*Dan Pi*), Rhizoma Atractylodis Macrocephalae (*Bai Zhu*), Sclerotium Poriae Cocos (*Fu Ling*), Radix Angelicae Sinensis (*Dang Gui*), Radix Albus Paeoniae Lactiflorae (*Bai Shao*), Radix Rubrus Paeoniae Lactiflorae (*Chi Shao*), and Bombyx Batryticatus (*Jiang Can*), 9g each, and Scolopendra Subspinipes (*Wu Gong*) and mix-fried Radix Glycyrrhizae (*Gan Cao*), 6g each.

ACUPUNCTURE & MOXIBUSTION: *He Gu* (LI 4), *Xing Jian* (Liv 2), *Zu Lin Qi* (GB 41), local points according to the location of the pain. Please see pattern #1 above.

ANALYSIS OF FORMULA: *He Gu* is the ruling point for diseases of the face and mouth. Draining it moves the qi and stops pain. Draining *Xing Jian* and *Zu Lin Qi* clears the liver and discharges heat. Draining all the local points quickens the network vessels and stops pain.

ADDITIONS & SUBTRACTIONS: Please see pattern #1 above.

4. PHLEGM STASIS IMPEDIMENT & OBSTRUCTION PATTERN

MAIN SYMPTOMS: Piercing one-sided face and head pain accompanied by heavy-headedness or pain leading to numbness and insensitivity, possible frequent vomiting at the time of pain, a possible slimy feeling in the mouth, a dark but pale tongue with glossy, slippery fur, and a choppy, possibly soggy, fine pulse

NOTE: This is not a commonly seen pattern in its pure form. However, phlegm and stasis may complicate any other pattern of this disease.

TREATMENT PRINCIPLES: Flush phlegm and free the flow of the network vessels

RX: *Er Chen Tang* (Two Aged [Ingredients] Decoction) & *Tong Qiao Huo Xue Tang* (Free the Flow of the Orifices & Quicken the Blood Decoction) with additions and subtractions

INGREDIENTS: Radix Ligustici Wallichii (*Chuan Xiong*) and Radix Angelicae Dahuricae (*Bai Zhi*), 15g each, Rhizoma Pinelliae Ternatae (*Ban Xia*), 12g, Semen Pruni Persicae (*Tao Ren*), Flos Carthami Tinctorii (*Hong Hua*), Radix Rubrus Paeoniae Lactiflorae (*Chi Shao*), Sclerotium Poriae Cocos (*Fu Ling*), Pericarpium Citri Reticulatae (*Chen Pi*), 9g each, Radix Glycyrrhizae (*Gan Cao*), 3g, cooked Rhizoma Zingiberis (*Sheng Jiang*), 2 slices

ANALYSIS OF FORMULA: *Ban Xia, Fu Ling, Chen Pi, Gan Cao*, and *Sheng Jiang* all transform phlegm. *Chuan Xiong* moves the qi and quickens the blood, transforms stasis and stops pain, especially in the head and face. *Bai Zhi* courses wind in the face, especially in the large intestine and stomach channels. *Tao Ren, Hong Hua, Chi Shao*, and *Chuan Xiong* quicken the blood, transform stasis, and stop pain.

ADDITIONS & SUBTRACTIONS: For severe pain, add nine grams of Rhizoma Typhonii Gigantei (*Bai Fu Zi*) and three grams of Herba Asari Cum Radice (*Xi Xin*). For fixed pain, add three grams each of Eupolyphaga Seu Opisthoplatia (*Tu Bie Chong*) and Radix Pseudoginseng (*San Qi*), powdered and taken with the strained decoction. For numbness and insensitivity, add nine grams of Rhizoma Typhonii Gigantei (*Bai Fu Zi*) and five grams of Fructus Gleditschiae Chinensis (*Zao Jiao*). For stubborn pain which resists treatment, add two grams each of Buthus Martensi (*Quan Xie*) with tail and Scolopendra Subspinipes (*Wu Gong*) and three grams of Bombyx Batryticatus (*Jiang Can*), powdered and taken with the strained decoction. For spleen qi vacuity, add nine grams of Rhizoma Atractylodis Macrocephalae (*Bai Zhu*) and 15 grams of Radix Astragali Membranacei (*Huang Qi*). For vomiting of foamy, clear, thin phlegm, add three grams of Herba Asari Cum Radice (*Xi Xin*) and six grams of dry Rhizoma Zingiberis (*Gan Jiang*). For poor appetite, indigestion, or nausea from taking this decoction, add nine grams each of Fructus Germinatus Hordei Vulgaris (*Mai Ya*) and Fructus Citri Aurantii (*Zhi Ke*). For concomitant liver depression or any qi stagnation, add nine grams each of Pericarpium Citri Reticulatae Viride (*Qing Pi*) and Rhizoma Cyperi Rotundi (*Xiang Fu*) and five grams of Fructus Meliae Toosendan (*Chuan Lian Zi*).

ACUPUNCTURE & MOXIBUSTION: *He Gu* (LI 4), *San Yin Jiao* (Sp 6), *Feng Long* (St 40), local points based on the location of the pain. Please see pattern #1 above.

ANALYSIS OF FORMULA: *He Gu* is the ruling point for diseases of the face. Draining it moves the qi and stops pain in the face. Draining *San Yin Jiao* quickens the blood and dispels stasis throughout the entire body, especially when combined with *He Gu*. These two points strongly move the qi and quicken the blood in the face. Draining *Feng Long* transforms phlegm, while draining all the local points quickens the network vessels and stops pain.

ADDITIONS & SUBTRACTIONS: Please see pattern #1 above.

5. PHLEGM FIRE HARASSING ABOVE PATTERN

MAIN SYMPTOMS: Short duration oppression and pain or burning, distention, and pain often provoked by eating, a desire for something chilled to put on the affected area, dry mouth but no desire to drink, heavy-headedness, chest and abdominal oppression and distention, occasional vomiting of phlegm drool, sour fluid, or bitter bile, a bitter taste in the mouth, irritability and impatience, a red tongue with slimy, yellow fur, and a bowstring, slippery, rapid pulse

TREATMENT PRINCIPLES: Transform phlegm and clear heat, free the flow of the network vessels and stop pain

RX: *Huang Lian Wen Dan Tang Jia Wei* (Coptis Warm the Gallbladder Decoction with Added Flavors)

INGREDIENTS: Radix Ligustici Wallichii (*Chuan Xiong*) and Rhizoma Corydalis Yanhusuo (*Yan Hu Suo*), 15g each, Sclerotium Poriae Cocos (*Fu Ling*), 12g, Rhizoma Pinelliae Ternatae (*Ban Xia*), Pericarpium Citri Reticulatae (*Chen Pi*), Fructus Immaturus Citri Aurantii (*Zhi Shi*), Caulis Bambusae In Taeniis (*Zhu Ru*), bile-processed Rhizoma Arisaematis (*Dan Nan Xing*), Rhizoma Gastrodiae Elatae (*Tian Ma*), and Radix Salviae Miltiorrhizae (*Dan Shen*), 9g each, Rhizoma Coptidis Chinensis (*Huang Lian*), 6g, Radix Glycyrrhizae (*Gan Cao*), 3g, and Fructus Zizyphi Jujubae (*Da Zao*), 3 pieces

ANALYSIS OF FORMULA: *Ban Xia*, *Fu Ling*, *Chen Pi*, and *Gan Cao* are the ingredients of *Er Chen Tang* (Two Aged [Ingredients] Decoction) which is the main formula in Chinese medicine for transforming phlegm. *Zhu Ru* and *Dan Nan Xing* clear heat and transform phlegm, while *Zhi Shi* strongly moves the qi to help flush the phlegm. *Huang Lian*, greatly bitter and cold, strongly drains fire and clears heat. When combined with the preceding medicinals, *Tian Ma* treats wind phlegm obstructing the network vessels. *Chuan Xiong*, *Dan Shen*, and *Yan Hu Suo* strongly quicken the blood and transform stasis due to phlegm obstructing the network vessels. They also stop pain.

ADDITIONS & SUBTRACTIONS: For severe heat, add nine grams of Radix Scutellariae Baicalensis (*Huang Qin*) and 5 grams of Concretio Silicea Bambusae (*Tian Zhu Huang*). For stomach heat, add nine grams of Rhizoma Anemarrhenae Asphodeloidis (*Zhi Mu*) and 20 grams of Gypsum Fibrosum (*Shi Gao*).

ACUPUNCTURE & MOXIBUSTION: *He Gu* (LI 4), *Feng Long* (St 40), *Nei Ting* (St 44), local points based on the location of the pain. Please see pattern #1 above.

ANALYSIS OF FORMULA: *He Gu* is the ruling point for diseases of the face. Draining it moves the qi, clears heat, and stops pain in the face. Draining *Feng Long* transforms phlegm. When *Feng Long* is combined with *Nei Ting*, a key point for internal heat, they clear heat and transform phlegm. Also, *He Gu* is well-known for treating pain and heat better in the lower jaw, while *Nei Ting* is preferred for treating pain and heat in the upper jaw. Draining all the local points quickens the network vessels and stops pain.

ADDITIONS & SUBTRACTIONS: Please see pattern #1 above. If heat is due to liver depression transforming fire, replace *Nei Ting* with *Xing Jian* (Liv 2).

6. QI VACUITY & BLOOD STASIS PATTERN

MAIN SYMPTOMS: Enduring facial pain, continuous aching and pain for a long time, piercing pain which is difficult to bear, localized pain which does not move around, a dark, stagnant facial complexion, scaly skin if stasis is severe, possible tics accompanying or following the pain, numbness following the pain, fear of wind, spontaneous perspiration, scanty qi, disinclination to speak, a low, faint voice, a pale white tongue with possible static macules or spots, and a deep, fine, weak pulse

TREATMENT PRINCIPLES: Boost the qi and quicken the blood, free the flow of the network vessels and stop pain

RX: *Shun Qi He Zhong Tang Jia Wei* (Normalize the Qi & Harmonize the Center Decoction with Added Flavors)

INGREDIENTS: Radix Astragali Membranacei (*Huang Qi*) and Radix Ligustici Wallichii (*Chuan Xiong*), 15g each, Radix Codonopsitis Pilosulae (*Dang Shen*), Rhizoma Atractylodis Macrocephalae (*Bai Zhu*), Radix Angelicae Sinensis (*Dang Gui*), Radix Albus Paeoniae Lactiflorae (*Bai Shao*), Radix Rubrus Paeoniae Lactiflorae (*Chi Shao*), Lumbricus (*Di Long*), and Fructus Viticis (*Man Jing Zi*), 9g each, Pericarpium Citri Reticulatae (*Chen Pi*) and mix-fried Radix Glycyrrhizae (*Gan Cao*), 6g each, Rhizoma Cimicifugae (*Sheng Ma*), 4.5g, and Radix Bupleuri (*Chai Hu*) and Herba Asari Cum Radice (*Xi Xin*), 3g each

ANALYSIS OF FORMULA: *Shun Qi He Zhong Tang Jia Wei* is a modification of *Bu Zhong Yi Qi Tang* (Supplement the Center & Boost the Qi Decoction). *Huang Qi, Dang Shen, Bai Zhu,* and mix-fried *Gan Cao* supplement the center and boost the qi. *Chai Hu* and *Sheng Ma* upbear the yang qi for better nourishment of the face. *Chen Pi* rectifies the qi, while *Dang Gui* harmonizes the blood. In addition, *Huang Qi, Dang Gui,* and *Bai Shao* nourish the blood to replenish the vessels, while *Dang Gui, Chuan Xiong,* and *Chi Shao* quicken the blood and dispel stasis. *Man Jing Zi* and *Xi Xin* stop pain, especially in the head and face. *Di Long* frees the flow of the network vessels and stops pain.

ADDITIONS & SUBTRACTIONS: If enduring disease has entered the network vessels, add six grams each of Buthus Martensis (*Quan Xie*), Scolopendra Subspinipes (*Wu Gong*), and Bombyx Batryticatus (*Jiang Can*).

If there is only blood stasis and no qi vacuity, replace *Shun Qi He Zhong Tang* with *Tao Hong Si Wu Tang* (Persica & Carthamus Four Materials Decoction) and *Zhi Jing San* (Stop Tetany Powder) with additions and subtractions: Radix Ligustici Wallichii (*Chuan Xiong*), Lumbricus (*Di Long*), Radix Rubrus Paeoniae Lactiflorae (*Chi Shao*), and Cortex Radicis Moutan (*Dan Pi*), 15g each, Bombyx Batryticatus (*Jiang Can*), 12g, Radix Angelicae Sinensis (*Dang Gui*), Semen Pruni Persicae (*Tao Ren*), and Flos Carthami Tinctorii (*Hong Hua*), 9g each, and Buthus Martensis (*Quan Xie*) and Scolopendra Subspinipes (*Wu Gong*), 6g each. For severe pain, add 1 gram of Borneolum (*Bing Pian*), powdered and swallowed with the decoction.

ACUPUNCTURE & MOXIBUSTION: *He Gu* (LI 4), *San Yin Jiao* (Sp 6), *Zu San Li* (St 36), local points based on the location of the pain. Please see pattern #1 above.

ANALYSIS OF FORMULA: *He Gu* is the ruling point for diseases of the face. Draining it moves the qi and stops pain in the face. Draining *San Yin Jiao* quickens the blood and dispels stasis in the whole body. These two points strongly move the qi and quicken the blood in the face. Supplementing *Zu San Li* supplements the center and boosts the qi. Draining all the local points quickens the network vessels and stops pain

ADDITIONS & SUBTRACTIONS: Please see pattern #1 above.

7. YIN VACUITY-YANG HYPERACTIVITY & BLOOD STASIS PATTERN

MAIN SYMPTOMS: Recurrent episodes of severe, fixed, burning hot, one-sided face and head pain, afternoon tidal heat, malar flushing, dizziness, tinnitus, low back and knee soreness and limpness, vexation and agitation, red eyes, a red tongue with scanty, possibly yellow and/or dry fur, and a bowstring, fine, rapid pulse

TREATMENT PRINCIPLES: Supplement the kidneys and enrich yin, clear heat and free the flow of the network vessels

RX: *Di Yuan Shi Gao Tang* (Rehmannia, Scrophularia & Gyspum Decoction)

INGREDIENTS: Uncooked Radix Rehmanniae (*Sheng Di*), Gypsum Fibrosum (*Shi Gao*), and Radix Scrophulariae Ningpoensis (*Xuan Shen*), 30g each, Radix Albus Paeoniae Lactiflorae (*Bai Shao*), 24g, Resina Myrrhae (*Mo Yao*), 15g, Radix Et Rhizoma Notopterygii (*Qiang Huo*), 6g, and Herba Asari Cum Radice (*Xi Xin*) and Rhizoma Gastrodiae Elatae (*Tian Ma*), 3g each

ANALYSIS OF FORMULA: *Sheng Di* cools the blood division, while *Shi Gao* clears the qi division. Together, they drain vacuity fire due to yin vacuity. *Xuan Shen* and *Bai Shao* help the preceding medicinals nourish yin and clear vacuity heat. *Mo Yao* quickens the blood and dispels stasis. *Qiang Huo, Xi Xin,* and *Tian Ma* free the flow of the network vessels and stop pain, especially in the upper part of the body.

ADDITIONS & SUBTRACTIONS: If one-sided, upper face pain is severe, add 15 grams of Radix Ligustici Wallichii (*Chuan Xiong*). If one-sided, lower face pain is severe, add 15 grams of Rhizoma Anemarrhenae Aspheloidis (*Zhi Mu*). If there are facial tics, add 15 grams of Ramulus Uncariae Cum Uncis (*Gou Teng*) and six grams of Scolopendra Subspinipes

(*Wu Gong*). If there are red eyes and tearing, add 15 grams of Flos Chrysanthemi Morifolii (*Ju Hua*) and nine grams of Radix Scutellariae Baicalensis (*Huang Qin*).

If there is yin vacuity with internal stirring of liver wind as evidenced by pronounced numbness and spasm of the affected area, use *Tian Ma Gou Teng Yin Jia Wei* (Gastrodia & Uncaria Drink with Added Flavors) instead: Radix Albus Paeoniae Lactiflorae (*Bai Shao*), 30g, Ramulus Loranthi Seu Visci (*Sang Ji Sheng*) and Caulis Polygoni Multiflori (*Ye Jiao Teng*), 20g each, Ramulus Uncariae Cum Uncis (*Gou Teng*) and Concha Haliotidis (*Shi Jue Ming*), 18g each, Radix Cyathulae (*Chuan Niu Xi*) and Herba Leonuri Heterophylli (*Yi Mu Cao*), 15g each, Sclerotium Pararadicis Poriae Cocos (*Fu Shen*) and Fructus Tribuli Terrestris (*Bai Ji Li*), 12g each, and Rhizoma Gastrodiae Elatae (*Tian Ma*), Fructus Gardeniae Jasminoidis (*Zhi Zi*), Radix Scutellariae Baicalensis (*Huang Qin*), Fructus Corni Officinalis (*Shan Zhu Yu*), and Cortex Eucommiae Ulmoidis (*Du Zhong*), 9g each.

ACUPUNCTURE & MOXIBUSTION: *He Gu* (LI 4), *Fu Liu* (Ki 7), *San Yin Jiao* (Sp 6), local points based on the location of the pain. Please see pattern #1 above.

ANALYSIS OF FORMULA: *He Gu* is the ruling point for diseases of the face. Draining it moves the qi and stops pain in the face. *Fu Liu* is the kidney channel water point. Supplementing it enriches yin and supplements the kidneys. *San Yin Jiao* is the intersection point of the leg three yin. Supplementing it supplements spleen, liver, and kidney yin. Draining all the local points quickens the network vessels and stops pain.

ADDITIONS & SUBTRACTIONS: Please see pattern #1 above.

REMARKS

1. Because most cases of trigeminal neuralgia are complicated by blood stasis entering the network vessels, worm or insect medicinals, such as Buthus Martensis (*Quan Xie*), Scolopendra Subspinipes (*Wu Gong*), Bombyx Batryticatus (*Jiang Can*), and Lumbricus (*Di Long*), are important in the treatment of this condition.

2. Whenever this condition is complicated by heat, patients should be advised not to eat spicy, hot, greasy, fried, fatty foods or to drink alcohol. When phlegm complicates this condition, patients should be advised not to eat greasy, oily foods, such as diary products and fried foods, or to eat foods which damage the spleen and engender fluids, such as excessive sugars and sweets, oranges, and tomatoes.

3. Whenever this condition is due to or aggravated by emotional stress, anger, or frustration, the patient should be counseled on stress reduction techniques, such as deep relaxation and aerobic exercise. Biofeedback therapy may also be very helpful.

4. Both internally administered Chinese medicinals and acupuncture are extremely effective for this problem. Therefore, one can use either. Unless the condition is unusually recalcitrant to treatment, it is usually not necessary to use both treatment modalities in combination.

5. When treating this condition with acupuncture, some Chinese practitioners look for strong needle sensation, especially at *Xia Guan* (St 7), *Jia Che* (St 6), *Si Bai* (St 2), and *Zan Zhu* (Bl 2), and then retain the needle for one hour per session. If one only uses acupuncture to treat this condition, two sessions per week should be considered the minimum, with three being better, at least for the first 2-3 weeks. Although *Xia Guan* (St 7) is specific for the second and third branches of the trigeminal nerve, it is also effective for treating the first branch. To help reduce pain, one can also needle *Nei Guan* (Per 6) through to *Wai Guan* (TB 5) and add ear *Shen Men* and *Shen Ting* (GV 24). Since this disease may affect more than a single branch, it is important to use adequate and appropriate local points according to the different nerves affected.

6. Contemporary Chinese doctors have experimented with a number of new Chinese medicinals to cure this unbearably painful disease. We like the following formula which integrates probably the most effective medicinals for this condition. It can be prescribed along with any other formula which treats the root pattern of the disease. The formula's name is *Yu Tong San* (Curing Pain Decoction): Rhizoma Typhonii Gigantei (*Bai Fu Zi*), 100g, Radix Ligustici Wallichii (*Chuan Xiong*), 200g, Radix Angelicae Dahuricae (*Bai Zhi*), 200g, Buthus Martensis (*Quan Xie*), 150g, and Bombyx Batryticatus (*Jiang Can*), 200g. Grind these medicinals into a fine powder and take 3 grams two times per day mixed with a small amount of warm alcohol. Ten days equal one course of treatment and 2-3 courses are usually suggested for best effect. This formula is a simple modification of *Qian Zheng San* (Lead to Symmetry Powder) with *Chuan Xiong* and *Bai Zhi* added. As we have seen above, these two medicinals are famous for treating the pain of trigeminal neuralgia. Alcohol is used for leading the medicinals both upward and into the network vessels.

7. Many Chinese formulas for the treatment of pain and especially that of trigeminal neuralgia use Secretio Moschi Moschiferi (*She Xiang*). Although *She Xiang* is a very effective and powerful medicinal, it is very expensive and often difficult to obtain. Therefore, for the treatment of pain, some Chinese doctors substitute the pair of Herba Asari Cum Radice (*Xi Xin*) and Borneolum (*Bing Pian*) for *She Xiang*.

8. To know which branch of the trigeminal nerve is affected, in addition to observing the course of the pain, one can use the following simple method. If there is pain when one press-

es *Zan Zhu* (Bl 2) with the finger, the first branch is affected. If there is pain when *Si Bai* (St 2) is pressed, the second branch is affected, and if there is pain when *Da Ying* (St 5) is pressed, the third branch is affected.

9. As mentioned above under pattern #1, many Chinese acupuncturists routinely use electroacupuncture for the treatment of all patterns of this disease.

71

Ulcerative Colitis

Ulcerative colitis (UC) is a chronic, non-specific, inflammatory, and ulcerative condition of the large intestine characterized by diarrhea, tenesmus, and pus and blood in the stools. Nonspecific in the preceding sentence means that no specific microbial entity is involved. Colitis may afflict patients at any age. However, most cases occur between the ages of 15-30 with a smaller peak between 50 and 70 years of age. The disease usually starts in the recto-sigmoid area and may then extend proximally until the entire colon is involved or it may attack the entire colon all at once. The usual manifestations are a series of attacks of bloody diarrhea of varying intensity and duration interspersed with periods of asymptomatic remission. Most often, attacks begin insidiously with increased urgency to defecate, mild lower abdominal cramps, and the appearance of blood and mucus in the stools. Eventually, there may be 10-20 bowel movements per day as well as severe cramps and rectal tenesmus. In that case, there may be fatigue, malaise, anemia, anorexia, and weight loss. Patients with long-standing, extensive ulcerative colitis have an increased risk of colon cancer. Extracolonic complications include peripheral arthritis, ankylosing spondylitis, sacroiliitis, posterior uveitis, erythema nodosum, pyoderma gangrenosum, episcleritis, and, in children, severely retarded growth and development.

The Western medical diagnosis of ulcerative colitis is based on the patient's history, their presenting signs and symptoms, and stool examination. This presumptive diagnosis is then usually confirmed by sigmoidoscopy. In certain difficult cases, colonoscopy and biopsy may aid in assessing the extent of the disease. The Western medical treatment of this disease consists of avoidance of raw fruits and vegetables and a dairyless diet as well as antidiarrheal agents, such as diphenoxylate, diordorized opium tincture, loperamide, and codeine, and corticosteriods such as Prednisone. Severe disease with more than 10 bloody bowel movements per day may require hospitalization. Emergency colectomy is indicated for massive hemorrhage, fluminating toxic colitis, or perforation.

In terms of prognosis, a rapidly progressive initial attack may be fatal in nearly 10% of patients. Patients who develop this disease after 60 years of age have an especially poor prognosis, with mortality from severe attacks exceeding 25%. Complete recovery after a single attack may occur in another 10%. Nearly one third of all patients with extensive ulcerative colitis ultimately require surgery, while patients with localized ulcerative proctitis have the best prognosis. The incidence of colon cancer is greatest when the entire colon is involved and the disease has lasted for more than 10 years independent of disease activity.

Chinese disease categorization: This disease is categorized as *xie xie*, diarrhea, *tong xie*, painful diarrhea, *chi bai li*, red and white dysentery, *jiu li*, enduring dysentery, *chang pi*, intestinal afflux, *bian xue*, hemafecia, and *chang bi*, intestinal impediment.

Disease causes: The six environmental excesses, the seven affects, unregulated eating and drinking, and taxation fatigue

Disease mechanisms: Damp heat evils invade the body from the outside or damp heat may be engendered internally due to over-eating hot, spicy, greasy, fried, fatty foods and drinking alcohol. If damp heat pours downward to the large intestine it may affect the intestine's conveyance and conduction, thus resulting in diarrhea. If damp heat brews and damages the network vessels, there may be hemafecia. Damp heat may also be caused by liver depression transforming heat and spleen vacuity engendering dampness internally. If this dampness and heat combine, they may also form damp heat. The causes of liver depression are mainly unfulfilled desires and anger. However, liver depression may be aggravated by blood vacuity and/or yang vacuity. Spleen vacuity in Western patients is most commonly due to over-eating sugars and sweets and uncooked, chilled foods, overthinking and especially worry and anxiety, too little exercise, too much fatigue, and prolonged or over-use of antibiotics. In addition, because of menstruation, gestation, and lactation, women are more prone to spleen vacuity than men, while both men's and women's spleens become vacuous and weak with age.

If spleen vacuity reaches kidney yang, spleen qi vacuity may evolve into a spleen-kidney dual vacuity. If blood and fluid loss damages yin, there may be a qi and yin dual vacuity. If damp heat, damp turbidity, or qi stagnation endure, they may become complicated by blood stasis. Likewise, either liver depression or spleen vacuity may also be complicated by food stagnation.

TREATMENT BASED ON PATTERN DISCRIMINATION:

1. LIVER EFFULGENCE-SPLEEN VACUITY WITH DAMP OBSTRUCTION PATTERN

MAIN SYMPTOMS: Episodes of diarrhea brought about by worry, anxiety, frustration, or anger, diarrhea most often accompanied by abdominal pain which subsides after passing stools, possible mucus or pus in the stools, possible rib-side, chest, or breast distention and pain, irritability, sighing, burping and belching, menstrual irregularities in females, torpid intake, fatigue, cold hands and feet, a pale or sallow facial complexion, a commonly fat, pale but dark tongue with white fur, and a fine, bowstring pulse

NOTE: This pattern is extremely common in Western clinical practice. However, it rarely presents as colitis without at least one other disease mechanism.

TREATMENT PRINCIPLES: Course the liver and resolve depression, fortify the spleen and overcome dampness

RX: *Xiao Yao San* (Rambling Powder) & *Tong Xie Yao Fang* (Essential Formula for Painful Diarrhea) with additions and subtractions

INGREDIENTS: Radix Bupleuri (*Chai Hu*), Radix Albus Paeoniae Lactiflorae (*Bai Shao*), Rhizoma Atractylodis Macrocephalae (*Bai Zhu*), Sclerotium Poriae Cocos (*Fu Ling*), and Radix Angelicae Sinensis (*Dang Gui*), 12g each, Radix Ledebouriellae Divaricatae (*Fang Feng*), 9g, and mix-fried Radix Glycyrrhizae (*Gan Cao*), 6g

ANALYSIS OF FORMULA: *Bai Zhu*, *Fu Ling*, and mix-fried *Gan Cao* fortify the spleen and dry and disinhibit dampness, thus treating earth vacuity. *Chai Hu* and *Bai Shao* course and harmonize the liver and resolve depression, thus treating wood repletion. Together, they harmonize the liver and spleen by supplementing the spleen and draining the liver. *Dang Gui* nourishes liver blood and helps *Chai Hu* and *Bai Shao* to prevent further liver depression. *Fang Feng* dispels wind in the intestines, overcomes dampness, and stops pain. *Bai Shao* and *Gan Cao* relax spasms and stop pain.

ADDITIONS & SUBTRACTIONS: For liver depression transforming heat, add nine grams each of Radix Scutellariae Baicalensis (*Huang Qin*), Fructus Gardeniae Jasminoidis (*Zhi Zi*), and Cortex Radicis Moutan (*Dan Pi*). For more pronounced spleen qi vacuity, add nine grams of Radix Codonopsitis Pilosulae (*Dang Shen*). For enduring heat damaging stomach fluids, add 12 grams of Tuber Ophiopogonis Japonici (*Mai Men Dong*). For concomitant blood stasis, add nine grams of Radix Rubrus Paeoniae Lactiflorae (*Chi Shao*) and 15 grams of Rhizoma Corydalis Yanhusuo (*Yan Hu Suo*). For qi stagnation tenesmus, add nine grams each of Radix Auklandiae Lappae (*Mu Xiang*) and Semen Arecae Catechu (*Bing Lang*). For marked blood vacuity, add 15 grams each of Radix Astragali Membranacei (*Huang Qi*) and Caulis Milletiae Seu Spatholobi (*Ji Xue Teng*). For concomitant damp heat, add nine grams of Radix Scutellariae Baicalensis (*Huang Qin*) and three grams of Rhizoma Coptidis Chinensis (*Huang Lian*). If there is damp heat stasis and stagnation, add 15 grams each of Herba Patriniae Heterophyllae Cum Radice (*Bai Jiang Cao*) and Caulis Sargentodoxae (*Hong Teng*). If there are cold limbs, add six grams of Ramulus Cinnamomi Cassiae (*Gui Zhi*) and/or dry Rhizoma Zingiberis (*Gan Jiang*). For frequent anger, depression, insomnia, and emotional tension, add 15 grams each of Caulis Polygoni Multiflori (*Ye Jiao Teng*) and Cortex Albizziae Julibrissinis (*He Huan Pi*). For night sweats, pale lips and nails, anger, and emotional tension, add 15 grams each of Semen Zizyphi Spinosae (*Suan Zao Ren*) and Sclerotium Pararadicis Poriae Cocos (*Fu Shen*). For anxiety and poor memory and concentration, add 12 grams each of Sclerotium Pararadicis Poriae Cocos (*Fu Shen*), Semen Biotae Orientalis (*Bai Zi Ren*), and Semen Zizyphi Spinosae (*Suan Zao Ren*). For mental confusion due to phlegm and stasis blocking the orifices of the heart, add nine grams each of Tuber Curcumae (*Yu Jin*) and Rhizoma Acori Graminei (*Shi Chang Pu*).

For liver-spleen disharmony with simultaneous cold (vacuity cold) and heat (damp heat), replace *Xiao Yao San* and *Tong Xie Yao Fang* with *Wu Mei Wan Jia Wei* (Mume Pills with Added Flavors): Radix Albus Paeoniae Lactiflorae (*Bai Shao*), 18g, Fructus Pruni Mume (*Wu Mei*) and Fructus Meliae Toosendan (*Chuan Lian Zi*), 12g each, Radix Angelicae Sinensis (*Dang Gui*), Cortex Phellodendri (*Huang Bai*), Radix Auklandiae Lappae (*Mu Xiang*), and Ramulus Cinnamomi Cassiae (*Gui Zhi*), 9g each, Radix Panacis Ginseng (*Ren Shen*), dry Rhizoma Zingiberis (*Gan Jiang*), Radix Lateralis Prarparatus Aconiti Carmichaeli (*Fu Zi*), and Rhizoma Coptidis Chinensis (*Huang Lian*), 6g each, Herba Asari Cum Radice (*Xi Xin*) and Fructus Zanthoxyli Bungeani (*Chuan Jiao*), 3g each. For mucus in the stools, add

21 grams of Semen Coicis Lachryma-jobi (*Yi Yi Ren*) and nine grams of Semen Plantaginis (*Che Qian Zi*). For hemafecia, add 15 grams each of Radix Sanguisorbae (*Di Yu*) and Herba Agrimoniae Pilosae (*Xian He Cao*).

ACUPUNCTURE & MOXIBUSTION: *Nei Guan* (Per 6), *Gong Sun* (Sp 4), *Zu San Li* (St 36), *Tian Shu* (St 25), *Tai Chong* (Liv 3)

ANALYSIS OF FORMULA: Supplementing *Zu San Li*, the master point of the abdomen, supplements the spleen, boosts the qi, and stops diarrhea, while draining *Tai Chong*, the source point of the liver, courses the liver and resolves depression. Draining *Nei Guan* helps *Tai Chong* to course the liver, stop abdominal pain, and quiet the spirit. In addition, with *Gong Sun* (Sp 4), it harmonizes the stomach and intestines, rectifies qi, and stops diarrhea. With even supplementing-even draining technique, *Tian Shu* locally harmonizes the intestines, rectifies the qi, and stops pain.

ADDITIONS & SUBTRACTIONS: For severe emotional tension, tendency to worry, anxiety, frustration, or anger, add *Si Shen Cong* (M-HN-1) and *Shen Ting* (GV 24). For cold symptoms, also moxa *Zu San Li* (St 36), *Tian Shu* (St 25), and *Shen Que* (CV 8). Use salt or ginger indirect moxibustion on *Shen Que*. For heat symptoms, add *Nei Ting* (St 44) and *He Gu* (LI 4). For severe spleen qi vacuity, add *Tai Bai* (Sp 3). For food stagnation, add *Xuan Ji* (CV 21) and *Liang Men* (St 21). For kidney qi or yang vacuity, add *Ming Men* (GV 4) with moxibustion. For yin vacuity, add *Fu Liu* (Ki 7). For liver depression transforming heat, subtract *Tai Chong* and *Nei Guan* and add *Xing Jian* (Liv 2) and *Yang Ling Quan* (GB 34). In case of hemafecia, delete *Tian Shu* and replace it with *San Yin Jiao* (Sp 6).

2. DAMP HEAT BREWING IN THE INTESTINES PATTERN

MAIN SYMPTOMS: Abdominal pain and diarrhea with pus and blood, burning heat around the anus, tenesmus, foul-smelling stools, possible fever, a bitter taste in the mouth, possible nausea and vomiting, yellow urine, a red tongue with slimy, yellow fur, and a slippery, rapid pulse

NOTE: This pattern often describes acute attacks of ulcerative colitis in which liver depression and spleen vacuity have been complicated by damp heat evils typically due to a combination of increased stress and faulty diet.

TREATMENT PRINCIPLES: Clear heat and dry dampness, regulate the qi and harmonize the blood

RX: *Bai Tou Weng Tang* (Pulsatilla Decoction) & *Bai Shao Tang* (Peony Decoction) with additions and subtractions

INGREDIENTS: Radix Pulsatillae Chinensis (*Bai Tou Weng*), 30g, Cortex Ailanthi Altissimi (*Chu Gen Bai Pi*), 15g, Cortex Phellodendri (*Huang Bai*), Cortex Fraxini (*Qin Pi*), Radix Albus Paeoniae Lactiflorae (*Bai Shao*), Radix Rubrus Paeoniae Lactiflorae (*Chi Shao*), Radix Angelicae Sinensis (*Dang Gui*), and Fructus Immaturus Citri Aurantii (*Zhi Shi*), 9g each, Rhizoma Coptidis Chinensis (*Huang Lian*), 6g, and Cortex Magnoliae Officinalis (*Hou Po*), 3g

ANALYSIS OF FORMULA: *Bai Tou Weng, Chu Gen Bai Pi, Huang Bai, Qin Pi*, and *Huang Lian* all clear heat, and eliminate dampness, resolve toxins and stop diarrhea. In addition, *Qin Pi* and *Chu Gen Bai Pi* secure the intestines and stop diarrhea by astringing. *Bai Shao, Dang Gui*, and *Chi Shao* harmonize the blood and stop bleeding. In addition, *Bai Shao* stops diarrhea. *Zhi Shi* and *Hou Po* rectifies the qi to stop pain and relax tenesmus.

ADDITIONS & SUBTRACTIONS: If heat is more than dampness as evidenced by more marked bleeding, add 12 grams of uncooked Radix Rehmanniae (*Sheng Di*), and nine grams each of Cortex Radicis Moutan (*Dan Pi*) and Radix Sanguisorbae (*Di Yu*). If dampness is more than heat as evidenced by more marked mucus, add 21 grams of Semen Coicis Lachryma-jobi (*Yi Yi Ren*), and nine grams each of Rhizoma Atractylodis (*Cang Zhu*) and Rhizoma Pinelliae Ternatae (*Ban Xia*), and six grams of Pericarpium Citri Reticulatae (*Chen Pi*). For tenesmus, add nine grams each of Radix Auklandiae Lappae (*Mu Xiang*) and Semen Arecae Catechu (*Bing Lang*). For damp heat stasis and stagnation, add 15 grams each of Herba Patriniae Heterophyllae Cum Radice (*Bai Jiang Cao*) and Caulis Sargentodoxae (*Hong Teng*). If heat has damaged fluids, add 12 grams each of Radix Glehniae Littoralis (*Sha Shen*) and Tuber Ophiopogonis Japonici (*Mai Men Dong*). If there is concomitant qi vacuity, add 15 grams of Radix Astragali Membranacei (*Huang Qi*) and nine grams of Radix Codonopsitis Pilosulae (*Dang Shen*). For food stagnation, add nine grams each of Massa Medica Fermentata (*Shen Qu*) and Fructus Crataegi (*Shan Zha*).

ACUPUNCTURE & MOXIBUSTION: *Shang Ju Xu* (St 37), *He Gu* (LI 4), *Nei Ting* (St 44), *Yin Ling Quan* (Sp 9), *San Yin Jiao* (Sp 6)

ANALYSIS OF FORMULA: Draining *Shang Ju Xu, He Gu*, and *Nei Ting* clears the yang ming, rectifies the qi in the intestines, and stops diarrhea. Draining *Yin Ling Quan* and *San Yin Jiao* disinhibits dampness and stops diarrhea. At the same time, *San Yin Jiao* cools the blood and stops bleeding.

ADDITIONS & SUBTRACTIONS: For fever, add *Qu Chi* (LI 11).

3. SPLEEN-STOMACH VACUITY WEAKNESS PATTERN

MAIN SYMPTOMS: Occasional loose stools or diarrhea, a

disease course enduring for many days, recurrent relapses, mucus in the stools and/or occassional blood, slight abdominal pain, increased bowel movements due to eating oily, slimy foods, undigested food in the stools, fatigue, lack of strength, reduced food intake, torpid intake, venter oppression and abdominal distention after meals, a pale or possibly sallow facial complexion, prolapse of the rectum if severe, a pale tongue with white fur, and a moderate (*i.e.*, slightly slow), fine, weak pulse

Note: This pattern rarely presents in this discrete form in colitis. However, spleen vacuity does complicate many cases of colitis.

Treatment principles: Fortify the spleen and boost the qi, harmonize the center and transform dampness

Rx: *Shen Ling Bai Zhu San Jia Jian* (Ginseng, Poria & Atractylodes Powder with Additions & Subtractions)

Ingredients: Radix Codonopsitis Pilosulae (*Dang Shen*), Sclerotium Poriae Cocos (*Fu Ling*), and Semen Coicis Lachryma-jobi (*Yi Yi Ren*), 15g each, Semen Nelumbinis Nuciferae (*Lian Zi*), Rhizoma Atractylodis Macrocephalae (*Bai Zhu*), and Radix Dioscoreae Oppositae (*Shan Yao*), 12g each, Semen Dolichoris Lablab (*Bai Bian Dou*) and Pericarpium Citri Reticulatae (*Chen Pi*), 9g each, and mix-fried Radix Glycyrrhizae (*Gan Cao*), 6g

Analysis of formula: *Dang Shen, Fu Ling, Lian Zi, Bai Zhu*, mix-fried *Gan Cao, Shan Yao,* and *Bai Bian Dou* supplement the center, boost the qi, and stop diarrhea. *Fu Ling* and *Yi Yi Ren* seep dampness, *Bai Bian Dou* transforms dampness, *Bai Zhu* and *Chen Pi* dry dampness. In addition, *Chen Pi* harmonizes the stomach. All contribute to stopping diarrhea and treating mucous in the stools.

Additions & subtractions: If heat has not yet been completely eliminated, add nine grams of Rhizoma Coptidis Chinensis (*Huang Lian*) and six grams of Radix Auklandiae Lappae (*Mu Xiang*). If diarrhea is severe, add 30 grams of Hallyositum Rubrum (*Chi Shi Zhi*) and nine grams of Semen Myristicae Fragrantis (*Rou Dou Kou*). If eating and drinking are devitalized, add nine grams of Endothelium Corneum Gigeriae Galli (*Ji Nei Jin*).

If spleen qi vacuity is severe and dampness is not pronounced, replace *Shen Ling Bai Zhu San* with *Bu Zhong Yi Qi Tang Jia Jian* (Supplement the Center & Boost the Qi Decoction with Additions & Subtractions): Radix Astragali Membranacei (*Huang Qi*) and Radix Puerariae (*Ge Gen*), 15g each, Radix Codonopsitis Pilosulae (*Dang Shen*), Rhizoma Atractylodis Macrocephalae (*Bai Zhu*), and Sclerotium Poriae Cocos (*Fu Ling*), 9g each, Fructus Amomi (*Sha Ren*) and Fructus Immaturus Citri Aurantii (*Zhi Shi*), 6g each, Rhizoma Cimicifugae (*Sheng Ma*), 4.5g, and Radix Bupleuri (*Chai Hu*), 3g

Acupuncture & moxibustion: *Zu San Li* (St 36), *Tian Shu* (St 25), *Yin Ling Quan* (Sp 9), *Shen Que* (CV 8)

Analysis of formula: Supplementing *Zu San Li* and *Shen Que* with moxibustion, warms the spleen, boosts the qi, and stops diarrhea. Supplementing *Tian Shu* with moxibustion scatters cold and secures the intestines to stop pain and diarrhea. Draining *Yin Ling Quan* disinhibits dampness to stop diarrhea.

Additions & subtractions: For blood in the stools, subtract *Zu San Li* and *Tian Shu* and add *San Yin Jiao* (Sp 6), *Pi Shu* (Bl 20), and *Ge Shu* (Bl 17). For severe bleeding, add *Yin Bai* (Sp 1) with moxibustion. For undigested food in the stools, add *Xuan Ji* (CV 21) and *Liang Men* (St 21). For lower abdominal pain or distention, add *Qi Hai* (CV 6). For severe qi vacuity, add *Tai Bai* (Sp 3). For concomitant blood vacuity, add *San Yin Jiao* (Sp 6) and *Ge Shu* (Bl 17).

4. Spleen-kidney dual vacuity pattern

Main symptoms: Repeated occurrences of diarrhea over a long period of time, very thin, loose stools, slippery desertion and incontinence if severe, occasional dark, purplish blood and pus mixed in with the stools, a somber white facial complexion, low back and knee soreness and coolness, lack of warmth in the four limbs, fear of cold, dread of chill, fatigue, lack of strength, lassitude of the spirit, torpid intake, a pale, fat, enlarged tongue with white fur, and a deep, fine pulse

Note: This pattern is mostly seen in the elderly or as a complication of long-term use of corticosteriods.

Treatment principles: Warm and supplement the kidneys and spleen, secure and astringe and stop diarrhea

Rx: *Fu Zi Li Zhong Wan* (Aconite Rectify the Center Pills) & *Si Shen Wan* (Four Spirits Pills) with additions and subtractions

Ingredients: Radix Codonopsitis Pilosulae (*Dang Shen*), 12g, Radix Lateralis Praeparatus Aconiti Carmichaeli (*Fu Zi*), Rhizoma Atractylodis Macrocephalae (*Bai Zhu*), Semen Myristicae Fragrantis (*Rou Dou Kou*), Fructus Psoraleae Corylifoliae (*Bu Gu Zhi*), Fructus Evodiae Rutecarpae (*Wu Zhu Yu*), and Pericarpium Citri Reticulatae (*Chen Pi*), 9g each, and dry Rhizoma Zingiberis (*Gan Jiang*), Fructus Schisandrae Chinensis (*Wu Wei Zi*), and mix-fried Radix Glycyrrhizae (*Gan Cao*), 6g each

Analysis of formula: *Dang Shen, Bai Zhu,* and mix-fried *Gan Cao* supplement the spleen to stop diarrhea. *Gan*

Jiang, Wu Zhu Yu, Fu Zi, and *Rou Dou Kou* warm the spleen to stop diarrhea. *Fu Zi* and *Bu Gu Zhi* warm the kidneys to stop diarrhea. *Chen Pi* and *Bai Zhu* dry dampness. *Rou Dou Kou* and *Wu Wei Zi* secure and astringe to stop diarrhea.

ADDITIONS & SUBTRACTIONS: For enduring, incessant diarrhea, add five grams of Rhizoma Cimicifugae (*Sheng Ma*), 15 grams of Radix Astragali Membranacei (*Huang Qi*), and 12 grams of Radix Puerariae (*Ge Gen*). For tenesmus and uneasy defecation, add nine grams of Radix Auklandiae Lappae (*Mu Xiang*). For fecal incontinence, add 12 grams each of Fructus Terminaliae Chebulae (*He Zi*) and Fructus Pruni Mume (*Wu Mei*). For pus and blood in the stools due to concomitant damp heat and blood stasis, add 12 grams each of Radix Pulsatillae Chinensis (*Bai Tou Weng*) and Radix Salviae Miltiorrhizae (*Dan Shen*) and 15 grams of Herba Patriniae Heterophyllae Cum Radice (*Bai Jiang Cao*). For only blood in the stools due to qi vacuity not containing, add 15 grams each of Terra Flava Usta (*Fu Long Gan*), Herba Agrimoniae Pilosae (*Xian He Cao*), and Rhizoma Bletillae Striatae (*Bai Ji*) and replace *Gan Jiang* with blast-fried Rhizoma Zingiberis (*Pao Jiang*). For severe abdominal distention, add nine grams each of Fructus Amomi (*Sha Ren*) and Radix Auklandiae Lappae (*Mu Xiang*). For undigested food in the stools, add nine grams each of Massa Medica Fermentata (*Shen Qu*), Fructus Germinatus Hordei Vulgaris (*Mai Ya*), and Fructus Crataegi (*Shan Zha*).

ACUPUNCTURE & MOXIBUSTION: *Ming Men* (GV 4), *Shen Que* (CV 8), *Tian Shu* (St 25), *Zu San Li* (St 36)

ANALYSIS OF FORMULA: Moxaing *Ming Men* warms and supplements kidney yang, while moxaing *Shen Que* warms and supplements the spleen. This combination is well-known for stopping diarrhea due to spleen-kidney vacuity. *Zu San Li* is the master point of the abdomen and the uniting point of the stomach channel. Supplementing it supplements the spleen and dries dampness, stops pain and stops diarrhea. Supplementing *Tian Shu,* the front *mu* or alarm point of the large intestine, with moxibustion secures and astringes the intestines and stops diarrhea. In case of blood in the stools, only moxa *Tian Shu* without needling it.

ADDITIONS & SUBTRACTIONS: For blood in the stools, subtract *Zu San Li* and add *San Yin Jiao* (Sp 6), *Pi Shu* (Bl 20), and *Ge Shu* (Bl 17). For severe bleeding, add *Yin Bai* (Sp 1) with moxibustion. For pus in the stools, add *Yin Ling Quan* (Sp 9) and *Nei Ting* (St 44) and replace *Zu San Li* with *Shang Ju Xu* (St 37). For mucus in the stools, add *Yin Ling Quan* (Sp 9) and *Feng Long* (St 40). For undigested food in the stools, add *Xuan Ji* (CV 21) and *Liang Men* (St 21). For lower abdominal pain or distention, add *Qi Hai* (CV 6). For severe qi vacuity, add *Tai Bai* (Sp 3). For concomitant blood vacuity, add *San Yin Jiao* (Sp 6) and *Ge Shu* (Bl 17).

5. STOMACH & INTESTINES PHLEGM RHEUM PATTERN

MAIN SYMPTOMS: Watery diarrhea with or without foamy mucus, abdominal distention, borborygmus, possible heart palpitations and/or shortness of breath, the sound of water sloshing in the stomach when the abdomen is jiggled or palpated, profuse saliva, scanty urination, a pale tongue with glossy, white fur, and a soft, slippery pulse

NOTE: This pattern mostly describes the complication of excessive phlegm rheum due to spleen loss of control over movement and transformation.

TREATMENT PRINCIPLES: Warm the middle and seep dampness

RX: *Ling Gui Zhu Gan Tang Jia Jian* (Poria, Cinnamon, Atractylodes & Licorice Decoction with Additions & Subtractions)

INGREDIENTS: Semen Lepidii Seu Descuraniae (*Ting Li Zi*) and Semen Arecae Catechu (*Bing Lang*), 18g each, Radix Stephaniae Tetrandrae (*Han Fang Ji*) and Fructus Citri Aurantii (*Zhi Ke*), 15g each, Sclerotium Poriae Cocos (*Fu Ling*), 12g, Fructus Zanthoxyli Bungeani (*Chuan Jiao*) and Rhizoma Atractylodis Macrocephalae (*Bai Zhu*), 9g each, mix-fried Radix Glycyrrhizae (*Gan Cao*), 6g, Fructus Zizyphi Jujubae (*Da Zao*), 5 pieces, and Ramulus Cinnamomi Cassiae (*Gui Zhi*), 3g

ANALYSIS OF FORMULA: *Ting Li Zi* and *Fu Ling* transform phlegm. *Ting Li Zi* strongly expels phlegm accumulation, while *Fu Ling* fortifies the spleen and seeps dampness. *Bing Lang* and *Han Fang Ji* disinhibit water and disperse swelling. They help the two first medicinals to expel phlegm accumulated in the stomach and intestines. *Zhi Ke* moves the qi to help to disperse phlegm. *Gui Zhi* frees the flow of yang and transforms qi to disperse phlegm. *Bai Zhu* supplements the center, boosts the qi, and treats the root to prevent further phlegm engenderment. *Da Zao* and *Gan Cao* harmonize all the other ingredients in this formula, especially protecting the stomach against the harsh, attacking nature of *Ting Li Zi.*

ADDITIONS & SUBTRACTIONS: For concomitant severe spleen qi vacuity, replace *Ting Li Zi* with Sclerotium Polypori Umbellati (*Zhu Ling*) and add nine grams each of Rhizoma Atractylodis (*Cang Zhu*) and Rhizoma Pinelliae Ternatae (*Ban Xia*) and 15 grams of Radix Astragali Membranacei (*Huang Qi*). For severe diarrhea, add nine grams each of Fructus Amomi (*Sha Ren*) and Pericarpium Citri Reticulatae (*Chen Pi*) and 15 grams of Terra Flava Usta (*Fu Long Gan*). For profuse phlegm, add nine grams each of Pericarpium Citri Reticulatae (*Chen Pi*) and Rhizoma Pinelliae Ternatae (*Ban Xia*). For vomiting of clear water, add nine grams each of Flos Inulae Racemosae (*Xuan Fu Hua*), Pericarpium Citri Reticulatae (*Chen Pi*), and Rhizoma Pinelliae Ternatae (*Ban Xia*). For abdominal fullness and distention, add six grams each of Radix Auklandiae Lappae (*Mu Xiang*) and Fructus Amomi (*Sha Ren*). For dizziness, add 12 grams of stir-fried Rhizoma Gastrodiae Elatae (*Tian Ma*).

ACUPUNCTURE & MOXIBUSTION: *Zu San Li* (St 36), *Tian Shu* (St 25), *Yin Ling Quan* (Sp 9), *Feng Long* (St 40)

ANALYSIS OF FORMULA: Supplementing *Zu San Li* supplements the spleen and boosts the qi, dries dampness and treats the root, thus preventing the further production of new phlegm. It also stops diarrhea. With even supplementing-even draining technique, *Tian Shu* rectifies the qi and disperses phlegm in the intestines, secures the intestines and stops diarrhea. Draining *Yin Ling Quan* disinhibits dampness, while draining *Feng Long* transforms phlegm.

ADDITIONS & SUBTRACTIONS: Please see the additions and subtractions of the two preceding patterns.

6. QI & YIN DUAL VACUITY PATTERN

MAIN SYMPTOMS: Enduring diarrhea, bleeding, or damaged yin due to corticosteriods, yellow, watery diarrhea, bright red blood, lassitude of the spirit, fatigue, lack of strength, possible shortness of breath, vexation and agitation, short, scanty urination, dry skin, dry mouth, red lips, malar flushing, vexatious heat in the five hearts, a crimson tongue with no or scanty fluids, and a fine, rapid pulse

TREATMENT PRINCIPLES: Clear heat, nourish yin, and stop diarrhea

RX: *Lian Mei Tang Jia Wei* (Coptis & Mume Decoction with Added Flavors)

INGREDIENTS: Radix Glehniae Littoralis (*Sha Shen*), Radix Dioscoreae Oppositae (*Shan Yao*), and Semen Dolichoris Lablab (*Bai Bian Dou*), 12g each, Herba Dendrobii (*Shi Hu*), Radix Albus Paeoniae Lactiflorae (*Bai Shao*), and Fructus Pruni Mume (*Wu Mei*), 9g each, Radix Panacis Ginseng (*Ren Shen*) and mix-fried Radix Glycyrrhizae (*Gan Cao*), 6g each, and Rhizoma Coptidis Chinensis (*Huang Lian*), 3-4.5g

ANALYSIS OF FORMULA: *Sha Shen* and *Shi Hu* nourish yin. *Bai Shao* nourishes the blood, restrains yin, and stops diarrhea. *Wu Mei* engenders fluids and stops diarrhea. *Shan Yao, Bai Bian Dou*, mix-fried *Gan Cao*, and *Ren Shen* supplement the spleen and boost the qi. In addition, *Ren Shen* engenders fluids. *Huang Lian* clears heat and eliminates dampness.

ADDITIONS & SUBTRACTIONS: For more pronounced qi vacuity with fatigue and anemia, add 15 grams of Radix Astragali Membranacei (*Huang Qi*). For concomitant night sweats, add 12 grams of Concha Ostreae (*Mu Li*) and nine grams of Fructus Schisandrae Chinensis (*Wu Wei Zi*). For more pronounced heat, add nine grams of Cortex Phellodendri (*Huang Bai*) and 15 grams of Flos Lonicerae Japonicae (*Jin Yin Hua*). For simultaneous qi stagnation, add 12 grams of Fructus Meliae Toosendan (*Chuan Lian Zi*) and nine grams of Radix Auklandiae Lappae (*Mu Xiang*). For hemafecia due to heat, add nine grams each of Radix Rubiae Cordifoliae (*Qian Cao Gen*) and Radix Sanguisorbae (*Di Yu*). For hemafecia due to qi vacuity, add 15 grams of Radix Astragali Membranacei (*Huang Qi*) and 12 grams of Herba Agrimoniae Pilosae (*Xian He Cao*). For marked dampness, add 21 grams of Semen Coicis Lachryma-jobi (*Yi Yi Ren*) and nine grams of Semen Plantaginis (*Che Qian Zi*).

ACUPUNCTURE & MOXIBUSTION: *Zu San Li* (St 36), *Tian Shu* (St 25), *Yin Ling Quan* (Sp 9), *Fu Liu* (Ki 7), *San Yin Jiao* (Sp 6)

ANALYSIS OF FORMULA: Supplementing *Zu San Li* fortifies the spleen, boosts the qi, and stops diarrhea. Supplementing *Tian Shu* secures the intestines to stop pain and diarrhea. Draining *Yin Ling Quan* disinhibits dampness to stop diarrhea. Supplementing *Fu Liu*, the metal-mother point of the kidneys, engenders fluids and nourishes true yin. With even supplementing-even draining technique, *San Yin Jiao* nourishes yin blood, cools the blood, and stops bleeding.

ADDITIONS & SUBTRACTIONS: For night sweats, add *Yin Xi* (Ht 6). For severe yin vacuity, add *Wei Shu* (Bl 21) and *Shen Shu* (Bl 23). For severe blood in the stools, subtract *Zu San Li* and *Tian Shu* and add *Pi Shu* (Bl 20) and *Ge Shu* (Bl 17). For undigested food in the stools, add *Xuan Ji* (CV 21) and *Liang Men* (St 21). For severe qi vacuity, add *Tai Bai* (Sp 3).

7. BLOOD STASIS OBSTRUCTING THE NETWORK VESSELS PATTERN

MAIN SYMPTOMS: Right-sided lower abdominal aching and pain or pain which is fixed in location, palpable lumps in the lower abdomen, purplish black blood clots expelled with the stools, a dark, purplish tongue or possible static macules or spots, and a deep, bowstring, choppy pulse

NOTE: Blood stasis typically only complicates other patterns of this disease. It does not usually present in this pure form on Western patients.

TREATMENT PRINCIPLES: Quicken the blood and transform stasis, move the qi and stop pain

RX: *Shao Fu Zhu Yu Tang Jia Jian* (Lesser Abdomen Dispel Stasis Decoction with Additions & Subtractions)

INGREDIENTS: Rhizoma Corydalis Yanhusuo (*Yan Hu Suo*), 12g, Radix Angelicae Sinensis (*Dang Gui*), Radix Rubrus Paeoniae Lactiflorae (*Chi Shao*), Pollen Typhae (*Pu Huang*), Feces Trogopterori Seu Pteromi (*Wu Ling Zhi*), and Resina Myrrhae (*Mo Yao*), 9g each, Radix Ligustici Wallichii (*Chuan Xiong*) and Fructus Foeniculi Vulgaris (*Xiao Hui Xiang*), 6g each, dry Rhizoma Zingiberis (*Gan Jiang*) and Cortex Cinnamomi Cassiae (*Rou Gui*), 3g each.

ANALYSIS OF FORMULA: *Yan Hu Suo, Dang Gui, Chi Shao, Pu Huang, Wu Ling Zhi, Mo Yao,* and *Chuan Xiong* all quicken the blood, transform stasis, and stop pain. In addition, *Pu Huang* and *Wu Ling Zhi* stop bleeding. *Xiao Hui Xiang, Gan Jiang,* and *Rou Gui* warm the spleen and stop diarrhea. *Xiao Hui Xiang* moves the qi and stops abdominal pain.

ADDITIONS & SUBTRACTIONS: For spasmodic pain, add 15 grams each of Radix Albus Paeoniae Lactiflorae (*Bai Shao*) and Radix Glycyrrhizae (*Gan Cao*). For severe blood in the stools, add 12 grams each of Radix Rubiae Cordifoliae (*Qian Cao Gen*), Fructus Immaturus Sophorae Japonicae (*Huai Hua Mi*), and Radix Sanguisorbae (*Di Yu*).

ACUPUNCTURE & MOXIBUSTION: *Zu San Li* (St 36), *Ge Shu* (Bl 17), *Pi Shu* (Bl 20), *Da Chang Shu* (Bl 25), *San Yin Jiao* (Sp 6)

ANALYSIS OF FORMULA: Even supplementing-even draining *Zu San Li* and *Pi Shu* rectifies the qi in the intestines, stops pain, and stops diarrhea. Draining *Ge Shu, Da Chang Shu,* and *San Yin Jiao* quickens the blood and transforms stasis in the intestines, stops abdominal pain and stops diarrhea.

ADDITIONS & SUBTRACTIONS: For severe bleeding, add *Yin Bai* (Sp 1) with moxibustion.

REMARKS

1. Most cases of ulcerative colitis in Western patients manifest a combination of two or more disease mechanisms or patterns. The two most common concomitant patterns in our experience are damp heat and liver-spleen disharmony. Depending on the severity of the condition, this may then be complicated by blood stasis, damaged fluids, blood vacuity, or yin insufficiency. If corticosteroids have been used for a long time, there may also be a dual yin and yang vacuity. The following is a complex formula for a combination of spleen vacuity, intestinal qi stagnation, damp heat, blood vacuity, blood stasis, and marked bleeding but no particular mucus: *San Shen San Bai Tang* (Three *Shens* & Three Whites Decoction): Rhizoma Corydalis Yanhusuo (*Yan Hu Suo*) and Radix Salviae Miltiorrhizae (*Dan Shen*), 15g, Fructus Tribuli Terrestris (*Bai Ji Li*), 12g, Radix Codonpsitis Pilosulae (*Dang Shen*), Radix Sophorae Flavescentis (*Ku Shen*), Cortex Radicis Dictamni Dasycarpi (*Bai Xian Pi*), Fructus Kochiae Scopariae (*Di Fu Zi*), Semen Arecae Catechu (*Bing Lang*), Radix Auklandiae Lappae (*Mu Xiang*), Herba Agrimoniae Pilosae (*Xian He Cao*), and Radix Sanguisorbae (*Di Yu*), 9g each. It is offered as a model of a complex formula for a complex combination of patterns.

For chronic UC due to liver depression, spleen vacuity, damp heat, blood stasis, blood vacuity, and damaged fluids, use *Li Chang Tang* (Rectify the Intestines Decoction): Radix Albus Paeoniae Lactiflorae (*Bai Shao*) and Rhizoma Atractylodis Macrocephalae (*Bai Zhu*), 15g each, Radix Bupleuri (*Chai Hu*), Cortex Phellodendri (*Huang Bai*), and Radix Sophorae Flavescentis (*Ku Shen*), 9g each, Fructus Immaturus Citri Aurantii (*Zhi Shi*), Radix Auklandiae Lappae (*Mu Xiang*), Fructus Pruni Mume (*Wu Mei*), and Radix Glycyrrhizae (*Gan Cao*), 6g each. If there is severe qi stagnation, add 9 grams of Cortex Magnoliae Officinalis (*Hou Po*). For severe blood stasis, add 15 grams of Rhizoma Corydalis Yanhusuo (*Yan Hu Suo*). For severe diarrhea, add 9 grams of Pericarpium Punicae Granati (*Shi Liu Pi*). For severe dampness, add 9 grams of Herba Agastachis Seu Pogostemi (*Huo Xiang*). For severe damp heat, add 3 grams of Rhizoma Coptidis Chinensis (*Huang Lian*) and 12 grams of Radix Pulsatillae Chinensis (*Bai Tou Weng*). For severe bleeding, add 9 grams of Radix Sanguisorbae Officinalis (*Di Yu*) and 15 grams of Flos Immaturus Sophorae Japonicae (*Huai Hua Mi*). For severe spleen qi vacuity, add 12 grams of Radix Codonopsitis Pilosulae (*Dang Shen*). For concomitant kidney yang vacuity, add 9 grams each of Fructus Psoraleae Corylifoliae (*Bu Gu Zhi*) and Semen Myristicae Fragrantis (*Rou Dou Kou*).

2. Ulcerative colitis is usually accompanied by hemafecia, a species of pathological bleeding. There are only four possible causes of pathological bleeding in Chinese medicine: 1) heat causing the blood to move frenetically outside its channels, 2) qi vacuity not containing the blood within its vessels, 3) stasis forcing the blood to move outside its pathways, and 4) traumatic injury severing the channels and vessels. In ulcerative colitis, only the first three disease mechanisms are involved. In order to stop bleeding, it is often necessary to add blood-stopping medicinals. However, when doing this, one should be careful to choose medicinals which stop bleeding for the right reason. For instance, if there is rectal bleeding due to heat, Radix Rubiae Cordifoliae (*Qian Cao Gen*), Fructus Immaturus Sophorae Japonicae (*Huai Hua Mi*), and Radix Sanguisorbae (*Di Yu*) are often used. When there is bleeding due to qi vacuity, Herba Agrimoniae Pilosae (*Xian He Cao*) and Terra Flava Usta (*Fu Long Gan*) are often the medicinals of choice. And for bleeding due to blood stasis, Radix Pseudoginseng (*San Qi*) and Pollen Typhae (*Pu Huang*) are often prescribed. Since there are often two or even three of the above causes at work in many patients with ulcerative colitis, one may frequently have to choose blood-stopping medicinals from more than a single category.

3. If either diarrhea or hemafecia continue for a long time, enduring disease may have damaged the kidneys, with the kidneys' loss of control over sealing and storing and the two yin. In that case, one should add astringent medicinals to the formula. These include Fructus Pruni Mume (*Wu Mei*), Fructus Schisandrae Chinensis (*Wu Wei Zi*), Fructus Terminaliae Chebulae (*He Zi*), and Fructus Myristicae Fragrantis (*Rou Dou Kou*). However, these should not be added if replete damp heat evils have not been dispelled.

4. Pus in the stools indicate dampness. When blood in the stools is due to heat forcing the blood to move frenetically outside its channels, the proportion of pus to blood tells one the predominance of dampness or heat. Therefore, when there are pus and blood in the stools, one should always ascertain whether there is more pus and less blood or more blood and less pus.

5. The color of the stools is one indicator of the presence of heat. In general, evil heat makes the stools dark, while spleen vacuity typically turns the stools lighter than normal. However, if the stools are lighter than normal in color but are a bright yellow or mustard color accompanied by either a foul smell or anal burning and irritation, this indicates a combination of spleen vacuity and damp heat. Dark-colored, greenish stools indicate depressive heat.

6. Enemas often play an important part in the adjunctive Chinese medical treatment of ulcerative colitis. Enemas made from decocted Chinese medicinals have the benefits of A) getting the medicine to the affected area and B) using strongly attacking, frequently bitter, cold medicines without damaging the spleen and stomach. For instance, for damp heat brewing and binding in the intestines, one can make an enema by decocting 15 grams each of Radix Herba Portulacae (*Ma Chi Xian*) and Radix Scutellariae Barbatae (*Ban Zhi Lian*) and nine grams each of Radix Sanguisorbae (*Di Yu*) and Cortex Phellodendri (*Huang Bai*). Allow the decocted liquid to cool to body temperature and then retain for 20 minutes to one half hour one or two times per day. Typically, such adjunctive retention enemas are composed of heat-clearing, dampness-eliminating, heat-clearing, toxin-resolving, blood-cooling, bleeding-stopping, blood-quickening, stasis-transforming, and/or securing and astringing medicinals. Spleen and kidney supplementing medicinals are not typically administer *per anum*.

7. If there is blood in the stools, needling *Tian Shu* (St 25) is inadvisable.

72

UROLITHIASIS

Urolithiasis refers to stones within the urinary tract. These are also called urinary calculi and nephrolithiasis. Approximately one in 1,000 adults are hospitalized in the U.S. per year due to urinary calculi, and urinary tract stones can be found in one percent of all autopsies. These calculi may range in size from microscopic crystalline foci to stones which are several centimeters in diameter. Eighty percent of calculi in the U.S. are composed of calcium. The remainder are formed from magnesium ammonium phosphate. Stones within the urinary tract form because of supersaturation of the urine with calculus-forming salts. Causes of such supersaturation include over-excretion of salt, urine acidity, and low urine volume. Magnesium ammonium phosphate stones indicate the presence of a urinary tract infection caused by urea-splitting bacteria. This type of stone mostly occurs in women. Unfortunately, studies have shown that patients passing a first CA calculus are likely of forming a second stone at a rate of 15% within the first year, 40% within five years, and 50% within 10 years.

Although many renal calculi are asymptomatic, they commonly cause pain, hematuria, urinary obstruction, and secondary infection. The pain associated with urolithiasis tends to be excruciating and intermittent. It typically originates in the flank or kidney area and radiates across the abdomen along the course of the ureter. Calculi in the bladder may cause suprapubic pain. GI symptoms commonly include nausea, vomiting, and abdominal distention and may obscure the urinary origin of this condition. Chills and fever are also common.

The Western medical diagnosis of urolithiasis mostly depends on its clinical symptoms. Differential diagnosis includes appendicitis, cholecystitis, peptic ulcer, prancreatitis, ectopic pregnancy, and dissecting aneurysm. A current history of a high protein diet and supplemental intake of vitamins C and D may help clarify the picture. Urine may be normal. However, macroscopic or microscopic hematuria are common, and pyuria with or without bacteria may also be seen. Crystalline substances may be identified in the sediment, and most urinary calculi are demonstrable on x-ray. Renal ultrasonography may be helpful, and noncontrast spiral CT scan is useful in emergency room evaluation of acute flank or abdominal pain.

According to Western medicine, small, solitary calculi uncomplicated by infection or obstruction require no specific therapy. The Western medical treatment of symptomatic calculi consists of antibiotic treatment of bacteria causing urinary tract infection and/or narcotics, such as morphine or meperidine, for the relief of pain. Shock wave lithotripsy is the usual therapy for symptomatic calculi which are located in the renal pelvis or the ureter and are less than two centimeters in diameter. Percutaneous nephrolithotomy may be used to remove larger renal calculi and ureteroscopy may be used for larger urethral calculi. Occasionally, uric acid calculi in the upper or lower urinary tract may be dissolved by prolonged alkalinization of the urine. In order to prevent recurrence of calculi, thiazide diuretics are prescribed for patients with hypercalciuria. For patients with hypocitruria, oral alkali, such as potassium citrate, are prescribed. Prophylaxis for those with hyperoxaluria varies. Patients with small intestine disease can be treated with a combination of low oxalate, low fat diet, calcium loading, and cholestryamine. In hyperuricosuria, intake of meat, fish, and poultry should be reduced and allopurinol may be prescribed. In general, patients with a history of urolithiasis should increase their water consumption.

CHINESE DISEASE CATEGORIZATION: The clinical symptoms of urolithiasis mostly fall under the categories of *shi lin*, stone strangury, *sha lin*, sand strangury, and *xue lin*, bloody strangury, *yao tong*, low back pain, *xiao fu tong*, lower abdominal pain, *fu zhang*, abdominal distention, e *xin*, nausea, and *ou tu*, vomiting.

DISEASE CAUSES: External contraction of evils, unregulated eating and drinking, internal damage by the seven emotions, excessive bedroom taxation

DISEASE MECHANISMS: Due to a damp hot environment, external contraction of wind, damp, heat evils, overeating acrid, hot, fatty, sweet foods, lack of constancy between anger and joy, or excessive bedroom taxation, damp heat may be produced which then results in the internal engenderment of fire toxins. If damp heat pours downward to the bladder and stews and steams fluids and humors, these may congeal and bind, thus forming stones. Damp heat may also damage the spleen, leading to spleen qi vacuity and/or consume and damage yin, leading to kidney yin vacuity. If spleen qi vacuity reaches the kidneys, both the spleen qi and kidney yang may become damaged. Of course, kidney vacuity may also be directly due to excessive sex and/or aging.

If the stones block and obstruct the urinary pathways, the urine will not be able to be excreted smoothly or freely. In addition, if sand and stones gather and accumulate, they will hinder the free flow of qi and blood, thus resulting in pain. However, anger and/or emotional depression may also cause qi stagnation which may evolve into blood stasis. Nausea and vomiting may be due to both damp heat evils obstructing the middle burner and chaos of the qi due to extreme pain associated with blood stasis leading to disharmony of the stomach. If the heat of damp heat evils damages the network vessels and causes the blood to move frenetically outside its pathways, there will be hematuria. Hematuria may also be caused by vacuity heat and spleen qi vacuity failing to contain the blood within its vessels.

TREATMENT BASED ON PATTERN DISCRIMINATION:

1. LOWER BURNER DAMP HEAT PATTERN

MAIN SYMPTOMS: Frequent, urgent, numerous urination accompanied by burning heat and piercing pain, yellow-red colored or turbid urine, choppy, stagnant, unsmooth urination or dribbling, possible stopping and starting or the passage of blood, pus, sand, or stones, extreme low back pain possibly radiating to the lower abdomen and the genitalia, cold and heat (*i.e.*, fever and chills), a bitter taste in the mouth, nausea and vomiting, possible constipation, slimy, white or yellow tongue fur, and a slippery, rapid pulse

NOTE: This pattern is mostly seen in the initial stage of urinary tract stones or during acute attacks.

TREATMENT PRINCIPLES: Clear heat and disinhibit dampness, free the flow of strangury and expel stones

RX: *Ba Zheng San Jia Jian* (Eight Correcting [Ingredients] Powder with Additions & Subtractions)

INGREDIENTS: Talcum (*Hua Shi*), Semen Plantaginis (*Che Qian Zi*), and Herba Lysimachiae Seu Desmodii (*Jin Qian Cao*), 30g each, uncooked Radix Rehmanniae (*Sheng Di*), 18g, Herba Polygoni Avicularis (*Bian Xu*) and Herba Dianthi (*Qu Mai*), 15g each, Cortex Phellodendri (*Huang Bai*), Semen Vaccariae Segetalis (*Wang Bu Liu Xing*), Semen Abutilonis Seu Malvae (*Dong Kui Zi*), and Radix Cyathulae (*Chuan Niu Xi*), 12g each, and Caulis Akebiae (*Mu Tong*) and Radix Glycyrrhizae (*Gan Cao*), 3g each

ANALYSIS OF FORMULA: *Che Qian Zi, Hua Shi, Bian Xu, Qu Mai, Dong Kui Zi,* and *Mu Tong* all clear heat and disinhibit dampness. *Hua Shi* and *Jin Qian Cao* free the flow of strangury and expel stones. *Sheng Di* cools the blood and enriches yin to prevent heat from damaging yin. *Wang Bu Liu Xing* and *Chuan Niu Xi* quicken the blood, transform stasis, and stop pain. *Gan Cao* harmonizes the other medicinals in this formula and relaxes spasm or cramping.

ADDITIONS & SUBTRACTIONS: For hematuria, add 12 grams each of Rhizoma Imperatae Cylindricae (*Bai Mao Gen*) and Herba Cephalanoploris Segeti (*Xiao Ji*) and nine grams of Cacumen Biotae Orientalis (*Ce Bai Ye*). For nausea and vomiting, add nine grams each of ginger-processed Caulis Bambusae In Taeniis (*Zhu Ru*) and Rhizoma Pinelliae Ternatae (*Ban Xia*). For alternating fever and chills, add nine grams each of Radix Bupleuri (*Chai Hu*) and Radix Scutellariae Baicalensis (*Huang Qin*). For severe spasmodic pain, add 15 grams each of Radix Albus Paeoniae Lactiflorae (*Bai Shao*) and Rhizoma Corydalis Yanhusuo (*Yan Hu Suo*) and increase the dosage of *Gan Cao* up to nine grams. *Yan Hu Suo* can itself be replaced with six grams each of Radix Auklandiae Lappae (*Mu Xiang*) and Rhizoma Cyperi Rotundi (*Xiang Fu*) if necessary. For profuse sand or stones which cannot flow out, add 15 grams each of Spora Lygodii Japonici (*Hai Jin Sha*) and Folium Pyrrosiae (*Shi Wei*) and increase the dosage of *Jin Qian Cao* up to 30 grams. In this case, the patient must be relatively strong and the stone less than 0.5mm in diameter. For constipation and yellow, scanty urine, add six grams of Radix Et Rhizoma Rhei (*Da Huang*) and 12 grams of Fructus Gardeniae Jasminoidis (*Zhi Zi*).

If the urine is yellow, turbid, and foul-smelling and there are red eyes, a bitter taste in the mouth, heart vexation, and easy anger plus a bowstring, slippery, rapid pulse, replace *Ba Zheng San* with *Long Dan Xie Gan Tang Jia Wei* (Gentiana Drain the Liver Decoction with Added Flavors): Herba Desmodii Styrachifolii (*Jin Qian Cao*), 15g, Endothelium Corneum Gigeriae Galli (*Ji Nei Jin*), uncooked Radix Rehmanniae (*Sheng Di*), and Radix Scutellariae Baicalensis (*Huang Qin*), 12g each, Fructus Gardeniae Jasminoidis (*Zhi Zi*), Caulis Akebiae (*Mu Tong*), Spora Lygodii Japonici (*Hai Jin Sha*), Rhizoma Alismatis (*Ze Xie*), Extremitas Radicis Angelicae Sinensis (*Dang Gui Wei*), Radix Bupleuri (*Chai Hu*), and Semen Plantaginis (*Che Qian Zi*), 9g each, Radix

Gentianae Scabrae (*Long Dan Cao*), 6g, and Radix Glycyrrhizae (*Gan Cao*), 3g.

If heat toxins have entered the blood and spread throughout the three burners, treat the branch in emergency by replacing *Ba Zheng San* with *Huang Lian Jie Du Tang* (Coptis Resolve Toxins Decoction) plus *Wu Wei Xiao Du Yin* (Five Flavors Disperse Toxins Drink): Flos Lonicerae Japonicae (*Jin Yin Hua*), Herba Taraxaci Mongolicii Cum Radice (*Pu Gong Ying*), and Herba Violae Yedoensitis Cum Radice (*Zi Hua Di Ding*), 15g each, Flos Chrysanthemi Indici (*Ye Ju Hua*) and Radix Scutellariae Baicalensis (*Huang Qin*), 12g each, Semen Semiaquilegiae (*Tian Kui Zi*), Cortex Phellodendri (*Huang Bai*), and Fructus Gardenisae Jasminoidis (*Zhi Zi*), 9g each, and Rhizoma Coptidis Chinensis (*Huang Lian*), 6g.

ACUPUNCTURE & MOXIBUSTION: *Jing Men* (GB 25), *Shen Shu* (Bl 23), *Wei Yang* (Bl 39), *Ran Gu* (Ki 2)

ANALYSIS OF FORMULA: The above formula is made up of two important combinations to clear heat and disinhibit dampness, free the flow of strangury, expel stones, and stop pain: *Jing Men* plus *Shen Shu* and *Wei Yang* plus *Ran Gu*. These points should be drained with strong stimulation or use electroacupuncture. Each session may last 1-3 hours, with 1-2 treatments per day.

ADDITIONS & SUBTRACTIONS: For extreme low back pain radiating to the lower abdomen and/or the genitalia, add *Shui Quan* (Ki 5), a key point for pain during the crisis of nephrolithiasis. After 30 minutes of strongly manipulating *Shui Quan*, replace it with *Jing Ling* (also named *Jing Ning*), an extrachannel point located on the dorsum of the hand, midway between the fourth and fifth metacarpal bones in a depression more or less 1.5 cun distal to the crease of the wrist. If there is marked urinary tract infection due to damp heat, add *Zhong Ji* (CV 3). If there is less pain but more urinary symptoms, replace *Wei Yang* and *Ran Gu* with *Pang Guang Shu* (Bl 28) and *Zhong Ji* (CV 3). After the crisis, if sand or small stones remain, replace *Wei Yang* and *Ran Gu* with *Zu San Li* (St 36) and continue treating once per day.

2. QI STAGNATION & BLOOD STASIS PATTERN

MAIN SYMPTOMS: Choppy, stagnant urination which dribbles and drips uneasily, blood clots within the urine or dark red blood, lower abdominal distention and pain or lancinating pain, possible excruciatingly severe low back pain, a normal or dark, purplish tongue or possible static macules or spots, and a deep, bowstring, possibly choppy pulse

TREATMENT PRINCIPLES: Move the qi and quicken the blood, free the flow of strangury and expel stones

RX: *Chen Xiang San* (Aquilaria Powder) plus *Xue Fu Zhu Yu Tang* (Blood Mansion Dispel Stasis Decoction) with additions and subtractions

INGREDIENTS: Semen Pruni Persicae (*Tao Ren*), uncooked Radix Rehmanniae (*Sheng Di*), Endothelium Corneum Gigeriae Galli (*Ji Nei Jin*), and Lignum Aquilariae Agallochae (*Chen Xiang*), 12g each, Flos Carthami Tinctorii (*Hong Hua*), Radix Angelicae Sinensis (*Dang Gui*), Radix Ligustici Wallichii (*Chuan Xiong*), Radix Rubrus Paeoniae Lactiflorae (*Chi Shao*), Radix Cyathulae (*Chuan Niu Xi*), Semen Arecae Catechu (*Bing Lang*), Sclerotium Rubrum Poriae Cocos (*Chi Fu Ling*), Fructus Foeniculi Vulgaris (*Xiao Hui Xiang*), and Radix Auklandiae Lappae (*Mu Xiang*), 9g each, Fructus Citri Aurantii (*Zhi Ke*), 6g, and Radix Glycyrrhizae (*Gan Cao*), 3g

ANALYSIS OF FORMULA: *Tao Ren, Hong Hua, Dang Gui, Chuan Xiong, Chi Shao,* and *Chuan Niu Xi* quicken the blood, transform stasis, and stop pain. *Chen Xiang, Bing Lang, Xiao Hui Xiang, Mu Xiang,* and *Zhi Ke* move the qi, especially in the lower burner, eliminate distention, and stop pain. *Sheng Di* cools the blood, nourishes yin, and stops bleeding. *Chi Fu Ling* clears and disinhibits dampness and heat, and *Ji Nei Jin* transforms stones.

ADDITIONS & SUBTRACTIONS: If blood stasis is marked or when pain is severe, add nine grams each of Resina Olibani (*Ru Xiang*) and Resina Myrrhae (*Mo Yao*). If there is chest oppression and rib-side pain, add 12 grams of Radix Albus Paeoniae Lactiflorae (*Bai Shao*), replace *Zhi Ke* with Fructus Immaturus Citri Aurantii (*Zhi Shi*) and raise its dose to nine grams, and add nine grams of Radix Bupleuri (*Chai Hu*). For blood clots within the urine, add three grams of Radix Pseudoginseng (*San Qi*), powdered and taken with the strained decoction. For hematuria, add 12 grams each of Rhizoma Imperatae Cylindricae (*Bai Mao Gen*) and Herba Cephalanoploris Segeti (*Xiao Ji*) and nine grams of Radix Sanguisorbae Officinalis (*Di Yu*). For profuse sand or stones, add 30 grams each of Herba Lysimachiae Seu Desmodii (*Jin Qian Cao*) and Semen Plantaginis (*Che Qian Zi*). For nausea or vomiting, add nine grams each of Rhizoma Pinelliae Ternatae (*Ban Xia*), uncooked Rhizoma Zingiberis (*Sheng Jiang*), and Pericarpium Citri Reticulatae (*Chen Pi*).

ACUPUNCTURE & MOXIBUSTION: Please see pattern #1 above.

3. SPLEEN-KIDNEY QI VACUITY PATTERN

MAIN SYMPTOMS: Somewhat red and choppy urination with dribbling and dripping that does not stop, recurrent attacks which come and go and which tend to be brought on by over-taxation, possible fine sand or stones expelled with the urine, possibly slightly painful urination with a hollow or empty feeling of pain which is better with pressure and worse with exertion or taxation, fatigue, abdominal distention, loose stools, low back and knee pain and limpness, lassitude of the spirit, lack of strength, a pale tongue, and a fine, weak pulse

Note: This pattern is mostly seen in those with enduring urinary tract stones which have not healed. In this case, evils have consumed and damaged the righteous qi.

Treatment principles: Fortify the spleen and boost the kidneys, supplement the qi and disperse stones

Rx: *Wu Bi Shan Yao Tang Jia Jian* (Incomparable Dioscorea Decoction with Additions & Subtractions)

Ingredients: Herba Lysimachiae Seu Desmodii (*Jin Qian Cao*) and Spora Lygodii Japonici (*Hai Jin Sha*), 30g each, Fructus Corni Officinalis (*Shan Zhu Yu*), 18g, cooked Radix Rehmanniae (*Shu Di*) and Radix Achyranthis Bidentatae (*Niu Xi*), 12g each, Radix Dioscoreae Oppositae (*Shan Yao*), Semen Cuscutae Chinensis (*Tu Si Zi*), Fructus Schisandrae Chinensis (*Wu Wei Zi*), Sclerotium Poriae Cocos (*Fu Ling*), Herba Cistanchis Deserticolae (*Rou Cong Rong*), Cortex Radicis Moutan (*Dan Pi*), Rhizoma Acori Graminei (*Shi Chang Pu*), Endothelium Corneum Gigeriae Galli (*Ji Nei Jin*), and Semen Plantaginis (*Che Qian Zi*), 9g each, and Radix Lateralis Praeparatus Aconiti Carmichaeli (*Fu Zi*) and Cortex Cinnamomi Cassiae (*Rou Gui*), 6g each

Analysis of formula: *Shu Di, Shan Zhu Yu, Niu Xi, Shan Yao, Tu Si Zi, Wu Wei Zi, Rou Cong Rong, Fu Zi*, and *Rou Gui* together supplement kidney qi, yin, and yang. *Shan Yao* and *Fu Ling* fortify the spleen and boost the qi. *Jin Qian Cao, Hai Jin Sha, Fu Ling, Che Qian Zi*, and *Ji Nei Jin* together disinhibit urination and disperse stones. *Shi Chang Pu* dries dampness and abducts turbidity. *Dan Pi* quickens the blood and transforms stasis.

Additions & subtractions: Without marked signs of cold, delete *Rou Gui* and *Fu Zi*. For pronounced fatigue due to spleen qi vacuity, add 15 grams of Radix Astragali Membranacei (*Huang Qi*) and nine grams of Radix Codonopsitis Pilosulae (*Dang Shen*). If concomitant blood stasis is pronounced, add 15 grams of Radix Salviae Miltiorrhizae (*Dan Shen*). For simultaneous hematuria, add 15 grams each of Herba Cephalanoploris Segeti (*Xiao Ji*) and Herba Cirsii Japonici (*Da Ji*) and nine grams of Radix Sanguisorbae (*Di Yu*).

Acupuncture & moxibustion: *Jing Men* (GB 25), *Shen Shu* (Bl 23), *Zu San Li* (St 36)

Analysis of formula: This formula is an empirical combination for supplementing the spleen and kidneys, freeing the flow of strangury, and expelling stones. Supplementing *Shen Shu* and *Zu San Li* supplements the spleen and kidneys, while draining *Jing Men* frees the flow of strangury and expels stones. One may also use electroacupuncture on *Jing Men* and *Shen Shu*. Treat once every three days.

Additions & subtractions: For occasional low back pain radiating to the lower abdomen and/or the genitalia, add *Shui Quan* (Ki 5). If there is frequent, urgent, difficult urination, add *Guan Yuan* (CV 4). If sand or small stones remain, add *Qi Hai Shu* (Bl 24) and *Pang Guang Shu* (Bl 28) with electroacupuncture. For severe spleen qi vacuity, add *Tai Bai* (Sp 3). For severe kidney qi vacuity, add *Tai Xi* (Ki 3). For stomach and abdominal distention, flatulence, reduced appetite, and nausea, add *Nei Guan* (Per 6) and *Gong Sun* (Sp 4).

4. Liver-kidney yin vacuity pattern

Main symptoms: Low back and knee pain and limpness, dizziness, tinnitus, tidal fever, night sweats, malar flushing, red lips, a dry mouth and parched throat, dribbling and dripping, uncrisp urination, possible discharge of sand or stones, a red tongue with scanty or no fur, and a deep, fine, rapid pulse

Note: In this pattern's case, mostly enduring damp heat has damaged and consumed yin and essence.

Treatment principles: Enrich yin and clear heat, boost the kidneys and disperse stones

Rx: *Yi Shen Pai Shi Tang Jia Jian* (Boost the Kidneys & Expel Stones Decoction with Additions & Subtractions)

Ingredients: Cooked Radix Rehmanniae (*Shu Di*), Spora Lygodii Japonici (*Hai Jin Sha*), Herba Pyrrosiae (*Shi Wei*), Rhizoma Alismatis (*Ze Xie*), and Talcum (*Hua Shi*), 30g each, processed Radix Polygoni Multiflori (*He Shou Wu*), 20g, Ramulus Loranthi Seu Visci (*Sang Ji Sheng*) and Cortex Radicis Moutan (*Dan Pi*), 15g each, and Radix Angelicae Sinensis (*Dang Gui*), Cortex Eucommiae Ulmoidis (*Du Zhong*), and Rhizoma Imperatae Cylindricae (*Bai Mao Gen*), 12g each

Analysis of formula: *Shu Di, He Shou Wu, Sang Ji Sheng, Dang Gui*, and *Du Zhong* supplement the liver and kidneys, nourish the blood and enrich yin. *Hai Jin Sha, Shi Wei, Ze Xie*, and *Bai Mao Gen* disinhibit urination and disperse stones. *Dan Pi* clears heat and quickens the blood.

Additions & subtractions: If there is effulgent fire, add nine grams each of Rhizoma Anemarrhenae Aspheloidis (*Zhi Mu*) and Cortex Phellodendri (*Huang Bai*). If there is heart vexation and heat in the hands, feet, and heart, add 12 grams of Tuber Asparagi Cochinensis (*Tian Men Dong*) and nine grams of Fructus Gardeniae Jasminoidis (*Zhi Zi*). If there are enduring, non-healing stones, add 15 grams of

Herba Lysimachiae Seu Desmodii (*Jin Qian Cao*) and nine grams of Endothelium Corneum Gigeriae Galli (*Ji Nei Jin*). If yin damage has reached yang, add nine grams each of Fructus Psoraleae Corylifoliae (*Bu Gu Zhi*), Herba Epimedii (*Yin Yang Huo*), and Rhizoma Curculiginis Orchioidis (*Xian Mao*). For simultaneous hematuria, add 15 grams each of Herba Cephalanoploris Segeti (*Xiao Ji*) and Herba Cirsii Japonici (*Da Ji*) and nine grams of Radix Sanguisorbae (*Di Yu*).

ACUPUNCTURE & MOXIBUSTION: *Jing Men* (GB 25), *Shen Shu* (Bl 23), *Tai Xi* (Ki 3)

ANALYSIS OF FORMULA: Supplementing *Shen Shu* supplements the kidneys, while draining *Jing Men* frees the flow of strangury and expels stones. One may also use electroacupuncture on *Jing Men* and *Shen Shu*. Using even supplementing-even draining technique on *Tai Xi* enriches kidney yin and disperse stones. It is also a main point for the treatment of urinary calculi. Treat once every three days.

ADDITIONS & SUBTRACTIONS: For occasional low back pain radiating to the lower abdomen and/or the genitalia, add *Shui Quan* (Ki 5). If frequent, urgent, difficult urination, add *Guan Yuan* (CV 4). If sand or small stones remain, add *Qi Hai Shu* (Bl 24) and *Pang Guang Shu* (Bl 28) with electroacupuncture. For concomitant spleen qi vacuity, add *Zu San Li* (St 36). For severe kidney yin vacuity, add *Fu Liu* (Ki 7).

5. KIDNEY YANG DEBILITY & DETRIMENT PATTERN

MAIN SYMPTOMS: Low back and knee soreness and limpness, fatigue, lack of strength, fear of cold, chilled limbs, frequent, numerous urination, forceless expulsion of urine, turbid, light-colored urine, possible terminal dribbling and/or slight pain, nocturia, possible occasional discharge of sand or stones, a somber white facial complexion, a pale tongue, and a deep, fine pulse

TREATMENT PRINCIPLES: Warm and supplement kidney yang, free the flow of strangury and disperse stones

RX: *Jin Gui Shen Qi Wan Jia Wei* (*Golden Cabinet* Kidney Qi Pills with Added Flavors)

INGREDIENTS: Herba Lysimachiae Seu Desmodii (*Jin Qian Cao*) and Spora Lygodii Japonici (*Hai Jin Sha*), 30g each, cooked Radix Rehmanniae (*Shu Di*), 15g, Fructus Corni Officinalis (*Shan Zhu Yu*), 12g, Radix Dioscoreae Oppositae (*Shan Yao*), Sclerotium Poriae Cocos (*Fu Ling*), Rhizoma Alismatis (*Ze Xie*), Radix Achyranthis Bidentatae (*Niu Xi*), and Fructus Immaturus Citri Aurantii (*Zhi Shi*), 9g each, Ramulus Cinnamomi Cassiae (*Gui Zhi*) and Radix Lateralis Praeparatus Aconiti Carmichaeli (*Fu Zi*), 6g each

ANALYSIS OF FORMULA: *Shu Di*, *Shan Zhu Yu*, *Shan Yao*, *Niu Xi*, *Gui Zhi*, and *Fu Zi* together supplement both the yin and yang of the kidneys. *Jin Qian Cao*, *Hai Jin Sha*, *Fu Ling*, *Ze Xie*, and *Zhi Shi* together disinhibit urination and disperse stones.

ADDITIONS & SUBTRACTIONS: If there are enduring, nonhealing stones, add nine grams of Endothelium Corneum Gigeriae Galli (*Ji Nei Jin*). For stones in the upper urinary tract, add 15 grams each of Radix Astragali Membranacei (*Huang Qi*), Radix Cyathulae (*Chuan Niu Xi*), and Radix Salviae Miltiorrhizae (*Dan Shen*). For stones in the lower urinary tract, add 15 grams of Semen Abutili Seu Malvae (*Dong Kui Zi*) and five grams of Caulis Akebiae (*Mu Tong*). For simultaneous hematuria, add 15 grams each of Herba Cephalanoploris Segeti (*Xiao Ji*) and Herba Cirsii Japonici (*Da Ji*) and nine grams of Radix Sanguisorbae (*Di Yu*). For severe kidney yang vacuity, add nine grams of Herba Epimedii (*Yin Yang Huo*). For concomitant spleen qi vacuity, add 15 grams of Radix Astragali Membranacei (*Huang Qi*), nine grams of Radix Codonopsitis Pilosulae (*Dang Shen*), and five grams each of Radix Bupleuri (*Chai Hu*) and Rhizoma Cimicifugae (*Sheng Ma*). For low back pain, add 12 grams each of Ramulus Loranthi Seu Visci (*Sang Ji Sheng*), Radix Dipsaci (*Xu Duan*), and Rhizoma Cibotii Barometsis (*Gou Ji*). For concomitant damp heat, add nine grams each of Cortex Phellodendri (*Huang Bai*), Rhizoma Anemarrhenae Asphodeloidis (*Zhi Mu*), and Semen Plantaginis (*Che Qian Zi*).

ACUPUNCTURE & MOXIBUSTION: *Jing Men* (GB 25), *Shen Shu* (Bl 23), *Tai Xi* (Ki 3), *Guan Yuan* (CV 4)

ANALYSIS OF FORMULA: Supplementing *Shen Shu* and *Guan Yuan* with moxibustion supplements the kidneys and invigorates yang. Draining *Jing Men* frees the flow of strangury and disperses stones. Even supplementation-even draining on *Tai Xi* boosts the kidney qi at the same time as it disperses stones. Electroacupuncture may also be used on *Jing Men* and *Shen Shu*. Treat once every three days.

ADDITIONS & SUBTRACTIONS: For occasional low back pain radiating to the lower abdomen and/or the genitalia, add *Shui Quan* (Ki 5). If there is frequent, urgent, difficult urination, add *San Yin Jiao* (Sp 6). If sand or small stones remain, add *Qi Hai Shu* (Bl 24) and *Pang Guang Shu* (Bl 28) with electroacupuncture. For concomitant spleen qi vacuity, add *Zu San Li* (St 36). For severe kidney yin vacuity, add *Fu Liu* (Ki 7).

REMARKS

1. Patients with kidney stones generally say that the pain associated with the movement of stones in the urinary tract is the worse pain they have ever experienced. Therefore, during acute attacks, everything possible should be done to pro-

mote pain relief. Electroacupuncture and ear acupuncture should both be employed. Each acupuncture session can last 1-3 hours. When strong stimulation is used, acupuncture is usually effective for relieving the pain of acute crises and, according to our experience, is even often more effective than Western medicine. In addition, intense, sharp, lancinating pain indicates blood stasis. Blood-quickening medicinals appropriate for the treatment of kidney stones accompanied by severe pain include Squama Manitis Pentadactylis (*Chuan Shan Jia*), Rhizoma Sparganii (*San Leng*), Rhizoma Curcumae Zedoariae (*E Zhu*), Spina Gleditschiae Chinensis (*Zao Jiao Ci*), Resina Olibani (*Ru Xiang*), and Resina Myrrhae (*Mo Yao*).

2. Patients with urolithiasis should generally drink a lot of water.

3. In China, Chinese medicinals combined with electroacupuncture and Western medications, such as atropine and dihydrochlorothiazide, are used conjunctively for the treatment of this condition in cases where the stones are less than one centimeter in diameter and there is no serious concomitant urinary tract infection. In that case, Chinese medicinals and Western drugs are given every day and electroacupuncture is given twice a week for 6-8 treatments. After a 1-2 week rest, a second course of treatment may be administered if necessary.

4. Obviously, several of the above patterns may present simultaneously. For instance, it is not uncommon to see patients with urolithiasis with liver-spleen disharmonies complicated by yin vacuity, damp heat, and blood stasis. In such cases, the practitioner should determine the relative proportion or importance of each pattern and create a combined treatment plan based on those proportions.

For kidney yin vacuity with damp heat, consider using *San Jin Hu Tao Tang* (Three Golds & Walnut Decoction): Herba Lysimachiae Seu Desmodii (*Jin Qian Cao*), 30-60g, uncooked Radix Rehmanniae (*Sheng Di*), 15g, Spora Lygodii Japonici (*Hai Jin Sha*), Radix Scrophulariae Ningpoensis (*Xuan Shen*), Folium Pyrrosiae (*Shi Wei*), Herba Dianthi (*Qu Mai*), Herba Plantaginis (*Che Qian Cao*), and Talcum (*Hua Shi*), 12g each, Tuber Asparagi Cochinensis (*Tian Men Dong*), Herba Polygoni Avicularis (*Bian Xu*), and Radix Achyranthis Bidentatae (*Niu Xi*), 9g each, Endothelium Corneum Gigeriae Galli (*Ji Nei Jin*), 6g, Caulis Akebiae (*Mu Tong*) and Radix Glycyrrhizae (*Gan Cao*), 4.5g each, and Semen Juglandis Regiae (*Hu Tao Ren*), 4 fruits.

Tong Lin Yi Shen Pei Shi Tang (Free the Flow of Strangury, Boost the Kidneys & Expel Stones Decoction) is a complex formula for kidney yang vacuity with damp heat: Herba Lysimachiae Seu Desmodii (*Jin Qian Cao*), Spora Lygodii Japonici (*Hai Jin Sha*), and Semen Plantaginis (*Che Qian Zi*), 30g each, Folium Pyrrosiae (*Shi Wei*), Semen Vaccariae Segetalis (*Wang Bu Liu Xing*), and Fructus Psoraleae Corylifoliae (*Bu Gu Zhi*), 15g each, and Radix Dipsaci (*Xu Duan*), Fructus Lycii Chinensis (*Gou Qi*), and cooked Radix Rehmanniae (*Shu Di*), 9g each.

5. A simple home remedy for reducing the excruciating pain during acute crises is to do acupressure at *Cheng Shan* (Bl 57) and *Wei Zhong* (Bl 40). These two points should be pressed strongly for 15-45 seconds. This is often sufficient to lower the pain for 1-3 hours. Occasionally, this manipulation can even promote the expulsion of urinary calculi.

6. Other effective pairs of points for treating renal colic with acupuncture include: *Shen Shu* (Bl 23) plus *Shui Dao* (St 28) or *Shen Shu* (Bl 23) plus *Gui Lai* (St 29), *Nei Guan* (Per 6) plus *San Yin Jiao* (Sp 6), and *Jing Men* (GB 25) plus *a shi* points. This latter combination may also be treated with electroacupuncture.

7. For Chinese ear acupuncture, use Kidney, Bladder, Urinary Tract, and Lumbus points.

8. Use of Caulis Akebiae (*Mu Tong*) long-term is forbidden since it may cause nephrotoxicity if Akebia has been substituted by Aristolochia Manchurensis.

9. The most commonly used Chinese medicinals for treating stone strangury and disinhibiting the urination in premodern formulas are: Herba Lysimachiae Seu Desmodii (*Jin Qian Cao*), Spora Lygodii Japonici (*Hai Jin Sha*), Folium Pyrrosiae (*Shi Wei*), Succinum (*Hu Po*), Herba Dianthi (*Qu Mai*), Semen Vaccariae Segetalis (*Wang Bu Liu Xing*), Talcum (*Hua Shi*), and Herba Polygoni Avicularis (*Bian Xu*). Typically, one or more of these medicinals is combined with other medicinals which eliminate dampness and disinhibit urination, such as Semen Abutili Seu Malvae (*Dong Kui Zi*), Semen Plantaginis (*Che Qian Zi*), Rhizoma Alismatis (*Ze Xie*), Rhizoma Dioscoreae Hypoglaucae (*Bei Xie*), and Caulis Akebiae (*Mu Tong*). Another important medicinal for the treatment of urinary calculi is Endothelium Corneum Gigeriae Galli (*Ji Nei Jin*) which is empirically known to transform stones. In most modern Chinese medicinal formulas, one will find Herba Lysimachiae Seu Desmodii (*Jin Qian Cao*) and Spora Lygodii Japonici (*Hai Jin Sha*), very often Succinum (*Hu Po*) and Endothelium Corneum Gigeriae Galli (*Ji Nei Jin*), and frequently Folium Pyrrosiae (*Shi Wei*) and Talcum (*Hua Shi*). Based on modern clinical experience, Radix Clematidis Chinensis (*Wei Ling Xian*) and Rhizoma Imperatae Cylindricae (*Bai Mao Gen*), 60g each, may also be used to disperse stones, and Semen Juglandis Regiae (*Hu Tao Ren*) is increasingly being used as an auxiliary medicinal to "lubricate" the urinary tract.

10. To help prevent stone formation from calcium, one

should avoid foods rich in calcium, including milk and dairy products. To prevent stone formation from urea, one should avoid foods rich in purine, such as brains, calf's sweetbreads, wild game, smoked meats, liver, fish (*e.g.*, sardines), caviar, shellfish, ripe cheese, strong black tea, coffee, chocolate, wine, and alcohol. To prevent stone formation from oxalic acid, one should avoid food rich in oxalate, such as chocolate, spinach, celery, cabbage, tomatoes, rhubarb, and asparagus.

BIBLIOGRAPHY

CHINESE LANGUAGE BIBLIOGRAPHY

"An Analysis of the Treatment Efficacy of *Qing Shang Quan Tong Tang* on Vascular Headaches" by Zhang Yue-mei & Fang Dong, *Hei Long Jiang Zhong Yi Yao (Heilongjiang Chinese Medicine & Medicinals)*, #2, 1995

"A Clinical Study of the Treatment of Systemic Lupus Erythmatosus by the Methods of Drying Dampness & Dispelling Stasis" by Xi Jin-shan, *He Nan Zhong Yi (Henan Chinese Medicine)*, #2, 1995

"A Clinical Survey of the Treatment of 12 Cases of Sjögren's Syndrome" by Hong Qing-xiang, *Shang Hai Zhong Yi Yao Za Zhi (Shanghai Journal of Chinese Medicine & Medicinals)*, #9, 1995

"A Clinical Survey of the Use of Hyperthyroid-leveling Decoction in the Treatment of 65 Cases of Hyperthyroidism" by Zhang Jun-zhao, Liu Shu-xian & Wu Qing-he, *Xin Zhong Yi (New Chinese Medicine)*, #1, 1995

"A Clinical Survey on the Treatment of 106 Cases of Hyperlipidemia with *Hua Tan Jiang Zhi Fang*" by Xu Hai-zheng, *Hu Nan Zhong Yi Za Zhi (Hunan Journal of Chinese Medicine)*, #3, 1994

"A Report on the Treatment of 86 Cases of Recalcitrant Headache with *Dang Gui Si Ni Tang Jia Jian*" by Jin Shao-xian & Zong Hui-min, *Tian Jin Zhong Yi (Tianjin Chinese Medicine)*, #6, 1993

"A Study of the Chinese Medicine Prevention of Relapse of Multiple Sclerosis" by Lu Xi *et al. Zhong Yi Za Zhi (Journal of Chinese Medicine)*, #7, 1995

"A Study of the Clinical Effectiveness of Treating 40 Cases of Rheumatoid Arthritis with a Traditional Experiential Formula" by Li Jie, *Tian Jin Zhong Yi (Tianjin Chinese Medicine)*, #5, 1995

"A Study of the Effectiveness of *Bi Zheng San* as the Main Treatment in 48 Cases of Rheumatoid Arthritis" by Guo Yan-lin *et al.*, *He Nan Zhong Yi (Henan Chinese Medicine)*, #2, 1995

"A Study of the Effectiveness of *Shen Ling Mai Dong Wu Wei Tang* in the Treatment of 68 Cases of Low Blood Pressure" by Jiang Zong-fa, *Si Chuan Zhong Yi (Sichuan Chinese Medicine)*, #9, 1995

"A Study of the Treatment Efficacy of Treating Paralysis Agitans by the Methods of Settling the Liver & Extinguishing Wind" by Cao Wen-lan, *Tian Jin Zhong Yi (Tianjin Chinese Medicine)*, #5, 1995

"A Survey of the Effectiveness of the Treatment of 280 Cases of Rheumatoid Arthritis with *Jian Gu Feng Shi Ye*" by Lin Wen-jun, *Xin Zhong Yi (New Chinese Medicine)*, #6, 1995

"A Survey of the Effectiveness of *Zhi Tong Ru Shen Tang* in the Treatment of 158 Cases of Bleeding Due to Internal Hemorrhoids" by Tang Yu-sen, *Gan Su Zhong Yi (Gansu Chinese Medicine)*, #1, 1995

"A Survey of the Treatment Effects of *Kang Lao San* as the Main Treatment in 2,139 Cases of Tuberculosis" by Li Shou-xin *et al.*, *Zhong Yi Za Zhi (Journal of Chinese Medicine)*, #10, 1994

"A Survey of the Treatment Efficacy of Treating 56 Cases of Irritable Bowel Syndrome with *Xiao Chai Hu Tang Jia Wei*" by Zhu Ke-qi & Huang Zhi-qiang, *Jiang Xi Zhong Yi Yao (Jiangxi Chinese Medicine & Medicinals)*, #10, 2000

"A Simple Treatise on the Disease Causes & Disease Mechanisms of Wasting & Thirsting" by Wu De-yong, *Hu Nan Zhong Yi Za Zhi (Hunan Journal of Chinese Medicine)*, #5, 2000

Bing Du Xing Ji Bing De Zhong Yi Zhi Liao (The Chinese Medical Treatment of Viral Diseases) by Ma Chao-ying & Li Yuan-shi, Shanghai University of Chinese Medicine Press, Shanghai, 1998

"Chen Tong-yun's Clinical Experiences & Thoughts on Treating Acne" by Liu Qing-deng, *Bei Jing Zhong Yi (Beijing Chinese Medicine)*, #6, 2000

"Clinical Observations of the Treatment of Common Acne with Herba Aloes" by Liu Ying *et al.*, *Si Chuan Zhong Yi (Sichuan Chinese Medicine)*, #12, 1998

"Experiences in Treating Chronic Colitis by Supporting the Righteous & Dispelling Evils" by Fei Qiu-yue, *Zhe Jiang Zhong Yi Za Zhi (Zhejiang Journal of Chinese Medicine)*, #2, 1994

"Experiences in the Treatment of 36 Cases of Migraine with *Xiong Qi Shao Zhi Tang*" by Huang Cheng-yun, *Hei Long Jiang Zhong Yi Yao (Heilongjiang Chinese Medicine & Medicinals)*, #5, 1996

"Experiences in the Treatment of 52 Cases of Senile Osteoporosis with *Qing E Wan Jia Wei*" by Shen Lin *et al.*, *Hu Bei Zhong Yi Za Zhi (Hubei Journal of Chinese Medicine)*, #3, 1994

"Experiences in the Treatment of Scleroderma with *Shen Qi Tang*" by Zhang Bing-zhang & Qiu Yong-liang, *Zhong Yi Za Zhi (Journal of Chinese Medicine)*, #5, 1995

"Experiences in the Treatment of Two Cases of Severe Pulmonary Tuberculosis" by Han Pei-rong, *Zhong Yi Za Zhi (Journal of Chinese Medicine)*, #9, 1995

"Experiences Treating Acute Stage Skin Damage in Systemic Lupus Erythmatosus by the Methods of Cooling the Blood & Resolving Toxins, Eliminating Dampness & Scattering Stasis" by Sun Feng-qin *et al.*, *Zhong Yi Za Zhi (Journal of Chinese Medicine)*, #8, 1995

Fang Ji Xue (A Study of Formulas & Prescriptions) by Xu Ji-qun *et al.*, Shanghai Science & Technology Press, Shanghai, 1986

Gu Fang Miao Yong (Ancient Formulas, Wondrous Uses) by Chen Bao-ming & Zhao Jin-xi, Science & Technology Press, Beijing, 1994

Han Ying Chang Yong Yi Xue Ci Hui (Chinese-English Glossary of Commonly Used Medical Terms) by Huang Xiao-kai, People's Health & Hygiene Press, Beijing, 1982

"Important Factors in the Treatment of Premenstrual Acne" by Yao Shi-an, *Zhong Yi Za Zhi (Journal of Chinese Medicine)*, #12, 1998

Jian Ming Zhong Yi Da Ci Dian (A Plain & Clear Dictionary of Chinese Medicine) compiled by the Research Institute, Guangzhou College of Chinese Medicine, People's Health & Hygiene Press, Beijing, 1986

Jin Yuan Si Da Yi Xue Jia Ming Zhu Ji Cheng (An Anthology of Famous Jin-Yuan Four Great Schools Medical Studies) edited by Ye Chuan & Jian Yi, Chinese National Chinese Medicine & Medicinal Press, Beijing, 1997

Jin Yuan Si Da Yi Xue Zhu Si Xiang Zhi Yan Jiu (A Study of Jin-Yuan Four Great Schools of Medicine's Thinking) edited by Li Cong-fu & Liu Bing-fan, People's Health & Hygiene Press, Beijing, 1983

"Jottings on the Acupuncture Treatment of Senile Dementia" by He Jun & Li Qiu-yang, *Tian Jin Zhong Yi (Tianjin Chinese Medicine)*, #3, 1993

Lao Nian Chang Xian Bing Zheng Fang Zhi Fa (The Prevention & Treatment of Commonly Seen Diseases in the Elderly) by Wu Jun-xi, Chinese National Chinese Medicine & Medicinal Press, Beijing, 1998

Lao Nian Qi Chi Dai Zheng De Zhong Yi Zhi Liao (The Chinese Medical Treatment of Senile Dementia) by Hu Long-cai, True China Book Publishers, Taipei, 1997

Lin Chuang Bian Zheng Shi Zhi Xue (A Study of the Clinical Basing of Treatment on Pattern Discrimination) by Liu Bin, Science, Technology & Literature Press, Beijing, 1992

Lin Chuang Zhong Yi Zheng Zhi Shou Ce (A Handbook of Clinical Chinese Medicine Confirmed Treatments) by Zhang Geng-yang *et al.*, Tianjin Science & Technology Press, Tianjin, 1999

Nan Ke Zheng Zhi Xin Fa (Male Department Proven Treatments & Heart Methods) by Cheng Shao-en *et al.*, Beijing Science & Technology Press, Beijing, 1991

Nan Zhi Bing De Liang Fang Miao Fa (Fine Formulas & Miraculous Methods for Difficult to Treat Diseases) by Wu Da-zhou & Ge Xiu-ke, Chinese National Chinese Medicine & Medicinal Press, Beijing, 1992

Nei Jing Jiang Yi (Inner Classic Teaching Materials) by Cheng Shi-de, Shanghai Science & Technology Press, Shanghai, 1985

Nei Ke Nan Zhi Bing De Zhong Yi Zhi Liao (Chinese Medical Treatment of Difficult to Treat Diseases in Internal Medicine) by Liu Dong-liang, People's Army Medical Press, Beijing, 1994

"Observations on the Clinical Use of Yin Fire Theory" by Zhang Qi & Long Jia-jun, *Zhe Jiang Zhong Yi Za Zhi (Zhejiang Journal of Chinese Medicine)*, #11, 2000

"Observations on the Effectiveness of Self-composed *Jiang Tang Yin* on the Treatment of 42 Cases of Diabetes Mellitus" by Xue Wen-sen, *Ji Lin Zhong Yi Yao (Jilin Chinese Medicine & Medicinals)*, #2, 1994

"Overeating Sugar & Sweets [Causes] Detriment & Damage to the Five Viscera" by Bu Lu-nuo & Bu Lu-ke, *Jiang Xi Zhong Yi Yao (Jiangxi Chinese Medicine & Medicinals)*, #1, 1995

"Progress on the Chinese Medical Medicinal Treatment of Rheumatoid Arthritis" by Li Zhong-nan, Wang Wei-sheng & Zhou Juan-xia, *Hu Bei Zhong Yi Za Zhi (Hubei Journal of Chinese Medicine)*, #5, 1995

Qi Nan Za Zheng Jing Xuan (A Carefully Chosen [Collection of] Strange, Difficult Miscellaneous Conditions) by Huang Yong-yuan, Guangdong Science & Technology Press, Guangzhou, 1996

Qian Jia Miao Fang (Ten Thousand Families' Wondrous Formulas) compiled by Li Wen-liang & Qi Qiang, People's Liberation Army Press, Beijing, 1985

Qin Bo Wei Yi Wen Ji (A Collection of Qin Bo-wei's Writings), Hunan Science & Technology Press, Changsha, 1991

"Recent Developments in the Treatment of Restless Leg Syndrome" by Zhang Bing-chun, *Shan Dong Zhong Yi Za Zhi (Shandong Journal of Chinese Medicine)*, #9, 1996

Shen Jing Jing Shen Ke Bing Zui Xing Zhong Yi Zhi Liao (The Newest Chinese Medical Treatments in Neurology-Psychiatry) by Liang Bing, Chinese Medicine Literature Press, Beijing, 1999

Shi Yong Zhen Jiu Tui Na Zhi Liao Xue (A Study of Practical Acupuncture-moxibustion & Tuina Treatments) by Xia Zhi-ping, Shanghai College of Chinese Medicine Press, Shanghai, 1990

Shi Yong Zhen Jiu Nei Ke Xue (A Study of Practical Acupuncture-moxibustion In Internal Medicine) by Cui Shu-gui *et al.*, White Mountain Press, Chen Yang, 1991

Shi Yong Zhong Guo Nan Xing Xue (Practical Chinese Male Sexual Diseases) by Jin Zhi-gang, Xue Yuan Press, Beijing, 1993

Shi Yong Zhong Yi Nei Ke Xue (A Study of Practical Chinese Medicine Internal Medicine) by Huang Wen-dong, Shanghai Science & Technology Press, Shanghai, 1985

Shi Yong Zhong Yi Zhen Duan Xue (A Study of Practical Chinese Medicine Diagnosis) by Deng Tie-tiao, Shanghai Science & Technology Press, Shanghai, 1995

Shi Yong Zhong Yi Shen Jing Bing Xue (A Study of Practical Chinese Medical Neurology) by Chen Jia-yang, Gansu Science & Technology Press, Lanzhou, 1989

"Supplementing the Qi, Quickening the Blood & Transforming Stasis Makes Life in the Treatment of Intracranial Bleeding" by Xu Du-cong, *Fu Jian Zhong Yi Yao (Fujian Chinese Medicine & Medicinals)*, #6, 2000

"The Acupuncture Treatment of 65 Cases of Migraine" by Bai Hui-min, *Tian Jin Zhong Yi Xue Yuan Xue Bao (Journal of the Tianjin College of Chinese Medicine)*, #2, 1996

"The Chinese Medicine & Medicinal Discrimination & Treatment of Allergic Rhinitis" by Zhang Xin-yi & Wei Shu-hua, *He Nan Zhong Yi (Henan Chinese Medicine)*, #6, 2000

"The Chinese Medicine Treatment of 33 Cases of Raynaud's Disease" by Liu Xiu-ru, *Bei Jing Zhong Yi (Beijing Chinese Medicine)*, #2, 1995

"The Integrated Chinese-Western Medical Treatment of 56 Cases of Subacute Systemic Lupus Erythmatosus" by Zhong Hong *et al.*, *Si Chuan Zhong Yi (Sichuan Chinese Medicine)*, #10, 1995

"The Integrated Chinese-Western Medical Treatment of 73 Cases of Systemic Lupus Erythmatosus" by Du Xu-lian & Fu Xin-li, *Shan Dong Zhong Yi Xue Yuan Xue Bao (Shandong College of Chinese Medicine Journal)*, #2, 1993

"The Lungs, Spleen & Kidneys Must Be Responsible for Allergic Rhinitis" by Zhu Yu-qin, *He Nan Zhong Yi (Henan Chinese Medicine)*, #6, 2000

"The Treatment of 13 Cases of Diabetic Polyneuritis with Modified *Bu Yang Huan Wu Tang*" by Guo Xia-xia & Liu Jia-yi, *Si Chuan Zhong Yi (Sichuan Chinese Medicine)*, #8, 1998

"The Treatment of 16 Cases of Acne with *Zhi Bai Di Huang Tang*" by Lin Zhen-zhong, *Si Chuan Zhong Yi (Sichuan Chinese Medicine)*, #9, 1998

"The Treatment of 19 Cases of Early Stage Parkinson's Disease by the Methods of Enriching the Kidneys & Extinguishing Wind" by Xing Li, *Tian Jin Zhong Yi (Tianjin Chinese Medicine)*, #4, 1995

"The Treatment of 21 Cases of Prostatic Hypertrophy with *Fu Fang Shu Fu Wan*" by Zeng Qing-pei, *Zhe Jiang Zhong Yi Za Zhi (Zhejiang Journal of Chinese Medicine)*, #1, 1994

"The Treatment of 24 Cases of Hyperthyroidism with *Xia Xuan Ping Kang Tang*" by Hong Zhi-hao & Chen Guo-yong, *Si Chuan Zhong Yi (Sichuan Chinese Medicine)*, #7, 2000

"The Treatment of 25 Cases of Chronic Prostatitis with Chinese Medicinals" by Cai Feng-jin, *Bei Jing Zhong Yi Za Zhi (Beijing Journal of Chinese Medicine)*, #1, 1994

"The Treatment of 26 Cases of Diabetes by the Methods of Boosting the Qi, Nourishing Yin & Quickening the Blood" by Li Yi, *Yun Nan Zhong Yi Zhong Yao Za Zhi (Yunnan Journal of Chinese Medicine & Chinese Medicinals)*, #1, 1997

"The Treatment of 28 Cases of Lumbar Disk Herniation with *Du Huo Ji Sheng Tang*" by Shi Chao, *Zhe Jiang Zhong Yi Za Zhi (Zhejiang Journal of Chinese Medicine)*, #2, 1994

"The Treatment of 28 Cases of Painful Wind Arthritis with *Tong Feng Jian*" by Fang Ju-zhi, *Shan Dong Zhong Yi Za Zhi (Shandong Journal of Chinese Medicine)*, #1, 1995

"The Treatment of 30 Cases of Diabetes Mellitus with Gao Hui-yun's Methods of Boosting the Qi & Nourishing Yin" by Liu Wen, *Hu Bei Zhong Yi Za Zhi (Hubei Journal of Chinese Medicine)*, #1, 1994

"The Treatment of 30 Cases of Hypertension with *Wu Cao Si Wu Tang*" by Zhang Jin-an & Zhang Xiao-hui, *Si Chuan Zhong Yi (Sichuan Chinese Medicine)*, #4, 1995

"The Treatment of 30 Cases of Neurovascular Headache with Acupuncture & Chinese Herbs" by Li Che-cheng & Xu Hui-min, *Hei Long Jiang Zhong Yi Yao (Heilongjiang Chinese Medicine & Medicinals)*, #1, 1996

"The Treatment of 30 Cases of Ulcerative Colitis with *Sheng Yang Yi Wei Tang*" by Ai Ying, *Hu Nan Zhong Yi Za Zhi (Hunan Journal of Chinese Medicine)*, #5, 1994

"The Treatment of 32 Cases of Type II Diabetes Mellitus with *Jia Wei Er Chen Tang*" by Zhang Xue-hong, *Zhe Jiang Zhong Yi Za Zhi (Zhejiang Journal of Chinese Medicine)*, #1, 1994

"The Treatment of 33 Cases of Irritable Bowel Syndrome with *Tong Xie Yao Fang*" by Yin Wei-che *et al.*, *Xin Zhong Yi (New Chinese Medicine)*, #3, 1998

"The Treatment of 35 Cases of Irritable Bowel Syndrome with *Xiao Yao San Jia Wei*" by Zheng Jia-yu, *Si Chuan Zhong Yi (Sichuan Chinese Medicine)*, #7, 2000

"The Treatment of 34 Cases of Prostatic Hypertrophy with *Hua Tan Ruan Jian Tang*" by Cao Guan-gen, *Zhe Jiang Zhong Yi Za Zhi (Zhejiang Journal of Chinese Medicine)*, #5, 1994

"The Treatment of 36 Cases of Scleroderma by Mainly Quickening the Blood & Transforming Stasis" by Zhen Chang-song, *Hu Bei Zhong Yi Za Zhi (Hubei Journal of Chinese Medicine)*, #4, 1995

"The Treatment of 38 Cases of Rheumatoid Arthritis with *Shen Qi Dang Di Si Teng Tang*" by Ge Bao-li, *Hei Long Jiang Zhong Yi Yao (Heilongjiang Chinese Medicine & Medicinals)*, #3, 1995

"The Treatment of 40 Cases of Post-Surgical Prostatic Hypertophy Urinary Incontinence with *Bu Zhong Yi Qi Tang Jia Wei*" by Li Zhi-qiang & Yang Jun, *He Nan Zhong Yi (Henan Chinese Medicine)*, #6, 2000

"The Treatment of 40 Cases of Rheumatoid Arthritis with Self-composed *Qing Bi Tang*" by Chen Yang-rong, *Fu Jian Zhong Yi Yao (Fujian Chinese Medicine & Medicinals)*, #6, 2000

"The Treatment of 42 Cases of Allergic Rhinitis with *Si Wu Tang Jia Wei*" by Li Guang-zhen, *Ji Lin Zhong Yi Yao (Jilin Chinese Medicine & Medicinals)*, #3, 1993

"The Treatment of 43 Cases of Diabetic Peripheral Neuropathy by the Methods of Boosting the Qi, Nourishing Yin & Transforming Stasis" by Ding Li-feng, *Si Chuan Zhong Yi (Sichaun Chinese Medicine)*, #3, 2000

"The Treatment of 42 Cases of Raynaud's Syndrome with Self-composed *Tong Mai Jie Jing San*" by Wu Yong & Wang Ji-xian, *Xin Zhong Yi (New Chinese Medicine)*, #3, 1995

"The Treatment of 45 Cases of Middle-aged Acne with Modified *Liu Wei Di Huang Wan*" by Lin Shao-jian, *Si Chuan Zhong Yi (Sichuan Chinese Medicine)*, #2, 1999

"The Treatment of 46 Cases of Chronic Fatigue Syndrome with Self-composed *Bu Gan Yi Qi Tang*" by Zhu Guang-wen, *Zhe Jiang Zhong Yi Za Zhi (Zhejiang Journal of Chinese Medicine)*, #11, 2000

"The Treatment of 46 Cases of Restless Leg Syndrome with *Huang Qi Wu Wu Tang Jia Wei*" by Wang Yu-xi, *Xin Zhong Yi (New Chinese Medicine)*, #1, 1998

"The Treatment of 50 Cases of Chronic Colitis with *Er Teng Qin Zhu Tang*" by Zhu Bo-lin, *Zhe Jiang Zhong Yi Za Zhi (Zhejiang Journal of Chinese Medicine)*, #5, 1994

"The Treatment of 50 Cases of Chronic Low Blood Pressure with *Zhi Gan Cao Tang Jia Jian*" by Chen Ya-jun, *Si Chuan Zhong Yi (Sichuan Chinese Medicine)*, #7, 1995

"The Treatment of 51 Cases of Bleeding Hemorrhoids with *Wu Hua Guo Jing Jie Tan Tang*" by Wang Can-tang, *Zhe Jiang Zhong Yi Za Zhi (Zhejiang Journal of Chinese Medicine)*, #5, 1995

"The Treatment of 52 Cases of Recalcitrant Migraines with *Huo Xue Hua Yu Xiao Tong Tang*" by Wang Xian-qi & Sun Qing, *Xin Zhong Yi (New Chinese Medicine)*, #7, 1996

"The Treatment of 54 Cases of Chronic Active Hepatitis with *Gan Fu San*" by Cheng Zhi-hong, *Si Chuan Zhong Yi (Sichuan Chinese Medicine)*, #7, 2000

"The Treatment of 58 Cases of Prostatic Hypertrophy with the Methods of Supplementing the Qi, Boosting the Kidneys & Dispelling Stasis" by Cui Xue-jiao, *Zhong Yi Za Zhi (Journal of Chinese Medicine)*, #4, 1994

"The Treatment of 64 Cases of Static Blood Headache with Self-composed *Zhu Yu Zhi Tong Tang*" by Sun Hai-long *et al.*, *Hei Long Jiang Zhong Yi Yao (Heilongjiang Chinese Medicine & Medicinals)*, #4, 1995

"The Treatment of 65 Cases of Allergic Rhinitis with *Jia Jian Xiao Chai Hu Tang*" by Kuang Nai-jia, Bi Guo-mei & Huang Ya-shan, *He Nan Zhong Yi (Henan Chinese Medicine)*, #5, 1995

"The Treatment of 68 Cases of Painful Wind Arthritis with *Xuan Bi Tang Jia Wei*" by Liu Hua, *Jiang Xi Zhong Yi Yao (Jiangxi Chinese Medicine & Medicinals)*, #10, 2000

"The Treatment of 71 Cases of Primary Onset Hypercholesterolemia with *Shu Tiao Zhi Tang*" by Zhang Jian-tang *et al.*, *Fu Jian Zhong Yi Yao (Fujian Chinese Medicine & Medicinals)*, #6, 2000

"The Treatment of 80 Cases of Hypotensive Dizziness with *Yi Qi Yang Yin Tang*" by Ji Yun-hai, *Si Chuan Zhong Yi (Sichuan Chinese Medicine)*, #7, 1995

"The Treatment of 80 Cases of Thrombotic External Hemorrhoids with *Shao Fu Zhu Yu Tang*" by Feng Zhen-long & Zhao Feng-ying, *Hu Bei Zhong Yi Za Zhi (Hubei Journal of Chinese Medicine)*, #3, 1994

"The Treatment of 100 Cases of Allergic Rhinitis with *Bu Zhong Yi Qi Tang Jia Wei*" by Feng Bi-qun & Lu Ji-sen, *Xin Zhong Yi (New Chinese Medicine)*, #6, 1995

"The Treatment of 105 Cases of Ulcerative Colitis with *Bai Cha Tang* as a Retention Enema" by Guo Pei-jun, *Bei Jing Zhong Yi Za Zhi (Beijing Journal of Chinese Medicine)*, #2, 1994

"The Treatment of 120 Cases of Allergic Rhinitis with *Suo Quan Wan Jia Jian*" by Chen De-jiang, *Yun Nan Zhong Yi Zhong Yao Za Zhi (Yunnan Journal of Chinese Medicine & Chinese Medicinals)*, #5, 1995

"The Treatment of 120 Cases of Irritable Bowel Syndrome Using *Shan Yao Che Qian Zi Tang*" by Chen Wei-di, *Shang Hai Zhong Yi Yao Za Zhi (Shanghai Journal of Chinese Medicine & Medicinals)*, #3, 1992

"The Treatment of 156 Cases of Irritable Bowel Syndrome with *Yi Min Tiao Chang Tang*" by Hong Zhe-ming, *Zhe Jiang Zhong Yi Za Zhi (Zhejiang Journal of Chinese Medicine)*, #3, 1998

"The Treatment of 226 Cases of Irritable Bowel Syndrome with *Jia Wei Zhu Shao Yin*" by Shen Wen-hua & Hu Wen-lei, *Zhe Jiang Zhong Yi Za Zhi (Zhejiang Journal of Chinese Medicine)*, #3, 1998

"The Treatment of 309 Cases of Diabetes Mellitus with a Combination of Acupuncture & *Xiao Ke Gao*" by Feng Ming-xiu *et al.*, *Zhong Yi Za Zhi (Journal of Chinese Medicine)*, #1, 1994

"The Treatment of Acne with Acupuncture Point Poking Treatment" by Shen Hong, *Zhe Jiang Zhong Yi Za Zhi (Zhejiang Journal of Chinese Medicine)*, #3, 1995

"The Treatment of Allergic Rhinitis Mainly by Moxibustion" by Zhang Gui-rong *et al.*, *Zhong Guo Zhen Jiu (Chinese National Acupuncture & Moxibustion)*, #4, 1995

"The Treatment of Chronic Prostatitis by Transforming Stasis & Disinhibiting Dampness" by Xia Zhi-bin, *Zhe Jiang Zhong Yi Za Zhi (Zhejiang Journal of Chinese Medicine)*, #2, 1994

"The Treatment of Periarthritis of the Shoulder with *Quan Xie Er Wu Gao*" by Song Ke-cheng & Zhang Sheng-ping, *Shan Dong Zhong Yi Za Zhi (Shandong Journal of Chinese Medicine)*, #3, 1995

"The Treatment of Post-herpetic Neuralgia Based on Pattern Discrimination" by Wang Tao, *Si Chuan Zhong Yi (Sichuan Chinese Medicine)*, #7, 2000

"The Treatment of Rheumatic Arthritis with *Jia Wei Ma Qian Zi Tang*" by Li Ying, *Shang Hai Zhong Yi Yao Za Zhi (Shanghai Journal of Chinese Medicine & Medicinals)*, #1, 1995

"The Treatment of Systemic Lupus Erythmatosus by the Methods of Cooling & Scattering the Blood, Enriching the Kidneys & Boosting Yin" by Fan Yong-sheng, *Zhong Yi Za Zhi (Journal of Chinese Medicine)*, #8, 1995

The Use of the Methods of Disinhibiting Dampness & Clearing Heat in Chronic Active Hepatitis" by Guo Peng & Kong Wei, *Shan Dong Zhong Yi Za Zhi (Shandong Journal of Chinese Medicine)*, #9, 1996

"The Use of *Yi Qi Zhu Yu Tong Mai Tang* in the Treatment of Diabetic Peripheral Neuropathy" by Xu Sheng-sheng, *Jiang Su Zhong Yi (Jiangsu Chinese Medicine)*, #3, 1999

"Thoughts on & Methods for Treating Rheumatoid Arthritis with Chinese Medicine & Medicinals" by Zhou Xue-ping, *Xin Zhong Yi (New Chinese Medicine)*, #1, 2001

"Treating Diabetes by Boosting the Qi, Enriching Yin & Draining Fire" by Luo Shan, *Bei Jing Zhong Yi (Beijing Chinese Medicine)*, #3, 1998

"Warming Yang & Boosting the Qi as the Main Method for Treating Allergic Rhinitis" by Wei Shu-hua, *He Nan Zhong Yi (Henan Chinese Medicine)*, #6, 2000

Xian Zai Nan Zhi Bing Zhong Yi Zhen Liao Xue (A Study of the Diagnosis & Treatment of Modern, Difficult to Treat Diseases) by Wu Jun-yu & Bai Yong-ke, Chinese Medicine Ancient Books Press, Beijing, 1993

Xing Bing Zheng Zhi (Sexual Diseases Patterns & Treatments [or Proven Treatments]) by Zhang Jian-bao, Chinese National Women's Press, Beijing, 1990

Yan De Xin Zhen Zhi Ning Nan Bing Mi Chi (A Secret Satchel of Yan De-xin's Diagnosis & Treatment of Knotty, Difficult to Treat Diseases) by Yan De-xin, Literary Press Publishing Co., Shanghai, 1997

Yi Nan Bing Zhong Yi Lin Zheng Zhi Nan (A Clinical Guide to the Treatment of Difficult Diseases in Chinese Medicine) by Jiang Ming, China Medical Press, Beijing, 1993

Yi Nan Zha Zheng Zhen Jiu Yan Fang Jing (A Selection of Proven Acupuncture & Moxibustion Formulas for Strange & Difficult Diseases) by Lun Xin *et al.*, Guangdong Science & Technology Press, Guangzhou, 2000

Yi Zong Jin Jian (The Golden Mirror of Ancestral Medicine) by Wu Qian *et al.*, People's Health & Hygiene Press, Beijing, 1985

Yu Xue Zheng Zhi (Static Blood Patterns & Treatments) by Zhang Xue-wen, Shanxi Science & Technology Press, Xian, 1986

Zhen Fa Jiu Fa Xe (A Study of Acupuncture & Moxibustion Methods) by Xi Yong-hong, Shanghai Science & Technology Press, Shanghai, 1985

Zhen Jiu Chu Fang Xue (A Study of Acupuncture & Moxibustion Prescriptions) by Wang Dai, Beijing Publishing Co., Beijing, 1990

Zhen Jiu Da Cheng (The Great Compendium of Acupuncture & Moxibustion) by Yang Ji-zhou, People's Health & Hygiene Press, Beijing, 1983

Zhen Jiu Xue (A Study of Acupuncture & Moxibustion) by Qiu Mao-liang *et al.*, Shanghai Science & Technology Press, Shanghai, 1985

Zhen Jiu Yi Xue (An Easy Study of Acupuncture & Moxibustion) by Li Shou-xian, People's Health & Hygiene Press, Beijing, 1990

Zhen Jiu Yi Xue You Ji (A Gathering of Case Studies of Acupuncture & Moxibustion) by Tian Cong-huo, Science & Technology Literature Press, Beijing, 1985

Zhong Guo Nan Ke Yi An (Chinese National Male Department Case Histories) by Zhang You-huan, Tianjin Technological Publishing Co., Tianjin, 1990

Zhong Guo Yi Xue Zhen Fa Da Quan (A Great Collection of Chinese Medical Diagnostic Methods) by Ma Zhong-xue, Shandong Science & Technology Press, Jinan, 1991

Zhong Guo Zhen Jiu Chu Fang Xue (A Study of Chinese Acupuncture & Moxibustion Prescriptions) by Xiao Shao-qing, Ningxia People's Press, Yinchuan, 1986

Zhong Guo Zhen Jiu Du Xue Liao Fa (Chinese Acupuncture & Moxibustion Single Point Treatment Method) by Chen De-cheng, Wang Fu-wen *et al.*, Kunlin Science & Technology Press, Changchun, 1992

Zhong Guo Zhen Jiu Dui Xue Liao Fa (Chinese Acupuncture & Moxibustion Paired Points Treatment Method), Chen De-cheng, Wang Fu-wen *et al.*, Kunlin Science & Technology Press, Changchun, 1998

Zhong Guo Zhen Jiu Pei Xue Liao Fa (Chinese Acupuncture & Moxibustion Point Combination Treatment Method) by Chen De-cheng, Wang Fu-wen *et al.*, Guizhou Science & Technology Press, Guiyang, 1995

Zhong Guo Zhong Yi Mi Fang Da Quan (A Great Compendium of Chinese National Chinese Medical Secret Formulas) edited by Hu Zhao-ming, Literary Propagation Publishing Co., Shanghai, 1992

Zhong Xi Yi Jie He Zhi Liao Pi Fu Bing Xing Bing (The Treatment of Dermatological Diseases with Integrated Chinese-Western Medicine) by Fan Rui-qiang, Guangdong People's Press, Guangzhou, 1996

Zhong Yi Bi Bing Da Quan (A Compendium of Chinese Medical Nose Diseases) by Lu Xiao-zuo & Jiang Xian-yang, Tianjin Science & Technology Press, Tianjin, 1995

Zhong Yi Bing Yin Bing Ji Xue (A Study of Chinese Medical Disease Causes & Disease Mechanisms) by Wu Dun-xu, Shanghai College of Chinese Medicine Press, Shanghai, 1989

Zhong Yi Er Bi Hou Ke Xue (A Study of Chinese Medicine Otonasolaryngology) by Tan Jing-shu, Hunan Science & Technology Press, Changsha, 1989

Zhong Yi Er Bi Yan Hou Kou Qiang Xue (A Study of Chinese Medicine E.N.T. & Stomatology) by Wang De-jian, People's Health & Hygiene Press, Beijing, 1994

Zhong Yi Ji Chu Li Lun (The Foundation Theories of Chinese Medicine) by Yin Hui-he, Shanghai Science & Technology Press, Shanghai, 1984

Zhong Yi Lin Chuang Ge Ke (Various Clinical Specialties in Chinese Medicine) by Zhang En-qin *et al.*, Shanghai College of Chinese Medicine Press, Shanghai, 1990

Zhong Yi Nei Ke Lin Chuang Shou Ce (A Clinical Handbook of Chinese Medicine Internal Medicine) by Gao Ying-sen *et al.,* People's Health & Hygiene Press, Beijing, 1996

Zhong Yi Nei Ke Lin Chuang Shou Ce (A Clinical Handbook of Chinese Medicine Internal Medicine) by Xia De-xin, Shanghai Science & Technology Press, Shanghai, 1989

Zhong Yi Nei Ke Xue (A Study of Chinese Medicine Internal Medicine) by Zhang Bo-yu, People's Health & Hygiene Press, Beijing, 1988

Zhong Yi Nei Ke Xun Lun (A New Theory of Chinese Medicine Internal Medicine) by Yin Hui-he, Shanxi Science & Technology Press, Taiyuan, 1983

Zhong Yi Nei Ke Zhen Zhuang Bian Zhi Shou Ce (A Handbook of Chinese Medicine Internal Medicine Symptom Discrimination & Treatment) by Fang Wen-xian, Liu Qing & Chu Xiu-jun, Chian Standard Press, Beijing, 1989

Zhong Yi Pi Fu Bing Zhen Liao (The Chinese Medical Diagnosis & Treatment of Skin Diseases) by Zhang Man-hua, Guangxi People's Publishing Co., Nanning, 1985

Zhong Yi Tong Zheng Zhen Liao Da Quan (A Great Collection of Treatments, Diagnosis & Patterns of Pain Conditions) by Wei Xu-xing *et al.,* China Medical Press, Beijing, 1992

Zhong Yi Yan Ke Xue (A Study of Chinese Medical Ophthalmology) by the Guangzhou College of Chinese Medicine, Shanghai Science & Technology Press, Shanghai, 1981

Zhong Yi Yan Ke Xue (A Study of Chinese Medical Ophthalmology) by Liao Pin-zheng, Shanghai Science & Technology Press, Shanghai, 1986

Zhong Yi Zhen Duan Xue (A Study of Chinese Medical Diagnosis) by Deng Tie-tao, People's Health & Hygiene Press, Beijing, 1994

Zhong Yi Zheng Hou Zhen Duan Zhi Liao Xue (A Study of Chinese Medicine Patterns, Diagnosis & Treatment) by Cheng Shao-en & Xiao Hong-sheng, Beijing Science & Technology Press, Beijing, 1993

Zhong Yi Zheng Zhuang Jian Bie Zhen Duan Xue (A Study of Chinese Medicine Symptoms & Differential Diagnosis) by Zhao Jin-ze, People's Health & Hygiene Press, Beijing, 1984

Zhong Yi Zhi Liao Xian Dai Nan Bing Ji Cheng (A Collection of Chinese Medicine Treatments for the Difficult Diseases of Modern Times) by Zhang Ren *et al.,* Wen Hui Press, Beijing, 1998

Zhong Yi Zhi Liao Xue (A Study of Chinese Medical Treatments) by Sun Guo-jie & Tu Jin-wen, Chinese Medicine & Medicinal Science & Technology Press, Beijing, 1990

"Zhu Liang-chun's Thoughts on the Treatment of Knotty, Difficult Diseases" by Wan Wen-rong, *Zhong Yi Za Zhi (Journal of Chinese Medicine)*, #1, 2000

ENGLISH LANGUAGE BIBLIOGRAPHY

260 Essential Chinese Medicinals by Bob Flaws, Blue Poppy Press, Boulder, CO, 1999

AARP Pharmacy Service Prescription Drug Handbook, 2nd edition, edited by Nancy J. Olins, HarperCollins Publishers, Inc., NY, 1992

"A Brief Report on Traditional Chinese Medical Education in China" by Li Wei-dong, *AATOM Newsletter,* American Association for Teachers of Oriental Medicine, Austin, TX, 1998

"ACE Inhibitors and Hydrochlorothiazide – Oral," www.healthcentral.com/mhc/top/001900.cfm

Acupuncture and Moxibustion Formulas & Treatments by Cheng Dan-an, trans. by Wu Ming, Blue Poppy Press, Boulder, CO, 1996

Aging & Blood Stasis: A New TCM Approach to Geriatrics by Yan De-xin, Blue Poppy Press, Boulder, CO, 2000

A Handbook of Chinese Hematology by Simon Becker, Blue Poppy Press, Boulder, CO, 2000

A Handbook of TCM Patterns & Their Treatments by Bob Flaws & Daniel Finney, Blue Poppy Press, Boulder, CO, 2000

A Handbook of Traditional Chinese Dermatology by Liang Jian-hui, trans. by Zhang Ting-liang & Bob Flaws, Blue Poppy Press, Boulder, CO, 1993

Alternative Medicine, The Definitive Guide by the Burton Goldberg Group, Future Medicine Publishing, Inc., Puyallup, WA, 1993

A Practical Dictionary of Chinese Medicine by Nigel Wiseman & Feng Ye, Paradigm Publications, Brookline, MA, 1998

"Anemia Due to Bone Marrow Failure" by Bruce M. Small, www.smbs.buffalo.edu/med/hem/failure.html

"Aplastic Anemia Answer Book," www.medic.med.uth.tmc.edu/ptnt/00001038.htm

"Blood-Cadmium Levels in Normotensive & Untreated Hypertensive Humans" by S.C. Glauser & E.M. Glauser, *Lancet*, #1, Apr. 1976

"Carpal Tunnel Syndrome" by Eric S. Fishman, www.continuousspeech.com/carpal-tunnel.html

"Carpal Tunnel Syndrome" by Keith W. Roach, http://uhs.bsd.uchicago.edu/~roach/carpal-tunnel.html

"Celiac Disease," www.niddk.nih.gov/health/digest/pubs/celiac/index.htm#1

"Cervical Myelopathy and Spinal Stenosis" by David Ben Eliyahu, www.chiroweb.com/archives/16/18/04.html

"Cervical Spondylosis," University of Maryland Medicine, http://umm.drkoop.com/conditions/ency/article/000436.htm

Chinese-English Manual of Commonly-used Prescriptions in Traditional Chinese Medicine edited by Ou Ming, Joint Publishing Co. Ltd, Hong Kong, 1989

Chinese-English Medical Dictionary, The Commercial Press Ltd. & People's Health & Hygiene Press, Hong Kong, 1988

Chinese-English Terminology of Traditional Chinese Medicine by Shuai Xue-zhong *et al.*, Hunan Science & Technology Press, Changsha, 1983

Chinese Herbal Medicine: Formulas & Strategies by Dan Bensky & Randall Barolet, Eastland Press, Seattle, 1990

Chinese Herbal Medicine: Materia Medica by Dan Bensky & Andrew Gamble, Eastland Press, Seattle, 1993

"Chronic Fatigue Syndrome: A Primer for Physicians and Allied Health Professionals" by Alan Gurwitt *et al.*, www.primenet.com/~camilla/cfs-prim.txt

"Chronic Hepatitis C: Current Disease Management," www.niddk.nih.gov/health/digest/pubs/chrnhepc.htm

"Chronic Thyroiditis (Hashimoto's Disease)," www.healthanswers.com.../overview.asp?id=endocrine+system&filename=000371.ht

"Diabetes Called Sure Fate for Obese People" by D. Satter, *Los Angeles Times*, Feb. 13, 1972

"Diet and the Geographical Distribution of Multiple Sclerosis" by B.W. Agranoff & D. Goldberg, *Lancet*, #7888, Nov. 1974

"Diverticulitis and Diverticulosis," www.sf.med.va.gov/4vets/handouts/divert.htm

"Do You Have Syndrome X?" http://onhealth.webmd.com/conditions/indepth/item/item,83798_1_1.asp

"Driving Out Demons and Snakes: *Gu* Syndrome and a Forgotten Clinical Approach to Chronic Parasitism" by Heiner Fruehauf, *The Journal of Chinese Medicine*, UK, #57, 1998

"Drug-induced End Stage Renal Disease" by P. Ronco & A. Flahault, *New England Journal of Medicine*, Vol. 331, #25, 1994

"Editor's Preface" by Yang Shou-zhong, *Extra Treatises Based on Investigation & Inquiry, A Translation of Zhu Dan-xi's Ge Zhi Yu Lun*, Blue Poppy Press, Boulder, CO, 1994

"Effect of Migration on Blood Pressure: The Yi People Study" by He J. *et al.*, *Epidemiology*, #2, Mar. 1991

Encyclopedia of Natural Medicine by J.E. Pizzorno & M.T. Murray, Prima Publishing, Rocklin, CA, 1991

"Endocrinology and Benign Prostatic Hypertrophy (BPH)," www.endo-society.org/pubaffai/factshee/bphyper.htm

English-Chinese Chinese-English Dictionary of Chinese Medicine by Nigel Wiseman, Hunan Science & Technology Press, Changsha, 1995

Essential Pathology, 2nd ed., edited by Emmanuel Rubin & John Farber, J.B. Lippincott Co., Philadelphia, 1995

"Facts About Carpal Tunnel Syndrome" by the American Academy of Orthopedic Surgeons, www.aaos.org/worldhtml/press/carpalfa.htm

"FMS: Fibromyalgia Syndrome" by Devin J. Starlanyl, www.sover.net/~devstar/fmsdef.htm

"Focus On Calcium Blockers and the Heart" by Lynn Wilson, www.pharminfo.com/pubs/msb/ccb_hrt.html

Fundamentals of Chinese Acupuncture by Andrew Ellis, Nigel Wiseman & Ken Boss, Paradigm Publications, Brookline, MA, 1988

Fundamentals of Chinese Medicine by Nigel Wiseman & Andrew Ellis, Paradigm Publications, Brookline, MA, 1985

"Genital Herpes," www.discoveryhealth.com/DH/ihtIH/WSDSC000/20726/10137.html

"Genital Herpes," www.info.gov.hk/aids/herpes.htm

"Genitourinary and Renal Disease: Benign Prostatic Hypertrophy (BPH)" by Mark A. Graber & Viviana Martinez-Bianchi, www.vh.org/Providers/ClinRef/FPHandbook/Chapter11/06-11.html

"Glomerular Filtration Impairment by Mercury from Dental 'Silver' Fillings in Sheep" by M.J. Vimy *et al.*, *The Physiologist*, #33, Aug. 1990

"Glomerulonephritis" by Burlington Urological Associates, PA, www.bua-pa.com/glomerulonephritis.html

Golden Needle Wang Le-ting: A 20th Century Master's Approach to Acupuncture by Yu Hui-chan & Han Fu-ru, trans. by Shuai Xue-zhong, Blue Poppy Press, Boulder, CO, 1997

"Gout," www.rheumatology.org/patients/factsheet/gout.html

"Gout," www.wellweb.com/INDEX/QGOUT.HTM

Harrison's Principles of Internal Medicine, 14th ed., edited by Braunwald, Isselbacher, Petersdorf *et al.*, McGraw-Hill Co., NY, 1997

"Herpes Information Center," www.herpes-coldsores-treatment-pictures.com/hsv/herpes_information.htm

"How to Help Your Sinus Problems," www.aafp.org/patientinfo/sinus.html

"Insulin Resistance and Endothelial Dysfunction" by S. J. Cleland *et al.*, *News Watch*, March 2000, www.ndei.org/newswatch/archives/date/2000/mar/032700d.html

"Interstitial Cystitis," www.bladder.org/interstitial%20cystitis.html

"Irritable Bowel Syndrome," www.broadwing.medunc.edu/medicine/fgidc

"Is Acupuncture Effective in the Treatment of Fibromyalgia?" by B.M. Berman, J. Ezzo, V. Hadhazy, & J.P. Swyers, *The Journal of Family Practice*, Mar. 1999

"Leukoplakia," www.healthgate.com/choice/uic/cons/mdx-books/sym/sym278.shtml

"Managing Migraine Today (II): Pharmacologic and Nonpharmacologic Treatment," JAMA Migraine Information Center, www.ama-assn.org/special/migraine.treatmnt/managmig/migdrug.htm

Manual of Dermatology in Chinese Medicine by Shen De-hui, Wu Xiu-fen & Nissi Wang, Eastland Press, Seattle, WA, 1995

Merritt's Textbook of Neurology edited by H. Merritt & L. Rowland, Lippincott, Williams and Wilkins, Baltimore, 1994

Mosby's Handbook of Pharmacology, 4th edition, by D. Bruce Clayton, The C.V. Mosby Co., St. Louis, MO, 1987

"New Migraine Drug Has Trigeminal Mechanisms of Action" by Neal Shankman, JAMA Migraine Information Center, www.amaassn.org/special/migraine/newsline/updates/021100b.htm

"Pain Treatment of Fibromyalgia by Acupuncture" by H. Sprott, S. Frank, & G. Hein, *Rheumatology International*, 1998

"Patient Guide to Tennis Elbow" by Ed McFarland & Leigh Ann Curl, www.med.jhu.edu/ortho/sports/tenelbow.htm
"Piriformis Syndrome" by M. Steckel, www.webgate.net/~welchiro/inj-piri.html

"Piriformis Syndrome" by ChiropracticCanada.com, www.acupuncture.ca/health%20info/piriformis%20syndrome.htm

Practical Therapeutics of Traditional Chinese Medicine by Yan Wu & Warren Fischer, Paradigm Publications, Brookline, MA, 1997

Practical Traditional Chinese Dermatology by Li Lin, trans. by Wang Tai, Peace Books, HaiFeng Publishing Co., Hong Kong, 1995

Principles of Neurology, 6th ed., by R. Adams & M. Victor, McGraw-Hill Co., NY, 1997

Seventy Essential Chinese Herbal Formulas by Bob Flaws, Blue Poppy Press, Boulder, CO, 2000

"Sinusitis," www.icondata.com/health/pedbase/files/SINUSITI.HTM

"Sinusitis," National Jewish Medical & Research Center, www.njc.org/MFhtml/SIN_MF.html

"Sinusitis," www.stjames.ie/nmic/commonupperrepiratory/curtsinu.html

"Spinal Diseases & Disorders: Cervical Disc Disease," UCLA Neurosurgery, www.neurosurgery.medsch.ucla.edu/Diagnoses/Spinal/SpinalDis_1.html

"Spinal Diseases & Disorders: Cervical Stenosis," UCLA Neurosurgery, http://neursun.medsch.ucla.edu/Diagnoses/Spinal/SpinalDis_2.html

"Syndrome X," www.syndrome-x.com

"Syndrome X and Insulin Resistance" by Pat Kendall, www.colostate.edu/Depts/CoopExt/PUBS/COLUMNNN/nn971022.htm

"Temporomandibular Joint Syndrome – TMJ," www.wellweb.com/INDEX/QTMJ.HTM

"Tennis Elbow – It's Not Just for Tennis Players" by David Higgins, www.hughston.com/hha/a.tennis.htm

Textbook of Natural Medicine by J.E. Pizzorno & M.T. Murray, John Bastyr College Publications, Seattle, WA, 1988

The Essential Guide to Prescription Drugs by James W. Long, Harper & Row, NY, 1990

The Heart & Essence of Dan-xi's Methods of Treatment by Zhu Dan-xi, trans. by Yang Shou-zhong, Blue Poppy Press, Boulder, CO, 1993

"The Male Reproductive System" by David L. Hoffman, www.healthy.net/library/books/hoffman/reproductive/prostate.htm

The Merck Manual, 17th edition, edited by Mark H. Beers & Robert Berkow, Merck Research Laboratories, Whitehouse Station, NJ, 1999

"The Role of Serotonin in Migraine" by Marilynn Larkin, JAMA Migraine Information Center, www.ama-assn.org/special/migraine/newsline/briefing/serotoni.htm

The Treatise on the Spleen & Stomach by Li Dong-yuan, trans. by Yang Shou-zhong, Blue Poppy Press, Boulder, CO, 1993

The Treatment of External Diseases with Acupuncture & Moxibustion by Yan Cui-lan & Zhu Yun-long, Blue Poppy Press, Boulder, CO, 1997

The Treatment of Disease in TCM, Vol. 1-7 by Philippe Sionneau & Lü Gang, Blue Poppy Press, Boulder, CO, 2000

"Thrombocytopenic Purpura" by Debra Symonette, www.emedicine.com/emerg/topic579.htm

"Treatment of Type I & Type II Diabetes" by P.H. Forsham, *Townsend Letter for Doctors*, #53, Dec. 1987

Understanding Acupuncture by Stephen J. Birch & Robert L. Felt, Churchill Livingstone, Edinburgh, 1999

"Urinary Incontinence in Adults: Clinical Practice Guideline" by the Urinary Incontinence Guideline Panel, AHCPR Pub. No. 92-0038, Rockville, MD, Mar. 1992

Webster's New World Dictionary of the American Language, The World Publishing Co, Cleveland & NY, 1966

"What Are the Drug Treatments for High Blood Pressure?" http://my.webmd.com/content/dmk/dmk_article_5462194

"What Causes Migraine?" JAMA Migraine Information Center, www.ama-assn.org/special/migraine/support/educate/causes.htm

French language bibliography

Grand Formulaire de Pharmacopée Chinoise (Great Formulary of Chinese Materia Medica) by Eric Marié, Editions Paracelse, 1991, Vitré, France, 1991

Pharmacopée Chinoise & Acupuncture: les traitements efficaces (Chinese Materia Medica & Acupuncture: The Effective Treatments) by Philippe Sionneau, Guy Trédaniel Editeur, Paris, 1996

Acupuncture: les points essentiels (Acupuncture: The Essential Points) by Philippe Sionneau, Guy Trédaniel Editeur, Paris, 2000

GENERAL INDEX

B

C

D

E

I

J

K

L

M

N

O

P

Q

X

Y

Z

Formula Index

D

E

F

G

H

J

K

L

T

W

X

Y

Z

OTHER BOOKS ON CHINESE MEDICINE AVAILABLE FROM:

BLUE POPPY PRESS

5441 Western Avenue, Suite 2, Boulder, CO 80301

For ordering 1-800-487-9296 PH. 303\447-8372 FAX 303\245-8362

Email: info@bluepoppy.com Website: www.bluepoppy.com

A NEW AMERICAN ACUPUNCTURE
By Mark Seem
ISBN 0-936185-44-9

ACUPOINT POCKET REFERENCE
by Bob Flaws
ISBN 0-936185-93-7

ACUPUNCTURE AND MOXIBUSTION FORMULAS & TREATMENTS
by Cheng Dan-an, trans. by Wu Ming
ISBN 0-936185-68-6

ACUPUNCTURE PHYSICAL MEDICINE: An Acupuncture Touchpoint Approach to the Treatment of Chronic Pain, Fatigue, and Stress Disorders
by Mark Seem
ISBN 1-891845-13-6

AGING & BLOOD STASIS: A New Approach to TCM Geriatrics
by Yan De-xin
ISBN 0-936185-63-5

BETTER BREAST HEALTH NATURALLY WITH CHINESE MEDICINE
by Honora Lee Wolfe & Bob Flaws
ISBN 0-936185-90-2

THE BOOK OF JOOK: Chinese Medicinal Porridges
by B. Flaws
ISBN 0-936185-60-0

CHANNEL DIVERGENCES Deeper Pathways of the Web
by Miki Shima and Charles Chase
ISBN 1-891845-15-2

CHINESE MEDICAL PALMISTRY: Your Health in Your Hand
by Zong Xiao-fan & Gary Liscum
ISBN 0-936185-64-3

CHINESE MEDICAL PSYCHIATRY A Textbook and Clinical Manual
by Bob Flaws and James Lake, MD
ISBN 1-845891-17-9

CHINESE MEDICINAL TEAS: Simple, Proven, Folk Formulas for Common Diseases & Promoting Health
by Zong Xiao-fan & Gary Liscum
ISBN 0-936185-76-7

CHINESE MEDICINAL WINES & ELIXIRS
by Bob Flaws
ISBN 0-936185-58-9

CHINESE PEDIATRIC MASSAGE THERAPY: A Parent's & Practitioner's Guide to the Prevention & Treatment of Childhood Illness
by Fan Ya-li
ISBN 0-936185-54-6

CHINESE SELF-MASSAGE THERAPY: The Easy Way to Health
by Fan Ya-li
ISBN 0-936185-74-0

THE CLASSIC OF DIFFICULTIES: A Translation of the Nan Jing
translation by Bob Flaws
ISBN 1-891845-07-1

CURING ARTHRITIS NATURALLY WITH CHINESE MEDICINE
by Douglas Frank & Bob Flaws
ISBN 0-936185-87-2

CURING DEPRESSION NATURALLY WITH CHINESE MEDICINE
by Rosa Schnyer & Bob Flaws
ISBN 0-936185-94-5

CURING FIBROMYALGIA NATURALLY WITH CHINESE MEDICINE
by Bob Flaws
ISBN 1-891845-08-9

CURING HAY FEVER NATURALLY WITH CHINESE MEDICINE
by Bob Flaws
ISBN 0-936185-91-0

CURING HEADACHES NATURALLY WITH CHINESE MEDICINE
by Bob Flaws
ISBN 0-936185-95-3-X

CURING IBS NATURALLY WITH CHINESE MEDICINE
by Jane Bean Oberski
ISBN 1-891845-11-X

CURING INSOMNIA NATURALLY WITH CHINESE MEDICINE
by Bob Flaws
ISBN 0-936185-85-6

CURING PMS NATURALLY WITH CHINESE MEDICINE
by Bob Flaws
ISBN 0-936185-85-6

A STUDY OF DAOIST ACUPUNCTURE & MOXIBUSTION
by Liu Zheng-cai
ISBN 1-891845-08-X

THE DIVINE FARMER'S MATERIA MEDICA A Translation of the Shen Nong Ben Cao
translation by Yang Shouz-zhong
ISBN 0-936185-96-1

THE DIVINELY RESPONDING CLASSIC: A Translation of the Shen Ying Jing from Zhen Jiu Da Cheng
trans. by Yang Shou-zhong & Liu Feng-ting
ISBN 0-936185-55-4

DUI YAO: THE ART OF COMBINING CHINESE HERBAL MEDICINALS
by Philippe Sionneau
ISBN 0-936185-81-3

ENDOMETRIOSIS, INFERTILITY AND TRADITIONAL CHINESE MEDICINE: A Laywoman's Guide
by Bob Flaws
ISBN 0-936185-14-7

THE ESSENCE OF LIU FENG-WU'S GYNECOLOGY
by Liu Feng-wu, translated by Yang Shou-zhong
ISBN 0-936185-88-0

EXTRA TREATISES BASED ON INVESTIGATION & INQUIRY: A Translation of Zhu Dan-xi's Ge Zhi Yu Lun
translation by Yang Shou-zhong
ISBN 0-936185-53-8

FIRE IN THE VALLEY: TCM Diagnosis & Treatment of Vaginal Diseases
by Bob Flaws
ISBN 0-936185-25-2

FU QING-ZHU'S GYNECOLOGY
trans. by Yang Shou-zhong and Liu Da-wei
ISBN 0-936185-35-X

FULFILLING THE ESSENCE: A Handbook of Traditional & Contemporary Treatments for Female Infertility
by Bob Flaws
ISBN 0-936185-48-1

GOLDEN NEEDLE WANG LE-TING: A 20th Century Master's Approach to Acupuncture
by Yu Hui-chan and Han Fu-ru,
trans. by Shuai Xue-zhong

A GUIDE TO GYNECOLOGY
by Ye Heng-yin,
trans. by Bob Flaws and Shuai Xue-zhong
ISBN 1-891845-19-5

A HANDBOOK OF TCM PATTERNS & TREATMENTS
by Bob Flaws & Daniel Finney
ISBN 0-936185-70-8

A HANDBOOK OF TRADITIONAL CHINESE DERMATOLOGY
by Liang Jian-hui, trans. by Zhang Ting-liang & Bob Flaws
ISBN 0-936185-07-4

A HANDBOOK OF TRADITIONAL CHINESE GYNECOLOGY
by Zhejiang College of TCM, trans. by Zhang Ting-liang & Bob Flaws
ISBN 0-936185-06-6 (4th edit.)

A HANDBOOK OF CHINESE HEMATOLOGY
by Simon Becker
ISBN 1-891845-16-0

A HANDBOOK OF MENSTRUAL DISEASES IN CHINESE MEDICINE
by Bob Flaws
ISBN 0-936185-82-1

A HANDBOOK of TCM PEDIATRICS
by Bob Flaws
ISBN 0-936185-72-4

A HANDBOOK OF TCM UROLOGY & MALE SEXUAL DYSFUNCTION
by Anna Lin, OMD
ISBN 0-936185-36-8

THE HEART & ESSENCE OF DAN-XI'S METHODS OF TREATMENT
by Xu Dan-xi, trans. by Yang Shou-zhong
ISBN 0-926185-49-X

THE HEART TRANSMISSION OF MEDICINE
by Liu Yi-ren, trans. by Yang Shou-zhong
ISBN 0-936185-83-X

HIGHLIGHTS OF ANCIENT ACUPUNCTURE PRESCRIPTIONS
trans. by Honora Lee Wolfe & Rose Crescenz
ISBN 0-936185-23-6

IMPERIAL SECRETS OF HEALTH & LONGEVITY
by Bob Flaws
ISBN 0-936185-51-1

INSIGHTS OF A SENIOR ACUPUNCTURIST
by Miriam Lee
ISBN 0-936185-33-3

KEEPING YOUR CHILD HEALTHY WITH CHINESE MEDICINE
by Bob Flaws
ISBN 0-936185-71-6

THE LAKESIDE MASTER'S STUDY OF THE PULSE
by Li Shi-zhen, trans. by Bob Flaws
ISBN 1-891845-01-2

Li Dong-yuan's TREATISE ON THE SPLEEN & STOMACH, A Translation of the Pi Wei Lun
trans. by Yang Shou-zhong
ISBN 0-936185-41-4

MASTER HUA'S CLASSIC OF THE CENTRAL VISCERA
by Hua Tuo, trans. by Yang Shou-zhong
ISBN 0-936185-43-0

MASTER TONG'S ACUPUNCTURE
by Miriam Lee
ISBN 0-926185-37-6

THE MEDICAL I CHING:
Oracle of the Healer Within
by Miki Shima
ISBN 0-936185-38-4

MANAGING MENOPAUSE NATURALLY with Chinese Medicine
by Honora Lee Wolfe
ISBN 0-936185-98-8

PAO ZHI: Introduction to Processing Chinese Medicinals to Enhance Their Therapeutic Effect
by Philippe Sionneau
ISBN 0-936185-62-1

PATH OF PREGNANCY, VOL. I, Gestational Disorders
by Bob Flaws
ISBN 0-936185-39-2

PATH OF PREGNANCY, Vol. II, Postpartum Diseases
by Bob Flaws
ISBN 0-936185-42-2

THE PULSE CLASSIC:
A Translation of the Mai Jing
by Wang Shu-he, trans. by Yang Shou-zhong
ISBN 0-936185-75-9

RECENT TCM RESEARCH FROM CHINA
by Bob Flaws and Charles Chase
ISBN 0-936185-56-2

SEVENTY ESSENTIAL CHINESE HERBAL FORMULAS
by Bob Flaws
ISBN 0-936185-59-7

SHAOLIN SECRET FORMULAS for Treatment of External Injuries
by De Chan, trans. by Zhang Ting-liang & Bob Flaws
ISBN 0-936185-08-2

STATEMENTS OF FACT IN TRADITIONAL CHINESE MEDICINE
by Bob Flaws
ISBN 0-936185-52-X

STICKING TO THE POINT 1: A Rational Methodology for the Step by Step Formulation & Administration of an Acupuncture Treatment
by Bob Flaws
ISBN 0-936185-17-1

STICKING TO THE POINT 2: A Study of Acupuncture & Moxibustion Formulas and Strategies
by Bob Flaws
ISBN 0-936185-97-X

A STUDY OF DAOIST ACUPUNCTURE
by Liu Zheng-cai
ISBN 1-891845-08-X

TEACH YOURSELF TO READ MODERN MEDICAL CHINESE
by Bob Flaws
ISBN 0-936185-99-6

THE SYSTEMATIC CLASSIC OF ACUPUNCTURE & MOXIBUSTION A translation of the Jia Yi Jing
by Huang-fu Mi, trans. by Yang Shou-zhong & Charles Chace
ISBN 0-936185-29-5

THE TAO OF HEALTHY EATING ACCORDING TO CHINESE MEDICINE
by Bob Flaws
ISBN 0-936185-92-9

THE TREATMENT OF DISEASE IN TCM, Vol I: Diseases of the Head & Face Including Mental/Emotional Disorders
by Philippe Sionneau & Lü Gang
ISBN 0-936185-69-4

THE TREATMENT OF DISEASE IN TCM, Vol. II: Diseases of the Eyes, Ears, Nose, & Throat
by Sionneau & Lü
ISBN 0-936185-69-4

THE TREATMENT OF DISEASE, Vol. III: Diseases of the Mouth, Lips, Tongue, Teeth & Gums
by Sionneau & Lü
ISBN 0-936185-79-1

THE TREATMENT OF DISEASE, Vol IV: Diseases of the Neck, Shoulders, Back, & Limbs
by Philippe Sionneau & Lü Gang
ISBN 0-936185-89-9

THE TREATMENT OF DISEASE, Vol V: Diseases of the Chest & Abdomen
by Philippe Sionneau & Lü Gang
ISBN 1-891845-02-0

THE TREATMENT OF DISEASE, Vol VI: Diseases of the Urogential System & Proctology
by Philippe Sionneau & Lü Gang
ISBN 1-891845-05-5

THE TREATMENT OF DISEASE, Vol VII: General Symptoms
by Philippe Sionneau & Lü Gang
ISBN 1-891845-14-4

THE TREATMENT OF EXTERNAL DISEASES WITH ACUPUNCTURE & MOXIBUSTION
by Yan Cui-lan and Zhu Yun-long, trans. by Yang Shou-zhong
ISBN 0-936185-80-5

160 ESSENTIAL CHINESE HERBAL PATENT MEDICINES
by Bob Flaws
ISBN 1-891945-12-8

630 QUESTIONS & ANSWERS ABOUT CHINESE HERBAL MEDICINE: A Workbook & Study Guide
by Bob Flaws
ISBN 1-891845-04-7

230 ESSENTIAL CHINESE MEDICINALS
by Bob Flaws
ISBN 1-891845-03-9